# Occupational Therapy Essentials for Clinical Competence

Third Edition

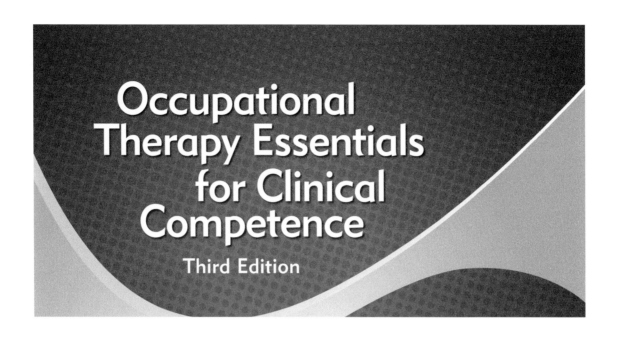


*Edited by*

Karen Jacobs, EdD, OTR/L, CPE, FAOTA
Clinical Professor & Program Director
On-Line Post-Professional Doctorate in Occupational Therapy (OTD) Program
Boston University
College of Health & Rehabilitation Sciences: Sargent College
Boston, Massachusetts

Nancy MacRae, MS, OTR/L, FAOTA
Associate Professor
Occupational Therapy Department
University of New England
Portland, Maine

Instructor's materials created by Mary Elizabeth Patnaude, MS, OTR/L and
Robin Newman, OTD, OTR/L, CLT, CDRS

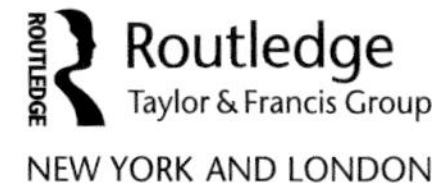


NEW YORK AND LONDON

*Occupational Therapy Essentials for Clinical Competence, Third Edition,* includes ancillary materials specifically available for faculty use. Included are Test Bank Questions and PowerPoint slides. Please visit www.routledge.com/9781630912475 to obtain access.

First published 2017 by SLACK Incorporated

Published 2024 by Routledge
605 Third Avenue, New York, NY 10158

and by Routledge
4 Park Square, Milton Park, Abingdon, Oxon OX14 4RN

*Routledge is an imprint of the Taylor & Francis Group, an informa business*



The child with the beaming smile and jovial personality in the top middle photo on the cover of this textbook is a child with Lowe syndrome. For more information, see lowesyndrome.org.



Library of Congress Cataloging-in-Publication Data

Names: Jacobs, Karen, editor. | MacRae, Nancy, editor.
Title: Occupational therapy essentials for clinical competence / edited by Karen Jacobs, Nancy MacRae ; instructor materials created by Mary Beth Patnaude and Robin Newman.
Description: Third edition. | Thorofare, NJ : SLACK Incorporated, [2017] | Includes bibliographical references and index.
Identifiers: LCCN 2017000331 (print) | ISBN 9781630912475 (hardcover : alk. paper)
Subjects: | MESH: Occupational Therapy | Clinical Competence--standards | Accreditation--standards
Classification: LCC RM735 (print) | NLM WB 555 | DDC 615.8/515--dc23
LC record available at https://lccn.loc.gov/2017000331

ISBN: 9781630912475 (hbk)
ISBN: 9781003525295 (ebk)

DOI: 10.4324/9781003525295

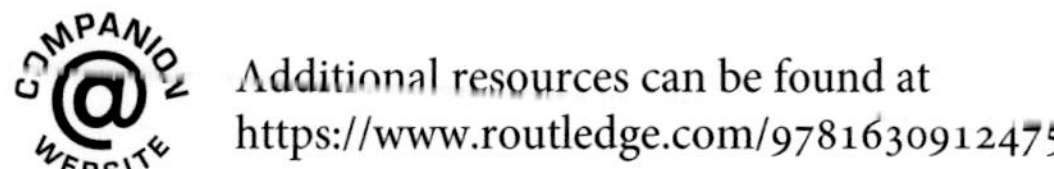

Additional resources can be found at
https://www.routledge.com/9781630912475

# Dedication

To our wonderful families and friends, who provide us with a support system; our students, past, current, and future; and our professional colleagues. They all continue to inspire and teach us. Our wish is for our students to become competent, confident, and compassionate practitioners of occupational therapy.

# Contents

*Occupational Therapy Essentials for Clinical Competence, Third Edition,* includes ancillary materials specifically available for faculty use. Included are Test Bank Questions and PowerPoint slides. Please visit www.routledge.com/9781630912475 to obtain access.

# Acknowledgments

We are grateful to Mary Beth Patnaude for creating the multiple-choice questions and to Robin Newman for making the PowerPoint slides for each chapter. Our thanks also go to SLACK Incorporated, and in particular, Brien and Jenn, for their ongoing support.

# About the Editors

*Karen Jacobs, EdD, OTR/L, CPE, FAOTA,* is a past president and vice president of the American Occupational Therapy Association (AOTA). She is a 2005 recipient of a Fulbright Scholarship to the University of Akureyri in Akureyri, Iceland; the 2009 recipient of the Award of Merit from the Canadian Association of Occupational Therapists (CAOT); the 2003 recipient of the Award of Merit from the AOTA; and recipient of the 2011 Eleanor Clarke Slagle Lectureship Award. The title of her Slagle lecture was *PromOTing Occupational Therapy: Words, Images, and Action.*

Dr. Jacobs is a clinical professor of occupational therapy and the Program Director of the online post-professional occupational therapy doctorate in occupational therapy program at Boston University. She has worked at Boston University for 34 years and has expertise in the development and instruction of online graduate courses.

Dr. Jacobs earned a doctoral degree at the University of Massachusetts, a Master of Science in Occupational Therapy at Boston University, and a Bachelor of Arts at Washington University in St. Louis, Missouri.

Dr. Jacobs' research examines the interface between the environment and human capabilities. In particular, she examines the individual factors and environmental demands associated with increased risk of functional limitations among populations of university- and middle school–aged students, particularly in notebook computing, use of tablets such as iPads (Apple), backpack use, and the use of games such as Wii Fit (Nintendo). Karen is presently part of an interprofessional demonstration project titled, Project Career: Development of an Interprofessional Demonstration to Support the Transition of Students With Traumatic Brain Injuries From Post-Secondary Education to Employment.

In addition to being an occupational therapist, Dr. Jacobs is also a certified professional ergonomist (CPE), the founding editor in chief of the international, interprofessional journal *WORK: A Journal of Prevention, Assessment & Rehabilitation* (IOS Press, The Netherlands), and a consultant in ergonomics, marketing, and entrepreneurship.

She is the proud mother of three children (Laela, Josh, and Ariel) and Amma (grandmother in Icelandic) to Sophie, Zachary, Liberty, and Zane. Her occupational balance is through travel, photography, kayaking, walking, co-writing children's books, and spending time with her family at Wakonda Pond.

*Nancy MacRae, MS, OTR/L, FAOTA,* is an associate professor at the University of New England (UNE), in Portland, Maine, where she has taught for 27 years. She has begun a 3-year process of phased-in retirement, where she teaches only one semester per school year. She is a past president of the Maine Occupational Therapy Association and a past director of the UNE occupational therapy program.

Nancy's work experience has been within the field of developmental disabilities, primarily mental retardation, across the lifespan. Her graduate degree is in adult education, with a minor in educational gerontology. Involvement in interprofessional activities at UNE allows her to mentor and learn with and from future health care practitioners and to model the collaboration our health care system needs. Scholarship has centered around aging and sexuality, documentation, professional writing, and interprofessional ventures. She has been a member of the editorial board of *WORK: A Journal of Prevention, Assessment & Rehabilitation* since its inception.

Nancy is the proud mother of two sons and a 17-year-old granddaughter. Occupational balance is maintained through participation in yoga, reading, walking, baking, and basket making, as well as volunteering within the community at a local school and working with caregivers of people with dementia. Travel plans have accelerated now that work is no longer full time.

# Contributing Authors

*Caroline Beals, MS, OTR/L (Chapters 46 and 54 )*
Assistant Clinical Professor
Health, Wellness, and Occupational Studies
University of New England
Biddeford, Maine

*Diane P. Bergey, MOT, OTR/L (Chapter 36)*
Belfast, Maine

*Caryn Birstler Husman, MS, OTR/L (Chapter 5)*
Director and Assistant Professor
Health, Wellness, and Occupational Studies
University of New England
Biddeford, Maine

*Roxie M. Black, PhD, OTR, FAOTA (Chapter 2)*
Professor Emerita of Occupational Therapy
University of Southern Maine
Lewiston-Auburn College
Lewiston, Maine

*Gail M. Bloom, OTD, MA, OTR/L (Chapter 50)*
Consultant
Andover, Massachusetts

*Jessica J. Bolduc, DrOT, MS, OTR/L (Chapters 17 and 25)*
University of New England
Mercy Hospital
Portland, Maine

*Alfred G. Bracciano, MSA, EdD, OTR/L, FAOTA (Chapter 34)*
Coordinator, Alaska Distance Pathway
Creighton University at University of Alaska Anchorage
Creighton University
Department of Occupational Therapy
Omaha, Nebraska

*Susan C. Burwash, PhD, MSc(OT), OTR/L, OT(C) (Chapter 55)*
Associate Professor and Chair
Department of Occupational Therapy
Eastern Washington University
Spokane, Washington

*Jane Clifford O'Brien, PhD, OTR/L, FAOTA (Chapters 24 and 30)*
Professor
Occupational Therapy Department
University of New England
Portland, Maine

*Marilyn B. Cole, MS, OTR/L, FAOTA (Chapter 15)*
Professor Emerita of Occupational Therapy
Quinnipiac University
Hamden, Connecticut

*Jeffrey L. Crabtree, OTD, MS, FAOTA (Chapter 38)*
Affiliate Research Scientist, Rehabilitation Research
Design & Disability (R2D2) Center
University of Wisconsin-Milwaukee
Associate Professor of Occupational Therapy and
Director, Community Mobility and Participation in
Society (COMPASS) Lab
Department of Occupational Therapy
School of Health and Rehabilitation Sciences
Indiana University
Indianapolis, Indiana

*Elizabeth W. Crampsey, MS, OTR/L, BCPR (Chapters 43 and 46 )*
Assistant Clinical Professor
Occupational Therapy
University of New England
Portland, Maine

*William R. Croninger, MA, OTR/L (Chapters 23 and 32)*
Staff Therapist
Maria Parham Medical Center
Henderson, North Carolina

*Danielle J. Cropley, MS, OTR/L (Chapter 22)*
Cary Medical Center
Professional Home Nursing
Caribou, Maine

*Laura Crossley-Marra, MS, OTR/L (Chapter 32)*
Occupational Therapist
Advocate Condell
Libertyville, Illinois

*Peter DaSilva, MSOT Class 2017 (Chapter 24)*
Occupational Therapy Department
University of New England
Portland, Maine

*Hailey C. Davis, MS, OTR/L (Chapter 13)*
Seaside Rehabilitation and Healthcare
Portland, Maine

*Betsy DeBrakeleer, COTA/L, ROH (Chapter 32)*
Biddeford, Maine

*Mary V. Donohue, PhD, OTL, FAOTA (Chapter 22)*
Semi-Retired, Clinical Professor
New York University
New York, New York
Member of New York State Board of Education for Licensure for Occupational Therapy
Associate Editor, *Occupational Therapy in Mental Health*
Vice Commodore of New York Sailing Club

*Nancy Doyle, OTD, OTR/L (Chapters 11 and 39)*
Lecturer in Occupational Therapy
Sargent College of Health and Rehabilitation Sciences
Boston University
Boston, Massachusetts

*Karen Duddy, OTD, MHA, OTR/L (Chapters 40 and 47)*
Supervisor of Occupational Therapy
Veterans Health Administration
Long Beach, California
Lecturer
Boston University Post-Professional Online Doctoral Program

*Verna G. Eschenfelder, PhD, OTR/L (Chapter 6)*
Assistant Professor of Occupational Therapy
University of Scranton
Scranton, Pennsylvania

*Thomas Fisher, PhD, OTR, CCM, FAOTA (Chapter 54)*
Professor and Chair
Department of Occupational Therapy
School of Health and Rehabilitation Sciences
Indiana University
Indianapolis, Indiana

*Erica A. Flagg, OT/L (Chapter 36)*
Knox Center
Union, Maine

*Kathleen Flecky, OTD, OTR/L (Chapter 8)*
Creighton University
Omaha, Nebraska

*Jan Froehlich, MS, OTR/L (Foreword and Chapters 9 and 10)*
Westbrook College of Health Professions
University of New England
Portland, Maine

*Liat Gafni Lachter, OTD, OTR/L (Chapter 41)*
Occupational Therapy Department
Sargent College of Health & Rehabilitation Sciences
Boston University
Boston, Massachusetts
Occupational Therapy Department
Faculty of Social Welfare and Health Sciences
University of Haifa
Haifa, Israel

*Heather Goertz, OTD, OTR/L (Chapter 8)*
Healthy Living Consultant
Omaha, Nebraska

*Michelle Goulet, MS, OTR/L (Chapter 21)*
Occupational Therapist
Northeast Rehabilitation Hospital Network
Salem, New Hampshire

*Elizabeth C. Hart, MS, OTR/L (Chapter 56)*
Occupational Therapist
Carol Woods Retirement Community
Chapel Hill, North Carolina

*Bevin Journey, MS, OTR/L (Chapter 28)*
Philadelphia, Pennsylvania

*Leanna W. Katz, MS, OTD, OTR/L (Chapter 38)*
Spaulding Rehabilitation Hospital
Boston, Massachusetts

*Rosalie M. King, DHS, OTR/L (Chapter 1)*
Associate Professor of Occupational Therapy (Retired)
University of Findlay
Findlay, Ohio

*Lisa Knecht-Sabres, DHS, OTR/L (Chapter 18)*
Professor
Occupational Therapy Program
Midwestern University
Downers Grove, Illinois

*Amy Lamb, OTD, OT/L, FAOTA (Chapters 44 and 56)*
Associate Professor
Eastern Michigan University
Dexter, Michigan
President of the American Occupational Therapy Association

*Barbara Larson, MA, OTR/L, FAOTA (Chapter 19)*
Independent Consultant, Work and Industry
Adjunct Faculty, Program in Occupational Therapy
The College of St. Scholastica
Duluth, Minnesota

*Kathryn M. Loukas, OTD, MS, OTR/L, FAOTA (Chapters 13, 28, and 33 )*
Department of Occupational Therapy
University of New England
Portland, Maine

*Sarah McKinnon, MS, OTR/L, BCPR, MPA (Chapter 51)*
Boston University
Partners Healthcare
Boston, Massachusetts

*Scott D. McNeil, OTD, MS, OTR/L (Chapter 33)*
Department of Occupational Therapy
University of New England
Portland, Maine

*Meghan McNierney, MSOT Class 2017 (Chapter 30)*
Occupational Therapy Department
University of New England
Portland, Maine

*Linda Miller, OT (C), OTD, CPE (Chapter 31)*
EWI Works International Inc.
Edmonton, Alberta, Canada

*Penelope Moyers Cleveland, EdD, OT/L, FAOTA (Chapter 53)*
Dean of Henrietta Schmoll School of Health and the Graduate College
St. Catherine University
St. Paul, Minnesota

*Julie Ann Nastasi, ScD, OTD, OTR/L, SCLV, FAOTA (Chapters 7, 37, and 45)*
Assistant Professor
University of Scranton
Scranton, Pennsylvania

*Robin Newman, OTD, OTR/L, CLT, CDRS (PowerPoints)*
Clinical Assistant Professor
Department of Occupational Therapy
Boston University Sargent College
Boston, Massachusetts

*Linda H. Niemeyer, OT, PhD (Chapter 47)*
Lecturer in Occupational Therapy
Sargent College of Health and Rehabilitation Sciences
Department of Occupational Therapy
Boston University
Boston, Massachusetts

*Claudia E. Oakes, OTR/L, PhD (Chapter 12)*
Department of Health Science
University of Hartford
West Hartford, Connecticut

*Jennifer O'Connor, MSOT Class 2017 (Chapter 24)*
Occupational Therapy Department
University of New England
Portland, Maine

*Megha Panchal, MSOT Class 2017 (Chapter 30)*
Occupational Therapy Department
University of New England
Portland, Maine

*Mary Elizabeth Patnaude, MS, OTR/L (Chapter 14 and Instructor's Manual)*
Assistant Clinical Professor
University of New England
Portland, Maine

*Michael E. Roberts, OTD, OTR/L (Chapter 26)*
Program Director, MSOT Program
Regis College
Weston, Massachusetts

*Regula H. Robnett, PhD, OTR/L, FAOTA (Chapter 25)*
Professor
Department of Occupational Therapy
University of New England
Portland, Maine

*Jan Rowe, DrOT, MPH, OTR/L, FAOTA (Chapter 52)*
Coordinator
Tourette Syndrome and Tic Disorders Program
Children's of Alabama
Department of Neurology
University of Alabama at Birmingham
TAA, Center of Excellence—Southeastern Consortium
Birmingham, Alabama

*Courtney Shufelt, MS, OTR/L (Chapter 29)*
Bangor, Maine

*Wendy B. Stav, PhD, OTR/L, SCDCM, FAOTA (Chapter 48)*
Nova Southeastern University
Ft. Lauderdale, Florida

*Barbara J. Steva, MS, OTR/L (Chapter 27 and Appendix E)*
Independent Contractor
Saco, Maine

*Christine Sullivan, OTD, OTR/L (Chapter 49)*
Associate Professor and Program Director
Occupational Therapy Assistant Program
Mercy College
Dobbs Ferry, New York

*Roseanna Tufano, LMFT, OTR/L (Chapter 16)*
Clinical Associate Professor of Occupational Therapy
Associate Chair of Occupational Therapy
Quinnipiac University
Hamden, Connecticut

*Rebecca Twinley, PhD, MSc, PGCAP, BSc(Hons), FHEA, HCPC (Chapter 3)*
Plymouth, United Kingdom

*Lori Vaughn, OTD, OTR/L (Chapter 20)*
Westfield State University
Westfield, Massachusetts

*John W. Vellacott, EdD, MEd, BA (Chapter 55)*
Independent Researcher
Spokane, Washington

*Nicole Villegas, OTD, OTR/L (Chapter 40)*
Occupational Therapist
Our House of Portland—
Neighborhood Housing and Care Program
Portland, Oregon

*Iris Wilbur-Kamien, MS, OTR/L (Chapter 52)*
Inpatient Occupational Therapist
Northeast Rehabilitation Hospital
Salem, New Hampshire

*Kristin Winston, PhD, OTR/L (Chapter 35)*
University of New England
Portland, Maine

*Patricia A. Wisniewski, MS, OTR/L, CPRP (Chapter 6)*
Faculty Specialist
University of Scranton
Scranton, Pennsylvania

# FOREWORD

The Third Edition of *Occupational Therapy Essentials for Clinical Competence* speaks as authentically as the preceding editions in articulating what is "essential" for competent occupational therapy practice. Students and faculty alike often call the text *Essentials* for short. This comprehensive text addresses what is "absolutely necessary and extremely important" (*Oxford Living Dictionary*, 2016) for occupational therapy practice in today's complex and ever-changing health care and human service arenas. The organization of the text around the finely crafted and compelling standards of practice established by the Accreditation Council for Occupational Therapy Education (ACOTE) 2011 Standards ensures all competencies for entry-level occupational therapy practitioners are addressed. Used alongside masterful teaching that supports application of theory to practice, clinical competence for entry-level occupational therapy generalists is developed and enhanced.

The text flows logically through nine sections that progressively build the learner's competence for clinical practice. Like the previous edition, Section I sets the stage by exploring the experience of flow and meaningful occupation, the impact of culture on occupation, and the interprofessional nature of education and practice as key constructs within occupational therapy. The addition of a chapter on "The Dark Side of Occupation" is timely. There is increasing awareness across the globe of human engagement in occupations that are harmful to each other and ourselves. This chapter calls upon occupational therapy practitioners and occupational scientists to be willing to explore, understand, and teach about the dark side of occupation so we can address this complexity in practice.

Section II addresses the basic tenets of occupational therapy beginning with an overview of the profession's history and philosophy; the *Occupational Therapy Practice Framework: Domain and Process, Third Edition* (American Occupational Therapy Association [AOTA], 2014); the meaning and dynamic of occupation; and occupational performance and health. Combined with subsequent chapters on effective communication; therapeutic use of self; teaching, learning, and health literacy; safety and support; and occupational performance in natural environments, the learner is well launched toward providing client-centered, occupation-based practice. An additional chapter on clinical reasoning optimizes practice by challenging the student to be a reflective practitioner. Section III solidly supports the application of occupational therapy theory in practice.

Screening, evaluation, and referral in each area of occupational performance in Section IV is complemented by formulation and implementation of intervention plans in Section V. Both sections support the Standards' call for the integration of frames of reference, models of practice, and available evidence in the provision of culturally relevant, occupation-based services that enhance occupational participation for both individuals and populations (AOTA, 2013).

Section VI, which addresses the context of service delivery, contains chapters on emerging areas of practice and telehealth, plus a new chapter on primary care. Each chapter facilitates the creative application of occupational therapy practice within the dynamic, ever-changing health and human services delivery system. The chapter on primary care eloquently highlights the distinctive value of occupational therapy practitioners in primary care and offers a team-based model for service delivery. Section VII positions the learner to understand the complexities of legislation and reimbursement in occupational therapy practice, as well as marketing, quality improvement, supervision, and the role of fieldwork. This section concludes with a chapter on leadership to promote the development of occupational therapists as critical leaders and agents of change in many facets of our global society. Our professional role in fostering occupational justice is highlighted.

Scholarship, as a significant and enduring factor in the evolution of our profession, is the focus of Section VIII. Competence as researchers, grant writers, and professional presenters is fostered to advance our body of knowledge, identify best practice, and generate ongoing inquiry in occupational therapy. The concluding section discusses professional ethics, values, and responsibilities and fosters adherence to the *Occupational Therapy Code of Ethics* in all our endeavors. Chapters on connecting with local and global resources, promoting occupational therapy, professional development, occupational therapy practitioner roles, conflict resolution, and advocacy in occupational therapy inspire creative and sound development of occupational therapy practice.

Both students and faculty alike find the structure and content of the text supports the achievement of clinical competence. Contributing authors are experienced and passionate practitioners, educators, and leaders in the field of occupational therapy who provide solid and practical overviews of each ACOTE Standard. Engaging, heartwarming, and inspiring examples of occupational therapy practice in a multitude of settings, including emerging areas of practice, are sprinkled throughout the text. While client-centered and occupation-based practice are at the heart of the text, an emphasis on evidence-based and theory-driven practice ensures the highest standards of practice are met. The clear and concise style in which each chapter speaks to the ACOTE Standards prepares students for entry-level practice. Key words, evidence-based research charts, self-assessments, and additional resources in each chapter effectively facilitate the teaching-learning process.

As the preamble to the ACOTE Standards states, "The rapidly changing and dynamic nature of contemporary health and human services delivery systems provides challenging opportunities for the occupational therapist to use knowledge and skills in a practice area as a direct care provider, consultant, educator, manager, leader, researcher, and advocate for the profession in the consumer" (AOTA, 2013).

Not only does the text prepare entry-level practitioners for the complex demands of today's health and human services delivery systems, but by adhering to the high standards established by ACOTE, it also fosters the development of occupational therapy practitioners who can contribute to AOTA's Vision 2025 "that occupational therapy maximizes health, well-being, and quality of life for all people, populations, and communities through effective solutions that facilitate participation in everyday living" (2017). *Occupational Therapy Essentials for Clinical Competence, Third Edition*, is an excellent vehicle for the development of what is not only "absolutely necessary" but "extremely important" for today's occupational therapy practitioner.

*—Jan Froehlich, MS, OTR/L*
Westbrook College of Health Professions
University of New England
Portland, Maine

## References

American Occupational Therapy Association. (2013). 2011 Accreditation Council for Occupational Therapy Education (ACOTE) standards and interpretive guide. Retrieved from http://www.aota.org/~/media/Corporate/Files/EducationCareers/Accredit%20/Standards/2011-Standards-and-Interpretive-Guide.pdf

American Occupational Therapy Association. (2014). Occupational therapy practice framework: Domain and process (3rd ed.). *American Journal of Occupational Therapy, 68*(Suppl. 1), S1-S48. doi:10.5014/ajot.2014.682006

American Occupational Therapy Association. (2017). *Vision 2025*. Retrieved from http://www.aota.org/AboutAOTA/vision-2025.aspx

*Oxford Living Dictionary*. (2016). Retrieved from https://en.oxforddictionaries.com/definition/essential

# Introduction

As you can see from the cover of this Third Edition, we are honoring our students from both of our respective universities because of all that they do to inspire us and from what we learn with and from them.

Occupation remains the core of this textbook as it does with our profession. All chapters are theory driven, evidence based, and client centered. It is with these threads in mind that we are pleased to offer this Third Edition in celebration of the 100th year of our profession.

We have expanded our concept of occupation to include a new chapter titled "The Dark Side of Occupation." It is imperative that our students and practitioners acknowledge that not all occupations are healthy. This realization can lead to a more realistic and individualized occupational therapy process, one that will facilitate the health and well-being of our clients. A second new chapter deals specifically with the practice area of primary care and occupational therapy's growing role within it. All other chapters have been revised and updated, and many have new authors whom we welcome to this Third Edition.

The Third Edition is again organized to address the current Accreditation Council for Occupational Therapy Education Standards. Additionally, the competency for practitioners, both occupational therapists and occupational therapy assistants, are addressed.

We hope that in using this text you will be inspired to be agents of change within the profession and to advocate for the roles of occupational therapy within interprofessional teams.

The language from the American Occupational Therapy Association's *Occupational Therapy Practice Framework: Domain and Process, Third Edition*, is the voice infused within each chapter. It is important to stress the necessity for occupational and social justice within our profession, as well as being actively engaged in our health care system to make health care available to all.

This Third Edition includes case studies for application of new knowledge. For instructors, PowerPoint presentations and multiple-choice questions for each chapter are available on www.routledge.com/9781630912475 .

*—Karen and Nancy*

# I

# Setting the Stage

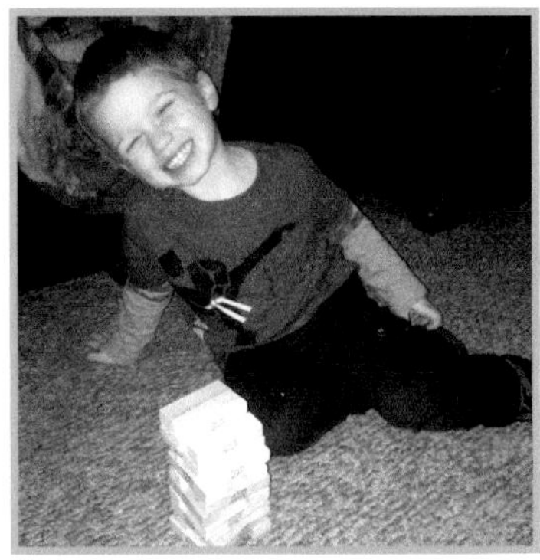

# 1

# The Experience of Flow and Meaningful Occupation

Rosalie M. King, DHS, OTR/L

**ACOTE STANDARDS EXPLORED IN THIS CHAPTER**

**B.3.6**

**KEY VOCABULARY**

- **Experience sampling method:** A research methodology designed to capture people's behaviors, thoughts, or feelings as they occur in real time.
- **Flow experience:** The mental state in which a person performing an activity is fully immersed in a feeling of energized focus, full involvement, and enjoyment in the process of the activity.
- **Meaningful occupation:** The ordinary, familiar things an individual does every day that are valued and have significance for that person.
- **Occupational therapy:** A health and wellness profession using occupation as both a means and an end in promoting participation, meaning, and satisfaction in all aspects of life.
- **Optimal experience:** Alternate term for *flow experience.*
- **Well-being:** Judging life as positive and satisfying.



Jacobs, K., & MacRae, N. (Eds.).
*Occupational Therapy Essentials for Clinical Competence, Third Edition* (pp. 3-11).

A review of the literature indicates a relationship between the characteristics of meaningful occupation and the experience of flow. Current literature within the occupational therapy profession frequently emphasizes the importance of using occupation, and, in doing so, practicing in a client-centered, holistic manner. Although there is a strongly held belief in the profession about the value of occupation, the need to provide supporting evidence still exists. In addition, there is a paucity of evidence available to assist occupational therapy practitioners in determining what is meaningful and enjoyable to the client, and the assignment of value and meaning to occupations is subjective (Csikszentmihalyi, 1997; Persson, Erlandsson, Eklund, & Iwarsson, 2001). People are not always able to articulate what is of particular value to them when asked directly. This review of the literature is an attempt to examine the characteristics of the concept of flow experiences and of occupations that contribute to the well-being of those we serve. In addition, because the flow construct is well established in the field of psychology, finding parallels would support the validity of the use of occupation and afford occupational therapists a larger body of knowledge upon which to build.

Flow, or optimal experience, is a construct studied in the discipline of social psychology and developed by Mihaly Csikszentmihalyi (1990). Flow describes a subjective state of consciousness in which one becomes totally immersed in the occupation or task at hand and from which the individual derives satisfaction and a sense of well-being. The theory has been well researched and clearly delineates the conditions that must be present for the flow experience to occur. A more thorough explanation of the construct will be developed to increase understanding of the prerequisite conditions for flow and the benefits to the person experiencing this state.

Occupational therapy has identified the importance of using meaningful occupation in interventions with client populations to increase motivation and success in achieving client goals. Christiansen, Backman, Little, and Nguyen (1999) spoke of the predominant perception that engagement in daily occupations serves to meet intrinsic and extrinsic needs and contributes to satisfaction and quality of life within the field. Founders of the profession of occupational therapy equated health and life satisfaction with balance in daily activities, a tenet we still espouse today. Yet it is true that a healthy balance varies from person to person, as does the idea of which activities and occupations are considered meaningful. Hammell (2004) also points out that occupational therapy theory tends to group occupations into the categories of self-care, leisure, and productivity, which can be limiting. Some occupations that might be meaningful do not appear to fall into these categories. This is further complicated by occupational therapy theories that do not clearly distinguish the difference between the terms *meaningful* and *purposeful*. If occupations are considered meaningful only if they are goal oriented and purposeful, occupations chosen by a practitioner during intervention might have meaning (not necessarily positive) but not be meaningful (Hammell, 2004).

Because there are activities and occupations an individual may consider important that do not result in optimal experience, the idea of examining and determining occupations that do result in flow for a given person does not provide a complete recipe for successful intervention. However, exploration of the concept of flow in relation to meaningful occupation bears consideration in terms of its potential to support the philosophical belief of occupational therapy and to learn more about how we might enable our clients to achieve a greater sense of well-being and life satisfaction.

## Methodology for Searching the Literature

A search of databases including the Cumulative Index to Nursing and Allied Health Literature (CINAHL), PsycINFO, OT Search, and the journal holdings of the American Occupational Therapy Association (AOTA) was conducted using the following key terms: *meaningful occupation*, *occupational therapy*, *well-being*, and *flow experience*. The term *optimal experience* was added to increase responses. In addition, a Google search was conducted using the same key words. Retrieved abstracts and articles, as well as references cited in some of the literature, led to an additional search using the term *experience sampling method*. The search yielded 44 articles, which were narrowed down to 33 for this review. Information that did not come from a peer-reviewed source was discarded.

## Review of the Literature

To address this topic, a review of the occupational therapy literature was conducted regarding the use of occupation and its role in contributing to life experience and satisfaction. Although the idea of participation in life through the activities and engagement in the occupations in which people take part every day is not new, its importance has been given greater emphasis as the occupational therapy profession attempts to reconnect with its roots. The psychology literature was consulted to examine optimal experience, or flow. The search yielded examples of studies conducted using the flow construct, which have been undertaken by researchers in various fields to include psychology, leisure, education, occupational therapy, technology, and business. Although flow is not a novel concept, especially in the discipline of psychology, little emphasis has been placed on it in the occupational therapy literature. Therefore, an exploration of both constructs seems to have merit, followed by an examination of the literature to look at a possible correlation between the two.

## The Importance of Meaningful Occupation

There has been a shift in the global view of health from that of absence of disease or impairment to one that supports the idea that true health has more to do with satisfaction, quality of life, and the pursuit of health (Zemke, 2004). Numerous accounts exist of individuals who have found new meaning in life after the onset of a traumatic illness or life-altering event, which has contributed to a greater sense of purpose and well-being. Dossey (1991, as cited in Bridle, 1999) talked about individuals not only seeking meaning in their lives and in their doing, but in their debility. Celebrities such as Michael J. Fox, Christopher Reeve, and countless others have talked openly about finding a new sense of purpose and meaning as a result of injury and illness.

Finding meaning in everyday occupations is important for all human beings. As occupational therapy practitioners, we are faced with the challenge of not only discerning which occupations a client values, but also aiding the individual in discovering new sources of meaning when previously valued occupations are no longer possible.

Christiansen (1999) highlighted the importance of occupations in contributing to one's sense of identity. He discussed the need human beings have to express themselves in a unique way that gives meaning to life, viewing engagement in occupations as a vehicle to fulfill that need. He also talked about the relationship between self and others in influencing this sense of identity, stating that we both affect others and are affected by them. Our identities are closely related to the things we do, as well as how we interpret what we do in the social context. In our analysis of events, human beings look for personal meaning, and if these events are deemed significant, we respond in an emotional way and are shaped by them. Our perceptions of life are subsequently formed as well. Therefore, Christiansen stated that identity plays an important role in promoting well-being and satisfaction in life. Having a sense of control and purpose gives meaning to individuals. Bridle (1999) also discussed identity in terms of the relationship between "being" and "doing" as a dimension of holism. Eakman and Eklund (2012) explored the role of personality in predicting well-being but found that occupations of meaning and value had greater influence on predicting satisfaction and meaning in life.

In a qualitative study that examined the relationship between occupation and its contribution to competence and identity, persons with serious mental illness engaged in woodworking occupations in two community settings (Mee, Sumsion, & Craik, 2004). All participants identified engagement in occupation as the mechanism to acquire skills, a sense of competence and purpose, and a personal sense of self-worth and identity. Hvalsøe and Josephsson (2003) found that their subjects with mental illness believed it was essential that occupations met their need to be engaged in various roles and that these occupations matched their personal preferences and interests for them to be of value. Use of occupations that are meaningful to people and that contribute to their sense of identity only underscore the importance of employing this in our intervention strategies with clients; in doing so, practitioners will be facilitating the fulfillment of a common basic need experienced by all human beings.

Yerxa (1998) examined the relationship between health and engagement in occupation, bringing in the idea of the importance of the human spirit. She identified some of the early theorists of the occupational therapy profession, such as Reilly and Meyer, who clearly saw the connection between involvement in everyday occupations and health. Yerxa cited research studies regarding some of the creative thinkers of the world, which revealed how little attention has been paid to the idea of work being a contributor to happiness, even if a given individual lacks close personal relationships. The point is made that the drive for autonomy is just as important as the impetus to get closer to other people. What is of greater significance is that the interests pursued are those that contribute to well-being and life satisfaction.

For many individuals, the occupation of work is a source of great meaning and satisfaction, regardless of health status (Kennedy-Jones, Cooper, & Fossey, 2005). In addition to the obvious practical benefits of working for a wage to sustain one's livelihood and one's family, the occupation of work is seen as an avenue to establish one's place in society, help form self-identity, and use and increase skills. Work was more frequently cited than leisure in numerous studies conducted to determine which everyday occupations resulted in optimal experiences, positive feelings, and satisfaction (Csikszentmihalyi, 1997; Csikszentmihalyi & LeFevre, 1989; Gerhardsson & Jonsson, 1996; Rebeiro & Polgar, 1999). Because many clients referred for occupational therapy services experience limitations in their ability to work, it is important to recognize the importance of any life changes that negatively affect this meaningful role. Occupational therapy intervention may involve helping clients to make adaptations so that they can resume the worker role or discover meaning through different occupations.

Effective occupational therapy intervention may require drawing on past occupations that once provided meaning for an individual. When asked why certain occupations were preferred, subjects in a study that elicited the perspectives of persons with mental illness identified occupations that had evoked positive feelings in the past (Hvalsøe & Josephsson, 2003). Knowledge of occupations that have been valued by the client may serve as an impetus to continue involvement or to reintroduce that occupation into one's life. Recently during a level II fieldwork placement in the community mental health system, my student discovered that one of her clients once derived satisfaction from needlework, but had stopped engaging in this leisure occupation. Inspired by that knowledge, the student provided materials for the client to participate in a similar occupation, which proved to be meaningful and, therefore, motivating.

The founders of occupational therapy strongly believed that health and well-being could be influenced by engagement in occupation (Schwartz, 2005). Schwartz gave the following examples of the meaning occupation held for these historical figures in occupational therapy. William Rush Dunton, Jr. found that crafts had a therapeutic effect on him personally and went on to further the Arts and Crafts movement as part of the intervention in children and adults with mental illness. Meyer and Slagle espoused the importance of habits and involvement in occupations as a way to deal with problems in living. Hall focused on the importance of work, rather than rest, as an avenue toward improved health. The profession, in some respects, has come full circle in recognizing the power of occupation. Therefore, it is imperative that we continue to learn how to unleash that power.

## The Concept of Flow

The theory of optimal experience based on the concept of flow was developed in the 1970s by Mihaly Csikszentmihalyi who said: "Flow [autotelic experience] is the way people describe their state of mind when consciousness is harmoniously ordered, and they want to pursue whatever they are doing for its own sake" (1990, p. 6). The experience is so enjoyable and absorbing that it becomes autotelic, meaning it is worth doing even if there is no tangible outcome (Csikszentmihalyi, 1999). Csikszentmihalyi wanted to understand the internal feeling state of individuals when they were doing what they enjoyed the most and to determine why they felt that way. He viewed this construct as a possible avenue to help improve quality of life. In addition, Csikszentmihalyi believed that the ability to experience flow, as well as hope and optimism, could be learned, which would in turn affect one's level of happiness (Csikszentmihalyi & Hunter, 2003). Whereas research has gathered information about the kinds of experiences (e.g., leisure, work, athletics, music, religious rituals, creative activities) that may result in flow, Csikszentmihalyi discussed the possibility of ordering one's consciousness so that any activity could result in flow and, thereby, enhance well-being (Csikszentmihalyi, 1990).

Regardless of the activity that generates the flow experience, people describe flow similarly across all cultures (Carlson & Clark, 1991; Moneta, 2004). When experiencing optimal flow, individuals become so immersed that they lose sense of time and feel joyful, motivated, creative, and intensely focused. There is a lack of self-consciousness, an escape from problems, and a clear sense of one's goal (Carlson & Clark, 1991; Csikszentmihalyi, 1990, 1999; Csikszentmihalyi & LeFevre, 1989; Gerhardsson & Jonsson, 1996; Jacobs, 1994; Rebeiro & Polgar, 1999). Process becomes more important than any outcome of this expenditure of psychic energy (Rebeiro & Polgar, 1999). It is also true that stress is an aspect of flow, the degree depending on the level of the challenge involved. Certain conditions must exist for flow to occur (Csikszentmihalyi, 1990; Gerhardsson & Jonsson, 1996; Jacobs, 1994; Persson, 1996; Rebeiro & Polgar, 1999):

- There must be a match between one's skills and the challenge of the activity.
- There must be clear short-term goals.
- The individual needs to feel he or she has control.
- The activity must provide immediate feedback.

Csikszentmihalyi identified the following contexts of challenge and skills: anxiety, flow, boredom, and apathy (Jacobs, 1994; McCormick, Funderburk, Lee, & Hale-Fought, 2005). In the anxiety context, the individual perceives the challenge of the activity as beyond one's capacity as compared with the skills the person possesses. Flow occurs when challenges and skills are equal, with the caveat that the activity or experience requires that the individual stretch beyond usual performance. Boredom occurs when the challenges are less than the skill level as perceived by the individual. Apathy occurs when both skills and challenges are perceived as below that of the individual's perception of his or her average capability and challenge (Jacobs, 1994).

The experience sampling method (ESM) was developed as an alternative to qualitative interviews to gather data about the flow experience of individuals as they occurred in natural contexts over time (Carlson & Clark, 1991; Csikszentmihalyi, 2003; Csikszentmihalyi & LeFevre, 1989; Farnworth, Mostert, Harrison, & Worrell, 1996; Jacobs, 1994). The instrument asks about challenges the subject is experiencing in the here and now to identify flow and gathers information about the subjective experience of the individual regarding the quality of experience and kind of activity in which he or she is engaged. Subjects wear an electronic device that beeps randomly throughout the day, and they are asked to complete an experience sampling form that addresses pertinent questions regarding what activities they were engaged in at the time as well as the perceived challenges and skills related to the task. This methodology for studying the experience of flow was seen as an improvement on other means of gathering these data (Farnworth et al., 1996). Time diaries have been used to collect similar data, but they do not necessarily provide direct access to the individual's internal experience, nor to the intensity of it. In addition, interviews have their limitations owing to selective remembering and the possibility that the subjects may skew their reports based on a desire to please the researcher in some way (Farnworth et al., 1996). Carlson and Clark (1991) highlighted the merits of this methodology as a valid way to record data to increase knowledge of how human beings are affected by ordinary activities.

To exemplify the use of the flow construct and the ESM of gathering data, some examples are given. Studies outside of the discipline of occupational therapy and within the profession are described.

In a study designed to predict boredom and anxiety in the lives of community mental health clients, McCormick et al. (2005) discovered that states of boredom and anxiety interfered with social and cognitive functioning. Through the use of the ESM, they learned that individuals with severe mental illness tend to have fewer challenges in their lives and spend most of their time engaged in activities below their skill level; this would be thought to result in boredom. However, that was not the subjective experience of the participants. Although their research indicated that there is little in the way of stimulating activity in the lives of persons with severe mental illness, it may well be that these individuals avoid anxiety by not seeking out more challenging situations. They concluded that for this population, understimulation and overstimulation could be problematic. Either way, these findings speak to the importance of balance between skills and challenge to promote well-being and quality of life.

To examine behaviors and habits that could be associated with happiness, Csikszentmihalyi and Hunter (2003) conducted a study of American youth using the ESM. As a premise, it was understood that events occurring outside of oneself have an effect on personal happiness, but one's values and interpretation of events also have an effect. Given the age of the subjects, weekdays were consumed with school or work activities. With regard to the time of day, the teens indicated a higher level of happiness at lunch and after school when they had free time. The activities with which the subjects were involved at a given time, as well as their companions, also had an effect on perceived happiness. The final results indicated that younger teens of lower socioeconomic groups were happier—they tended to spend less time alone and more time in high-challenge/high-skill activities, which resulted in flow. The ESM allowed researchers to capture information about what was meaningful and fulfilling to this population.

Jacobs (1994) used the ESM to examine optimal flow experiences and job satisfaction in occupational therapy practitioners. Most of her subjects worked in physical rehabilitation settings and reported experiencing flow a relatively small percentage of time (average of 5.24 times per week). As expected, flow experiences occurred most often during the intervention process. Her intent was to gain information to enable practitioners to develop and apply strategies to enhance flow experiences for occupational therapists while at work, and to enable them to facilitate this experience for their clients. In her article, she reiterates the suggestions made by Csikszentmihalyi (1990) regarding how this might be accomplished.

Persson (1996) used the concepts of play and flow theories to examine the occupational process with a creative activity group for clients with chronic pain. The aim of this study was to look at theory that would emphasize a "doing" perspective and to see if the chosen theories could be used to study this process. Many of the components of both theories are congruent. The results indicated that the concepts of play and flow are useful in this context. Subjects experienced the creative activities as both serious and playful, as well as enjoyable, although frustrating at times (Persson, 1996). Some typical characteristics of flow experiences were reported by the subjects while they were engaged in the activity, including statements that pain was sometimes forgotten. Persson gave an example describing "how a meaningful activity and its possibilities and demands can arouse the energy and intention for the actor when he/she at first enters into it with skepticism" (p. 40).

Subjects with schizophrenia were engaged in a study by Gerhardsson and Jonsson (1996) designed to explore intrinsic motivation and flow experience. The participants were observed during selected activities of personal interest at three different times, followed by a semi-structured interview immediately after each session. The content of the interview was designed to learn about the subject's experience of the activity and to compare his or her report with the observation report, which was based on elements of the flow experience. If the participant had experienced the activity previously, the chances of flow increased. Overall, the results suggested that the elements of the flow theory are useful in describing which aspects of a particular occupation have a therapeutic effect on an individual (Gerhardsson & Jonsson, 1996).

Csikszentmihalyi and LeFevre (1989) used the ESM in a study with adult workers to discern any differences in the quality of experience for these individuals while they were engaged in work versus leisure. Quality was measured in terms of the match of challenges and skills, as well as level of happiness, satisfaction, creativity, and motivation. Although it might seem unlikely, more subjects appeared to experience flow-like conditions while at work as opposed to when engaged in leisure pursuits. The researchers hypothesized that it may be that during free time people just need to relax and recuperate from an intense workday, or that they are unable to direct their psychic energy when time is not organized and structured. It was suggested that if people realized that they actually derived more benefits from work than they had previously thought, it might result in a reevaluation of any negative perceptions they held about their jobs. In addition, it might be that a more conscious use of leisure activities could result in experiences more conducive to flow during free time.

The explosion of technology to include social media has resulted in increasing numbers of individuals using the Internet. Online learning, researching, shopping, and gaming have become meaningful occupations for many individuals, and occupational therapists need to be mindful of this development. In exploring the literature, a significant number of researchers have conducted studies that examine the flow experience in relation to Internet use and web design. Skadberg and Kimmel (2004) found that two primary factors contributed to optimal experience or flow: attractiveness and the interactivity of the website. One of their most important discoveries was that telepresence (loss of awareness, intense focus) was the greatest measure of flow. Furthermore, optimal experience was associated with the context of the situational interaction in addition to gathering information on a particular topic. Pace (2004) found that informants in his study experienced time distortion, escape from concerns, and decreased awareness of the physical and social environment while they were engaged online.

Playing online games has become a valued leisure activity for many people. Flow is encouraged through online gaming in that the player receives immediate feedback, experiences enjoyment, and the activity requires concentration (Chiang, Lin, Cheng, & Liu, 2011). Teng and Huang (2012) found that skill and challenge predicted flow when subjects were engaged in gaming. Online games produce a cognitive state that facilitates flow, and players can begin at a simpler level and advance to more challenging levels, thereby increasing mastery (Cowley, Charles, Black, & Hickey, 2008). Researchers investigating what motivated customers to continue online gaming or remain loyal to a particular game found that having an optimal experience/flow experience was the greatest factor (Choi & Kim, 2004; Lee & Tsai, 2010). Flow theory plays a significant role in research related to information technology (Teng & Huang, 2012).

Through a critical review of the literature, York and Wiseman (2012) found evidence supporting the use of gardening to enhance well-being. For individuals who value gardening, this occupational behavior setting offers a feeling of stability and safety, which are key components of occupational therapy intervention (York & Wiseman, 2012). To further explore the relationship between meaningful occupation and flow, a mixed methods study was conducted in 2015 to determine if avid gardeners experienced flow while engaged in this occupation (King, Hess, Matanick, Vorst, & Wagner, 2015). An online survey with quantitative questions based on Csikszentmihalyi's components of flow was disseminated to 93 individuals who were master gardeners or garden club members, resulting in a 39% return. Most of the respondents engaged in gardening at home in a solitary environment, although some also pursued this occupation in community gardens. The Likert scale responses indicated participants experienced components of flow 64% of the time averaged over the eight flow-related questions with responses of "Always" or "Very Often." The components of flow that yielded the highest percentages of affirmation were those indicating worrying less, experiencing enjoyment/reward, having clear goals, and feeling their engagement was automatic. Qualitative data were gathered regarding the respondents' primary reasons for gardening and the value it held for them. They stated gardening provided the following:

- A connection with nature
- Stress reduction and relaxation
- Exercise
- An opportunity to gain related knowledge
- Satisfaction
- The benefits of having healthy produce if a vegetable gardener

Overall, survey results pointed to engagement in the occupation of gardening as providing meaning, life satisfaction, and contributing to quality of life while often producing a flow experience (King et al., 2015).

## Discussion

Early theorists as well as current scholars in the field of occupational therapy discuss skill acquisition and providing the "just-right challenge" when planning and implementing interventions for those we serve (Carlson & Clark, 1991; Mee et al., 2004; Yerxa, 1998). One of the most important criteria in producing flow is that skills must match the challenge of the activity and that there should be a certain degree of tension. An individual should have to stretch his or her capacity to expand, grow, and actualize potential. The work of Csikszentmihalyi and LeFevre (1989) in breaking down the ratio of skills to challenge into the contexts of anxiety, boredom, flow, and apathy provides a lens through which the occupational therapist might analyze occupational choices and occupational behavior when designing effective interventions for clients (Carlson & Clark, 1991). Another important requirement for facilitating flow is that the goals of the activity or occupation must be clear and distinct. Christiansen (1999) equated occupation with "goal-directed activity in the context of living" (p. 553), and elaborated by saying that because an individual imagines the outcome if a goal is met, that goal becomes a source of motivation. Setting achievable goals based on client input to increase motivation is inherent in occupational therapy practice.

The concept of balance in life as a determinant of health has been germane to the field of occupational therapy since its inception. Yerxa (1998) cited leaders in the profession, to include Meyer and Reilly, as espousing the merits of a healthy balance. Csikszentmihalyi, too, saw the value of balance when he discussed the need for a match between perceived skills and the challenge of activities in the environment (Yerxa, 1998). Law (2007) saw the relevance of Csikszentmihalyi's work to occupational therapy just as her colleagues had (Carlson & Clark, 1991; Yerxa, 1998).

Christiansen (1999), in discussing the power of occupation, proposed that we create meaning in our lives through the things we do. Csikszentmihalyi (1990) devoted a chapter to the subject of meaning, stating that "creating meaning involves bringing order to the contents of the mind by integrating actions into a unified flow experience" (p. 216). Meaningful lives require challenging goals of significance that must be pursued with resolve to produce harmony (Csikszentmihalyi, 1990). Engelhardt (1983) echoed the perspective of founders of the profession by describing occupational therapists as custodians of meaning. Studies designed to validate the importance of meaningful occupation, including some cited in this chapter, have provided evidence that what we do in everyday life has a profound effect on life satisfaction and well-being. However, what is meaningful to one individual may not be to another (Persson et al., 2001). For occupational therapy interventions to be successful, we must learn which occupations are of value to clients because the concepts of purpose and meaning are central to therapeutic outcomes (Farnworth et al., 1996). To underscore the powerful effect the discovery of a meaningful occupation can have on an individual, Csikszentmihalyi (1997) described a woman with chronic schizophrenia who had been hospitalized for more than 10 years. In a period of study using the ESM, she reported having positive moods several times that occurred when she was caring for her fingernails. Based on those findings, the staff in the facility enlisted the aid of a professional manicurist to teach the client skills that resulted in the woman giving manicures to other clients. Not only did her mood improve, but she was able to be discharged to the community where she eventually took up the trade and became self-sufficient within a year.

Despite the similarities between the concept of flow and the philosophy of occupational therapy with respect to the value of meaningful occupation, Csikszentmihalyi's work has not been used to provide evidence in support of our work. The flow construct has been researched and utilized in the fields of psychology, leisure, education, and business. However, there was little to be found in the occupational therapy literature that referenced flow, and much of the evidence was produced more than a decade ago, primarily outside of the United States. It would appear that we have not taken advantage of a well-researched body of work that has considerable merit, but we have the opportunity to do so. On a macro level, the flow construct could serve to validate the importance of the role of occupational therapy in facilitating health, well-being, and quality of life. On a micro level, Csikszentmihalyi's theory could enable us to determine what is, in fact, meaningful occupation as we intervene with clients on a day-to-day basis.

## Summary

The literature clearly indicates a relationship between meaningful occupation and the concept of flow. The studies described exemplify how one might use Csikszentmihalyi's work and methodology to provide further evidence on the value of occupation. Flow "is highly relevant to occupational science because it documents an everyday phenomenon that importantly relates to, among other things, happiness, self-esteem, work productivity, the enjoyment of leisure, and life satisfaction" (Carlson & Clark, 1991, p. 239).

Embracing Csikszentmihalyi's theory and capitalizing on the extensive body of evidence that has been produced primarily outside of the occupational therapy profession would lend credence to our own body of knowledge. The degree to which the relationship between these two constructs needs to be investigated is beyond the scope of this chapter. Occupational therapists need to engage in the meaningful occupation of producing evidence to validate what we do and to increase our understanding of how we can best intervene to facilitate successful outcomes for our clients who are depending on us to assist them with improving quality of life.

## Student Self-Assessment

1. List some of your favorite occupations. What are some of your usual feelings when engaged in these pursuits?
2. Do you think you experience flow when participating in any of these occupations? Which ones?
3. Evaluate your favorite occupations in terms of Csikszentmihalyi's conditions of flow. Do any of these pursuits meet his criteria for flow? If so, which ones? If not, which ones? Why or why not?
4. Review the challenge and skills contexts discussed on pages 6 and 7. Identify an activity or occupation in which you experience (a) anxiety, (b) boredom, and (c) apathy. How do these subjective feelings affect your motivation and sense of well-being?

## Evidence-Based Research Chart

| Topic | Evidence |
|---|---|
| Occupational therapy and meaningful occupation | Bridle, 1999; Christiansen, 1999; Christiansen, Backman, Little, & Nguyen, 1999; Eakman & Eklund, 2012; Engelhardt, 1983; Hammell, 2004; Hvalsøe & Josephsson, 2003; Kennedy-Jones, Cooper, & Fossey, 2005; Law, 2007; Mee, Sumsion, & Craik, 2004; Persson, Erlandsson, Eklund, & Iwarsson, 2001; Schwartz, 2005; Yerxa, 1998; York & Wiseman, 2012; Zemke, 2004 |
| Theory of flow | Csikszentmihalyi, 1990, 1997, 1999, 2003; Csikszentmihalyi & Hunter, 2003; Csikszentmihalyi & LeFevre, 1989 |
| Studies about flow | Chiang, Lin, Cheng, & Liu, 2011; Choi & Kim, 2004; Cowley, Charles, Black, & Hickey, 2008; Lee & Tsai, 2010; McCormick, Funderburk, Lee, & Hale-Fought, 2005; Moneta, 2004; Pace, 2004; Skadberg & Kimmel, 2004; Teng & Huang, 2012 |
| Flow and occupational therapy | Carlson & Clark, 1991; Farnworth, Mostert, Harrison, & Worrell, 1996; Gerhardsson & Jonsson, 1996; Jacobs, 1994; King, Hess, Matanick, Vorst, & Wagner, 2015; Persson, 1996; Rebeiro & Polgar, 1999 |

5. Discuss any parallels you see between the experience of flow and occupations that are meaningful to individuals. How could you apply this to occupational therapy practice?
6. Do you think it is possible to experience flow while engaged in an activity or occupation even if all of Csikszentmihalyi's conditions are not met?

## References


Bridle, M. J. (1999). Are doing and being dimensions of holism? *American Journal of Occupational Therapy, 53*(6), 636-639.

Carlson, M. E., & Clark, F. A. (1991). The search for useful methodologies in occupational science. *American Journal of Occupational Therapy, 45*(3), 235-241.

Chiang, Y., Lin, S., Cheng, C., & Liu, E. (2011). Exploring online game players' flow experiences and positive affect. *The Turkish Online Journal of Educational Technology, 10*(1), 106-114.

Choi, D., & Kim, J. (2004). Why people continue to play online games: In search of critical design factors to increase customer loyalty to online contents. *CyberPsychology & Behavior, 7*(3), 11-23.

Christiansen, C. H. (1999). The 1999 Eleanor Clarke Slagle lecture: Defining lives: Occupation as identity: An essay on competence, coherence, and the creation of meaning. *American Journal of Occupational Therapy, 53*(6), 547-558.

Christiansen, C. H., Backman, C., Little, B. R., & Nguyen, A. (1999). Occupations and well-being: A study of personal projects. *American Journal of Occupational Therapy, 53*(1), 91-100.

Cowley, B., Charles, D., Black, M., & Hickey, R. (2008). Toward an understanding of flow in video games. *ACM Computers in Entertainment, 6*(2), 20.1-20.27.

Csikszentmihalyi, M. (1990). *Flow: The psychology of optimal experience.* New York, NY: HarperCollins.

Csikszentmihalyi, M. (1997). *Finding flow: The psychology of engagement with everyday life.* New York, NY: Basic Books.

Csikszentmihalyi, M. (1999). If we are so rich, why aren't we happy? *American Psychologist, 54*(10), 821-827.

Csikszentmihalyi, M. (2003). Happiness in everyday life: The uses of experience sampling. *Journal of Happiness Studies, 4*(2), 185-199.

Csikszentmihalyi, M., & Hunter, J. (2003). Happiness in everyday life: The uses of experience sampling. *Journal of Happiness Studies, 4,* 185-199.

Csikszentmihalyi, M., & LeFevre, J. (1989). Optimal experience in work and leisure. *Journal of Personality and Social Psychology, 56*(5), 815-822.

Eakman, A. M., & Eklund, M. (2012). The relative impact of personality traits, meaningful occupation and occupational value on meaning in life and life satisfaction. *Journal of Occupational Science, 19*(2), 165-177.

Engelhardt, T. (1983). Occupational therapists as technologists and custodians of meaning. In G. Kielhofner (Ed.), *Health through occupation* (pp. 139-144). Philadelphia, PA: F. A. Davis Company.

Farnworth, L., Mostert, E., Harrison, S., & Worrell, D. (1996). The experience sampling method: Its potential use in occupational therapy research. *Occupational Therapy International, 3*(1), 1-17.

Gerhardsson, C., & Jonsson, H. (1996). Experience of therapeutic occupations in schizophrenic subjects: Clinical observations organized in terms of the flow theory. *Scandinavian Journal of Occupational Therapy, 3*(4), 149-155.

Hammell, K. (2004). Dimensions of meaning in the occupations of daily life. *Canadian Journal of Occupational Therapy, 5*(71), 296-305.

Hvalsøe, B., & Josephsson, S. (2003). Characteristics of meaningful occupations from the perspective of mentally ill people. *Scandinavian Journal of Occupational Therapy, 10*(2), 61-71.

Jacobs, K. (1994). Flow and the occupational therapy practitioner. *American Journal of Occupational Therapy, 48*(11), 989-996.

Kennedy-Jones, M., Cooper, J., & Fossey, E. (2005). Developing a worker role: Stories of four people with mental illness. *Australian Occupational Therapy Journal, 52*(2), 116-126.

King, R., Hess, S., Matanick, N., Vorst, M., & Wagner, E. (2015). Gardening as a meaningful occupation and its relationship to flow [unpublished master's thesis]. Findlay, OH: The University of Findlay.

Law, M. (2007). Occupational therapy: A journey driven by curiosity. *American Journal of Occupational Therapy, 61,* 599-602.

Lee, M., & Tsai, T. (2010). What drives people to continue to play online games? An extension of technology model and theory of planned behavior. *International Journal of Human-Computer Interaction, 26*(6), 601-620.

McCormick, B. P., Funderburk, J. A., Lee, Y. K., & Hale-Fought, M. (2005). Activity characteristics and emotional experience: Predicting boredom and anxiety in the daily life of community mental health clients. *Journal of Leisure Research, 37,* 236-253.

Mee, J., Sumsion, T., & Craik, C. (2004). Mental health clients confirm the value of occupation in building competence and self-identity. *British Journal of Occupational Therapy, 67*(5), 225-233.

Moneta, G. (2004). The flow experience across cultures. *Journal of Happiness Studies, 5*(4), 115-121.

Pace, S. (2004). The roles of challenge and skill in the flow experiences of Web users. *Issues in Informing Science and Information Technology, 1,* 341-358.

Persson, D. (1996). Play and flow in an activity group—A case study of creative occupations with chronic pain patients. *Scandinavian Journal of Occupational Therapy, 3*(1), 33-42.

Persson, D., Erlandsson, L., Eklund, M., & Iwarsson, S. (2001). Value dimensions, meaning, and complexity in human occupation—A tentative structure for analysis. *Scandinavian Journal of Occupational Therapy, 8*(1), 7-18.

Rebeiro, K. L., & Polgar, J. M. (1999). Enabling occupational performance: Optimal experiences in therapy. *Canadian Journal of Occupational Therapy, 66*(1), 14-22.

Schwartz, K. (2005). The history and philosophy of psychosocial occupational therapy. In E. Cara & A. MacRae (Eds.), *Psychosocial occupational therapy: A clinical practice* (2nd ed., pp. 61-68). Florence, KY: Delmar Cengage Learning.

Skadberg, Y., & Kimmel, J. (2004). Visitor's flow experience while browsing a web site: Its measurement, contributing factors and consequences. *Computers in Human Behavior, 20*(3), 403-422.

Teng, C., & Huang, C. (2012). More than flow: Revisiting the theory of four channels of flow. *International Journal of Computer Games Technology,* 1-9. doi:10.1155/2012/724917

Yerxa, E. J. (1998). Health and the human spirit for occupation. *American Journal of Occupational Therapy, 52*(6), 412-418.

York, M., & Wiseman, T. (2012). Gardening as an occupation: A critical review. *British Journal of Occupational Therapy, 75*(2), 76-84.

Zemke, R. (2004). The 2004 Eleanor Clarke Slagle lecture: Time, space, and the kaleidoscopes of occupation. *American Journal of Occupational Therapy, 58*(6), 608-620.

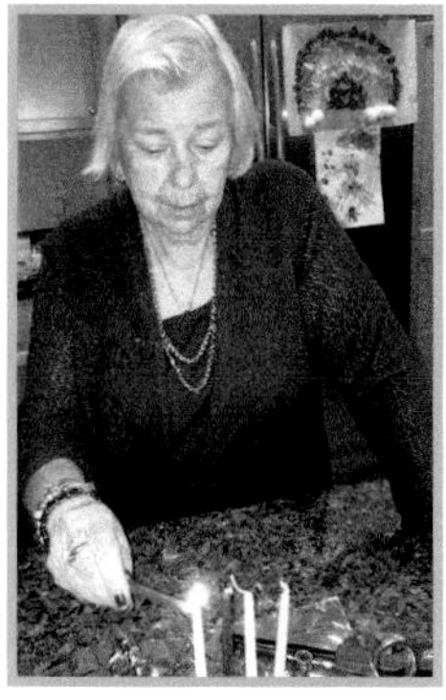

# 2

# Cultural Impact on Occupation

Roxie M. Black, PhD, OTR, FAOTA

**ACOTE STANDARDS EXPLORED IN THIS CHAPTER**

B.1.4–B.1.6, B.2.9, B.4.0, B.4.2, B.4.4, B.4.7, B.5.0, B.5.1

**KEY VOCABULARY**

- **Cultural competence:** The process of actively developing and practicing cultural self-awareness, knowledge, and skill when interacting with someone culturally diverse from oneself.
- **Cultural effectiveness:** The process of interacting with someone culturally different from oneself, with self-awareness, knowledge, and skill, while engaging in critical reflection both during and following the interaction.
- **Culturally sensitive assessment tools:** Tools and surveys that add questions that elicit information about the client's cultural beliefs and practices related to health care.
- **Culture:** The sum total of a way of living that influences the behavior(s) of a group of people.
- **Occupational justice:** The rights of people to have access to and opportunity to engage in meaningful occupations.



Jacobs, K., & MacRae, N. (Eds.).
*Occupational Therapy Essentials for Clinical Competence, Third Edition* (pp. 13-28).

The concept of culture is deeply embedded, yet readily visible, in occupational therapy. It is addressed in multiple standards from the Accreditation Council for Occupational Therapy Education (ACOTE); identified in the *Occupational Therapy Practice Framework* (American Occupational Therapy Association [AOTA], 2014), as a vital context when assessing and developing interventions with occupational therapy clients; is addressed in multiple occupation-based models of practice (Christiansen & Baum, 1997; Dunn, Brown, & McGuigan, 1994; Iwama, 2006; Law, Cooper, Strong, Stewart, Rigby, & Letts, 1996; Schkade & Schultz, 2003); examined in relation to ethical practice in the *Occupational Therapy Code of Ethics*; addressed in the Centennial Vision; and found in numerous occupational therapy books and other publications. Cultural competency is a vital aspect of occupational therapy education and practice.

The concept of culture, however ubiquitous in occupational therapy documents, is quite complex. This chapter defines culture; discusses its relevance to occupational therapy practitioners, educators, and researchers; speaks to the concepts of bias and prejudice and how they impact practice; addresses its importance in developing assessment tools and examining marginalized populations; and discusses its relevance in culturally effective care.

## Culture Defined

Iwama (2004) described culture as a "slippery concept, taking on a variety of definitions and meanings, depending on how it has been socially situated and by whom" (p. 1). Some people may define "having culture" as being sophisticated and knowledgeable, whereas the term *culture* might connote racial and ethnic differences to others. A much broader definition of culture is:

> The sum total of a way of living, including values, beliefs, standards, linguistic expression, patterns of thinking, behavioral norms, and styles of communication that influence the behavior(s) of a group of people that is transmitted from generation to generation. It includes demographic variables such as age, gender, and place of residence, status variables such as social, educational, and economic levels, and affiliation variables. (Black & Wells, 2007, p. 5)

In addition, culture is learned. Because it is transmitted to others and following generations, aspects of one's culture—including attitudes, values, and behaviors—can be examined, changed, and/or adapted to meet the requirements of changing current times and contexts.

**Student Activity 1**

After reading the definition of culture, examine and write down how you would describe yourself considering all the aspects listed. This is your cultural self. Share with a friend, family member, or classmate.

As is evident in the preceding complex definition, culture is all encompassing and influences multiple aspects of a person's life, including occupational behaviors and occupational choices. For example, the occupation of eating breakfast varies between different cultural groups. The time we rise in the morning, the food we choose to eat (or do not eat), the utensils we use (or do not use), what time of the day we eat, how much time we take to have a meal, whether we stand or sit, and whether we eat alone or with others are all influenced by one's cultural group and expectations.

Not only are we influenced by the culture into which we are born (family, community, society), we are also affected by the subcultures to which we choose to belong. These may include groups from our church, synagogue, or temple; our college and occupational therapy program; our cohort of friends; our biking or hiking group; or our gym companions. Because each of these subgroups holds certain values and expectations that we choose to share, they also influence our behaviors and choices. Sometimes the expectations of these various cultural groups are in conflict with one another. For example, as an occupational therapy student, the faculty of your occupational therapy program may expect you to study for several hours a day or night, whereas your family or roommates may have expectations that you will be home for dinner each evening. Your occupational choice will depend on what you determine is most important to you at that time given the context of the situation.

What is meaningful and important is culturally determined and influences occupational behaviors, choices, and performance for not only each of us, but also for each client with whom we work. Recognizing the extent of cultural influence on behavior is vital for understanding the context within which our clients live and work. Therefore, "culture represents one of the most important issues facing occupational therapy today" (Iwama, 2004, p. 1).

## Multiple Levels of Cultural Influence

As occupational therapy students and practitioners, including occupational therapy assistants, occupational therapists, educators, and researchers, culture influences us and our occupational choice on many levels, just as it does the people with whom we work. These levels begin with each of us personally, and move through several levels to the global level (Figure 2-1). We briefly examine each of these levels in this section of the chapter.

## Personal Influences

Each of us develops from a particular social location. This means that our place of birth, year of birth, birth order, gender and sexual identity, class, family structure, ability, religion, and ethnicity all influence who we are at birth, our values and interests as we age, and, in many cases, who we will become as adults. All of these cultural characteristics influence our behavior or what we do: our occupations. For example, I was born just after the end of World War II and raised in a rural state by working-class parents. I was raised to believe in hard work, the importance of education (which my parents were unable to acquire yet knew the value of), the importance of helping others, and the love of family and nature. All of these values influence what I choose to do today, from teaching in an occupational therapy program, to spending important time with family and friends, to one of my favorite pastimes—gardening.

Most of us are taught our cultural values by members of our families, friends, mentors, teachers, and spiritual leaders. We also learn cultural lessons that may not always be to our best interest from the media, such as the standard of feminine beauty, the importance of wealth, and the value of commodities. Often the messages learned from these various groups/people conflict, and we must choose what best meets our needs. For example, we may come from a large Italian family where the message of "Mangia! Mangia!" ("Eat! Eat!") rings in our ears, yet the print and electronic media constantly tell us that being painfully thin is the true vision of beauty in the United States. Or our peer group enjoys playing at the beach, lying in the sun, and developing a deep, rich tan, whereas the message from the health community is that getting too much sun can lead to health issues. What do we do? Each of us is a unique and complex cultural being, so we will make occupational choices based on what we value, or what is important to us at that time. For these reasons, each person must be viewed as an individual.

This is also true of the people with whom we work as occupational therapy practitioners. Although there may be cultural similarities among members of a particular group, we cannot assume each member of the group holds the same beliefs, values, and occupational interests, and we cannot treat each member of a group in the same way. Certainly not all of the students in a given academic program perform the same, learn in the same manner, study the same way, or enjoy the same topics, even though the majority may be all White women as they are in academic programs in the state of Maine. Therefore, it is imperative that the faculty understand each student as an individual, just as occupational therapy practitioners must view each client as an individual.

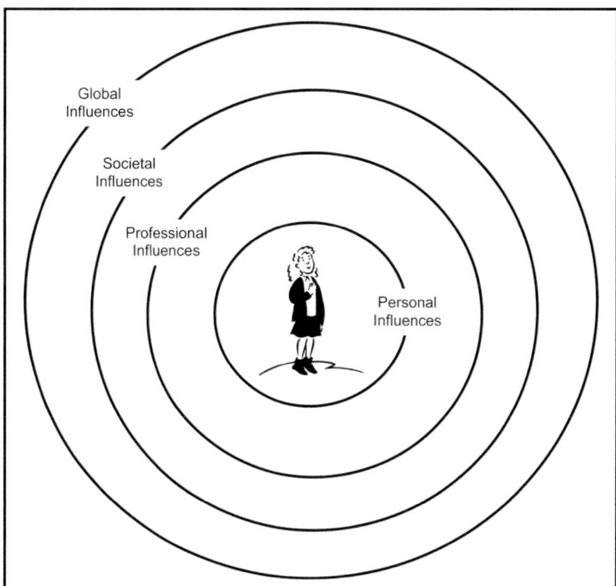


**Figure 2-1.** Cultural levels of influence.

One reason that there is such individuality within a group or subgroup is that culture can be learned as well as unlearned. Although we are taught certain values as children, as we develop and experience more of life, we sometimes reject or modify those earlier teachings and assume other values. For instance, we may have been taught negative things about a certain race or ethnicity, or that older people are cranky and helpless, or that women are emotional and weak, or that motorcyclists are all hoodlums. But our life experiences and/or education have refuted those lessons, and we may now perceive members of those groups in different ways. As we mature, we may choose a spiritual path or lifestyle that is different from that of our parents or cultural group, or we may move into a different socioeconomic class—an experience that may change our perception of our world and the people in it. These changing beliefs and values will alter our occupational choices and patterns, and demonstrate the dynamic nature of our cultural influences and reemphasize the importance of learning about people's individual and personal cultures as we work with them. Not only are we influenced by our personal beliefs and values, but also what we learn as occupational therapists affects our beliefs and behaviors as well.

## Professional Influences: Culture and Occupational Therapy

The concept of culture is embedded in our profession and has been since we first began recognizing clients as individuals with unique needs. The very first set of standards for occupational therapy emphasized the importance of providing treatment to each client as an individual (*Standards of the National Society for the Promotion of Occupational Therapy*, 1925). Although a client's "cultural influences" may not have been the language used at that time, as we sought to understand each unique client's interests, beliefs, and needs, we were actually examining aspects of his or her culture. Over the past nine decades we have continued to view each recipient of occupational therapy services as an individual, although many concepts within the field have developed and changed. Some of the more current notions and language related to occupational therapy and culture are identified in the following text.

## Culture and the *Occupational Therapy Practice Framework*

Several educational standards refer to culture as being part of the context of a client's life. That language derives from the *Framework* (AOTA, 2014), which describes the domain of occupational therapy practice "which outlines the profession's purview and the areas in which its members have an established body of knowledge and expertise" (p. S3). Occupational therapy recognizes the importance of the context of a person's life to support engagement in occupation. The *Framework* states that "[c]ontext refers to a variety of interrelated conditions within and surrounding the client [that] exert a strong influence on performance" (AOTA, 2014). This document identifies two environmental and four contextual conditions that an occupational therapy practitioner must consider when working with a client. One of these is culture. The *Framework* defines culture as the "customs, beliefs, activity patterns, behavior standards, and expectations accepted by the society of which the individual is a member" (AOTA, 2014).

The *Framework* (AOTA, 2014) not only identifies the domain of occupational therapy practice and the process by which we provide interventions, but it also guides practice. As such, this document highlights the importance of considering the culture of the people with whom we work, and mandates that we consider the clients' cultural influences on their occupational choices and performance.

## Client-Centered Care

Another important concept in occupational therapy theory and practice that supports cultural consideration of clients is client-centered care. This notion arose from Rogers's (1951) theoretical belief that a client is a partner in the client/therapist dyad and should and must be part of the decision-making process regarding his or her own treatment. The occupational therapy practitioner must respect the client, recognize the client as the first authority on what he or she needs, and try to see the world through the client's eyes as well as through those of the authoritative health professional. Since the early 1990s, occupational therapists have adopted Rogers's ideas and have been redefining them to support and frame occupational therapy practice (Law, 1998; Law, Baptiste, & Mills, 1995; Pollack, 1993; Sumsion, 1993, 1999). Many of these authors suggest that for client-centered care to occur, the occupational therapy practitioner must understand the client's medical, social, and occupational history as well as his or her beliefs and values so that the client and practitioner can collaboratively determine an intervention approach that is meaningful to the client. In other words, the practitioner must understand the client's culture and the cultural influences on his or her performance. Understanding another's culture is one aspect of cultural competence and part of culturally competent care. I had previously made the argument that client-centered care must, by its definition, be culturally competent care (Black, 2005). Recently, however, there has been a call for a critical review of client centered care, and researchers have discovered that the concept, although still espoused in occupational therapy literature, is inconsistently practiced in reality due to current contexts and values that problematize true client-centered care (Gupta & Taff, 2015; Hammell, 2013; Njelesani, Teachman, Durocher, Hamdani, & Phelan, 2015).

## Cultural Competence

In an earlier edition of this text, I argued for the need for culturally competent care (Black, 2014). "For good outcomes in health care, cultural competence is needed at the individual, team, organizational, and systemic levels" (Srivastava, 2007, p. 23). Although "cultural competence" is often used when talking about race and ethnicity, the changing demographics of the United States ensures a greater increase in the multiple diversities of our clients. Diversity is apparent in race and ethnicity, in class and socioeconomic levels, in age and ability, in religion and political views, in lifestyle choices, and in gender and sexual identity. If we understand culture to incorporate all of the preceding and more, then cultural competence is appropriate when working with all people, not just those who are racially or ethnically different from ourselves (Black, 2005).

Within the occupational therapy literature, cultural competence is described "as the process of actively developing and practicing appropriate, relevant, and sensitive strategies and skills in interacting with culturally different persons" (AOTA Multicultural Task Force, 1995). An often-used definition from Cross, Bazron, Dennis, and Isaacs (1989) states that cultural competence is "a set of congruent behaviors, attitudes, and policies that come together in a system, agency, or among professionals and enable that system, agency, or those professionals to work effectively in cross-cultural situations" (p. 13). As might be extrapolated from these definitions, cultural competence is more than just understanding the culture of our clients. It incorporates three distinct characteristics:

cultural self-awareness, cultural knowledge, and cross-cultural skills (Black & Wells, 2007).

*Cultural self-awareness* may be the most important of the three characteristics of cultural competence (Black & Wells, 2007; Harry, 1992; Lynch & Hanson, 1998). It means recognizing yourself as a cultural being who sees the world through a unique cultural lens. This awareness assists us in knowing where we fit in the sociocultural matrix of the dominant culture, especially if we are a person of color, a woman, poor, old, physically or mentally impaired, or have a sexual identity other than heterosexuality. Being culturally self-aware means recognizing our privileged status if we are part of the dominant culture, acknowledging our biases and prejudices, and knowing how, from where, and from whom we learned these.

It is extremely important to do the hard work of cultural self-exploration because knowing ourselves in this way will make us more sensitive when working with a client who is culturally different from ourselves. Without that awareness, unexplored biases may become a barrier when working with certain clients with a culture different from our own, and may lead to ineffective, unethical, or inappropriate interventions. In the worst case, it might lead to discriminatory behaviors that might harm the client in some way.

*Cultural knowledge*, the second characteristic of cultural competence, is the information we gather about a client's culture, which includes customs, traditions, body language, values, beliefs about health and wellness, and the meaning of illness. It may mean learning a little of their language if it differs from our own. Trying to speak to people in their own language connotes respect for them and—in my experience—is always appreciated. In addition, cultural knowledge includes understanding the sociocultural "status" of this person's culture, and understanding the oppression and discrimination she or he might face. Taking the time to learn about a client's culture is vital in establishing rapport and providing client-centered care.

The third characteristic of cultural competence, *cross-cultural skill*, is what differentiates cultural competence from cultural sensitivity. To develop this skill, you must actively engage in communicating and interacting with others who differ from yourself. You must be willing to "put yourself out there," to be open to differing ideas and beliefs, and to make mistakes (Black, 2002; Black & Wells, 2007). You must also learn how to recover from those mistakes. Successful cross-cultural communication means understanding nonverbal communication as well as negotiating conflict. All three of these characteristics—cultural self-awareness, cultural knowledge, and cross-cultural skill—must be developing or in place to provide culturally competent care.

For occupational therapy practitioners to understand the client's perspective of his or her illness or condition, we need to learn to ask the right questions through a culturally sensitive assessment approach, which will be discussed later in this chapter, and to listen carefully to the answers. We cannot assume that a culturally diverse client believes and thinks the same way we do. Therefore, it is important to constantly ask for clarification of ideas and meaning. Assuming that we understand what the client means without clarification can result in miscommunication and inadequate or poor intervention.

### Culture and Occupational Justice

*Occupational justice* is a fairly new term found in occupational therapy literature that connotes that individuals have a right to access and engage in meaningful occupations. "Occupational injustices exist when, for example, participation is barred, confined, segregated, prohibited, undeveloped, disrupted, alienated, marginalized, exploited, or otherwise devalued" (Whiteford & Townsend, 2011, p. 69). Much of the literature on occupational justice and injustice has been written outside of the United States about groups of people who are socially oppressed. However, the terminology and ideas are increasingly and appropriately used in this country as well, as many individuals and groups in the United States are also barred from engaging in activities that have meaning for them. Prisoners, street people and the homeless, people with mental illness, and others in institutions are a few examples. Many of these individuals come from a sociocultural background that differs from that of the occupational therapy practitioners who work with them—the majority of whom are White, middle-class, and highly educated women. To recognize occupational injustices and to provide the best interventions, occupational therapy practitioners will have to provide effective client-centered and culturally competent care as meaningful occupations are culturally defined.

## Societal Influences

The next level of cultural influence is the societal level. Every society has its own cultural beliefs and customs. Lewis (2002) writes that "culture is constructed by humans to communicate and create community" (p. 13). In the United States, we are guided by the principles of the U.S. Constitution, which extol the value of and rights to freedom, equality, and the pursuit of happiness for all. However, the dominant culture of the United States includes English-speaking, White, middle-class, heterosexual people who have become the "standard" by which others are measured, and most of us recognize that those constitutional promises are realized by more members of the dominant group than by the nondominant members of our society. Those of us who fall within the dominant categories have more privilege than others and easier access to goods and services (Kendall, 2012; McIntosh, 1988).

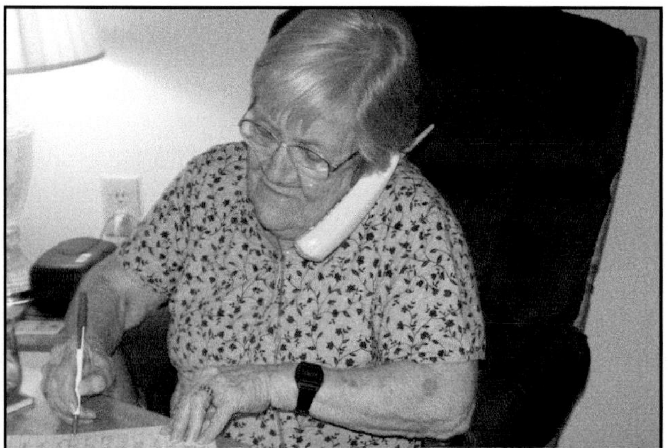

**Figure 2-2.** Enjoying the solitary occupation of doing a crossword puzzle while socially interacting with a friend on the telephone.

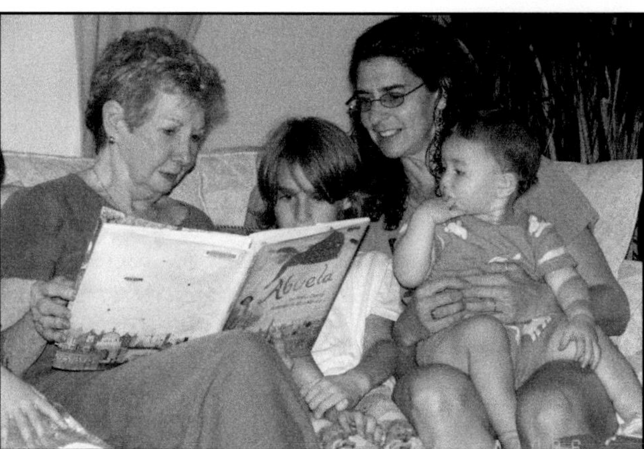


**Figure 2-3.** Enjoying family time by reading a favorite story to grandchildren.

Therefore, although all citizens of the United States may be governed by the same principles and beliefs, our experiences and perceptions of our world may differ because of our cultural characteristics and the societal hierarchy within our country. Our opportunities will differ from one another, leading to varied choices and occupational behaviors. For example, the daily activities of a widowed 79-year-old White woman living in low-income housing in a small city in the northeast region of the United States may differ significantly from that of a Puerto Rican woman of the same age living with her daughter and her family in the same geographical area. The first woman may be far more isolated, especially in the winter. Her occupations may include watching favorite television shows, doing crossword puzzles, reading biographies and nonfiction literature, talking on the telephone with family and friends, and doing light housework. Because she cannot afford a car, this woman rarely leaves her housing development, having to rely on others to take her grocery shopping or to do errands. Her children and grandchildren call often and see her regularly every few weeks or so. Nevertheless, she keeps busy, and although sometimes lonely, is fairly satisfied with her life (Figure 2-2).

The second woman, who is nearly the same age as our first example, comes from Puerto Rico, with a cultural background where it is common for older individuals to live with extended family and where being an older adult has value. She continues to have an important place in this family, and her occupations reflect that. She often cooks and helps to clean up after meals, assists with laundry and babysitting for the older children, and has become a confidante to her granddaughter. She watches her favorite television shows with the family in the evenings and is included in family excursions on the weekends. She reads to the younger children and tells them stories of their parents and grandparents and of times in the "old country." Although she goes to bed fairly exhausted in the evening, and sometimes wishes for a little more time to herself, this woman is also quite satisfied with her life (Figure 2-3).

Both of these women live full, but very different, lives. If we were to receive them as clients in our practice, we could not effectively work with them in the same way, nor could we expect their occupations to be alike just because they are women in their 70s living in the same region of the United States. The life of each woman is influenced by societal expectations, yet their personal and family cultures allow them to be individuals, and they must be respected as such.

Within the health professions, our behaviors are influenced not only by the larger societal expectations, but also by federal and state rules and regulations and our organizations' codes of ethics. Among these regulations are the *National Standards for Culturally and Linguistically Appropriate Services in Health Care* (U.S. Department of Health and Human Services, 2000). This collective set of 14 mandates, guidelines, and recommendations was developed to inform, guide, and facilitate required and recommended practices related to culturally and linguistically appropriate health services for health care organizations and their employees. As occupational therapy practitioners, these standards will help guide our work with people and groups that are culturally diverse.

## Global Influences

The broadest level of cultural influence on occupations, and perhaps the least apparent for many, comes from the larger, global world. Often, many people are ethnocentric and exclusionary, and do not seem interested in what is going on outside of his or her own country; nor do they believe they are affected by events beyond their shores. Yet, there is an impact on each of us. There is an old saying that goes something like this: The flutter of a butterfly's wings in one part of the world can spawn a hurricane in another. Our occupations may change in significant or subtle ways owing to events happening around the world.

The continuing war in Iraq, for instance, has changed the occupations of not only the men and women from the United States who are fighting overseas, but also those of their families and friends who spend more time writing letters or emails, searching for and sending appropriate gifts, or—in the worst case—going to hospitals or funeral homes. Returning veterans with and without injuries struggle to pursue pre-deployment occupations and may have difficulty resuming roles that once were easy for them. Families continue to work at adjusting to the return of these men and women. Others who did not have friends or family members who were deployed may have spent more time watching newscasts, reading newspapers and news magazines, or campaigning for favorite politicians as a result of the conflicts. Many of us engaged in new occupations as a direct result of the war.

When the tsunami hit Indonesia and Sri Lanka in 2005, many from the United States traveled there to help, began campaigns to send supplies or money as aid, or, again, stayed glued to their television sets to watch the latest news or increased the amount of time they spent reading newspapers and other news to follow the event.

The earthquake in Japan in March 2011, which caused damage at the Fukushima nuclear facility, brought officials from the United States to examine the structure. As the evening television news, newspapers, and blogs published information in the United States on a daily basis for months about the effects and the cleanup of the disaster, politicians and lawmakers in the United States worked diligently to develop new policies to try to avert the same kind of man-made disaster in this country (Lyman, 2011). Again, many people in this country engaged in new occupations as a result of an event on the other side of the world.

Before the prevalence of new technology, people could ignore what was happening outside of their own communities or country. With television, social networking sites, and print media in most homes in the United States today and with email, smartphones, instant messaging, and other technological advances in communication, people not only know what is going on around the world, but also have knowledge of events as they occur (Black & Wells, 2007). As a result, because we are more aware of world events, we become a more active part of our global culture and may choose to act on those events.

In summary, the multiple levels of cultural influences affect each of us in unique ways, shaping our own identities, the identities of the people with whom we work, and the manner in which we engage in occupational pursuits. How we understand and use this important information informs and guides our occupational therapy practice.

# Culturally Effective Occupational Therapy Practice

## *Defining Cultural Effectiveness*

Cultural effectiveness is a notion that advances the concept and practice of cultural competence. Although it incorporates the three major characteristics of cultural competence—cultural self-awareness, knowledge, and cultural skill—it additionally requires cross-cultural interactions where critical reflection and consideration of the context are vital aspects of the practitioner's practice (Wells, Black, & Gupta, 2016). This type of reflection is reminiscent of Schon's (1983) description of reflection in action, and reflection on action. The practitioner reflects on the interaction as it is happening, and following the interaction critically analyzes and reviews the effectiveness and personal skill she displayed to determine what changes, if any, should be considered to improve the next cross-cultural interaction. More information can be found about this concept in Wells, Black, and Gupta (2016).

As outlined by the *Framework*, the occupational therapy "process includes evaluation, intervention, and outcome monitoring" (AOTA, 2014). Perhaps the most important of these steps is evaluation, which includes selecting and administering the most appropriate assessment tool(s) to determine the needs of the client. Although there is a multitude of evaluation tools from which occupational therapy practitioners may choose, it is important for occupational therapy students and practitioners to also consider the best culturally sensitive assessment tool as part of their assessment "tool box."

## *The Impact of Prejudice and Discrimination on Culturally Effective Care*

Prejudice is an erroneous judgment, usually negative, held against people based on incomplete or faulty information (Bennett, 1995) and results in bias, which is an opinion made without adequate basis. People are not born biased or prejudiced, but unfortunately many of us in the United States have been taught to have negative opinions about certain groups of people. Although some people are clear about and may voice these negative beliefs, many people are unaware of their biases. For some, these attitudes turn to discriminatory actions. Although prejudicial attitudes may be deplorable, it is discrimination that is the social problem (Black & Wells, 2007) that may affect effective occupational therapy practice.

### Case Study

Casey is a novice occupational therapist, in her first year of practice, and has just been assigned to begin a gross motor group in the public school where she is employed. The group becomes filled with six first- and second-graders, four boys and two girls. All of the children are active and seem happy to be in the group, and they all display various motor problems. Jeffy is unique in that he is quite obese, but he tries to engage as much as the other children. Casey's supervisor decides to observe the group after 3 weeks and is surprised to note that although Casey is using good clinical reasoning and is setting up appropriate therapeutic and fun activities for the children, her interaction with Jeffy differs from that with the other children. With him she appears more critical and impatient, and in that session she wasn't observed giving Jeffy as much positive feedback as she did the others. When asked about this in a later private session with her supervisor, Casey seemed surprised about her behavior. However, as they continued to discuss this issue, Casey began to cry, admitting that her mother and brother were extremely obese, and she found it very difficult to be with them. Both Casey and her supervisor began to explore if she held a bias against all people who are obese, and if so, they would begin a plan of how she might overcome this bias or learn how to not let it affect her practice.

## *Bias Against Obesity*

Much has been written and known about racism, sexism, heterosexism, classism, and other areas of bias, but until recently, many of us have not thought about the general bias around obesity. Obesity is a significant health and social problem in the United States. More than 72% of adults in the United States are classified as either overweight or obese, and 18.4% of adolescents and 30% of children ages 2 to 11 years are obese (Ogden, Carroll, Kit, & Flegal, 2012). The United States has been described as experiencing an "obesity crisis." Obesity has been identified by Flanagan (1996) as the "last bastion of prejudice" and is one of the last forms of accepted prejudice.

Numerous studies document prejudice in both the general and medical population against those who are obese with attitudes that view adults and children who are obese as physically unattractive and undesirable; as responsible for their weight due to some character flaw such as laziness, gluttony, or lack of self-control; and are assumed to lack self-discipline, be less conscientious, less competent, sloppy, disagreeable, and emotionally unstable (Puhl & Brownell, 2001). Is it possible that Casey (in the Case Study) is feeling some bias toward Jeffy? Maybe so.

Although there is limited research on attitudes toward obesity in occupational therapy (Vroman & Cote, 2011), there are a growing number of publications about occupational therapy and obesity. AOTA (2011) has identified childhood obesity as an "emerging niche" for occupational therapy and in 2013 published a Position Paper about obesity and occupational therapy. Additionally, occupational therapy practitioners and researchers have shared information about a variety of interventions used with children and adults who are obese (Bacon et al., 2012: Haracz, Ryan, Hazelton, & James, 2013; Lau, Stevens, & Jia, 2013; McLain, 2011; Pizzi, 2013). As effective occupational therapists, however, we must all be engaged in critical reflection of our own attitudes and behaviors when working with this population of clients.

### Student Activity 2

Have you, one of your friends, or a family member been discriminated against because of obesity? Describe what happened. How did you, and the other person, feel and react? Upon reflection, can you think of a positive way to respond in that situation? You may be working with clients who are obese. Think about how you might respond to them.

## *Culturally Sensitive Assessment Tools*

One aspect of culturally effective care is to consider a client's culture and beliefs as part of the assessment process. As outlined by the *Framework*, the occupational therapy process includes evaluation, intervention, and "the process of targeting outcomes" (AOTA, 2014). Perhaps the most important of these steps is evaluation, which includes selecting and administering the most appropriate assessment tool(s) to determine the needs of the client. Although there is a multitude of evaluation tools from which occupational therapy practitioners may choose, it is important for occupational therapy students and practitioners to consider the best culturally sensitive assessment tool as part of their assessment "tool box." Many occupational therapy assessment tools have been developed for, and are biased toward, the sociocultural norms of a White, middle-class population, and have incorporated Western values, ethics, theories, and standards as part of their development. Although some have taken culture into consideration, notably the Loewenstein Occupational Therapy Cognitive Assessment battery (Josman, Abdallah, & Engel-Yeger, 2011), the Canadian Occupational Performance Measure (Fisher, 2005), and the Assessment of Motor and Process Skills (Buchan, 2002), most have not been standardized for ethnic populations (Black & Wells, 2007). Because these assessments are not so standardized, the results of these tests may be less than optimal and could be unproductive or even harmful when administered to some individuals.

Table 2-1.

**Culturally Sensitive Assessment Models, Tools, and Questionnaires**

| Authors | Instrument |
|---|---|
| Black & Wells, 2007 | Cultural Information Questionnaire<br>Opening statement<br>Questions about current illness<br>Health beliefs and practices<br>Cultural beliefs and values |
| Leininger, 1988 | The Sunrise Model<br>Cultural values and lifeways<br>Religious, philosophical, and spiritual beliefs<br>Economic factors<br>Educational factors<br>Technological factors<br>Kinship and social ties<br>Political and legal factors |
| Levin, Like, & Gottlieb, 2000 | The ETHNIC tool<br>E: Explanation (How do you explain your illness?)<br>T: Treatment (What treatment have you tried?)<br>H: Healers (Have you sought any advice from folk healers?)<br>N: Negotiate (mutually acceptable options)<br>I: (Agree on) intervention<br>C: Collaboration (with patient, family, and healers) |
| Dobbie, Medrano, Tysinger, & Olney, 2003 | The BELIEF tool<br>B: Health beliefs (What caused your illness/problem?)<br>E: Explanation (Why did it happen at this time?)<br>L: Learn (Help me understand your belief/opinion.)<br>I: Impact (How is this illness/problem impacting your life?)<br>E: Empathy (This must be very difficult for you.)<br>F: Feelings (How are you feeling about it?) |

Adapted from Dobbie, A. E., Medrano, M., Tysinger, J., & Olney, C. (2003). The BELIEF instrument: A preclinical teaching tool to elicit patients' health beliefs. *Family Medicine, 35,* 316-319.

For example, there are limited mental health data for the Somali population owing to the lack of appropriate assessment tools (Bhui et al., 2003). Somalis do experience mental health symptoms but traditionally believe that these symptoms are related to spirit possession (Lewis, 1998), and they endure this emotional discomfort in a somewhat fatalistic manner. Using a culturally sensitive approach to assessment might help practitioners more deeply understand the beliefs of this population of clients, resulting in more effective intervention.

The *Framework* (AOTA, 2014) suggests beginning the evaluation process by using an occupational profile, which would include gathering information "that describes the client's occupational history and experiences, patterns of daily living, interests, values, and needs." This is a client-centered and collaborative approach that guides intervention. Adding specific questions that elicit information about the client's cultural beliefs and practices related to health care will enrich and deepen the understanding that the therapist has of the client, and will strengthen the therapist/client relationship.

There are several culturally sensitive assessment tools that the occupational therapist can choose from. These include the approach used by Black and Wells (2007), entitled *Eliciting Cultural Information in Clinical Interactions* (p. 258). The authors suggest beginning with an opening paragraph that clearly explains the purpose of the questions, followed by questions regarding the client's current illness, questions regarding health beliefs and practices, and questions regarding cultural beliefs and values (Table 2-1). Using these questions to help expand the narrative and life history of the client "allows the provider to frame the problems and limitations in a cultural context" (Black & Wells, 2007, p. 257).

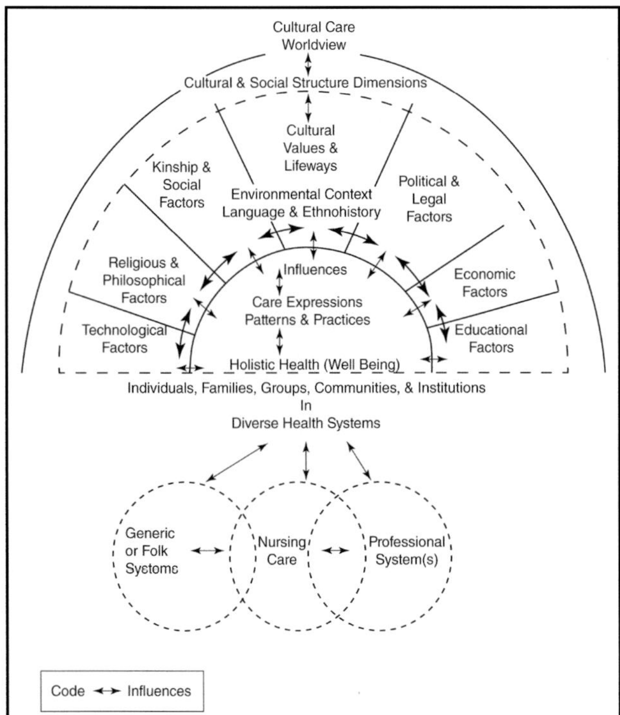


**Figure 2-4.** Leininger's Theory of Culture Care Worldview Image. (Reprinted with permission from http://www.madeleine-leininger.com/cc/sunrise.pdf)

Other culturally sensitive tools and models include the Sunrise Model by Leininger (1988), the ETHNIC Cultural Assessment (Levin, Like, & Gottlieb, 2000), and the BELIEF Cultural Assessment (Dobbie, Medrano, Tysinger, & Olney, 2003; see Table 2-1).

Madeleine Leininger, the nurse educator who developed much of the theory related to transcultural nursing (1988), believed that the intake or interview questions that should be asked of a client be broadly conceived, and cover the following areas:

- Cultural values and lifeways
- Religious, philosophical, and spiritual beliefs
- Economic factors
- Educational factors
- Technological factors
- Kinship and social ties
- Political and legal factors

The Sunrise Model, which developed from Leininger's theory (Leininger & McFarland, 2002; Figure 2-4), has been applied in nursing practice for years and provides an interesting approach that could be adopted by other health care professionals, including occupational therapy practitioners. The ETHNIC (Levin et al., 2000) and BELIEF (Dobbie et al., 2003) assessments are similar culturally relevant interviewing instruments that address clients' beliefs and perspectives about their illness and/or health condition (see Table 2-1). Both are useful in identifying cultural beliefs and values and enhancing occupational therapy assessment that would support and influence culturally effective client-centered practice.

### Student Activity 3

After reviewing some of the culturally sensitive assessment tools, choose some of the pertinent questions that you would add to your occupational profile to elicit information about a client's culture, and practice asking those questions with a peer.

As well as identifying and using an effective culturally sensitive assessment tool, practitioners must be aware of some of the cultural characteristics that have the potential to become barriers to effective cross-cultural interactions.

## Cultural Characteristics That Affect Effective Cross-Cultural Interactions

There are many unique characteristics and beliefs that individuals from various cultures may possess that, if not examined, may interfere with effective client-centered and culturally effective care. As a point of illustration, this chapter briefly examines three of these characteristics: self-concept, perceptions of power and authority, and temporal issues.

### *Self-Concept*

In North America and much of Europe, the notion of self-concept was thought to be about the individual, where identity is developed as something unique and differentiated from others, often referred to as *individualism* (Brewer & Gardner, 2004). Cross-cultural research, however, identified another approach to the development of self-concept and identity—one that relied on a social identity that "reflects internalizations of the norms and characteristics of important reference groups and consists of cognitions about the self that are consistent with that group identification" (Brewer & Gardner, 2004, p. 68). This type of identity is called *collectivism*. Although few people develop a sense of self apart from others (Brewer & Gardner, 2004), and every person is unique, in many cultures, belief systems and ideals strongly emphasize one or the other of these approaches.

### Individualism

Banks (1997) states, "individualism as an ideal is extreme in the United States core culture" (p. 9). In an individualistic society, the focus is on "I" rather than on the family, group, or community. People are taught to be strong and tough and take care of themselves, and seeking out help or advice from others is sometimes seen as weakness. Consider the icons in traditional American culture that represent this ideal: the strong, independent "Marlboro Man" and heroes like John Wayne. Independence and autonomy are valued, and people who are ill or disadvantaged are often told to "tough it out" or "pull themselves up by their bootstraps." The Protestant work ethic, with the belief that hard work is morally good and that sloth is sinful, has contributed to the individualistic ideal (Banks, 1997). "Doing" something is more important than talking, and practicality and efficiency are important values for people from these cultures. The individualism is often future-oriented, resulting in a sense of comfort with change (Lattanzi & Purnell, 2006).

When working with someone who holds individualistic beliefs, the occupational therapy practitioner must remember the following concepts:

- Illness is a major threat to this person's independence.
- It is important to consult the person on every decision so he or she will have some sense of control.
- This person will appreciate "working hard" toward recovery.
- It is important to respect the person's privacy.
- Seek permission before entering this person's space.
- Set individual goals to increase independence.

Because many of the values of occupational therapy were developed from a Western, individualistic ideal (Iwama, 2006), working with a client with these values should not cause much conflict with the majority of U.S. practitioners.

### Collectivism

Many Eastern cultures, including the Chinese and Japanese, have more of a collectivist worldview. People from these cultures generally develop the identity of the larger society, and self-concept and identity focus on the "we." One is expected to be committed first to the family and group and then to self (Banks, 1997). Interdependence is valued, and decisions are usually made by group consideration rather than individually. Health may be measured by one's ability to function within the group. Human interaction is valued over time, and cooperation is important. The past and tradition are important and authority is respected (Lattanzi & Purnell, 2006).

When working with people with a collectivist viewpoint, practitioners will want to consider the following:

- Practitioners may seek someone who knows the client to introduce them.
- Once rapport is established, the practitioner may be expected to provide all the answers as the authority figure.
- It will be important to work closely with family and group members regarding decisions about the client's interventions.
- Remember to emphasize the team approach to effective and safe care.

## Perceptions of Power and Authority

Another characteristic that is culturally determined is one's perception of power and authority. The way in which people view authority figures and the power inherent within those positions often influences relationships and occupational behaviors. The perception of personal power is the sense of one's ability to affect the environment, which allows one to feel good about oneself and to believe that he or she is important, and for others to recognize his or her worth (Glasser, 1984). Personal power affects our own sense of authority and our ability to control others. It is often internalized and unconscious.

The perception of power informs one's degree of the acceptance of inequality. For instance, if we accept the inequality of power, authority, and privilege as a given, then we will not see ourselves as having the need or power to change it. If we do not accept inequality as a given, and instead believe that everyone should be treated equally, we perceive a need for change in an unequal context. Geert Hofstede's (1980, 2001) research with people from 40 different nations resulted in a description of *power distance*, which is "the extent to which the less powerful members of organizations and institutions (like the family) accept and expect that power is distributed unequally" (Clearly Cultural, n.d., para. 1). Hofstede identifies the difference in high power distance and low power distance cultures, stating that "the basic issue involved, which different societies handle differently, is human inequality" (2001, p. 79).

### High Power Distance Cultures

High power distance defines a culture in which inequality is accepted. Members of the culture believe that each person has a rightful place, and that superiors and subordinates treat each other differently and do not mix socially. Members of these cultures do not challenge power and authority (Hofstede, 1980, 2001). It is important to recognize these cultural characteristics in occupational therapy practice because they will affect the relationship that practitioners have with diverse clients. When working with people from high power distance cultures, one must consider the following:

- They are more conscious of the hierarchy in the health care system.
- They will want to know their place in that hierarchy and how the health care facility works.
- They may relate to people differently based on age, gender, and professional role.
- Authority is important to them, and they will tend to look to the professional for decisions and directions.
- It may be important for practitioners to share their credentials and accomplishments with the client so that authority may be established.
- It may be more difficult to provide a client-centered approach to interventions because of the expectation that the authority figure (the practitioner) will make the decisions.
- It may be more difficult to develop an empowered or participatory power relationship with the client.

### Low Power Distance Cultures

In low power distance cultures, the majority of the members feel that any inequality in the society should be minimized. Members believe in equal rights and that the existence of hierarchy is only for the convenience of accomplishing tasks in an organization. Many people from low power distance cultures believe that education increases power and that people can move within this fluid system (Hofstede, 1980). With the client from a low power distance culture, consider the following:

- This person will expect to be treated on an equal basis and may want to be treated as a peer when not in a professional role.
- He or she may challenge authority and, in turn, expect to be challenged; this is seen as a sign of respect.
- It is important to keep this client apprised of the progress of therapy.
- This client is usually a good candidate for client-centered occupational therapy.

Hofstede developed a power distance index (PDI), which determined the relative power distance of various nations (Clearly Cultural, n.d.). Of interest, Austria has a PDI of 11 (very low), whereas Malaysia's PDI is 104 (very high). Many Central American countries and the Philippines fall in the 90s, the PDI of Arab nations is 80, and the United States falls somewhere in the middle with a PDI of 40 (Clearly Cultural, n.d.). Occupational therapy practitioners must be aware of and recognize this important cultural characteristic in their clients for effective cross-cultural interactions.

## Temporal Issues

Although the characteristics previously identified are culturally defined and important to recognize, one aspect that causes a tremendous amount of difficulty in business and health care is the difference in the concept of time between the employer and employee and therapist and client. All cultures have unique concepts of time, and much has been written about this cultural characteristic. Although several authors discuss the difference between future, present, and past temporal orientations (Bonder, Martin, & Miracle, 2002; Lattanzi & Purnell, 2006) and its impact on health care, this section of the chapter addresses the relationship of monochronic and polychronic time and how it may affect cross-cultural interactions.

### Monochronic Time

There are cultures and people who perceive time as linear and can do only one thing at a time. These monochronic people are schedule dominated, tending to live by the clock. They see the world in segmented compartments and even tend to sequence communications as well as tasks (O'Hara-Devereaux & Johansen, 1994). According to O'Hara-Devereaux and Johansen, these individuals would be disinclined to interrupt a telephone conversation to greet a third person. Efficiency and convenience are important factors for monochronic people (Table 2-2).

Within a therapeutic relationship with a monochronic patient, consider the following:

- The client may not be interested in a holistic approach.
- The client will be interested in information about schedules, interventions, and time of discharge.
- The practitioner must follow the schedules as closely as possible; inform the client if you must be late to the appointment.
- If the client is highly stressed, give him or her permission to relax; schedule time for relaxation.

### Polychronic Time

In contrast to the preceding characteristics, a polychronic person can accomplish multiple activities at the same time and will not cut a discussion short if "out of time," according to his or her schedule. "Polychronic time is open-ended; completing the task or communication is more important than adhering to a schedule" (O'Hara-Devereaux & Johansen, 1994, p. 37). These people can and often will carry on several conversations simultaneously. Polychronic people are relationship dominated; their strength is an emphasis on interactions with others and they enjoy nonlinear, creative tasks.

Table 2-2.

## Common Temporal Differences

| Monochronic Cultures | Polychronic Cultures |
|---|---|
| Do one thing at a time | Do many things at once |
| Concentrate on a task | Highly distractible; accepts interruptions |
| Time commitments (such as deadlines and schedules) are taken seriously | Time commitments to be achieved only if possible |
| Low context; needs information | High context; has information |
| Committed to the task | Committed to people |
| Religious adherence to plans | Changes plans often and easily |
| Follows rules of privacy and consideration; doesn't want to disturb others | More concerned with relations (families, friends, colleagues) than with privacy |
| Emphasizes promptness | Bases promptness on the relationship |

Adapted from Hall, E. T., & Hall, M. R. (1990). *Understanding cultural differences: Germans, French, and Americans.* Boston, MA: Nicholas Brealey Publishing and from O'Hara-Devereaux, M., & Johansen, R. (1994). *Globalwork: Bridging distance, culture, and time.* San Francisco, CA: Jossey-Bass.

Within a therapeutic setting, remember the following:

- Developing rapport and a comfortable relationship with the client is primary.
- Always relate to the person in some way before and during the intervention.
- Expect there to be family and friends in the treatment room.
- You may have to remind the client about the schedule and follow-up home activities.

As occupational therapy practitioners, providing effective cross-cultural care is vital when working with diverse clients. Being aware of the characteristics identified previously and addressing them with the client in an effort to minimize misunderstandings will move the practitioner toward cultural competence and the client to a place of trust, both of which will result in more effective and respectful care.

## Research Evidence on Culture, Cultural Competence, and Culturally Effective Care

Over the past decade, there has been a significant increase in the occupational therapy literature on issues of culture, cultural competence, and culturally competent care (Black & Wells, 2007; Bonder & Martin, 2013; Gray & McPherson, 2005; Kirsh, Trentham, & Cole, 2006; Pooremamali, Persson, & Eklund, 2011; Stedman & Thomas, 2011; Wells et al., 2016). However, several of the articles written continue to be concept papers or descriptions of programs. Although this body of literature provides significant value in developing dialogue in this area, there is limited reported research on the importance of the knowledge of culture, on aspects of cultural competence, and on the effectiveness of culturally competent care in occupational therapy practice.

Some notable exceptions include the developing research literature on cultural safety (Gerlach, 2012; Gray & McPherson, 2005; Jull & Giles, 2012; Stedman & Thomas, 2011). Cultural safety emphasizes relationships of trust in which the patient determines whether the care is safe. For occupational therapy practitioners, this is about positive attitudinal change that enables occupational therapists to "offer a more appropriate and effective service to clients from diverse cultures" (Gray & McPherson, p. 34). Another area of research includes studies that examine the efficacy of education on the development of cultural competence (Musolino et al., 2009; Suarez-Balcazar et al., 2009; Velde, Wittman, & Mott, 2007), whereas a third research focus examines the occupational lives of immigrants and refugees (Black, 2011; Hon, Sun, Suto, & Forwell, 2011; Martins & Reid, 2007; Nayar, Hocking, & Giddings, 2012; Suto, 2009).

These developing areas of study are exciting, but there continues to be a need for further research in occupational therapy practice to provide the evidence that supports culturally competent and/or culturally effective care. According to the Center on an Aging Society, "cultural competence is not an isolated aspect of medical care, but an important component of overall excellence in health care delivery" (2004, p. 11). Providing "excellence in health care delivery" is an important goal of

## Evidence-Based Research Chart

| Topic | Issue | Evidence |
|---|---|---|
| Culture | Cultural safety | Gerlach, 2012; Gray & McPherson, 2005; Jull & Giles, 2012; Whiteford, 2012 |
| | Western viewpoints and occupational identity | Bourke-Taylor & Hudson, 2005; Rudman & Dennhardt, 2008 |
| Culturally effective/ competent care | Responses from therapists | Beagan et al., 2013: McFarland & Mixer, 2012; Stedman & Thomas, 2011 |
| | Responses from clients | Kirsh, Trentham, & Cole, 2006 |
| Cultural competence | Of occupational therapy practitioners | Munoz, 2007; Saurez-Balcazar et al., 2009; Wray & Mortenson, 2011 |
| | Of occupational therapy students | Humbert et al., 2011; McAllister, Whiteford, Hill, Thomas, & Fitzgerald, 2006; Murden et al., 2008; Rasmussen, Lloyd, & Wielandt, 2005; Taylor-Ritzler et al., 2008 |
| | Educational pedagogy to develop cultural competence | Ekelman, Bello-Haas, Bazyk, & Bazyk, 2003; Price et al., 2005; Taylor-Ritzler et al., 2008; Velde, Wittman, & Mott, 2007 |
| | Cultural competence assessment tools and models | Balcazar, Suarez-Balcazar, & Taylor-Ritzler, 2009; Kumas-Tan, Beagan, Loppie, MacLeod, & Frank, 2007 |

occupational therapy practice, but we must increase the amount of research that is completed and published to provide evidence to further support this aspect of our practice. Selected studies from occupational therapy literature are included in the Evidence-Based Research Chart.

## References


American Occupational Therapy Association. (2014). Occupational therapy practice framework: Domain and process (3rd ed.). *American Journal of Occupational Therapy, 68*(Suppl. 1), S1-S48. doi:10.5014/ajot.2014.682006

American Occupational Therapy Association. (2011). Emerging niche: Childhood obesity. Retrieved from http://.aota.org/Practice/Children-Yourth/Emerging-Niche/Childhood-Obesity.aspx

American Occupational Therapy Association Multicultural Task Force. (1995). *Definition and terms*. Bethesda, MD: AOTA Press.

Bacon, N., Farnworth, L., & Boyd, R. (2012). The use of the Wii Fit in forensic mental health: Exercise for people at risk of obesity. *British Journal of Occupational Therapy, 25*(2), 61-68.

Balcazar, F. E., Suarez-Balcazar, Y., & Taylor Ritzler, T. (2009). Cultural competence: Development of a conceptual framework. *Disability and Rehabilitation, 31*(14), 1153-1160.

Banks, J. A. (1997). Multicultural education: Characteristics and goals. In J. A. Banks & C. A. M. Banks (Eds.), *Multicultural education: Issues and perspectives* (3rd ed., pp. 3-31). Boston, MA: Allyn and Bacon.

Beagan, B. L., Chiasson, A., Fiske, C. A., Forseth, S. D., Hosein, A. C., Myers, M. R., & Stang, J. E. (2013). Working with transgender clients: Learning from physicians and nurses to improve occupational therapy practice. *Canadian Journal of Occupational Therapy, 80*(2), 82-91.

Bennett, C. K. (1995). *Multicultural education: Issues and perspectives* (3rd ed.). Newton, MA: Allyn and Bacon.

Bhui, K., Abdi, A., Abdi, M., Pereira, S., Dualeh, M., Robertson, D. ... Ismail, H. (2003). Traumatic events, migration characteristics, and psychiatric symptoms among Somali refugees: Preliminary communication. *Social Psychiatry and Psychiatric Epidemiology, 38*, 35-43.

Black, M. (2011). From kites to kitchens: Collaborative community-based occupational therapy with refugee survivors of torture. In F. Kronenberg, N. Pollard, & D. Sakellariou (Eds.), *Occupational therapy without borders. Vol. 2: Towards an ecology of occupation-based practice* (pp. 217-225). Edinburgh, Scotland: Churchill Livingstone Elsevier.

Black, R. M. (2002). *The essence of cultural competence: Listening to the voices of occupational therapy students*. Unpublished dissertation. Cambridge, MA: Lesley University.

Black, R. M. (2005). Intersections of care: An analysis of culturally competent care, client centered care, and the feminist ethic of care. *WORK: A Journal of Prevention, Assessment & Rehabilitation, 24*(4), 409-422.

Black, R. M. (2014). Cultural impact on occupation. In K. Jacobs, N. MacRae, & K. Sladyk (Eds.), *Occupational therapy essentials for clinical competence* (2nd ed., pp. 11-24). Thorofare, NJ: SLACK Incorporated.

Black, R. M., & Wells, S. A. (2007). *Culture and occupation: A model of empowerment in occupational therapy*. Bethesda, MD: AOTA Press.

Bonder, B., & Martin, L. (2013). *Culture in clinical care: Strategies for competence* (2nd ed.). Thorofare, NJ: SLACK Incorporated.

Bonder, B., Martin, L., & Miracle, A. (2002). *Culture in clinical care*. Thorofare, NJ: SLACK Incorporated.

Bourke-Taylor, H., & Hudson, D. (2005). Cultural differences: The experience of establishing an occupational therapy service in a developing community. *Australian Journal of Occupational Therapy, 52*(3), 188-198.

Brewer, M. B., & Gardner, W. (2004). Who is this 'We?' Levels of collective identity and self representations? In M. J. Hatch & M. Schultz (Eds.), *Organizational identity: A reader*. New York, NY: Oxford University Press.

Buchan, T. (2002). The impact of language and culture when administering the Assessment of Motor and Process Skills: A case study. *British Journal of Occupational Therapy, 65*(8), 371-373.

Center on an Aging Society. (February, 2004). *Cultural competence in health care: Is it important for people with chronic conditions?* Issue Brief No. 5. Georgetown University. Retrieved from http://ihcrp.georgetown.edu/agingsociety/pubhtml/cultural/cultural.html

Christiansen, C., & Baum, C. (Eds.). (1997). *Occupational therapy: Enabling function and well-being* (2nd ed.). Thorofare, NJ: SLACK Incorporated.

Clearly Cultural (n.d.). Retrieved from http://www.clearlycultural.com/geert-hofstede-cultural-dimensions/power-distance-index/

Cross, T., Bazron, B., Dennis, K., & Isaacs, M. (1989). *Towards a culturally competent system of care* (Vol. 1). Washington, DC: Georgetown Center.

Dobbie, A. E., Medrano, M., Tysinger, J., & Olney, C. (2003). The BELIEF instrument: A preclinical teaching tool to elicit patients' health beliefs. *Family Medicine, 35*, 316-319.

Dunn, W., Brown, C., & McGuigan, A. (1994). The ecology of human performance: A framework for considering the effect of context. *American Journal of Occupational Therapy, 48*, 595-607.

Ekelman, B., Bello-Haas, V. D., Bazyk, J., & Bazyk, S. (2003). Developing cultural competence in occupational therapy and physical therapy education: A field immersion approach. *Journal of Allied Health, 32*(2), 131-137.

Fisher, S. (2005). The Canadian Occupational Performance Measure: Does it address the cultural occupations of ethnic minorities? *British Journal of Occupational Therapy, 68*(5), 224-234.

Flanagan, S. A. (1996, June 12). Obesity: The last bastion of prejudice. Presented at the Allied Health Sciences Session of the 13th Annual Meeting of the American Society for Bariatric Surgery, Quebec City, Canada.

Gerlach, A. J. (2012). A critical reflection on the concept of cultural safety. *Canadian Journal of Occupational Therapy, 79*(3), 151-158.

Glasser, W. (1984). *Take effective control of your life*. New York, NY: Harper and Row.

Gray, M., & McPherson, K. (2005). Cultural safety and professional practice in occupational therapy: A New Zealand perspective. *Australian Occupational Therapy Journal 52*, 34-42.

Gupta, J., & Taff, S. D. (2015). The illusion of client-centred practice. *Scandinavian Journal of Occupational Therapy, 22*(4), 244-251.

Hammell, K. R. W. (2013). Client-centred practice in occupational therapy: Critical reflections. *Scandinavian Journal of Occupational Therapy, 20*(3), 174-181.

Haracz, K., Ryan, S., Hazelton, M., & James, C. (2013). Occupational therapy and obesity: An integrative literature review. *Australian Occupational Therapy Journal, 60*(5), 356-365.

Harry, B. (1992). Developing cultural self awareness: The first step in values clarification for early interventionists. *Topics in Early Childhood Special Education, 12*, 333-350.

Hofstede, G. (1980). *Culture's consequences: International differences in work-related values*. Thousand Oaks, CA: Sage Publications.

Hofstede, G. (2001). *Culture's consequences: Comparing values, behaviors, institutions and organizations across nations* (2nd ed.). Thousand Oaks, CA: Sage Publications.

Hon, C., Sun, P., Suto, M., & Forwell, S. J. (2011). Moving from China to Canada: Occupational transitions of immigrant mothers of children with special needs. *Journal of Occupational Science, 18*(3), 223-236.

Humbert, T. K., Burket, A., Deveney, R., & Kennedy, K. (2011). Occupational therapy students' perspectives regarding international cross-cultural experiences. *Australian Occupational Therapy Journal, 59*(3), 225-234.

Iwama, M. (2004). Meaning and inclusion: Revisiting culture in occupational therapy. (Guest editorial). *Australian Occupational Therapy Journal, 51*(1), 1-2.

Iwama, M. (2006). *The KAWA model: Culturally relevant occupational therapy*. Montreal, Canada: Churchill Livingston.

Josman, N., Abdallah, T. M., & Engel-Yeger, B. (2011). Using the LOTCA to measure cultural and sociodemographic effects on cognitive skills in two groups of children. *American Journal of Occupational Therapy, 65*(3), e29-e37.

Jull, J. E. G., & Giles, A. R. (2012). Health equity, Aboriginal peoples and occupational therapy. *Canadian Journal of Occupational Therapy, 79*, 70-76.

Kendall, F. (2012). *Understanding white privilege: Creating pathways to authentic relationships across race* (2nd ed.). New York, NY: Routledge.

Kirsh, B., Trentham, B., & Cole, S. (2006). Diversity in occupational therapy: Experiences of consumer who identify themselves as minority group members. *Australian Occupational Therapy Journal, 53*, 302-313.

Kumas Tan, Z., Beagan, B., Loppie, C., MacLeod, A., & Frank, B. (2007). Measures of cultural competence: Examining hidden assumptions. *Academic Medicine, 82*(6), 548-557.

Lattanzi, J. B., & Purnell, L. D. (2006). *Developing cultural competence in physical therapy practice*. Philadelphia, PA: F. A. Davis Company.

Lau, C., Stevens, D., & Jia J. (2013). Effects of an occupation-based obesity prevention program for children at risk. *Occupational Therapy in Health Care, 27*(2), 163-175.

Law, M. (Ed.). (1998). *Client-centered occupational therapy*. Thorofare, NJ: SLACK Incorporated.

Law, M., Baptiste, S., & Mills, J. (1995). Client-centered practice: What does it mean and does it make a difference? *Canadian Journal of Occupational Therapy, 62*, 250-257.

Law, M., Cooper, B., Strong, S., Stewart, D., Rigby, P., & Letts, L. (1996). The person-environment-occupation model: A transactive approach to occupational performance. *Canadian Journal of Occupational Therapy, 63*, 9-23.

Leininger, M. (1988). Leininger's theory of nursing: Cultural care diversity and universality. *Nursing Science Quarterly, 1*(4), 152-160.

Leininger, M., & McFarland, M. R. (2002). *Transcultural nursing: Concepts, theories, research and practice* (3rd ed.). New York, NY: McGraw-Hill.

Levin, S. J., Like, R. C., & Gottlieb, J. E. (2000). ETHNIC: A framework for culturally competent clinical practice. *Patient Care, 9* (special issue), 188.

Lewis, I. M. (1998). *Saints and Somalis: Popular Islam in a clan-based society*. Lawrenceville, NJ: Red Sea Press.

Lewis, J. (2002). *Cultural studies: The basics*. London, England: Sage Publications.

Lyman, E. S. (2011). Surviving the one-two nuclear punch: Assessing risk and policy in a post-Fukushima world. *Bulletin of the Atomic Scientists, 67*(5), 47-54.

Lynch, E. W., & Hanson, M. J. (1998). *Developing cross-cultural competencies: A guide for working with children and their families* (2nd ed.). Baltimore, MD: Paul H. Brookes Publishing Co.

Martins, V., & Reid, D. (2007). New-immigrant women in urban Canada: Insights into occupation and sociocultural context. *Occupational Therapy International, 14*(4), 203-220.

McAllister, L., Whiteford, G., Hill, B., Thomas, N., & Fitzgerald, M. (2006). Reflection in intercultural learning: Examining the international experience through a critical incident approach. *Reflective Practice: International and Multidisciplinary Perspectives, 7*(3), 367-381.

McFarland, M. R., & Mixer, S. J. (2012). Ethnonursing: A qualitative research method for studying culturally competent care across disciplines. *International Journal of Qualitative Methods, 11*(3), 259-279.

McIntosh, P. (1988). *White privilege and male privilege: A personal account of coming to see correspondences through work in women's studies* (Working Paper No. 189). Wellesley, MA: Wellesley College, Center for Research on Women.

McLain, A. (2011). *The effectiveness of occupational therapy in preventing childhood obesity in the school setting.* Retrieved from http://commons.pacificu.edu/otpeds/13

Munoz, J. P. (2007). Culturally responsive caring in occupational therapy. *Occupational Therapy International, 14*(4), 256-280.

Murden, R., Norman, A., Ross, J., Sturdivant, E., Kedia, M., & Shah, S. (2008). Occupational therapy students' perceptions of their cultural awareness and competency. *Occupational Therapy International, 15*(3), 191-203.

Musolino, G. M., Babitz, M., Burkhalter, S. T., Thompson, C., Harris, R., Ward, R. S., & Chase-Cantarini, S. (2009). Mutual respect in healthcare: Assessing cultural competence for the University of Utah interdisciplinary health sciences. *Journal of Allied Health, 38*(2), 54E-62E(9).

Nayar, S., Hocking, C., & Giddings, L. (2012). Using occupation to navigate cultural spaces: Indian immigrant women settling in New Zealand. *Journal of Occupational Science, 19*(1), 62-75.

Njelesani, J., Teachman, G., Durocher, E., Hamdani, Y., & Phelan, S. K. (2015). Thinking critically about client-centred practice and occupational possibilities across the life-span. *Scandinavian Journal of Occupational Therapy, 22*(4), 252-259.

Ogden, C. L., Carroll, M. D., Kit, B. K., & Flegal, K. M. (2012). Prevalence of obesity and trends in body mass index among US children and adolescents, 1999-2010. *Journal of the American Medical Association, 307*(5), 483-490.

O'Hara-Devereaux, M., & Johansen, R. (1994). *Globalwork: Bridging distance, culture and time.* San Francisco, CA: Jossey-Bass.

Pizzi, M. (2013). Special issue of obesity and the role of occupational therapy. *Occupational Therapy in Health Care, 27*(2), 75-77.

Pollack, N. (1993). Client centered assessment. *American Journal of Occupational Therapy, 47,* 298-301.

Pooremamali, P., Persson, D., & Eklund, M. (2011). Occupational therapists' experience of working with immigrant clients in mental health care. *Scandinavian Journal of Occupational Therapy, 18*(2), 109-121.

Price, E. G., Beach, M. C., Gary, T. L., Robinson, K. A., Gozu, A., Palacio, A., ... Cooper, L. A. (2005). A systematic review of the methodological rigor of studies evaluating cultural competence training of health professionals. *Academic Medicine, 80*(6), 578-586.

Puhl, R., & Brownell, K. D. (2001). Bias, discrimination, and obesity. *Obesity Research, 9*(12), 788-805.

Rasmussen, T. M., Lloyd, C., & Wielandt, T. (2005). Cultural awareness among Queensland undergraduate occupational therapy students. *Australian Journal of Occupational Therapy, 52*(4), 302-310.

Rogers, C. (1951). *Client-centered care.* Boston, MA: Houghton-Mifflin.

Rudman, D. L., & Dennhardt, S. (2008). Shaping knowledge regarding occupation: Examining the cultural underpinnings of the evolving concept of occupational identity. *Australian Journal of Occupational Therapy, 55*(3), 153-162.

Schkade, J. K., & Schultz, S. (2003). Occupational adaptation. In E. Crepeau, E. Cohn, & B. A. B. Schell (Eds.), *Willard and Spackman's occupational therapy* (10th ed., pp. 200-203). Philadelphia, PA: Lippincott.

Schon, D. (1983). *The reflective practitioner.* New York, NY: Basic Books.

Srivastava, R. (2007). *The healthcare professional's guide to clinical cultural competence.* Toronto, Ontario, Canada: Elsevier Canada.

*Standards of the National Society for the Promotion of Occupational Therapy.* (1925). (Available from the AOTA Wilma L. West Library, Bethesda, MD).

Stedman, A., & Thomas, Y. (2011). Reflecting on our effectiveness: Occupational therapy interventions with Indigenous clients. *Australian Occupational Therapy Journal, 58,* 43-49.

Suarez-Balcazar, Y., Rodawoksi, J., Balcazar, F., Taylor-Ritzler, T., Portillo, N., Barwacz, D., & Willis, C. (2009). Perceived levels of cultural competence among occupational therapists. *American Journal of Occupational Therapy, 63*(4), 498-595.

Sumsion, T. (1993). Reflections on . . . Client-centered practice: The true impact. *Canadian Journal of Occupational Therapy, 60*(1), 6-8.

Sumsion, T. (Ed.). (1999). *Client-centered practice in occupational therapy: A guide to implementation.* New York, NY: Churchill Livingstone.

Suto, M. (2009). Compromised careers: The occupational transition of immigration and resettlement. *WORK: A Journal of Prevention, Assessment & Rehabilitation, 32,* 417-429.

Taylor-Ritzler, T., Valcazar, F., Dimpfl, S., Suarez-Balcazar, Y., Willis, C., & Schiff, R. (2008). Cultural competence training with organizations serving people with disabilities from diverse cultural backgrounds. *Journal of Vocational Rehabilitation, 29*(2), 77-91.

U.S. Department of Health and Human Services Office of Minority Health. (2000). *National standards for culturally and linguistically appropriate services in health care.* Washington, DC: Author.

Velde, B. P., Wittman, P. P., & Mott, V. W. (2007). Hands-on learning in Tillery. *Journal of Transformative Education, 5*(1), 79-92.

Vroman, K., & Cote, S. (2011). Prejudicial attitudes toward clients who are obese: Measuring implicit attitudes of occupational therapy students. *Occupational Therapy in Health Care, 25*(1), 77-90.

Wells, S. A., Black, R. M., & Gupta, J. (2016). *Culture and occupation: Effectiveness in practice, education, and research* (3rd ed.). Bethesda, MD: AOTA Press.

Whiteford, G. E. (2012). Other worlds and other lives: A study of occupational therapy student perceptions of cultural difference. *Occupational Therapy International, 2*(4), 291-313.

Whiteford, G., & Townsend, E. (2011). Participatory occupational justice framework (POJF 2010): Enabling occupational participation and inclusion. In F. Kronenberg, N. Pollard, & D. Sakellariou (Eds.), *Occupational therapies without borders* (Vol. 2, pp. 65-84). Edinburgh, Scotland: Churchill Livingstone Elsevier.

Wray, E. L., & Mortenson, P. A. (2011). Cultural competence in occupational therapists working in early intervention therapy programs. *Canadian Journal of Occupational Therapy, 78*(3), 180-186.

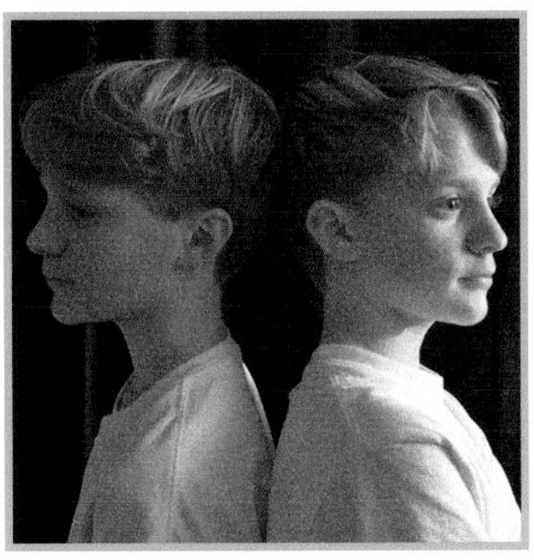

# 3

# The Dark Side of Occupation

Rebecca Twinley, PhD, MSc, PGCAP, BSc(Hons), FHEA, HCPC

**ACOTE STANDARDS EXPLORED IN THIS CHAPTER**

B.1.5, B.2.2, B.2.4, B.2.7

**KEY VOCABULARY**

- **Dark side of occupation:** Occupations that remain unexplored—such as those that are health compromising, damaging, and deviant—and which therefore challenge the pervasive belief in a causal relationship between occupation and health.
- **Occupational perspective:** Perceiving humans as occupational beings and understanding the links among their occupations, health, and well-being, within context.
- **Occupations:** The things people do every day that are subjectively experienced as well as contextually dependent and influenced.
- **People:** Those who occupational therapy practitioners work with and provide occupational therapy services to—either as individuals, in groups, or as part of communities.
- **Subjective experience:** A person's private and lived experience of internal and external events, including the way he or she experiences occupations and the world. It is subjective because individuals have no way of knowing whether other people are having the same experience when exposed to the same external stimuli (occupational experience, for instance).



Jacobs, K., & MacRae, N. (Eds.).
*Occupational Therapy Essentials for Clinical Competence, Third Edition* (pp. 29-36).

This chapter explores the dark side of occupation—a concept developed in response to growing awareness that there are aspects of people's subjective experience of occupation that have yet to be explored from an occupational perspective. An explanation of the dark side of occupation is provided, followed by consideration of how and where you can identify occupations that could be analyzed and understood from this conceptual perspective. The power of occupation is highlighted to facilitate your ability to consider the importance of appreciating people's subjective experience of occupation. For you to understand and begin to deliberate some of the ways in which the dark side of occupation can be implemented into your work, I offer possibilities for occupational therapy education, practice, and research. Comments from practitioners and educators are included to demonstrate the current perspective regarding implementing the dark side of occupation. The student self-assessments are intended to prompt you to examine examples of the ways in which people do not always do things that are perceived (by others) as positive and productive as they engage in health-compromising occupations.

## Naming the Dark Side of Occupation

I was asked to consider naming this concept something else because of concern with using the phrase "dark side," which has been assumed to be suggestive of something to do with witchcraft or the dark arts. I reflected at length regarding the use of this phrase and, to be very clear, naming this concept the dark side of occupation was primarily because it derived from my perception that the dark side portrays something less known: occupations that remain unexplored and uncovered and are left in the dark. Largely, such occupations are those that can have damaging or problematic impacts upon people's health. In 2012, Addidle and I published a paper with the sole intention of highlighting that some of the things people do may not always be understood or subjectively experienced as positive, productive, prosocial, or health giving. We asked readers to consider the suggestion that:

> ... the definition of occupation needs to include aspects of doing that are not deemed as prosocial, healthy, or productive... Debatably, these antisocial occupations may hold meaning for people that engage in them and might even be done for the purpose of relaxation, creativity, celebration and entertainment (Ferrell et al., 2008). (Twinley & Addidle, 2012, pp. 202-203)

Subsequent to this, in 2013, I published a paper with the intent of proposing "the dark side of occupation" as a concept for consideration by occupational therapy practitioners and occupational scientists alike. We will all work with people who do things that we might not approve of; this does not mean we can ignore these occupations and what they mean to the person doing them. Use of this term is not about labeling what others do, and is certainly not about labeling what others do as either good or bad, based upon subjective judgments and perceptions. Rather, my use of this term is to represent and to prompt consideration of occupations that remain underexplored from an occupational perspective. As someone who advocates to understand the subjective experience of occupation, I would not label another person's occupation as "dark" (either in its form, function, value, or meaning) because my opinion is subjective, as is my experience (and reality) as an occupational being. Indeed, I might regard some of my occupations as "dark" in nature that another person might not. However, there are some things that people do—and which they find meaning and purpose in—that are indisputably health compromising, harmful, maladaptive, antisocial, or illegal. As an illustration, and to return to the concern that it might be assumed that I am suggesting the need for an occupational perspective of witchcraft, the dark arts, or the occult, the following questions are posed: "Do we have one yet?" and "Why is this concerning?" There are people in every society who engage in some form of magical, spiritual, or religious practice (including the various denominations, cults, and sects to which some people belong); you may have already worked with such people, be working with some now, or work with some in the future. Surely, an appreciation of their subjective experience of occupations that are connected to their practices and beliefs would enable a richer understanding and evaluation of them as an occupational being. A willingness to explore the range of people's occupations that contribute to who they are and to their experience of health and well-being has the potential to challenge our professional and ethical practice, in addition to our personal judgments regarding what we do and do not approve of. Therefore, I believe there is very real value in instigating an occupational understanding of occupations that are not inherently healthy or positive or productive (and it is important to note this suggestion is from a Western perspective of productivity). For such reasons, the key intention of this chapter is to recommend a shift in current occupation-based research, practice, and education to examine, understand, and teach about the overlooked dark side of occupation.

## Identifying the Dark Side of Occupation

Occupation is the core concept of the occupational therapy profession and its philosophical foundations. Accordingly, founding occupational scientists intended to establish a science of occupation that would inform and enhance occupational therapy practice (Pierce, 2014,

p. 1). There is an imperative consensus among occupational therapy practitioners and occupational scientists that occupation is complex and multidimensional; it is, therefore, constantly defined and debated. This means that the understanding of what constitutes occupation is ever-evolving and, importantly, it is responsive to innovative conceptual developments.

Until recent years, the focus of occupational therapy and occupational science literature has been upon occupations as positive and the links to good health and well-being. Reference to what is considered "the dark side of occupation" is something that has only subtly been present in the literature. For example, in her thought-provoking paper entitled "Promise," Pierce (2012) suggested occupational science can increase its social relevance by describing self-damaging, deviant, or disrupted occupations. In 2011, Kiepek and Magalhães presented their synthesis of literature regarding addictions and impulse-control disorders as occupation. They describe how problematic engagement in activities can include those that are part of our daily interactions with others in our sociocultural environments, such as: "... gambling, sex, Internet use, shopping, substance use, eating, work, and exercise" (Kiepek & Magalhães, 2011, p. 255). Previously, Lentin (2002, p. 143) demonstrated that—by not focusing on health-promoting occupations—it is possible to explore and understand how "... engagement in occupations and activities can be traumatic to humans."

## *Activities of Daily Living*

Consider the chapter by Nastasi, who discusses the areas of occupation, as outlined by the American Occupational Therapy Association (AOTA) in 2014. Now reconsider these by thinking about occupations that could be understood from the conceptual perspective of the dark side of occupation. Think through scenarios when people perform activities that compromise their ability to care for themselves but that still constitute the things they regularly do, often on a daily basis. Examples include over- or undereating (please see the case studies where these are explored in more detail), alcohol use, drug use (see Kiepek & Magalhães, 2011), and perverse (as perceived by others) or addictive sexual activity. Each of these are typically performed in the home but are certainly not limited to this environmental context. The following discussion of the seven areas of occupation is intended to further prompt your thoughts on this.

## *Instrumental Activities of Daily Living*

Instrumental activities that are completed both at home and in the community could include compulsive shopping, excessive self-medication (of prescribed medications), dangerous (reckless) driving, and participating in cults, sects, or religions that are perceived as harmful or negatively extreme.

## *Rest and Sleep*

When do those glorious activities of rest and sleep become unproductive or disturbed? It could be argued they do when a person overengages in them; people who are perceived to rest too much are socially viewed as being lazy or idle. In contrast, sleep disturbances are known to be experienced by individuals with alcohol or other drug use, abuse, and dependence. Whatever the cause of sleep disturbance, it affects a person's ability to actively participate in activities during the hours of the day that are meant to be their waking hours.

## *Education*

Education is an interesting area of occupation to consider. Can a person engage in too much education? Globally, many societies place high value on formal education and level of educational attainment, so much so that children are expected to perform and produce pleasing results—often from as young as 4 years old. In the United States, the No Child Left Behind Act (U.S. Department of Education, 2001) emphasized the accountability public schools had for broadening children's educational achievements. An implication of this was the emphasis upon test scores and academic achievement over physical education, play, and artistic and creative activities. Although still in place for the 2016-2017 academic year, No Child Left Behind has been replaced by the Every Student Succeeds Act; this gives states more power to maintain accountability, which involves monitoring how successful their public schools are (The White House, 2015). Unfortunately, due to the accountability movement, "Play and play environments... must promise measurable positive effects on test scores, otherwise they are replaced with academically focused programs" (Sutterby & Frost, 2013, p. 306).

## *Work*

Work, by its very nature, is not always productive, yet people engage in this form of productivity because they are expected to, they need to, or they want to. The dark side of work can include the stress and demands placed upon workers to perform and the unhealthy activities some people engage in to produce good results. Unfortunately, workplace environments can become unsafe for some people who become victims of workplace violence or harassment, which can be physical, psychological, or sexual in nature. This aspect of people's occupational lives is something that is largely hidden due to the silencing nature of much of this form of violence (Holmes, Rudge, Perron, & St-Pierre, 2012).

### Play

Activities that provide enjoyment, excitement, or entertainment are certainly not always harmless. Play can be performed by children in ways that intentionally exclude other children from participating. Indeed, bullying at school can be perpetrated by groups or individuals, and can include leaving a peer out of games or activities (Lodge, 2014). People of all ages can participate in video/computer game playing, which can be fun and prosocial; yet video/computer game play also has negative aspects, such as that it can become addictive (Gentile et al., 2011). At the extreme, the dark side of play is enacted by adults who use pretend play (including games with rules) to manipulate and abuse children (Child Welfare Information Gateway, 2013).

### Leisure

The way in which adults play, or spend their non-work time, is varied. How much do we really know about the dark side of people's leisure occupations? This can include those instances where healthy leisure pursuits can become unhealthy (such as overexercising). Then there are unhealthy, harmful, or high-risk leisure pursuits that people are motivated to do. Conversely, leisure boredom leads to risky behavior (Wegner, 2011).

### Social Participation

A person's interactions with others may not always be socially desirable or acceptable. A contemporary and internationally relevant example of this is the existence of countries that have previously had, or continue to have, criminal laws prohibiting marriage and consensual sexual activity by lesbian, gay, bisexual, transgender, or intersex people (United Nations, n.d.). In the United States, there are still states that have anti-sodomy laws, even though they were ruled unconstitutional by the U.S. Supreme Court in 2003.

## Appreciating the Subjective Experience of Occupation

Categories have their use; they can be helpful for students to use, and to structure their learning around, when examining occupation. Categories also have their limitations, including the expectations that categorization (or labeling) can place upon occupations, in terms of what is performed; where, how, and why it is performed, and with whom. Just like definitions, categories are simultaneously inclusive and exclusive. The widely accepted and long-held assertion that human occupation is complex (Hersh, Lamport, & Coffey, 2005; Wilcock, 1999) reflects the understanding that people's capacities are immense. This, in turn, should lead us to critically reflect upon categorizing occupation which, as we know, is subjectively experienced. Hammell cites Pierce (2001) and logically articulates this point:

> The belief that all occupations are divisible into the three categories of self-care, work, and play (Kielhofner, 2002) or self-care, productivity, and leisure (Creek, 2003; Townsend & Polatajko, 2007) is viewed as particularly problematic (Hammell, 2009); these categories have been portrayed as "simplistic, value laden, decontextualized, and insufficiently descriptive of subjective experience" (Pierce, 2001, p. 252). Hammell (2009, p. 107)

For such a reason, I advocate seeking to understand the subjective experience of occupation, including the dark side of occupation. I am not suggesting that it is our role to promote people's engagement in occupations that may not be healthy or contribute to their well-being. Rather, it is suggested that we can contribute toward promoting an improved state of health and well-being for people by genuinely understanding their subjective experience of occupation, and their unique priorities for what they want to do, be, become, and have a sense of belonging to—the very dimensions of occupation (Hammell, 2004).

## The Power of the Dark Side (of Occupation)

Historically, occupational therapy has experienced many calls for a return to its founding beliefs, and to focus on the profession's core concept of occupation (Christiansen & Baum, 1997; Molineux, 2004; Reilly, 1962; Shannon, 1977; Twinley & Morris, 2014). There is a very clear-cut reason for this: such commentators are expressing the necessity to focus on, appreciate, use, and scrutinize the power of occupation—that is, to be committed to an occupational perspective of people (as occupational beings), their health, and their well-being. From these perspectives, occupation is deemed to have therapeutic power to improve the health of individuals, groups, and communities. Progressively, more is becoming known about this power and the potential that occupation holds to enhance, rebuild, restore, maintain, or strengthen people's daily lived experience. This is important and there are areas—such as restorative occupations—that still need to be explored in greater depth. Still, far less is known about the power of the dark side of occupation in people's daily lives. From my work and that of others that have offered an occupational perspective (as discussed in this chapter), and learning from other disciplines that have explored health-compromising, antisocial, or unproductive occupations, I suggest this needs to be developed. Just as Darth Vader warned Luke Skywalker in *Star Wars: Episode VI: Return of the Jedi* (1983): "You underestimate the power of the Dark Side."

## Implementing the Dark Side of Occupation

I remain keen to explore and to encourage discussion about the ways in which some consideration of the dark side of occupation can be incorporated into theory, education, practice, and research. To assist with understanding how this could be achieved, I am thankful for my colleagues at Plymouth University and particularly for Amelia Di Tommaso based in Australia who gathered the perspectives from those who might be responsible for implementing the dark side of occupation into their work. Excerpts from these discussions are included in the remainder of this section.

### *Education*

In 2013, I asserted that: "... we do not sufficiently ask that they [students] consider the impact of non-health-giving, antisocial or unproductive occupations upon an individual and his/her daily routine" (p. 302). Equally, some of the educator perspectives that were gathered affirmed this:

- "... most of our text books, the way we teach, and talk about occupation, it's all fairly positive. That it impacts on health, and for me going through university I didn't really realize that there could be occupations that people did that were 'bad' for them but that as a therapist we just skim over the top of them."
- "... if we don't acknowledge and work with all occupations how can we truly be occupation-focused? This is why dark side conversations need to continue."

Ideas for implementation into preregistration education included use of case studies in which individuals engage in the dark side of occupation; one educator recommended: "... using PBL triggers that encourage the debate around the need for belonging to a social group like, for instance, a gang, and having acceptance within that, and how this relates to the dark side." There was some consensus that discussing the dark side of occupation should fall within the remit of "... teaching an overall view of occupation." Opportunities within the curriculum were noted, such as:

- "We discuss occupation from the outset, and when we talk about the lifespan, and socializing, and introducing the variety of occupations people engage in. We can also be open to having ethical debates around client choice versus our perception of what is healthy and what may provide a sense of well-being."
- "Educators need to have an awareness of this so they can provide a forum for students to discuss occupations in their entirety, so they consider possibilities like, for example, working with someone who chooses to spend their money on gambling (like the lottery or bingo) and enjoys this and its meaning to them."
- "There is potential to integrate practice placements that expose students to the dark side of occupations in the sense of occupations that may not be life-fulfilling... such as probation, or drug and alcohol services. And it's not just about working with those people but encouraging reflection of the things they do that are not generally perceived as life-fulfilling."

To understand the nature of occupation in its entirety, students are encouraged to question what they read, hear, and observe regarding occupational therapy practice; this begins with the curriculum design of pre-registration (or entry level) occupational therapy programs. For instance, ACOTE Standard B.2.7 requires all students are able to "demonstrate task analysis in areas of occupation" (AOTA, 2011, p. 20); it does not stipulate that these occupations must only be positive, health-enhancing ones.

### *Practice*

Occupational therapy practitioners could consider the dark side of occupation by asking the same questions they have been about healthy, legal, productive, and daily occupations. For instance, what do such occupations mean to the individuals, groups, and communities doing them? Why do they do these things? What does it feel like? Who else is involved? How much importance or value did they have? In what context are they experienced? Understanding the totality of each person's subjective experience of occupation necessitates expansion of the focus solely upon occupations that lead to good health and/or well-being.

In November 2015, Di Tommaso facilitated the Reclaiming Occupation As Means (ROAM; see link under Electronic Resources) Australian Capital Territory Community of Practice group discussion regarding the dark side of occupation with occupational therapy students and practitioners. The group members granted permission to have their anonymous comments shared with others. Their opinions in response to first reading about the dark side of occupation included comments such as:

- "Before reading this, I never really thought about occupation as a bad thing. I have always advocated for the power of occupation and using occupation in practice, and the only time I ever really came up against it in practice was people, for example, smoking and being in hospital."
- "... it challenged the current view on occupation... Thinking that it was always a good thing."

The group agreed that this perspective compels occupational therapy practitioners to examine their values and were in agreement that a person's experience of the dark side of occupation is subjective, based on their own value judgments, and those of others. For example, one commented:

- "... people might think smoking is bad but others think that it's good or they smoke themselves."

Importantly, there was consideration of the fact that there are many sides to occupation:

- "I think that if you only see occupation as being positive that's a very sort of black and white view of the world, and that no one action or thing is only positive; that all things can have negative consequences as well, because doing one thing means, for example, that you are not doing something else."

They also considered the environmental impact of engaging in an occupation perceived as positive, highlighting how an occupation such as knitting requires certain resources to be used and exploited:

- "... knitting, that's making something, so that's a nice thing to be doing, and it's creative and it might be making a scarf that is going to keep you or someone else warm... But in order for the yarn to be existing, then a lot of other things need to have happened beforehand, and a lot of those might have involved transport... Some of those things are not necessarily good for the environment... how was the wool made, how were the needles made?"

In terms of identifying the dark side of occupation with the people they work with, they were supportive of people's right to choose what they do. The group was mindful of the implications of placing their own values and judgments upon this, particularly when the subjective experience of occupation is a private one:

- "... You might be treating someone you consider to be an upstanding citizen and frown upon someone who is smoking because legislation is going that way, but the other person might be doing dark things behind closed doors."

They were also mindful of what constitutes safe and ethical practice, and what their role and responsibility is when people want to, or are known to be, engaging in harmful or dangerous occupations. The general consensus was that there are external factors that influence and direct their practice with others:

- "I think we have become such a risk adverse society and profession, so it's not always about what's good for the client, but the workplace or society."

However, they understood it was their role to promote health through occupation and so, in instances where people are known to engage in occupations that are health compromising, they suggested their role involved:

- "... getting to know a person and understanding why they do what they do; the meaning or need behind [it]."
- "I guess you have to try and reframe it to them and get them to see how it could be destructive to their recovery essentially."
- "We can only provide the education and support but they can still make that decision."

## Research

Occupational therapy research is vital to the contemporary practice of occupational therapy. Contemporary practice has a complex nature, which is further compounded by the contexts in which it takes place (Baptiste, 2010). Research that explores the complexity of occupation can have clinical relevance for occupational therapy practice. For example, exploring the value and meaning of engagement in occupations drives the aim of enabling occupation. Research that explores the value and meaning of the dark side of occupation—to include the problematic engagement in everyday activities—has the potential to contribute to our understanding of what enables and what hinders occupation. Greber (2013) proffered his opinion on this, stating:

> As occupational therapy has matured and diversified, the relationship between occupation and meaning has become as fundamental to the profession as the relationship between occupation and health. Hence, we are now in a better position to understand the meaning offered by health-compromising occupations, yet without a sufficient exploration of this "dark side," we remain unable to adequately incorporate this understanding into our practice. (p. 658)

Research could therefore explore occupations that are perceived as any combination of negative, harmful, unhealthy, health compromising, antisocial, maladaptive, addictive, risky, immoral, or disruptive. It may well be that they have not been explored because of their very nature and form; there are, of course, ethical and practical considerations. Still, I hope researchers are not dissuaded by the ethical approval procedures they must satisfy in an attempt to study such occupations.

## Summary

Expanding your understanding of occupation by considering the dark side of occupation means that you are open to challenging the pervasive belief in the causal relationship between occupation and health. It also places you in a position that recognizes people find value and meaning in, for example, health-compromising, deviant, and destructive occupations. In your work with individuals, groups, and communities, it is crucial to appreciate the subjective experience of occupation, and the context within which occupation is experienced.

**Case Study 1**

Being productive is very important to Faye. She finds it difficult to allow herself to engage in restful or leisure activities, believing that this would make her "lazy" and that she does not deserve to enjoy herself. Fearful about the painful thoughts and emotions that might emerge if she has time to stop and think, Faye makes sure that there are no gaps in her routine. In addition to her job role as a mechanic, Faye also volunteers for a range of charities in her spare time. People often question whether Faye is overcommitting herself; however, she brushes this off, saying that she likes feeling useful.

Faye usually turns down invitations to social events that involve food and has lost touch with many of her friends. She is lonely and spends a chunk of her evenings on pro-anorexia websites. Faye feels accepted and understood by the friends she has made through these online communities. Faye gains satisfaction from posting her eating disorder achievements and getting acknowledgment from others for her hard work and also enjoys participating in the more light-hearted discussions.

Faye walks long distances, often taking a more circuitous route than required to get to her destination. She stands when on public transport, even if there are seats available. Faye has multiple gym memberships, and uses different gyms to avoid raising suspicion of overexercise.

Faye regularly weighs herself and checks her appearance whenever she passes a reflective surface. Losing weight gives her a sense of mastery and achievement. Faye feels proud of herself, seeing weight loss as tangible evidence of her self-control.

**Case Study 2**

Carol works as a cleaner. She is often late for work and struggles to concentrate because she is so tired. People often find that snacks go missing from their desks, and they suspect that Carol is eating their food.

Carol likes going grocery shopping at the end of the day when food items are being reduced. She knows the time that each shop reduces their prices and is skilled at haggling with the shop assistants. Buying food at a significantly reduced price—particularly as a result of bartering—gives Carol a sense of satisfaction. It is also a necessity; Carol is in debt and spends a significant proportion of her income on binge food. Sometimes, Carol shoplifts. She finds this exciting and tells herself that the shops would be throwing the food away at the end of the day anyway.

Carol regularly buys shoes, clothing, and homeware online, even though she doesn't need or use them. At the time, she thinks it will cheer her up but the feeling doesn't last. Most of what Carol buys remains unopened and takes up a lot of space in her flat. As a result, Carol has limited space available for engaging in other hobbies and interests.

Carol spends her evenings bingeing and vomiting, which disrupts her sleep pattern. Carol cannot remember the last time she watched TV "live." She binges while watching programs online, and pauses to purge. She is often awake for most of the night and sleeps during the day. Carol has never experienced the same sense of release or enjoyment from any other occupation. This also helps Carol to numb her feelings.

## Student Self-Assessment

Consider your own engagement in the dark side of occupation when working through these.

1. Reflecting on the examples above, think about how the occupations mentioned in the case studies may influence an individual's:
   - Occupational identity
   - Time use and routine
   - Social network and relationships
2. What could the appeal be of maintaining performance of these occupations?
3. What might it be like for someone to give up these occupations?
4. As an occupational therapy practitioner, how could you start a conversation about the dark side of occupation? What kinds of questions might you ask to gain a collaborative understanding of the meaning and value of an individual's engagement in the dark side of occupation?
5. In Cowan and Sørlie's practice experience, some people choose to describe their eating disorder behaviors as "dark occupations." Which occupational therapy model(s) could you use to guide your understanding of an individual's self-disclosed engagement in "dark occupations"? Where would the dark side of occupation fit into this framework/model?

## Acknowledgments

The two composite case studies were kindly provided by two occupational therapists, Mary Cowan and Clarissa Sørlie, working in an Eating Disorders Service in the United Kingdom. The case studies are based on their combined clinical experience in eating disorders and are not singular individuals. Please note that the case study examples contain descriptions of eating disorder behaviors.

## Electronic Resources

The Dark Side of Occupation: https://thedarksideofoccupation.wordpress.com/

https://www.facebook.com/reclaimingoccupationasmeans?fref=ts

## Evidence-Based Research Chart

| Topic | Evidence |
|---|---|
| Addictions | Helbig & McKay, 2003; Kiepek & Magalhães, 2011; Knis-Matthews, 2010; Martin, Bliven, & Boisvert, 2008 |
| Alcohol use | Andersson et al., 2012; Gill et al., 2011; McQueen & Allan, 2006 |

## References


American Occupational Therapy Association. (2011). *2011 Accreditation Council for Occupational Therapy Education (ACOTE®) Standards and Interpretive Guide (effective July 31, 2013) August 2015 Interpretive Guide Version.* Retrieved from http://www.aota.org/-/media/Corporate/Files/EducationCareers/Accredit/Standards/2011-Standards-and-Interpretive-Guide.pdf

American Occupational Therapy Association. (2014). Occupational therapy practice framework: Domain and process (3rd ed.). *American Journal of Occupational Therapy, 68*(Suppl. 1), S1-S48. doi:10.5014/ajot.2014.682006

Andersson, C., Eklund, M., Sundh, V., Thundal, K., & Spak, F. (2012). Women's patterns of everyday occupations and alcohol consumption. *Scandinavian Journal of Occupational Therapy, 19*(3), 225-238.

Baptiste, S. (2010). Enabling communication in a person-centred, occupation-focused context. In M. Curtin, M. Molineux, & J. Supyk-Mellson (Eds.), *Occupational therapy and physical dysfunction: Enabling occupation* (6th ed., pp. 151-160). London, England: Churchill Livingstone.

Child Welfare Information Gateway. (2013). *Parenting a child who has been sexually abused: A guide for foster and adoptive parents.* Retrieved from https://www.childwelfare.gov/pubPDFs/f_abused.pdf

Christiansen, C. H., & Baum, C. (Eds.). (1997). *Occupational therapy: Enabling function and well-being* (2nd ed.). Thorofare, NJ: SLACK Incorporated.

Gentile, D. A., Choo, H., Liau, A., Sim, T., Li, D., Fung, D., & Khoo, A. (2011). Pathological video game use among youths: A two-year longitudinal study. *Pediatrics, 127*(2), e319-e329.

Gill, J., Maclean, F., Renton, L., & O'May, F. (2011). Occupational therapy graduates of 2009: Knowledge and attitudes relating to their role in the area of alcohol misuse. *British Journal of Occupational Therapy, 74*(4), 168-175.

Greber, C. (2013). Re: The dark side of occupation: A concept for consideration. *Australian Occupational Therapy Journal, 60*(6), 458-459.

Hammell, K. W. (2004). Dimensions of meaning in occupations of daily life. *Canadian Journal of Occupational Therapy, 71*(5), 296-305.

Hammell, K. W. (2009). Self-care, productivity, and leisure, or dimensions of occupational experience? Rethinking occupational "categories." *Canadian Journal of Occupational Therapy, 76*(2), 107-114.

Helbig, K., & McKay, E. (2003). An exploration of addictive behaviours from an occupational perspective. *Journal of Occupational Science, 10*(3), 140-145.

Hersh, G. I., Lamport, N. K., & Coffey, M. S. (2005). *Activity analysis: Application to occupation* (5th ed.). Thorofare, NJ: SLACK Incorporated.

Holmes, D., Rudge, T., Perron, A., & St-Pierre, I. (2012). Introduction. In D. Holmes, T. Rudge, & A. Perron (Eds.), *(Re)thinking violence in health care settings: A critical approach* (pp. 1-20). Surrey, United Kingdom: Ashgate Publishing Limited.

Kiepek, N., & Magalhães, L. (2011). Addictions and impulse-control disorders as occupation: A selected literature review and synthesis. *Journal of Occupational Science, 18*(3), 254-276.

Knis-Matthews, L. (2010). The destructive path of addiction: Experiences of six parents who are substance dependent. *Occupational Therapy In Mental Health, 26*(3), 201-340.

Lentin, P. (2002). The human spirit and occupation: Surviving and creating a life. *Journal of Occupational Science, 9*(3), 143-152.

Lodge, J. (2014). *Helping your child stop bullying: A guide for parents.* Australian Institute of Family Studies. Retrieved from https://aifs.gov.au/cfca/publications/helping-your-child-stop-bullying-guide-parents

Martin, L. M., Bliven, M., & Boisvert, R. (2008). Occupational performance, self-esteem, and quality of life in substance addictions recovery. *OTJR: Occupation, Participation and Health, 28*(2), 81-88.

McQueen, J., & Allan, L. (2006). The role of occupation in behaviour change for alcohol abusers. *International Journal of Therapy and Rehabilitation, 13*(8), 342.

Molineux, M. (2004). Occupation in occupational therapy: A labour in vain? In M. Molineux (Ed.), *Occupation for occupational therapists* (pp. 1-14). Oxford, United Kingdom: Blackwell Publishing Ltd.

Pierce, D. (2012). Promise. *Journal of Occupational Science, 19*(4), 298-311.

Pierce, D. (2014). Occupational science: A powerful disciplinary knowledge base for occupational therapy. In D. Pierce (Ed.), *Occupational science for occupational therapy* (pp. 1-10). Thorofare, NJ: SLACK Incorporated.

Reilly, M. (1962). Occupational therapy can be one of the great ideas of 20th century medicine. *American Journal of Occupational Therapy, 16*, 1-9.

Shannon, P. D. (1977). The derailment of occupational therapy. *American Journal of Occupational Therapy, 31*(4), 229-234.

Sutterby, J. A., & Frost, J. (2013). Creating play environments for early childhood: Indoors and out. In B. Spodeck & O. N. Saracho (Eds.), *Handbook of research on the education of young children* (2nd ed., pp. 305-322). London, England: Routledge.

Twinley, R. (2013). The dark side of occupation: A concept for consideration. *Australian Occupational Therapy Journal, 60*(4), 301-303.

Twinley, R., & Addidle, G. (2012). Considering violence: The dark side of occupation. *British Journal of Occupational Therapy, 75*(4), 202-204.

Twinley, R., & Morris, K. (2014). Editorial: Are we achieving occupation-focussed practice? *British Journal of Occupational Therapy, 77*(6), 275.

United Nations. (n.d.). *Fact sheet: LGBT rights: Frequently asked questions.* Retrieved from https://www.unfe.org/system/unfe-7-UN_Fact_Sheets_v6_-_FAQ.pdf

U.S. Department of Education. (2001). *No child left behind act.* Retrieved from http://www2.ed.gov/policy/elsec/leg/esea02/beginning.html#sec2

Wegner, L. (2011). Through the lens of a peer: Understanding leisure boredom and risk behaviour in adolescence. *South African Journal of Occupational Therapy, 41*(1), 18-24.

The White House. (2015). *White House report: The every student succeeds act.* Retrieved from https://www.whitehouse.gov/the-press-office/2015/12/10/white-house-report-every-student-succeeds-act

Wilcock, A. A. (1999). Reflections on doing, being and becoming. *Australian Occupational Therapy Journal, 46*(1), 1-11.


## Suggested Reading


Chang, E. (2008). Drug use as an occupation: Reflecting on Insite, Vancouver's supervised injection site. *Occupational Therapy Now, 10*(3), 21-23.

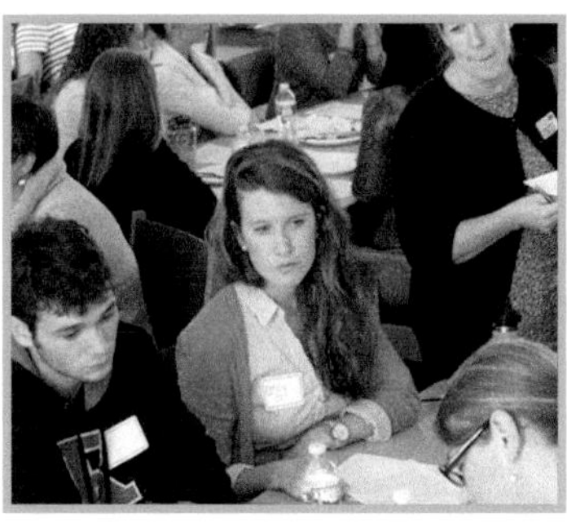

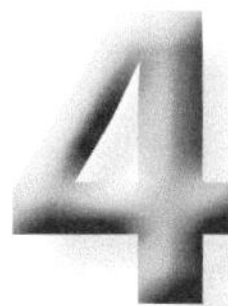

# Interprofessional Education and Practice
## A Current Necessity for Best Practice

*Nancy MacRae, MS, OTR/L, FAOTA*

**ACOTE STANDARDS EXPLORED IN THIS CHAPTER**

Preamble, B.5.21

**KEY VOCABULARY**

- **Interprofessional:** A group of professionals for which communication is collaborative, goals are shared, and all are responsible for team efforts (MacRae & Dyer, 2005).
- **Interprofessional education:** "... When two or more professions learn with, from, and about each other to improve collaboration and the quality of care" (Center for the Advancement of Interprofessional Education, 2010).
- **Interprofessional practice:** Interprofessional implementation of interprofessional intervention.



Jacobs, K., & MacRae, N. (Eds.).
*Occupational Therapy Essentials for Clinical Competence, Third Edition* (pp. 37-42).

Interprofessional education (IPE) now has a place in many occupational therapy programs and continues to gain popularity (Reeves, Tassone, Parker, Wagner, & Simmons, 2012). Although occupational therapists have been engaged in practice with other professions from the beginning of our profession (Jacobs, 2012), the extent to which this has occurred and how effective such collaboration efforts have been depended on a number of factors. Some of these factors included the context or type of practice, the experience and cooperative and collaborative nature of the practitioner, and administrative support.

With the increased complexity of practice and the interwoven goals for meeting the Triple Aim (improved care and outcomes for client, better health for the population, and lower per-capita costs, promulgated by the Institute for Healthcare Improvement in 2008) and the Affordable Care Act, instituted in 2010, there has been a renewed effort to educate aspiring occupational therapy practitioners about how to be effective and efficient members of an interprofessional team (Reeves et al., 2012). This emphasis on being an effective interprofessional team member is reflected in the 2012 Accreditation Council for Occupational Therapy (ACOTE) Standards: first in the ACOTE Preamble and then in Standard B.5.21. It is also reflected in the committee's 2015 paper on the *Importance of Interprofessional Education in Occupational Therapy Curricula* (2015).

In its 2001 report, the Institute of Medicine first called for professionals to be educated about working collaboratively. Both the United States and Canada have seen this skill as a necessity, and have created collaboratives to facilitate this call for action and identify the skills necessary for interprofessional practice (IPP).

The U.S. version, created in 2010 by the Interprofessional Education Collaborative, devised core competency domains for collaborative practice. The domains consist of the following (Interprofessional Education Collaborative Expert Panel, 2011):

- Values/ethics for IPP
- Roles/responsibilities
- Interprofessional communication
- Teams and teamwork

This report also produced a learning continuum, which is composed of exposure (introduction) to immersion (development) to competence (entry to practice), and was founded on reflection, learning, and formative assessment (Core Competencies for Interprofessional Practice, 31). Building teamwork competencies was stressed, as was transforming ways of knowing, from absolute to transitional, to independent, and to contextual (Medical University of South Carolina, 2007).

The Canadian Interprofessional Health Collaborative (2010) also devised a national interprofessional competency framework consisting of the following six competency domains:

1. Interprofessional communication
2. Patient-/client-/family-/community-centered care
3. Role clarification
4. Team functioning
5. Collaborative leadership
6. Interprofessional conflict resolution

Although the U.S. and Canadian versions present some differences, the primary purpose of preparing professionals to work in an interprofessional manner to facilitate clients' improvement and health is clearly paramount. The currently accepted definition of IPE is "when two or more professions learn with, from, and about each other to improve collaboration and the quality of care" (Centre for the Advancement of Interprofessional Education, 2010). This definition differentiates the term *interprofessional*, where communication is collaborative, goals are shared, and all are responsible for team efforts, from that of *multiprofessional*, where team members share client information but decisions are made independently (MacRae & Dyer, 2005).

Ethics of interprofessional efforts need to be considered. Frodeman (2010) has detailed intellectual ethics as generosity, confidence, humility, flexibility, and integrity being critically important for team functioning. Besides the ethical components of interprofessional teams, relationship-centered care has become a prominent goal. This concept, developed from a feminist ethic, encourages teams to always individualize intervention and to exhibit the following interdependent characteristics of mindfulness, diversity of mental models, heedful interaction, a mixture of lean and rich communication, as well as social and task-oriented interactions, mutual respect, and trust. Such an approach can facilitate an atmosphere of collaboration and mutual support (Safan, Miller, & Beckman, 2006, p. S.12).

For IPE endeavors to be successful, they need to be fully supported by the administration, and faculty also need to be involved and feel a sense of ownership. Effective IPE programs have occurred when they are not dictated by the administration but instead developed and embraced by faculty (Graybeal, Long, Scalise-Smith, & Zeibig, 2010). IPE courses can be elective, which initially helps maneuver around scheduling difficulties, but a combination of elective and mandatory classes elevates IPE to a higher status. Faculty members are not the only ones who can develop IPE. Students, families, and clients can also be involved in co-developing educational activities (Abu-Rish et al., 2012), which may make them more meaningful and relevant.

## Application of Interprofessional Education and Interprofessional Practice

There are many ways that students/practitioners can learn about IPP. Efforts to inform can begin prior to, during, or after professional socialization. What is critical is the creation of opportunities to practice the components of IPP. To gain the skills necessary to be a fully participating and effective team member, a person must be capable of clear communication. This involves both clearly articulating and actively listening. An understanding of the parameters of your profession and those of others with whom you will likely work helps teams to gain a holistic perspective of a client and how his or her challenges can be effectively and respectfully addressed by the appropriate profession. It also shows when and how to effectively refer to other professions. Being able to explain your professional viewpoint without using acronyms or words others will not understand becomes paramount, as does the need to question anything that is not understood. This type of clarity and questioning can break down professional barriers and strengthen the confidence of an interprofessional team. This same kind of plain language also applies to communication with clients and central team members, who need to comprehend their medical situations (Stableford, 2015).

With the health care system becoming more complex, one profession cannot adequately address most clients' concerns. Drinka and Clark (2000) contend that interprofessional teams are needed when clients present "wicked problems." A client with a clear-cut problem, such as a hip fracture, for which there is an established clinical protocol or pathway, would not require the time and expertise of an interprofessional team. However, an older adult with multiple diagnoses, some chronic and some acute, needs the focus of an interprofessional team to help decipher the most appropriate care for the best client outcomes.

Safety issues and achieving positive client outcomes have been particularly important goals as accountability has become more pronounced, not only in health care, but also throughout society. Having more than one profession assuming responsibility for the totality of care/intervention for a client increases the likelihood that areas will not be missed and errors will not occur. Instituting a rotating leadership of the team can ensure responsibility as a team member, dedication to problem solving, and creating the best plan of intervention for the client. It can also minimize hierarchy and power differentiation by encouraging everyone's voice to be heard.

## Health Literacy

Health literacy is essential when decisions about such issues as surgery or life-sustaining efforts or medication schedules, precautions, or following prescribed routines need to be made by the client. Health literacy is the ability to understand verbal and written materials. Understanding what is at stake is required for the individual to make the best decisions for him- or herself. Furthermore, ensuring that clients understand—without patronization or being made to feel ashamed about their poor literacy—is important for teams to consider. Consistent use of plain language among team members facilitates the use of such language with clients (Smith & Gutman, 2011; Stableford, 2015).

## Interprofessional Education Development

Students can be placed in IPE teams at the initiation of their health care career education. They can truly learn with, from, and about each other from discussing a case. As students gain more information about their profession they can begin to formulate more holistic and detailed intervention plans. Finally, they can be provided with opportunities to first watch experienced practitioners model intervention and then to provide it themselves. This type of trajectory follows adult education principles that facilitate student learning and immediate application (Cross, 1984; Knowles, 1980). Reflection on all of these potential experiences allows students to analyze their skills and areas for change, and to begin to integrate and think about how best to apply what has been learned.

Some applied IPE examples are:

- Students from one profession teach students from another profession; nursing students teaching occupational therapy students about taking blood pressures and pulses and occupational therapy students teaching physician assistant students about adaptive equipment are examples of one profession teaching another.
- Use of Readers Theater, where interprofessional faculty or student players read a health-related script to an interprofessional audience of students, with considerable time allowed after the reading to discuss the issues that were highlighted during the production, exemplifies multiple professions exploring one relevant topic (MacRae & Pardue, 2007).
- Collaboration with medical centers, where students can be exposed to other professional roles in the hospital environment via specific learning activities, including videoconferencing technology (Sheldon et al., 2012), exemplifies partnership of academia and a specific medical community.

- Two professions can develop person-centered health care communication skills using evidence-based principles and shared learning methods (Cavanaugh & Cohen-Konrad, 2012), which exemplifies two professional student groups learning with and from each other.
- Community volunteer or service learning efforts at such sites as shelters for homeless men can provide simple interventions (an example is foot care) for a group of homeless men, thus providing a service to a specific community program.
- Students can provide an interprofessional fall prevention program in the community, which uses a generic syllabus and student reflective narratives and is delivered by students from a number of professions to a group of independent-living older adults (Gray & MacRae, 2012), exemplifies interprofessional health care students participating in an academic/community partnership.
- The Interprofessional Geriatric Education Program, coordinated by the University of New England Physician Assistant department, is a program in which physician assistant, occupational therapy, and physical therapy students and dental externs learn from each other and their older adult teachers by using interprofessional assessment and participation in rounds, the Objective Standardized Clinical Exams student evaluation method, and reflective journals (MacRae, 2012). This is an example of interprofessional students collaborating with the community in providing services to older adults.
- Thomas Jefferson University's Health Mentors Program is a 2-year person-centered team-based curriculum, which involves medical nursing, occupational therapy, physical therapy, pharmacy, and couple and family therapy students. Students work and learn together as a team and complete four learning modules where they produce a comprehensive life history, wellness plan, assessment of patient safety, and a close look at self-management support and healthy behavior (personal communication, S. Kerns & A. Herge, December 7, 2012). This is an example of IPE centering on a specific client.
- A transcultural, interprofessional health mission experience in Ghana for building cultural proficiency among individual University of New England students and their teams through intense cultural immersion, including students from nursing, pharmacy, physician assistant, physical therapy, and occupational therapy departments, exemplifies a health mission to another country, with services provided by interprofessional students (Morton, 2012).
- Camp Hand to Hands is a program developed by the Medical University of South Carolina for children with hemiplegic cerebral palsy and unilateral motor weakness. Occupational and physical therapy students use constraint-induced movement therapy to remediate the effects of "learned non-use." In a modified camp environment, children receive 6 hours of specific task training each day over 5 consecutive camp days. Students plan the theme-based camp activities, review the research evidence about pediatric constraint-induced movement therapy, learn principles of such therapy, and practice handling and other treatment techniques. Each child works with one occupational therapy student and one physical therapy student for a 2:1 ratio (personal communication, P. Coker-Bolt, December 28, 2012). This is an example of two sets of professional students working to devise and provide an intensive constraint-induced movement therapy camp to children with hemiplegic cerebral palsy and unilateral muscle weakness.

Collaborative research is another venue for learning more about interprofessionalism and potentially can broaden the scope of outcomes.

Each of these strategies and examples target improving knowledge and understanding of professional roles (own and others), collaboration, client care, care models, quality improvement, safety, and cultural competence (Abu-Rish et al., 2012). A pilot study on in-service learning in the community provides the "most value in learning with students from other professions . . ." (Buff et al., 2016, p. 161).

The interprofessional case study on the following page demonstrates how a complex client case can be handled by an interprofessional team. Read the case and consider the questions.

## Summary

As these examples show, many educational and experiential efforts are underway to assist future occupational therapy practitioners in developing effective teamwork skills, all to enhance the quality of intervention and outcomes for clients. Embracing both IPE and IPP concepts adds value to team approaches and helps to ensure quality care and positive client outcomes while minimizing medical errors. The occupational therapy profession needs to continue to encourage entry-level and experienced practitioners to understand the importance of collaboration and to continue to refine their team and problem-solving skills to enhance the value and quality of the ever-increasing complexity of care they provide to their clients.

## Case Study

Lori is a 35-year-old woman with paraplegia that resulted from a recent spinal cord injury, secondary to a motor vehicle accident. In the car accident, Lori sustained T9-T12 fractures, leaving her without the use of or feeling in her legs, dysfunctional bowel and bladder control, and chronic back pain.

Prior to the accident, Lori tended to prioritize work and wellness. Fiercely independent and highly motivated, Lori initially approached her rehabilitation as another fitness regimen. While occasionally admitting to sadness at the loss of full functioning, Lori presented as realistic and hopeful in her outlook. She fully intends to return to work and is already planning the necessary steps to achieve that goal in the near future.

Ryan, Lori's husband of 5 years, is a computer animation filmmaker. Currently unemployed, he drives a cab on weekends to help with household expenses. Ryan's calm demeanor makes it appear that, like Lori, he has accepted her situation and will do what is needed. He is present at all medical and rehab sessions and takes pride in his partner's independence. He respects her desire to call the shots in her recovery.

Lori recently transitioned from working with ambulatory rehab to a new outpatient center located in a private practice near her home. Her current rehab program focuses on transfer training, advanced wheelchair skill training, and upper extremity strength training and other activities of daily living. She has experienced painful bed sores that became infected while hospitalized. She hopes to learn how to avoid further skin breakdowns through frequent movement and the use of over-the-counter antibiotic ointments. Additionally, her mouth is often very dry and she has a few canker cores, which she has never had before, and her jaw is frequently sore.

Lori strives to be independent and seeks to gain more independence such as fully dressing and bathing herself. She has learned to manage upper body hygiene, grooming, and dressing, and she can independently self-catheterize to empty her bladder. However, she needs help with showering, bathing, lower body dressing, and managing her bowel program.

Since the accident, Lori has gained back weight she previously lost because of her former exercise routine. Remembering her pre-injury relationship with exercise has made her uncharacteristically depressed; her primary care physician prescribed a low-dose antidepressant to elevate her mood, but Lori states that chocolate, kettle corn, binge-watching TV, and the occasional cigarette seem to help more than the medication.

The couple has talked about having the remaining vehicle modified for her to drive. She has asked to have her home assessed in preparation for a state-of the-art motorized wheelchair.

Lori had never been one to take even aspirin. Now she and Ryan must manage a range of medications including those for blood pressure, spasticity, chronic pain and neuropathy, sleep, and bowel movements. Lori is worried that the medications will make her drowsy and sometimes listless. She acknowledges that she doesn't always take them as prescribed.

The couple has done well relationally given the strains of Lori's health changes, but Ryan worries about what the future holds for them as a family, one with children, which they had planned to have. Their social and love lives have been suspended until Lori feels more in control of her situation.

**Consider the following questions:**

1. Given the issues that this couple faces, individually and as a couple, identify and explain the role(s) that occupational therapy can play as part of the interprofessional health team.
2. What other professions need to be involved in intervention? Why?
3. Explain how you will interface with the team to maximize the occupational therapy scope of practice in a client- and relationship-centered approach to this case.
4. What additional information about this case do you need?
5. What barriers may limit further improvement?
6. What topics may be more difficult to discuss?
7. Identify the barriers and opportunities to Lori's health and well-being.

Adapted from and used with permission from the University of New England's Interprofessional Team Immersion project (2015).

## Evidence-Based Research Chart

| Topic | Evidence |
|---|---|
| Interprofessional competencies | Canadian Interprofessional Health Collaborative, 2010; Interprofessional Education Collaborative Expert Panel, 2011 |
| Interprofessional learning models | Cavanaugh & Cohen-Konrad, 2012; Gray & MacRae, 2012; MacRae, 2012; Morton, 2012; Sheldon et al., 2012 |
| Health literacy | Smith & Gutman, 2011; Stableford, 2015 |

## Student Self-Assessment

1. Choose one of the following topics and, in a small group, design an IPE program.
   - ◊ Fall prevention program
   - ◊ Diabetes education program
   - ◊ Sexuality program for developmentally disabled teenagers
   - ◊ Energy conservation program for adults recovering from stroke
2. Discuss the challenges of working with other students and deciding which professions should do what in your chosen program.
3. How might the development of the program have gone more smoothly?
4. What did you learn about yourself and the team as a result of this exercise?

## References


Abu-Rish, E., Kim, S., Choe, L., Varpio, L., Malik, E., White, A. A., ... Zierler, B. (2012). Current trends in interprofessional education of health sciences students: A literature review. *Journal of Interprofessional Care, 26*(6), 444-451.

Buff, S. M., Jenkins, K., Kern, D., Worrall, C., Howell, D., Martin, K., ... Blue, A. (2015). Interprofessional service-learning in a community setting: Findings from a pilot study. *Journal of Interprofessional Care, 29*(2), 159-161.

Canadian Interprofessional Health Collaborative. (2010). *A national interprofessional competency framework*. Vancouver, British Columbia, Canada: Canadian Interprofessional Health Collaborative.

Cavanaugh, J. T., & Cohen-Konrad, S. (2012). Fostering development of effective person-centered healthcare communication skills: An interprofessional shared learning model. *WORK, 41*(3), 293-301.

Centre for the Advancement of Interprofessional Education. (2010). *Interprofessional Education: A definition*. Retrieved from www.caipe.org.uk/us/defining-ipe

Cross, K. P. (1984). *Adults as learners*. San Francisco, CA: Jossey-Bass Publishers.

Drinka, J. K., & Clark, G. P. (2000). *Health care teamwork: Interdisciplinary practice and teaching*. Westport, CT: Auburn House.

Frodeman, R. (2010). Ethics of interprofessionalism. In R. Frodeman, J. T. Klein, & C. Mitcham (Eds.), *Oxford handbook of interdisciplinarity*. Oxford, United Kingdom: Oxford University Press.

Gray, B., & MacRae, N. (2012). Building a sustainable academic-community partnership: Focus on fall prevention. *WORK, 41*(3), 261-267.

Graybeal, C., Long, R., Scalise-Smith, D., & Zeibig, E. (2010, Fall). The art and science of interprofessional education. *Journal of Allied Health, 39*(3, part 2), 232-237.

Importance of interprofessional education in occupational therapy curricula. (2015). *American Journal of Occupational Therapy, 69*, 6913410020p1-6913410020p14. doi:10.5014/ajot2015.691S02

Interprofessional Education Collaborative Expert Panel. (2011). *Core competencies for interprofessional collaborative practice: Report of an expert panel*. Washington, DC: Interprofessional Education Collaborative.

Institute of Medicine. (2001). *Crossing the quality chasm: A new health system for the 21st century*. Washington, DC: National Academies of Science.

Jacobs, K. (2012). Promoting occupational therapy: Words, images, and actions. *American Journal of Occupational Therapy, 66*(6), 652-671.

Knowles, M. S. (1980). *The modern practice of adult education: From pedagogy to andragogy*. Chicago, IL: Association Press, Follett Publishing Company.

MacRae, N. (2012), Turf, team, and town: A geriatric interprofessional education program. *WORK, 41*(3), 285-292.

MacRae, N., & Dyer, J. (2005). Collaborative teaching models for health professionals. *Occupational Therapy in Health Care, 19*(3), 93-103.

MacRae, N., & Pardue, K. T. (2007). Use of readers theater to enhance interdisciplinary geriatric education. *Educational Gerontology, 33*(6), 529-526.

Medical University of South Carolina. (2007). *Creating collaborative care (C3): A quality enhancement plan (QEP)*. Charleston, SC: Author.

Morton, J. (2012). Transcultural healthcare immersion: A unique interprofessional experience poised to influence collaborative practice in cultural settings. *WORK, 41*(3), 303-312.

Reeves, S., Tassone, M., Parker, K., Wagner, S., & Simmons, B. (2012). Interprofessional education: An overview of key developments in the past three decades. *WORK, 41*(3), 233-245.

Safan, D. G., Miller, W., & Beckman, H. (2006). Organizational dimensions of relationship-centered care. *Journal of General Internal Medicine, 21*(Suppl. 1), S9-S15.

Sheldon, M., Cavanaugh, J. T., Croninger, W., Osgood, W., Robnett, R., Seigle, J., & Simonson, L. (2012). Preparing rehabilitation healthcare providers in the 21st century: Implementation of interprofessional education through an academic-clinical site partnership. *WORK, 41*(3), 269-275.

Smith, D. L., & Gutman, S. A. (2011). Health literacy in occupational therapy practice and research. *American Journal of Occupational Therapy, 65*(4), 367-369.

Stableford, S. (2015). Health literacy and clear health communication: Teaching and writing so older adults understand. In R. H. Robnett & W. C. Chop (Eds.), *Gerontology for the health care professional* (3rd ed., pp. 323-336). Burlington, MA: Jones and Bartlett Learning.

# II

# Basic Tenets of Occupational Therapy

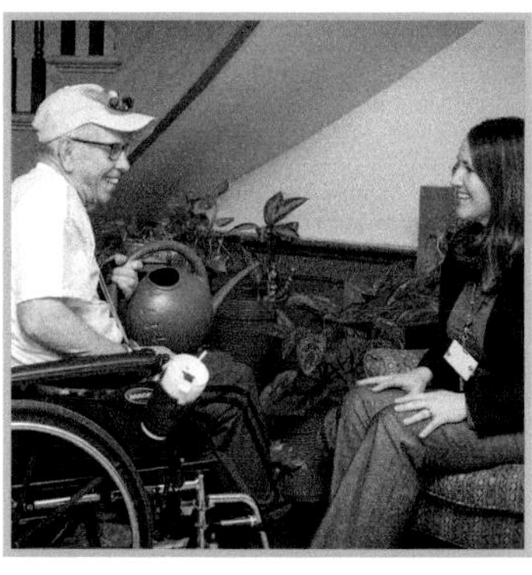

# 5

# History and Philosophy

Caryn Birstler Husman, MS, OTR/L

**ACOTE STANDARDS EXPLORED IN THIS CHAPTER**

B.2.1, B.3.4, B.3.6

**KEY VOCABULARY**

- **Humanism:** Philosophy that emphasizes the value of humans.
- **Moral treatment:** A humanistic treatment for people with mental illness.
- **Occupation:** Meaningful and purposeful human engagement.
- **Rehabilitation movement:** Provided opportunities for people with disability and injury to regain function and health.
- **Wellness:** Positive state of health.



Jacobs, K., & MacRae, N. (Eds.).
*Occupational Therapy Essentials for Clinical Competence, Third Edition* (pp. 45-54).

Contemporary occupational therapy is a complex and varied practice. Although the untrained eye at first may be unable to recognize the connections among occupational therapies in all forms, therapists understand that the golden thread is occupation. Occupation has been described as work, work-like activities, and recreation (Meyer, 1977). Occupation has been related to concepts such as activity, task, and environment, as well as more complex notions, including social and temporal contexts (Crepeau, Cohn, & Schell, 2009). Put simply, occupation is meaningful and purposeful human engagement. Bing (1981) further called occupation the "union between the mind and the body." Faust (1979) went so far as to say that life itself is the process of engagement in occupation.

Occupational therapy is the application of occupation as a therapeutic modality (Nelson, 1997). Occupation itself has the power to facilitate change and growth in a person. Within occupational therapy, occupation is the process as well as the goal (Gray, 1998). Occupational therapy practitioners seek to apply the core values of the profession: altruism, equality, freedom, justice, dignity, truth, and prudence (Peloquin, 2007) to improve performance in daily occupations through occupation. Let us explore how the profession has evolved, from its earliest roots to the diverse contemporary practice it has become through the influences of historical context, historical movements, innovative health care providers, and the progression of the medical field.

## Moral Treatment

The earliest use of occupation in therapy can be found in *moral treatment*, a term first used by the French physician Philippe Pinel in 1801. Moral treatment described a revolutionary treatment for individuals with mental illness based upon humanism: the belief that all humans have inherent value. Prior to that time, people who had mental illnesses were subjected to terrible living conditions and horrifying "treatments." These treatments were informed by the idea that individuals with mental illnesses were influenced by negative supernatural forces. Alternately, the practice of moral treatment included patient respect, care for basic needs, and routines of typical daily activities, physical exercise, and work (Bing, 1981). Patients with mental illness were offered a variety of occupations, including exercise, work, religious services, and diversional leisure. Occupations were provided in the context of routine to provide the stability the patients needed to begin recovery (Peloquin, 1989). This early practice of moral treatment and the participation in daily occupations that were included resulted in drastically improved mental health for patients previously thought to be beyond help.

William Tuke was an early adopter of moral treatment. In the late 18th century, he founded the York Retreat in England in response to deplorable conditions at the York Hospital. He applied the concepts of moral treatment by infusing a wide range of occupations into patients' daily lives. His grandson, Samuel Tuke, recorded the successes of moral treatment in *The Retreat* in 1813. This work, along with Pinel's writings, sparked implementation of reforms in hospitals across England and America that included a strong emphasis on daily occupations (Bing, 1981).

Throughout the early 19th century, hospitals and asylums were founded that applied the philosophy of moral treatment. In these treatment centers, patients received humane treatment and engaged in physician-prescribed routines of work and leisure (Peloquin, 1989). Moral treatment became an effective means for recovery from mental illness, and its effectiveness is attributed in part to the comprehensive program of daily occupations (Bockoven, 1971). The implementation of moral treatment paved the way for the use of occupation as a healing modality and set a course for the emerging profession of occupational therapy.

## Arts and Crafts Movement

Another factor that influenced the development of the use of occupation in therapy was the Arts and Crafts Movement of the early 19th century. The Arts and Crafts movement was a cultural phenomenon in the United States that promoted the benefits of occupation. During this time in American history, industrialization resulted in mass production of low quality products and excessive materialism (Levine, 1981). In addition, industrialization altered the cultural landscape: People moved out of traditional family farming cultures and into cities in search of work (Peloquin, 1989), thereby eroding their connection with previously held meaningful occupations. John Ruskin, the father of the movement, believed that machination and factory work resulted in deep unhappiness. He alleged that reliance on machines, poor working conditions, and displacement of human skill caused a deterioration of physical health as well as the common complaints of disease, anxiety, and fatigue. American society responded by adopting a "do-it-yourself" mentality and making products by hand. Proponents of the Arts and Crafts movement advocated for a return to a meaningful lifestyle, which included farming, using natural materials, and producing and purchasing items that were simple in design. For many, the Arts and Crafts movement symbolized a return to human dignity and quality of life, as well as a return to occupations of handicraft (Levine, 1981).

At the same time, the medical profession was building a scientific foundation for treatment of disease. Although this allowed for new treatment of disease, some physicians were unsatisfied with a reductionist view of health and were inspired by the Arts and Crafts movement to investigate the effects of human occupation. Three such physicians were Herbert J. Hall, Adolf Meyer, and William Rush Dunton, Jr. (Levine, 1981).

Herbert J. Hall used work as an alternative to bed rest and created sheltered workshops where patients designed and created useful products to be sold in local shops. Hall promoted the workshops to provide opportunities to earn a living through the production of handmade objects, provide spiritual support to professional craftsmen, and employ people with physical and mental disabilities (Levine, 1981).

Adolf Meyer was a leader in the medical profession of his day. Meyer collaborated with social worker Julia Lathrop to bring craftwork to chronically mentally ill patients (Levine, 1981). He believed that providing patients with opportunities to work, plan, create, and learn how to use materials facilitated balance between work, play, rest, and sleep. He stated that a balance between these four factors helped promote achievement in healthy harmony with human nature. Meyer went on to present the first organized model of occupational therapy in 1921. His lecture, "The Philosophy of Occupational Therapy," was the first article in the *Archives of Occupational Therapy* (Meyer, 1977).

William Rush Dunton, Jr., was a psychiatrist who recommended exercise, work, and recreation for his patients with mental illness. He promoted goal-directed occupations and structured his patients' occupations through the use of arts and crafts. He sought training in craftsmanship so that he could provide education in the production of crafts that interested his patients (Peloquin, 1991a).

As the health benefits of craftwork became apparent to the medical community, the philosophy of the Arts and Crafts movement was applied to meet the rehabilitation goals of patients with both physical and mental disabilities. Furthermore, arts and crafts became a central focus of early occupational therapy practice. Early therapists recognized that healthy individuals used arts and crafts occupations to maintain and improve their health (Levine, 1981). The philosophy of humanism was also applied to realize the healing that arts and crafts could bring to less fortunate individuals, and those with chronic illnesses and disabilities.

## National Society for the Promotion of Occupational Therapy: Early Pioneers of Occupational Therapy

With recognition of the immense therapeutic value of occupation, made evident through moral treatment and the values of the Arts and Crafts movement, leaders in the emerging field sought to found occupational therapy as a distinct profession. In 1917, a small group gathered for the first meeting of the National Society for the Promotion of Occupational Therapy (NSPOT). The founders were a diverse collection of doctors, nurses, and craftsmen whose ideas regarding occupational therapy and health shaped the foundation of the complex practice it has become. Although each founder brought his or her unique perspective, they shared a common philosophy: Engagement in occupation facilitated health and healing. During the early 20th century, the founders worked to describe what distinguished occupational therapy from other types of treatment, determine the type of education that would be suitable for occupational therapists, and carve out the role of occupational therapy in the medical realm (Peloquin, 1991a). The following passages provide insight into how George Edward Barton, William Rush Dunton, Jr., Eleanor Clarke Slagle, Susan C. Johnson, Thomas B. Kidner, Susan Elizabeth Tracy, and Herbert J. Hall—each of the pioneers of occupational therapy—helped to shape the profession in its early evolution.

George Edward Barton was an architect with background knowledge in nursing and medicine. Following foot surgery, he experienced paralysis and was treated at a solarium where he experienced the healing effect of occupation. He believed that occupation could provide mental as well as physical benefit. Barton asserted that individuals could become self-sufficient and productive through occupational therapy. He contended that occupational therapy should provide clients with a means to work and support themselves despite illness and disability. Barton saw a strong connection between the medical field and occupation, and recommended occupation should be prescribed and taught by a medical professional trained in occupation (i.e., an occupational nurse). He called for a thorough evaluation before the prescription of occupational therapy and for the therapist to monitor occupation's effects. He further believed that occupation could enhance medical prescriptions via by-products of the occupation, such as exposure to beneficial chemicals in an industrial plant (Peloquin, 1991a).

William Rush Dunton, Jr., was a psychiatrist who was president of the NSPOT in 1917. He asserted that occupational therapy was the continuation of moral treatment. Dunton extolled the merits of occupation, stating it was vital to human life (Peloquin, 1991b). He believed that the power of occupation lies in its ability to give purpose to the patient, rather than to make marketable products (Peloquin, 1991a). Dunton strongly believed that occupational therapists should be medical professionals, and created a training program for nurses based on the work of Susan Tracy. Dunton described three distinct types of occupation: invalid occupation, occupational therapy, and vocational training. Invalid occupation was defined as a diversion to provide respite from illness. Occupational therapy was intended to restore

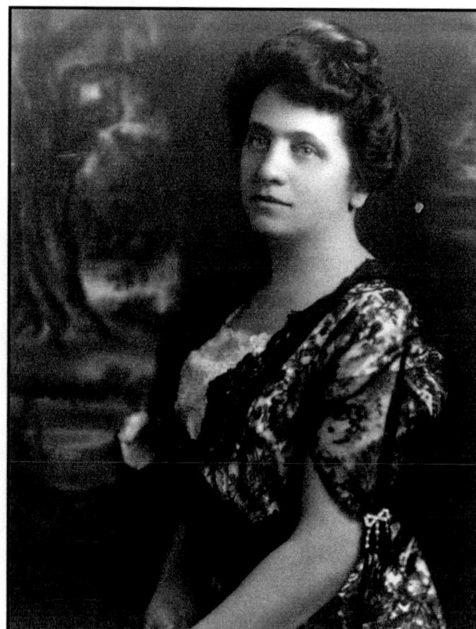

**Figure 5-1.** Eleanor Clarke Slagle. (Courtesy of the Archive of the American Occupational Therapy Association, Inc.)

function that was lost through physical or mental illness. Vocational training was viewed as a means to provide restoration of function for people who had disabilities. Dunton also recommended occupational engagement for well people, being the first to recognize occupation's role in health maintenance (Peloquin, 1991b).

Eleanor Clarke Slagle (Figure 5-1) became a strong leader in the burgeoning profession of occupational therapy. She was elected vice president at the first meeting of the NSPOT and, over time, held every office. She was instrumental in the training of nurses, attendants, and occupational therapists; she created a 3-week training courses for nurses and founded the Henry B. Favill School of Occupations (Peloquin, 1991b). As she provided intervention, she noted that teaching occupation was a distinct form of therapy (Licht, 1967). Slagle believed that a physician should prescribe the medical outcome, but the occupational therapist should be independent in determining the specific occupation that would meet the patient's needs. Slagle's unique contribution to the profession included the application of habit training to chronically ill patients. She found that by using daily occupations in a routine fashion, significantly ill patients could begin to show progress (Peloquin, 1991b). As the profession progressed, Slagle held several offices of the American Occupational Therapy Association (AOTA) and assisted in the formation of the first list of qualified therapists (Punwar & Peloquin, 2000). She was such a strong leader in the field of occupational therapy and a pioneering woman that her contribution was honored by the presence of Eleanor Roosevelt and Adolf Meyer at her retirement party. Furthermore, the AOTA honored her by creating an annual Honorary Guest Lectureship in her name, henceforth known as the Eleanor Clarke Slagle Lectureship (Schwartz, 2009) and commonly known to contemporary therapists as the "Slagle."

Susan C. Johnson was a high school teacher of the arts who believed in the healing power of occupation. She demonstrated that engagement in occupation could facilitate health, morality, and self-sufficiency for inmates in hospitals and almshouses. Johnson contributed greatly to occupational therapy through her focus on the education of practitioners and the process of teaching occupations to patients. She published several articles regarding training of occupational practitioners and the role of occupational therapy within the hospital setting. Johnson asserted that occupational therapists needed education in psychology, teaching methodology, and medical practice. She viewed the path of the occupational practitioner as between that of an educator and that of a nurse (Peloquin, 1991b).

Thomas B. Kidner was a Canadian architect who was committed to the health and rehabilitation of soldiers returning from war and people injured in industrial accidents. He believed in the power of occupation to cure patients, and that the therapeutic value was paramount to other applications—such as the generation of income. He argued that the value of occupation was in the process rather than the product. Kidner was a strong leader in the NSPOT as it evolved into the AOTA, and he served as president for six terms. During his tenure, standards for occupational therapy education were set. At that time, a training course of 6 hours daily for a minimum of 12 months was required. Occupational therapy education was further required to include psychology, anatomy, kinesiology, orthopedics, mental diseases, tuberculosis, and general medical concerns in addition to handicrafts (Peloquin, 1991b).

Susan Elizabeth Tracy is considered an incorporator of the profession even though she was not in attendance at the first meeting of the NSPOT due to her strong influence on the early shaping of the profession. Tracy was a nurse who recognized the healing power of occupation in her patients and promoted a holistic definition of the word "cure" that included emotional state. Tracy was one of the first educators of occupational therapy and wrote several books, including the landmark *Studies of Invalid Occupations: A Manual for Nurses and Attendants* (1912). Tracy asserted that occupational therapy should be included in the realm of medication, and occupation should be prescribed by physicians. She felt that the occupational needs of very sick patients should be attended to by a nurse, but that less ill individuals could be served by non-medically trained individuals who had compassion and a desire to help others. Tracy focused on the purpose and quality of objects made by patients, rather than the ability to earn money through their production. Tracy was one of the first to educate medical professionals in teaching occupations to patients. She also promoted adaptation of occupations to meet the abilities of the client and wrote specifically about how to teach individuals who had physical disabilities or limitations in movement. Tracy even noted the healing effect of occupational therapy on the practitioner who provided the service (Peloquin, 1991a).

Herbert J. Hall is also considered an influential "near-founder" of occupational therapy (Peloquin, 1991b, p. 738). He studied the use of occupation for individuals with neurasthenia at Harvard University in 1906. He believed in the power of using one's hands to create products, the potential for occupation to provide peace of mind, and the strong influence of work on happiness. He believed that industry should be created to hire, and thus meet the occupational needs of, people who had disabilities (Peloquin, 1991b). Hall believed in the medical prescription of occupation and called occupational therapy the "science of prescribed work" (as quoted in Peloquin, 1991b).

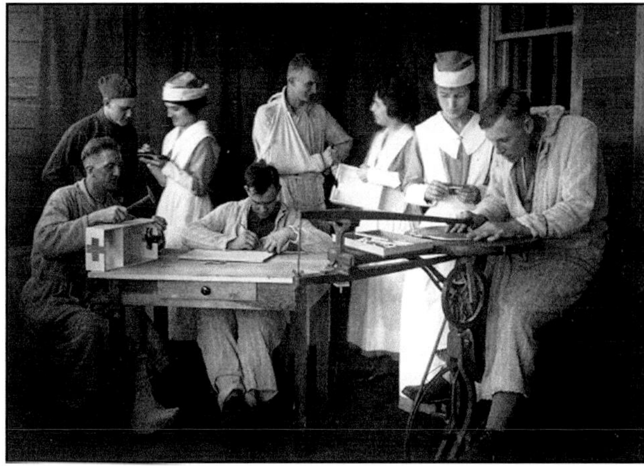

**Figure 5-2.** Reconstruction aides. (Courtesy of the Archive of the American Occupational Therapy Association, Inc.)

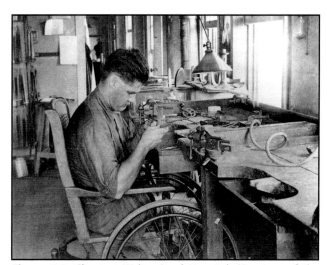

**Figure 5-3.** Client at Walter Reed Hospital. (Courtesy of the Archive of the American Occupational Therapy Association, Inc.)

## World War I

William Rush Dunton, Jr., indicated that World War I was a turning point for the early profession. He believed that the war caused therapists to refine their ideals and demonstrate their purpose in the medical field (Peloquin, 1991b). Additionally, the war altered the makeup of the population that occupational therapists served. Before World War I, occupational therapists worked primarily with individuals who had mental illnesses. However, large numbers of soldiers returned from the war with physical disabilities, thus creating a new treatment milieu for occupational therapists (Punwar & Peloquin, 2000).

Occupational therapists were initially not recognized as part of the treatment team on the battlefield. Dr. Frankwood Williams, a military psychiatrist, was the first to recognize the utility of occupational therapy in the war zone (Punwar & Peloquin, 2000). Although he was unable to convince his superiors to enlist occupational therapists, he found openings for civilian workers, known as *scrub-aides* or *reconstruction aides* (Figure 5-2), and convinced a small group of occupational therapy workers to join the medical team under this guise (Peloquin, 1991b). Some reconstruction aides were artists or craftsmen who received short wartime courses to provide a modicum of medical background. Small numbers of reconstruction aides were occupational therapists. All were women, reflecting the cultural idea that women were best suited to inspire and provide refuge for the all-male military (Peloquin, 1991b).

The occupational reconstruction aides used what materials they could find to assist men stricken with neuroses from the war horrors they had seen. Through woodwork and metalwork, the aides provided opportunities for diversion and healing. The aides were well recognized for their positive impact on the soldiers, and the power of occupation began to receive wide support (Low, 1992). As the war continued, occupational reconstruction aides began to use occupation for physical rehabilitation, recommend work adaptations, and create assistive devices to promote independence in daily tasks such as self-care (Peloquin, 1991b).

The war years had a profound effect on the profession. Perhaps the greatest effect the war had on occupational therapy was the increase in the population served. Following the success of rehabilitating injured soldiers in the field, occupational therapy gained new acceptance and was widely prescribed in the expanding numbers of Army and Navy hospitals (Woodside, 1971; Figure 5-3). During the war, occupational therapy began to distinguish itself from nursing, as there were few nurses who attended strictly to the medical needs of injured patients. The relationship between the occupational therapist and the patient became understood as part of the curative aspect of therapy. The war experience also helped to solidify the view that the value of occupation lies not just in the product, but also in the process of engagement. Occupational therapy's role in returning patients to functional tasks became evident. In addition, the process of adapting and modifying tasks and equipment to facilitate function in an individual with a physical disability began to take hold (Peloquin, 1991b). During this period, occupational therapy literature began to embrace scientific advances, and the leaders in the field recognized that therapists required intensive education that went beyond handicrafts to include emphasis on the medical model (Levine, 1981; Peloquin, 1991b).

## Post-War Boom

The 1920s heralded another advancement in the practice of occupational therapy. The economic boom of the 1920s resulted in a significant increase in the number of hospitals and, in turn, a greater need for occupational therapists (Cole & Tufano, 2008). Legislation also increased the need for occupational therapy, moving the practice from volunteer status to a medical service. The Smith-Bankhead Bill of 1920 established the basis for federal vocational rehabilitation by emphasizing that people with disabilities could be rehabilitated through vocational training (Woodside, 1971). The Federal Industrial Rehabilitation Act of 1923 required hospitals to employ occupational therapists to rehabilitate patients following industrial accidents and illnesses. By the end of the 1920s, occupational therapy was formally recognized as a medical ancillary service (Rerek, 1971). Occupational therapy was now required through physical prescription, and medical record-keeping standards were developed (Quiroga, 1995).

With the increase in occupational therapy services provided in the hospital setting, the AOTA looked toward the American Medical Association to assist in the establishment of standards for training institutions and accreditation of educational facilities. Susan Cox Johnson and Elizabeth Upham Davis sought to standardize educational requirements, create a means of professional development for practitioners, and further research the medical conditions for which occupational therapy was prescribed. In 1923, the *Minimum Standards for Courses of Training in Occupational Therapy* was adopted by the AOTA by a unanimous vote. The standards addressed prerequisites for admission and the length and content of courses (Quiroga, 1995).

By the mid-1920s, the official scope of occupational therapy included the use of activity to facilitate recovery from illness or injury and to socialize individuals with chronic illnesses. Occupations were used to prepare for future employment and improve the mental well-being of the sick. The process of engagement in occupation was valued more than the product, and the selection of occupations was based on individual interests, abilities, and need. The ability to teach patients and provide a positive relationship and outlook were valued traits in the therapist (Levine, 1981).

## The Great Depression and World War II

The expansion and gains of occupational therapy were halted with the stock market crash of 1929 and the depression that followed, causing a decline in health care services overall (Rerek, 1971). Budget cuts enacted due to the Depression and the National Economy Act of 1933 resulted in decreased occupational therapy jobs and closing of clinics and occupational therapy schools (Hopkins & Smith, 1993). Therefore, when World War II began, the profession was not prepared to meet the needs of soldiers on the battlefield or at home. Because occupational therapists did not reach military status during World War I, funding was not available to provide service during World War II, which resulted in a shortage of occupational therapists. During World War II, there were 12 individuals in the U.S. Army working in occupational therapy, only 8 of whom were registered therapists (Hopkins & Smith, 1993). As veterans returned home, few facilities were available for rehabilitation or long-term care, and institutions for community reintegration did not exist. Veterans and their families soon sought the care they deserved, and the government responded (Rerek, 1971). Among the changes was the elevation of occupational therapists to military status (Messick, 1947). Funding for occupational therapy was provided through the New Deal (Cole & Tufano, 2008), which provided Social Security income for people who had disabilities, and the GI Bill, which provided funding for vocational training. Furthermore, the Vocational Rehabilitation Act and amendments of 1943 allowed for the payment of medical services, including occupational therapy (Harvey-Krefting, 1985). Recognizing the health care system's inability to respond to the number of wounded veterans returning from the war, society pushed for the rehabilitation movement.

## Rehabilitation Movement

The rehabilitation movement occurred from 1942 to 1960 (Punwar & Peloquin, 2000). The movement began by recognizing that, with proper care and rehabilitation, individuals with disabilities could be independent and contributing members of the community (Mosey,

1971). Rehabilitative occupational therapy consisted primarily of technical intervention, including training and fitting of prosthetics and orthotics, activities of daily living, and resistive exercises to improve strength. At this time, occupational therapy was practiced with little connection to theory or guiding models of practice. Education was increasingly medically based, and therapy became more specialized and deficit focused (Punwar & Peloquin, 2000).

In the 1950s, the profession responded to the growing need for rehabilitation by expanding to include the first occupational therapy assistants. In 1958, the first training program for occupational therapy assistants began, consisting of 3 months of education focused on mental health intervention. Education expanded to include other areas of occupational therapy practice in the 1960s (Punwar & Peloquin, 2000). Leaders in the profession added to the knowledge base through the application of psychoanalytic and sensory motor frames of reference. Advances in neurology led to new treatment techniques, including Rood's sensorimotor reflex model and Bobath's Neurodevelopmental Therapy (Cole & Tufano, 2008).

## The 1960s

The 1960s were an era of great social and political change in the United States. Advances in technology and changes in the family structure altered the professional and social landscape. The U.S. government made health care available to citizens who were economically disadvantaged or disabled through the enactment of Medicare and Medicaid legislation (Coombs, 2005). The Community Mental Health Act of 1963 expanded the breadth of mental health services to include a variety of levels and venues of service (Cole & Tufano, 2008).

During the 1960s, the field of medicine was becoming increasingly advanced and specialized. Survival rates for individuals with injuries and infants with severe medical conditions skyrocketed, resulting in significantly larger populations of people living with disabilities. Occupational therapy showed a significant movement toward specialization as well, with new focus on advanced practice areas such as hand therapy, spinal cord injury rehabilitation, and sensory integration. New practice areas such as schools, clinics, and community settings emerged. In addition, occupational therapy responded to the new social challenges of substance abuse and addiction and the increasing prevalence of stress-related illness (Punwar & Peloquin, 2000).

## The 1970s and 1980s

As the medical advances of 1970s and 1980s continued to quicken in pace, medical care itself became increasingly expensive. A trend of hospitalization for only the most significant treatment and deinstitutionalization for individuals with mental illnesses and intellectual disabilities resulted (Punwar & Peloquin, 2000). Occupational therapists quickly noted the value of working outside of the medical system, and the shift toward the community model began. The 1975 Education for All Handicapped Children Act ensured that children with disabilities received public education and marked the entrance of occupational therapy into the public school system as a related service (P.L. 94-142).

Philosophically, a holistic view of the client and an occupational focus was called forth by leaders in the field, such as Kielhofner and Burke (1980), who developed the Model of Human Occupation, one of the most widely used models of practice today. The profession also began to shift its scope of practice to include wellness and disease prevention (Punwar & Peloquin, 2000).

On an organizational level, the AOTA sought to unify the profession through the development and refinement of the *Uniform Terminology of Occupational Therapy*. This document delineated the roles of the occupational therapist and clarified knowledge of occupation by introducing the concepts of performance components and performance areas. The document also provided terminology for uniform documentation (Cole & Tufano, 2008).

During this era, occupational therapy education continued to become more in-depth and refined. Increasing numbers of graduate programs were founded to meet the needs of occupational therapy practitioners entering an increasingly broad field of practice (Punwar & Peloquin, 2000). The economic challenges of providing medical care ushered in an age when justification for services and accountability for outcomes emerged (Cole & Tufano, 2008). The AOTA sought to address this need for knowledge and validation of therapeutic intervention through research (Punwar & Peloquin, 2000). Standardized assessment also emerged as a justification for service. State regulation of licensure was adopted to ensure the quality of therapists practicing across the United States (Cole & Tufano, 2008).

## The 1990s

During the late 20th century, the expense of medicine and increasing numbers of chronically ill individuals continued to tax the economic system. The right of individuals to make their own decisions regarding their health care entered the social consciousness, while at the same time health management organizations were developed to determine what services would be rendered to people with medical insurance (Punwar & Peloquin, 2000).

The profession of occupational therapy responded with a movement into health care services rendered in the home and rehabilitation in nursing facilities. The Individuals with Disabilities Education Act of 1990 ensured public education and services, including occupational therapy, to assist students in accessing their education (U.S. Department of Education, n.d.; P.L. 108-446). The Americans with Disabilities Act (ADA) of 1990 also increased the need for occupational therapists (U.S. Equal Employment Opportunity Commission, n.d.). The ADA prohibited discrimination of people with disabilities and addressed architectural barriers and environmental modification to ensure that all buildings were accessible to people of all abilities (U.S. Equal Employment Opportunity Commission, n.d.). ADA compliance, environmental modification, advocacy for those with disabilities, and quality of life constituted new areas of practice for occupational therapists (Punwar & Peloquin, 2000).

In the 1990s, theoretical foundations for practice and clinical reasoning were recognized as highly important facets of occupational therapy practice, most notably with the development of a framework for clinical reasoning through the work of Mattingly and Fleming (1994). In addition, occupational performance–focused models added to the practice knowledge, including, among others, the Canadian Model of Occupational Performance (1991) and Person-Environment-Occupational Performance Model (Punwar & Peloquin, 2000). Furthermore, a new field of scientific inquiry known as *occupational science* was developed to examine the nature of occupation itself (Clark et al., 1991) and to provide basic scientific knowledge regarding occupation from which the practice of occupational therapy could draw (Yerxa et al., 1990).

Education continued to move forward in the 1990s as well. Prior to this time, advanced degrees in occupational therapy were not available. Therefore, academics held degrees in related fields (Clark et al., 1991). To move the profession forward academically, an advanced clinical doctorate was developed to feature an emphasis on advanced occupational therapy practice (Pierce & Peyton, 1999). The first post-professional clinical doctorate was offered in 1994 at Nova Southeastern University. Creighton University went on to create the first entry-level occupational therapy doctorate. Entry-level and post-professional programs continue to proliferate at universities, such as Boston University and Washington University, among others (Griffiths & Padilla, 2006; Jacobs, personal communication, January 26, 2013).

## Occupational Therapy in the 21st Century

With the entrance into the 21st century, society began to focus more on health and wellness promotion and the prevention of disease. The definition of health as the ability to live a full and productive life despite physical or societal limitations became recognized by such institutions as the World Health Organization (Schwartz, 2009). Occupational therapy scholars project that the profession will develop further into the areas of health promotion, disease prevention, and preventative occupation with a variety of innovative treatment foci (Scaffa & Reitz, 2014). The AOTA identified key practice areas that are expected to flourish given the movement toward proactive health including therapy for older adults, amelioration of health care disparities, obesity management, quality of life, and technology (Health and Wellness, 2016).

In response to the reorientation toward healthy living as occupational therapy nears its 100-year anniversary, the Centennial Vision for the profession was developed. This vision connects with the founding philosophy regarding the value of occupation, and it further expands the definition of occupation by including the social context. The vision also promotes the prevention and dissolution of barriers to participation in occupation. The Centennial Vision calls for continued research and validation of the therapeutic interventions. Furthermore, the vision acknowledges that occupation is an integral vehicle for the health of all people throughout the global community (Schwartz, 2009).

In the 21st century, leaders in the profession again sought to increase the standard for professional education. In 2007, educational institutions were required to phase out remaining baccalaureate occupational therapy degrees and provide post-baccalaureate or entry-level master's degrees. This change addressed the need for advanced clinical reasoning, a high level of knowledge across a wide therapeutic milieu, a depth of knowledge in research, and autonomous practice in a variety of settings (Griffiths & Padilla, 2006). During this time, an emphasis on evidence-based practice has also grown. The AOTA developed practice guidelines to assist contemporary occupational therapists in addressing current practice areas including home modifications, treatments for neurodegenerative diseases, low vision, productive aging, traumatic brain injury, stroke, driving and community mobility, work-related injuries, early childhood, sensory integration, promotion of mental health, and autism (Practice Guidelines, 2016).

During this second decade of the 21st century, occupational therapists are called to connect with our heritage. Practitioners, educators, and students alike strive to blend science with humanism (Schwartz, 2009) and expound the value of occupation as a health-promoting

## Evidence-Based Research Chart

| Topic | Evidence |
|---|---|
| Occupation | Crepeau et al., 2009; Gray, 1998; Nelson, 1997; Peloquin, 2007; Pierce, 2000; Yerxa et al., 1990 |
| Moral treatment | Bing, 1981; Bockoven, 1971; Peloquin, 1989 |
| Reconstruction aide | Low, 1992; Peloquin, 1991b; Punwar & Peloquin, 2000 |
| Community model | Punwar & Peloquin, 2000; Scaffa & Reitz, 2014 |

and disease-preventing force. We aim to elevate our professional status through education and research and by acting as leaders in social and medical arenas (Baum, 2006). Furthermore, occupational therapy practitioners are called to promote our philosophy and profession among people we encounter in everyday life, as well as through interprofessionalism, scholarship, and social media (Jacobs, 2012). Occupational therapy practitioners and students promote the profession through Occupational Therapy Global Day of Service. We continue to strive for the best possible education by providing education with an occupation focus (Pierce, 2000) and expanding knowledge with PhD programs focused specifically on occupational therapy and occupational science. As our theoretical knowledge is ever expanding, we must also work to connect theories and research with practice (Pierce, 2000). We must all the while hold close our humanistic roots that remind us that all people deserve the ability to live healthy and productive lives within their scope of interest and ability. Occupational therapy facilitates this core value for the people we serve.

## Student Self-Assessment

1. Describe moral treatment and its influence on the use of occupation in therapy. How do you think the philosophy continues to influence contemporary practitioners?
2. Explain the impact of the Arts and Crafts movement on the development of the profession. What influence do you think crafts and handiwork has on occupational therapy today?
3. Name the founders of the NSPOT and the key contributions of each.
4. Explain the effect of World War I on the profession.
5. Describe the rehabilitation movement. Did the movement limit or facilitate growth for occupational therapists?
6. Describe the shift from the medical model to the community model. In what ways did the shift change occupational therapy?
7. Explain the tenets of the Centennial Vision for occupational therapy. How will you apply these to your future practice?
8. What current historical and cultural influences do you think will affect the continued development of occupational therapy?

## References


Baum, M. C. (2006). Presidential Address, 2006: Centennial challenges, millennium opportunities. *American Journal of Occupational Therapy, 60*(6), 609-616.

Bing, R. K. (1981). Eleanor Clarke Slagle Lectureship—1981. Occupational therapy revisited; A paraphrastic journey. *American Journal of Occupational Therapy, 35*(8), 499-517.

Bockoven, J. S. (1971). Occupational therapy—A historical perspective. Legacy of moral treatment—1800s to 1910. *American Journal of Occupational Therapy, 25*(5), 223-225.

Clark, F. A., Parham, D., Carlson, M. E., Frank, G., Jackson, J., Pierce, D., Wolfe, R. J., & Zemke, R. (1991). Occupational science: Academic innovation in the service of occupational therapy's future. *American Journal of Occupational Therapy, 45*(4), 300-310.

Cole, M. B., & Tufano, R. (2008). *Applied theories in occupational therapy: A practical approach*. Thorofare, NJ: SLACK Incorporated.

Coombs, J. G. (2005). *The rise and fall of HMO's: An American health care revolution*. Madison, WI: The University of Wisconsin Press.

Crepeau, E. B., Cohn, E. S., & Schell, B. A. B. (2009). *Willard and Spackman's occupational therapy* (11th ed.). Philadelphia, PA: J. B. Lippincott.

Faust, L. (1979). Therapy and function: An issue of professional direction. *American Journal of Occupational Therapy, 33*(11), 725-727.

Gray, J. M. (1998). Putting occupation into practice: Occupation as ends, occupation as means. *American Journal of Occupational Therapy, 52*(5), 354-364.

Griffiths, Y., & Padilla, R. (2006). National status of the entry-level doctorate in occupational therapy (OTD). *American Journal of Occupational Therapy, 60*(5), 540-550.

Harvey-Krefting, L. (1985). The concept of work in occupational therapy: A historical review. *American Journal of Occupational Therapy, 39*(5), 301-307.

Health and Wellness. (2016). Retrieved from http://www.aota.org/Practice/Health-Wellness.aspx

Hopkins, H. L., & Smith, H. D. (1993). *Willard and Spackman's occupational therapy* (8th ed.). Philadelphia, PA: J. B. Lippincott.

Jacobs, K. (2012). PromOTing occupational therapy: Words, images, and actions (Eleanor Clarke Slagle Lecture). *American Journal of Occupational Therapy, 66*, 652-671.

Kielhofner, G., & Burke, J. (1980). A model of human occupation, part 1: Conceptual framework and content. *American Journal of Occupational Therapy, 34*, 572-581.

Levine, R. (1981). The influence of the arts and crafts movement on the professional status of occupational therapy. *American Journal of Occupational Therapy, 41*(4), 248-254.

Licht, S. (1967). The founding and founders of the American Occupational Therapy Association. *American Journal of Occupational Therapy, 21*(5), 269-277.

Low, J. F. (1992). The reconstruction aides. *American Journal of Occupational Therapy, 46*(1), 38-43.

Mattingly, C., & Fleming, M. (1994). *Clinical reasoning: Forms of inquiry in a therapeutic practice.* Philadelphia, PA: F. A. Davis Company.

Messick, H. E. (1947). The new women's medical specialist corps. *American Journal of Occupational Therapy, 1*(5), 298-300.

Meyer, A. (1977). The philosophy of occupation therapy. *American Journal of Occupational Therapy, 31*(10), 639-642.

Mosey, A. C. (1971). Involvement in the rehabilitation movement 1942-1960. *American Journal of Occupational Therapy, 25*(5), 234-236.

Nelson, D. L. (1997). Why the profession of occupational therapy will flourish in the 21st century. *American Journal of Occupational Therapy, 51*(1), 11-24.

Peloquin, S. M. (1989). Moral treatment: Contexts reconsidered. *American Journal of Occupational Therapy, 43*(8), 537-544.

Peloquin, S. M. (1991a). Occupational therapy service: Individual and collective understandings of the founders, part 1. *American Journal of Occupational Therapy, 45*(4), 352-360.

Peloquin, S. M. (1991b). Occupational therapy service: Individual and collective understandings of the founders, part 2. *American Journal of Occupational Therapy, 45*(8), 733-744.

Peloquin, S. M. (2007). A reconsideration of occupational therapy's core values. *American Journal of Occupational Therapy, 61*(4), 474-478.

Pierce, D. (2000). Occupational by design: Dimensions, therapeutic power and creative process. *American Journal of Occupational Therapy, 55*, 249-259.

Pierce, D., & Peyton, C. (1999). A historical cross-disciplinary perspective on the professional doctorate in occupational therapy. *American Journal of Occupational Therapy, 53*, 64-71.

Practice Guidelines. (2016). Retrieved from http://www.aota.org/Practice/Researchers/practice-guidelines.aspx

Punwar, A. J., & Peloquin, S. M. (2000). *Occupational therapy principles and practice* (3rd ed.). Baltimore, MD: Lippincott Williams and Wilkins.

Quiroga, V. A. M. (1995). *Occupational therapy: The first 30 years, 1900 to 1930.* Bethesda, MD: AOTA Press.

Rerek, M. D. (1971). The depression years—1929-1941. *American Journal of Occupational Therapy, 25*(5), 231-233.

Scaffa, M. E., & Reitz, S. M. (2014). Occupational therapy in community-based practice settings (2nd ed.). Philadelphia, PA: F. A. Davis Company.

Schwartz, K. B. (2009). Reclaiming our heritage: Connecting the founding vision to the centennial vision. *American Journal of Occupational Therapy, 63*(6), 681-690.

Tracy, S. E. (1912). *Studies of invalid occupations: A manual for nurses and attendants*. Boston, MA: Whitcomb and Barrows.

U.S. Department of Education. (n.d.). *Individuals with disabilities education act.* Retrieved from http://idea.ed.gov

U.S. Equal Employment Opportunity Commission. (n.d.). *Americans with disabilities act (ADA): 1990-2002.* Retrieved from http://www.eeoc.gov/ada

Woodside, H. H. (1971). The development of occupational therapy 1910-1929. *American Journal of Occupational Therapy, 25*(5), 226-230.

Yerxa, E. J., Clark, F., Frank, G., Jackson, J., Parham, D., Pierce, D., Stein, C., & Zemke, R. (1990). An introduction to occupational science: A foundation for occupational therapy in the 21st century. *Occupational Therapy in Health Care, 6*(4), 1-18.

## Suggested Readings

The Education of Handicapped Children Act of 1975. (P. L. 94-142).

Yerxa, E. J. (1980). Occupational therapy's role in creating a future climate of caring. *American Journal of Occupational Therapy, 34*, 533.

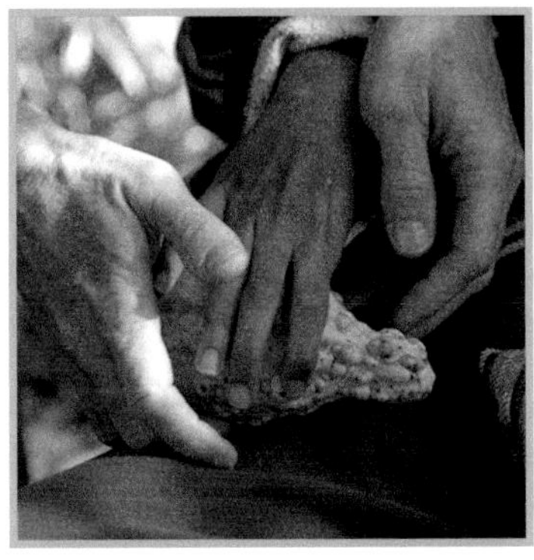

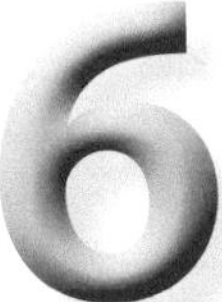

# The Occupational Therapy Practice Framework
## Domain and Process, Third Edition

Verna G. Eschenfelder, PhD, OTR/L and Patricia A. Wisniewski, MS, OTR/L, CPRP

**ACOTE STANDARDS EXPLORED IN THIS CHAPTER**

Preamble

**KEY VOCABULARY**

- **Client factors:** The physiological and psychological aspects that reside within a client and body structures that may affect occupational performance (American Occupational Therapy Association [AOTA], 2014).
- **Context and environment:** Contextual and environmental influences both internal and external to a client that influence occupational performance including physical and social environment and cultural, personal, temporal, and virtual context (AOTA, 2014).
- **Occupations:** Common occupations people may engage in include activities of daily living, instrumental activities of daily living, rest and sleep, education, work, play, leisure, and social participation (AOTA, 2014).
- **Performance patterns:** A client's habits, routines, rituals, and roles that support engagement, participation, and health (AOTA, 2014).
- **Performance skills:** Actions or elements of actions that can be observed when an individual participates in meaningful occupation (AOTA, 2014).



Jacobs, K., & MacRae, N. (Eds.).
*Occupational Therapy Essentials for Clinical Competence, Third Edition* (pp. 55-68).

The *Occupational Therapy Practice Framework: Domain and Process, Third Edition*, is an official document of the American Occupational Therapy Association (AOTA). It is designed to summarize constructs that define and guide occupational therapy practice and to articulate the profession's contribution to the promotion of health and participation of people, organizations, and populations through engagement in occupation (AOTA, 2014). This chapter provides a review of the *Framework* as it relates to the scope and delivery of occupational therapy services and as it is applied to the case of an occupational therapy client. The reader is encouraged to refer to the *Framework* (AOTA, 2014). Included in this chapter is a description of the evolution of the *Framework* and the ways in which it contributes to and supports the language of the profession. By the end of the chapter, the reader should understand basic factors that led to the development of the *Framework*, recognize the interrelatedness of the domain and process of the *Framework*, and begin to apply this knowledge to the delivery of occupational therapy practice. With guidance from an instructor, the student will apply the *Framework* to a hypothetical case study involving a client named Marie to facilitate understanding of the complexity inherent in the *Framework*.

## Evolution of a Language for Occupational Therapy

From the profession's beginning, occupational therapists have placed great emphasis on the relationship between active engagement in occupation and an individual's health and well-being (Fidler & Fidler, 1978; Meyer, 1922). Toward the middle of the 20th century, the profession became increasingly aligned with the medical model of practice that involved a more reductionistic approach to treating clients. While this alignment with medicine led to a number of advancements for the profession, occupational therapists became increasingly focused on limiting impairment while there was less emphasis placed on occupation as a means and end to the therapeutic process. Over the past several decades, leaders in the profession have increased efforts to better articulate the importance of occupation as a unique contribution of the profession for the clients occupational therapists treat (Bing, 1981; Gilfoyle, 1984).

This most recent paradigm shift for the profession has resulted in a return to occupational therapy's holistic roots that place value on the relationship between occupation and health. In 1979, the Representative Assembly of the AOTA developed the *Uniform Terminology* document, which sought to unify occupational therapy under one set of guidelines (Punwar, 1994). The Second Edition of *Uniform Terminology* was published in 1989 and set out to advance a commonly defined language for the profession. In 1994, the AOTA published *Uniform Terminology, Third Edition* (UT-III), which further expanded the document to incorporate contextual aspects of performance (AOTA, 1994). The UT-III provided definitions and a structure for the practice of occupational therapy. Five years later, the Commission on Practice of the AOTA determined the need to develop a document that retained the initial intent of UT-III, but better reflected current occupational therapy practice. This effort resulted in the First Edition of the *Occupational Therapy Practice Framework: Domain and Process* in 2002. This original framework was organized into domain and process sections, with an emphasis on the interrelatedness of both components. The authors of the original framework placed great importance on occupation as the cornerstone for the profession (AOTA, 2002). Leaders in the profession recognized the need to improve on this original framework in an attempt to refine the document's domains, more clearly describe the process of evaluation and intervention, and place greater emphasis on the impact of occupational engagement on health (AOTA, 2008; Gutman, Mortera, Hinojosa, & Kramer, 2007). The *Occupational Therapy Practice Framework: Domain and Process, Second Edition* (OTPF-2), was published in 2008 and was designed to articulate occupational therapy's contribution to promoting the health and participation of individuals, organizations, and populations through engagement in occupation (AOTA, 2008). The fit between the OTPF-2 and the World Health Organization's *International Classification of Functioning, Disability and Health* was noted. The authors described the change in focus from "consequences of disease" to "components of health and participation in activities of life" (p. 4) of the *International Classification of Functioning, Disability and Health* as it related to the OTPF-2 focus on "supporting health and participation in life through engagement in occupation" (AOTA, 2008, p. 660).

Just as occupational therapy is an evolving profession, the framework must also evolve. In 2012, the Commission on Practice began the process of reviewing and updating the OTPF-2. As a part of this process, the Commission on Practice sought feedback from occupational therapists and stakeholders to guide revisions to the OTPF-2. The *Occupational Therapy Practice Framework: Domain and Process, Third Edition,* was published in 2014. The following sections describe the domain and process of occupational therapy as described in the current *Framework* as applied to the activity of tending a home vegetable garden.

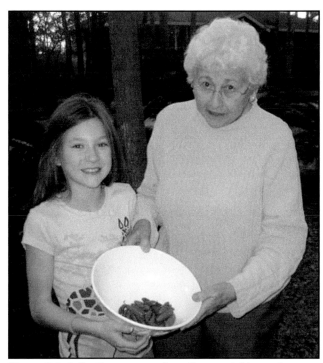

**Figure 6-1.** Collecting peppers from the vegetable garden.

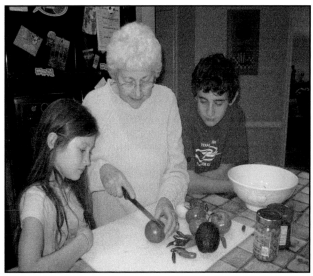

**Figure 6-2.** Preparing a meal for the family using vegetables from the garden.

# The Domain of Occupational Therapy

The domain of occupational therapy provides a common language used to describe the scope of occupational therapy practice. The domains are categorized into five groups that include occupations, client factors, performance skills, performance patterns, and contexts and environments. In the following paragraphs, the domains of the *Framework* are applied to the activity of tending to a home vegetable garden (Figure 6-1).

## *Occupations*

The *Framework* identifies the following eight occupations in which individuals, organizations, and populations engage on a regular basis: activities of daily living (ADLs), instrumental activities of daily living (IADLs), rest and sleep, education, work, play, leisure, and social participation (AOTA, 2014). ADLs typically include basic activities required of a person to support personal health and well-being, such as bathing and showering, bowel and bladder management, dressing, eating, feeding, functional mobility, personal device care, personal hygiene and grooming, sexual activity, and toilet hygiene.

IADLs refers to activities that support occupational performance in context. These activities are typically more complex in nature and include care of others; care of pets and child rearing; shopping; preparing meals (Figure 6-2); management of home, finances, and health; along with participation in religious observances. Additional IADLs, which are often necessary for successful occupational engagement, include communication management, community mobility, and maintenance of safety. Using the activity of planting a vegetable garden as an example, a gardener establishes and maintains a garden throughout the growing season, uses gardening tools safely to prevent injury, and eventually can use the produce to prepare healthy meals.

The occupation of rest and sleep includes "activities related to obtaining restorative sleep that supports healthy active engagement in other occupations" (AOTA, 2014, p. S20). Restful sleep is imperative for productive engagement in occupations requiring attention, judgment, motor processing, and safety. For an individual to participate in the activity of gardening, the person must be rested to maintain the energy and focus necessary to safely participate in planning and performing related tasks. Education includes formal and informal education, as well as activities that promote exploration of personal interests. These activities are considered necessary for learning and participating in one's learning environment (AOTA, 2014, p. S20). A gardener, for example, might use experience and new knowledge obtained by reading publications or accessing informative media broadcasts to decide what to plant and how to obtain a bountiful harvest. Thereafter, the gardener might then choose to share his or her successful tips with others.

Work occupations involve activities in which one engages for the purpose of gaining some form of remuneration, including volunteer activities (Mosey, 1996). The *Framework* identifies employment interests and pursuits, employment seeking and acquisition, job performance, preparation and adjustment for retirement, and exploration and participation in volunteer opportunities

Table 6-1.

**AREA OF OCCUPATION ASSOCIATED WITH PLANTING A HOME VEGETABLE GARDEN**

| |
|---|
| **Activities of Daily Living** |
| Dressing: donning a long-sleeved top and shorts, gardening gloves, and a sun hat |
| Functional mobility: walking on a soft uneven terrain, bending down, and stepping over obstacles |
| Personal hygiene: washing and drying hands thoroughly after planting vegetables in the garden |
| **Instrumental Activities of Daily Living** |
| Home establishment and management: spacing plants according to growing needs |
| Safety and emergency maintenance: operating a garden tiller according to the directions in a safe manner to prevent injury |
| **Education** |
| Informal: reading gardening magazines, attending gardening education seminars, researching gardening tips online, and sharing gardening expertise with others |
| **Work** |
| Job performance: planting vegetables and watering the plants |
| Volunteer participation: growing and sharing produce with local community soup kitchens or food pantries |
| **Play** |
| Play exploration: including children by structuring play opportunities in the garden, such as digging for worms, watering the plants, and digging holes or creating roads with toy bulldozers and backhoes |
| **Leisure** |
| Leisure participation: hobby |
| **Social Participation** |
| Community: contributing to a community garden |
| Family: gardening with family members to share enjoyable experiences |
| Peer/friend: sharing produce with friends and neighbors |

as activities that compose work occupations. Gardening can be work if the harvest is sold as a means to support one's family, or it can be considered volunteer work if the gardener offers his or her services to support the upkeep of a local community garden.

Play, which is often regarded as the work of childhood, is described as play exploration and play participation occupations in the *Framework* (AOTA, 2014). Play can be described as any spontaneous or organized activity, the primary goal of which is to provide enjoyment or diversion (Parham & Fazio, 1997). A garden can be a place for children to explore and play. Numerous games and unplanned activities can be engaging and entertaining, such as digging for treasure, collecting different sized and colored rocks, and playing hide-and-seek behind plants.

Leisure is "a nonobligatory activity that is intrinsically motivated and engaged in during discretionary time, that is, time not committed to obligatory occupations such as work, self-care, or sleep" (Parham & Fazio, 1997, p. 250). The authors of the *Framework* divide leisure activities into leisure exploration and leisure participation (AOTA, 2014). Feeling a breeze against your skin, smelling the scents of nature, and listening to nature's sounds are some of the appealing aspects that make gardening a relaxing leisure interest.

Mosey (1996) provides the definition of social participation used in the *Framework* as "organized patterns of behavior that are characteristic and expected of an individual or a given position within a social system" (p. 340). Social participation is an occupation that is organized by the contexts in which and the people with whom an individual might interact while participating in a particular activity (AOTA, 2014). Gardeners often share their hobby and leisure interests with others. Gardening can be a co-occupation among family members, friends, or a community who help with maintaining the garden or preparing the harvest for eating by washing, cooking, freezing, or canning the produce.

Table 6-1 summarizes the areas of occupation associated with planting a vegetable garden. Although rest and sleep are not included in the activity of gardening, they are necessary for a person to fully engage in the occupation. A person must be rested to safely focus on related activities and tasks or operate equipment such as a garden tiller.

## Client Factors

Client factors are abilities, qualities, or characteristics that dwell within the person, a group, or a population and influence occupational performance (AOTA, 2014, p. S7).

Table 6-2.

## Client Factors Associated With Planting a Home Vegetable Garden

**Values**

Nurturing living things to share with others, providing a sustainable food source, pesticide-free gardening that supports a healthy lifestyle, and enjoying a pleasurable activity outdoors

**Beliefs**

Hard work will produce a sense of personal accomplishment and a high yield of vegetables, and homegrown vegetables taste better than store bought and are more economical

**Spirituality**

Leisure activity that offers an outlet for stressful life experiences, feeling connected with nature, and gaining a sense of enjoyment from nurturing plants throughout the growing cycle

**Body Structures**

- The brain and associated structures (lobes of the brain, midbrain, cerebellum, brainstem, and cranial nerves) that control all thought processes related to decision making, sensory interpretation, movement, and emotions
- Structures of the eyes and associated muscles and glands, and ears (external, middle, and internal ear components) to see objects and hear sounds in the environment
- Structures related to speech (mouth, pharynx, and larynx) if gardening with others
- Cardiovascular system to regulate heart rate and blood flow that sustains activity
- Immunological system to protect the body from infection if the skin is not intact and comes in contact with contaminated soil or other substances
- Respiratory system in relation to physical endurance and voice functions
- Structures related to movement including the muscles of the head, neck, arms, hands, trunk, and legs
- Skin functions to protect the body from injury or infection

**Body Functions**

- Mental functions: higher level cognitive, attention, memory, perception, mental functions of sequencing complex movement, consciousness, temperament and personality, and energy and drive
- Sensory functions: seeing, hearing, vestibular, smell, proprioceptive, and touch functions, as well as sensitivity to pain, temperature, and pressure
- Neuromusculoskeletal and movement-related functions: joint mobility and stability
- Muscle functions: muscle power, muscle tone, and muscle endurance
- Movement functions: motor reflexes, involuntary movement reactions, control of voluntary movement, and gait patterns
- Cardiovascular, hematological, immunological, and respiratory system functions
- Voice and speech functions; digestive, metabolic, and endocrine system functions; genitourinary and reproductive functions: dependent on social context and individual self-care needs
- Skin and related structure functions

Information compiled from American Occupational Therapy Association. (2014). Occupational therapy practice framework: Domain and process (3rd ed.). *American Journal of Occupational Therapy, 68*(Suppl. 1), S1-S48.

Client factors are categorized into values, beliefs, and spirituality; body structures; and body functions. Values, beliefs, and spirituality arise from and are embedded in an individual's personal, social, and cultural context. They influence a client's motivation to engage in occupations and give meaning to life (AOTA, 2014, p. S7). Body functions refer to the physiological functions of the body, whereas body structures refer to the anatomical parts of the body (AOTA, 2014, p. S7). Occupational therapy practitioners must consider the interrelated nature of body functions and body structures when addressing a client's occupational participation. Table 6-2 identifies client factors associated with planting a vegetable garden. Client factors are specific to a particular individual and depend on the context and environment in which the gardening activity is performed.

## Performance Skills

Fisher (2006) defines performance skills as observable, concrete, goal-directed actions clients use to engage in daily life occupations (p. 375). The performance skills of the *Framework* have been classified into motor skills, process skills, and social interaction skills that are

Table 6-3.

**Performance Skills Associated With Planting a Home Vegetable Garden**

| |
|---|
| **Motor Skills** |
| Bends, kneels, reaches, grasps gardening tools, grips seeds, transports vegetable plants, coordinates fingers to compact soil around each vegetable plant, coordinates both upper extremities to hold and place each vegetable plant, uses gardening tools (hoe, shovel, long-handled cultivator, and spading fork), maintains balance, adjusts body posture, steps over vegetable plants, calibrates muscle power when handling each vegetable plant, uses smooth controlled movements when watering vegetable plants, persists with physical activity over a period of time, pushes and pulls soil with a hoe, paces self over the course of the activity |
| **Process Skills** |
| Adjusts pace over the course of the activity; attends to the planning and planting phases of gardening; completes planting a garden; chooses what vegetable plants to include, what gardening tools to use, how deep to dig each hole, and how much water each vegetable plant needs; uses each garden tool as intended; handles garden equipment (tiller), shovel, and hoe safely; follows directions on each seed packet and how to safely operate gardening equipment (tiller); initiates and terminates each step throughout the planning and planting phases; continues the activity throughout the duration of the task; sequences each step in planning and planting vegetable garden in a logical manner; finds, gathers, and returns required garden tools and materials to complete the activity; organizes and plans space requirements for plants; navigates garden to avoid stepping on plants; plans rest and water breaks; adjusts or accommodates performance if obstacles are encountered such as compacted soil, space restrictions, or inclement weather; correctly identifies each vegetable plant |
| **Social Interaction Skills** |
| Communicates and engages with others in order to obtain information and secure resources and supplies; seeks assistance and advice needed to successfully participate in the gardening activity; interacts with others when sharing the garden harvest |

interrelated within and among each of the five domains. Performance skills encompass various combinations of body structures and body functions that underlie an individual's ability to participate in occupations and activities (AOTA, 2014, p. S25). Table 6-3 presents specific examples of motor, process, and social interaction performance skills that might be associated with planting a home vegetable garden.

### Performance Patterns

Performance patterns refer to the habits, routines, roles, and rituals that often serve as the impetus for engagement in occupations. Performance patterns, such as fulfillment of roles and participation in rituals, are commonly associated with occupations deemed most meaningful to individual clients (Eschenfelder, 2005). Client factors, performance skills, and context and environment shape the performance patterns of individuals over time (AOTA, 2014). Table 6-4 identifies examples of how performance patterns might relate to planting a vegetable garden as an organized activity.

### Context and Environment

People engage in occupations within a particular context and environment. There exists much interaction and interdependence between context and environment factors and other domains of the *Framework*. The environment is composed of elements considered external to the client, such as the physical or nonhuman environment and the social environment. Contexts are thought of as being both within and surrounding the individual (AOTA, 2014, p. S9). Components of the context and environment domain include the physical environment, social environment, cultural contexts, personal contexts, temporal contexts, and virtual contexts (AOTA, 2008). Table 6-5 describes contextual and environmental factors that play a role in supporting or hindering the ability to plant a vegetable garden in one's backyard.

## The Process of Occupational Therapy

The process of occupational therapy outlines the way in which occupational therapists provide services to clients. It is a nonlinear, dynamic process that requires knowledge, experience, and clinical and professional reasoning on the part of the occupational therapist (Schell & Schell, 2007). Crucial to successful occupational therapy practice is the collaboration required between the client and the therapist. To the extent possible, given the client's current capacities and abilities and his or her personal meanings, the client's needs and desired outcomes must

Table 6-4.

**Performance Patterns Associated With Planting a Home Vegetable Garden**

| Performance Patterns Associated With Planting a Home Vegetable Garden |
|---|
| **Habits** |
| Applies sunscreen, dons sun hat, puts gardening gloves on, buys seedlings or plants from seed depending on preference |
| **Routines** |
| Gathers all materials, tools, and equipment; prepares the soil for planting; plants seeds; waters the seeds; plants vegetable plants; waters each vegetable plant as it is planted; cleans all tools and equipment; puts extra material, tools, and equipment away; washes up |
| **Roles** |
| Spouse, parent, grandparent, or friend wanting to grow and share his or her vegetables |
| **Rituals** |
| Canning vegetables using recipes passed through generations |

Table 6-5.

**Context and Environment Associated With Planting a Home Vegetable Garden**

| Context and Environment Associated With Planting a Home Vegetable Garden |
|---|
| **Cultural** |
| Cultivating one's own food, sharing or selling produce |
| **Personal** |
| Age, gender, and experience planting a vegetable garden |
| **Temporal** |
| Seasonal factors affecting gardening |
| **Virtual** |
| Using the computer to research plants, gardening tips, plant diseases, or how to design a garden to maximize yield based on landscape and individual plant requirements (sun exposure, shade, soil drainage) |
| **Physical** |
| A sunny area in the backyard that is spacious enough with favorable growing conditions |
| **Social** |
| Sharing vegetables with others, sharing planting space as part of a co-op, or selling produce at a local farmer's market |

be central to the process of occupational therapy. The process of occupational therapy begins with evaluation, which is ongoing throughout the process; intervention planning, implementation, and intervention review follow; and the process concludes or is renegotiated based on focus, selection, and measurement of outcomes that support health and participation in life through engagement in occupation (AOTA, 2014).

## Evaluation

Clinical reasoning, which includes constant reflection and renegotiation of aggregate information obtained throughout the process of occupational therapy, is fundamental to successful occupational therapy practice (AOTA, 2014; Hinojosa, Kramer, & Crist, 2010). To address specific activities and the occupational demands of clients, occupational therapists must understand the context of the targeted activity or occupation along with the needs of the client. During the occupational therapy process, therapists must consider activity demands in terms of the relevance to the client, the objects used or required, the physical environment, the social environment, the cultural context, and the sequencing and timing of thoughts and actions (AOTA, 2014, p. S12). In addition, the therapist must also analyze and continuously assess required actions and performance skills, body functions, and body structures related to occupational performance (AOTA, 2014, p. S32). The *Framework* describes an occupation-based evaluation as consisting of the occupational profile and analysis of occupational performance (AOTA, 2014). Section IV of this text examines the evaluation

## Case Study: Marie's Story

Marie is a 68-year-old woman who lives with her husband of 48 years in a small ranch-style home in Florida. Marie has two married daughters and two grandchildren, all living nearby. Early onset dementia was diagnosed when Marie was 55 years old. Marie retired at age 57 secondary to complications associated with a decline in memory, word finding difficulties, and mood fluctuations.

Since her diagnosis, Marie has responded promisingly to medical intervention that helped to improve some of her symptoms. In addition, Marie adhered to a daily routine to help keep her mind active and reduce anxiety by doing familiar things she enjoyed, which is believed to have helped her to maintain her current level of function. Marie cares for her two grandchildren, ages 8 and 12, during the summer and after school during the school year. Marie has been gardening for more than 30 years and continues to tend to her vegetable garden on a daily basis, often including her granddaughters in a variety of gardening tasks. Marie is proud that she is able to donate vegetables to the local food bank and enjoys the annual ritual of making homemade spaghetti sauce to freeze, canning crushed tomatoes, and pickling a variety of fresh vegetables with members of her family. On the weekends, Marie goes to the senior center for bingo and attends church faithfully on Sunday mornings with her husband.

Over the past year, Marie's family has been noticing a decline in her mental and physical skills that affect her ability to independently and safely participate in her usual daily occupations. Marie's family reports the greatest impact to her ability to attend to conversations with others, pay household bills, balance the family checkbook, and remember special ingredients from favorite recipes. Especially worrisome is that Marie leaves appliances turned on or unattended for periods of time. Last month, while helping her mother balance her checkbook, Marie's daughter found that she made mathematical errors, omitted entering bills that were paid, or forgot to write checks for bills entered in the ledger. As a result, the checkbook was in disarray, which indicated inconsistencies in not paying bills on time or paying bills more than once. Physically, Marie is experiencing greater difficulty in daily occupations that require gross motor coordination including ambulation inside and outside the home.

Recently, Marie experienced a fall that led to a right proximal humeral fracture that required an open reduction internal fixation to stabilize the upper extremity. Marie is right-hand dominant and has experienced functional limitations, which have significantly impaired her ability to complete basic ADLs. Marie's family reports that she is experiencing severe bouts of depression, which they think are related to the disruption in her daily routine and participation in meaningful activities, such as caring for her grandchildren and gardening. Marie's family also reports that she is spending the majority of her time in bed, neglecting her ADLs, and experiencing periods of emotional lability. In addition, her family expresses concerns regarding Marie's insight into her decline in occupational performance. Marie was referred to occupational therapy home health services for evaluation and treatment upon discharge from the acute care setting.

process in detail. The following paragraphs describe the occupational profile and analysis of occupational performance and apply the related information to the case study of Marie.

### Occupational Profile

The *Framework* defines the occupational profile as "a summary of the client's occupational history and experiences, patterns of daily living, interests, values, and needs" (AOTA, 2014, p. S44). The occupational therapist uses a client-centered approach by collaborating with the client to discover those occupations most important and meaningful to the individual client. For occupational therapists, the client-centered approach focuses on occupations and barriers to occupational engagement rather than dysfunction alone. After collecting profile data, the occupational therapist views the information; identifies the client's strengths, limitations, and needs; and develops a working hypothesis regarding possible reasons for identified problems and concerns (AOTA, 2014).

Table 6-6 lists questions that the occupational therapist addresses to obtain information for the occupational profile. In the case study of Marie, the occupational therapist will seek to understand her personal occupational history, which includes meaningful occupations and roles, and concerns that she has regarding her ability to engage in personally meaningful occupations such as care of others and tending to her vegetable garden. The occupational therapist might include information from Marie as well as from close family members to obtain the most accurate and currently relevant information. From the information provided in the case study, the occupational therapist might find that Marie sees herself as unable to participate in her role of grandmother and friend because she has not been able to garden and care for her grandchildren. Marie may also indicate that she is having trouble bathing and dressing, and that not completing these tasks makes it hard for her to feel "up to" going outside and being in her garden or participating in activities with family and friends.

Table 6-6.

## Questions Addressed During the Occupational Profile

- Who is the client and what services are being sought?
- What are the client's occupational concerns?
- Which areas of occupation and daily life roles are successful and which are problematic for the client?
- Which contexts and environments contribute to occupational engagement?
- What is the client's occupational history and what is the associated meaning?
- What are the priorities and desired outcomes of the client, as related to occupational performance?

Information compiled from American Occupational Therapy Association. (2014). Occupational therapy practice framework: Domain and process (3rd ed.). *American Journal of Occupational Therapy, 68*(Suppl. 1), S1-S48.

Table 6-7.

## Steps Used to Analyze Occupational Performance

- Identify areas of occupation and context(s) that need to be addressed
- Observe and evaluate the client's performance during occupationally relevant activities
- Select appropriate assessments related to the *Framework* domains
- Interpret the assessment data to determine factors that support or inhibit occupational performance
- Explore strengths and limitations related to occupational performance
- Collaborate with the client to create goals that address the client's desired outcomes
- Identify appropriate outcome measures of intervention
- Identify potential intervention approaches based on best practice and existing evidence

Information compiled from American Occupational Therapy Association. (2014). Occupational therapy practice framework: Domain and process (3rd ed.). *American Journal of Occupational Therapy, 68*(Suppl. 1), S14.

### Analysis of Occupational Performance

The analysis of occupational performance may include interviews, observations, review of records, occupation-based activity analysis, and direct assessment of specific client factors (AOTA, 2014). For an occupational therapist working in collaboration with Marie, the occupational therapist would use information collected during the occupational profile. If Marie indicates that bathing is a barrier that prohibits engagement in a desired occupation such as gardening, the occupational therapist would analyze the task of bathing further and develop interventions accordingly. The occupational therapist may also modify gardening activities to observe and analyze Marie's performance during this adapted activity to compensate for limited range of motion and poor gross motor coordination. The occupational therapist will consider specific assessments that can be used to support the therapy plan and measure outcomes. In collaboration with Marie, the occupational therapist will create goals and intervention strategies to address Marie's specific wants and needs. Table 6-7 identifies steps that occupational therapists use to analyze occupational performance.

## *Intervention*

The use of occupation-based interventions is central to authentic occupational therapy practice. Included here is the idea that occupation can be used as an end or as a means for occupational therapy (Nelson, 1996; Trombly, 1995). The occupational therapist, in collaboration with the client, plans, implements, and continuously reviews the occupational therapy intervention. Occupational therapists must continuously utilize and update information gathered during the evaluation process and renegotiate the intervention plan and targeted outcomes during the process of occupational therapy. Although intervention will be discussed in detail in Section V of this text, the following paragraphs will describe each phase of the intervention process in relation to the case study involving Marie.

### Intervention Plan

During intervention planning, the occupational therapist sets measurable goals and selects an intervention approach based on his or her knowledge base, theory, and evidence. Table 6-8 shows an outline of intervention planning, developed collaboratively with clients, as described in the *Framework*. Approaches to occupation-based

Table 6-8.

## Planning the Intervention

The occupational therapy practitioner must do the following:

- Develop objectives and measurable goals that include a time frame for goal achievement
- Select occupational therapy intervention approaches that are theoretically sound and based on best available evidence
- Identify service delivery mechanisms that best fit the client's needs and available resources
- Develop and continuously update a plan for discharge based on the client's needs and progress
- Select outcome measures that appropriately reflect the client's desired outcomes
- Make recommendations for health and community-based referral and follow-up as needed

Adapted from American Occupational Therapy Association. (2014). Occupational therapy practice framework: Domain and process (3rd ed.). *American Journal of Occupational Therapy, 68*(Suppl. 1), S15.

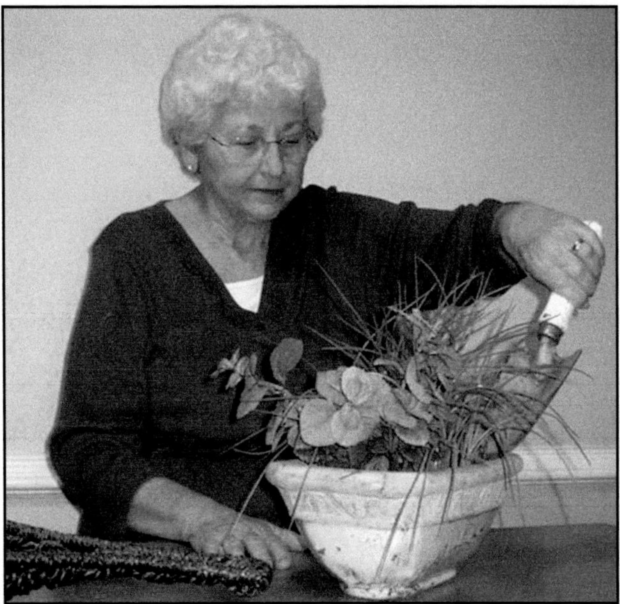

**Figure 6-3.** Planting a tabletop herb garden.

intervention include creating or promoting occupation, establishing or restoring a skill that has not yet developed or has been impaired, maintaining performance that has been gained or is at risk due to progression of a disease or illness, modifying context and environmental factors or activity demands, and preventing disability for clients who are at risk for occupational performance problems (AOTA, 2014, p. S33). The intervention-planning phase also must include initial discharge-planning needs, selection of outcome measures, and plans for making recommendations or referrals that will enhance the client's outcomes (AOTA, 2014).

When planning an intervention for Marie, goals of therapy might relate to restoration of her ability to bathe and dress safely and independently or with a defined level of assistance. Marie might also benefit from modifying the activity demands of gardening to allow her to participate in this self-determined and meaningful occupation (Figure 6-3). Due to Marie's decline in cognitive status, creating a chart to help organize bills that need to be paid, using a calculator, or appointing an assistant to balance the family checkbook could help Marie maintain her role in managing the household finances. In the kitchen, reminders could be posted on the refrigerator or doorways to check for appliances left on or she can safely use recipes of favorite foods to continue to provide for her family during mealtimes. Discharge needs for Marie will include continued evaluation of Marie's ability to maintain safety, which should include a home safety assessment, family education, and recommendations for additional supervision or assistance in the home to complete more complex or risk-laden tasks. Outcome measures should relate to Marie's expressed desires and be based on assessment and reassessment of Marie's occupational performance skills and performance patterns over time. In addition, any recommendations or instructions provided during Marie's transition home should be written out as a reference for later use or as a reminder, and a referral to a gerontologist who specializes in dementia should be considered.

### Intervention Implementation

Intervention implementation is the process of putting the intervention plan into action. The occupational therapist uses therapeutic use of self and therapeutic use of occupations and activities during this phase of intervention (AOTA, 2014, p. S15). The occupational therapist is responsible for directing, monitoring, and supervising the implementation of intervention in a safe and efficacious manner (Schultz-Krohn & Pendleton, 2013). The type of intervention to be used and the way in which the occupational therapist monitors the client's response according to ongoing assessment and reassessment must also be determined (AOTA, 2014, p. S15).

Occupations and activities used during Marie's occupational therapy intervention may include ADLs such as bathing, grooming, and dressing; IADLs related to her role as grandmother such as baking cookies (Figure 6-4); and a modified leisure activity such as tabletop gardening. Marie's therapy process will likely include the types of interventions described in Table 6-9. Marie might require fabrication of a fracture brace or splint following

Table 6-9.

**Types of Occupational Therapy Intervention**

| Type and Purpose | Examples |
|---|---|
| ***Occupation-based intervention:*** the client engages in specifically selected, client-directed occupations that enhance participation and match goals (AOTA, 2014). | • Completing bathing, dressing, and morning hygiene using adaptive devices and compensatory techniques<br>• Attending a class on gardening<br>• Baking cookies that she can share with others |
| ***Preparatory methods:*** "the occupational therapist selects directed methods and techniques that prepare the client for occupational performance. These methods are used in preparation for or concurrently with purposeful and occupation-based activities" (AOTA, 2014, p. S29-S30). | • Providing splints needed to support and facilitate safe movement<br>• Providing strengthening and range of motion exercises<br>• Providing sensory stimulation to promote alertness and orientation |
| ***Education:*** "the occupational therapist shares information with the client and others involved that supports engagement in occupations" (AOTA, 2014, p. S30). | • Providing information on the healing process for bone fracture and the impact on occupational performance<br>• Providing information on dementia and how to monitor for changes and impact on occupational performance<br>• Educating caregivers on compensatory techniques |
| ***Advocacy:*** "the occupational therapist promotes occupational justice and empowering the client to utilize resources that enable participating in life" (AOTA, 2014, p. S30). | • Collaborating with the client's family members to inquire about community resources for respite care<br>• Researching community services available to older individuals that may support Marie's nurturing personality, such as participating in a day program where she can share her garden produce and skill of cooking |

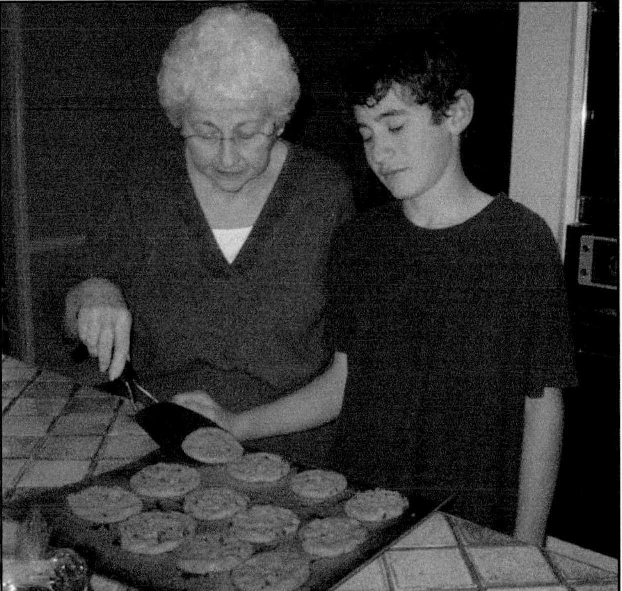

**Figure 6-4.** Baking cookies with grandson.

her upper arm fracture. She also may be issued adaptive devices and asked to practice using these devices to help her perform ADLs and other desired activities. As a part of her occupational therapy intervention, Marie might also engage in practicing how to gather ingredients for baking cookies and then actually bake cookies with supervision or assistance by the occupational therapist or family members.

### Intervention Review

Intervention review is described in the *Framework* as "the continuous process of reevaluating and reviewing the intervention plan, the effectiveness of its delivery and the progress toward outcomes" (AOTA, 2014, p. S16). During this ongoing phase, the occupational therapist reevaluates the plan to determine its effectiveness in leading to achievement of desired outcomes. Modifications to the plan are made to improve effectiveness of intervention as the client's occupational performance changes or as new information is uncovered. Intervention review is crucial in determining the need for continued changes to the types or approaches of intervention being used (see Table 6-9). In addition, intervention review also helps occupational therapists determine when intervention should be discontinued and what recommendations or referrals should be made.

## Outcomes

Achievement of outcomes that support the client's health and participation in life through engagement in occupation is central to occupational therapy practice. Outcomes are the end result of the occupational therapy process and serve to describe the value and impact of occupational therapy intervention for clients (AOTA, 2014). Outcome measures must be selected early and modified as needed during the evaluation and intervention phases of the occupational therapy process. The outcome measures that are selected should be congruent

## Evidence-Based Research Chart

| *Framework* Topic | Evidence | Area of Practice |
|---|---|---|
| ADLs, Rest and Sleep, Education, and Work | Weaver, 2015 | Autism spectrum disorder |
| ADLs | Rao, Chou, Bursley, Smulofsky, & Jezequel, 2014 | Alzheimer disease |
| ADLs, Play, Education | Dunn, Cox, Foster, Mische-Lawson, & Tanquary, 2012 | Pediatrics |
| ADLs | Mennem, Warren, & Yuen, 2012 | Low vision |
| ADLs | Sackley et al., 2012 | Rehabilitation |
| IADLs | Ciro, Anderson, Hershey, Prodan, & Holm, 2015 | Mild cognitive impairment |
| IADLs, Performance Skills Performance Patterns, Context and Environment, Activity Demands, and Client Factors | Gibson, D'Amico, Jaffe, & Arbesman, 2011 | Mental health |
| IADLs | Orellano, Colón, & Arbesman, 2012 | Geriatrics |
| IADLs, ADLs, Leisure, Work, Social Participation | Stav, Hallenen, Lane, & Arbesman, 2012 | Geriatrics, wellness |
| Rest/Sleep | Brown, Swedlove, Berry, & Turlapati, 2012 | Pediatrics |
| Rest/Sleep | Gibbs & Klinger, 2011 | Rehabilitation |
| Play | Wilkes, Cordier, Bundy, Docking, & Munro, 2011 | Pediatrics |
| Education | Reid, Chiu, Sinclair, Wehrmann, & Naseer, 2006 | Pediatrics |
| Work | Darragh, Harrison, & Kenny, 2008 | Workplace, ergonomics |
| Work | Paquette, 2008 | Work rehabilitation |
| Work, Performance Skills, Client Factors, Outcome Process (of OTPF-2) | Schene, Koeter, Kikkert, Swinkels, & McCrone, 2007 | Mental health, workplace, treatment efficacy |
| Leisure | Ball, Corr, Knight, & Lowis, 2007 | Geriatrics |
| Leisure, Play, Intervention Process | Kolehmainen et al., 2011 | Pediatrics |
| Leisure | Wensley & Slade, 2012 | Wellness |
| Social Participation and Occupational Performance | Wolf, Chuh, Floyd, McInnis, & Williams, 2014 | Rehabilitation |
| Social Participation | Donohue, Hanif, & Berns, 2011 | Mental health |
| Social Participation | Griswold & Townsend, 2012 | Pediatrics |
| Social Participation | Price, Stephenson, Krantz, & Ward, 2011 | Rehabilitation, community based |

with the client's desired goals. The occupational therapist must consider the appropriateness of subjective or qualitatively assessed outcomes as well as more quantitatively measurable outcomes, based on the client's individual condition and situation. The movement toward establishing an evidentiary basis for occupational therapy has made significant gains. Although occupational therapists continue to be challenged in this regard, the Evidence-Based Research Chart identifies published research related to the *Framework*. While this chart contains only a fragment of available articles, it does serve as a starting point for those interested in investigating the aspects of the *Framework*.

## Student Self-Assessment

1. Use the *Framework* to identify the effects of early onset dementia and the recent fall and arm fracture on Marie and her family.

2. Identify the occupations that have been affected by Marie's fall.
3. Identify the performance skills and client factors that are related Marie's ability to prepare a small, tabletop herb garden.
4. Describe how the recent fracture may affect Marie's performance patterns.
5. Describe how context and environment factors may hinder or support Marie's recovery.
6. Develop a list of questions that you would use to facilitate completion of an occupational profile for Marie.
7. Identify the types of occupational therapy intervention that you would consider using with Marie during early, mid, and later phases of treatment.
8. Consider how the domains of the *Framework* relate to the evaluation, intervention, and outcome processes associated with occupational therapy services for Marie.

## Electronic Resources

American Occupational Therapy Association:

*Occupational Therapy Practice Framework: Domain and Process*: http://ajot.aota.org/article.aspx?articleid=1860439

Official Documents: https://www.aota.org/practice/manage/official.aspx

Position Paper—*Occupational Therapy's Perspective on the Use of Environments and Contexts to Support Health and Participation in Occupations*: http://ajot.aota.org/article.aspx?articleid=1865188

Statement—*The Philosophical Base of Occupational Therapy*: http://ajot.aota.org/article.aspx?articleid=1865199

World Health Organization—*International Classification of Functioning, Disability and Health*: http://www.who.int/classifications/icf/training/icfchecklist.pdf

## References

American Occupational Therapy Association. (1994). Uniform terminology for occupational therapy (3rd ed.). *American Journal of Occupational Therapy, 48,* 1047-1054.

American Occupational Therapy Association. (2002). Occupational therapy practice framework: Domain and process. *American Journal of Occupational Therapy, 56,* 609-639.

American Occupational Therapy Association. (2008). Occupational therapy practice framework: Domain and process (2nd ed.). *American Journal of Occupational Therapy, 62,* 625-683.

American Occupational Therapy Association. (2014). Occupational therapy practice framework: Domain and process (3rd ed.). *American Journal of Occupational Therapy, 68*(Suppl. 1), S1-S48. doi:10.5014/ajot.2014.682006

Ball, V., Corr, S., Knight, J., & Lowis, M. J. (2007). An investigation into the leisure occupations of older adults. *British Journal of Occupational Therapy, 70,* 393-400.

Bing, R. K. (1981). Occupational therapy revisited: A paraphrastic journey: 1981 Eleanor Clarke Slagle Lecture. *American Journal of Occupational Therapy, 35,* 499-518.

Brown, C., Swedlove, F., Berry, R., & Turlapati, L. (2012). Occupational therapists' health literacy interventions for children with disordered sleep and/or pain. *New Zealand Journal of Occupational Therapy, 59,* 9-17.

Ciro, C. A., Anderson, M. P., Hershey, L. A., Prodan, C. I., & Holm, M. B., (2015). Instrumental activities of daily living performance and role satisfaction in people with and without mild cognitive impairment: A pilot project. *American Journal of Occupational Therapy, 69.* doi:10.5014/ajot.2014.015198

Darragh, A. R., Harrison, H., & Kenny, S. (2008). Effect of an ergonomics intervention on workstations of microscope workers. *American Journal of Occupational Therapy, 62,* 61-69.

Donohue, M. V., Hanif, H., & Berns, L. W. (2011). An exploratory study of social participation in occupational therapy groups. *Mental Health Special Interest Section Quarterly, 34,* 1-3.

Dunn, W., Cox, J., Foster, L., Mische-Lawson, L., & Tanquary, J. (2012). Impact of a contextual intervention on child participation and parent competence among children with autism spectrum disorders: A pretest–posttest repeated-measures design. *American Journal of Occupational Therapy, 66,* 520-528.

Eschenfelder, V. G. (2005). Shaping the goal setting process in occupational therapy: The role of meaningful occupation. *Physical and Occupational Therapy in Geriatrics, 23,* 67-82.

Fidler, G. S., & Filder, J. W. (1978). Doing and becoming: Purposeful action and self-actualization. *American Journal of Occupational Therapy, 32,* 305-310.

Fisher, A. (2006). Overview of performance skills and client factors. In H. Pendelton & W. Schultz-Krohn (Eds.), *Pedretti's occupational therapy: Practice skills for physical dysfunction* (6th ed., pp. 372-402). St. Louis, MO: Mosby-Elsevier.

Gibbs, L. B., & Klinger, L. (2011). Rest is a meaningful occupation for women with hip and knee osteoarthritis. *Occupational Therapy Journal of Research, 31,* 143-150.

Gibson, R. W., D'Amico, M., Jaffe, L., & Arbesman, M. (2011). Occupational therapy interventions for recovery in the areas of community integration and normative life roles for adults with serious mental illness: A systematic review. *American Journal of Occupational Therapy, 65,* 247-56.

Gilfoyle, E. M. (1984). Transformation of a profession: 1984 Eleanor Clarke Slagle Lecture. *American Journal of Occupational Therapy, 38,* 575-584.

Griswold, L. A., & Townsend, S. (2012). Assessing the sensitivity of the evaluation of social interaction: Comparing social skills in children with and without disabilities. *American Journal of Occupational Therapy, 66,* 709-717.

Gutman, S. A., Mortera, M. H., Hinojosa, J., & Kramer, P. (2007). Revision of the Occupational Therapy Practice Framework. *American Journal of Occupational Therapy, 61,* 119-126.

Hinojosa, J., Kramer, P., & Crist, P. (2010). Evaluation: Where do we begin? In J. Hinojosa, P. Kramer & P. Crist (Eds.), *Evaluation: Obtaining and interpreting data* (3rd ed., pp. 1-20). Bethesda, MD: AOTA Press.

Kolehmainen, N., Francis, J. J., Ramsay, C. R., Owen, C., McKee, L., Ketelaar, M., & Rosenbaum, P. (2011). Participation in physical play and leisure: Developing a theory- and evidence-based intervention for children with motor impairments. *BMC Neurology, 11,* 100.

Mennem, T. A., Warren, M., & Yuen, H. K. (2012). Brief report—preliminary validation of a vision-dependent activities of daily living instrument on adults with homonymous hemianopia. *American Journal of Occupational Therapy, 66,* 478-482.

Meyer, A. (1922). The philosophy of occupational therapy. *Archives of Occupational Therapy, 1,* 1-10.

Mosey, A. C. (1996). *Applied scientific inquiry in the health professions: An epistemological orientation* (2nd ed.). Bethesda, MD: AOTA Press.

Nelson, D. L. (1996). Therapeutic occupation: A definition. *American Journal of Occupational Therapy, 50,* 775-782.

Orellano, E., Colón, W. I., & Arbesman, M. (2012). Effect of occupation- and activity-based interventions on instrumental activities of daily living performance among community-dwelling older adults: A systematic review. *American Journal of Occupational Therapy, 66*, 292-300.

Paquette, S. (2008). Return to work with chronic lower back pain: Using an evidence-based approach along with the occupational therapy framework. *WORK, 31*, 63-71.

Parham, L. D., & Fazio, L. S. (Eds.). (1997). *Play in occupational therapy for children.* St. Louis, MO: Mosby-Elsevier.

Price, P., Stephenson, S., Krantz, L., & Ward, K. (2011). Beyond my front door: The occupational and social participation of adults with spinal cord injury. *Occupational Therapy Journal of Research, 31*, 81-88.

Punwar, A. J. (1994). *Occupational therapy: Principles and practice* (2nd ed.). Baltimore, MD: Williams and Wilkins.

Rao, A. K., Chou, A., Bursley, B., Smulofsky, J., & Jezequel, J. (2014). Systematic review of the effects of exercise on activities of daily living in people with Alzheimer's disease. *American Journal of Occupational Therapy, 68*, 50-56. doi:10.5014/ajot.2014.009035

Reid, D., Chiu, T., Sinclair, G., Wehrmann, S., & Naseer, Z. (2006). Outcomes of an occupational therapy school-based consultation service for students with fine motor difficulties. *Canadian Journal of Occupational Therapy, 73*, 215-224.

Sackley, C. M., Burton, C. R., Herron-Marx, S., Lett, K., Mant, J., Roalfe, A. K. ... Feltham, M. G. (2012). A cluster randomised controlled trial of an occupational therapy intervention for residents with stroke living in UK care homes (OTCH): Study protocol. *BioMedCentral Neurology, 12*, 52.

Schell, B. A. B., & Schell, J. W. (Eds.). (2007). *Clinical and professional reasoning in occupational therapy.* Philadelphia, PA: Lippincott Williams and Wilkins.

Schene, A. H., Koeter, M. W., Kikkert, M. J., Swinkels, J. A., & McCrone, P. (2007). Adjuvant occupational therapy for work-related major depression works: Randomized trial including economic evaluation. *Psychological Medicine, 37*, 351-362.

Schultz-Krohn, W., & Pendleton, H. M. (2013). Application of the *Occupational Therapy Practice Framework* to physical dysfunction. In W. Schultz-Krohn & H. M. Pendleton (Eds.), *Pedretti's occupational therapy: Practice skills for physical dysfunction* (7th ed., pp. 28-54). St. Louis, MO: Elsevier-Mosby.

Stav, W. B., Hallenen, T., Lane, J., & Arbesman, M. (2012). Systematic review of occupational engagement and health outcomes among community-dwelling older adults. *American Journal of Occupational Therapy, 66*, 301-310.

Trombly, C. A. (1995). Occupation: Purposefulness and meaningfulness as therapeutic mechanisms: 1995 Eleanor Clarke Slagle Lecture. *American Journal of Occupational Therapy, 49*, 960-972.

Weaver, L. L. (2015). Effectiveness of work, acticities of daily living, education, and sleep interventions for people with autism spectrum disorder: A systematic review. *American Journal of Occupational Therapy, 69.* doi:10.5014/ajot.2015.017962

Wensley, R., & Slade, A. (2012). Walking as a meaningful leisure occupation: The implications for occupational therapy. *British Journal of Occupational Therapy, 75*, 85-92.

Wilkes, S., Cordier, R., Bundy, A., Docking, K., & Munro, N. (2011). A play-based intervention for children with ADHD: A pilot study. *Australian Occupational Therapy Journal, 58*, 231-240.

Wolf, T. J., Chuh A., Floyd, T., McInnis K., & Williams E. (2014). Effectiveness of occupation-based interventions to improve areas of occupation and social participation after stroke: An evidence-based review. *American Journal of Occupational Therapy, 69.* doi:10.5014/ajot.2015.012195

## Suggested Reading

American Occupational Therapy Association. (2014). Occupational therapy practice framework: Domain and process (3rd ed.). *American Journal of Occupational Therapy, 68*(Suppl. 1), S1-S48. doi:10.5014/ajot.2014.682006

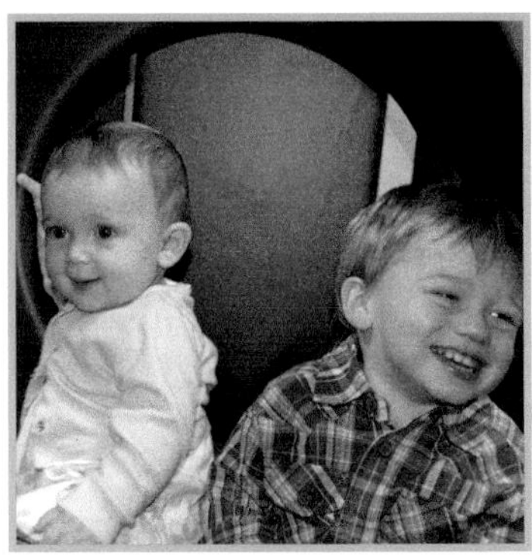

# 7

# Meaning and Dynamic of Occupation and Activity

*Julie Ann Nastasi, ScD, OTD, OTR/L, SCLV, FAOTA*

**ACOTE STANDARDS EXPLORED IN THIS CHAPTER**

B.2.2, B.2.4, B.2.7

**KEY VOCABULARY**

- **Activity:** A specific task that is completed for an end result.
- **Co-occupations:** Activities that involve the social interaction of two or more persons.
- **Groups:** Multiple individuals not limited to but including families, colleagues, or classmates.
- **Occupational performance:** The ability to complete an occupation or activity successfully.
- **Occupations:** Everyday activities that are purposeful and meaningful to persons, groups, or populations.
- **Persons:** Recipients of occupational therapy services, such as clients, spouses, partners, families, siblings, caregivers, employers, teachers, and other relevant individuals.
- **Populations:** Groups within communities or similar locations that have a commonality such as, but not limited to, brain injury, diabetes, refugees, or prisoners of war who receive occupational therapy services.



Jacobs, K., & MacRae, N. (Eds.).
*Occupational Therapy Essentials for Clinical Competence, Third Edition* (pp. 69-83).

This chapter will explore the meaning and dynamics of occupation and activity. An overview of the history of occupation will be provided, as well as an in-depth analysis of occupation, which is the core of the profession of occupational therapy. By the end of the chapter, you will be able to understand how occupations encompass everyday activities in which persons, groups, and populations participate. You will be able to distinguish the areas of occupation, performance skills, performance patterns, activity and occupational demands, contexts and environments, and client factors as they relate to occupational performance.

## Investigation of Occupation

The profession of occupational therapy is thought to have emerged from the moral treatment that occurred during the late 18th and early 19th centuries (Reed, Hocking, & Smythe, 2013). During moral treatment, a humane approach was adopted for individuals with mental illness (Wilcock, 2001). This included addressing the physical, temporal, and societal aspects of the environment to facilitate the individual's participation in occupations (Kielhofner, 2009). Over time, occupational therapy has expanded and now addresses persons, groups, and organizations in a variety of contexts and environments (American Occupational Therapy Association [AOTA], 2014).

Occupational therapy was officially named as a profession in 1917 when George Barton, William Dunton, Eleanor Clark Slagle, Susan Cox Johnson, Thomas Kidner, and Isabel Newton met in Clifton Springs, New York, and produced a certificate of incorporation for the National Society for the Promotion of Occupational Therapy. The National Society for the Promotion of Occupational Therapy remained the name of the association until 1921, when the membership voted and changed the name to the American Occupational Therapy Association (O'Brien & Hussey, 2012). The AOTA continues to be our profession's national association. The AOTA plays a vital role in ensuring the growth and the future of our profession.

The concepts of occupation and using occupation for health and wellness date back prior to the naming of the profession of occupational therapy. Human occupations have existed since the beginning of time. For example, stories of occupation for health have been found in the Bible (Reed, Smythe, & Hocking, 2013). Wilcock's (2001) *Occupation for Health, Volume 1,* identified "the fall of humankind" in Genesis where "people were condemned to work for their survival and health" after eating the forbidden fruit (p. 30). Other Bible passages identified in the book include Deuteronomy's "accounts of people cultivating and harvesting grain, olives and grapes" (Wilcock, 2001, p. 33). Attention was given to how different occupations contributed to society. Reitz (2010) shared stories of the early philosophers, Pythagoras and Thales, using music as a therapeutic modality. Reitz (2010) also identified how the Chinese in 2600 B.C. used activities for prevention and treatment. Occupations and activities play a vital role in the health and participation of persons, groups, and populations (AOTA, 2014) both prior to the naming of the profession and since the official incorporation of the profession.

## Occupation Versus Activity

"Occupations are central to a client's identity and sense of competence and have particular meaning and value to that client" (AOTA, 2014, p. S5). Occupations are complex and have multiple dimensions to them while activities typically refer to a specific task. Occupations may require persons, groups, or populations to complete many activities within an occupation. The definitions of occupation vary, but generally they encompass the concepts of an activity or activities that are purposeful and meaningful with some type of goal as the end result. The *Occupational Therapy Practice Framework: Domain and Process, Third Edition*, states that "occupations can involve the execution of multiple activities" (AOTA, 2014, p. S6). In practice, occupational therapy practitioners often use the terms *occupation* and *activity* interchangeably.

## Meaning and Dynamics of Occupation and Activity

Occupations and activities can range from very simple to very complex in nature. It is the occupational therapist's role to select "occupations and activities as primary methods of intervention" (AOTA, 2014, p. S11). This is done through the client-therapist collaborative process of evaluation, intervention, and outcomes. During the evaluation, the occupational therapist creates an occupational profile where the occupational therapist gains an understanding of the client's occupational history and experiences. The client identifies the problems and concerns that are affecting his or her ability to complete occupations and activities. The occupational therapist then analyzes the client's occupational performance. Occupational performance refers to "the act of doing and accomplishing a selected action, activity, or occupation that results from the dynamic transaction among the client, the context, and the activity" (AOTA, 2014, p. S43). The occupational therapist and the occupational therapy assistant then work with the client to improve the client's engagement in occupations or activities. Client factors include values, beliefs, spirituality, body functions, and body structures that play a role in the client's occupational performance, as well as the environment or context where the activity takes place, and the demands of the activity. In the next sections, the dynamics and meaning of occupation will further be explored.

## Occupations

"Occupations are various kinds of life activities in which individuals, groups, or populations engage including activities of daily living, instrumental activities of daily living, rest and sleep, education, work, play, leisure, and social participation" (AOTA, 2014, p. S19). Specific activities associated with each category are discussed below and in the *Framework* (AOTA, 2014). Refer back to Chapter 6 for more information on the *Framework*.

### Activities of Daily Living

Activities of daily (ADLs) are activities that are typically oriented toward caring for one's self. These activities are typically performed prior to leaving one's home, but are not restricted to being performed in the home. See Table 7-1 for the activities and their definitions from the *Framework* and an example of the activities. See Chapters 18 and 26 for additional information on ADLs.

### Instrumental Activities of Daily Living

Instrumental activities of daily living (IADLs) are more complex than ADLs. They typically are completed at home and in the community. By nature, they require more complex interactions and may involve other persons, groups, or populations. See Table 7-2 for the activities and their definitions from the *Framework* and an example of the activities. See Chapters 18 and 26 for additional information on IADLs.

### Rest and Sleep

Rest and sleep refer to all of the activities related to supporting restorative rest and sleep to participate in occupations (AOTA, 2014). Rest and sleep include rest, sleep preparation, and sleep participation. During rest, the client refrains from activities and relaxes in a quiet, calm environment. To successfully fall asleep, the client may complete the activities of sleep preparation and sleep participation. Sleep preparation includes the routines performed prior to going to bed (e.g., grooming, changing clothes). During sleep participation, the client takes care of the needs of others to be able to sleep through the night. This may mean giving a baby a bottle so the baby will not wake during the night. Finally, after completing the other activities successfully, the client obtains the goal of sleep (Figure 7-4). See Table 7-3 for the activities and their definitions from the *Framework* and an example of the activities. See Chapters 21 and 29 for additional information on rest and sleep.

### Education

Education refers to activities that are needed for learning and participating in an educational environment (AOTA, 2014). This includes formal education participation, informal personal education needs or interest exploration, and informal personal education participation. See Table 7-4 for the activities and their definitions from the *Framework* and an example of the activities. See Chapters 19 and 27 for additional information on education.

### Work

Work refers to employment and volunteer activities. This includes employment interests and pursuits, employment seeking and acquisition, job performance, retirement preparation and adjustment, volunteer exploration, and volunteer participation (AOTA, 2014). Occupational therapy practitioners work with clients on all aspects of paid and voluntary work. See Table 7-5 for the activities and their definitions from the *Framework* and an example of the activities. See Chapters 19 and 27 for additional information on work.

### Play

Play refers to activities that are planned or unplanned that provide enjoyment or entertainment (AOTA, 2014). Play is divided into play exploration and play participation. The activity of play is typically associated with children (Figures 7-8 and 7-9). See Table 7-6 for the activities and their definitions from the *Framework* and an example of the activities. See Chapters 20 and 28 for additional information on play.

### Leisure

Leisure activity might be considered the play of adults. It is intrinsically motivating and engaging activity that is completed in free time. Leisure is divided into leisure exploration and leisure participation. See Table 7-7 for the activities and their definitions from the *Framework* and an example of the activities. See Chapters 20 and 28 for additional information on leisure.

Table 7-1.

## Activities of Daily Living

| Activity and Definition | Example of Activities |
|---|---|
| ***Bathing/showering:*** "obtaining and using supplies; soaping, rinsing, and drying body parts; maintaining bathing position; and transferring to and from bathing positions" (AOTA, 2014, p. S19). | Jane turns on the water and enters the shower. In the shower, Jane obtains her shampoo, conditioner, and body wash. She uses the products to clean her hair and body. Jane maintains her balance throughout the activity, and then turns off the water once she has finished bathing herself. Jane dries herself off and then exits the shower. |
| ***Dressing:*** "selecting clothing and accessories appropriate to time of day, weather, and occasion; obtaining clothing from storage area; dressing and undressing in a sequential fashion; fastening and adjusting clothing and shoes; and applying and removing personal devices, prosthetic devices, or splints" (AOTA, 2014, p. S19). | Rosie selects the outfit that she is going to wear to work. She considers the weather and selects an outfit that is appropriate to wear. Rosie then obtains the clothes, put the clothes on in the correct order, and fastens items. At the end of the day, Rosie undresses from her work clothes and changes into sleep wear. |
| ***Feeding:*** "setting up, arranging, and bringing food [or fluid] from the plate or cup to the mouth; sometimes called self-feeding" (AOTA, 2014, p. S19). | Sam's mom places Sam in the high chair. Sam reaches for the cookie, and eats the cookie (Figure 7-1). |
| ***Functional mobility:*** "moving from one position or place to another (during the performance of everyday activities), such as in-bed mobility, wheelchair mobility, and transfers" (AOTA, 2014, p. S19). | Mike broke his leg and is unable to walk on it. He has learned how to move from one position to another without using his one leg. He transfers in and out of bed with a sliding board to his wheelchair. He also uses the sliding board to transfer to the car, toilet, and shower. |
| ***Personal device care:*** "using, cleaning, and maintaining personal care items, such as hearing aids, contact lenses, glasses, orthotics, prosthetics, adaptive equipment, glucometers, and contraceptive and sexual devices" (AOTA, 2014, p. S19). | Janice rinsed her contact lenses and stored them in the case her doctor provided. |
| ***Personal hygiene and grooming:*** "obtaining and using supplies; removing body hair; applying and removing cosmetics; washing, drying, combing, styling, brushing, and trimming hair; caring for nails; caring for skin, ears, eyes, nose; applying deodorant; cleaning mouth; brushing and flossing teeth; and removing, cleaning, and reinserting dental orthotics and prosthetics" (AOTA, 2014, p. S19). | Wesley brushes his teeth before bed (Figure 7-2). |
| ***Sexual activity:*** "engaging in activities that result in sexual satisfaction and/or meet relational or reproductive needs" (AOTA, 2014, p. S19). | Dave had a total hip replacement and maintained his total hip precautions during sexual intercourse. |

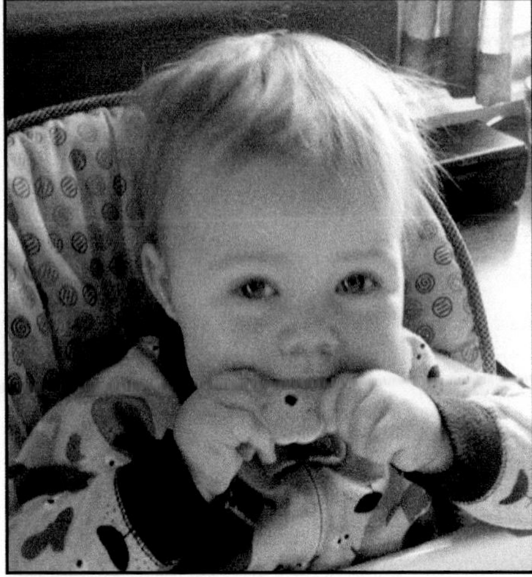

**Figure 7-1.** Infant eating a cookie.

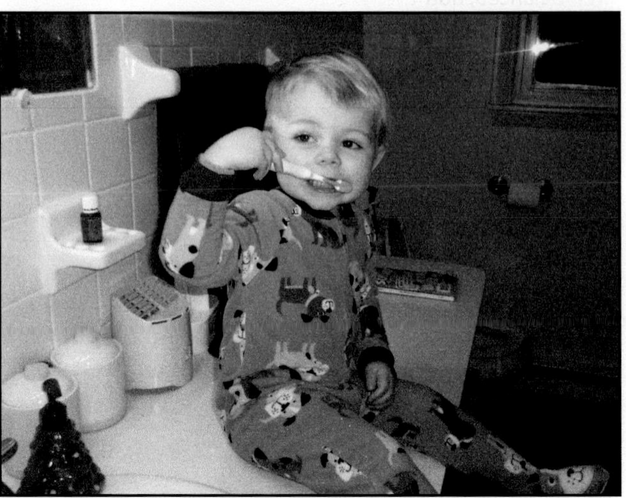

**Figure 7-2.** Toddler brushing his teeth before bed.

Table 7-2.

## Instrumental Activities of Daily Living

| Activity and Definition | Example of Activities |
|---|---|
| ***Care of others:*** "arranging, supervising, or providing care for others" (AOTA, 2014, p. S19). | John cares for his wife Beth who has dementia. He watches over her so she is able to remain at home. When he is unable to supervise her, he arranges for a visiting nurse to come to their house. |
| ***Care of pets:*** "arranging, supervising, or providing the care for pets and service animals" (AOTA, 2014, p. S19). | Bill feeds his dog twice a day. He walks his dog before and after work, and has a doggie door so his dog can go into the fenced-in area in the backyard. |
| ***Child rearing:*** "providing care and supervision to support the developmental needs of a child" (AOTA, 2014, S19). | Michelle takes her daughter Lucy to the beach. Michelle places Lucy in a tent to protect her from the sun and puts her daughter in a robe to stay warm. See Figure 7-3 to see Lucy's needs supported at the beach. |
| ***Communication management:*** "sending, receiving, and interpreting information using a variety of systems and equipment, including writing tools, telephones, keyboards, audiovisual recorders, computers or tablets, communication boards, call lights, emergency systems, Braille writers, telecommunication devices for deaf people, augmentative communication systems, and personal digital assistants" (AOTA, 2014, p. S19). | Erin checks her work e-mail account multiple times a day and returns e-mails as appropriate to the senders. Erin also sends new e-mails out when she needs to contact co-workers at different locations in different time zones. |
| ***Driving and community mobility:*** "planning and moving around in the community and using public or private transportation, such as driving, walking, bicycling, or accessing and riding in buses, taxi cabs, or other transportation systems" (AOTA, 2014, p. S19). | Jen took a taxi to the train station and then rode the train to work. |
| ***Financial management:*** "using fiscal resources, including alternate methods of financial transaction, and planning and using finances with long-term and short-term goals" (AOTA, 2014, p. S19). | Aaron opted to pay for his bills online to reduce mailing expenses. |
| ***Health management and maintenance:*** "developing, managing, and maintaining routines for health and wellness promotion, such as physical fitness, nutrition, decreasing health risk behaviors, and medication routines (AOTA, 2014, p. S19). | Patrick placed all of his medications into a pillbox that organized his medications for the week. He removes his medications on a daily basis from the organizer. |
| ***Home establishment and management:*** "obtaining and maintaining personal and household possessions and environment, including maintaining and repairing personal possessions and knowing how to seek help or whom to contact (AOTA, 2014, p. S19). | James called the roofer to repair the leak in his roof. |
| ***Meal preparation and cleanup:*** "planning, preparing, and serving well-balanced, nutritional meals and cleaning up food and utensils after meals" (AOTA, 2014, p. S20). | Kate gathered the ingredients from the refrigerator and her shelves to bake a chicken. After preparing and making the chicken, she carved the chicken and served it to her family. After the meal, she cleaned the roasting pan and supplies she used to make the chicken. |
| ***Religious and spiritual activities and expression:*** "participating in religion... and engaging in activities that allow a sense of connectedness to something larger than oneself" (AOTA, 2014, p. S20). | Luke attends church services every Sunday. |
| ***Safety and emergency maintenance:*** "knowing and performing preventative procedures to maintain a safe environment; recognizing sudden, unexpected hazardous situations; and initiating emergency action to reduce the threat to health and safety" (AOTA, 2014, p. S20). | Mrs. Smith heard the fire alarm go off in her classroom. She gathered her students and led them safely out of the building to the location where they were supposed to wait until the building was cleared for re-entry. |
| ***Shopping:*** "preparing shopping lists; selecting, purchasing, and transporting items; selecting method of payment; and completing money transactions; included are Internet shopping and related use of electronic devices such as computers, cell phones, and tablets" (AOTA, 2014, p. S20). | Mary made a list of groceries that she needed from the local supermarket. At the supermarket, she gathered all of the items on her list and proceeded to the cash register where she paid for her groceries. |

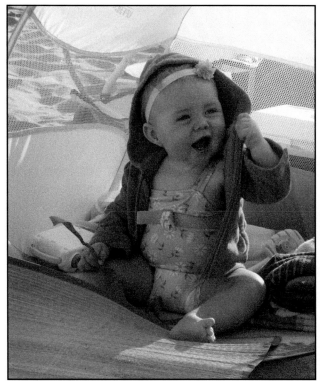

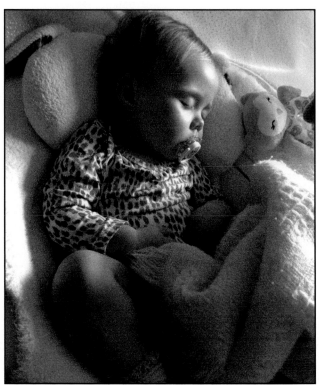

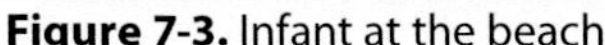
**Figure 7-3.** Infant at the beach.

**Figure 7-4.** An infant sleeping.

Table 7-3.

## Rest and Sleep

| Activity and Definition | Example of Activities |
|---|---|
| ***Rest:*** "engaging in quiet and effortless actions that interrupt physical and mental activity resulting in a relaxed state" (AOTA, 2014, p. S20). | Sarah sits in her recliner, closes her eyes, and listens to the sounds of waves crashing outside of her balcony. |
| ***Sleep preparation:*** "engaging in routines that prepare the self for a comfortable rest" and "preparing the physical environment for periods of unconsciousness" (AOTA, 2014, p. S20). | Ashley brushes her teeth and changes into her sleep wear prior to falling asleep. |
| ***Sleep participation:*** "taking care of personal needs for sleep, such as cessation of activities to ensure onset of sleep, napping, dreaming, sustaining a sleep state without disruption, and performing nighttime care of toileting needs and hydration" (AOTA, 2014, p. S20). | Sean stops drinking at 7 p.m. to ensure that he does not wake to go to the bathroom during the night. Right before going to bed, Sean goes to the bathroom one last time to void his bladder. This routine allows Sean to sleep through the night. |

Table 7-4.

**EDUCATION**

| Activity and Definition | Example of Activities |
|---|---|
| ***Formal education participation:*** "participating in academic, nonacademic, extracurricular, and vocational educational activities" (AOTA, 2014, p. S20). | Heather and Kelly are studying to be occupational therapists. In school, they researched a topic that they were interested in. They submitted their research to their state occupational therapy association and presented the findings of their research at the state conference (Figure 7-5). |
| ***Informal personal education needs or interests exploration (beyond formal education):*** "identifying topics and methods for obtaining topic-related information or skills" (AOTA, 2014, p. S20) | Kristen is knitting a scarf for the first time; she knitted the length that she desired for the scarf. Kristen went on her computer and looked up a video online on how to end the scarf. Kristen watched the video and then completed her scarf. |
| ***Informal personal education participation:*** "participating in informal classes, programs, and activities that provide instruction or training in identified areas of interest" (AOTA, 2014, p. S20). | Mariah has a family member with low vision. One of Mariah's classmates attended a low-vision seminar and shows her how to use a closed-circuit television while simulating low vision (Figure 7-6). |

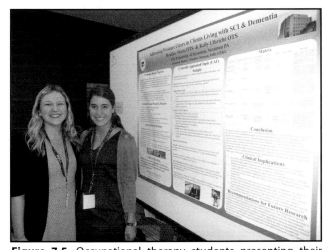


**Figure 7-5.** Occupational therapy students presenting their research at a state conference.

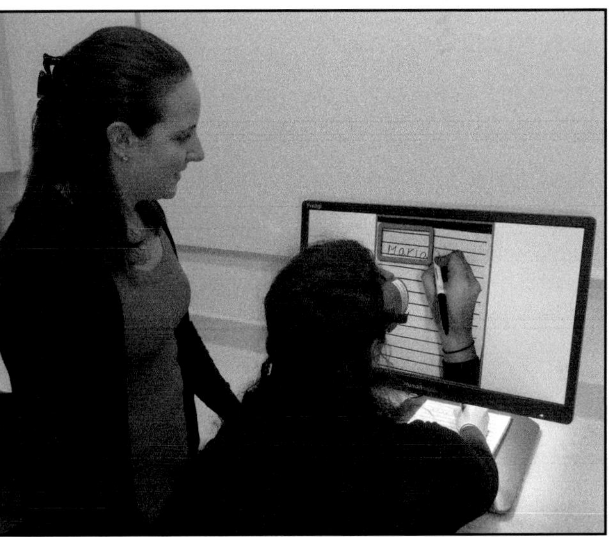


**Figure 7-6.** A classmate teaches another classmate how to write using a closed-circuit television.

## Social Participation

Social participation consists of behaviors that are expected of persons as a member of society. Social participation takes place at the peer/friend, family, and community levels. Behaviors and expectations vary depending with whom the person is interacting. See Table 7-8 for the activities and their definitions from the *Framework* and an example of the activities. See Chapters 22 and 30 for additional information on social participation.

## Summary

Persons, groups, and populations are involved in different occupations. Knowing and understanding the occupations helps occupational therapy practitioners to identify relevant areas to address with clients. Occupation can be used as an end or as a means during therapy (Trombly, 2011). Occupation-as-end refers to persons completing an occupation for the sake of being able to complete the occupation. Occupation-as-means refers to using different occupations to build performance skills and patterns needed to achieve a specific occupational performance related to the client's goals. The next sections will further explore performance skills and performance patterns.

Table 7-5.

**WORK**

| Activity and Definition | Example of Activities |
|---|---|
| ***Employment interests and pursuits:*** "identifying and selecting work opportunities based on assets, limitations, likes, and dislikes relative to work" (AOTA, 2014, p.S20). | Jake participates in a transition program. He and other high school students attend a class where they identify the types of activities that they like to do and those that they do not. Based on their likes and dislikes, they look up jobs that match their desires. |
| ***Employment-seeking and acquisition:*** "advocating for oneself; completing, submitting, and reviewing appropriate application materials; participating in interviews and following up afterward; discussing job benefits; and finalizing negotiations" (AOTA, 2014, p. S20). | Colleen flips through an occupational therapy magazine and cuts out an ad for a position that she would like. Colleen reviews and completes the materials that she needs to submit for the position. Colleen attends her interview and sends a thank you note after the interview. The employer calls Colleen and offers her the position. Colleen negotiates her pay and benefits and sets up her start date. |
| ***Job performance:*** "performing the requirements of a job, including work skills and patterns; time management; relationships with co-workers, managers, and customers; leadership and supervision; creation, production, and distribution of products and services; initiation, sustainment, and completion of work; and compliance with work norms and procedures" (AOTA, 2014, p. S20). | Mary Ann is an administrative assistant for an occupational therapy program. Part of her job is to answer the telephone (Figure 7-7). |
| ***Retirement preparation and adjustment:*** "determining aptitudes, developing interests and skills, and selecting appropriate avocational pursuits, and adjusting lifestyle in the absence of the worker role" (AOTA, 2014, p. S20). | Janet plans to retire at the end of the school year. She thinks about what activities she would like to participate in after retiring. She knows that she likes to work out, and plans to work out daily. She also likes quilting and decides that she will enroll in some quilting classes. |
| ***Volunteer exploration:*** "determining community causes, organizations, or opportunities for unpaid work in relationship to personal skills, interests, location, and time available" (AOTA, 2014, p. S21). | Mary Alice retired from the local elementary school and is exploring the possibility of volunteering at her old school. She would like to assist the teachers by volunteering in their classrooms and providing extra help to children who need one-on-one help. She contacts the principal to see if any of the teachers would like a volunteer. |
| ***Volunteer participation:*** "performing unpaid work activities for the benefit of identified selected causes, organizations, or facilities" (AOTA, 2014, p. S21). | Jack volunteers at the local hospital. He visits the patients in their rooms and drops off the daily newspaper to patients who would like to read it. |

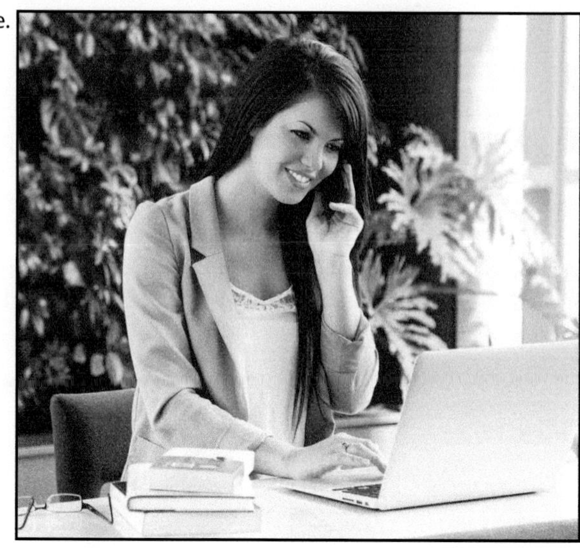

**Figure 7-7.** An administrative assistant answers the phone.

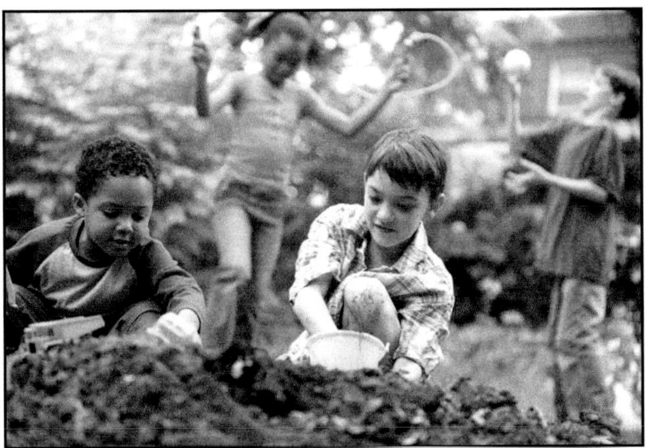

**Figure 7-8.** Children playing.

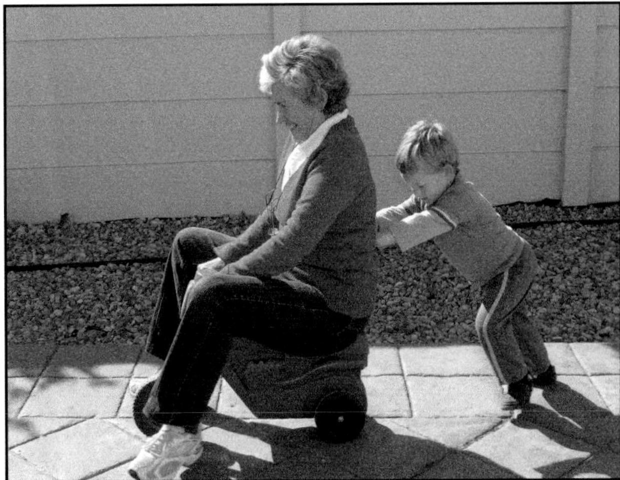

**Figure 7-9.** Grandmother playing with child.

Table 7-6.

**PLAY**

| Activity and Definition | Example of Activities |
|---|---|
| ***Play exploration:*** "identifying appropriate play activities, including exploration play, practice play, pretend play, games with rules, constructive play, and symbolic play" (AOTA, 2014, p. S21). | Tommy searches his playroom for toys to play with. He thinks that he wants to play doctor, so he looks for his toy stethoscope and doctor bag. |
| ***Play participation:*** "participating in play; maintaining a balance of play with other occupations; and obtaining, using, and maintaining toys, equipment, and supplies appropriately" (AOTA, 2014, p. S21). | Lauren invites her friend Stephanie over to play a board game. Lauren gets the game from the closet and sets it up for them to play. After playing the game, Lauren packs up the game and returns it to the closet. |

Table 7-7.

**LEISURE**

| Activity and Definition | Example of Activities |
|---|---|
| ***Leisure exploration:*** "identifying interests, skills, opportunities, and appropriate leisure activities" (AOTA, 2014, p. S21). | Joe's co-worker goes fishing on the weekends and invites him to join him. Joe thinks he would like fishing since he likes the outdoors, is pretty athletic, and likes fish. Joe goes to a local sporting goods store and looks into what equipment he will need to go fishing with his co-worker. |
| ***Leisure participation:*** "planning and participating in appropriate leisure activities; maintaining a balance of leisure activities with other occupations; and obtaining, using, and maintaining equipment and supplies as appropriate" (AOTA, 2014, p. S21). | Lucy likes yoga and participates in a yoga class 2 nights a week. When she is not in yoga class, she incorporates some of the breathing techniques into her daily activities. |

Table 7-8.

| Social Participation | |
|---|---|
| **Activity and Definition** | **Example of Activities** |
| ***Community:*** "engaging in activities that result in successful interaction at the community level" (AOTA, 2014, p. S21). | Mike and Julie attend a fundraiser. |
| ***Family:*** "engaging in activities that result in successful interaction in specific required and/or desired familial roles" (AOTA, 2014, p. S21). | Grandma invites her whole family over for Sunday pasta suppers and chocolate cake. |
| ***Peer/friend:*** "engaging in activities at different levels of interaction and intimacy, including engaging in desired sexual activity" (AOTA, 2014, p. S21). | Courtney started dating Chris, and they had their first kiss under the maple tree on their college campus. |

## Performance Skills

Performance skills are "goal-directed actions that are observable as small units of engagement in daily life occupations" (AOTA, 2014, p. S7). These include motor skills, process skills, and social interaction skills. Motor skills encompass the abilities to align, stabilize, position, reach, bend, grip, manipulate, coordinate, move, lift, walk, transport, calibrate, flow, endure, and pace. Process skills encompass the abilities to pace, attend, heed, choose, use, handle, inquire, initiate, continue, sequence, terminate, search/locate, gather, organize, restore, navigate, notice/respond, adjust, accommodate, and benefit. Social interaction skills encompass the abilities to approach/start, conclude/disengage, produce speech, gesticulate, speak fluently, turn toward, look, place self, touch, regulate, question, reply, disclose, express emotion, disagree, thank, transition, time response, time duration, take turns, match language, clarify, acknowledge and encourage, empathize, heed, accommodate, and benefit (AOTA, 2014). Deficits or deficiencies in performance skills can hinder and prevent successful participation in occupations. See Table 7-9 for the performance skills and their definitions from the *Framework* and an example of the skills.

## Performance Patterns

Performance patterns are the habits, rituals, roles, and routines that persons, groups, or populations engage in during their occupations and activities. Habits are automatic behaviors that are engaged in, whereas rituals are symbolic actions that have meaning. Habits are only found at the person level. Rituals, roles, and routines are found at the person, group, and population levels. Rituals are completed because of the cultural, social, or spiritual meaning of the action or behavior. Roles, like rituals, also have a social aspect. Roles are formed based on societal expectations and how persons, groups, or populations define the societal expectations while routines create order and a sequence for occupations (AOTA, 2014). Routines may be created to promote healthy occupations and activities to participate in while avoiding occupations or activities that have negative effects on persons, groups, and populations. See Table 7-10 for the performance patterns and their definitions from the *Framework* and an example of the skills.

## Activity and Occupational Demands

Every activity or occupation has certain requirements that are needed for the activity or occupation to be completed. Activity and occupational demands refers to the objects and their properties, space demands, social demands, sequence and timing, required actions and performance skills, required body functions, required body structures, and the relevance and importance to a client for an activity (AOTA, 2014). The demands are specific to a specific activity. As occupational therapy practitioners, we pay a lot of attention to the activity and occupational demands when working with our clients. Occupational therapy practitioners are skilled at grading and adapting the activity and occupational demands to allow the client to successfully complete the activity. For example, Mary enjoys going to her grandson's football games. Mary recently had a total hip replacement, and needs to maintain her total hip precautions. Mary and her occupational therapist discussed the activity and occupational demands required for Mary to go to the football games. Mary will need to use her cane and bring a cushion to sit on at the stadium (objects and properties). Mary will need to walk 200 yards from the parking lot to the open stadium on a paved path using her cane and carrying her cushion (space demands). Mary will need to be aware of the kids and families also going to the game while she walks to and from the stadium and while seated in the bleachers (social demands).

Table 7-9.

## Performance Skills

| Performance Skills and Definitions | Example of Performance Skills |
|---|---|
| ***Motor skills:*** "occupational performance skills observed as the person interacts with and moves task, objects, and self around the task environment" (AOTA, 2014, p. S25). | Sue reaches up to the cabinet door, and she grabs the handle on the door to pull it open. Sue opens the cabinet and grabs a cup from within the cabinet. |
| ***Process skills:*** "occupational performance skills observed as a person (1) selects, interacts with, and uses task tools and materials; (2) carries out individual actions and steps; and (3) modifies performance when problems are encountered" (AOTA, 2014, p. S25). | Allison has low vision and cannot see objects in her environment. Allison uses the back of her hand to feel her counter surface and guide herself to her refrigerator. Allison organizes the objects in her refrigerator so they are easy to find. Allison opens and smells her milk to ensure she doesn't drink spoiled milk. Allison knows the shape of the milk bottle so she can identify it from other bottles. |
| ***Social interaction skills:*** "occupational performance skills observed during the ongoing stream of a social exchange" (AOTA, 2014, p. S26). | Tim gets upset when other students bump into him in line at school. His occupational therapist taught him to go to the end of the line so he can watch his classmates and to take deep breaths when students bump into him. Tim lines up at the end of the line and practices deep breaths when students bump into him. |

Table 7-10.

## Performance Patterns

| Performance Patterns and Definitions | Example of Performance Patterns |
|---|---|
| ***Habits:*** "specific, automatic behaviors performed repeatedly, relatively automatically, and with little variation" (AOTA, 2014, p. S27). | ***Person:*** Jill automatically locks the door to her home immediately after entering. |
| ***Rituals:*** "symbolic actions with spiritual, cultural, or social meaning contributing to....and reinforcing values and beliefs" (AOTA, 2014, p. S27). | ***Person:*** The Jones family has a special birthday celebration plate that is used as the birthday person's dinner plate on his or her birthday. The plate has been used from generation to generation.<br>***Group or Population:*** XYZ company holds an annual New Year's Eve party for all of its employees. |
| ***Roles:*** "sets of behaviors expected by society and shaped by culture and context that may be further conceptualized and defined" (AOTA, 2014, p. S27). | ***Person:*** Grandmother of four grandchildren ranging from 2 to 14 years of age.<br>***Group or Population:*** Mothers Against Drunk Driving fights to stop drunk driving. |
| ***Routines:*** "patterns of behavior that are observable, regular, and repetitive and that provide structure for daily life" (AOTA, 2014, p. S27). | ***Person:*** Everyday Julie goes into work, unlocks the office and file cabinets, turns on the copy machine, drops off her coat, and pulls her files for the day.<br>***Group or Population:*** Every fall, people are reminded that they should get their annual flu shot. |

Mary's occupational therapist recommends that Mary arrives early to the games, and then waits until the stadium has almost cleared to avoid people bumping into Mary as she walks along the path (sequencing and timing). Mary will need strength and endurance to travel the 200-yard distance in both directions, as well as remain aware of her total hip precautions (required actions and performance skills, required body functions, and required body structures).

## Contexts and Environments

The contexts and environments in which occupations take place may facilitate or hinder occupational performance. Occupational therapists analyze the contexts and environments to support persons' abilities to learn and perform (AOTA, 2015). The environment refers to the physical and social aspects, whereas the contexts refer to the cultural, personal, temporal, and virtual aspects (AOTA, 2014). The physical environment and social environment were first addressed in the area of activity and occupational demands in this chapter. The physical environment includes the built and non-built objects that persons, groups, and populations interact with while the social environment includes the relationships of the persons, groups, and populations. When the physical environment is built using concepts of universal design, it promotes occupational performance of all (Ringaert, 2003). Buildings without ramps or elevators hinder the participation of persons who are unable to ambulate. Social aspects may also facilitate or hinder occupational performance. Persons with family members who are able to assist them allow for a supportive environment. Persons without supports or with negative supports may have fewer opportunities to participate in activities and occupations that require more than one person.

Cultural, personal, temporal, and virtual contexts also may facilitate or hinder occupational performance. Cultural aspects are customs and beliefs held by society; for instance in the United States, people stand for the national anthem and men remove their hats. Personal aspects refer to the specifics about the person, group, or population. This may be the age, gender, socioeconomic status, and educational status of the person, group, or population. The temporal aspects refer to time—the amount of time until a certain period in life, the amount of time to complete an activity or occupation, a specific date or time of day, etc. Finally, virtual aspects are communications without physical presence. This is achieved through computers, tablets, radios, telephones, cell phones, etc. Understanding the contexts helps identify how the contexts may be used to facilitate or how they may hinder occupational performance. One client may benefit from using applications on a tablet; however, this client may not have access to using or purchasing a tablet. Another client may come from a culture where family members step in and provide for the client all of the assistance needed to allow the client to complete occupations and activities.

## Client Factors

"Client factors are specific abilities, characteristics, or beliefs that reside within the person and that influence performance in occupations" (AOTA, 2014, p. S7). Client factors include the values, beliefs, and spirituality of the person, group, or population. They also include the body functions and body structures that play a role in occupational performance. Occupational therapists gather information about client factors during the evaluation. Knowing and understanding the values, beliefs, and spirituality of the person as well as the current status of the person's body functions and body structures helps provide a holistic picture of the person as well as an appropriate treatment plan. Persons, groups, and populations are complex and transactional relationships occur between occupations, performance skills, performance patterns, activity and occupational demands, contexts and environments, and client factors. Understanding all of these areas allows occupational therapy practitioners to assist persons in living a life of occupational balance.

## Occupational Balance

Occupational balance has been one of the tenets of occupational therapy since its foundation (Backman, 2004). Originally, occupational balance was considered a balance among different daily occupations that promoted well-being and health (Anaby, Backman, & Jarus, 2010). However, because of its complexity, definitions of occupational balance differ (Wagman, Hakansson, & Bjorklund, 2012). Current definitions define occupational balance as "a balance of engagement in occupation that leads to well-being" (Wilcock, 2006, p. 343). As occupational therapy practitioners, we need to work with our clients for them to obtain their unique occupational balance. Coordinating time and occupation enhances well-being (Pemberton & Cox, 2015). If a client is not getting enough sleep, it can lead to inability to complete other occupations. By obtaining an understanding of the client's occupations during the evaluation stage, interventions to allow for occupational balance during the treatment stage can take place to allow for health and wellness. Occupational therapy practitioners should also explore the dark side of occupation during the evaluation stage. Refer back to Chapter 3 for more information on the dark side of occupation. By understanding disruptive and destructive occupations, occupational therapy practitioners will gain a deeper understanding of the client, thus allowing the practitioners to develop appropriate intervention plans (Twinley, 2013).

## Task Analysis to Formulate an Intervention Plan

As occupational therapy practitioners who use occupation as the basis of our intervention plans, we have a lot to ponder. Whereas occupations and activities seem simple to the untrained eye, occupational therapists and occupational therapy assistants are constantly analyzing occupations and activities to maximize our clients' occupational performance. Intervention plans must address occupations, performance skills, performance patterns, activity and occupational demands, contexts and environments, and client factors to maximize the success for our clients. Typical interventions include the use of occupation and activities, preparatory methods and tasks, education and training, advocacy, and group interventions (AOTA, 2014). Occupational therapy practitioners use the therapeutic use of self and therapeutic use of occupations and activities to accomplish this. Purposeful activities use activities that develop the client's skills for occupational engagement. Occupation-based interventions use engagement in specific occupations to match the client's goals for occupational performance in specific occupations. All activities should be goal directed, purposeful, and meaningful to the client.

When approaching the intervention, the occupational therapist will choose one or more of the following approaches: create, promote, establish, restore, maintain, modify, or prevent. See Table 7-11 for the intervention approaches and their definitions from the *Framework* and an example of the intervention approach.

## Summary

Occupations and activities are complex and multidimensional. By understanding all of the dimensions of occupation and activity, we are able to maximize occupational performance for our clients. Our clients are persons, groups, and populations. While occupational therapy has traditionally had a large impact at the person level, it is also extremely influential in working at group and population levels. Occupational therapy has distinct value and contributes to "health, well-being, and participation in life" (AOTA, 2014, p. S17). As our profession continues to grow, we will continue to maximize all of our clients' lives, helping them to live life to the fullest.

### Case Study

An occupational therapy student at a low vision clinic prepares to see a new client. The prescription the student receives states the client is a 68-year-old woman with macular degeneration. The prescription states to evaluate and treat the client for decreased participation in occupations and activities. The student knows that macular degeneration affects central vision.

This is the student's first client with macular degeneration. The student retrieves a copy of the *Framework* to review occupations that might be effected by deficits in the central visual field.

During the occupational profile, the student listens to the client and documents the client's occupational history and areas of concern for the client. The student notices that the client did not mention a number of reading activities. The student asks the client about health management, shopping, and financial management. The client thanks the student for asking about these areas, as the client forgot to mention them. The client reports problems with reading medication bottles, prices on items at the store, and seeing the numbers on financial statements.

Using the *Framework* as a guide, the student was able to prompt the client on occupations typically affected by macular degeneration.

## Student Self-Assessment

1. Select an ADL or IADL that you complete on a regular basis.
   - What are the activity and occupational demands for it?
   - How would the demands differ if you were unable to walk?
   - What approach would you use to obtain occupational performance in it?
   - Why?
2. Using the activity selected for the first question, describe two other environments or contexts that the activity could be completed in.
   - How would the activity be the same in environments or contexts?
   - How would it be different in those environments or contexts?

Table 7-11.

## Intervention Approaches

| Approaches and Definitions | Example of Approaches |
|---|---|
| ***Create, promote:*** "an intervention approach that does not assume a disability is present or that any aspect would interfere with performance. This approach is designed to provide enriched contextual and activity experiences that will enhance performance for all people in the natural contexts of life" (AOTA, 2014, p. S33). | Create a transition class for high school seniors to promote exploration of vocations and education programs. |
| ***Establish, restore:*** "an intervention approach designed to change client variables to establish a skill or ability that has not yet developed or to restore a skill or ability that has been impaired" (AOTA, 2014, p. S33). | Develop a craft class for individuals with low vision and blindness that develops other sensory skills (hearing function, vestibular function, taste, smells, proprioceptive function, touch, and temperature/pressure) through the participation in different craft activities. |
| ***Maintain:*** "an intervention approach designed to provide supports that will allow clients to preserve the performance capabilities they have regained, that continue to meet their occupational needs, or both. The assumption is that without continued maintenance intervention, performance would decrease, occupational needs would not be met, or both, thereby affecting health, well-being, and quality of life" (AOTA, 2014, p. S33). | Provide a low vision support group to individuals with low vision and blindness to maintain functional independence. |
| ***Modify:*** "an intervention approach directed at finding ways to revise the current context or activity demands to support performance in the natural setting, [including] compensatory techniques, [such as]… enhancing some features to provide cues or reducing other features to reduce distractibility" (AOTA, 2014, p. S33). | Use a box mix to reduce the number of steps to make brownies. |
| ***Prevent:*** "an intervention approach designed to address clients with or without a disability who are at risk for occupational performance problems. This approach is designed to prevent occurrence or evolution of barriers to performance in context. Interventions may be directed at client, context, or activity variables" (AOTA, 2014, p. S33). | Prevent repetitive strain injuries by teaching stretching techniques and training the person to take breaks prior to feeling pain. |

## Evidence-Based Research Chart

| Topic | Evidence |
|---|---|
| Occupational balance | Anaby, Backman, & Jarus, 2010; Backman, 2004; Pemberton & Cox, 2015; Twinley, 2013; Wagman, Hakansson, & Bjorklund, 2012 |
| Occupation-based practice | AOTA, 2014, 2015; Baker, Jacobs, & Tickle-Degnen, 2003; DeGrace, 2003; Fisher, 2003; Lysaght & Wright, 2005; Moll et al., 2015; Nelson & Mathiowetz, 2004; Pemberton & Cox, 2015; Reed, Hocking, & Smythe, 2013; Reed, Smythe, & Hocking, 2013 |

## Electronic Resources

American Occupational Therapy Association: www.aota.org

Society for the Study of Occupation: USA: www.sso-usa.org

## References


American Occupational Therapy Association. (2014). Occupational therapy practice framework: Domain and process (3rd ed.). *American Journal of Occupational Therapy, 68*(Suppl. 1), S1-S48. doi:10.5014/ajot.2014.682006

American Occupational Therapy Association. (2015). Occupational therapy's perspective on the use of environments and contexts to facilitate health, well-being, and participation in occupations. *American Journal of Occupational Therapy, 69*(Suppl. 3), 1-13.

Anaby, D., Backman, C., & Jarus, T. (2010). Measuring occupational balance: A theoretical exploration of two approaches. *Canadian Journal of Occupational Therapy, 77*, 280-288.

Backman, C. (2004). Occupational balance: Exploring relationships among daily occupations and their influence on well-being. *Canadian Journal of Occupational Therapy, 71*, 202-209.

Baker, N., Jacobs, K., & Tickle-Degnen, L. (2003). A methodology for developing evidence about meaning in occupation: Exploring the meaning of work. *OTJR: Occupation, Participation and Health, 23*, 57-66.

DeGrace, B. (2003). Occupation-based and family-centered care: A challenge for current practice. *American Journal of Occupational Therapy, 57*, 347-350.

Fisher, A. (2003). Why is it so hard to practice as an occupational therapist? *Australian Occupational Therapy Journal, 50*, 193-194.

Kielhofner, G. (2009). *Conceptual foundations of occupational therapy practice* (4th ed.). Philadelphia, PA: F. A. Davis Company.

Lysaght, R. & Wright, J. (2005). Professional strategies in work-related practice: An exploration of occupational and physical therapy roles and approaches. *American Journal of Occupational Therapy, 59*, 209-217.

Moll, S., Gewurtz, R., Krupa, T., Law, M., Lariviere, N., & Levasseur, M. (2015). "Do-live-well": A Canadian framework for promoting occupation, health, and well-being. *Canadian Journal of Occupational Therapy, 82*(1), 9-23.

Nelson, D. & Mathiowetz, V. (2004). Randomized controlled trials to investigate occupational therapy research questions. *American Journal of Occupational Therapy, 58*, 24-34.

O'Brien, J., & Hussey, S. (2012). *Introduction to occupational therapy*. St. Louis, MO: Elsevier Mosby.

Pemberton, S., & Cox, D. (2015). Synchronisation: Co-ordinating time and occupation. *Journal of Occupational Science, 22*(3), 291-303.

Reed, K., Hocking, C., & Smythe, L. (2013). The meaning of occupation: Historical and contemporary connections between health and occupation. *New Zealand Journal of Occupational Therapy, 60*, 38-44.

Reed, K., Smythe, L., & Hocking, C. (2013). The meaning of occupation: A hermeneutic (re)view of historical understanding. *Journal of Occupational Science, 20*, 253-261.

Reitz, S. M. (2010). Historical and philosophical perspectives of occupational therapy's role in health promotion. In M. E. Scaffa, S. M. Reitz, & M. A. Pizzi (Eds.), *Occupational therapy in the promotion of health and wellness* (pp. 1-21). Philadelphia, PA: F. A. Davis Company.

Ringaert, L. (2003). Universal design of the built environment to enable occupational performance. In L. Letts, P. Rigby, & D. Stewart (Eds.), *Using environments to enable occupational performance* (pp. 97-115). Thorofare, NJ: SLACK Incorporated.

Trombly, C. (2011). Occupation: Purposeful and meaningfulness as therapeutic mechanisms. In R. Padilla & Y. Griffiths (Eds.), *A professional legacy*. Bethesda, MD: AOTA Press.

Twinley, R. (2013). The dark side of occupation: A concept for consideration. *Australian Occupational Therapy Journal, 60*, 301-303.

Wagman, P., Hakansson, C., & Bjorklund, A. (2012). Occupational balance as used in occupational therapy: A concept analysis. *Scandinavian Journal of Occupational Therapy, 19*, 322-327.

Wilcock, A. (2001). *Occupation for health* (Vol. I). London, United Kingdom: British Association and College of Occupational Therapists.

Wilcock, A. (2006). *An occupational perspective of health*. Thorofare, NJ: SLACK Incorporated.

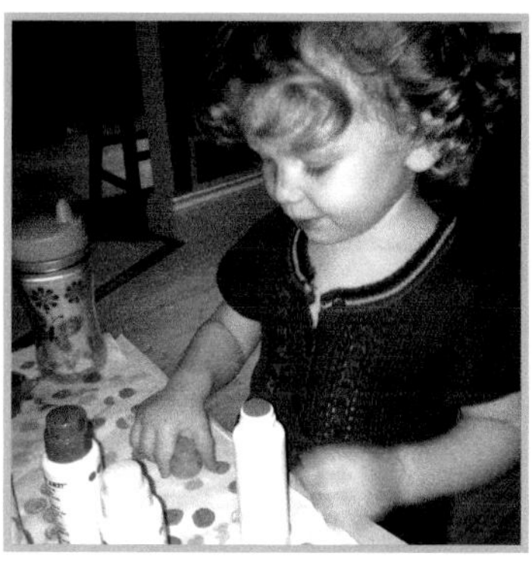

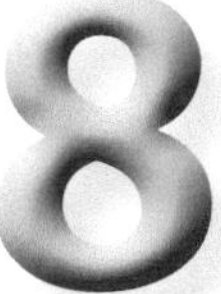

# Occupational Performance and Health

*Kathleen Flecky, OTD, OTR/L and Heather Goertz, OTD, OTR/L*

**ACOTE STANDARDS EXPLORED IN THIS CHAPTER**

B.2.5, B.2.6

**KEY VOCABULARY**

- **Body functions and structures:** "The physiological functions of body systems, including psychological functions (World Health Organization [WHO], 2001, p. 65) and the anatomical parts of the body such as organs, limbs, and their components" (WHO, 2001, p. 111).
- **Disability:** "Dynamic interaction between an individual (with a health condition) and that individual's contextual factors (environmental and personal factors" (WHO, 2001, p. 190).
- **Environmental factors:** "Physical, social and attitudinal environment in which people live and conduct their lives" (WHO, 2001, p. 22).
- **Function:** "Positive aspects of the interaction between an individual (with a health condition) and the individual's contextual factors (environmental and personal factors)" (WHO, 2001, p. 190).
- **Health:** "Aiming for a balance of physical, mental, and social well-being attained through valued occupation" (Wilcock, 2006, p. 112); state of complete physical, mental and social well-being and not merely the absence of health (WHO, 1946).

*(continued)*



Jacobs, K., & MacRae, N. (Eds.).
*Occupational Therapy Essentials for Clinical Competence, Third Edition* (pp. 85-98).

## KEY VOCABULARY (CONTINUED)

- **Health promotion:** "[T]he process of enabling people to increase control over, and to improve, their health. To reach a state of complete physical, mental, and social well-being, an individual or a group must be able to identify and realize aspirations, to satisfy needs, and to change or cope with the environment" (WHO, 1986, as cited in American Occupational Therapy Association [AOTA], 2014, p. S42).
- **Impairments:** "Problems in body function or structure as a significant deviation or loss" (WHO, 2001, p. 15).
- ***International Classification of Functioning, Disability and Health*** **(ICF):** "Unified and standard language and framework for the description of health and health-related states" (WHO, 2001, p. 3).
- **Occupational performance:** "The act of doing and accomplishing a selected activity or selected occupation that results from the dynamic transaction among the client, the context, and the activity" (AOTA, 2014, p. S43).
- **Participation:** "Involvement in a life situation" (WHO, 2001, p. 19).
- **Personal factors:** "Particular background of an individual's life and living, and comprise features of the individual that are not part of the health condition or health status" (WHO, 2001, p. 23).
- **Wellness:** "An active process through which individuals become aware of and make choices toward a more successful existence" (Hettler, 1984, p. 1117, as cited in AOTA, 2014, p. S34).

What does it mean to be healthy and well? Occupational therapy professionals generally view persons as more than their disease processes. Two people can have the same disease or condition and differ widely in terms of physical, mental, social, and spiritual well-being. An individual's state of health is considered within the context of his or her ability to participate in needed and desired roles and to meet occupational lifestyle goals and tasks. Disease, illness, injury, and trauma can create occupational disruption that may lead to conditions of impairment, dysfunction, and disability.

Occupational therapy professionals analyze information about diseases, impairments, and other health conditions in terms of how these health states affect performance in life's roles and routines (Hansen & Atchinson, 2011). We value a perspective of health that includes the consideration of one's ability to participate in meaningful occupations. According to Wilcock (2005), an occupational perspective of health encompasses "aiming for a balance of physical, mental, and social well-being attained through valued occupation" (p. 112).

This chapter discusses health, disease, and disability within the context of occupational functioning and performance. In addition, the effects of physical and mental health, inheritable diseases, predisposing genetic conditions, disability, disease processes, and injury on the individual will be analyzed in terms of health and health promotion.

Health perspectives from a sampling of occupational therapy students have been provided to begin this chapter. In 2015, the AOTA reported an enrollment of 28,598 students in occupational therapy programs across America (AOTA, 2015a). Our profession's philosophy of education stated the importance of students and occupational therapy professionals working with clients to foster health and well-being (AOTA, 2015b). As occupational therapy students embrace concepts of health and disease, it is important to understand that health and disease are complex and that there is much more information about these concepts that exists beyond the scope of this chapter. This section introduces the discussion by exposing students to different viewpoints of health and disease.

Let us begin this discussion by reviewing a survey about occupational therapy students' opinions of health and disease characteristics. They were not given health definitions prior to completing the survey. The students granted permission to have their comments shared with others when asked the following questions:

- Describe health.
- Describe your personal characteristics of occupational performance when you are healthy.
- Have you ever had a major disease or illness? If yes, explain.
- Describe your personal characteristics of occupational performance when you were affected by disease or illness.

The following sidebars highlight four students' views related to health, disease, and occupational performance. Following these views is a description of several themes identified through analysis of the students' narratives.

### Shelly's View

Health is mind, body, and spiritual wellness. I have balance in my life between work, school, friends, self-care, and leisure. When I let one take over, I usually stress about the others. If I allow time for everything, I feel I have a better handle on my life and I do a better job at each individual component. I have not experienced a major disease or illness.

### Joseph's View

Health is physical, mental, and emotional balance and general wellness. I feel more productive, I can multitask, and I feel pretty confident in the work I am completing. I had chronic pain and depression. It was harder to complete schoolwork on time, and sometimes I just did the bare minimum. I slept a lot more, and sometimes my occupations didn't seem important. Reading, cooking, and exercising were discontinued in favor of sleep.

### Elisa's View

Health is a state of being at an optimal weight, not having high blood pressure, exercising, eating right, and having no illness or disease. When I am healthy, I can function at a high level, perform at my best, focus, be sweet to others, and feel good about myself. I had atrioventricular nodal reentrant tachycardia. I needed help getting out of bed. I felt dependent on others and paid closer attention to how everyone treated me.

### Amber's View

Health is the physical absence of disease or sickness with a mental balance and stability. I have more energy and motivation, I work toward goals, and I have a balance of occupations and leisure when I am healthy. I have Crohn's disease. The following are some characteristics of my occupational performance when I am ill: lack of energy and motivation, preoccupation with being physically ill and knowing that occupational performance is limited, difficulty focusing on working hard at school and balancing that with a social life, all while I feel that I can't physically and mentally perform up to my potential.

As the student narratives reveal, health and wellness are multidimensional concepts that include physical, emotional, social, and spiritual aspects. Definitions of health vary individually depending on one's personal values, cultural beliefs, societal values, and experiences. Other factors that influence our conceptualizations of health, as well as what it means to be ill or disabled, may include age, sex, race, ethnicity, socioeconomic status, and current and past medical status. In summary, terms such as *health* and *well-being* are difficult to define because they are personally and socially constructed. They have evolved over time as society has revised notions of health, disease, and disability. For example, the constructs of health, as described by these occupational therapy students, represented the following characteristics as shown in Table 8-1.

An awareness of your view of health constructs is vital to understanding how you will collaborate with your clients. Imagine standing in line at a grocery store behind a person in a wheelchair. Do you consider this person to be impaired? Why or why not? The answers to these questions are based largely on perceptions and life experiences and not necessarily on the unique lived experience of that person. An exploration of personal presuppositions and assumptions, beliefs, values, experiences, and historical perspectives, as well as asking and clarifying client views, will enhance your professional skills at analyzing the effects of health and disease on occupational performance.

This chapter does not seek to examine every different view of health, but it introduces the concept of health by discussing historical perspectives of health, impairment, disease, and disability. For you to appreciate the complexity of health and disease, we have chosen to examine the historical views of impairments. Whether you have learned to recognize impairment as just a normal part of daily life or whether you feel sorry for the lady next door because she walks so slowly and painfully, occupational therapy professionals recognize that society has classified and categorized persons who are different from the norm. The consequences of these categorizations is that experts have identified and defined who is impaired, diseased, or disabled rather than the people being categorized. Lack of attention to personal experiences of persons with impairments, diseases, and disabilities has led to marginalization, stigmatization, and exclusion (Depoy & Gilson, 2004; Oliver, 2009). It is necessary to recognize that contemporary perceptions of health, impairments, diseases, and disabilities exist within a historical context; where we are today is based largely on where we have been. Therefore, three predominant health models are described in the next section, and these illustrate how persons have been viewed as different, atypical, or abnormal owing to disease, impairment, and disability. Historical background is provided with these models of health to show how perspectives of health and disability are influenced by the cultural, social, spiritual, economic, and political contexts.

Table 8-1.

**STUDENT SURVEY RESPONSES**

| Student Survey Categories | Disease Thematic Characteristics | Health Thematic Characteristics | Occupational Performance Characteristics |
|---|---|---|---|
| Responses from 24 occupational therapy students | Difficulty completing work on time<br>Increased sleep<br>Occupations do not seem important<br>Lack of energy and motivation<br>Preoccupation with being physically ill<br>Easily frustrated<br>Dependent on others | Well-being of physical or bodily, mental, spiritual, and emotional health<br>An absence of disease<br>A harmonious state<br>All of the above | Balanced life<br>Alert<br>Well rested<br>Productive<br>Energetic<br>Active<br>Motivated<br>Goal oriented<br>Happier<br>Determined |

## Historical Perspectives on Health and Disability

Throughout the history of Western civilization, the predominant cultural and religious values along with social, political, and economic contexts influenced how persons with disease, impairment, and disability were viewed by society (Altman, 2001; Stiker & Sayers, 2000). A multitude of health perspectives have been advanced to define and describe health, but this section focuses on three predominant models: the religious, medical, and social perspectives, as identified in Table 8-2.

Prior to the Enlightenment Era of the 1600s, disablement or abnormality in general—whether due to illness, injury, disease, or mental or physical impairment—was based on a religious model of disability (Stiker & Sayers, 2000). Within the religious approach, personal impairments and limitations were attributed to moral or supernatural causes. Illnesses and disease were manifestations of either sinfulness or a special spiritual relationship with higher powers or with God (Braddock & Parish, 2001). With increased scientific and medical knowledge and with the influence of industrialization, atypicality was increasingly viewed as an individual affliction that limited one's ability to be a productive member of society. The impairment or disease required one to be fixed or restored through the care of others (Llewellyn & Hogan, 2000; Oliver, 2009). Charitable and medical care systems either rehabilitated the disabled for the purpose of returning them to society or confined them to custodial care within institutions (Braddock & Parish, 2001; Llewellyn & Hogan, 2000).

Initially, the occupational therapy profession was grounded in the social charitable movements of the early 20th century (Quiroga, 1995). The use of arts and crafts activities and habit training were incorporated into the everyday lives of those persons considered unproductive because of physical and mental impairments. During World War I and World War II, occupational therapy flourished within the milieu of the medical model of disablement by treating those with physical and mental disabilities (Quiroga, 1995). Our profession aligned with the medical model, which explained health, disease, and illness as bodily entities intrinsic to the person and treatable through either remediation or compensation for the effects of disease or injury (Kielhofner, 2009).

By the 20th century, medical diagnostic classification systems were created to categorize illnesses, diseases, and conditions based on health conditions, impairments, and limitations. Further advancement in medicine increased the survival rate for those with illness, injury, disease, impairment, and disability, which led to progressively more complex delineation of medical diagnoses and categories (Longmore & Umansky, 2001; Oliver, 2009). Health, ability, and disability became a function of one's individual health condition status rather than the capacity or opportunity to participate in desired life activities. Moreover, social, economic, and political policies based on these classifications created a climate of exclusion from participation from work and other valued life experiences for persons who had certain health conditions or impairments (Altman, 2001; Falk, 2001; Longmore & Umansky, 2001).

More recently, civil rights and social movements in Western societies advocating for self-determination and equal opportunity for all persons influenced both the development of a rights-based model of disability and the disability movement. Furthermore, legislation and disability advocacy and activism promoted a conceptual shift in disability as a medical construct to disability as a social construct (Donoghue, 2003; Oliver, 2009). In contrast to the medical model of disability, an individual with a disability was considered impaired or limited not based on individual attributes, but by an unaccommodating environment and society (Gill, 2001; Mercer &

Table 8-2.

## Health Models

| Features | Religious Model | Medical Model | Social Model |
|---|---|---|---|
| Views of health | Individual<br>Based on spiritual or supernatural factors<br>A reward for living a good life or a punishment for sinfulness | Individual<br>Based on intrinsic biological factors<br>Biological interactions and processes lead to health or ill health | Individual and environmental<br>Based on interaction of intrinsic and extrinsic factors<br>Social and physical environments influence health |
| Views of disability | Afflictions due to either sinfulness and deviancy, or impairments that indicated a special relationship with higher powers | Impairments and disability are a result of disease, illness, injury, and other abnormal health conditions; impairments are the cause of disability | Social, economic, and political factors create disability along with individual characteristics |

Barnes, 2010). Disability is often rhetorically constructed in negative language, such as what disability is not, rather than what disability is (Dolmage, 2014). Through the advocacy effort to enhance opportunities for participation in society, provisions for protective legislation and resources were established to prevent discrimination based on disability (Albrecht, Seelman, & Bury, 2001; Hahn, 1993).

## World Health Organization Classifications

The need for a universal classification system for increasingly complex medical categorizations and consequences of health, disease, and disability led to the development of the family of WHO classifications. As part of this classification system, the *International Classification of Impairments, Disabilities and Handicaps* (ICIDH) was developed in an effort to create a universal framework to describe the consequences of disease and disorders that included definitions of impairment, disability, and handicap (WHO, 2001).

In the new millennium, the WHO recognizes the importance of revisions to the ICIDH constructs of impairment, disability, and handicap to include a more comprehensive view of health that reflects both medical and social models of health and disability (WHO, 2001). It encompasses components of health for all persons, not just those with disease, illness, or disability. According to the *International Classification of Functioning, Disability, and Health* (ICF), elements of health, functioning, disease, and disability, termed *health conditions*, are organized according to two dimensions: body structures and function as one dimension, and activities and participation as a second dimension (WHO, 2001).

Moreover, contextual factors, including personal and environmental factors, are significant components of health, functioning, and disability. Health and functioning are affected by contextual factors in an interactive and dynamic manner to impact health and functioning, and biological, personal, and sociocultural dimensions are included in a more holistic picture of health. In this way, these dimensions are linked in a nonlinear manner to demonstrate the impact of change of one dimension on another (WHO, 2001; Figure 8-1).

Body functions and structures in ICF denote the anatomy, physiology, and psychology of the body systems in terms of degree of impairment or problems in body structure or function (WHO, 2001). The ICF recognizes that health and disability are not only internal to the individual, but also involve factors that define the ability to function and participate in life situations. Activities are defined as actions or tasks being executed by an individual, whereas participation describes the level of involvement of an individual in performing actions and tasks in everyday life (WHO, 2001). Examples of activities and participation are shown in Table 8-3.

Contextual factors are recognized as an important aspect of health, functioning, and disability. The ICF was developed to blend a medical model of disability with a socioecological model. Instead of classifying health, disease, and disability only as intrinsic aspects of the individual, these domains are viewed as having intrinsic and extrinsic components that have multiple interactions with the environment (WHO, 2001). Therefore, contextual factors involve both environmental and personal factors. The ICF views environmental factors as extrinsic to the individual, such as the physical and social environment, but personal factors are considered intrinsic to the individual and include features such as age, sex, genetics, personality, education, sociocultural background, and life experiences (WHO, 2001). Examples of personal and

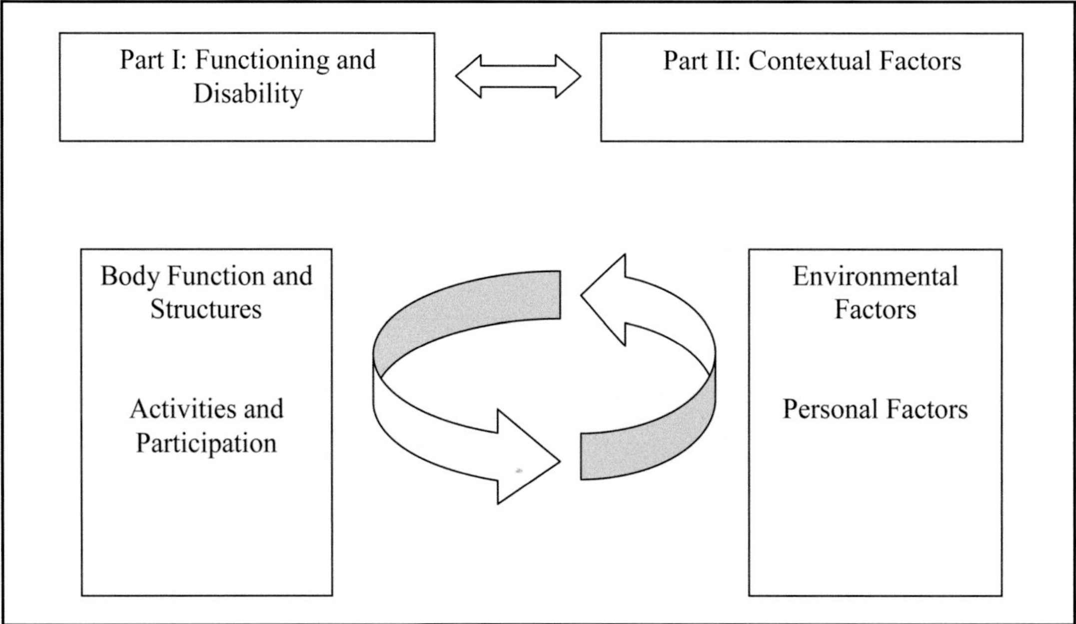


**Figure 8-1.** Multidimensional aspects of health and functioning. (Adapted from World Health Organization. [2001]. *International Classification of Functioning, Disability and Health*. Geneva, Switzerland: Author.)

Table 8-3.

## International Classification of Functioning, Disability and Health Activities and Participation

- Learning and applying knowledge (e.g., school occupations)
- General tasks and knowledge (e.g., coordinating multiple tasks)
- Communication
- Mobility
- Self-care
- Domestic life (e.g., obtaining a place to live)
- Interpersonal interactions and relationships
- Major life areas (e.g., work occupations)
- Community, social, and civic life

Adapted from World Health Organization. (2001). *International Classification of Functioning, Disability and Health*. Geneva, Switzerland: Author.

environmental factors from the ICF are shown in Table 8-4. The ICF is updated yearly and revisions are available on the WHO website (WHO, 2014).

The interactions among body structures, body functioning, personal factors, and environmental factors are evident in the way genetics and the environment influence the nature of human disease. For example, in the United States, racial and ethnic groups display differences in incidence, progression, and severity of disease. Although there are differences in genetic frequencies that contribute to these disparities, most of the differences are due to the effects from the physical and social environment (Race, Ethnicity, and Genetics Working Group, 2005).

Disease and illness are components of health that reflect the interplay of factors intrinsic and extrinsic to the individual. Genetics, biology, personality, temperament, age, and sex affect the potential to experience disease and illness. Environmental factors, including physical and sociocultural aspects, can interact with intrinsic factors in both positive and negative ways to tip the balance toward health and well-being or toward

Table 8-4.

**International Classification of Functioning, Disability and Health Personal and Environmental Factors**

| Personal Factors | Environmental Factors |
|---|---|
| Sex, age, other health conditions, coping style, social background, education, profession, past experience, character style | Products, relationships, institutions, social norms, culture, built environment, political factors, nature |

Adapted from World Health Organization. (2001). *International Classification of Functioning, Disability and Health.* Geneva, Switzerland: Author.

ill health (AOTA, 2014; Edelman, Kudzma, & Mandle, 2013). Alternatively, having a disease, illness, or disability does not by necessity mean that an individual is disabled or has limited opportunities to engage in meaningful occupations (Altman, 2001; AOTA, 2014).

## International Classification of Functioning, Disability and Health and Occupational Performance

The *Occupational Therapy Practice Framework: Domain and Process, Third Edition* (AOTA, 2014), has much in common with the ICF, with its emphasis on health and functioning as related to participation in life tasks and activities. Both frameworks provide a shared language regarding the domains of health, functioning, disability, participation, and activity (AOTA, 2014; WHO, 2001). In the *Framework*, body function and body structures as described in the ICF are situated within client factors. In addition, the ICF conceptualizes activities and participation as centrally located within areas of occupation. Finally, ICF environmental factors are congruent with the framework constructs of context (AOTA, 2014; WHO, 2001). Both the *Framework* and the ICF acknowledge the central role of participation and the environment as contributors to health and disability (AOTA, 2014; WHO, 2001). The *Framework* further asserts that the essence of occupational engagement is a vital link to health and participation. Occupational performance becomes an interactive and dynamic engagement of an individual within environments that support and/or inhibit health and well-being (AOTA, 2014). There have been articles related to use of ICF and concepts of occupational performance (Forget & Higgins, 2014; Kristensen, 2015; Schaaf et al., 2015; Stewart et al., 2014).

## Importance of Occupation in Relation to Health

In order to promote health, it is necessary to discover the occupations that are meaningful to the individual in the community. Personal motivation is reflective of an established meaning in life and the roles and routines of one's lifestyle. Referring back to the occupational therapy student narratives of health, the students who indicated that they were healthy used self-descriptors such as *active, motivated, energetic,* and *goal oriented.* However, when students commented on disease characteristics, they used self-descriptors that included the terms *unmotivated, exhausted,* and *preoccupied.* It is possible for illness to be exacerbated or reduced depending on our ability to participate in meaningful occupations (Bridle, 1999). In addition, it is possible for individuals with terminal illness to maintain well-being when they are actively engaged in occupations (Lyons, Orozovic, Davis, & Newman, 2002; OTAL Occupational Therapy Australia Ltd., 2015).

Consider how you feel when you are ill. How does being ill change your daily routines and your lifestyle? Occupational therapy professionals play a key role in health promotion with individuals in the community through promoting healthy lifestyles, incorporating occupation into existing health programs, and advocating for community and individual needs. It is important to remember that health promotion is an approach that "does not assume a disability is present or that any factors would interfere with performance" (Brownson & Scaffa, 2001, p. 657). AOTA identifies various interventions that may enhance the occupational therapist's and occupational therapy assistant's role in health promotion. Examples of health promotion interventions include advocating for safe playgrounds, promoting policies that support economic self-determination for all persons, and training business personnel about disability etiquette (AOTA, 2014; Brownson & Scaffa, 2001).

Health promotion is relevant within the context of occupational performance because the effects of illness and disease are influenced by environmental factors, and such factors influence personal health. Individuals rely on community supports and resources for optimal performance. Partnerships in health are critical for the overall well-being of individuals in community with others. Healthy People 2010, now updated to Healthy People 2020, a joint document developed by the U.S. Public Health Service and the U.S. Department of Health and Human Services (2000), encourages partnerships in health and delineates core health objectives to increase quality and years of healthy life and to eliminate health disparities.

## Partnerships for Health: Health Promotion and Disease Prevention

Health promotion from an occupational perspective involves not only the prevention and reduction of illness, injury, trauma, and disability, but also the enhancement of health and well-being of all persons through the promotion of healthy lifestyle practices and healthy communities (AOTA, 2013, 2014).

Acknowledging Wilcock's (1998) occupational perspective relating to health and occupational performance is essential. She articulated that, for health and well-being to be present in individuals and communities alike, the following must occur for engagement in occupation (p. 123):

- Have meaning and be balanced between capacities
- Provide optimal opportunity for desired growth in individuals or groups
- Be flexible enough to develop and change according to context and choice
- Be compatible with sustaining ecology and sociocultural values

Occupational therapists and occupational therapy assistants should be mindful of the preceding qualities to improve the effects of health and disease on clients' performance. We also encourage practitioners to ask many questions until they arrive at a comfortable knowledge of the occupational profile of their clients. It is through such questioning or interviews that we develop a trusting relationship between the practitioner and client. Mutual interview is preferred to honor collaboration with occupational therapists, occupational therapy assistants, and clients. Hence, the practitioner is sharing stories and examples of his or her own experiences to guide the client toward sharing his or her experiences. Some other traits that we have found to be transforming in the practitioner-client relationship are to recognize that health and/or disease is a normal part of the client's life and to look for the client's strengths and positive health indicators rather than focusing on disease specifics.

Occupational therapists and occupational therapy assistants are in a position to advocate for health promotion regardless of a person's current impairment. For instance, imagine that you are working with a client who has a wrist fracture and a long history of major depressive disorder. She is also obese and inactive. The physician referral calls for upper extremity rehabilitation, including strengthening, functional and home safety assessments, and a medication maintenance plan. However, you, the practitioner, know that more services are necessary to improve this person's overall health. Therefore, you request and are granted additional referrals for nutrition and activity planning that will promote healthy living at home. Partnering with other professionals and seeking external resources would be necessary for this client's well-being.

We have worked collaboratively with multiple organizations and agencies including school systems, nonprofits, businesses, and institutions as consultants and trainers in health promotion. We have chosen three case studies to help you better understand perspectives of health and disability. In these examples, composites of persons have been used and client names and identifying information have been removed. You will meet Carrie, Salvatore, and Thomas, who exemplify the effects of health, disease, and disability on occupational performance within their own cultural context.

## Summary

This chapter examined health as a dynamic process that is ever-changing based on the individual, his or her occupational performance, and the environment. You should be able to discuss the importance of health, disease, and disability from multiple perspectives both intrinsic and extrinsic to the person. Persons are more than their disease processes, as explained through the occupational therapy perspective and the WHO's ICF framework. We encourage occupational therapy students to continue learning about health promotion and disability along with the effects occupational performance can have on well-being. Understanding the role of occupation in health promotion is necessary early on in your education, such that you may appreciate the complexity of health when collaborating and advocating for and with clients.

## Case Study: Carrie's Story

Carrie is an artist who experienced a stroke several years ago. She currently is not able to work as a mortgage broker at a bank owing to frequent seizures and difficulties in speaking. Carrie uses her work as an artist as a means to support herself and as an expression of her feelings and experiences as a person with a disability. Carrie is a mentor and partner with occupational therapy students who are learning about environmental strengths and barriers to persons with disabilities who are participating in their local arts and entertainment venues. As Carrie and the students visit an art gallery to investigate physical and social barriers and make recommendations, they realize that the staff has not been trained in disability etiquette. Carrie also notes that the gallery brochure, labels for exhibits, and other signage would not be accessible to persons with visual concerns. The students and Carrie discuss with the staff that if disability etiquette staff training and minor signage changes were put in place, the gallery would be more welcoming to all persons, not just persons without disabilities.

This case is an example of how the physical and social environments can interact with individual capacities and abilities in a way that promotes exclusion and marginalization by limiting access and participation to certain individuals. Due to her experiences, disability training, and previous interactions with persons with disabilities, Carrie had an increased awareness and knowledge of potential problems that persons might encounter in enjoying the gallery offerings. The occupational therapy students were skilled in analyzing client personal factors, environmental factors, and activity demands in terms of how these interact with client occupations. Together, Carrie and the students discussed how the contexts or interrelated environmental conditions, such as the physical, personal, social, cultural, and attitudinal aspects of the gallery, affect a visitor's ability to both gain access and fully engage in desired activities.

## Case Study: Salvatore's Story

Below is a letter that Salvatore wrote about his experience with West Nile virus. West Nile virus is spread by infected mosquitoes and can cause serious, life-altering, and even fatal disease.

Hello Family and Friends,

Get ready for this: I am now an official number at the CDC—one of over 30 cases this year. I have seen the West Nile virus and I have survived! Twenty days ago, I began feeling a bit tired, and my tummy was out of sorts. One morning I woke up with the worst headache I've ever had. It not only hurt inside but also outside! I had no desire to eat and the couple times I did it squirted right back out one end or the other. I was getting chills that had my teeth chattering. My mouth was desert-dry! My coffee cup felt so heavy! My weight had lessened and my thermal output was heightened to 101 degrees. On trip 2 to the doctor, I found out I had lost the ability to sign my name. Sonya, my wife, got me loaded into the car for another trip to the emergency room. They got me in quick while doctor number 3 got me one of those glorious IVs heated to perfection.

He ordered up a CAT and spinal tap and then sent me home to wait for results. The weekend passed by and I began feeling a little bit better every day, but the external tenderness persisted. I came home at lunch and had to stay. My doctor finally called at 4:45 p.m. on Friday and said the results were positive for West Nile. She couldn't understand why I was so happy. I said, "Mystery finally solved. Now you can get me healed." I hadn't been out of the house in 2 weeks except for work, so I went and enjoyed watching high school football on a glorious late summer evening, played games on my computer, and then looked at e-mails around 1 a.m. and stumbled upon these messages that Sonya "The Wise, Well-Connected, Always-By-My-Side, Fleet-of-Foot, Medically Savvy, Persistent, Morbid, Well-Stashed, and Truthful" had been circulating. I guess Salvatore "The Night Owl" is back!

Thanks for your prayers,

Salvatore

Salvatore's story exemplifies the need for external support. In this case, his wife was his primary health advocate. There were many unknowns about his condition (i.e., diagnosis, unexplainable symptoms), along with many occupations that motivated him to heal. Health literacy—the degree to which individuals have the capacity to obtain, process, and understand the basic health information and services needed to make appropriate health decisions—was a factor in this case (U.S. Department of Health and Human Services, 2000).

## Case Study: Thomas's Story

Health and wellness services can be population specific. Many communities focus on population-specific care for cohorts including adolescents, refugees, or HIV/AIDS survivors. Thomas's story comes from a class of occupational therapy students that served as mentors through a community-based course.

Occupational therapy students participated in a service-learning experience that involved developing a health promotion program with teenagers. Their semester-long efforts resulted in the "Health Through Photography" project. This project's goal was to empower teenagers to develop a new skill of photography while learning about healthy lifestyles through a camera's lens. Thomas, a quiet, polite teen, expressed some potential interest in photography. The teens took photos of numerous health objects and settings and brought this all together in an art portfolio for which they earned high school art credit. The concentrated effort toward health promotion encouraged Thomas to develop a trusting relationship with a group of college students while exploring various environments. The neighborhood, the city's downtown, and a college fitness center were some examples of the locations visited. During such visits, Thomas learned the importance of nutrition, physical fitness, hygiene, and environments on healthy lifestyles. He increased his trust in others and developed confidence in acquiring new skills (i.e., photography). His school then acknowledged this new skill by asking him to be the photographer for a special event at the end of the semester. Figures 8-2 and 8-3 are samples of this project.

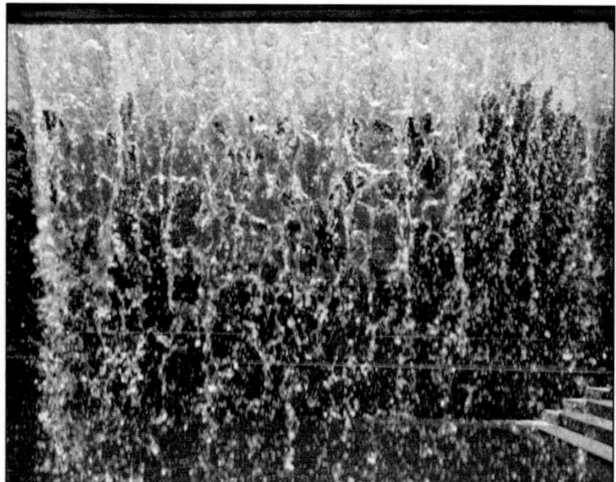

**Figure 8-2.** This waterfall photo was taken by a teen who was exploring environmental influences on health.

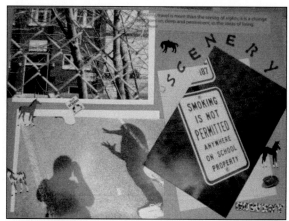


**Figure 8-3.** A page from the portfolio designed collaboratively by high school students and occupational therapy students.

For this project, the students chose an adolescent-specific population because there are numerous health risks facing youth (e.g., mental illness, asthma, sexually transmitted diseases, obesity). The most common causes of disability, disease, and premature death may result from adolescents' individual choices and behaviors. Thomas is an example of the success that health promotion can have on an individual's occupational performance even in the absence of disease.

## Student Self-Assessment

1. The ICF provides a framework that describes functioning as an interaction between health conditions and the environment. Compare and contrast an occupational perspective of health with perspectives within the ICF.
2. Going back to Carrie's case study, what are strategies that Carrie and the students could suggest to the gallery owners that have the potential to enhance participation and occupational engagement in this cultural venue? Many strategies can enhance participation for all persons, not just people with disabilities. How could the strategies you described in Question 1 be beneficial for others?
3. Going back to Salvatore's case study, how is the health status of Salvatore influenced by his occupations? If health and illness are dynamic and viewed as a continuum of interaction among many factors, which factors seem to facilitate health for Salvatore? Which are barriers to health?
4. Going back to Thomas's case study, explain the importance of population-specific interventions for the occupational therapy profession. How does

## Evidence-Based Research Chart

| Topic | Evidence |
|---|---|
| Health, participation, and wellness | Anderson et al., 2013; Baum, 2003; Braden et al., 2012; Foster, Galjour & Spengel, 2015; Goldworth, 2005; Hammell, 2015; Hull et al., 2015; Letts et al., 2011; Shaw & MacKinnon, 2004; Stav, Hallenen, Lane, & Arbesman, 2012; Suarez-Balcazar, 2005; Wilcock, 1993, 2005 |
| Health promotion and occupational therapy | Duque, 2004; Mallinson, Fischer, Rogers, Ehrlich-Jones, & Chang, 2009; Matuska, Giles-Heinz, Flinn, Neighbor, & Bass-Haugen, 2003; Orellano-Colon, Varas-Diaz, Bernal, & Mountain, 2014; Schepens et al., 2015; Scriven & Atwal, 2004; Thibodaux, 2005; Turcotte, Carrier, Desrosiers, & Levasseur, 2015 |
| Prevention of disease, injury, and disability | Clark et al., 1997; Hogan et al., 2013; Kroll, Jones, Kehn, & Neri, 2006; Michaud, Murray, & Bloom, 2001; Nakasato & Carnes, 2006; Schepens et al., 2015; Turcotte et al., 2015 |
| Disability constructs | Breen, Wildy, Saggers, Millsteed, & Raghavendra, 2011; Donoghue, 2003; Gitlow & Flecky, 2005; Hammell, 2015; Llewellyn & Hogan, 2000; Lutz & Bowers, 2005; Mitra, 2006; Taylor, 2005; Temple, McLeod, Gallinger, & Wright, 2001; Vrkljan, 2005 |
| *International Classification of Functioning, Disability and Health* | Battaglia et al., 2004; Cramm, Aiken, & Stewart, 2012; Grill, Stucki, Boldt, Joisten, & Swoboda, 2005; Hemmingsson & Jonsson, 2005; Kuijer, Brouwer, Preuper, Groothoff, & Dijkstra, 2006; Pettersson, Pettersson, & Frisk, 2012; Stamm, Cieza, Machold, Smolen, & Stucki, 2006 |
| Health promotion and partnerships | Hemming & Langille, 2006; Hodge & Nandy, 2011; King, Tucker, Baldwin, & LaPorta, 2006; Suarez-Balcazar et al., 2005; Young, Patterson, Wolff, Greer, & Wynne, 2015 |
| Occupational performance despite impairment | Bedell, Cohn, & Dumas, 2005; Chan, 2004; Hammell, 2015; Kirsh, Cockburn, & Gewutz, 2005; Reid, 2002; Rice & Thomas, 2000; Schenker, Coster, & Parush, 2005; Wilkins, Jung, Wishart, Edwards, & Norton, 2003 |

health promotion benefit individuals who are not affected by a specific disease or impairment? If you were Thomas, how might your thinking about your abilities have changed through the "Health Through Photography" project?

5. As indicated in this chapter, student self-examination of their perceptions about health and disease enhances their understanding of occupational performance in relationship to health. Return to the student health survey. Compare and contrast your health experiences with the student responses. What interactions have you had with persons with different health conditions? How did you respond to these differences? How have the concepts discussed in this chapter enhanced your understanding about differences related to health, disease, and disability?
6. Encourage students to explore diversity in health, disease, and disability. Ask them to complete a health application in another language. For example, you may access a form for health insurance in Spanish at https://www.healthcare.gov/language-resource/.
7. Review concepts and definitions from the ICF framework and compare definitions of activity and participation to the *Framework* definitions of activity, occupation, and participation.
8. Give examples of personal and environmental factors that affect occupational performance, function, and participation.

## Electronic Resources

Community Campus Partnerships for Health: www.ccph.info

Disability History Museum: www.disabilitymuseum.org

Health Literacy Consulting: www.healthliteracy.com

Office of Disease Prevention and Health Promotion: http://health.gov/

World Health Organization and ICF link: www.who.int/en or www.who.int/classifications/icf/e

## References

Albrecht, G. L., Seelman, K. D., & Bury, M. (2001). Introduction: The formation of disabilities studies. In G. L. Albrecht, K. D. Seelman, & M. Bury (Eds.), *Handbook of disabilities studies* (pp. 1-8). Thousand Oaks, CA: Sage Publications.

Altman, B. M. (2001). Disability definitions, models, classification schemes, and application. In G. L. Albrecht, K. D. Seelman, & M. Bury (Eds.), *Handbook of disability studies* (pp. 97-122). Thousand Oaks, CA: Sage Publications.

American Occupational Therapy Association. (2013). Occupational therapy in the promotion of health and well-being. *American Occupational Therapy Association, 67*(6), S47-S58.

American Occupational Therapy Association. (2014). Occupational therapy practice framework: Domain and process (3rd ed.). *American Journal of Occupational Therapy, 68*(Suppl. 1), S1-S48. doi:10.5014/ajot.2014.682006

American Occupational Therapy Association. (2015a). *Academic programs annual data: Academic year 2014-2015*. Retrieved from http://www.aota.org/-/media/corporate/files/educationcareers/educators/2014-2015-annual-data-report.pdf

American Occupational Therapy Association. (2015b). Philosophy of occupational therapy education. *American Journal of Occupational Therapy, 69*(Suppl. 3), 6913410052p1-6913410052p2. doi:10.5014/ajot.2015.696S17

Anderson, L. L., Humphries, K., McDermott, S., Marks, B., Sisarak, J., & Larson, S. (2013). The state of the science of health and wellness for adults with intellectual and developmental disabilities. *Intellectual and Developmental Disabilities, 51*(5), 385-398. doi:10:1352/1934-9556.51.5.385

Battaglia, M., Russo, E., Bolla, A., Chiusso, A., Bertelli, S., Pellegri, A., et al. (2004). *International Classification of Functioning, Disability and Health* in a cohort of children with cognitive, motor, and complex disabilities. *Developmental Medicine and Child Neurology, 46*(2), 98-106.

Baum, C. M. (2003). Participation: Its relationship to occupation and health. *OTJR: Occupation, Participation and Health, 23*(2), 46-47.

Bedell, G. M., Cohn, E. S., & Dumas, H. M. (2005). Exploring parents' use of strategies to promote social participation of school-age children with acquired brain injuries. *American Journal of Occupational Therapy, 59*, 273-284.

Braddock, D. L., & Parish, S. L. (2001). An institutional history of disability. In G. L. Albrecht, K. D. Seelman, & M. Bury (Eds.), *Handbook of disability studies* (pp. 11-68). Thousand Oaks, CA: Sage Publications.

Braden, C. A., Cuthbert, J. P., Brenner, L., Hawley, L., Morey, C., Newman, J., Staniszewski, K., & Harrison-Flex, C. (2012). Health and wellness characteristics of persons with traumatic brain injury. *Brain Injury, 26*(11), 1315-1327. doi:10.3109/02699052.2013

Breen, L. J., Wildy, H., Saggers, S., Millsteed, J., & Raghavendra, P. (2011). In search of wellness: Allied health professionals' understandings of wellness in childhood disability services. *Disability and Rehabilitation, 33*(10), 862-871. doi:10.3109/096388.2010.520799

Bridle, M. J. (1999). Are doing and being dimensions of holism? *American Journal of Occupational Therapy, 53*(6), 636-639.

Brownson, C. A., & Scaffa, M. E. (2001). Occupational therapy in the promotion of health and the prevention of disease and disability statement. *American Journal of Occupational Therapy, 55*(6), 656-660.

Chan, S. C. C. (2004). Chronic obstructive pulmonary disease and engagement in occupation. *American Journal of Occupational Therapy, 58*, 408-415.

Clark, F., Azen, S. P., Zemke, R., Jackson, J., Carlson, M., Mandel, D., et al. (1997). Occupational therapy for independent-living older adults. A randomized controlled trial. *Journal of the American Medical Association, 278*(16), 1321-1326.

Cramm, H., Aiken, A. B., & Stewart, D. (2012). Perspectives on the International Classification of Functioning, Disability, and Health: Child and Youth Version (ICF-CY) and occupational therapy practice. *Physical and Occupational Therapy in Pediatrics, 32*(4), 388-403.

Depoy, E., & Gilson, S. F. (2004). *Rethinking disability: Principles for professional and social change*. Belmont, CA: Brooks/Cole.

Dolmage, J. T. (2014). *Disability rhetoric*. Syracuse, NY: Syracuse University Press.

Donoghue, C. (2003). Challenging the authority of the medical definition of disability: Analysis of the resistance to the social constructionist paradigm. *Disability and Society, 18*, 199-208.

Duque, R. L. (2004). Health promotion and the values of occupational therapy. *WFOT Bulletin, 49*, 5-8.

Edelman, C. L., Kudzma, E. C., & Mandle, C. L. (Eds.). (2013). *Health promotion throughout the lifespan* (8th ed.). St. Louis, MO: Mosby-Elsevier.

Falk, G. (2001). *Stigma: How we treat outsiders*. Amherst, NY: Prometheus Books.

Forget, N. J., & Higgins, J. (2014). Comparison of generic patient-reported outcome measures used with upper extremity musculoskeletal disorders: Linking process using the *International Classification of Functioning, Disability and Health (ICF)*. *Journal of Rehabilitation Medicine, 46*(4), 327-334. doi:10.2340/16501977-1784

Foster, T., Galjour, C., & Spengel, S. (2015). Investigating holistic wellness dimensions during older adulthood: A factor analytic study. *Journal of Adult Development, 22*, 239-247. doi:10.1007/s10804-015-9215-4

Gill, C. J. (2001). Divided understandings: The social experience of disability. In G. L. Albrecht, K. D. Seelman, & M. Bury (Eds.), *Handbook of disability studies* (pp. 351-372). Thousand Oaks, CA: Sage Publications.

Gitlow, L., & Flecky, K. (2005). Integrating disability studies concepts into occupational therapy education using service learning. *American Journal of Occupational Therapy, 59*(5), 546-553.

Goldworth, A. (2005). Disease, illness, and ethics. *Cambridge Quarterly of Healthcare Ethics, 14*(3), 346-351.

Grill, E., Stucki, G., Boldt, C., Joisten, S., & Swoboda, W. (2005). Identification of relevant ICF categories by geriatric patients in an early post-acute rehabilitation facility. *Disability and Rehabilitation, 27*(7-8), 467-473.

Hahn, H. (1993). The politics of physical differences: Disability and discrimination. In M. Nagler (Ed.), *Perspectives on disability* (2nd ed., pp. 37-42). Palo Alto, CA: Health Markets Research.

Hammell, K. W. (2015). Quality of life, participation and occupational rights: A capabilities perspective. *Australian Occupational Therapy Journal, 62*(2), 78-85. doi:10.1111/1440-1630.12183

Hansen, R. A., & Atchinson, B. (2011). *Conditions in occupational therapy: Effect on occupational performance* (4th ed.). Baltimore, MD: Lippincott Williams and Wilkins.

Hemming, H. E., & Langille, L. (2006). Building knowledge in literacy and health. *Canadian Journal of Public Health, 97*(Suppl. 2), S31-S36.

Hemmingsson, H., & Jonsson, H. (2005). An occupational perspective on the concept of participation in the International Classification of Functioning, Disability and Health—Some critical remarks. *American Journal of Occupational Therapy, 59*(5), 569-576.

Hettler, W. (1984). Wellness: The lifetime goal of a university experience. In J. D. Matarazzo, S. M. Weiss, J. A. Herd, N. E. Miller, & S. M. Weiss (Eds.), *Behavioral health: A handbook of health enhancement and disease prevention* (p. 1117). New York, NY: Wiley.

Hodge, F. S., & Nandy, K. (2011). Predictors of wellness and American Indians. *Journal of Health Care for the Poor and Underserved, 22*(3), 791-803. doi:10.1353/hpu.2011.0093

Hogan, V, K., Culhane, J. F., Crews, K., J., Mwaria, C. B., Rowley, D. L., et al. (2013). The impact of social disadvantage on preconception health, illness, and well-being: An intersectional analysis. *American Journal of Health Promotion, 27*(3), eS32-eS42.

Hull, A., Holliday, S. B., Eickhoff, C., Rose-Boyce, M., Sullivan, P., & Reinhard, M. (2015). The Integrative Health and Wellness Program: Development and use of a complementary and alternative medicine clinic for veterans. *Alternative Therapies in Health and Medicine, 21*(6), 12-21.

Kielhofner, G. (2009). *Conceptual foundations of occupational therapy* (4th ed.). Philadelphia, PA: F. A. Davis Company.

King, G. A., Tucker, M. A., Baldwin, P. J., & LaPorta, J. A. (2006). Bringing the life needs model to life: Implementing a service delivery model for pediatric rehabilitation. *Physical and Occupational Therapy in Pediatrics, 26*(1-2), 43-70.

Kirsh, B., Cockburn, L., & Gewutz, R. (2005). Best practice in occupational therapy: Program characteristics that influence vocational outcomes for people with serious mental illness. *Canadian Journal of Occupational Therapy, 72*, 265-279.

Kristensen, H. K. (2015). Achieving a holistic perspective in stroke rehabilitation: An overview of the use of the ICF by Danish physiotherapists and occupational therapists. *International Journal of Therapy and Rehabilitation, 22*(10), 460-469. doi:10.12968/ijtr.2015.22.10.460

Kroll, T., Jones, G. C., Kehn, M. E., & Neri, M. T. (2006). Barriers and strategies affecting the utilization of primary preventive services for people with physical disabilities: A qualitative inquiry. *Health and Social Care in the Community, 14*(4), 284-293.

Kuijer, W., Brouwer, S., Preuper, H. R., Groothoff, J. W., Geertzen, J. H., & Dijkstra, P. U. (2006). Work status and chronic low back pain: Exploring the International Classification of Functioning, Disability and Health. *Disability and Rehabilitation, 28*(6), 379-388.

Letts, L., Edwards, M., Berenyi, J., Moros, K., O'Neill, C., O'Toole, C., et al. (2011). Using occupations to improve quality of life, health and wellness, and client and caregiver satisfaction for people with Alzheimer's disease and related dementias. *American Journal of Occupational Therapy, 65*, 497-504. doi:10.5014/ajot.2011.002584

Llewellyn, A., & Hogan, K. (2000). The use and abuse of models of disability. *Disability and Society, 15*(1), 157-165.

Longmore, P., & Umansky, L. (2001). *The new disability history: American perspectives (History of disability)*. New York, NY: New York University Press.

Lutz, B. J., & Bowers, B. J. (2005). Disability in everyday life. *Qualitative Health Research, 15*(8), 1037-1054.

Lyons, M., Orozovic, N., Davis, J., & Newman, J. (2002). Doing, being, becoming: Occupational experiences of persons with life-threatening illnesses. *American Journal of Occupational Therapy, 56*(3), 285-295.

Mallinson, T., Fischer, H., Rogers, J. C., Ehrlich-Jones, L., & Chang, R. (2009). The issue is human occupation for public health promotion: New directions for occupational therapy practice with persons with arthritis. *American Journal of Occupational Therapy, 63*, 220-226.

Matuska, K., Giles-Heinz, A., Flinn, N., Neighbor, M., & Bass-Haugen, J. (2003). Outcomes of a pilot occupational therapy wellness program for older adults. *American Journal of Occupational Therapy, 57*(2), 220-224.

Mercer, G., & Barnes, C. (2010). *Exploring disability: A sociological introduction*. Malden, MA: Polity Press.

Michaud, C. M., Murray, C. J., & Bloom, B. R. (2001). Burden of disease: Implications for future research. *Journal of the American Medical Association, 285*(5), 535-539.

Mitra, S. (2006). The capability approach and disability. *Journal of Disability Policy Studies, 16*(4), 236-247.

Nakasato, Y. R., & Carnes, B. A. (2006). Health promotion in older adults: Promoting successful aging in primary care settings. *Geriatrics, 61*(4), 27-31.

Oliver, M. (2009). *Understanding disability: From theory to practice* (2nd ed.). New York, NY: Palgrave Macmillan.

Orellano-Colon, E. M., Varas-Diaz, N., Bernal, G. & Mountain, G. A. (2014). Achieving ecological validity of occupational based interventions for healthy aging. *Physical and Occupational Therapy in Geriatrics, 32*(4), 368-380. doi:10.3109/02703181.2014.955623

OTAL Occupational Therapy Australia Ltd. (2015). Position Statement: Occupational therapy in palliative care. *Australian Occupational Therapy Journal, 62*(6), 459-461. doi:10.1111/1440-1630.12264

Pettersson, I., Pettersson, V., & Frisk, C. (2012). ICF from an occupational therapy perspective in adult care: An integrative literature review. *Scandinavian Journal of Occupational Therapy, 19*, 260-273.

Quiroga, V. A. M. (1995). *Occupational therapy: The first 30 years: 1900 to 1930*. Bethesda, MD: AOTA Press.

Race, Ethnicity, and Genetics Working Group. (2005). The use of racial, ethnic, and ancestral categories in human genetics research. *American Journal of Human Genetics, 77*(4), 519-532.

Reid, D. T. (2002). Critical review of the research literature of seating interventions: A focus on adults with mobility impairments. *Assistive Technology, 14*, 118-129.

Rice, M. S., & Thomas, J. J. (2000). Perceived risk as a constraint on occupational performance during hot and cold water pouring. *American Journal of Occupational Therapy, 54*, 525-532.

Schaaf, R. C., Cohn, E. S., Burke, J., Dumont, R., Miller, A., & Mailloux, Z. (2015). Linking sensory factors to participation: Establishing intervention goals with parents for children with autism spectrum disorder. *American Journal of Occupational Therapy, 69*(5), 1-8. doi:10.5014/ajot.2015.018036

Schenker, R., Coster, W. J., & Parush, S. (2005). Neuroimpairments, activity performance and participation in children with cerebral palsy mainstreamed in elementary schools. *Developmental Medicine and Child Neurology, 47*(12), 808-814.

Schepens Neimiec, S. L., Carlson, M., Martinez, J., Guzman, L., Mahajan, A., & Clark, F. (2015). Developing occupation-based preventive programs for late-middle-aged Latino patients in safety-net health systems. *American Journal of Occupational Therapy, 69*(6), 6906240010. doi:10.5014/ajot2015.015958

Scriven, A., & Atwal, A. (2004). Occupational therapists as primary health promoters: opportunities and barriers. *British Journal of Occupational Therapy, 67*(10), 424-429.

Shaw, L., & MacKinnon, J. (2004). A multidimensional view of health. *Education for Health, 17*(2), 213-222.

Stamm, T. A., Cieza, A., Machold, K. P., Smolen, J. S., & Stucki, G. (2006). An exploration of the link of conceptual occupational therapy models and the International Classification of Functioning, Disability and Health. *Australian Occupational Therapy Journal, 53*(1), 9-17.

Stav, W. B., Hallenen, T., Lane, J., & Arbesman, M. (2012). Systematic review of occupational engagement and health outcomes among community-dwelling older adults. *American Journal of Occupational Therapy, 66*, 301-310. doi:10.5014/ajot.2012.003707

Stewart, D., Samrai, B., Stark, S., Carswell, A., McIntyre, A., & Hemmingsson, H. (2014). WFOT survey about the use and utility of the *International Classification of Functioning, Disability and Health (ICF)*. *WFOT Bulletin, 68*, 9-25.

Stiker, H. J., & Sayers, W. (Trans.). (2000). *A history of disabilities (Corporealities: Discourses of disability)*. Ann Arbor, MI: University of Michigan Press.

Suarez-Balcazar, Y. (2005). Empowerment and participatory evaluation of a community health intervention: Implications for occupational therapy. *OTJR: Occupation, Participation and Health, 25*(4), 133-142.

Suarez-Balcazar, Y., Hammel, J., Helfrich, C., Thomas, J., Wilson, T., & Head-Ball, D. (2005). A model of university-community partnerships for occupational therapy scholarship and practice. *Occupational Therapy in Health Care, 19*, 47-70.

Taylor, R. R. (2005). Can the social model explain all of disability experience? Perspectives of persons with chronic fatigue syndrome. *American Journal of Occupational Therapy, 59*(5), 497-506.

Temple, L. K., McLeod, R. S., Gallinger, S., & Wright, J. G. (2001). Essays on science and society. Defining disease in the genomics era. *Science, 293*(5531), 807-810.

Thibodaux, L. R. (2005). Habitus and the embodiment of disability through lifestyle. *American Journal of Occupational Therapy, 59*(5), 507-515.

Turcotte, P., Carrier, A., Desrosiers, J., & Levasseur, M. (2015). Are health promotion and preventions integrated into occupational therapy practice with older adults having disabilities? Insights from six community health settings in Quebec, Canada. *Australian Occupational Therapy Journal, 62*, 56-67. doi:10.1111/1440-1630.12174

U.S. Department of Health and Human Services. (2000). *Healthy people 2010: Volume 1: Understanding and improving health. Objectives for improving health* (2nd ed.). Washington, DC: U.S. Government Printing Office.

Vrkljan, B. H. (2005). Dispelling the disability stereotype: Embracing a universalistic perspective of disablement. *Canadian Journal of Occupational Therapy, 72*(1), 57-59.

Wilcock, A. A. (1993). Biological and sociocultural aspects of occupation, health and health promotion. *British Journal of Occupational Therapy, 56*(6), 200-203. doi:10.1177/030802269305600605

Wilcock, A. A. (1998). *An occupational perspective of health*. Thorofare, NJ: SLACK Incorporated.

Wilcock, A. A. (2005). Occupational science: Bridging occupation and health. *Canadian Journal of Occupational Therapy, 72*(1), 5-12.

Wilcock, A. (2006). *An occupational perspective of health* (2nd ed.). Thorofare, NJ: SLACK Incorporated.

Wilcock, A. A. (2015). *An occupational perspective of health* (3rd ed.). Thorofare, NJ: SLACK Incorporated.

Wilkins, S., Jung, B., Wishart, L., Edwards, M., & Norton, S. G. (2003). The effectiveness of community-based occupational therapy education and functional training programs for older adults: A critical literature review. *Canadian Journal of Occupational Therapy, 70*, 214-225.

World Health Organization. (1946). Preamble to the Constitution of the World Health Organization. *Official Records of the World Health Organization, 2*, p. 100. Retrieved from http://who.int/about/definitions/en/print.html

World Health Organization. (1986). *The Ottawa Charter for Health Promotion*. First International Conference on Health Promotion, Ottawa. Retrieved from http://www. who.int/healthpromotion/conferences/previous/ottawa/en/print.html

World Health Organization. (2001). *International classification of functioning, disability, and health (ICF). Short version*. Geneva, Switzerland: Author.

World Health Organization. (2014). *ICF updates*. Retrieved from http://www.who.int/classifications/icfupdates/en/

Young, S., Patterson, L., Wolff, M., Greer, Y., & Wynne, N. (2015). Empowerment, leadership, and sustainability in a faith-based partnership to improve health. *Journal of Religious Health, 54*, 2086-2098. doi:10.1007/s10943-014-9911-6

## Suggested Readings

American Occupational Therapy Association. (2015). Occupational therapy's perspective on the use of environments and contexts to facilitate health, well-being, and participation in occupations. *American Journal of Occupational Therapy, 69*(Suppl. 3), 6913410050. doi:10.514/ajot.64S57

Bases C. G. (2014). What's bad about wellness? What the disability rights perspective offers about the limitations of wellness. *Journal of Health Politics, Policy and Law, 39*(5), 1035-1066. doi:10.1215/03616878-2813695

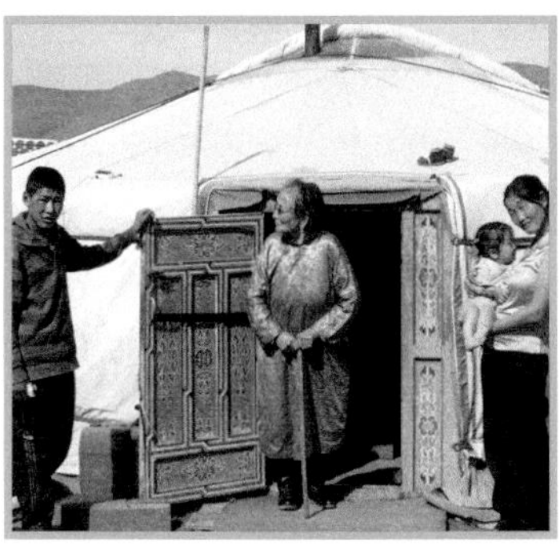

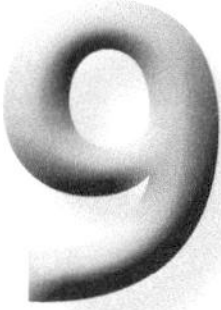

# EFFECTIVE COMMUNICATION

*Jan Froehlich, MS, OTR/L*

**ACOTE STANDARDS EXPLORED IN THIS CHAPTER**

B.5.20, B.5.21

**KEY VOCABULARY**

- **Cultural competence:** A process of gaining self-awareness, knowledge and awareness of others, and skill in communicating with diverse groups of people (Black & Wells, 2007).
- **Effective communication:** The artful interplay between listening and speaking with attention to both verbal and nonverbal communication, coupled with an awareness and sensitivity to human diversity.
- **Interprofessional collaboration:** Two or more health or social care professions actively working together to provide services or solve problems (Zwarenstein & Reeves, 2006).
- **Nonverbal communication:** Communication through eye contact, tone of voice, facial expression, body language, and posture.
- **Reflective listening:** A process of listening to both the verbal and emotional content of a speaker and verbalizing both the feelings and attitudes sensed behind the spoken words to the speaker (Davis, 2011).



Jacobs, K., & MacRae, N. (Eds.).
*Occupational Therapy Essentials for Clinical Competence, Third Edition* (pp. 99-132).

The importance of communication competency in the provision of quality health care has been increasingly recognized (Alpert, 2011; Boschma et al., 2010; IOM, 2000; Joint Commission, 2015; Lingard et al., 2008; O'Sullivan, Chao, Russell, Levine, & Fabiny, 2008; Reisdorff et al., 2006; Sargent, MacLeod, & Murray, 2011; Sutcliffe, Lewton, & Rosenthal, 2004; Taylor, 2008). Furthermore, evidence shows that single communication actions can affect health outcomes (Robinson & Heritage, 2006). Effective communication is essential to the occupational therapy process, yet communicating well with a wide range of clients, patients, family, significant others, members of the interprofessional team, and the public can be challenging.

Every occupational therapy practitioner, like every human, has undoubtedly experienced many successes and failures in communication. Nonetheless, much can be learned about how to make the communication process increasingly effective. The artful interplay between listening and speaking, coupled with awareness and sensitivity to human diversity, is at the heart of effective communication. For some occupational therapy practitioners, listening comes more easily than speaking. For others, sharing information may come easily, whereas listening is the greater challenge. For still others, the greater challenge is to communicate with confidence and ease when they are with someone from a background that is different from their own. Additional communication challenges faced by all health professionals include mastery of effective interprofessional team communication and conflict resolution, as well as thoughtful integration of technology and documentation in health care communication.

## The Challenge to Truly Listen

As Alpert (2011) noted, "the commonest failure in communicating information is the result of inattentive or inaccurate listening" (p. 381). Listening has been ranked as the most important behavior of health professionals by clients (Harris & Templeton, 2001). Client-centered therapy requires good listening (Law, Baptiste, & Mills, 1995). Only when the therapist can listen well enough to his or her clients to understand what their real concerns are can client-centered therapy occur. Naturally, attentive listening is also essential for effective interprofessional collaboration (Sargeant, Loney, & Murphy, 2008; Sargent et al., 2011).

Whereas listening appears to be a simple skill, it has many complexities that are worth exploring. On a basic level, listening involves learning to not interrupt the individual to whom we are listening. In everyday interactions between people, interruptions are frequent (Jackins, 1981). This occurs because as humans, we all want and need to be listened to. Not surprisingly, it is also true that as humans, we all need and want to listen to others. Sometimes, we find ourselves in professional and/or personal relationships where there is a natural balance between listening and being listened to. Other times, we find ourselves in relationships in which we are the listener or the talker most of the time. Unless these are client/therapist relationships in which we expect to be the primary listener, imbalanced relationships may be fraught with tension and misunderstandings. Additionally, the functioning of interprofessional teams will be in jeopardy when there is no balance between listening and talking among members. Essential information may not be imparted or heard if listening and speaking roles are not shared (Sargent et al., 2008, 2011).

In many communication exchanges, if examined closely, we will find there is often frequent interrupting going on in the communication process. This occurs in interactions between interprofessional team members, clients and practitioners, supervisors and supervisees, friends, family members, and peers of any kind. Interruptions often take the form of telling one's own story, opinion, similar experience, or giving unsought advice. These interruptions often arise as an inherent need for reciprocity. However, when one considers the frequent interruptions that characterize human conversations, step number one in becoming an effective communicator is first noticing how much we interrupt others as we communicate, and step two is to stop doing this. Unfortunately, this may be easier said than done. It may be particularly challenging to do this, unless we know that we too will get a turn to be listened to without interruption. Listening partnerships with peers can assist with this challenge.

## Overview of Listening Partnerships

Studies show that the communications skills of health professionals do not necessarily improve over time or with clinical experience (Fallowfield et al., 2002; Fellowes, Wilkinson, & Moore, 2004). Health professional communication skills can improve with formal communication skills training. Whereas lectures appear to have limited use in teaching communication skills, effective methods include small and large group discussion, role play, videotapes, feedback, skill practice, multidisciplinary panels, Objective Structured Clinical Examination, interactive theater, and listening partnerships (Berkhof, van Rijssen, Schellart, Anema, & van der Beek, 2011; Boschma et al., 2010; Froehlich & Nesbit, 2004; Froehlich, Pardue, & Dunbar, 2016; Harmsen et al., 2005; O'Sullivan et al., 2008; Sargeant et al., 2011; Shield, Tong, Tomas, & Beesdine, 2011).

Froehlich and her colleagues have used listening partnerships extensively in small group seminars on culturally responsive communication for more than 20 years (Froehlich & Nesbit, 2004; Froehlich et al., 2016), and occupational therapy students and faculty have generally found them to be an invaluable learning tool. Listening partnerships, which involve taking turns listening and speaking with a peer for a mutually agreed-on amount of time, are borrowed from the theory and practice of co-counseling, also known as *reevaluation counseling* (Jackins, 1981; Kauffman & New, 2004). Taking turns listening allows listeners to develop better and better mental focus. Knowing one will have a turn to be listened to can enable one to listen better. As new occupational therapy practitioners noted about the value of listening partnerships:

- "Practicing the art of listening through listening partnerships truly taught me how to 'be in the moment.' Too often, I would catch my mind wandering during daily conversations with friends and family rather than be fully devoted to the exchange at hand. These assignments not only showed me the importance of truly hearing and listening to a person, they allowed me to refine my effective communication skills for my personal life and clinical practice."
- "These partnerships have taught me multiple tools that I carry with me to this day and know that I will carry and take with me throughout my professional career. Being able to listen to my clients as well as coworkers makes for a better, safer, and more effective environment."

## Communication and Cultural Competence Surveys

Prior to practicing listening partnerships, the reader is encouraged to complete the Froehlich Communication Survey (Figure 9-1) and the Cultural Awareness and Action Survey (Figure 9-2). Both surveys were tested on students, who rated the surveys favorably. A number of students indicated that simply by completing the communication survey, they became communicators who were more aware. Refinement and content validity of the communication survey was established by a panel of experts from the disciplines of psychology, counseling, nursing, social work, and medical education. Froehlich, Pardue, and Dunbar (2016) found the tool had good test–re-test reliability and strong internal consistency (Cronbach alpha, .847).

## Evaluation of Listening Partnerships

Using the Froehlich communication survey in a pre-test/post-test design, listening partnerships were introduced and evaluated in an interprofessional undergraduate course, Introduction to the Health Professions (Froehlich et al., 2016). The authors found listening partnerships had a significant influence on student perceptions of their verbal and nonverbal communication skills on 16 of 25 survey items. Of particular note, repeated practice with listening partnerships was shown to increase student perceptions of their ability to listen with compassion. This is a significant finding because many health educators question whether the important attribute of compassion can be learned or improved upon. Only with repeated practice with listening partnerships throughout the semester, compared with a control group, which practiced listening partnerships in two class sessions, did student ratings of their ability to listen with compassion show a significant improvement.

## Engaging in Listening Partnerships

Because it is not possible to become a better communicator without intentional practice, once both surveys are completed, the learner is encouraged to proceed to practicing listening partnerships with a peer or peers who are also reading this text. Pairs are ideal, but small groups can work as well. Meeting with different partners for each meeting over the course of several weeks is recommended for optimal skill development. Then, establishing an agreement to meet with the same person on a regular basis (a regular listening partner) can further enhance the development of effective communication skills. In addition, these partnerships will only go well if the listener keeps time and notifies the speaker when time is up, and if both parties can agree to two kinds of confidentiality:

1. Nothing said in the listening partnership will be shared with anyone outside the listening partnership with the person's name attached.
2. Once a listening partnership is completed, the listener needs permission from the speaker to bring up anything said in the listening partnership.

This chapter is arranged into three sections: enhancing interpersonal communication skills; culturally responsive communication; and intra- and interprofessional teamwork, technology, and other communication challenges. Focused questions are provided for listening partnerships.

## Froehlich Communication Survey

**Name:**

Developing effective interpersonal communication is an ongoing process. The purpose of this survey is to help you identify your strengths, areas for improvement, and goals related to effective interpersonal communication. Please circle the number that best reflects your agreement with the following statements so you can clarify where you need to work to be a more effective communicator.

| | | |
|---|---|---|
| 1 | Strongly Disagree | Much Improvement Needed |
| 10 | Strongly Agree | Little Improvement Needed |

I can listen without interrupting.
1 2 3 4 5 6 7 8 9 10

I can keep my mind free of distractions while listening.
1 2 3 4 5 6 7 8 9 10

I can allow for silences.
1 2 3 4 5 6 7 8 9 10

When appropriate, I can offer steady eye contact while listening.
1 2 3 4 5 6 7 8 9 10

I am aware of body language while listening.
1 2 3 4 5 6 7 8 9 10

My posture and facial expression show interest and caring.
1 2 3 4 5 6 7 8 9 10

I don't fidget while listening.
1 2 3 4 5 6 7 8 9 10

I can build rapport with others.
1 2 3 4 5 6 7 8 9 10

I appropriately maintain confidentiality.
1 2 3 4 5 6 7 8 9 10

I can maintain compassion while listening.
1 2 3 4 5 6 7 8 9 10

I use open- and closed-ended questions to determine someone's concerns and goals.
1 2 3 4 5 6 7 8 9 10

I can effectively use restatement, summaries, and clarification in a conversation.
1 2 3 4 5 6 7 8 9 10

I can identify, reflect, and validate emotional and verbal content in a conversation.
1 2 3 4 5 6 7 8 9 10

I can maintain mental focus when listening to someone who is upset.
1 2 3 4 5 6 7 8 9 10

I can convey hopefulness.
1 2 3 4 5 6 7 8 9 10

I can use humor effectively.
1 2 3 4 5 6 7 8 9 10

I can judge when to use touch during conversations.
1 2 3 4 5 6 7 8 9 10

I can judge when to redirect someone or help someone get their attention off their distress in a conversation.
1 2 3 4 5 6 7 8 9 10

I can judge when someone is ready to hear information or advice.
1 2 3 4 5 6 7 8 9 10

I am clear, concise, and confident when I speak.
1 2 3 4 5 6 7 8 9 10

I can give, receive, and solicit constructive feedback including appreciation of others and myself.
1 2 3 4 5 6 7 8 9 10

I can be appropriately assertive in interactions with others.
1 2 3 4 5 6 7 8 9 10

I communicate well on teams by listening to multiple perspectives and sharing mine.
1 2 3 4 5 6 7 8 9 10

I understand the importance of seeking an interpreter when I don't understand the language of a client.
1 2 3 4 5 6 7 8 9 10

I can communicate effectively with people from different cultural groups.
1 2 3 4 5 6 7 8 9 10

**Score: /250**

**Communication skills I want to be better at (progress reported on goals in post-survey):**

**1.**

**2.**

**3.**

**Thanks for your time.**



**Figure 9-1.** Froehlich Communication Survey.

## Cultural Awareness and Action Survey

**Name:**

The journey toward cultural competence is a deeply enriching process that is is fueled by building relationships with people from diverse backgrounds. The purpose of this survey is to help you identify your strengths, areas for improvement, and goals related to cultural awareness, cultural humility and cultural effectiveness. Please circle the number that best reflects your agreement with the following statements so you can clarify action steps you need to take to become increasingly culturally aware and effective in building relationships across cultural lines.

| | | |
|---|---|---|
| 1 | Strongly Disagree | Much Improvement Needed |
| 10 | Strongly Agree | Little Improvement Needed |

I am aware that culture encompasses many human experiences related to gender, race, class, ethnicity, disability status, sexual orientation, religion, etc.
1 2 3 4 5 6 7 8 9 10

I am aware of my own ethnic heritage (national origin of my ancestors).
1 2 3 4 5 6 7 8 9 10

I am aware of why my ancestors came to this country, or if I am indigenous, I am aware of my tribal heritage.
1 2 3 4 5 6 7 8 9 10

I am aware of the historical context, strengths, and challenges of being an immigrant in my country.
1 2 3 4 5 6 7 8 9 10

I am aware of the historical context, strengths, and challenges of being a refugee in my country.
1 2 3 4 5 6 7 8 9 10

I am aware of the historical context, strengths, and challenges of being indigenous of Native American Heritage.
1 2 3 4 5 6 7 8 9 10

I am aware of the historical context, strengths, and challenges of being African Heritage.
1 2 3 4 5 6 7 8 9 10

I am aware of the historical context, strengths, and challenges of being Asian Heritage.
1 2 3 4 5 6 7 8 9 10

I am aware of the historical context, strengths, and challenges of being Arab Heritage.
1 2 3 4 5 6 7 8 9 10

I am aware of the historical context, strengths, and challenges of being Latina/Latino Heritage.
1 2 3 4 5 6 7 8 9 10

I am aware of the historical context, strengths, and challenges of being Pacific Island Heritage.
1 2 3 4 5 6 7 8 9 10

I am aware of the historical context, strengths, and challenges of being White European Heritage.
1 2 3 4 5 6 7 8 9 10

I am aware of the historical context, strengths, and challenges of being Jewish or Jewish Heritage.
1 2 3 4 5 6 7 8 9 10

I am aware of the historical context, strengths, and challenges of being Catholic or Catholic Heritage.
1 2 3 4 5 6 7 8 9 10

I am aware of the historical context, strengths, and challenges of being Muslim or Muslim Heritage.
1 2 3 4 5 6 7 8 9 10

I am aware of the historical context, strengths, and challenges of being Buddhist or Buddhist Heritage.
1 2 3 4 5 6 7 8 9 10

I am aware of the historical context, strengths, and challenges of being Protestant or Protestant Heritage.
1 2 3 4 5 6 7 8 9 10

I am aware of the historical context, strengths, and challenges of being Hindu or Hindu Heritage.
1 2 3 4 5 6 7 8 9 10

I am aware of the history, strengths, and challenges of being an atheist or agnostic.
1 2 3 4 5 6 7 8 9 10

I am aware of the historical context, strengths, and challenges of being currently or raised poor.
1 2 3 4 5 6 7 8 9 10

I am aware of the historical context, strengths, and challenges of being currently or raised working class.
1 2 3 4 5 6 7 8 9 10

I am aware of the historical context, strengths, and challenges of being currently or raised middle or professional class.
1 2 3 4 5 6 7 8 9 10

I am aware of the historical context, strengths, and challenges of being currently or raised upper class.
1 2 3 4 5 6 7 8 9 10

I am aware of the historical context, strengths, and challenges of being a homeless person.
1 2 3 4 5 6 7 8 9 10

I am aware of the historical context, strengths, and challenges of being female.
1 2 3 4 5 6 7 8 9 10

I am aware of the historical context, strengths, and challenges of being male.
1 2 3 4 5 6 7 8 9 10

*(continued)*

## Cultural Awareness and Action Survey (continued)

I am aware of the historical context, strengths, and challenges of being gay.
1 2 3 4 5 6 7 8 9 10

I am aware of the historical context, strengths, and challenges of being lesbian.
1 2 3 4 5 6 7 8 9 10

I am aware of the historical context, strengths, and challenges of being bisexual.
1 2 3 4 5 6 7 8 9 10

I am aware of the historical context, strengths, and challenges of being transgendered or queer.
1 2 3 4 5 6 7 8 9 10

I am aware of the historical context, strengths, and challenges of being a person with a visible disability.
1 2 3 4 5 6 7 8 9 10

I am aware of the historical context, strengths, and challenges of being a person with a hidden disability.
1 2 3 4 5 6 7 8 9 10

I am aware of the historical context, strengths, and challenges of being a large person.
1 2 3 4 5 6 7 8 9 10

I am aware of the historical context and stigma associated with mental illness.
1 2 3 4 5 6 7 8 9 10

I am aware of the historical context, strengths, and challenges of being an older adult.
1 2 3 4 5 6 7 8 9 10

I am aware of the historical context, strengths, and challenges of being an adult.
1 2 3 4 5 6 7 8 9 10

I am aware of the historical context, strengths, and challenges of being a parent.
1 2 3 4 5 6 7 8 9 10

I am aware of the historical context, strengths, and challenges of being a young adult (approximately 21 to 30 years old).
1 2 3 4 5 6 7 8 9 10

I am aware of the historical context, strengths, and challenges of being a teen (approximately 13 to 20 years old).
1 2 3 4 5 6 7 8 9 10

I am aware of the historical context, strengths, and challenges of being a young person (12 years old and under).
1 2 3 4 5 6 7 8 9 10

I am aware of the historical context, strengths, and challenges of speaking English as a second language.
1 2 3 4 5 6 7 8 9 10

I attempt to learn languages other than my first language.
1 2 3 4 5 6 7 8 9 10

I am aware of biases and prejudices within myself and my family toward other groups.
1 2 3 4 5 6 7 8 9 10

I refrain from acting on biases and prejudices I have toward other groups.
1 2 3 4 5 6 7 8 9 10

I value relationships with people from cultures different from my own.
1 2 3 4 5 6 7 8 9 10

I am comfortable interacting with people from groups different from my own.
1 2 3 4 5 6 7 8 9 10

I can remember my goodness as a human even when I mistakes in interactions with people from different groups.
1 2 3 4 5 6 7 8 9 10

I take action when I notice that someone is being hurtful or oppressive to another human.
1 2 3 4 5 6 7 8 9 10

I am aware of the impact of sociocultural determinants and poverty on health.
1 2 3 4 5 6 7 8 9 10

I understand that listening to different viewpoints does not mean I agree.
1 2 3 4 5 6 7 8 9 10

**Score: /500**

**Three action steps I can take to further develop my cultural knowledge, awareness, and effectiveness:**

**1.**

**2.**

**3.**

**Additional Comments:**

**Thanks for your time.**



**Figure 9-2.** Cultural Awareness and Action Survey.

Whereas some partnership questions are more relevant for enhancing communication skills with clients/patients and others are more relevant for good interprofessional team communication, most partnership topics will enhance not only professional, but also personal communication skills. Besides potential listening partnership questions, time allotments are recommended for initial listening partnerships (Tables 9-1 through 9-3). Naturally, the learners may increase or decrease the suggested questions and session times as they see appropriate. Discussion/journal prompts are also provided, so that at the end of each listening partnership, pairs will have an opportunity to reflect both orally and in writing about what they have learned from their exchange and to provide feedback to each other on their communication skills. Journaling will offer an opportunity for students to express and clarify their thinking. Murphy (2004) found focused reflection and articulation actually promotes clinical reasoning. Furthermore, Elbow (2000) has documented that journaling can enhance writing skills—another critical form of communication for occupational therapists.

## Listening Partnerships on Enhancing Interpersonal Communication Skills

### *Not Interrupting*

Starting with a 1-minute-each-way exchange of listening is often enough for an initial listening partnership. Because many of us are not used to being given another person's full attention, it may feel quite awkward to have someone listen to us without interrupting. On the other hand, others of us will feel a great sense of relief to finally have someone listen to us without interruption. It may also feel very hard to listen without saying anything for 1 "whole" minute. We may want to say things to reassure the other person or to give him or her advice or to let him or her know we have been through a similar experience so he or she knows that we are indeed listening. As hard as it may be, it is important to simply listen and say nothing in this first listening partnership and to then discuss how it went afterward with your partner. Students report that in this initial listening partnership, they learn to "bite their tongue" before they speak. Increased awareness of the pattern of interrupting in conversations occurs immediately. It will be important to take turns listening not only during the formal listening partnership, but also to be mindful of shared, equal time during discussions as well. Discussions will differ from the partnerships in that no one will be timing the shared exchanges.

#### Practitioner Examples: Not Interrupting

- Bethany found that learning to not interrupt a client is invaluable in every practice setting. For example, a client experiencing agitation, frustration, or anger often redirects him- or herself when someone truly listens to him or her. The previously listed behaviors are demonstrated when a client has a lot to say and does not understand how to express these internal thoughts. Allowing a client to speak freely without interruption often allows the client to guide his or her mind to the real problem.
- While working on an inpatient psychiatric unit, Julie was able to learn firsthand what it was like to have a conversation without even speaking. Julie was working with Mark, who was suffering from drug addiction. Julie introduced herself and explained her role as Mark's occupational therapist and her role in his plan of care, but before Julie could explain any further, Mark began describing his dilemmas and family problems, and before the session was over, Mark had solved his problems without advice. "Well, I guess all I needed to do was just think it all through," said Mark. Even though Julie did not offer professional advice or problem solving, Mark was able to think through his thoughts and actions without being interrupted and took charge of his own problem-solving strategies.
- While working in home care, Claire found meetings with the interprofessional team to be invaluable. Unless she overlapped in a treatment session or did a co-treat with physical therapy or nursing, she felt a certain degree of isolation in home care. Team meetings were most informative when people listened to each other with minimal interrupting so that each perspective could be heard.

### *Nonverbal Communication*

This leads us to the next important skill necessary for effective communication. In addition to learning to not interrupt, one needs to learn effective nonverbal communication (Davis, 2011; Mueller, 2010; Taylor, 2008). Tone of voice, posture, body language, touch, eye contact, and facial expressions often speak louder than our words to the person we are assisting. The more we can show we care about the person who is speaking, the more he or she is likely to open up and share what is on his or her mind and heart. Eye contact is a good place to begin. Offering our eye contact to someone who is sharing what is on his or her mind is one important way to let the person know you are there and you are listening. This can be hard for the beginning practitioner to do—especially if making eye contact was not done much in one's family of origin or cultural group. As many people speak and share what is on their

Table 9-1.

# Interpersonal Communication Skills: Potential Listening Partnership Questions and Discussion/Journal Prompts

| Interpersonal Communication Skills | Potential Listening Partnership Questions (Each speaker decides on which questions he or she would like to answer.) | Discussion/Journal Prompts |
|---|---|---|
| Not interrupting (1 minute each way) | 1. Why do you want to be an occupational therapist?<br>2. What were communication patterns like in your family?<br>3. Are you more comfortable listening or speaking? | • What was it like to listen and be listened to for 1 minute without interrupting?<br>• Discuss if you would have preferred more or less time of for your partner to say anything.<br>• What kind of nonverbal communication did you use? |
| Nonverbal communication (2 minutes each way) | 1. What have you noticed about your nonverbal communication?<br>2. What is it like to make eye contact as a listener or a speaker?<br>3. What have you noticed about the nonverbal communication of others?<br>4. Have there been times when you did not feel listened to because of someone's nonverbal behavior?<br>5. What kinds of nonverbal communication have enabled you to open up to a friend, family member, or professional? | • Was this listening partnership any easier than the first one?<br>• Were you conscious of your nonverbal behavior as you were the listener?<br>• What did your partner do well in terms of nonverbal communication?<br>• Were you able to continue practicing not interrupting? |
| Asking questions: Allowing for silences (5 minutes each way) | 1. What is new and good in your life?<br>2. What is hard or challenging in your life right now? Or where do you need a hand? Tell me more.<br>3. Describe experiences with good and poor communication with health care providers. | • What went well in this listening partnership?<br>• What could have made it even better for both individuals?<br>• Discuss if there was an opportunity to allow for silence. |
| Listening to and validating emotions (5 minutes each way) | 1. What was emotional expression like in your family as your were growing up?<br>2. Were there any gender differences in the expression of emotion?<br>3. What do you currently do when you feel upset? Is there anyone you can turn to if you need to cry?<br>4. What have you noticed when you have had a chance to laugh, cry, shake, or rage? Have you been able to listen to someone when he or she cried hard?<br>5. Which emotions are the easiest for you to listen to?<br>6. Discuss what it is like to maintain mental focus when someone is upset. Can you do this when someone is upset at you?<br>7. What is it like to give and receive validation? | • Would you feel comfortable venting painful emotion with your listening partner?<br>• What do you anticipate it will be like to listen to future clients who share painful emotion?<br>• What positive feedback and suggestions for improvement can you offer your listening partner at this point? |
| Self-awareness and life stories (15 minutes or more each way) | 1. What are some pleasant memories of your childhood?<br>2. What are some pleasant memories of elementary school?<br>3. What did you love to play?<br>4. Who did you like to play with?<br>5. What was difficult or challenging about your childhood within your family, school, or neighborhood? | • What made this partnership go well?<br>• What could have made it even better?<br>• Could you have talked longer?<br>• What was it like to listen for 15 minutes?<br>• Were you able to stay in roles as listener and speaker?<br>• Were you able to allow for silences?<br>• Were there emotions shared? If so, were the listener and speaker comfortable with the emotions shared? |

*(continued)*

Table 9-1 (continued).

## Interpersonal Communication Skills: Potential Listening Partnership Questions and Discussion/Journal Prompts

| Interpersonal Communication Skills | Potential Listening Partnership Questions (Each speaker decides on which questions he or she would like to answer.) | Discussion/Journal Prompts |
|---|---|---|
| Restatement, reflection, clarification, and summaries in listening to life stories (15 minutes or more each way) | 1. What are some pleasant memories of your adolescence?<br>2. What was your favorite activity?<br>3. Talk about your first job<br>4. What was difficult or challenging about being an adolescent within your family, school, church, community, or neighborhood?<br>5. What is/was great/challenging about being a young adult? What is great/challenging about being an adult? | • Was it helpful to continue to discuss life stories?<br>• Did you use restatement, reflection, clarification, summarizing, or validation as you listened to your partner?<br>• If so, did it work well from your partner's point of view?<br>• Discuss times when you felt validated by a listener and why. |
| Redirection (5 minutes each way) | 1. Share a time when you wanted to redirect someone and were or were not successful.<br>2. Do you recall a time when you were redirected in a conversation? What was this like? | • What do you anticipate it will be like to redirect clients in your future practice?<br>• What clients in what types of situations will be harder to redirect? |
| Giving, receiving, and soliciting feedback (10 minutes each way) | 1. Share positive and negative experiences with receiving feedback.<br>2. How can you welcome constructive feedback?<br>3. What strategies can you use to solicit constructive feedback? | • Discuss if you have been videotaped interacting with others and whether or not you are ready to implement this in a listening partnership. |

minds, they themselves do not maintain eye contact, but it is important for them to know that if they do look out, the listener's gaze is available. With practice in listening partnerships, this skill can be obtained very quickly. With that said, it is important to note that for some occupational therapy clients, too much eye contact might interfere with the therapy relationship. This may be true of people from some cultural groups and some people with disabilities. The observant practitioner will pay attention to what works and does not work in offering eye contact.

Beyond eye contact, the facial expression of an effective listener will show approval, respect, and interest toward the person sharing. A relaxed, confident attitude toward the speaker will enable the person to share his or her concerns. Some of us are not aware of what our facial expressions communicate to others. We may convey an attitude of tension and criticism without being aware of this. Seeking feedback on our facial expressions from those who will give us honest feedback on how we are perceived will assist us in refining our nonverbal communication. Again, listening partnerships are a good way to seek feedback and refine our nonverbal communication skills. Lastly, it is essential to recognize that everyone has a unique nonverbal language. One person may make only brief eye contact, so when he or she chooses to hold your gaze it is worth noting. In addition, increased awareness of nonverbal language can be transferred into understanding the body language of group members.

Understanding tone is a crucial element to understanding the person in a listening partnership, as well as any client. Much of the time the word "affect" is used to describe a client's presentation. However, it is essential to know that each person's tone, affect, and emotional state are ever changing. When someone is speaking, it is essential to listen to the tone embedded within his or her words. At times, people's words may not match their affect. Ask yourself why that may be. Specific medications often mask emotion or cause emotional liability. Being aware of potential reasons why a person's words are not matching his or her demeanor may help guide practitioners in a direction of more holistic and encompassing therapy.

### Practitioner Examples: Effective Nonverbal Communication

- Marie was working with a client with dementia who was a fluent speaker of English, but began to speak her first language, Italian. Although Marie did not understand Italian, the more she offered her

Table 9-2.

## Culturally Responsive Communication: Potential Listening Partnership Questions and Discussion/Journal Prompts

| Culturally Responsive Communication | Potential Listening Partnership Questions (Each speaker decides on which questions he or she would like to answer.) | Discussion/Journal Prompts |
|---|---|---|
| The Journey toward cultural competence | 1. Were you ever a minority in your neighborhood, school, church, or social situation as you were growing up? If so, what was this like?<br>2. Were there ever times that you felt mistreated as a member of a particular group? What was this like? | • What was it like to dialogue about diversity?<br>• How much time did your need for this partnership?<br>• Discuss times that you made friends with someone from a different ethnic, cultural, or religious group. |
| Gender | 1. What is great about being male/female?<br>2. What is challenging about being male/female?<br>3. What do you not like about your own gender?<br>4. When have you stood up to sex oppression?<br>5. When have you been an effective ally to the other sex? | • What was it like to dialogue about gender?<br>• Were you able to listen to your partner without interrupting?<br>• What would it be like to ask these questions of someone of the other gender who is not a listening partner? |
| Sex and sexual orientation | 1. While you were growing up, what attitudes were communicated to you about sex by family, clergy, teachers, and friends? Were you able to talk openly with anyone?<br>2. Share your experiences with people who are gay, lesbian, bisexual, transgendered, and/or queer.<br>3. If you feel comfortable doing so, talk about your own sex and sexual identity. What is great and what has been hard? | • If you have a friend who is gay, lesbian, bisexual, transgendered, or queer, what would it be like to ask him or her what it has been like to be his or her identity?<br>• What do you and your listening partner appreciate about each other? |
| Disability | 1. Talk about a disability you currently have or an accident, injury, or disability you had in the past, describing both positive and challenging aspects to your situation.<br>2. Share all your experiences, both positive and challenging, with people with disabilities. | • What disability would be the hardest for you to have or to work with and why?<br>• Have you noticed any students with disabilities on your campus? What would it be like to reach out to this person or people? |
| Oppression and size | 1. What do you appreciate about your own body?<br>2. Share thoughts about how to interrupt oppression based on size. | • Discuss if large women and men feel comfortable talking with you about their oppression.<br>• What would help you appreciate your own body more? |
| Age differences | 1. Have you ever been mistreated for being a particular age?<br>2. Talk about the age group you have the hardest time relating to and share experiences with that group.<br>3. What concerns you about growing older?<br>4. How would you like to be treated as an elder? | • Would you like to have a regular listening partner at this point?<br>• What have you noticed about yourself as a listener and talker now that you have engaged in many listening partnerships? |
| Religion and spirituality | 1. Describe your religious/spiritual heritage and current practices.<br>2. What are the strengths of your religious heritage and what are any challenges or hardships that are part of your religious/spiritual background?<br>3. What has it been like to develop relationships from people of other religious/spiritual backgrounds? | • What do you want to know about other religions or spiritual practices? |

(continued)

Table 9-2 (continued).

**Culturally Responsive Communication: Potential Listening Partnership Questions and Discussion/Journal Prompts**

| Culturally Responsive Communication | Potential Listening Partnership Questions (Each speaker decides on which questions he or she would like to answer.) | Discussion/Journal Prompts |
|---|---|---|
| Ethnicity and culture | 1. What is your cultural/ethnic background?<br>2. Why did you or your ancestors come to the United States?<br>3. What are you proud of and what are challenges related to your cultural heritage?<br>4. What makes you proud of your nation of origin and how would you like your nation of origin to be different? | • Discuss any changes you have noted in your listening partnerships and how they could be improved on. |
| Classism | 1. Share what you feel comfortable sharing about your parents' educational level and their work.<br>2. Did your family have enough, more than enough, or less than enough when you were growing up? Did this change?<br>3. What are the strengths and challenges associated with your class background?<br>4. Have you ever encountered anti-Semitism? If so, talk about it. Did you stand up against it or did anyone else? What do you remember about the Holocaust and the economic scapegoating of Jews? | • What was it like to talk about class background?<br>• Were there taboos in your family regarding discussion of money and class? |
| Racism | 1. How has racism affected you?<br>2. What is your earliest memory of noticing someone with a skin color other than yours?<br>3. Scan all your memories of racial groups different from your own (Native Americans, Asians, Latinos/Latinas, Arabs, People of African Heritage, People of European Heritage, etc.).<br>4. Talk about a time that you witnessed racism. Did you stand up against racism? If so, what was it like? If not, what held you back from taking a stand against racism when you witnessed it? | • What conditions enable you to talk freely about racism?<br>• What has it been like, overall, to engage in listening partnerships on diversity? |
| Interpreters, cultural brokers, and health literacy | 1. Share any experiences you have had communicating with people who do not speak your first language. | • Discuss experiences using interpreters and cultural brokers and what you know about cultural literacy. |

eye contact and a warm facial expression, the more animated her client became. Family reported they hadn't seen that level of animation in a long time. Eventually, she grabbed Marie's arm and was ready to walk again. She hadn't walked without her walker in many weeks. Marie attributes her client's progress to her skilled nonverbal communication.

- Tillie worked with a Sudanese woman who began to share that she had lost nine children in the war in her country. She found that simply by leaning in and showing her caring nonverbally, the woman began to speak in her mother tongue and started to sob about her loss. Tillie found that it didn't matter that she didn't understand the words her client spoke, she just listened. Her client was then ready to engage in therapy.

## Asking Questions: Allowing for Silences

Beyond learning not to interrupt and learning to provide effective nonverbal communication, the artful communicator learns to ask relevant questions to draw out the speaker. Robinson and Heritage (2006) found

Table 9-3.

## Intra- and Interprofessional Teamwork, Technology, and Other Communication Challenges: Potential Listening Partnership Questions and Discussion/Journal Prompts

| Interprofessional Teamwork, Technology, and Other Communication Challenges | Potential Listening Partnership Questions (Each speaker decides on which questions he or she would like to answer.) | Discussion/Journal Prompts |
|---|---|---|
| Intra- and interprofesssional teamwork | 1. Talk about your experiences on teams. What has made teams function poorly or well?<br>2. Talk about any interprofessional experiences you have had. | • Discuss what you have done or can do to ensure teams you are on function well.<br>• Discuss what questions you have about the roles and responsibilities of other health care professionals and how you will learn about other professions. |
| Assertiveness, conflict resolution, and teamwork | 1. Are you able to assert yourself? Do you tend be passive and quiet or aggressive in situations of conflict?<br>2. How was conflict handled in your family as you were growing up?<br>3. Talk about times when you successfully handled conflict.<br>4. What is challenging for you in situations of conflict? How would you like to handle conflict differently? | • Discuss any goals you might have regarding assertive communication.<br>• Discuss a conflict you did not handle well and identify how you might handle it differently now.<br>• Discuss the potential role of taking turns listening to resolve conflict. |
| Other challenging communication | 1. Describe any communication challenges you have faced (aggression, power dilemmas, resistance, avoidance, etc.).<br>2. What did you do that was effective and what could you have done differently? | • Who can you turn to for support when you encounter a communication challenge?<br>• What has it been like to offer support to a peer around communication challenges? |
| Technology and health care communication | 1. How have technology and social media enhanced your interpersonal communication?<br>2. Discuss whether technology and social media have interfered with interpersonal communication.<br>3. How has technology enhanced or detracted from professional communication? | • Discuss your vision for how technology can further enhance professional communication.<br>• What is the longest time you have gone without the use of technology or social media and what was this like? What do you think about taking breaks from technology? |

that physicians who began with open-ended general inquires—"What can I do for you today?" or "Tell me what going on" compared with physicians who initiated visits with close-ended requests for confirmation of symptoms or conditions were more positively evaluated by their clients in the affective-relational dimension of communication. The literature on motivational interviewing emphasizes the skillful use of open-ended questions, yet also identifies a place for closed-ended questions (Rollnick, Miller, & Butler, 2008). A good open-ended question to begin listening partnerships with is "What is new and good?" Many of us go through much of our lives with our attention on our worries and frustrations rather than on what is going well in our lives. It is useful to take a few moments to notice what is going well in our lives. There may be times when it is hard to come up with something new and good in our lives, yet the client listener will give the speaker time to think about something that is new and good. Equally important follow-up questions to "What is new and good?" are "What is upsetting or challenging in your life?" or "Where do you need a hand?" A flexible communicator may notice that some people are more responsive to being asked to share a "rose and thorn"—a rose being something going well and a thorn being something challenging, or similarly a "joy and a concern."

As we try out these questions, we may note the speaker pauses or runs out of things to say. Many beginning listeners have a hard time allowing for silences and feel compelled to say something when a speaker pauses. In fact, when we allow for silences, the person talking often has more to say with no more prompting than simply having a listener at hand who can stay relaxed around silences. Much "magic" occurs around grief and loss related to disability when the practitioner can pause for silence. The client can fill the space with what weighs heavily on him or her. After allowing for a few seconds of silence, if the speaker is struggling with what else to say, the simple phrase, "Tell me more" or "What else?" may be all that the speaker needs to hear to continue talking about what is on his or her mind.

### Practitioner Example: Allowing for Silences

- I was working in an outpatient pediatric clinic and had been treating a young boy, Lucas, for gravitational insecurity. We had been working together for a few weeks when I had the opportunity to consult with both his mother and father after a treatment session. I simply asked, "How are things going?" At first, their responses were broad, but as I allowed for silence, Lucas's parents began to express new concerns they had not yet shared with me. I learned that Lucas had only slept in his own bed a handful of times throughout his life—which was tiresome and frustrating for both him and his parents. I collaborated with the family to incorporate this new information into a revised plan of care.

## *Listening to and Validating Emotions*

As listening partners feel increasingly comfortable with each other, more and more emotions may be shared. Emotions are neither good nor bad; they just are. However, it has been found that expression of emotions can decrease stress and tension and foster reevaluation of one's situation. Crying can release grief and depression; laughter can release fear, tension, and embarrassment; yawning can release physical tension and exhaustion; trembling and shaking can release fear; and raging can release anger and indignation (Jackins, 1981).

Despite the emotional healing and reevaluations that can occur with emotional release, other than young children, most humans are inhibited from emotional expression. Although this varies among different cultural groups, many of us grew up in households where emotions were not welcome or where only certain emotions were allowed. In some families, it was acceptable for women to show grief and sadness and for men to show their anger. Others of us learned to only express our emotions privately, and others grew up in families where they were encouraged to express a whole range of emotion. For occupational therapy practitioners to be effective with a wide range of clients, it is important for them to be comfortable listening to a wide range of emotional expression. In addition, they may find it helpful to vent to a good listener so they can think more flexibly about each new situation they are in.

As we listen to clients, patients, and colleagues share emotions, validation can be very important. When it seems appropriate, letting a person know that it is not only "okay" to vent, but also that it will help him or her think through his or her situation more clearly is often helpful. Further validation can be offered with statements such as, "That sounds awful" or "I am sorry you had to experience…" Naturally, there will be other times when what is most important is assisting someone in getting his or her attention off his or her feelings or his or her distresses. This will be discussed further in the section on redirection.

### Practitioner Examples: Listening to and Validating Emotions

- Marie was assisting a gentleman with dementia in transitioning to a new residence. He had incontinence and started to cry and stated, "I am so embarrassed that I wet my pants in front of you." Marie shared that it was not his fault and he cried more. She reassured him that it is okay to cry, that this is a big change for him.
- Jen was working in a skilled nursing facility with Rachel, a 78-year-old woman who was experiencing episodes of incontinence. Rachel was embarrassed by these episodes and cried each time they occurred. Jen sat by Rachel's side and said, "I am here to help. This is my job. Let's try to think of some strategies to help decrease these episodes. I know I am not a doctor but I know of a few tricks to help. I can't tell you that I understand, but let me try." From then, Rachel was open to strategies and techniques to assist with the episodes. Jen listened to Rachel's emotions, which were affecting and limiting her ability to participate in rehab.
- Ali was conducting an evaluation in response to a referral for a 4-year-old girl, Mila, with signs of sensory integration difficulties and resistance to transitions; consequently, Mila had some challenging behaviors. She used a variety of evaluation tools and after an hour was able to draw preliminary conclusions about her new client. Ali discussed the session with Mila's mother and invited her to express any questions or concerns. Mila's mother began to share her anxiety and exasperation with the situation. As she continued to speak, she became more visually

frustrated. Ali validated her emotions and assured her that occupational therapy could help Mila engage with her environment and transition appropriately.

- Claire noticed that one of her coworkers, Sal, looked withdrawn and distressed. She approached Sal and asked if she was all right and Sal began to cry as she shared that she and her husband had decided to get a divorce. Claire expressed that she could only imagine how hard this was for Sal and offered her listening ear for several minutes. After Sal vented for a few minutes, Claire joked around with her to help her get her attention off her distress so they both could get back to work.

These vignettes illustrate how listening to the emotions of both clients and coworkers can be helpful. When practitioners listen to clients' emotions, they can dig deeper into treatment plans that truly will make a difference in each individual's life. Emotions allow practitioners to see a person at a moment where he or she needs assistance and we as practitioners need to provide this help. Taking into consideration job and productivity demands, when one can take a few minutes to listen to the emotions of our coworkers or interprofessional team members, we may serve to improve the quality of care they can offer.

## *Self-Awareness and Life Stories*

Occupational therapy practitioners generally listen to pieces of our client's life story, yet on some occasions we listen to long narratives about the difficulties of our client's life (Kielhofner, 2008). To listen well to life stories, it helps to first have opportunities to share and reflect upon our own life story (Davis, 2011). Because our lives are filled with both wonderful experiences and many hardships, it may only feel safe to share certain pieces of our life story with certain people. Each person gets to choose what he or she feels safe sharing with whom. A good way to begin to share life stories is to reflect on positive memories from childhood first. As increased safety is created within listening partnerships, it will be useful to share some of the things that were hard when we were young. The more relaxed our listening partner is in listening to the hardships we have endured, the more we will be able to share with him or her. Additionally, the more our listening partner can listen to a range of emotional experiences, the more we will feel comfortable sharing the difficulties we have faced. Lastly, it is important to be aware that everyone has more depth than meets the eye. No one ever fully knows the life or unique experiences of to whom he or she is speaking. Practitioners should understand and evaluate their own personal limits so that they can be prepared to hear things that are distressing.

### Practitioner Examples: Listening to Life Stories

- Claire was working in home care and asked her client to share a little of her life history. Her client, in her 90s, began, "When I was born in 1924, and my parents owned a farm..." Claire knew she had to think fast. She did not have time to hear her client's full life story, so she validated several of her memories and then asked her to share more about her current situation and her current goals.
- When working on an inpatient psychiatry unit, Linda, an occupational therapy practitioner, approached one of her clients who rarely spoke and appeared shaken. When asked about what was bothering her, her client proceeded to tell her fragments of her life story—details of the unspeakable horrors done unto her by her ex-husband.

As illustrated in each of these practice examples, life stories can come out in unexpected ways. When asking a question, even a simple one, occupational therapy practitioners need to be prepared for how to address unexpected challenges or emotional releases by clients. Claire quickly realized she needed to skillfully use redirection after validating her older client's memories. As Linda's situation illustrates, an occupational therapy practitioner may be the first individual a survivor of abuse feels comfortable disclosing this aspect of her life history. Recommendations for seeking support after listening to a client's trauma are becoming increasingly noted in the field of social work and is relevant for occupational therapy practitioners (Bell, Kulkarni, & Dalton, 2003).

## *Restatement, Reflection, Clarification, and Summaries in Listening to Life Stories*

In addition to learning to ask relevant questions, the skilled communicator offers restatement, reflection, clarification, and summaries so the listener knows he or she is being listened to and to validate his or her experiences (Davis, 2011; Rollnick et al., 2008). Restatement, or stating back almost exactly what the speaker has said, is used when the listener wants the speaker to know that a very important piece of information he or she shared has been clearly heard. It is often used as a question so the client can report whether or not the listener heard exactly what was being communicated. For example, one out of many events a client shared about his or her adolescence may have been, "Things were so bad that I ran away from home." Using restatement, the listener might say, "Things were that bad at home that you ran away?" This invites the speaker to confirm the information and to say more. Many of us use restatement without even thinking about it in our everyday conversations. Naturally, restatement can be overused, and if so, it can be annoying to anyone speaking. The beginning listener will want to begin to notice when he or she uses restatement in everyday interactions, as well as listening partnerships, and evaluate its effectiveness.

A more complex skill is reflective listening. In reflective listening,the listener listens not only to the content being shared, but also for the emotions that underlie that content (Davis, 2011; Rollnick et al., 2008). This requires the listener be very attentive to not only what a person is sharing verbally, but also to what is being shared nonverbally. Nonverbal communication, including tone of voice, posture, facial expression, and eye contact, gives us great insight into what a person might be feeling. When our speaker pauses, it may be helpful to reflect back to him or her both the content of what he or she said and the emotions that we detected. For example, if in sharing her life story, our listening partner looks sad and discloses she felt left out in high school because she did not make the cheerleading squad, you might reflect this back by saying, "It sounds like it was really hard for you when you didn't make the cheerleading squad."

Reflection such as this may invite an outpouring of even more emotion than our partner had previously shared. The beginning listener often refrains from such reflective questions exactly for this reason. He or she knows his or her speaker will feel more emotion if such a statement is made. Yet, this type of statement conveys a real empathy for what our partner has experienced and may deepen the trust within the listening partnership. Furthermore, as was noted earlier, despite all the societal taboos on crying, release of old grief and resentments can clear up our thinking and compel our lives forward in a positive direction (Jackins, 1981).

Natural follow-ups to the listening skill of reflection are clarification and summarization. As we listen closely to our listening partner, we may notice he or she has shared a great deal of information. Clarification and summarizing involve identifying the key issues the individual has expressed and focusing the individual on what is most important or most significant (Davis, 2011; Rollnick et al., 2008). Often, there will be a ring in the voice of the speaker as they discuss their most significant experiences. The skilled listener listens for this "ring" and refers back to the content that generated the "ring" for clarification and more information. Restatement, reflection, clarification, and summarizing can each be a powerful form of validation as a patient/client or peer shares pieces of his or her life story and experiences.

### Practitioner Example: Restatement, Reflection, Clarification, and Summaries in Listening to Life Stories

- Clarice was in the hospital for a decompressive laminectomy surgery. She was being evaluated by her occupational therapy practitioner, Ali, for functional mobility and to determine the most appropriate setting for her upon discharge from acute care. This type of evaluation was typically straightforward and brief. As Ali and Clarice discussed her history, Clarice became weepy-eyed and emotional. Clarice began sharing with Ali an extensive life story—how she had been battling cancer for 10 years, her consequential deteriorated health, and how her medical complications weighed on her family. Ali spent over an hour at Clarice's bedside listening to her story. Having no medical complications, children, or comparable experience of her own, Ali could only listen, reflect, and clarify what Clarice was sharing with her. Ali could see the comfort on Clarice's face from sharing her story and knowing she was heard. It wasn't mobility training Clarice needed at that moment, but a caring human presence to truly listen to her.

## Redirection

Practitioners must build rapport with their clients, develop individualized plans of care, and carry out treatment plans while acting in accordance with heavy caseloads demands, productivity requirements, and time constraints. As was noted in the section on life stories, it is befitting for practitioners to develop tactful and tasteful methods for redirecting or concluding conversations with clients at appropriate times (Taylor, 2008). This may mean interrupting a client/patient while he or she shares his or her experiences, getting a distracted client to focus on therapy tasks at hand, or it may mean assisting a client in getting his or her attention off his or her distress.

It requires assertiveness on the part of the practitioner to redirect a client. Workload demands necessitate excellent time management and assertiveness skills of all health practitioners. It can be difficult to convey caring for clients/patients in the context of high productivity demands, yet practitioners can reach for artful and caring ways to redirect clients when time is up or it is time for a new task. Additionally, the practitioner can help a client get his or her attention off his or her distress by asking questions such as what did you have for breakfast today, what is your favorite color, stating a phone number backward, notice objects of a particular color in the room, or asking what someone is looking forward to.

### Practitioner Examples: Redirection

- Ali describes her first fieldwork rotation in an acute care setting—it was a fast-paced environment that required prioritization and time management skills:

  > I quickly learned that my friendly disposition made it difficult to end conversations once they progressed from clinical relevance to being sociable. For me, one of the most effective methods to politely end a conversation was to say, "Thank you for your time today Mrs. Smith. I've enjoyed chatting with you, but unfortunately, I have some other business to attend to." My clients appreciated the few minutes of extra time and understood I had other responsibilities.

- Julie was working in a skilled nursing facility when she met John, a 43-year-old man with a traumatic brain injury from a fall as well as a right cerebral vascular accident resulting in left hemiparesis. John wanted to tell Julie his life story when he saw her each day. Julie quickly learned that this gentleman needed to be redirected to continue his skilled treatment session. Social cues were difficult for John to understand secondary to his brain injury and stroke, but Julie was able to redirect John by looking him in the eye and explaining how important it was to focus on the task at hand. Julie stated that "Each time we complete an activity together, I want you to tell me one aspect of your life." John agreed and was able to continue with therapy.

## *Giving, Receiving, and Soliciting Feedback*

The following beautiful story on giving feedback was found on the Internet Cello Society Forum:

> ### Pablo Casals (1876-1973) Finding the Good to Praise
>
> Pablo Casals, one of the greatest cellists of all time, revolutionized cello technique, thrilled millions of music lovers, dozens of composers to write works for his instrument, and composed for the cello himself. However, his supreme contribution may be in the thousands of students he inspired.
>
> Casals loved his students. In an age when critics were looking for one wrong note on which to condemn a young performer, Casals looked for the good in cellists under his tutelage. An example was Gregor Piatigorsky (1903-1976) who would in time become one of the great cello master performers. As a young man, Piatigorsky was eager to play for the renowned Casals, but when the opportunity arrived, he unfortunately turned into a bundle of nerves. Botching every movement, he doggedly plowed through works of Bach, Beethoven, and Schumann—knowing he disgraced himself.
>
> But no. To Piatigorsky's amazement, at the end of the last piece, Casals burst into applause and praise. He even leaned over and embraced the confused Piatigorsky, who knew that he had done poorly. How could this great man stoop to such patronizing praise?
>
> In time, Piatigorsky's talents were evident to all, and as a fellow world-class performer, he developed a friendship with Casals. One night after the two had play duets for hours, Piatigorsky mustered the courage to confront Casals about that "undeserved praise" of long ago.
>
> Casals hadn't forgotten the private performance, and he responded intensely: He quickly grabbed his cello and played a phrase from the very Beethoven sonata that Piatigorsky had blundered through. "Listen!" he shouted. "Didn't you play this fingering? It was novel to me . . . It was good ... and here, didn't you attack that passage with up-bow, like this?" On and on he went, recalling the good in Piatigorsky's "inadequate" presentation. He concluded with words that Piatigorsky never forgot: "And for the rest, leave it to the ignorant and stupid who judge by counting only the faults. I can be grateful, and so must you be, for even one note, one wonderful phrase."
>
> Casals words haunt me. How easy to see what's wrong rather than what's right or worthy of praise. (The Apostle) Paul tells us to think about what is excellent, admirable, or praiseworthy. I suggest we take that a step further and talk about talents or actions or qualities that meet those qualifications.
>
> Almost anyone can tell someone what he's doing wrong, rather than what he's doing right. I do this all too often myself—with colleagues, with students, with my children, even with my wife. How much better life would be if I could learn the secret of Pablo Casals—the ability to inspire others by telling them the truth about what they do well. (Kavanaugh, 1995, pp. 21-22)

It is human to be challenged with giving, receiving, and soliciting feedback. This story about Pablo Casals offers insight into the value of positive feedback. Psychologists have determined that although human lives tend to be filled with more positive than negative events, unless we have worked on the mental discipline of focusing on the positive, the human mind gravitates toward negative concerns (Rozin & Royzman, 2001). Thus, for many of us, receiving feedback with any hint of criticism can weigh heavy on our hearts and minds. With this in mind, it is often helpful to balance positive with negative feedback with a greater emphasis on what a person has done well rather than areas for improvement.

In situations where one is receiving critical feedback that is not balanced with what one has done well, there may be an opportunity to request positive feedback in addition to negative feedback. This requires assertiveness on the part of the individual soliciting feedback as well as a good assessment of whether or not it makes sense in that situation to do so. There are occasions where it is important to just accept critical feedback with a thank you. This is easier said than done, but becomes easier with practice. Having a place to vent to someone other than the person giving critical feedback can be extremely useful in clarifying one's mind about next steps. It may make sense to let a supervisor, peer, or client know that you can integrate feedback better when it is balanced with positives and negatives.

### Practitioner Example: Giving, Receiving, and Soliciting Feedback

- Jordon was a new practitioner working in physical rehabilitation. As a single mother, she had been struggling more than usual with balancing work demands with parenting her 4-year-old daughter because her daughter recently had become ill. After her first 2 weeks of work, Jordon's supervisor called her into her office to let her know that her documentation was not as timely as it needed to be. Jordon was upset because this was the first feedback of any kind she had received from her supervisor. She worked very hard to be the best practitioner she could be and had received much praise from the interprofessional team and her clients. Nonetheless, she could see her supervisor's point. She apologized for not getting her documentation in on time and thanked her supervisor for the feedback stating she would get it in on time in the future. She then let her supervisor know that she worked hard and it would be helpful to hear some positive feedback on her work as well.

It took assertiveness for Jordon to request some positive feedback from her supervisor. Some supervisors will be able to respond to such a request; others will not. Even if her supervisor cannot meet Jordon's request for a balance between positive and negative feedback, Jordon may feel better about herself knowing she did ask for acknowledgment of what she does well. Assertiveness and conflict resolution will be further addressed later in this chapter.

## Listening Partnerships for Culturally Responsive Communication

### *The Journey Toward Cultural Competence*

As humans, we are much more alike than we are different. Yet the societies that we live in tend to emphasize our differences in the areas of gender, race, class, culture, religion, physical ability/disability, country or origin, languages, body size, sexual orientation, etc. (Rothenberg, 1998; Royeen & Crabtree, 2006). All of us have intersecting identities—we may be African heritage, a female lawyer, and have a physical disability, or a be a working class, Jewish man who is truck driver. Each identity is significant and the intersection of identities is also significant. The reader is referred to the work of Balcazar, Suarez-Balcazar, Taylor-Ritzler, and Keys (2010) for a thorough analysis of the nexus of race, culture, and disability in rehabilitation.

Although some of us may feel proud of our different identities, many of us are mistreated and made to feel badly about our differences through prejudice, discrimination, social conditioning, and oppression. Jackins (1997) defines oppression as, "the systematic mistreatment of a group of people by the society and/or by another group of people who serve as agents of the society, with the mistreatment encouraged or enforced by society and its culture" (p. 151). Internalized oppression occurs when groups of oppressed people begin to believe the negative messages, lies, and misinformation the society has placed on them. They invalidate not only themselves, but other members of their group (Kauffman & New, 2004). This process, also called *horizontal violence*, has received significant attention in the nursing field to address the phenomenon of nurses mistreating other nurses (St-Pierre & Holmes, 2008).

As listening partners begin to feel comfortable with each other, they will find it useful to explore diversity within themselves. In doing so, they can look at both what has been positive about being a member of a particular group and what has been challenging about being a member of a particular group. Ultimately, by engaging in this type of self-examination with a supportive listener, they can heal from any mistreatment they have endured as members of different groups and take fuller pride in all aspects of themselves (Brown & Mazza, 1997). In addition, as a number of scholars have pointed out, engaging in this type of self-reflection is an important step on the journey of becoming a culturally competent practitioner (Black & Wells, 2007; Campinha-Bacote, 2011). Dean (2001) reminds us that becoming culturally competent truly is a journey and exposes the myth that cultural competence is ever achieved.

Campinha-Bacote (2011) and Black and Wells (2007) emphasize that one cannot be responsive and sensitive to diversity in others if one has not looked at diversity within oneself. Therefore, the next several listening partnerships will give the reader many opportunities to explore diversity within themselves and learn about diversity within their peers. Additionally, as Campinha-Bacote (2011) suggests, encounters with people from different groups greatly breaks down barriers that exist between groups. Thus, the reader is encouraged to explore how to facilitate encounters and use attentive listening with people from many different groups to build relationships. Finally, because knowledge gathering is an essential component of cultural competence, many sources are cited in this chapter for additional information on human diversity.

## Gender

When men and women begin to talk about gender in listening partnerships, they often have quite a bit to say on the subject. It can be challenging in listening partnerships to listen without sharing our experiences. An important question for the listener to always consider is, "Is what I am saying helping my partner to continue to do most of the talking?" The beauty of listening partnerships is that both individuals agree to take turns listening to one another. Knowing you will have a turn to be heard enables many a beginner listener to refrain from sharing his or her life story while listening to the life story of another. Yet the question always arises, might it not be helpful for me to share my life story with the person I am listening to while I am listening? The answer is "sometimes." Sometimes when we are listening to someone share his or her life story, it reminds us of similar experiences of our own. We feel eager to let the speaker know that we have been through something similar. On occasion, by sharing a little bit about our experience that is similar to the person speaking, we enable him or her to keep sharing about his or her experience. What we need to be mindful of is not turning this into our own turn. Again, knowing that we will get our chance when our listening partner has finished telling his or her story can enable us to wait for our turn. Another important fact to keep in mind is listening does not mean agreement. We can listen to someone for a long time and not agree with what he or she is saying.

The forces of gender oppression attempt to ascribe rigid roles to both men and women (Froehlich, Hamlin, Loukas, & MacRae, 1992). Both groups are mistreated by gender oppression, but in different ways. Some of the key features of women's oppression include the assumption that women are less intelligent or less capable than men, lower pay for equal work (Froehlich, 2005; MacRae, 2005), preoccupation with appearance, lack of pay or recognition for the significant work of mothering (Crittenden, 2001, Pierce & Frank, 1992; Primeau, 1992), violence and sexual abuse, limited access to positions of influence within businesses and governments, discrediting for being too emotional, and the assumption that mothering and care giving are our ultimate contributions.

The society has only recently begun to recognize that men are also oppressed—not by women but by society as a whole (Jackins, 1999). Socialization to be violent and competitive begins early in the lives of boys within the family, and it is reinforced in the media. At an early age, boys learn they may be called upon to kill other men for their country. In preparation for this role, boys are systematically humiliated when they show their grief or tenderness, causing them to be hardened early. Men are also socialized to believe they can only have closeness with one significant partner and that sex is the ultimate closeness. Boredom and substance use are more prevalent among men (Corvinelli, 2005). Lastly, the worker role weighs heavily on men. Mossakowski (2009) found that the association between being out of the work force and depressive symptoms was stronger for men than women.

Even though individual families work hard to break this conditioning for men and women, society continues to oppress us in these ways. As was mentioned previously, one of the worst consequences of oppression is internalized oppression. Once we internalize gender conditioning about ourselves, we oppress ourselves and members of our own group.

Listening partnerships offer an opportunity to free ourselves from internalized oppression—especially when we can first share about our experiences with someone from a similar background (i.e., women with women and men with men). By listening well to each other's experience, we can challenge and dispel the internalization of oppression. After we have shared with someone from a similar background, it is often rich and rewarding to hear the perspective from other groups. Additionally, a number of occupational therapy scholars offer rich readings on the experiences of men and women in occupational therapy (Flinn, Sanders, Yen, Sommerich, & Lavender, 2013; Javaherian, Krabacher, Andriacco, & German, 2007; Palmadottir, 2009; Peloquin & Ciro, 2013; Sterling & Nayar, 2013).

### Practitioner Examples: Communicating With Awareness and Sensitivity to Gender

- Ali was working in a hospital when she had a new evaluation on the intensive care unit. She approached the darkened room, knocked on the door, and quietly entered the room. Her new client, Li, was laying in bed with a battered, swollen face and bruised arms, with blood still under her fingernails. According to Li's chart, her live-in boyfriend beat her up the night before after having one too many drinks. Li suffered bruises, broken bones, and displaced teeth. The first session was composed mainly of an interview and test of standing tolerance. Li was very honest with her practitioner and disclosed intimate details about the past night's events and her relationship with her abuser. Li was born and raised in China and had come to the states for college. She was a full-time student and lived with her boyfriend, unbeknownst to her family back home. Li confessed that this was not the first time her boyfriend abused her. She refused to call her parents or friends in the area for help and planned on returning to her apartment after discharge. Ali struggled with her own convictions that Li needed additional help and should leave her abusive relationship. However, Ali was aware that Li's situation had complexities that she did not fully understand and that Li had the right to autonomy and the freedom to make her own choices. Ali could only offer herself as a resource and work with the interprofessional team in making appropriate referrals for support around domestic violence.

- Claudette, an 86-year-old French Canadian Catholic woman, was being seen in her home after a mild stroke. Her occupational therapy practitioner noted that she was extremely modest in allowing assistance with self-care. Across several occupational therapy visits, Claudette discussed the recent loss of her husband and shared that he had been abusive physically and sexually to her and that she had been sexually abused as a child. She also shared proudly that one night when he husband was very drunk, she shaved a cross on his chest, When he awoke, he thought it was a sign from God and the drinking and abuse stopped for a while.

Men are not inherently dominating, but boys learn at an early age that it will be their job to dominate and control women. Although many men resist the pull to reenact violence they endured as boys, there is a tendency to reenact childhood violence on intimate partners as adults (Stagg et al., 2003; Whitfield, Anda, Dube, & Felitti, 2003). The reader is referred to the work of Javaherian, Krabacher, Andriacco, and German (2007) and *Occupational Therapy Services for Individuals Who Have Experienced Domestic Violence* (American Occupational Therapy Association [AOTA], 2011b) for more guidance on the occupational therapy role in addressing the complexities of domestic violence.

## Sexual and Gender Diversity

Regardless of one's sexual orientation, we all grow up with some confusions and embarrassments about sex and sexuality. In attempting to communicate with us about sex when we were young, family members, clergy, and teachers did their best to share helpful information, but generally also shared some embarrassment, awkwardness, and perhaps even misinformation. Because sexuality is a part of life many occupational therapy practitioners address in their interventions with clients, it is important to work toward increasing comfort with the subject so open communication can occur.

In addition, increased comfort with the subject of human sexuality will most likely increase one's comfort in discussing sexual orientation. A number of occupational therapy practitioners have identified that homophobia is a barrier to gay, lesbian, bisexual, transgendered, and queer (GLBTQ) individuals in receiving optimum occupational therapy services (Beagan et al., 2013; Jackson, 2000; Kelly, 2000; Kingsley & Molineux, 2000). Although much progress has been made in eliminating gay oppression (e.g., the recent legalization of gay marriage in the United States), suicide among gay, lesbian, and bisexual adolescents continues to be a public health concern (Kitts, 2005). Because gay oppression continues to threaten the security of people who are GLBTQ, many choose not to be "out" about their sexual identity in their communities. Therefore, as occupational therapy practitioners, it is important for heterosexuals not to make assumptions about the sexual orientation of people with whom they are interacting.

Listening partnerships between two individuals who are GLBTQ can provide a safe place for venting about and discrimination or hurtful experiences. Internalized oppression, which places divisions between them can be challenged. It will be useful for heterosexual people to get together with other heterosexual people to talk about all their experiences with individuals who are GLBTQ so they are less awkward in relating to them. As increased safety is gained, it will be richly rewarding for people who are GLBTQ to be able to share about their experiences with heterosexuals and for heterosexuals to be strong allies for individuals who are GLBTQ in combating gay oppression.

### Practitioner Examples: Communicating With Awareness and Sensitivity to Sexual and Gender Diversity

- Sarah was working on an inpatient psychiatric unit when she met Alex, a transgendered female. Alex was screaming and yelling at the nursing staff and was very difficult to redirect. Sarah was nervous to begin the initial evaluation with Alex so she approached her gently. Alex agreed to speak with Sarah in a private room. Alex began to cry when Sarah asked why she was so upset. Alex cried out that she was "male trapped in a female's body." Alex stated that she wanted to have a baby before she became a man, but no one around her supported her decision. Sarah decided to help Alex make a pros and cons list to attempt to help Alex with this decision. When Alex began sobbing again, Sarah touched Alex's hand, knowing that no contact was supposed to be made between practitioner and client on the psychiatric unit but Sarah knew that a simple touch could mean a world of difference to Alex. When Alex wiped her tears and looked at Sarah and said "Thanks," Sarah knew she had made the right decision.

- Larry, a 36-year-old gay man, was dying of AIDS. Gary shared with Claire, his occupational therapist, that his biggest wish was for his family to accept his partner, but they never did accept him. In the end, Larry's family also did not honor Larry's wishes for his partner to inherit any of his belongings. His occupational therapist noted that now that gay marriage is legal in Maine, other people who are GLBTQ will have greater protections than Larry did.

Sarah's story, shared in Chapter 10 on therapeutic use of self, is repeated here because of the sensitivity Sarah demonstrated in communicating with her transgendered client. Claire, obviously, also created a great deal of safety for Larry to open up about his struggles as a gay man.

## *Disability*

Some studies have shown that occupational therapy practitioners tend to have positive attitudes toward people with disabilities, yet there is still room for improvement (Coffey, 2001; White & Olson, 1998). Occupational therapy practitioners who have had people with disabilities in their lives as friends or family members tend to have the most positive attitudes toward people with disabilities (Benham, 1988). People with positive attitudes toward people with disabilities easily notice the shared humanity between themselves as able-bodied people and their friends with disabilities.

The inclusion movement has created many more opportunities for people with disabilities and able-bodied people to form relationships. People from the United States can be particularly proud of the Americans' with Disabilities Act (ADA) of 1990. Enacting a law that ensures people with disabilities receive reasonable accommodations in employment, telecommunications, transportation, and public services has increased the inclusion of people with disabilities the United States. Despite these advances, discrimination and oppression toward people with disabilities persists and is magnified at the intersection of race and disability (Clay, Seekins, & Castillo, 2010). The field of disabilities studies and occupational therapy literature on disabilities promises to further break stereotypes about people with disabilities and move us toward even greater inclusion of people with disabilities in all facets of society (Balcazar et al., 2010; Clay et al., 2010; Craddock, 1996a, 1996b; Frantis, 2005; Garci & Mandich, 2005; Hemsley, Balandin, & Worrall, 2011; Kielhofner, 2005; Phelan, 2011; Shinton & Mairs, 2009).

### Practitioner Example: Communicating With Awareness and Sensitivity to Disability

- Jen worked on an acute rehabilitation floor for amputees and burn clients when she met Bill. Bill had just had a left above-knee amputation secondary to poor circulation. Bill owned a local pizza shop and now had to deal with questioning how he was going to be able to go home and work to support his family "with only one leg." Jen assumed that Bill was going to experience a tough battle with losing his identity when he lost his leg. She knew it was her role as his occupational therapy practitioner to create adaptations and modifications to his house and workplace prior to his discharge home to assist Bill in keeping and even changing or adapting his identity. Jen helped Bill plan out certain changes that needed to be made and Bill had a surprisingly positive response to planning by stating, "I have been a planner my whole life." Jen learned from Bill not to make assumptions about disability and identity.

In addition to communicating with awareness and sensitivity to disability, occupational therapy practitioners often need to address complex communication needs of clients with neurological impairments. Hemsley, Balandin, and Worrall (2011) found some nurses perceive communicating with people with complex communication needs takes too much time, while others find that spending more time in communication and using adaptive communication techniques are efficient practices that improve care. Speech and language pathologists and occupational therapy practitioners often have specialized training in communicating with people with complex communication needs and can play a significant role in assisting other professionals to increase their skill and comfort in communicating with our clients with complex communication needs.

Autism is coined *autism spectrum disorder* because it runs on a continuum. People with autism may be mildly or severely affected by the condition. It is characterized by difficulty with social interactions and impaired verbal and nonverbal communication. It is important for practitioners to be mindful that although their clients may not be able to communicate with words, they can express their needs, wants, feelings, and ambitions. Attentiveness to nonverbal communication is paramount with any client who has difficulty with verbal communication.

### Practitioner Example: Communicating With Awareness and Sensitivity to Complex Communication Needs

- Tyler is a 3-year-old boy attending a school for children with autism. He has sensory-seeking behaviors and is nonverbal. He is just beginning to use a picture exchange system for communication. His one-on-one behavioral health professional expressed concerns to the occupational therapy practitioner about figuring out what Tyler needs or wants because of his lack of communication. The occupational therapy practitioner established rapport with Tyler, observed his preferences and dislikes, and used her therapeutic use of self to effectively communicate with him. By observing his behavior, she was able to determine the best methods for communication for both her and the behavioral health professional to use. The consultation allowed the behavioral health professional to feel more confident when working with Tyler.

## *Oppression and Size*

The cult of thinness transverses much of the globe and perpetuates that notion that only thin people are attractive and worthy. As a result, both large females and males of all ages are mistreated for their size and many internalize self-hatred because of negative societal attitudes. Although males experience oppression because of their size, females face harsher judgment, targeting, and blame because we live in societies that are dominated by men who perpetuate the stereotype that a women's attractiveness, with thin equaling attractive, is her most important characteristic. As Vroman (2016) points out, after race, size is the most stigmatizing physical characteristic. Mold and Forbes (2013) cite numerous studies that have shown that health professionals act out negative stereotypes on large patients/clients and this affects their willingness to seek the care of a health professional and also affects overall health and well-being. It behooves all health care practitioners to reach for the appreciation of themselves and their own bodies exactly as they are to appreciate and work well with clients who are large. Exploration of attitudes toward one's own weight and the weight of large people is best accomplished with other people who are not targeted by fat oppression. It is deeply offensive to large people to listen to people who are thin or even a little overweight be preoccupied with what is wrong with their bodies in their presence.

### Practitioner Example: Communicating With an Awareness and Sensitivity Around Oppression Related to Size

- Loretta shared with her occupational therapy practitioner that she doesn't care to interact with most health practitioners because they are clueless about what it means to be a large woman. They are all full of advice she has already heard or researched herself about how to lose weight. She has spent her lifetime trying to diet and lose weight and health professionals act like they are sharing new information with her. She appreciates her occupational therapy practitioner for providing a listening ear and expressing confidence in her while not pretending she has any solutions. She also appreciates how her occupational therapy practitioner conveys that she thinks Loretta is beautiful just the way she is. Their relationship compels Loretta to want to work in occupational therapy toward increased independence with multiple sclerosis.

## *Age Differences*

It is actually great to be any age we are. Yet the societies we live in parcel out respect differentially according to age. Young people, teenagers, young adults, and older adults experience less respect than adults in their 30s and 40s. Although adults in their 30s and 40s experience greater respect than people of other ages, they tend to be overburdened with work and family responsibilities. Thus, there are certain hardships associated with being any age.

Because many occupational therapy practitioners work with individuals across the lifespan, reflecting on our experiences with people of all ages may help us build on any positive experiences we had and leave behind any negative experiences. In particular, examining any mistreatment we have experienced as a young person can assist us in being mindful of not perpetuating disrespect toward other young people.

Although all human communication is complex, communication with young people has an added complexity because few children like to sit down and talk about their concerns. Because play is the primary occupation of children, listening through play or "play-listening" is an effective communication process with children (Cohen, 2002; Greenspan, 1998; Wipfler, n.d.). One of the primary tenets of play-listening is to turn the table on the power dynamic where adults are always in charge and offer time-limited opportunities for a young person to take the lead in play and have the adult follow.

### Practitioner Example: Communicating With Awareness and Sensitivity to Children

- Some practitioners have the misconception that just because children are young they lack the knowledge and insight to contribute to their own plans of care. In my experience, many children can acknowledge what is difficult for them and aid in their own treatment. I worked with John, a young boy with incoordination problems. He was hesitant to begin therapy. I used playful listening to better understand what intrigued John. I could use this information to create an environment that promoted success without making John feel like he was working. John was able to take the lead in constructing an obstacle course. He became proud of what he was making and was willing to work hard to complete the course while simultaneously challenging his coordination. Feeling empowered, John continued to provide input during therapy.

## Religion and Spirituality

Religion and spirituality can be a powerful source of hope, inspiration, connection, and meaning in people's lives. Yet at the same time, humanity remains divided around religion. People are oppressed for their particular religious or spiritual beliefs, wars continue to be fought based on these differences, and some religious and spiritual traditions enforce hurtful rigidities upon its participants.

Egan and Swedersky (2003) noted that despite considerable literature describing the potential place of spirituality in occupational therapy practice, many occupational therapy practitioners felt uncomfortable with the concept of spirituality in practice. Over a decade later, Morris and colleagues (2014) found that occupational therapy practitioners were generally open to incorporating religion and spirituality into practice, but the vast majority felt their educational programs did not prepare them for this complex endeavor. The scholarship on religion and spirituality in occupational therapy is increasing and can inform practitioners on incorporating religion and spirituality into practice (Levin & Prince, 2011; Smith-Gabai & Ludwig, 2011). Listening partnerships can help occupational therapy practitioners become more comfortable discussing religion and spirituality. As we become more aware of any strengths and challenges associated with our own religious or spiritual heritage, the more we can listen to others and appreciate the strengths and challenges of their traditions.

### Practitioner Example: Communicating With Awareness and Sensitivity to Religion and Spiritual Beliefs

- I have found that honoring clients' religious and spiritual beliefs is crucial for the delivery of effective treatment in all settings. Incorporating spirituality and religion into treatments and interactions can either make or break a person's involvement with therapy. Involving these beliefs allows clients to feel honored and respected. If we as practitioners try to take religion and spirituality out of a person's daily activities, we are asking them to change as a person on the inside and out. If one of our clients watches the rosary at 10 a.m., we should respect that routine and schedule their therapy for before or after the rosary hour. I have noticed that in the elderly population, spirituality and religion are very important to their everyday routines and their souls.

## Ethnicity and Culture

We all have a rich cultural heritage that is important to recognize. The United States historically forced people to give up their cultural/ethnic heritage in favor of assimilating and becoming an "American." People have lost connections with their language and many fine cultural traditions as a result of assimilation. As with religion and spirituality, as we each deepen our awareness and appreciation of our cultural/ethnic heritage, we can appreciate the cultural heritage of others. This will be important in occupational therapy interactions with people from diverse backgrounds (Awaad, 2003; Black, 2002; Black & Wells, 2007; Chiang & Carlson, 2003; Darnell, 2002; Forwell, Whiteford, & Dyck, 2001; Iwana, 2003; Odawara, 2005; Piven & Duran, 2014; Pooremamali, Eklund, Ostman, & Persson, 2012; Richardson, 2004; Suarez-Balcazar et al., 2009; Velde & Wittman, 2001; Whiteford & St. Clair, 2002; Wittman & Velde, 2002). For those of us who identify as citizens of the United States, it is also important to fully claim this identity and any nuances related to being from a particular part of the United States.

In occupational therapy practice, attentive listening to determine a meaningful context for engagement in occupation can change the way an intervention session is heading. People from different cultures have different habits, routines, and rituals that we as therapists have to try to understand and honor and continuously learn about every day. Listening to understand about differences is essential.

### Practitioner Examples: Communicating With Awareness and Sensitivity to Culture

- Julie notes that working in an acute rehabilitation setting in a large urban area opened up opportunities to work with people from a variety of different cultural and ethnic backgrounds. Listening to what was most important to each individual gave her insight into many cultures. Creating a cooking group with an Indian woman and having her cook a meal from her culture enhanced her occupational performance because she felt more at home.
- Claire noted many cultural variances as she worked in home care. In working with a Cambodian child, Claire was impressed with the involvement of the extended family in care for the child. Interdependence and collective decisions appeared highly valued.

When she was referred to work with a Sudanese man, she discovered that only another male could touch a Sudanese male and work with him on personal care. When she worked with a Muslim man in prison for a wrist injury, she was impressed with his strong self-advocacy for accommodations around food restrictions and fasting during Ramadan.

- Claire was working with a 28-year-old Chicano man who sustained severe injuries to his right arm in an car accident. When his family was present for occupational therapy, he cried about the pain in his arm and identified his pain level as 8 on a pain scale. An hour or so later, when he was only in the presence of the medical team, he showed no emotion and identified his pain level as a 3.

## Classism

Jackins (1990) describes how classism has existed as long as humans have functioned in organized societies. The vicious classism that existed under slavery gave way to a slightly less vicious form of classism under feudalism. Despite a few attempts at alternatives, feudalism was eventually replaced by capitalism, or owning/working class societies worldwide. Under capitalism, a small percentage of the population owns and controls most of the wealth and means of production, while the rest of the population works for a living. In the United States, the top 20% of households own more than 84% of the wealth, while the bottom 40% owns 0.3% (Fitz, 2015). The United States continues to be the wealthiest and most unequal nation of the world (Sherman, 2015).

The working class has many subdivisions that include the middle class, blue/pink collar workers (or what has been traditionally thought of as the working class), working poor people, and unemployed people. None of the divisions between classes is clear-cut. People can often identify with more than one class background, so individual stories become more meaningful than labels associated with class background.

As Hawes (1996) points out, class society permeates everything and the contradictions of capitalism are manifested in the lives of all individuals. People within the working class are often pitted against one another—the middle class is given extra privileges and more status than working class and poor people in exchange for carrying out oppressive roles. An example of this dynamic is Jewish people, who transcend all classes, yet have historically been used by owning class leaders as scapegoats. They have been made to appear as the controllers of wealth and power by the owning class so whenever working class people organize and fight their own oppression, they target Jews rather than the actual owning class (Jackins, 1990). Jewish oppression persists in the forms of stereotyping, denial of anti-Semitism, and continued scapegoating of Jewish people.

Regardless of their class background, most occupational therapy practitioners function in the middle class as professionals. Yet class is very fluid under capitalism. Job cuts, disability, medical issues, divorce, single parenting, etc., can change one's socioeconomic class status virtually overnight. Increased awareness related to class will be beneficial to future occupational therapy practitioners on both a personal and professional level (Baum, McGeary, Pankiewicz, Braford, & Edwards, 1996; Bottomley, 2001; CDC, 2011; Finlayson, Baker, Rodman, & Hertzberg, 2002; Froehlich, 2005; Humphry, 1995; Neufeld & Lysack, 2004; Padilla, Gupta, & Liotta-Kleinfeld, 2004; Tryssenaar, Jones, & Lee, 1999; VanLeit, Starrett, & Crowe, 2006; Von Zuben, Crist, & Mayberry, 1991; Watson & Duncan, 2010). For the occupational therapy practitioner who was raised poor or working class, talking about class can promote pride in one's heritage and assist the transition to the middle class. For the occupational therapy practitioner who was raised middle class, talking about class can increase awareness of the strengths and challenges present in middle-class life. Sensitivity and awareness of class can promote open communication and caring relationships between professional occupational therapy practitioners and clients of all class backgrounds.

### Practitioner Examples: Communicating With Awareness and Sensitivity to Class

- John was a homeless man who came to a long-term rehabilitation facility due to increased Korsakoff disease, and he was also exhibiting parkinsonian symptoms. John required constant support and assistance because he was not able to return to the shelter from where he came. Julie, his occupational therapy practitioner, was working with John for about a month when she realized that he did not have any clothes; he had been in hospital gowns since admission. John did have a few visitors who would bring him snacks and candy but never clothes. Julie was torn. Was she able to bring in old clothes from her basement for John so he was more comfortable? Was it her place? Julie battled with the idea until she decided to bring in extra clothes for John and wrote his name on the tags and assisted him with dressing. Julie knew that she would not want to see her own father, uncle, or grandfather living in hospital gowns for this long. John could not take the smile off of his face as he received his new clothes. "Thank you—thank you, I can't believe it," said John to Julie as she walked out the door.
- In home care, Jan worked with many clients who struggled economically. When Paul shared his struggle to pay his bills and feed his family after his back injury, Jan acknowledged that the economic system is unfair and that it is not his fault that he is having a hard time. She also acknowledged that she

can't fully imagine what it would be like to be in his shoes. Paul appreciated this acknowledgment.

It is often difficult for practitioners to witness the poverty some of our clients endure. Julie's kind actions and respectful interactions made a difference in not only John's life, but also in Julie's life because she knows she did the right thing by bringing in clothing for John. Even though she is middle class, Jan's awareness and sensitivity to poverty and struggle enhanced her therapeutic relationships with poor and working class clients.

No matter what someone's socioeconomic class background, humans often have an object, a place in nature, a house, or something else that symbolizes "home." When conducting home safety evaluations or working on discharge planning, it is crucial to remain unbiased of the person's living environment. As long as the person's environment is safe, the therapist should remember that this is "home" to the client, regardless of the way it appears to the practitioner.

## *Racism*

There is really only one human race, yet racism would have us believe otherwise. Racism is a vicious form of classism whereby people of color (also known as the people of the global majority) are treated as less than White people. In terms of global economics, people who reside in the southern hemisphere of the world are mostly people of color, tend to be the poorest people in the world, and are also the global majority (Powell & Udayakumar, 2006). The United States, founded on the enslavement of people of African heritage and the genocide of Native American people, continues to struggle with enduring effects of racism and internalized racism.

Many of the effects of racism on people of color, particularly those of African heritage, are obvious in terms of media stereotyping, racial profiling, poverty, violence, lack of access to higher education (Alexander, 2012), poor access to health care, and poor health (CDC, 2011). The Black Lives Matter movement in the United States offers tremendous hope toward ending racism. Occupational therapy practitioners have contributed powerful scholarship toward dismantling racism within occupational therapy (Beagan & Etowa, 2009; Black, 2002; Black & Wells, 2000; Cena, McGruder, & Tomlin, 2002; Clay et al., 2010; David, 1995; Evans, 1992; Matlala, 1993; Nelson, 2007; Odawara, 2005).

The effects of racism on White people is also damaging, but in different and less obvious ways. It is damaging for White people to grow up in a society where they are bombarded with negative stereotypes about people of color and told they cannot be close to people of color. No White child was born racist, but when White children first learn about race, they are often confronted with awkwardness and guilt on the part of White adults who are challenged to communicate about race. They grow up to be young adults and adults who also feel bad about racism and awkward about discussing it (Jackins, 2002). The implicit association test shows that even people who think they are not racist tend to carry unaware racist attitudes (Greenwald, Poehlman, Uhlmann, & Banaji, 2009). Listening partnerships on racism can foster new awareness about racism, assist in healing from internalized racism, and deepen relationships between White people and people of color.

### Practitioner Examples: Communicating With Awareness and Sensitivity to Race

- Tonia, a Black occupational therapy practitioner, shared with her supervisor, Claire, that one of her clients with an acquired brain injury made a racial slur in her presence and refused to work with her. Claire shared how sorry she was that Tonia ever had to hear a racial slur and asked what Tonia wanted her to do. Tonia felt validated by Claire's response and shared that she did not want to work with this particular client. Claire immediately reassigned the client to a White occupational therapy practitioner who agreed to do what she could to challenge his racism.
- While working in an inpatient psychiatric unit, Julie was introduced to racism in ways she had never seen before. She heard clients scream racial slurs and saw them cause a scene because their nurse or roommate was Black. Julie found it useful to offer apologies and a listening ear to colleagues and clients who experienced overt racism. She also experienced prejudice in other ways. A client of hers was of Hispanic descent and would not work with Julie because she was White. Because racism affects people of every background, it is important to work on creating a safe environment for all clients and staff.
- In her work with Passamaquoddy people, Jan learned to be a listener more than a talker. She found that Passamaquoddy people were more comfortable just "being" and "being silent" rather than needing to fill time and space with lots of talking and constant activity.

## *Interpreters, Cultural Brokers, and Health Literacy*

Occupational therapy practitioners are increasingly working with clients from different ethnic backgrounds with differing spoken languages. While interpreter services are increasingly available in many practice settings, a newer concept in enhancing communication between people of differing cultural groups is the concept of a cultural broker. Cultural brokers serve not only as interpreters when there are language barriers, but they also serve to help health practitioners understand subtle and not-so-subtle cultural differences that can impact health outcomes. A complimentary development in health communication is increasing recognition of the significance of health literacy. Health literacy is the concept of ensuring that verbal and written health information is presented at a level that is understandable to clients. A systematic analysis by Berkman, Sheridan, Donahue, Halpern, and Crotty (2011) shows health literacy is highly correlated with health outcomes. All health care professionals need to refrain from the overuse of jargon and integrate health literacy and cultural competence in health interactions. Occupational therapists are no exception to this rule.

### Practitioner Examples: Communicating Using Interpreters and Cultural Brokers

- In working on with people of Native American heritage, Deb noted that her clients were often quiet and reserved around her. She filled in the silences with questions and chit-chat. Fortunately, one Native American woman served as a cultural broker and cared enough about Deb and her work to let her know that she was alienating people on the reservation with all her questions and chatter. Deb appreciated the feedback and modified her behavior by allowing for long silences and learning to just be, rather than speak and ask questions. Occupational therapy interventions proceeded much more smoothly with Deb's modified communication style.
- Marie was working with a young Sudanese child with developmental disabilities. A Sudanese interpreter was brought in for a family meeting, but he happened to be from a Sudanese tribe that was at war with the family's tribe. He was immediately dismissed and phone interpreter services were used until an acceptable match was found. The interprofessional team found that making minimal eye contact with the interpreter allowed him to perform his services optimally.

# Intra- and Interprofessional Teamwork, Technology, and Other Communication Challenges

## *Intra- and Interprofessional Teamwork*

The Interprofessional Education Collaborative Expert Panel report (2011) identified competencies for effective interprofessional health care within the four domains of values and ethics, roles and responsibilities, interprofessional communication, and interprofessional teamwork or team-based care. While values and ethics are addressed in Section IX, this section will further address interprofessional communication/teamwork and explore understanding professional roles as they relate to our professional standard that occupational therapy practitioners "effectively communicate and work interprofessionally with those who provide services to individuals, organization, and/or populations in order to clarify each member's responsibility in executing an intervention plan" (AOTAa, 2011, p. 6).

Understanding the roles and responsibilities of interprofessional team members is best accomplished when educational programs infuse this information in their curriculums (Konrad & Browning, 2012; Pardue, 2013). Understanding intraprofessional roles is equally important. Costa, Molinsky, and Sauerwald (2012) cite numerous studies that demonstrate the value of collaborative, intraprofessional education not only in the classroom and but also during fieldwork involving occupational therapy and occupational therapy assistant students. An essential educational component for all occupational therapy practitioners is learning about the distinct roles and responsibilities and the supervisory process between a registered occupational therapist and a certified occupational therapy assistant. AOTA's (2014) *Guidelines for Supervision, Roles, and Responsibilities During the Delivery of Occupational Therapy Services* is an essential guideline for understanding the complexities of these responsibilities.

Being grounded in the roles and responsibilities of intra- and interprofessional team members is an important starting point for building effective intra- and interprofessional teamwork and communication. However, as Curtis et al. (2011) noted, complex variables such as hierarchical relationships, increasing workload, differing perceptions, language differences, as well as prior experience, pose conflict and barriers to effective interprofessional communication and teamwork. Dillon (2001) highlighted the challenges presented by intraprofessional teamwork, or teamwork within a given profession. Meade, Brown, and Trevan-Hawke (2005) found that maintaining collegial relationships with coworkers, teamwork, and gaining respect and recognition from others were among the top factors contributing to job satisfaction among occupational therapy practitioners.

## *Assertiveness, Conflict Resolution, and Teamwork*

Conflict occurs both between members of a particular group and between people from different groups As was noted, internalized oppression or horizontal violence plays a role in conflict as members of oppressed groups mistreat each other (i.e., women vs. women, poor people targeting other poor people, nurses vs. other nurses and nursing staff, occupational therapists vs. occupational therapy assistants). Obviously, conflict between people across different groups (i.e., doctors and nurses, men and women, occupational and physical therapists, and different religious groups) also continues to be a challenge. Fortunately, increased awareness of the experiences of people from groups other than our own, combined with increased awareness of the mechanism of internalized oppression or horizontal violence, can begin to decrease conflict and assist in its resolution (Brown & Mazza, 1997).

Many of us have negative associations with conflict, yet in reality, conflict can be an opportunity for increased communication, brainstorming, problem solving, and new learning. Negative associations with conflict often stem from our early experiences with conflict in our families and can be reevaluated in listening partnerships. When we free ourselves from some of the negative emotions associated with early conflict, we can more skillfully handle conflict in the present (Brown & Mazza, 1997).

Each conflict one encounters requires flexible, on-the-spot thinking. When appropriate, the skilled communicator knows how to use both assertiveness and listening as conflict resolution tools. It is important to remember that listening does not mean agreement. Listening means seeking to understand another point of view. If the reader has practiced the listening partnerships in this chapter, he or she may be ready to not only listen to someone he or she is in conflict with, but also to assert that the reader him- or herself deserves to be listened to as well. It may be necessary to teach the party one is in conflict with to listen without interruption.

Finding our voice in situations of conflict can be particularly challenging in hierarchical relationships or relationships between members of oppressed and oppressor or dominant groups. Davis (2011) underscores the challenges women face in asserting themselves in the presence of men. Sometimes it works to vent aggressive feelings we have toward an individual with a supportive listening partnership and noting whether this person reminds us of someone from our past can clear our mind so we can act assertively in the present (Brown & Mazza, 1997).

Studies have shown that occupational therapy practitioners (Landa-Gonzalez, 2008; Scheirton, Mu, & Lohman, 2003) and nurses (Curtis et al., 2011), both female-dominated professions, have difficulty asserting themselves in interprofessional, hierarchical relationships. Ethical or internal dilemmas often arise during practice. Practitioners may ask questions such as, "Should I tell the doctor about this change in status?" When a client's safety has potential to be compromised, there is no negotiating of reporting this to someone higher up in the specific organization. Practitioners who truly advocate for their clients will own the emotion of concern for their clients' well-being and will go to a source where they know the problem will be addressed.

Similarly, certified occupational therapy assistants may feel barriers in communicating with occupational therapists. Dillon (2001) conducted a phenomenological study on the relationships between 22 pairs of occupational therapists and occupational therapy assistants. Themes that emerged from interviews highlighted the importance of mutual respect, two-way communication, and professionalism in every aspect of the job as essential to effective occupational therapist/certified occupational therapy assistant relationships. Communication themes that emerged included becoming familiar with each other's communication styles, having in-person communication, communicating openly, and providing each other with regular feedback. These individuals indicated that building effective intraprofessional relationships required concerted effort, but ultimately allowed them to provide a higher quality of occupational therapy services and feel a greater sense of personal satisfaction in their work.

Improved assertiveness can enhance both intra- and interprofessional communication. Davis (2011) describes the work of Bower and Bower in identifying a process (DESC) for asserting oneself that involves the following steps:

- Describing the specific behavior that is bothersome
- Expressing how this behavior made you feel
- Specifying the desired changes in behavior
- [Sharing the] consequences that will occur as a result of the behavioral change

Curtis et al. (2011) suggest a graded approach to assertiveness for nurses that is also relevant for occupational therapists:

- Level I: Express initial concern with an "I" statement
- Level II: Make an inquiry or offer a solution
- Level III: Ask for an explanation
- Level IV: A definitive challenge demanding a response

Another form of assertive communication generated from the nursing profession is use of Introduction, Situation, Background, Assessment, and Recommendation (ISBAR). ISBAR has been validated as an effective way to improve the clarity and content of clinically based communication (Marshall et al., 2009).

On a positive note, it may be that interprofessional communication is improving. The Joint Commission (2013) tracks sentinel events in health care, or "unexpected occurrences involving death or serious physical or psychological injury, or the risk thereof." The Commission's 2015 report showed that 563/887 sentinel events in 2013 were due to communication errors—second only to human factors as a root cause of medical errors. Communication as a root cause of sentinel errors had dropped to third place behind human factors and leadership by the second quarter of 2015 (Joint Commission, 2015).

### Practitioner Examples: Assertiveness, Conflict Resolution, and Teamwork

- Conflict within a professional team can stimulate improved communication and generate novel ideas. People with differing ideas can offer a variety of solutions to a problem. For example, I was working as part of an interprofessional team in an acute care setting. Our client had just experienced a severe stroke. She was nonverbal, dependent in all activities of daily living, and was beginning to form contractures of the upper and lower extremities. Each team member had specific concerns for how to prevent these contractures. Each practitioner's viewpoint was slightly different based on his or her professional and clinical backgrounds, but each team member shared the same goal of providing client-centered care. As we worked out our differing opinions, the team ultimately chose splints and orthotics that were best suited for the client.
- Working in a skilled nursing facility has taught me how important assertiveness is to ensure that my patients are receiving the best care that can be provided from everyone involved in their plan of care. I have learned that being an advocate for my clients has allowed me to be an advocate for myself in making sure that I am doing what is right for my clients. Assertiveness is crucial in working in health care and with many other professionals who have vast knowledge. When responsibility increases, assertiveness must increase. My responsibility is to my clients. When I walk by a room and notice that a client with severe chronic obstructive pulmonary disease is unhooked from the oxygen machine, I assume responsibility to find out why it is unhooked and make sure that staff understands the importance of the oxygen being on her at all times. I find that I intuitively use ISBAR for communication—Judy, who has severe chronic obstructive pulmonary disease, was experiencing dizziness and shortness of breath while lying in bed. I checked her oxygen and noted that she was at 79% oxygen on 3 L of oxygen. I immediately contacted the nurse, stating the situation, providing background on the client, and stated that I recommend getting blood oxygen levels from the client to see if there is an underlying problem. I used my professional opinion to speak with the nurse and I was open to listening to her recommendations and assisting her with finding a solution to this problem.

Each of these clinical examples highlights the importance of assertiveness, interprofessional teamwork, and conflict resolution. Once the reader has learned to listen well to others, it might be important to assert that others learn to listen to you. For example, using the DESC formula you might say:

- Describe: I have noticed you interrupt me when I am trying to speak.
- Express: I am bothered when I don't get to complete a thought.
- Specify: How about if you listen to me for 5 minutes without saying anything?
- Consequence: Then I will listen to you for 5 minutes without interruption and we might find our relationship works better.

## *Other Challenging Communication*

Although communicating across cultural differences and hierarchical relationships can be challenging, there are many additional challenges that occupational therapy practitioners will encounter in their practice. Based on extensive interviews with occupational therapy practitioners, Taylor (2008) has identified the following categories of inevitable interpersonal events of therapy:

- Expressions of strong emotion
- Intimate self-disclosures
- Power dilemmas
- Nonverbal cues
- Crisis points
- Resistance and reluctance
- Boundary testing
- Empathic breaks
- Emotionally charged therapy tasks and situations
- Limitations of therapy
- Contextual inconsistencies

While effective listening can play a role in handling interpersonal events, the inquisitive occupational therapy practitioner will seek multiple strategies for addressing these interpersonal events and is encouraged to read Taylor's book *The Intentional Relationship Model: Occupational Therapy and Use of Self* (2008). In addition to offering a listening ear in some challenging encounters, because these encounters can be distressing to the occupational therapy practitioner, seeking an opportunity to be listened to may be equally important. Whether hearing a life story of illness, trauma, and loss or feeling slighted or disrespected by a colleague, client, or interprofessional team member, it is important for an occupational therapist to practice self-care. Venting to a supervisor or person who cares can make a significant difference in the practitioner's ability to proceed effectively after challenging communication encounters.

### Practitioner Example: Handling Communication Challenges

- Hazel was a new practitioner working in an inpatient psychiatric unit and approached a 16-year-old girl, Maribeth, to see if she was interested in participating in occupational therapy. Maribeth proceeded to scream and utter profanities at Hazel and insisted that she leave her room. Hazel calmly left her room and sought support from her supervisor, who encouraged Hazel not to take Maribeth's behavior personally and informed her that it was not uncommon for agitated clients to respond in this way. Hazel checked in with Maribeth the next day, and Maribeth was eager to participate in occupational therapy.

## *Technology and Health Care Communication*

Whether typed or handwritten, journaling is a form of communication that facilitates an individual's independent thought process; it can enhance clarity of thought and writing skills (Elbow, 2000). If the reader has engaged in journaling while reading this chapter, his or her writing skills may have improved—particularly if he or she had the opportunity to share journals and feedback with a partner.

Many practitioners are currently expected to write clear and concise notes using technology for documentation and other forms of health communication. Although technology facilitates communication in a multitude of ways, the mindful practitioner will continually evaluate whether technology is enhancing or inhibiting effective communication (Mueller, 2010). Nonverbal communication can be compromised when the practitioner needs to log notes while engaged in a conversation with a client. Lost nonverbal communication can contribute to declining rapport, which may in turn result in poor interpersonal communication and the loss of important health information. Nonetheless, some overworked practitioners are finding that communication technology reduces the stress of too much paperwork.

Although some clients may not disclose any information about themselves if the practitioner is using a computer, others may feel that what they are saying is significant because the practitioner is typing their words on a computer. Younger clients exposed to technology may be more responsive to a therapist who uses technology. Dialogue among interprofessional teams can aid in generating creative solutions regarding how to best integrate technology with health care communication.

Although smartphone technology, email, and social media have enabled increased communication and connection between humans, they also present barriers when the use of such forms of communication become addictive and a substitute for face-to-face human communication. Young people who have grown up with smartphones and social media appear to be particularly vulnerable to overuse of these technologies and may find listening partnerships with their cell phones turned off to be particularly useful.

### Practitioner Example: Technology and Health Care Communication

- Marie was working with a 90-year-old retired lobsterman who noted her computer and said, "Get that damn thing out of here. If I see that again you can take yourself and your computer out of here for good." Marie quickly put the computer away and focused her attention so she could remember what her client shared. Another 102-year-old man responded to her computer similarly, "That's the problem with today's world. People are more interested in that than people." Marie validated his perspective and closed the computer once again. In contrast, when she worked work with children with disabilities, she found they were intrigued by technology and it was a great asset to the therapy relationship.

## Summary

As Ueland (2006) stated, "When we are listened to, it creates us, makes us unfold and expand. Ideas actually begin to grow within us and come to life." More than 20 years of experience teaching occupational therapy students to use listening partnerships for the enhancement of their communication skills has enabled me to witness the unfolding and expansion of my students. Students who have had the opportunity to engage in multiple listening partnerships report in journals and papers that not only do they become much better listeners, but they also become more confident as thinkers, speakers, and writers. Although they initially find it difficult to stay in the role as listener or speaker, over time, this becomes natural. Students generally report that as the class progresses they notice how much others do not listen and many decide to teach friends and family to listen to them.

In addition, listening partnerships focused on diversity have a positive impact on students' awareness and comfort with human diversity within themselves and their peers. Often times, students from oppressed groups find enough caring, trust, and safety in their listening partnerships to vent about their experiences of mistreatment and discrimination. Students from dominant groups, such as heterosexual, gentile, White middle

## Evidence-Based Research Chart

| Topic | Components | Evidence |
|---|---|---|
| Interprofessional and intraprofessional teamwork | Conflict resolution and assertiveness | Curtis et al., 2011; Landa-Gonzalez, 2008; Marshall et al., 2009; Meade, Brown, & Trevan-Hawke, 2005; St-Pierre & Holmes, 2008; Sargeant, Loney, & Murphy, 2008; Sargent, MacLeod, & Murray, 2011; Scheirton, Mu, & Lohman, 2003 |
| | Occupational therapist and assistant relationships | AOTA, 2014; Costa, Molinsky, & Sauerwald, 2012; Dillon, 2001 |
| Culturally competent communication: The process | Awareness/knowledge/skills | Awaad, 2003; Black, 2002; Black & Wells, 2000, 2007; Campinha-Bacote, 2011; Chiang & Carlson, 2003; Iwana, 2003; Odawara, 2005; Royeen & Crabtree, 2006; Velde & Wittman, 2001; Whiteford & St. Clair, 2002*; Wittman & Velde, 2002 |
| Culturally competent communication: Self-awareness and knowledge of others | Life story/narrative | Black & Wells, 2007; Davis, 2011; Frank, 1995; Frantis, 2005; Kielhofner, 2008; Taylor, 2008 |
| | Sex | AOTA, 2011b; Crittenden, 2001; Flinn, Sanders, Yen, Sommerich, & Lavender, 2013; Froehlich, 2005; Froehlich, Hamlin, Loukas, & MacRae, 1992; Jackins, 1999; Javaherian et al., 2007*; MacRae, 2005; Mossakowski, 2009*; Palmadottir, 2009; Peloquin & Ciro, 2013; Pierce & Frank, 1992; Primeau, 1992; Sterling & Nayar, 2013 |
| | Sex and sexual orientation | Jackson, 1995; Kelly, 2000; Kinglsey & Molineux, 2000; Kitts, 2005 |
| | Disability | Balcazar et al., 2010; Benham, 1988*; Clay, Seekin, & Castillo, 2010; Coffey, 2001*; Craddock, 1996a, 1996b; Frantis, 2005; Garci & Mandich, 2005; Hemsley, Balandin, & Worrall, 2011*; Kielhofner, 2005; Phelan, 2011; Shinton & Mairs, 2009; White & Olson, 1998* |
| | Oppression and size | Mold & Forbes, 2013; Vroman, 2016 |
| | Age differences | Bottomley, 2001; Cohen, 2002; Greenspan, 1998; Wipfler, n.d. |
| | Religion and spirituality | Egan & Swedersky, 2003; Farrar, 2001*; Levin & Prince, 2011; Morris et al., 2014; Smith-Gabai & Ludwig, 2011 |
| | Ethnicity and culture | Awaad, 2003; Balcazar et al., 2010; Black & Wells, 2007; Campinha-Bacote, 2011; Campos, 2007; Chiang & Carlson, 2003; Darnell, 2002; Dean, 2001; Iwana, 2003; Odawara, 2005; Piven & Duran, 2014; Pooremamali, Eklund, Ostman, & Persson, 2012; Richardson, 2004; Suarez-Balcazar et al., 2009; Swider, 2002; Velde & Wittman, 2001; Whiteford & St. Clair, 2002; Whitley, Everhart, & Wright, 2006; Wittman & Velde, 2002 |
| | Class | Bottomley, 2001; CDC, 2011*; Finlayson, Baker, Rodman, & Hertzberg, 2002*; Fitz, 2015; Froehich, 2005; Galbraith, 2003; Hawes, 1996; Humphry, 1995; Neufeld & Lysack, 2004; Padilla, Gupta, & Liotta-Kleinfeld, 2004; Sherman, 2015; Tryssenaar, Jones, & Lee, 1999; Van Leit, Starrett & Crowe, 2006*; Watson & Duncan, 2010 |
| | Race | Balcazar et al., 2010; Beagan & Etowa, 2009*; Black, 2002; Cena, McGruder, & Tomlin, 2002*; Clay, Seekin, & Castillo, 2010; David, 1995*; Evans, 1992; Greenwald, Poehlman, Uhlmann, & Banaji, 2009*; Matlala, 1993; National Research Council, 2003; Nelson, 2007; Powell & Udayakumar, 2006; Van Ryn & Fu, 2003 |

*(continued)*

## Evidence-Based Research Chart (continued)

| Topic | Components | Evidence |
|---|---|---|
| Health literacy | | Barrett & Puryear, 2006; Berkman, Sheridan, Donahue, Halpern, & Crotty, 2011* |
| Interprofessional communication and teamwork | | Froehlich, Pardue, & Dunbar, 2016; Ingram, Sabo, Rothers, Wennerstrom, & de Zapien, 2008; Konrad & Browning, 2012; Zwarenstein & Reeves, 2006 |
| Listening skills | Nonverbal and verbal communication | Alpert, 2011; Browning & Waite, 2010; Davis, 2011; Fisher, Emerson, Firpo, Ptak, Wonn, & Bartolacci, 2007*; Froehlich & Nesbit, 2004; Jackins, 1981; Kauffman & New, 2004; Robinson & Heritage, 2006*; Rollnick, Miller, & Butler, 2008; Taylor, 2008 |
| Written communication | Journaling | Elbow, 2000; Murphy, 2004* |

*= Research papers. Papers without * are conceptual papers.

class men and women, report that they have been deeply enriched by the stories of students of color, students from countries outside the United States, students with disabilities, students raised poor and working class, and students who are Jewish or Buddhist. Male and female students are riveted by what each other has to say about their experiences. The occupational therapy student who applies weekly time and practice to listening partnerships will make great steps toward becoming an effective, culturally competent communicator, a necessity for forming effective relationships with clients, family, significant others, interprofessional team members, and the public.

## Acknowledgments

Case vignettes were provided by Marie C. Roy, LCSW, OTR/L; Bethany Augustoni, MS, OTR/L; Julie Eldredge, MS, OTR/L; and Ali Arsenault, MS, OTR/L.

## Student Self-Assessment

The following activities will help the student consolidate his or her skills in effective communication. These activities can be done in both listening partnerships and in a journal format.

1. Complete the communication and cultural competence surveys (see Figures 9-1 and 9-2) again and reflect on how your communication skills have changed as a result of reading this chapter and completing some of the listening exercises. Describe to a peer or in a journal any changes you have noticed in your listening skills, with attention to both verbal and nonverbal behavior. Have peers, family, or coworkers given you any feedback on your communications skills? If so, what have they said? Have you noticed any changes in your ability to express your ideas verbally and in writing? If so, describe these changes.
2. What in particular stands out in your mind with regard to journaling and engaging in listening partnerships on diversity? Can you identify some next steps with regard to becoming a culturally competent communicator? If so, what are they?
3. Describe your thoughts regarding the concept of internalized oppression and reflect upon any of your own struggles with self-invalidation and invalidation of members of your own group.
4. Have you attempted to teach other people to refrain from interrupting you or others as they are speaking? If so, what has this been like?
5. Have you used either listening or the DESC approach to conflict resolution? If so, what were your results? If not, discuss your feelings about potentially using either of these approaches.

## References

Alexander, M. (2012). *The new Jim Crow: Mass incarceration in the age of colorblindness.* New York, NY: The New Press.

Alpert, J. (2011). Some simple rules for effective communication in clinical teaching and practice environments. *American Journal of Medicine, 124*(5), 381-382.

American Occupational Therapy Association. (2011a). Accreditation Council for Occupational Therapy Education (ACOTE®) standards. *American Journal of Occupational Therapy, 66*(6), 1-45.

American Occupational Therapy Association. (2011b). Occupational therapy services for individuals who have experienced domestic violence. *American Journal of Occupational Therapy, 65,* S32-S45. doi:10.5014/ajot.2011.65S32

American Occupational Therapy Association. (2014). Guidelines for supervision, roles, and responsibilities during the delivery of occupational therapy services. *American Journal of Occupational Therapy, 68*(Suppl. 3), S16-S22. doi:10.5014/ajot.2014.686S03

Awaad, T. (2003). Culture cultural competency, and occupational therapy: A review of the literature. *British Journal of Occupational Therapy, 66*(8), 356-362.

Balcazar, F., Suarez-Balcazar, Y. Taylor-Ritzler, T., & Keys, C. B. (Eds.). (2010). *Race, culture and disability: Rehabilitation science and practice*. Sudbury, MA: Jones and Bartlett Publishers.

Barrett, S. E., & Puryear, J. S. (2006). Health literacy: Improving quality of care in primary care settings. *Journal of Health Care for the Poor and Underserved, 17*(4), 690-697.

Baum, C., McGeary, T., Pankiewicz, R., Braford, T., & Edwards, D. (1996). An activity program for cognitively impaired low-income inner city residents. *Topics in Geriatric Rehabilitation, 12*(2), 54-62.

Beagan, B. L., Chiasson, A., Fiske, C. A., Forseth, S. D., Hosein, A. C., Myers, M. R., & Stang, J. E. (2013). Working with transgender clients: Learning from physicians and nurses to improve occupational therapy practice. *Canadian Journal of Occupational Therapy, 80*(2), 82-91.

Beagan, B. L., & Etowa, J. (2009). The impact of everyday racism on the occupations of African Canadian women. *Canadian Journal of Occupational Therapy, 76*(4), 285-293.

Bell, H., Kulkarni, S., & Dalton, L. (2003). Organizational prevention of vicarious trauma. *Families in Society, 84*(4), 463-470. doi:10.1606/1044-3894.131

Benham, P. K. (1988). Attitudes of occupational therapy personnel toward persons with disabilities. *American Journal of Occupational Therapy, 42*, 305-311.

Berkhof, M., van Rijssen, J., Schellart, A. J. M., Anema, J. R., & van der Beek, A. J. (2011). Effective training strategies for teaching communication skills to physicians: An overview of systematic reviews. *Patient Education Counseling, 84*(2), 152-162.

Berkman, N. D., Sheridan, S. L., Donahue, K. E. Halpern, D. J., & Crotty, K. (2011). Low health literacy and health outcomes: and updated systematic review. *Annals of Internal Medicine, 155*(2), 97-107. doi:10.1059/0003-4819-155-2-201107190-00005

Black, R. M. (2002). Occupational therapy's dance with diversity. *American Journal of Occupational Therapy, 56*, 140-148.

Black, R. M., & Wells, S. A. (2000). *Cultural competency for health professionals*. Bethesda, MD: AOTA Press.

Black, R. M., & Wells, S. A. (2007). *Culture and occupation: A model of empowerment for occupational therapy*. Bethesda, MD: American Occupational Therapy Association.

Boschma, G., Einboden, R., Groening, M., Jackson, C., MacPhee, M. Marshall, H., ... Roberts, E. (2010). Strengthening communication education in an undergraduate nursing curriculum. *International Journal of Nursing Education Scholarship, 7*(1), 1-14.

Bottomley, J. M. (2001). Health care and homeless older adults. *Topics in Geriatric Rehabilitation, 17*(1), 1-21.

Brown, C. R., & Mazza, G. J. (1997). *Healing into action: A leadership guide for creating diverse communities*. Washington, DC: National Coalition Building Institute.

Browning, S., & Waite, R. (2010). The gift of listening: JUST listening strategies. *Nursing Forum, 45*(3), 150-158.

Campinha-Bacote, J. (2011). Delivering patient-centered care in the midst of a cultural conflict: The role of cultural competence. *Online Journal of Issues in Nursing, 16*(2), manuscript 5.

Campos, C. (2007). Addressing cultural barriers to the successful use of insulin in Hispanics with type 2 diabetes. *Southern Medical Journal, 100*(8), 812-820.

Cena, L., McGruder, J., & Tomlin, G. (2002). Representations of race, ethnicity, and social class in case examples in the *American Journal of Occupational Therapy. American Journal of Occupational Therapy, 56*, 130-139.

Centers for Disease Control and Prevention. (2011). *CDC health disparities and inequality report: United States*. Retrieved from http://www.cdc.gov/mmwr/pdf/other/su6001.pdf

Chiang, M., & Carlson, G. (2003). Occupational therapy in multicultural contexts: Issues and strategies. *British Journal of Occupational Therapy, 66*(12), 559-567.

Clay, J., Seekins, T., & Castillo, J. (2010). Community infrastructure and employment opportunities for Native Americans and Alaska Natives. In F. E. Balcazar, Y. Suarez-Balcazar, T. Taylor-Ritzler, & C. B. Keys (Eds.), *Race, culture and disability: Rehabilitation science and practice*. Sudbury, MA: Jones and Bartlett Publishers.

Cohen, L. J. (2002). *Playful parenting*. New York, NY: Ballantine Publishing Group.

Coffey, D. M. (2001). "The experience of being an occupational therapist with a disability": What about being a student? *American Journal of Occupational Therapy, 55*, 352.

Costa, D., Molinsky, R., & Sauerwald, C. (2012). Collaborative interprofessional education with occupational therapy and occupational therapy assistant students. *OT Practice, 17*(21), CE-1.

Corvinelli, A. (2005). Alleviating boredom in adult males recovering from substance use disorder. *Occupational Therapy in Mental Health, 21*(2), 1-11.

Craddock, J. (1996a). Responses of the occupational therapy profession to the perspective of the disability movement, part 1. *British Journal of Occupational Therapy, 59*(1), 17-24.

Craddock, J. (1996b). Responses of the occupational therapy profession to the perspective of the disability movement, part 2. *British Journal of Occupational Therapy, 59*(2), 73-78.

Crittenden, A. (2001). *The price of motherhood: Why the most important job in the world is still the least valued*. New York, NY: Henry Holt and Company.

Curtis, K., Tzannes, A., & Rudge, T. (2011). How to talk to doctors: A guide for effective communication. *International Nursing Review, 58*, 13-20.

Darnell, R. (2002). Occupation is not a cross-cultural universal: Some reflections from an ethnographer. *Journal of Occupational Science, 9*(1), 5-11.

David, P. A. (1995). Service provision to black people: A study of occupational therapy staff in physical disability teams within social services. *British Journal of Occupational Therapy, 58*(3), 98-102.

Davis, C. M. (2011). *Patient practitioner interaction: An experiential manual for developing the art of health care* (5th ed.). Thorofare, NJ: SLACK Incorporated.

Dean, R. G. (2001). The myth of cross-cultural competence. *Families in Society, 82*(6), 623-630.

Dillon, T. (2001). Practitioner perspectives: effective intraprofessional relationships in occupational therapy. *Occupational Therapy In Health Care, 14*(3/4), 1-15.

Egan, M., & Swedersky, J. (2003). Spirituality as experienced by occupational therapists in practice. *American Journal of Occupational Therapy, 57*(5), 525-533.

Elbow, P. (2000). *Everyone can write: Essays toward a hopeful theory of writing and teaching writing*. New York, NY: Oxford Press.

Evans, J. (1992). What occupational therapists can do to eliminate racial barriers to healthcare access. *American Journal of Occupational Therapy, 46*, 676-766.

Fallowfield, L., Jenisn, V., Farewell, V., Saul, J., Duffy, A., & Eves, R. (2002). Efficacy of a cancer research UK communication skills training model for oncologists: A randomized controlled trial. *The Lancet, 359*(9307), 650-656.

Farrar, J. E. (2001). Addressing spirituality and religious life in occupational therapy. *Physical and Occupational Therapy in Geriatrics, 18*(4),65-85.

Fellowes, D., Wilkinson, S., & Moore, P. (2004). Communication skills training for health care professionals working with cancer patients, their families and/or careers. *Cochrane Database Systematic Review*, (2), CD003751.

Finlayson, M., Baker, M., Rodman, L., & Hertzberg, G. (2002). The process and outcomes of a multimethod needs assessment at a homeless shelter. *American Journal of Occupational Therapy, 56*, 313-321.

Fisher, G. S., Emerson, L., Firpo, C., Ptak, J., Wonn, J., & Bartolacci, G. (2007). Chronic pain and occupation: An exploration of the lived experience. *American Journal of Occupational Therapy, 61*, 290-303.

Fitz, N. (2015). *Economic inequality: It is far worse than you think*. Retrieved from http://www.scientificamerican.com/article/economic-inequality-it-s-far-worse-than-you-think/

Flinn, S. R., Sanders, E. B., Yen, W., Sommerich, C. M., & Lavender, S. A. (2013). Empowering elderly women with osteoarthritis through hands-on exploration of adaptive equipment concepts. *Occupational Therapy International, 20*(4), 163-172. doi:10.1002/oti.1348

Forwell, S. J., Whiteford, G., & Dyck, I. (2001). Cultural competence in New Zealand and Canada: Occupational therapy students' reflections on class and fieldwork curriculum. *Canadian Journal of Occupational Therapy, 68*(2), 90-103.

Frank, G. (1995). Life histories in occupational therapy clinical practice. *American Journal of Occupational Therapy, 50*, 251-263.

Frantits, L. E. (2005). Nothing about us without us: Searching for the narrative of disability. *American Journal of Occupational Therapy, 59*, 577-579.

Froehlich, J., Pardue, K., & Dunbar, D. S. (2016). Evaluation of a communication survey and interprofessional education curriculum for undergraduate health professional students. *Health and Interprofessional Practice, 2*(4), eP1082.

Froehlich, J. (2005). Steps toward dismantling poverty for working poor women. *Work: A Journal of Prevention, Assessment and Rehabilitation, 24*(4), 401-408.

Froehlich, J. Hamlin, R. B. Loukas, K. M., & MacRae, N. (1992). Special issue on feminism as an inclusive perspective. *American Journal of Occupational Therapy, 46*, 967-1044.

Froehlich, J., & Nesbit, S. (2004). The aware communicator: Dialogues on diversity. *Occupational Therapy in Health Care, 18*(1/2), 171-182.

Galbraith, J. K. (2003). Why Bush likes a bad economy. *Progressive, 67*(October), 26-29.

Garci, T. H., & Mandich, A. (2005). Going for gold: Understanding occupational engagement in elite-level wheelchair basketball athletes. *Journal of Occupational Science, 12*(3), 170-175.

Greenspan, S. (1998). *The child with special needs*. Reading, MA: Perseus Books.

Greenwald, A. G., Poehlman, T. A., Uhlmann, E., & Banaji, M. R. (2009). Understanding and using the Implicit Association Test: III. Meta-analysis of predictive validity. *Journal of Personality and Social Psychology, 97*(1), 17-41.

Harmsen, H., Bernsen, R., Meeuwesen, L., Thomas, S., Dorrenboom, G., Pinto, D., & Bruijnzeels, M. (2005). The effect of educational intervention on intercultural communication: Results of a randomized controlled trial. *British Journal of General Practice, 55*, 343-350.

Harris, S. R., & Templeton, E. (2001). Who's listening? Experiences of women with breast cancer in communicating with physicians. *The Breast Journal, 7*(6), 444-469.

Hawes, D. (1996). Against postmodernism: A Marxist perspective. *British Journal of Occupational Therapy, 59*(3), 131-132.

Hemsley, B., Balandin, S., & Worrall, L. (2011). Nursing the patient with complex communication needs: Time as a barrier and a facilitator to successful communication in hospital. *Journal of Advanced Nursing, 68*(1), 116-126. doi:10.1111/j/1365 2648.2011.05722.x

Humphry, R. (1995). Families who live in chronic poverty: Meeting the challenge of family-centered services. *American Journal of Occupational Therapy, 49*, 687-693.

Ingram, M., Sabo, S., Rothers, J., Wennerstrom, A., & de Zapien, J. G. (2008). Community health workers and community advocacy: Addressing health disparities. *Journal of Community Health, 33*(6), 417-424.

Institute of Medicine. (2000). In Kohn, L. T., Corrigan, J. M., & Donaldson, M. L. (Eds.), *To err is human—Building a safer health system*. Washington, DC: Natiaonal Academies Press.

Interprofessional Education Collaborative Expert Panel. (2011). *Core competencies for interprofessional collaborative practice: Report of an expert panel*. Washington, DC: Interprofessional Education Collaborative.

Iwana, M. (2003). The issue is: Toward a culturally relevant epistemologies in occupational therapy. *American Journal of Occupational Therapy, 57*, 582-588.

Jackins, H. (1981). *The art of listening*. Seattle: WA: Rational Island Publishers.

Jackins, H. (1990). *Logical thinking about a future society*. Seattle: WA: Rational Island Publishers.

Jackins, H. (1997). *The list*. Seattle: WA: Rational Island Publishers.

Jackins, H. (1999). *The human male: A men's liberation draft policy*. Seattle, WA: Rational Island Publishers.

Jackins, T. (2002). *Working together to end racism: Healing from the damagecaused by racism*. Seattle: WA: Rational Island Publishers.

Jackson, J. (1995). Sexual orientation: Its relevance to occupational science and the practice of occupational therapy. *American Journal of Occupational Therapy, 49*, 669-679.

Jackson, J. (2000). Understanding the experience of non-inclusive occupational therapy clinics: Lesbians' perspectives. *American Journal of Occupational Therapy, 54*(1), 26-35.

Javaherian, H., Krabacher, V., Andriacco, K., & German, D. (2007). Surviving domestic violence: Rebuilding one's life. *Occupational Therapy in Health Care, 21*(3), 35-59.

Joint Commission. (2013, March). *Comprehensive accreditation manual for hospitals. Sentinel events (SE)*. CAMH Update 1.

Joint Commission. (2015). *Sentinel event data: Root causes by event type*. Retrieved from http://www.tsigconsulting.com/tolcam/wp-content/uploads/2015/04/TJC-Sentinel-Event-Root_Causes_by_Event_Type_2004-2014.pdf

Kauffman, K., & New, C. (2004). *Co-counselling: The theory and practice of re-evaluation counseling*. New York, NY: Brunner-Routledge.

Kavanaugh, P. (1995). *Spiritual moments with the great composers*. Grand Rapids, MI: Zondervan. Retrieved from www.cello.org/heaven/mbarchs/jan31/casals.htm

Kelly, G. (2000). Rights, ethics and the spirit of occupation. *British Journal of Occupational Therapy, 58*(4), 176.

Kielhofner, G. (2005). Special issue: Disability studies. *American Journal of Occupational Therapy, 61*, 481-600.

Kielhofner, G. (2008). *Model of human occupation* (3rd ed.). Philadelphia, PA: Lippincott Williams and Wilkins.

Kingsley, P., & Molineux, M. (2000). True to our philosophy? Sexual orientation and occupation. *British Journal Of Occupational Therapy, 63*(5), 205-210.

Kitts, R. (2005). Gay adolescents and suicide: Understanding the association. *Adolescence, 40*(159), 621-628.

Konrad, S. C., & Browning, D. M. (2012). Relational learning and interprofessional practice: Transforming health education for the 21st century. *Work: A Journal of Prevention, Assessment and Rehabilitation, 41*(3), 247-251.

Landa-Gonzalez, B. (2008). To assert or not to assert: Conflict management and occupational therapy students. *Occupational Therapy In Health Care, 22*(4), 54-70.

Law, M., Baptiste, S., & Mills, J. (1995). Client-centered practice: What does it mean and does it make a difference? *Canadian Journal of Occupational Therapy, 62*, 250-257.

Levin, J., & Prince, M. F. (2011). Judaism and health: Reflections on an emerging scholarly field. *Journal of Religion and Health, 50*(4), 765-777.

Lingard, L., Regehr, G., Orser, B., Reznick, R., Baker, G. R., Doran, D., ... Whyte, S. (2008). Evaluation of a preoperative checklist and team briefing among surgeons, nurses, and anesthesiologists to reduce failures in communication. *Archives of Surgery, 143*(1), 12-17.

MacRae, N. (2005). Women and work: A ten year retrospective. *Work: A Journal of Prevention, Assessment and Rehabilitation, 24*(4), 331-340.

Marshall, S., Harrison, J., & Flannigan, B. (2009). The teaching of a structured tool improves the clarity and content of interprofessional clinical communication. *Quality and Safety in Health Care, 18*, 137-140.

Matlala, M. R. (1993). Race relations at work: A challenge to occupational therapy. *British Journal of Occupational Therapy, 56*(12), 434-436.

Meade, L., Brown, G. T., & Trevan-Hawke, J. (2005). Female and male occupational therapists: A comparison of their job satisfaction level. *Australian Occupational Therapy Journal, 52*, 136-148.

Mold, F., & Forbes, A. (2013). Patients' and professionals' experiences and perspectives of obesity in health-care settings: a synthesis of current research. *Health Expectations, 16*(2), 119-142.

Morris, D., Stecher, J., Briggs-Peppler, K., Chittenden, C., Rubira, J., & Wismer, L. (2014). Spirituality in occupational therapy: Do we practice what we teach? *Journal of Religion & Health, 53*(1), 27-36. doi:10.1007/s10943-012-9584-y

Mossakowski, K. N. (2009). The influence of past unemployment duration on symptoms of depression among young women and men in the United States. *American Journal of Public Health, 99*(10), 1826-1832.

Mueller, K. (2010). *Communication from the inside out: Strategies for the engaged professional*. Philadelphia, PA: F. A. Davis Company.

Murphy, J. (2004). Using focused reflection and articulation to promote clinical reasoning: an evidence-based teaching strategy. *Nursing Education Perspectives, 25*(2), 226-231.

National Research Council. (2003). *Unequal treatment: Confronting racial and ethnic disparities in health care*. Washington, DC: The National Acadamies Press. Retrieved from http://www.nap.edu/catalog.php?record_id=10260

Nelson, A. (2007). Seeing white: A critical exploration of occupational therapy with indigenous Australian people. *Occupational Therapy International, 14*(4), 237-255. doi:10.1002/oti

Neufeld, S., & Lysack, C. (2004). Allocation of rehabilitation services: Who gets a home evaluation. *OT Practice, 9*(16), CE1-CE8.

Odawara, E. (2005). Cultural competency in occupational therapy: Beyond a cross-cultural view of practice. *American Journal of Occupational Therapy, 59*, 325-334.

O'Sullivan, P. Chao, S., Russell, M., Levine, S., & Fabiny, A. (2008). Development and implementation of an objective structured clinical examination to provide formative feedback on communication and interpersonal skills in geriatric training. *Journal of the American Geriatric Society, 56*, 1730-1735.

Padilla, R., Gupta, J., & Liotta-Kleinfeld, L. (2004). Occupational therapy and social justice: A school-based example. *Occupational Therapy Practice, 9*(16), CE1-CE8.

Palmadottir, G. (2009). The road to recovery: Experiences and occupational lives of Icelandic women with breast cancer. *Occupational Therapy in Health Care, 23*(4), 319-335. doi:10.3109/07380570903242433

Pardue, K. T. (2013). Not left to chance: Introducing an undergraduate interprofessional education curriculum. *Journal of Interprofessional Care, 27*(1), 98-100.

Peloquin, S. M., & Ciro, C. A. (2013). Self-development groups among women in recovery: Client perceptions of satisfaction and engagement. *American Journal of Occupational Therapy, 67*(1), 82-90. doi:10.5014/ajot.2013.004796

Phelan, S. K. (2011). Constructions of disability: A call for critical reflexivity in occupational therapy. *Canadian Journal of Occupational Therapy, 78*(3), 164-172.

Pierce, D., & Frank, G. (1992). A mother's work: Two levels of feminist analysis of family-centered care. *American Journal of Occupational Therapy, 46*, 972-980.

Piven, E., & Duran, R. (2014). Reduction of non-adherent behaviour in a Mexican-American adolescent with type 2 diabetes. *Occupational Therapy International, 21*(1), 42-51. doi:10.1002/oti.1363

Pooremamali, P., Eklund, M., Ostman, M., & Persson, D. (2012). Muslim Middle Eastern clients› reflections on their relationship with their occupational therapists in mental health care. *Scandinavian Journal of Occupational Therapy, 19*(4), 328-340.

Powell, J. A., & Udayakumar, S. P. (2000). *Race, poverty and globalization*. Retrieved from http://www.globalexchange.org/resources/econ101/globalization

Primeau, L. A. (1992). A woman's place: Unpaid work in the home. *American Journal of Occupational Therapy, 46*, 981-988.

Reisdorff, E. J., Hughes, M. J., Castaneda, C., Carlson, D. J., Donohue, W. A., Fediuk, T. A., & Hughes, W. P. (2006). Developing a valid evaluation for interpersonal and communication skills. *Academy of Emergency Medicine, 13*(10), 1056-1061.

Richardson, P. (2004). How cultural ideas help shape the conceptualization of mental illness. *Mental Health Occupational Therapy, 9*(1), 5-8.

Robinson, J. D., & Heritage, J. (2006). Physicians' opening questions and patients' satisfaction. *Patient Education and Counseling, 60*(3), 279-285.

Rollnick, S., Miller, W. R., & Butler, C. (2008). *Motivational Interviewing in health care: helping patients change behavior*. Guilford Press

Rothenberg, P. S. (1998). *Race, class and gender in the United States: An integrated study* (4th ed.). New York, NY: St. Martin Press.

Royeen, M., & Crabree, J. L. (2006). *Culture in rehabilitation: From competency to proficiency*. Upper Saddle River, NJ: Pearson-Prentice Hall.

Rozin, P., & Royzman, E. B. (2001). Negativity bias, negativity dominance, and contagion. *Personality and Social Psychology Review, 5*(4), 296-320.

St-Pierre, I., & Holmes, D. (2008). Managing nurses through disciplinary power: A Foucauldian analysis of workplace violence. *Journal of Nursing Management, 16*(3), 352-359.

Sargeant, J., Loney, E., & Murphy, G. (2008). Effective interprofessional teams: "Contact is not enough" to build a team. *Journal of Continuing Education in the Health Professions, 28*(4), 228-234.

Sargent, J., MacLeod, T., & Murray, A. (2011). An interprofessional approach to teaching communication skills. *Journal of Continuing Education in the Health Professions, 31*(4), 265-267.

Scheirton, L., Mu, K., & Lohman, H. (2003). Occupational therapists' responses to practice errors in physical rehabilitation settings. *American Journal of Occupational Therapy, 57*, 307-314.

Sherman, E. (2015). *America is the richest and most unequal nation*. Retrieved from http://fortune.com/2015/09/30/america-wealth-inequality/

Shield, R. R., Tong, I., Tomas, M., & Besdine, R. W. (2011). Teaching communication and compassionate care skills: An innovative curriculum for pre-clerkship medical students. *Medical Teacher, 33*, e408-e416.

Shinton, E., & Mairs, H. (2009). Working in mental health and deafness. *British Journal of Occupational Therapy, 72*(4), 180-182.

Smith-Gabai, H., & Ludwig, F. (2011). Observing the Jewish Sabbath: A meaningful restorative ritual for modern times. *Journal of Occupational Science, 18*(4), 347-355.

Stagg, S. J., Sheridan, D., Jones, R. A., Whitfield C. L., Anda, R. F., Dube, S. R., & Felitti, V. J. (2003). Violent childhood experiences and the risk of intimate partner violence in adults: Assessment in a large health maintenance organization. *Journal of Interpersonal Violence, 8*(2), 166-185.

Sterling, K., & Nayar, S. (2013). Changes to occupation for Indian immigrant men: Questions for practice. *New Zealand Journal of Occupational Therapy, 60*(2), 21-26.

Suarez-Balcazar, Y., Rodawoski, J., Balcazar, F., Taylor-Ritzler, T., Portillo, N., Barwacz, D., et al. (2009). Perceived levels of cultural competence among occupational therapists. *American Journal of Occupational Therapy, 63*, 498-505.

Sutcliffe, K. M., Lewton, E., & Rosenthal, M. M. (2004). Communication failures: An insidious contributor to medical mishaps. *Academic Medicine, 79*(2), 186-194.

Swider, S. M. (2002). Outcome effectiveness of community health workers: An integrative literature review. *Public Health Nursing, 19*(1), 11-20.

Taylor, R. (2008). *The intentional relationship model: Occupational therapy and use of self.* Philadelphia, PA: F. A. Davis Company.

Tryssenaar, J., Jones, E. J., & Lee, D. (1999). Occupational performance needs of a shelter population. *Canadian Journal of Occupational Therapy, 66*(4), 188-196.

Ueland, B. (2006). *The art of listening.* Retrieved from http://traubman.igc.org/listenof.htm

VanLeit, B., Starrett, R., & Crowe, T. K. (2006). Occupational concerns of women who are homeless and have children: An occupational justice critique. *Occupational Therapy in Health Care, 20*(3/4), 47-62. doi:10.1300/J003v20n03_04

Van Ryn, M., & Fu, S. S. (2003). Paved with good intentions: Do public health and human service providers contribute to racial/ethnic disparities in health? *Journal Information, 93*(2).

Velde, B. P., & Wittman, P. P. (2001). Helping occupational therapy students and faculty develop cultural competence. *Occupational Therapy in Health Care, 13*(3/4), 23-32.

Von Zuben, M. V., Crist, P. A., & Mayberry, W. (1991). A pilot study of differences in play behavior between children of low and middle socioeconomic status. *American Journal of Occupational Therapy, 45*, 113-118.

Vroman, K. G. (2016). Childhood and adolescent obesity. In J. W. Solomon & J. C. O'Brien (Eds.), *Pediatric skills for occupational therapy assistants* (pp. 277-298). St. Louis, MO: Elsevier.

Watson, R., & Duncan, E. M. (2010). The "right" to occupational participation in the presence of chronic poverty. *WFOT Bulletin, 62*, 26-32.

White, M. J., & Olson, R. S. (1998). Attitudes toward people with disabilities: A comparison of rehabilitation nurses, occupational therapists, and physical therapists. *Rehabilitation Nursing, 23*(2), 126-131.

Whiteford, G., & St.-Clair, V. W. (2002). Being prepared for diversity in practice: Occupational therapy students' perceptions of valuable intercultural learning experiences. *British Journal of Occupational Therapy, 65*(3), 129-137.

Whitfield, C. L., Anda, R. F., Dube, S. R., & Felitti, V. J. (2003). Violent childhood experiences and the risk of intimate partner violence in adults: Assessments in a large health maintenance organization. *Journal of Interpersonal Violence, 18*(2), 165-185.

Whitley, E. M., Everhart, R. M., & Wright, R. A. (2006). Measuring return on investment of outreach by community health workers. *Journal of Health Care for the Poor and Underserved, 17*(1), 6-15.

Wittman, P., & Velde, B. P. (2002). Attaining cultural competence, critical thinking and intellectual development: A challenge of occupational therapists. *American Journal of Occupational Therapy, 56*(4), 453-456.

Wipfler, P. (n.d.). *Build connection with your child through play: Playlistening.* Retrieved from http://www.handinhandparenting.org/news/56/64/Playlistening

Zwarenstein, M., & Reeves, S. (2006). Knowledge translation and interprofessional collaboration: Where the rubber of evidence-based care hits the road of teamwork. *Journal of Continuing Education in the Health Professions, 26*(1), 46-54.

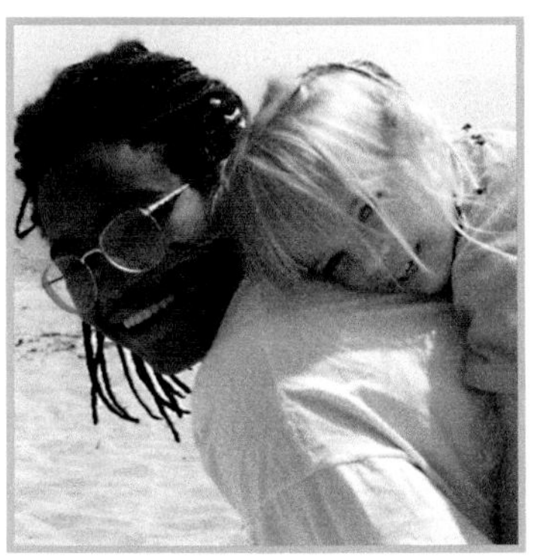

# 10

# THERAPEUTIC USE OF SELF

*Jan Froehlich, MS, OTR/L*

**ACOTE STANDARDS EXPLORED IN THIS CHAPTER**

B.5.7

**KEY VOCABULARY**

- **Caring:** A set of feelings, attitudes, and actions that convey respect, hope, and care toward others.
- **Client-centered practice:** A partnership between a client and practitioner that serves to empower a client toward reaching goals of his or her own choosing.
- **Compassion:** A feeling of sorrow for the pain of another combined with the desire and actions to alleviate suffering.
- **Countertransference:** When one person, usually the practitioner, accepts the role the client has placed on him or her.
- **Effective communication:** The artful interplay between listening and speaking coupled with awareness and sensitivity to human diversity.
- **Empathy:** A process of reaching for true understanding of the experiences and feelings of another person.
- **Transference:** When one person, usually the client, places a role on another, usually the practitioner.



Jacobs, K., & MacRae, N. (Eds.).
*Occupational Therapy Essentials for Clinical Competence, Third Edition* (pp. 133-147).

*Jody, the occupational therapist, has tried many strategies with Annabelle, but none have motivated her to get out of bed. Exasperated, Jody says, "How about if I wear my wedding dress to work tomorrow, will you get out of bed for me then?" Jody wears her wedding dress to the nursing home the next day, and sure enough, Annabelle chuckles as she gets out of bed and engages in occupational therapy interventions related to her self-care.*

## Caring

One of the most rewarding aspects of being an occupational therapy practitioner is that we get to care for our clients. Every time we show our caring toward our clients, we are using ourselves as a therapeutic tool. Sometimes, therapeutic use of self is the most profound aspect of the therapy process or conversely, if we have not achieved therapeutic use of self with a given client, the most expert techniques may be ineffective. Taylor, Lee, Kielhofner, and Ketkar (2009) found that more than 80% of survey respondents rated therapeutic use of self as the most important determinant of the outcome of therapy. Graybeal (2007) cites significant evidence that the therapeutic alliance matters most in predicting psychotherapy outcomes.

Jody was able to inspire Annabelle to engage in occupational therapy because she cared enough about her to try something as outlandish as wearing her wedding dress to work to get Annabelle out of bed. Allowing ourselves to care for our clients comes naturally to many occupational therapy practitioners. We chose occupational therapy as our profession because we wanted to make a difference in the lives of clients in need of our services. We show our caring for our clients in a variety of ways. On a most basic level, occupational therapy practitioners are required to care for our clients by providing technically competent occupational therapy services that are based on sound judgment. Beyond providing technically competent care, some practitioners show their caring by spending time creating adaptive equipment for their clients or engaging in research on a particular occupational therapy intervention or assessment instrument. Others, like Jody, have a talent for bringing humor to the occupational therapy relationship. Still others deepen the therapeutic relationship by allowing themselves to cry right alongside their clients as tragedies and losses are expressed and faced. Many offer deep hope to clients who find little meaning and hope in their lives.

Obviously, there are a multitude of different ways that occupational therapists and certified occupational therapy assistants show caring for their clients and the way we show our caring is in part related to our personality. There is no one right way to care for our clients. Often, caring occurs right from the start in a therapy relationship, and many times, it deepens over the course of the therapy relationship. Other times, we initially may find ourselves not being able to notice we like or care for a particular client, yet we offer our care just the same. Paradoxically, we can care about people even if we do not feel like we like them.

To elucidate the nature and importance of caring in occupational therapy, the 60th American Occupational Therapy Association (AOTA) conference theme was on caring. At that conference, Gilfoyle (1980) identified the importance of knowledge, skill, and attitudes in caring. She emphasized how important it is to truly know who our client is—what a person's strengths, limitations, and needs are and what will enable them to grow and change. In addition, she felt knowledge must include the ability to know how to respond to another person's needs and to know your own abilities and limitations as a practitioner. Flexibility was identified as a key skill in caring as we continually assess and reassess our effectiveness. Patience, honesty, trust, humility, hope, and courage were identified as the attitudes we bring to caring.

King (1980) challenged therapists to provide both effective and creative caring in occupational therapy. Like Gilfoyle, she also emphasized the importance of knowledge in caring, yet she highlighted the importance of the practitioner's engagement in independent thinking and examination of the broad issues related to therapy. Generating creative alternatives in occupational therapy were stressed as a deep form of caring.

A few years later, Devereaux (1984) described occupational therapy practitioners as specialists in making caring and connection happen. She highlighted seven elements of the caring, therapeutic relationship: belief in the dignity and worth of the individual, belief in an innate potential for change and growth, effective communication, humor, values, touch, and competence. Many other scholars have applied their own fresh thinking to therapeutic use of self and caring in occupational therapy. Peloquin (2002, 2003) and Abreu (2011) have emphasized empathy in therapeutic relationships. Many practitioners have contributed to the development of client-centered practice in occupational therapy (Law, 1998). Black and Wells (2007) stand out for inspiring occupational therapy practitioners to develop cultural competence. Schwartzberg (2002) has articulated the nature of interactive reasoning in occupational therapy. Tickle-Degnen (2002) has interwoven the principles of client-centered practice and therapeutic use of self with the use of evidence-based research. Black (2005) draws an intersection of caring among client-centered practice, culturally competent care, and the feminist ethic of caring. Taylor (2008) has developed an intentional relationship model for occupational therapy practitioners.

## Compassion

Compassion is a close relative to caring in health care. The discourse on optimal health care in nursing, medicine, and social work literature places compassion at the center. Although occupational therapy literature does emphasize caring and therapeutic use of self, Thomas and Menage (2016) note an absence of occupational therapy scholarship that specifically addresses compassion. Drawing from the nursing literature, Crawford, Brown, Kvangarsnes, and Gilbert (2014) emphasize kindness as the core concern of compassion and define it as "an awareness of or sensitivity to the pain or suffering of others that results in taking verbal, nonverbal, or physical action to remove, reduce, or alleviate the impact of such affliction" (p. 3591), Sinclair and colleagues (2016) analyzed semistructured interviews of adult patients with cancer and from this identified multiple themes related to compassionate care and propose a slightly different definition of compassion: "a virtuous response that seeks to address the suffering and needs of a person through relational understanding and action" (p. 198). Both definitions support the health care practitioner in choosing from a vast range of compassionate verbal, nonverbal, and physical actions to address the needs of a given client. However, a client who responds better to humor than empathy might appreciate emphasizing a relational approach.

Although occupational therapy literature does not specifically address compassion, both definitions of compassion describe what we as occupational therapy practitioners offer our clients/patients. For example, Randall Espinsosa, a hand surgeon, beautifully praises both certified occupational therapy assistants and registered occupational therapists for their compassionate care in remote, war-torn areas of Iraq:

> As we conducted clinics in dusty tents near the Syrian border, I was deeply moved every time that I watched the occupational therapists and occupational therapy assistants create or fabricate complex dynamic, static, or hinged splints using materials carried in their rucksacks, salvaged items from community care packages, motor pool parts, with a coffee pot, and bath basin for a warming pan. I could only watch with heartfelt awe and admiration, every time that I witnessed any of these individuals touch, console, comfort, and gently work with these victims of war, through the pain of recovery, especially with the many seriously wounded and frightened Iraqi children. The experience called to mind was like watching skilled artisans at work, subjecting every facet of their constructions to passion for detail and perfection. (2008, p. 104)

In addition to emphasizing what actions we can take to alleviate our clients' suffering, an important dimension to occupational therapy is that we also strongly support our clients in taking action to reduce their own suffering. As Thomas and Menage (2016) advocate, it is time for occupational therapy practitioners to enter the discourse on compassion to shed light on the compassion that already exists within our practice and to contribute to its evolving conceptualization in health care.

## Complexity of the Therapeutic Relationship

Devereaux's seven elements of a caring and the therapeutic relationship are still important today and can be expanded upon by the rich contributions of scholars from within and outside of occupational therapy. Each of these elements, with the addition of compassion, will be now be explored from the perspective of multiple scholars. This will be done in the context of occupational therapy clinical examples drawn from the author's own clinical experience and that of her occupational therapy colleagues in Northern New England so that readers can gain an increasing appreciation and understanding of the complexity of therapeutic use of self in occupational therapy.

### *Belief in the Dignity and Worth of the Individual: Respect*

> *The first client I (J.F.) worked with on an inpatient psychiatric unit was Kenny, a 15 year old who had stabbed his mother to death. He was psychotic at the time and believed his mother was poisoning him. As a new occupational therapy practitioner, I found it a little challenging to notice I liked this client, but I could offer my care and respect. As his life story unfolded before me, I never doubted that when the entire situation was taken into account, that he had done his best. I grew to like this client over time, yet right from the beginning, I cared about his well-being. Occupational therapy sessions aimed at boosting his self-confidence regarding his ability to master a variety of age-appropriate social, leisure, and prevocational activities were effective.*

The most effective occupational therapy practitioners approach their clients with an attitude of deep respect and belief in the dignity and worth of every individual. Respect can be offered even when we do not feel like we like somebody. This respect generally acknowledges that the client we are assisting has probably been through many difficulties in his or her life and has done his or her best with the cards he or she has been dealt.

Jackins (1993) expresses this well in the following quote: "Every single human being, when the entire situation is taken into account, has always, at every moment, done the very best that he or she could do, and so deserves neither blame nor reproach from anyone, including self" (p. 3).

A caring and compassionate attitude that communicates respect is one that separates people from their problems, behaviors, and distresses. In my work with Kenny, not only did I offer respect, but in my mind, I also made a sharp distinction between who he is and what his problems and distresses were at that time. I held a mental picture of him as a smart, caring boy who had had many hard experiences in his lifetime. Yet at the same time, I did not forget that in a distressed and psychotic state, he had killed his mother. I did not respect his distress.

Not confusing our clients with their distresses or problems is a crucial element in maintaining respect for a client and for enhancing the therapeutic use of self. I worked with a young woman, Martha, who after experiencing whiplash from a car accident had bilateral wrist and foot drop that was a conversion disorder. In other words, her physical disability was in her mind. Her paralysis followed no neurological pattern. She was dependent on others for all her self-care needs including toileting. My gut response to this situation was judgmental. However, I quickly checked that response at the door and replaced it with an attitude of respect for her as a human, not for her distresses. I assumed that when the entire situation was taken into account that this woman was doing her best. Therapy proceeded well, because I could separate Martha as a human being from her problems or distresses. Using a physical rehabilitation approach and a caring and compassionate attitude, Martha regained complete independence with her self-care and decided it was time to begin exploring childhood trauma in psychotherapy.

Besides not confusing our clients with their distresses or problems, we also need to not confuse our clients with people whom they remind us of. Transference is the process when one person places a role on another because he or she reminds the individual of a significant relationship from his or her own past. Countertransference is when one person accepts the role that has placed on him or her. Both are handled by reflection on the part of the practitioner combined with skillful communication and limit setting when appropriate with the client (Schwartzberg, 2002).

*Ella was working on an inpatient psychiatric unit when she met Sean, a man battling with alcoholism. During a group treatment session, Sean began discussing his threatening actions and feelings toward his two daughters, ages 23 and 16, as well as his wife to whom he had been married to for 27 years. Ella began feeling anger toward this man because of the way he was describing what he has said and done to these women, but also because she had experienced an alcoholic parent. She knew that Sean had a disease and that she needed to take a deeper look into Sean to learn who he was as a person, separate from the alcoholism and negative behavior, and separate from her experiences with an alcoholic father, to create a successful treatment plan for this man.*

A supportive listener, counselor, or supervisor can aid in addressing transference and countertransference or any other situation when a practitioner finds it hard to care for or respect a given client. When a practitioner finds he or she cannot work therapeutically or show compassion for a particular client, it is important address this with a supervisor and, in some cases, find a different practitioner for that client.

## Belief in Our Clients' Innate Potential for Change and Growth

*I worked with Alice for several months on an inpatient psychiatric unit. She was lethally suicidal (attempted to hang herself) as she recalled the trauma of sexual abuse in her early life. The team and I worked with her and were able to separate Alice from her distresses and problems. She was a very intelligent, witty, attractive young woman, yet she battled with irrational thoughts in her mind that she was no good and should die. We communicated our belief in Alice that she could face the trauma of her past and move on to a brighter future. With plenty of psychotherapy, occupational therapy, expressive therapy, and assistance from a social worker, Alice was able to reconstruct a new life. After discharge from a long hospitalization, she completed a bachelor's degree and a master's degree and worked as a victim's advocate for years, before marrying and becoming a mother of two children.*

*Meili was from China and lived with her husband, her husband's family, and her newborn baby. She was hospitalized on my unit for multiple serious suicide attempts and postpartum depression. She was frequently told by her husband's family that her depression was nonexistent and that her character was "weak." Meili would come to groups on my inpatient psychiatry unit but rarely would she speak. During individual treatments, we would ask her to try and use simple mantras or phrases that began with "I am." Meili was unable to identify any of her strengths with the exception of her ability to draw. "We know that you do not believe in yourself" we would tell her, "so we will do that for you until you have that strength." Meili, through intensive occupational therapy, and collaborative psychiatric efforts, was discharged home with a plane ticket back to China with her husband and newborn baby. On the last day in our unit she came to us and said, "Thank you, I am strong."*

*Ali inherited a young client, Lily, when she began a fieldwork rotation at a pediatric outpatient clinic. Lily had been coming to the clinic because she had gravitational insecurity and general developmental delays. Ali first observed Lily using the clinic's suspended equipment and obstacle course. Lily was extremely hesitant exploring new equipment and negotiating different floor surfaces. She requested help from Ali when climbing on and off the equipment despite having the physical capabilities to do so independently. Ali began providing unconditional positive regard toward Lily's potential to conquer the clinic's equipment. Over the weeks, Lily came in for treatment with a newfound confidence to try things she had been so afraid to do before. By the end of their time together, Lily was jumping from a loft into a ball pit with safety and without hesitation. Ali had believed in Lily's potential for growth and in turn, Lily believed it, too.*

Each of these case vignettes illustrates how important our belief in our client's ability to have a better life is. Psychiatric rehabilitation literature (Anthony, 1993; Anthony, Cohen, Farkas, & Gagne, 2002) provides us with a compelling picture of the power of believing in our clients' with psychiatric challenges ability to recover. The recovery perspective, which assumes psychiatric clients can find new meaning and hope in their lives, can be used in pediatrics and physical rehabilitation as well.

It appears that many occupational therapy practitioners intuitively offer hope to our clients, even those with the most disabling conditions. The simple statement that we frequently use in occupational therapy, "You can," is a strong contradiction to the despair that many people with disabilities feel about their ability to gain or regain function, occupation, meaning, and purpose in their lives. We may need to follow this statement with a reminder that it may take a great deal of work to achieve particular goals a client has identified (Figure 10-1).

Many clients experiencing any form of depression often have lost sight of the worth they hold within their own world. Believing in them takes on a new complexity and looms as an exhausting task to those who are struggling to remember who they are or what value they still hold. Providing clients with verbal confirmation that someone else believes in them allows individuals time to focus their remaining energy elsewhere. When we notice we are not feeling hopeful about a particular client who we are working with, it is useful for us to seek supervision so we can explore any personal roadblocks to being hopeful about particular clients.

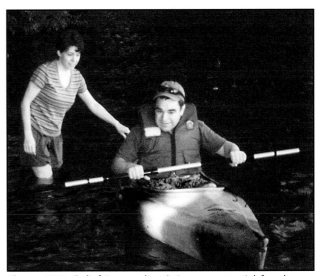

**Figure 10-1.** Belief in our client's innate potential for change and growth.

## Effective Communication

### Listening and Empathy

*Claire worked on general medical acute, inpatient unit. She introduced herself to her client, Robert, to let him know she would work with him in the afternoon. Robert perceived Claire's kind attention and began right then to talk about his situation. He was a chiropractor who had a son who had been in a car accident and needed extensive rehabilitation. Unable to find life worth living with his disability, his son committed suicide. Robert felt betrayed by his son and shameful that this could have happened to him, a man so knowledgeable about disability. He had never told anyone his son had killed himself prior to this moment with Claire. He cried heavily with Claire and she gently touched his shoulder and let him cry for a while. She thanked him for sharing his difficult story and said she would be back later. As she was leaving, a nurse came in and Robert said, "That is the best damn occupational therapist I have ever met."*

Claire was able to listen with compassion not only to Robert's story, but also to all the emotions that accompanied them. She was able to know Robert in ways he had never shared with anyone before. Caring and compassion can both be expressed through listening. One of the most profound actions that a practitioner may offer his or her clients is the gift of listening and paying attention so we can reach for the true knowing that Gilfoyle (1980) described.

As Schwartzberg (2002) suggests, the practitioner's job is to facilitate the flow of communication and to validate the person as the meaning and the content come forth. If we return to Alice, my client who was lethally suicidal, over time, more and more of her trauma experiences were shared with members of the treatment team who could listen to what she endured and all the emotions that accompanied those experiences, while validating her for surviving her childhood. As Isham (2006) stated, "Listening is an attitude of the heart, a genuine desire to be with another, which both attracts and heals."

Empathy is closely linked to caring and compassion. It is an important part of the listening process. Abreu (2011) describes empathic interactions as one of the most important factors in occupational therapy interventions. Peloquin (2002, 2003) described empathy as a process of reaching for both the hands and the heart of our client. In doing so, we enter the experience of our clients through a communication partnership that is often deeply moving and inspiring. This partnership changes both the client and the practitioner. Claire will never forget her time with Robert, nor will I forget my time with Alice. Alice expressed deep grief, fear, and anger as her life story unfolded. I was able to listen to her well by allowing myself to enter her experience and shed a few tears of my own, voice my own indignation at what had occurred, while laughing with relief that it was all in the past. This level of empathy deepened the effectiveness of the occupational therapy process. Yet, as much as I allowed myself to enter Alice's experience as I listened to her, I was also able to remind both of us the abuse was in the past and she had survived.

In a systematic review on interventions to cultivate empathy among medical students and physicians, Kelm, Womer, Walter, and Feudtner (2014) found 66% of reviewed studies reported a significant increase in empathy. A variety of approaches to teaching empathy were used, yet communication skills were often emphasized. Chapter 9 on effective communication provides the reader with a process for becoming an increasingly effective communicator.

## Client-Centered Therapy and Patient-Centered Therapy

*Janey, a 4-year-old girl at a center for children with disabilities, had hypoglossia-hypodactylia, which presented with the absence of hands and feet. She was a brilliant and determined little girl who was eager to participate in the world by using all kinds of utensils and craft tools. Bilateral activities were extra challenging for Janey, but 6 months into therapy, she expressed with vehemence that she really wanted to use scissors. With some trial and error, her occupational therapy practitioner, Marie, created a custom scissor block, with mounted spring-loaded scissors angled so gravity assisted in cutting. This scissor block enabled Janey to use one residual limb to stabilize the paper and the other to actively cut. When she saw the scissor block and tried it for the first time, Marie said, "She lit up like a Christmas tree." Despite being a shy girl, she proclaimed to everyone in her class, "Look at me, look at what I can do!" She wanted to cut paper grass for spring baskets for all eight of her peers.*

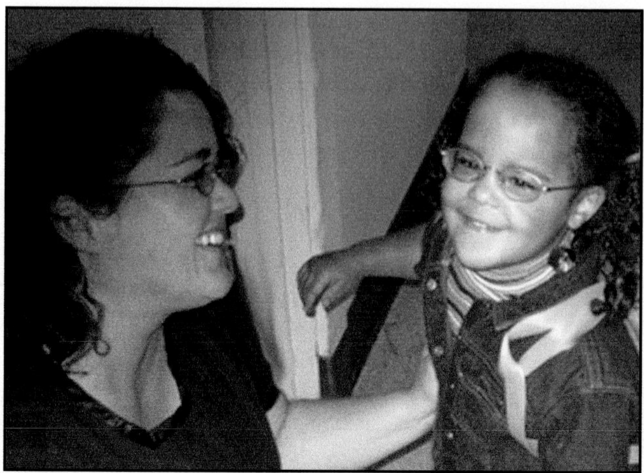

**Figure 10-2.** Client-centered therapy.

Client-centered occupational therapy has been defined as "an approach to service which embraces a philosophy of respect for, and partnership with, people receiving services" (Law, Baptiste, & Mills, 1995, p. 253). Canadian occupational therapy practitioners have developed and disseminated seminal thinking about the nature of client-centered practice in occupational therapy. The key concepts of client-centered practice include respect for clients, clients have the ultimate responsibility for decisions about occupations and occupational therapy, person-centered communication with an emphasis on provision of information, physical comfort and emotional support, facilitation of client participation in all aspects of occupational therapy, flexible and individualized occupational therapy service delivery, enabling clients to solve occupational performance issues, and a focus on the person-environment-occupation relationship (Law, 1998; Figure 10-2).

It would appear obvious that Marie engaged in client-centered occupational therapy that empowered Janey to achieve her goals. Tickle-Degnen (2002) describes the client-centered relationship as involving the formation of two types of relationship bonding: rapport building and a working alliance. The working alliance is formed when clients and practitioners collaborate with one another to develop common goals and as they develop a sense of shared responsibility for working on tasks that are involved in achieving those goals. For a practitioner to ascertain what a client's true concerns are and therefore be client-centered, he or she must be able to first build rapport and then listen well enough to accurately know what these concerns are. Marie quickly bonded with Janey as they instantly took a great liking to one another. They saw each other 5 days a week for 2 years. The working alliance between them was strong because Marie was deeply respectful and listened well to Janey's wishes and goals, which besides using scissors included working with markers, feeding herself with a spoon, and learning to hang onto a swing independently.

Noting that health care reform in the United States emphasizes patient-centered care, Mroz, Pitonyak, Fogelberg, and Leland (2015) highlight the similarities and differences between client- and patient-centered care and advocate for occupational therapy practitioners to hold a strong place in the national dialogue about how to best enact patient-centered care. All that we have learned about client-centered practice can be infused into patient-centered care.

*Randy had been given the diagnosis of a rare disease whose symptoms presented similarly to a spinal cord injury. With little known about his prognosis, occupational and physical therapy worked collaboratively by providing extensive upper and lower extremity strengthening exercises and adaptive equipment to work toward his goal of walking once around the rehabilitation gym. One day, while working with another client, I saw Randy standing with a walker. The physical therapist had a gait belt and Therabands around him and was assisting him in taking his first steps. His upper body stood tall and his hands grasped firmly around the walker. The people present in the gym watched in awe as Randy began taking supported steps to complete is goal of walking around the rehabilitation gym. "Keep pushing me, keep pushing me," he said through his tears "I know what it is like to work hard, and this was all I wanted."*

As Jackins (1993) stated, "Happiness is the overcoming of obstacles on the way to a goal of one's own choosing" (p. 34). Learning as a practitioner to adapt to a client's goal while incorporating site-specific protocol can often be a challenging task. However, a client's goal can be embedded within the foundation of the practice setting. For Randy, it would have been hard to justify the goal of "walking"; however, by using the right upper extremity strengthening exercises and adaptations, the goals of independent dressing, feeding, and leisure could be addressed in conjunction with Randy's goal of walking around the gym. The more occupational therapy practitioners can truly listen to their clients to find out what their real goals and concerns are, the more they will be able to engage in client-centered occupational therapy that is satisfying to their clients. Not surprisingly, a number of studies have reported that client satisfaction does increase when therapists truly use a client-centered approach (Calnan et al., 1994; Henbest & Fehrsen, 1992; Wasserman, Inui, Barriatua, Carter, & Lippincott, 1984). However, as Maitra and Erway (2006) demonstrated, there is still a gap between occupational therapy practitioners' perception of their use of client-centered therapy and client's perceptions of how involved they were in decisions about occupational therapy. As occupational therapy practitioners continue to refine their communication skills, client-centered therapy will be more readily achieved.

## Humor

*Florence was attempting to get her client Carla who had mild mental retardation and depression to increase her engagement in self-care and social activities in her residence. Carla was so unmotivated one day that she opened the door to allow Florence into her apartment and then began walking back to her bedroom stating she wasn't going to cook today, she was just going to lie down. Florence ran ahead of her and got in her bed before Carla could lie down. Carla laughed and said, "OK, what are we cooking today?"*

*Julie was working with Maria, an 89-year-old woman with late-stage dementia causing Maria to live in the past and demonstrate an inability to grasp reality. Maria was very hard to motivate and to participate in therapy outside of her bedroom because of her increased confusion and her nonsensical speech at times. Maria's family brought in* The Sound of Music *soundtrack to play while Maria was in bed or relaxing in her chair. Julie pressed play on the CD player and began to dance and yodel to the "Goat Herd" song. Before she knew it, Maria was by her side dancing, smiling, and singing along while holding Julie's hands.*

Like Jody, Florence and Julie conveyed their caring and compassion by using humor to break their clients' depressed state. Physician and clown Patch Adams states that the greatest success in health care involves caring for others and that fun is as important as love (Adams & Mylander, 1993). He finds that humor contributes to the success of many professional and social relationships because we deepen connections when we laugh together. The therapeutic value of humor and laughter has been noted by many health professionals. Laughter increases the secretion of catecholamines and endorphins, natural chemicals in the brain that make people feel good. Laughter also enhances immune function by decreasing cortisol secretion. Although when we initially laugh, our heart rate and blood pressure rise, as our arteries relax, both of these lower resulting in a general relaxation response. After a hearty laugh, this therapeutic response can last up to 45 minutes (Adams & Mylander, 1993).

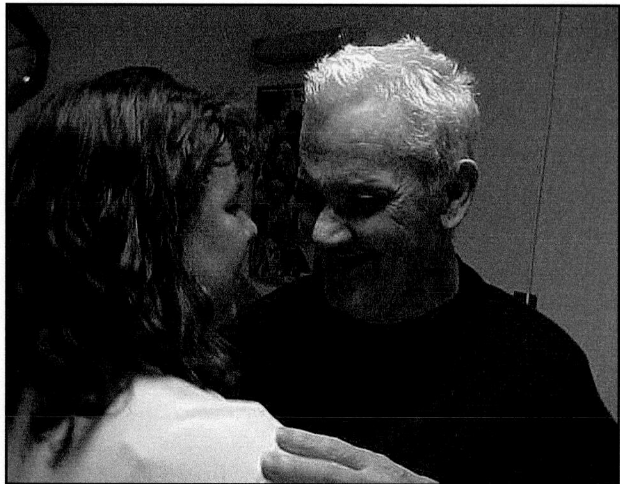

**Figure 10-3.** Humor.

Dunbar et al. (2011) found that social laughter is correlated with an elevated pain threshold.

Adams and Mylander (1993) suggest we all learn to cultivate our sense of humor by paying closer attention to what makes ourselves and those around us laugh. Workshops on humor and health care are well worth attending so we can learn to bring laughter to even the most trying and difficult situations we encounter as occupational therapy practitioners. Ultimately, we will enhance and deepen our relationships in occupational therapy by cultivating our own sense of humor (Figure 10-3).

## Values

*At his mother's insistence, John, a young adult man with schizoaffective disorder, was receiving home health occupational therapy to increase his participation in daily routines and to work with him in becoming more independent. An initial interview using the Canadian Occupational Performance Measure revealed the most important goal for John was going to the gym to increase his strength and endurance. His second most important goal was learning some social skills so he could make friends. Goals important to his mother, but less important to John, were learning to cook, managing his money, and finding an apartment. The second week into therapy, Florence, his occupational therapy practitioner, successfully assisted John in establishing a routine of working out at one of the local gyms three times a week. Other goals were eventually achieved as they became important to John.*

Altruism, equality, freedom, justice, dignity, truth, and prudence are the core values of occupational therapy (AOTA, 2015), and they provide the foundation for a caring, therapeutic relationship. In the case of John, Florence valued John's own freedom of choice regarding his engagement in occupation, and because of this, she was successful with him and client-centered therapy was achieved. Each core value of occupational therapy has significant implications for how we relate to our clients. The reader is referred to Chapter 50 on ethics for a review of the meaning of each of these values and is reminded of the commitment we make to upholding these values as occupational therapists.

## Touch

*Marie works with children with severe developmental disabilities. One of the greatest aspects of her job is that she gets to be physically close with young people day in and day out while helping them be active participants in the world. They rely on her physical presence and caring touch for external support in order to explore textures, to activate switches connected to toys, to experience movement by bouncing on a ball or riding a horse, to be in water or to use a paintbrush or a spoon. They experience great joy and exuberance with many of these occupations. Marie finds that there is a touch that is custodial such as wiping a mouth or nose, and then there is a whole other kind of touch that is affectionate, playful, and facilitates experiencing the world. There is also touch that is comforting and consoling and it is often more acceptable to give this kind of touch to young children.*

*Sarah was working on an inpatient psychiatric unit when she met Alex, a transgendered female. Alex was screaming and yelling at the nursing staff and was very difficult to redirect. Sarah was nervous to begin the initial evaluation with Alex so she approached her gently. Alex agreed to speak with Sarah in a private room. Alex began to cry when Sarah asked why she was so upset. Alex was a "male trapped in a female's body." Alex stated that she wanted to have a baby before she became a man, but no one around her supported her decision. Sarah decided to help Alex make a pros and cons list to attempt to help Alex with this decision. When Alex began sobbing again, Sarah touched Alex's hand, knowing that no contact was supposed to be made between practitioner and patient on the psychiatric unit but Sarah knew that a simple touch could mean a world of difference to Alex. When Alex wiped her tears and looked at Sarah and said "Thanks," Sarah knew she had made the right decision.*

As humans, we all need close physical contact. Young people instinctively seek out large amounts of physical closeness and touch. Infants often protest loudly when they are not held. It is only as we mature through childhood that we become resigned to less and less physical contact and loving touch. In adolescence, human closeness becomes less available, and in many societies, it becomes sexualized. In the United States, the sexualization of closeness has resulted in increased homophobia or fear of closeness with someone of the same gender. The net result has been less physical closeness and touch for many people (D'Arc, 2003).

Despite some of the societal taboos on closeness, health care workers often have opportunities to use touch in thoughtful and caring ways as Marie and Sarah described. Purtilo and Haddad (2002) speak of touching privileges that are granted to health professionals. Comforting touch, such as Claire touching Robert's shoulder, has particular legitimacy and may speak more loudly than the kindest words. Yet on the other hand, some health care professionals may provide only functional touching because of concerns about a client's misinterpretation of their touch. Through extensive interviews, Chang (2001) identified that touch has physical, emotional, social, and spiritual dimensions. Hertenstein, Holmes, McCullough, and Keltner (2009) found that even blindfolded subjects could decode the emotions behind touch. The work of Kim and Buschmann (1999) demonstrates that touch can lower anxiety levels and decrease episodes of dysfunctional behavior in patients with dementia. Guided by our ethics as a practitioner and paying close attention to the nonverbal and verbal communication of our clients, occupational therapy practitioners can determine what is appropriate and therapeutic touch.

*Carol, a 65-year-old woman who had experienced a stroke, exhibited global aphasia and a right neglect. She was aware of her deficits and would frequently get frustrated. She was given many proprioceptive cues to bring attention to her right side. These cues were much more effective when accompanied with understanding tones and kind touch. Carol would be unresponsive or become agitated when people talked with her in a way she found offensive.*

Touch, although often used solely as a comfort measure, is also used in transfers, Neurodevelopmental Treatment, and for proprioceptive purposes. When touch is used with the well-being of the client in mind, it can act as a powerful catalyst in promoting physical and emotional safety (Figure 10-4).

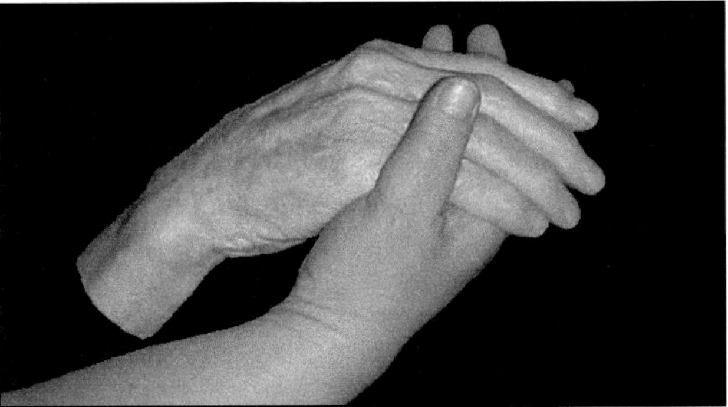

**Figure 10-4.** Touch.

## Competence

*Dom worked in a rehabilitation hospital with an elderly gentleman, William, who was recovering from a stroke. William was despondent and shut down. Doctors and practitioners could not engage him in therapy routines. Aware of how withdrawn William was, Dom went into his room and got down on his knees near his bed and said, "I can hardly imagine how hard this is for you. I know it has been hard for you to want to participate in therapy. What did you enjoy doing in the past?" The gentleman mentioned he used to enjoy reading and writing and that some of his poetry had been published. As Dom listened to William, he decided that he was going to the library to check out his book. He brought it into work with him the next day and read to William one of his own poems about living life well. Dom read the first few sentences and William recited the rest from memory. He closed the book and with gratitude and said, "Thank you for reminding me that I want to live." He got up and began to engage in occupational therapy.*

Many of the chapters in this text address the development of theoretical, technical, and practical competence in the delivery of occupational therapy services. As Devereaux (1984) pointed out, this is one of the most fundamental aspects of the occupational therapy relationship. Every client deserves an occupational therapy practitioner who is technically competent. In addition, every client also deserves a practitioner who is competent in developing a therapeutic relationship. Dom's work with William beautifully demonstrates such competence.

Taylor (2008) has developed an intentional relationship model to assist practitioners in refining their interpersonal competence with clients. She proposes that practitioners tend to adopt a preferred mode of relating to and caring for their clients. These modes include advocating, collaborating, empathizing, encouraging, instructing, and problem solving. Although practitioners tend to have a preference for a particular mode, nonpreferred modes can be developed and enhanced. In the example above, Dom exemplifies an encouraging mode with William. By reading some of William's own poetry about the value of life, Dom has encouraged William to move forward in his own life and in therapy.

As Taylor notes, every practitioner is presented with inevitable interpersonal events where we are challenged to relate effectively with our clients. The most effective practitioners are able to handle inevitable interpersonal events by shifting modes in their practice. For example, when clients are admitted to a hospital, they are not functioning at their highest performance capacity. Not only is their inner drive and volition low, but they are also experiencing a disruption in their everyday habituation (Kielhofner, 2008). Thus, as a practitioner, it is essential to remain flexible in thought and action rather than rigid in routine. Becoming stuck in the use of only one mode, for example, instructing mode, causes interactions with clinicians to be seen as a hierarchy rather than a collaborative approach to treatment. Yet with other patients, such as a client who is experiencing mania, it may be important to use a mode that provides balance to a chaotic mind. Thus, the intentional relationship model and its modes remain a dynamic part of the therapeutic use of self and can be used in conjunction with concrete practice models.

*John was a truck driver who had recently had an above-the-knee amputation. He had a sense of humor that was hard to understand at times, and although his intentions were well meant he would often make inappropriate sexual innuendos and comments. It was not long before I figured out that John's rough-around-the-edges personality was seeking praise, humor, and someone to match his outspoken comments. It took me a while to understand that working with John required a lot of mode shifting. It was important to be instructing when he had crossed a line. However, it was also essential that he saw that his practitioners were also multifaceted people just like himself. He responded well to brief uses of empathy but would then seek a collaboration mode when trying to decide which adaptive equipment would work best upon discharge.*

Cultural competence is also a critical ingredient in competent therapeutic use of self. Black (2005) has found that much of the literature on cultural competence agrees that a culturally competent individual exhibits cultural self-awareness, knowledge of diverse groups, and skill in relating to diverse groups of people. Obviously, cultural competence is an ongoing process as health care providers continually learn new information about different cultures, so an open mind and willingness to learn is also essential. The following example illustrates a practitioner's willingness to reevaluate her work with someone from a different culture.

*Kazuki, a Japanese man in his late 60s, found himself at my acute rehabilitation hospital after a bilateral knee replacement. He was in incredible shape and was always willing to push himself. Kazuki spoke no English and we needed a translator to communicate. This was often hard because crucial information got lost within translation. Upon initial evaluation, I was going through home management tasks when he stated he did not even go into the kitchen. He was quick to participate in exercises that required extreme strength, often wanting to do exercises other clients found too difficult. I spent many sessions addressing dressing but rarely did he show interest. One day, when doing a shower activities of daily living assessment, his wife came and took over. She began dressing him and stated that she did all the housework and usually helped him with whatever he needed. It was at this moment that I had to backtrack. I began to realize that I had pushed my own agenda as a practitioner, without understanding the unique cultural differences that defined Kazuki's routines.*

Often times within specific practice settings it is easy to lose site of the differences in cultural values when site protocol wants everything done in a similar way. Individual cultural practices, values, or traditions do not inhibit the therapy process. Often times they open different venues for carrying out more individually relevant occupation-based interventions. Chapter 2 on culture more fully addresses cultural competence and Chapter 9 on effective communication will guide the reader through a process of becoming a culturally sensitive communicator.

## Therapeutic Use of Self in Group Work

*Bethany was working with Sara, a 19-year-old woman from Colombia. She was sensitive, reserved, and caring, Sara came to the unit after a suicide attempt following the loss of her mother. During a group session about simple pleasures in a life, another member brought up food. There was a pause in the group that was soon filled by Sara's crying. The entire dynamic of the group shifted in that moment. A moment that had previously only brushed the surface of human emotion quickly turned to one that encompassed depth. Sara continued crying and explained how had she followed through with her suicide attempt she never would have been able to eat another meal. She went on to explain that even the things humans find so simple can behold so much meaning when there is a threat of it being taken away.*

Bethany's story is an example of how compassionate listening and empathy is not only essential in individual interactions but also in the facilitation of group dynamics. It is important to allow individuals within a group to be a part of a healing process for another group member. In Sara's case, the members of the group listened with patience, understanding, and empathy. By doing this, Sara's peers not only gave her the gift of their listening and attention, they gave themselves feelings of satisfaction and worth by knowing they had helped her.

Although caring, listening, and empathy will enhance therapeutic use of self as a group leader, Bethany's success in this group situation was also based on her group leadership skills including an understanding of group development, fostering mutual support, and handling challenging group and individual behaviors.

## Group Development

Groups often take on a life of their own and group dynamics can be complex. A number of theorists have described group development, yet perhaps Tuckman's (1965, 1977) ideas are most well known. He identified five stages to group development including forming, storming, norming, performing, and adjourning. In the forming stage, group members are often somewhat anxious as they become acquainted with one another and become more aware of the nature and the purpose of the group. They are often very dependent on the group leader. In the storming stage, conflict occurs as group members challenge the rules, expectations, tasks, and leadership of the group. During the norming stage, these conflicts are resolved and relationships deepen as the group learns to work together. The performing stage occurs when group members work together on mutually agreed-on goals in a manner that is supportive and growth promoting. Attention to the adjourning phase or the termination of a group is important for consolidation of gains made in a group.

Based on her work in leading groups primarily composed of women, Schiller (2003) constructed a relational model of group development that is somewhat different. The relational model has a stronger emphasis on the development of relationships within groups, and consequently, the stage of conflict is replaced by one of challenge and change. It includes the following stages: preaffiliation, establishing a relational base, mutuality and interpersonal empathy, challenge and change, and separation. Similar to Tuckman's forming stage, in the preaffiliation stage, group members are somewhat anxious and determining with whom they can relate and be close. During the stage of establishing a relational base, group members seek out friendship and support and begin to share openly about themselves. During the phase of mutuality and interpersonal empathy, trust is deepened and group members take greater risks in sharing their experiences. Commonalities are noted and empathy for each other is experienced. The challenge and change stage occurs when group members feel safe enough with each other to challenge each other, yet at the same time maintain connections and relationships. The separation stage is identified as an important part of the overall group, and time is spent on reviewing both positive and challenging experiences in the group and saying goodbye. Schiller finds her model of group development occurs not only in groups that are all women, but also in groups that have both men and women in them when the leader adopts a relational perspective. The relational perspective intentionally fosters caring and connection between group members.

## Fostering Mutual Support

Occupational therapy practitioners may find some of the groups that they lead follow the relational model of group development and others follow Tuckman's model. This may have to do with the practitioner's leadership style, the focus of the group, or it may have to do with the membership of a particular group. Regardless, practitioners will be effective group leaders with many different kinds of groups when they can foster mutual support within their groups as Bethany did. When it is possible, the formation of groups is made easier when the leader or orchestrator of the group uses a relational approach by getting to know members on an individual as well as a group basis. Many individuals adapt their behavior in order to take on a group role that they as an individual may not demonstrate. When working on an acute inpatient psychiatry unit, for example, groups will run more smoothly when individuals feel that the clinician has made an effort to understand them prior to attending a group.

As the group leader or facilitator models therapeutic use of self with each client in a group, he or she can at the same time support group members in relating to each other therapeutically as well. Bethany achieved this and enabled group members to play a profound role in empowering each other.

For clients in a group to play an empowerment role with each other, it is useful to establish group norms at the beginning of a group regarding confidentiality and respect. In addition, group members can be taught the importance of truly listening to each other without interrupting. A useful guideline for groups is no one person is permitted to speak twice unless each person in the group has had a chance to speak once. It is the group leader's job to ensure every voice is heard in a group. It is generally tedious for all group members when one group member tends to dominate with his or her ideas or experiences. A simple way to intervene in this situation is to simply thank the group member who is dominating for speaking and then asking what other group members think about a given subject. Giving each group member a particular amount of time to speak on a particular topic or experience can assist group members in truly getting to know each other and, therefore, develop empathy and support.

Supporting the leadership development of group members by giving them specific tasks and responsibilities will enhance group member empowerment as well. Group member tasks and responsibilities may include leading an opening circle or an icebreaker, sharing thoughts on a reading, or organizing clean-up or refreshments.

## *Handling Challenging Group and Individual Behaviors*

> *The first group I (Bethany) ever led began with a poem. I was working on an acute inpatient psychiatry unit and had spent the previous night preparing. I figured the more prepared I was the less that could go wrong. After reading the poem to begin the group, I asked what the members had thought about it. Instantly one of my clients said, "I thought it was stupid." Initially I was taken aback, almost offended. I had tried so hard to do well and had come up short. After asking her why she felt that way, I attempted to listen carefully to her response. When I put my own ego aside, I realized that she made good and insightful points. This particular member seemed shocked that I went on to validate what she said. After that moment, she felt free to speak within the group. However, this time her comments were kind. Creating a safe space for clients often involves the practitioner coming out of his or her comfort zone. No preparation will ever prepare for what others are going to say. Ultimately, there is powerlessness over others; however, the control lies in the way practitioners choose to respond to group members' reactions.*

Julie handled criticism from her group member artfully. By listening to her client's concerns, she validated her perspective and the group was able to move forward. This approach does not always work. There is much to learn about how to flexibly and effectively handle challenging group behaviors such as criticism or attacks toward the group leader or facilitator, group member conflict, the silent nonparticipating group member, the hostile group member, and other forms of disruptive behavior. Using the intentional relationship model will facilitate appropriate mode shifting to handle challenging group behaviors (Taylor, 2013). Vroman (2013) also offers excellent insights into managing challenging group behavior. Based on many years of leading a variety of groups, the following are good general guidelines for leading groups so that conflict is productive and empowerment of group members occurs:

- Whenever possible, involve the group in determining group norms.
- Listen, listen, listen to find out where people are coming from.
- Be respectful of people, but not any negative patterns of behavior.
- When a group member is very challenging, you can always ask the group to take a break or discuss a particular topic in pairs while you discuss with that person what you need from him or her so he or she can stay in your group.
- When workable, use humor to assist in conflict resolution.
- Do not assume that someone who appears not to be participating is not gaining things from your group.
- Use work or discussion in pairs to foster new interconnections.
- Allow a range of behaviors that are not disruptive or distracting.
- Always remember as a group leader that you have the right to ask someone to leave your group if he or she is making it impossible for you to lead.

Humor is a very important tool in Julie's occupational therapy toolbox. When working on an inpatient psychiatric unit, Julie used humor in most if not all of her treatments, when deemed appropriate. When conducting a group on positive affirmations, patients voiced their strong opinion on how this was "the dumbest worksheet ever" and "Really? We are not 5 years old." Julie knew that she was stuck and had to think of something quick to say. "OK, I know this is pretty silly but give me a chance. If you fill these out and discuss them with me, I will get you all ice cream." After that, the 10 members of the group sat quietly filling out the sheets and completed a very detailed discussion on positive affirmations. Julie was validating the patients' responses, and in doing so, the patients felt as though she was "on their side and understood them."

The reader is referred to the work of Yalom and Leszcz (2005) for an overview of integrating psychotherapy principles in the leadership of groups. O'Brien and Solomon's (2013) *Occupational Analysis and Group Process*, Cole's (2012) *Group Dynamics in Occupational Therapy*, and Schwartzberg, Howe, and Barnes' (2008) *Groups: Applying the Functional Group Model* are recommended for an understanding of the theoretical underpinnings of group work in occupational therapy.

## Summary

Ultimately, in caring, compassionate, therapeutic relationships we bring together our minds and our hearts. Every time we think about how to offer our assistance to

## Evidence-Based Research Chart

| Topic | Issue | Evidence |
|---|---|---|
| Caring | Knowledge, skills, and attitude | Devereaux, 1984; Gilfoyle, 1980; King, 1980; Peloquin, 2002 |
| Compassion | | Espinosa, 2008; Sinclair et al., 2016; Thomas & Menage, 2016 |
| Competence | Cultural | Black, 2005; Black & Wells, 2007 |
| | Interpersonal | Taylor, 2008 |
| Effective communication | Empathy | Abreu, 2011; Davis, 2011; Kelm, Womer, Walter, & Feudtner, 2014; Peloquin, 2002; Taylor, 2008 |
| | Listening | Jackins, 1981; Rollnick, Miller, & Butler, 2008; Schwartzberg, 2002; Taylor, 2008 |
| | Client-centered | Calnan et al., 1994*; Henbest & Fehrsen, 1992*; Law, 1998; Law, Baptiste, & Mills, 1995; Maitra & Erway, 2006*; Tickle-Degnen, 2002; Wasserman, Inui, Barriatua, Carter, & Lippincott, 1984* |
| | Patient-centered | Mroz, Pitonyak, Fogelberg, & Leland, 2015 |
| Group work | Group development | Cole, 2012; O'Brien & Solomon, 2013; Schiller, 2003; Schwartzberg, Howe, & Barnes, 2008; Taylor, 2013; Tuckman, 1965; Tuckman & Jensen, 1977; Vroman, 2013; Yalom & Leszcz, 2005 |
| Humor | Therapeutic effects | Adams & Mylander, 1993; Dunbar et al., 2011* |
| Respect | Belief in the dignity and worth of our clients | Devereaux, 1984 |
| Therapeutic relationships | Evidence on significance | Graybeal, 2007*; Taylor, Lee, Kielhofner, & Ketkar, 2009* |
| Touch | Comforting and functional | Chang, 2001*; Hertenstein, Holmes, McCullough, & Keltner, 2009*; Kim & Buschman, 1999*; Purtilo & Haddad, 2002 |
| Values | Altruism, equality, freedom, justice, dignity, truth, and prudence | AOTA, 2015 |

*Evidence-based research.

our clients so their lives go better, we are caring for that individual. Much can be learned about how to enhance therapeutic use of self in occupational therapy by continually refining our technical, cultural, and interpersonal competence. In doing so, we need to recommit to the core values of occupational therapy and hold firm to our belief in the dignity and worth of the individual and our belief in an innate potential for change and growth. We need to continually refine our use of compassion, empathy, touch, humor, and listening as important aspects of client-centered practice. The novice and experienced occupational therapy practitioner alike can expect to experience many successes and to make mistakes as they attempt to build rapport and a working alliance with their clients. As Gilfoyle (1980) suggested, skill in caring is achieved by continually assessing and reassessing our practice. Having opportunities to reflect on these experiences with supportive peers and/or a supervisor will prove invaluable in refining therapeutic use of self in occupational therapy.

## Student Self-Assessment

Use the following questions to either guide a discussion with a peer or to guide your thoughts in a journal regarding therapeutic use of self in occupational therapy.

1. Describe what caring means to you and how you will use caring in occupational therapy.
2. Can you respect someone even if you do not like him or her? What do you think of the Jackins' (1993) quote, "Every single human being, when the entire situation is taken in to account, has always, at every

moment, done the very best that he or she could do, and so, deserves neither blame nor reproach from anyone, including self" (p. 3)?

3. What will it be like to offer hope to your future occupational therapy clients? Are there some people you will find it difficult to be hopeful about? Has it been helpful to you when someone offered you his or her hope? If so, discuss this time.
4. Describe a time you noticed you felt empathy for someone or that someone felt empathy for you.
5. Have you ever been assisted in pursuing a goal of your own choosing? Describe what was and was not effective in this situation.
6. Pay attention to what makes you laugh and what makes other people laugh and journal about this on a daily basis for a week. Do you have any new insights about humor from this exercise? How confident are you about using humor as an occupational therapist?
7. What is your own comfort level with touch? Describe how this varies in different situations.
8. In friendships, do you tend to be an encourager, empathizer, instructor, problem solver, advocate, or collaborator? Describe a situation when you functioned in one of these interpersonal modes.
9. Describe a time when you have interacted with someone from a different cultural group. Did you gain any new insights from this interaction? Once you know what your future clinical site will be, find out about the different ethnic populations served by your site and do some research to become better informed about those groups.
10. Describe how a group that you have participated in followed either Tuckman's or Schiller's model of group development.

## Acknowledgments

Thank you to Marie C. Roy, LCSW, OTR/L; Bethany Augustoni, MS, OTR/L; Julie Eldredge, MS, OTR/L; and Ali Arsenault, MS, OTR/L, for enriching this chapter with their case vignettes from clinical practice.

## References


Abreu, B. C. (2011). Accentuate the positive: Reflections on empathic interpersonal interactions. *American Journal of Occupational Therapy, 65*, 623-634. doi:10.5014/ajot.2011.656002

Adams, P., & Mylander, M. (1993). *Gesundheit: Bringing good health to you, the medical system, and society through physician service, complementary therapist, humor and joy*. Rochester, VT: Healing Arts Press.

American Occupational Therapy Association. (2015). Occupational therapy code of ethics (2015). *American Journal of Occupational Therapy, 69*(Suppl. 3).

Anthony, W. A. (1993). Recovery from mental illness: The guiding vision of the mental health service system in the 1990s. *Psychosocial Rehabilitation Journal, 16*(4), 11-23.

Anthony, W., Cohen, M., Farkas, M., & Gagne, C. (2002). *Psychiatric rehabilitation* (2nd ed.). Boston, MA: Center for Psychiatric Rehabilitation.

Black, R. M. (2005). Intersections of care: An analysis of culturally competent care, client centered care, and the feminist ethic of care. *WORK, 24*(4), 409-422.

Black, R. M., & Wells, S. A. (2007). *Culture and occupation: A model of empowerment for occupational therapy*. Bethesda, MD: American Occupational Therapy Association.

Calnan, M., Katsouyiannopoulos, V., Ovcharov, V. K., Prokhorskas, R., Ramic, H., & Williams, S. (1994). Major determinants of consumer satisfaction with primary care in different health systems. *Family Practice, 11*(4), 468-478.

Chang, S. O. (2001). The conceptual structure of physical touch in caring. *Journal of Advanced Nursing, 33*(16), 820-827.

Cole, M. B. (2012). *Group dynamics in occupational therapy: The theoretical basis and practice application of group intervention* (4th ed.). Thorofare, NJ: SLACK Incorporated.

Crawford, P., Brown, B., Kvangarsnes, M., & Gilbert, P. (2014). The design of compassionate care. *Journal of Clinical Nursing, 23*(23-24), 3589-3599.

D'Arc, J. (2003). *Allies to gay/lesbian/bisexual/transgendered workshop*. China Lake, Maine.

Davis, C. M. (2011). *Patient practitioner interaction: An experiential manual for developing the art of health care* (5th ed.). Thorofare, NJ: SLACK Incorporated.

Devereaux, E. B. (1984). Occupational therapy's challenge: The caring relationship. *American Journal of Occupational Therapy, 38*, 791-798.

Dunbar, R. I. M., Baron, R., Frangou, A., Pearce, E., van Leeuwin, E. J. C., Stow, J., Partridge, G., & van Vugt, M. (2011). Social laughter is correlated with an elevated pain threshold. *Proceedings of the Royal Society: Biological Sciences, 279*(1731), 1161-1167.

Espinosa, R. A. (2008). Heroes in hand therapy: OTRs and COTAs on the frontline. *Journal of Hand Therapy, 21*(2), 104-105. doi:10.1197/j.jht.2007.10.016

Gilfoyle, E. M. (1980). Caring: A philosophy for practice. *American Journal of Occupational Therapy, 34*, 517-521.

Graybeal, C. T. (2007). Evidence for the art of social work practice. *Families in Society, 88*(4), 513-523.

Henbest, R. J., & Fehrsen, G. S. (1992). Patient-centeredness: Is it applicable outside the West? Its measurement and effect on outcomes. *Family Practice, 9*, 311-317.

Hertenstein, M. J., Holmes, R., McCullough, M., & Keltner, D. (2009). Communication of emotion via touch. *Emotion, 9*(4), 566-573. doi:10.1037/a0016108

Isham, J. (2006). *Quotes of the heart*. Retrieved from http://www.heartquotes.net/Listening.html

Jackins, H. (1981). *The art of listening*. Seattle: WA: Rational Island Publishers.

Jackins, H. (1993). *Quotes*. Seattle, WA: Rational Island Publishers.

Kelm, Z., Womer, J., Walter, J. K., & Feudtner, C. (2014). Interventions to cultivate physician empathy: A systematic review. *BMC Medical Education, 14*(1), 219.

Kielhofner, G. (2008). *Model of Human Occupation: Theory and application* (4th ed.). Philadelphia, PA: Lippincott Williams and Wilkins.

Kim, E. J., & Buschmann, M. T. (1999). Effect of expressive physical touch on patients with dementia. *International Journal of Nursing Studies, 36*(3), 235-243.

King, L. J. (1980). Creative caring. *American Journal of Occupational Therapy, 34*, 522-534.

Law, M. (1998). *Client-centered occupational therapy*. Thorofare, NJ: SLACK Incorporated.

Law, M., Baptiste, S., & Mills, J. (1995). Client-centered practice: What does it mean and does it make a difference? *Canadian Journal of Occupational Therapy, 62*, 250-257.

Maitra, K. K., & Erway, F. (2006). Perception of client-centered practice in occupational therapists and their clients. *American Journal of Occupational Therapy, 60*, 298-310.

Mroz, T. M., Pitonyak, J. S., Fogelberg, D., & Leland, N. E. (2015). Client centeredness and health reform: Key issues for occupational therapy. *American Journal of Occupational Therapy, 69*(5), 6905090010p1-6905090010p8.

O'Brien, J. C., & Solomon, J. W. (2013). *Occupational analysis and group process*. St. Louis, MO: Elsevier Mosby.

Peloquin, S. (2002). Reclaiming the vision of reaching for heart as well as hands. *American Journal of Occupational Therapy, 56*, 517-526.

Peloquin, S. (2003). The therapeutic relationship: manifestations and challenges in occupational therapy. In E. B. Crepeau, E. S. Cohn, & B. A. Boyt Schell (Eds.), *Willard and Spackman's occupational therapy* (10th ed., pp. 157-170). Philadelphia, PA: Lippincott Williams and Wilkins.

Purtilo, R., & Haddad, A. (2002). *Health professional and patient interaction* (6th ed.). Philadelphia, PA: W. B. Saunders Co.

Rollnick, S., Miller, W. R., & Butler, C. (2008). *Motivational Interviewing in health care: helping patients change behavior*. Guilford Press

Schiller, L. Y. (2003). Women's group development from a relational model and a new look at facilitator influence on the group. In A. Mullender & M. B. Cohen (Eds.), *Gender and groupwork* (pp. 16-40). London, England: Routledge Press.

Schwartzberg, S. (2002). *Interactive reasoning in the practice of occupational therapy*. Upper Saddle River, NJ: Pearson Education, Inc.

Schwartzberg, S. L., Howe, M. C., & Barnes, M. A. (2008). *Groups: Applying the functional group model*. Philadelphia, PA: F. A. Davis Company.

Sinclair, S., McClement, S., Raffin-Bouchal, S., Hack, T. F., Hagen, N. A., McConnell, S., & Chochinov, H. M. (2016). Compassion in health care: An empirical model. *Journal of Pain and Symptom Management, 51*(2), 193-203.

Taylor, R. (2008). *The intentional relationship model: occupational therapy and use of self*. Philadelphia, PA: F. A. Davis Company.

Taylor, R. (2013). Therapeutic use of self: applying the intentional relationship model in group therapy. In J. C. O'Brien & J. W. Solomon (Eds.), *Occupational analysis and group process* (pp. 36-52). St. Louis, MO: Elsevier Mosby.

Taylor, R. R., Lee, S. W., Kielhofner, G., & Ketkar, M. (2009). Therapeutic use of self: A nationwide survey of practitioners. *American Journal of Occupational Therapy, 63*, 198-207.

Thomas, Y., & Menage, D. (2016). Reclaiming compassion as a core value in occupational therapy. *British Journal of Occupational Therapy, 79*(1), 3-4.

Tickle-Degnen, L. (2002). Evidence-based practice forum: Client-centered practice, therapeutic relationship, and the use of research evidence. *American Journal of Occupational Therapy, 56*, 470-479.

Tuckman, B. (1965). Developmental sequence in small groups. *Psychological Bulletin, 63*, 384-399.

Tuckman, B., & Jensen, M. (1977). Stages of small-group development revisited. *Group Organizational Management, 2*(4) 419-427.

Vroman, K. (2013). Managing and facilitating groups. In J. C. O'Brien & J. W. Solomon (Eds.), *Occupational analysis and group process* (pp. 63-74). St. Louis, MO: Elsevier Mosby.

Wasserman, R. C., Inui, T. S., Barriatua, B. S., Carter, W. B., & Lippincott, B. A. (1984). Pediatric clinician's support for parents makes a difference: An outcome-based analysis of clinician-parent interaction. *Pediatrics, 74*(6), 1047-1053.

Yalom, I., & Leszcz, M. (2005). *The theory and practice of group psychotherapy* (5th ed.). New York, NY: Basic Books.

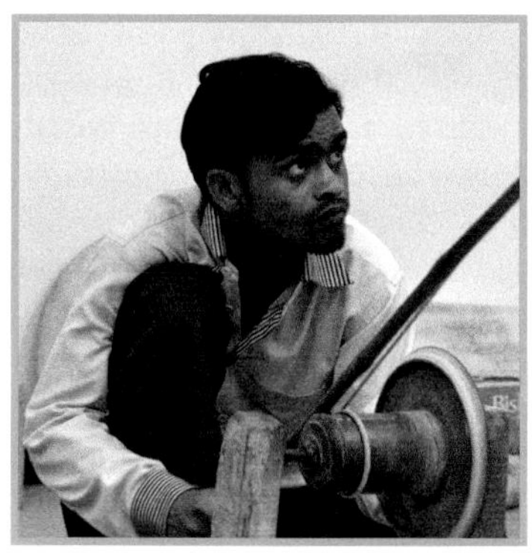

# 11

# Teaching, Learning, and Health Literacy

*Nancy Doyle, OTD, OTR/L*

**ACOTE STANDARDS EXPLORED IN THIS CHAPTER**

B.5.4, B.5.18–B.5.21

**KEY VOCABULARY**

- **Health literacy:** Ability to find, understand, and use information to make health-related decisions.
- **Learner characteristics:** Features of a learner that may influence his or her learning experience and retention of information.
- **Teaching-learning process:** Interactive work of a teacher and student with the end goal of increasing the student's knowledge or skill.
- **Transfer of learning:** Ability to apply what one has learned in a different context or occupation.



Jacobs, K., & MacRae, N. (Eds.).
*Occupational Therapy Essentials for Clinical Competence, Third Edition* (pp. 149-160).

Occupational therapy's main focus is on "achieving health, well-being, and participation in life through engagement in occupation" (American Occupational Therapy Association [AOTA], 2014, p. S4) at all client levels: individuals, groups, and populations. Our work affords many active teaching and learning opportunities regarding occupation, health, well-being, and participation (AOTA, 2014). For example, we may teach an individual one-handed adaptations for gardening, a company about promoting occupational balance within its organization, and populations who are homeless about strategies to address and alleviate occupational deprivation. In each scenario and at each client level, we must strive to provide the most effective and efficient teaching-learning process for our clients. Just as in all areas of occupational therapy practice, our challenge is to provide not only the best clinical intervention but also the best education possible guided by theory, based in evidence, and infused with our clinical reasoning (AOTA, 2014, 2015).

When we look at education in occupational therapy, we must consider a variety of audiences and contexts. There are three main teaching audiences in occupational therapy: students, practitioners, and clients. The latter may include individual clients as well as their family members, significant others, caregivers, and community. All audiences can be at individual, group, organization, community, or population levels. Teaching contexts are highly varied. We teach students in the classroom and in fieldwork settings, practitioners in post-professional and continuing education courses, and clients and those around them in a variety of clinical and community settings. Yet despite the differences in learners and contexts, there are four commonalities that we can discuss in relation to the teaching-learning process for all: the learners' characteristics, the process of learning, teaching theories and methods, and assessment of learning. In this chapter, we highlight the teaching, learning, and health literacy of occupational therapy clients. However, similar considerations can be extended to occupational therapy students and practitioners.

## Occupational Therapy Research on Teaching and Learning

Although there has been recent recognition that, like all areas of practice, the educational experiences we provide must be client-centered (Sharry, McKenna, & Tooth, 2002) and evidence-based (AOTA, 2007b; Bondoc, 2005; Stern, 2005), we are still working to build a body of evidence specific to occupational therapy education. This includes education for three main groups: students, continuing education of practitioners, and education of clients. There is a growing body of literature about how to educate occupational therapy students (Crist, Scaffa, & Hooper, 2010). Less is written about evidence-based continuing education strategies for occupational therapy practitioners. With regard to client education, some of the literature is often focused on specific conditions, such as for clients with stroke (Gustafsson, Hodge, Robinson, McKenna, & Bower, 2010) or for individuals with traumatic brain injury (Radomski, Davidson, Voydetich, & Erickson, 2009). Other researchers have begun to discuss the importance of educating occupational therapy students and practitioners about specific teaching strategies to facilitate efficacious client learning in all areas of practice (Carrier, Levasseur, Bedard, & Desrosiers, 2012; DeCleene & Ridgway, 2013; Greber, Ziviani, & Rodger, 2007a, 2007b, 2011). Until all three areas of education research are firmly established within our profession, we must use the best available evidence and theories from not only occupational therapy but also allied health and general education literatures. In doing so, we can provide the most evidence-based and effective teaching-learning experiences possible.

What is critical is that as we educate students, professionals, and clients, we study and document our efforts to contribute to the scholarship of teaching and learning (AOTA, 2009; Carrier et al., 2012). These efforts will add to the occupational therapy literature on how to best provide learning opportunities for students, clients, family, significant others, colleagues, other health providers, and the general public. By doing so we will help achieve the Centennial Vision to become a powerful force supporting the health and wellness of individuals, groups, and populations by working to meet their occupational needs (AOTA, 2007a, 2014).

## Occupational Therapy Education and the *Practice Framework*

The elements of the teaching-learning process are easily embedded in the *Occupational Therapy Practice Framework* (AOTA, 2014) process, which guides all occupational therapy practice. For example, as we develop clients' occupational profiles and analyze their occupational performance, we can also gather information about their learning needs and characteristics. As we establish a therapeutic relationship with the client, we promote an open environment where genuine goals for both occupational participation and learning can be discussed and collaboratively formulated. The learning process and teaching methods we select for each client are then embedded in the occupational therapy intervention we provide. And just as the intervention strategies are guided by theory

**Case Study**

You are on your first home health visit with a woman who is returning home after a hip and knee replacement. The purpose of this visit is to assess and provide client education about the safety of her environment. You provide the client with a pamphlet about occupational therapy and home safety and falls prevention. The client sets it aside immediately, stating that her eyes are tired and she will review it later when she can find her glasses. However, during the first few minutes of the visit, you notice and comment on some beautifully embroidered pillows. The client makes them and shows you her current project, demonstrating how she sews without glasses or any signs of fatigue.

You then ask the client to show you around her home. During the tour, you learn about this client's attitude, social supports, and patterns of occupational engagement. She has a very positive attitude to staying healthy, being active, and spending time with an extensive network of family and friends. You also notice that she has very few books or other reading material in her home. Additionally, you notice several physical safety hazards that warrant adaptation or modification.

Based on her interaction with the informational pamphlet and the lack of reading materials in the home, you realize that reading might be a challenge for your client. With your client's permission, you take photos of the physical safety issues around the home. At the end of the tour, you print out copies of these photos. With your client's help, you draw on them to indicate where a throw rug should be removed, where grab bars should be installed, and where furniture or decorations can be moved to ensure more direct and clear walkways throughout the home. She comments how helpful these images are, and says how excited she is to make these changes so that she—as well as her grandchildren and older friends—will be safer walking through her home.

and evidence, so are the teaching-learning process and methods we select. Finally, assessing what has been learned can be included seamlessly in the review of the occupational therapy intervention and outcomes.

Occupational therapists guide the development of an appropriate teaching-learning process to "design experiences to address the needs of the client" (Accreditation Council for Occupational Therapy Education [ACOTE], 2012, p. 26), in collaboration with the client and any occupational therapy assistants. Occupational therapy assistants can collaborate with the occupational therapist to "identify appropriate educational methods" and "use the teaching-learning process" (ACOTE, 2012, p. 26). Together, occupational therapy practitioners can then communicate this teaching-learning plan to other professionals who are providing services to the same clients, thereby promoting effective interprofessional work where each member's "responsibility in executing an intervention plan" (ACOTE, 2012, p. 26) is clear and coordinated.

## Learner Profile

For the educator or clinician to engage in the teaching-learning process with students or clients, it is helpful to first identify and understand the characteristics of the learner—something we may describe as the learner profile. Two main questions guide the development of these profiles:

1. What are the clients' learning needs?
2. What are the learners' characteristics?

First, we must determine with clients and their significant others what they need to know. Then, we work to understand characteristics of the learners that will help us in developing the most successful learning experience possible. These profiles consider the specific abilities, readiness, and motivation of the learners. They also include evaluation of the developmental and literacy levels of the learners, their contexts and cultures, and any other supports or barriers to learning. The process of understanding these learner characteristics is easily embedded in the process of developing a client's occupational profile. By working through the evaluation stage of the occupational therapy process (AOTA, 2014), we will come to understand the client's occupations, occupational desires and barriers, and learning needs and characteristics.

### *Learner Needs*

To create successful learning experiences for our clients, we must first work with them to determine their learning needs. These are what information, processes, adaptations, habits, and routines the client needs to achieve or enhance his or her occupational goals. For example, if a client is recovering from a rotator cuff tear and has a goal to return to cooking daily meals for his or her family, he or she may have a need to learn one-handed adaptations in the kitchen and recipe short cuts. If a business is working with an occupational therapy practitioner to reduce work-related injuries, learning needs may include ergonomic information and education about the importance of new work habits, such as regular rest and stretch breaks. If an occupational therapy practitioner is contributing to public health efforts to combat childhood obesity, he or she may provide education about occupational balance as well as the importance of providing not only discussion of but also actual opportunities within a program for building new routines that incorporate physical activity, healthy cooking and eating, and rest and leisure occupations. Once learning needs such as these have been determined, other learner characteristics can be examined to plan the best client education possible.

## Learner Abilities

As we assess a client, we are looking for his or her abilities, strengths, and challenges. Included in this assessment are abilities for learning. Perhaps the client has strong visual skills but difficulty with multistep directions. Or the client self-regulates attention levels well but has difficulty hearing. As you assess the client factors, performance skills, and performance patterns, many of the same abilities, strengths, and challenges you note in occupational performance will also affect the client's ability to learn.

In addition to learning abilities that would be evaluated during the occupational therapy process (AOTA, 2014), additional considerations may include cognitive and learning styles. Although both style types will benefit from continued basic and applied research to better understand the constructs and their application in educational settings (Coffield, Moseley, Hall, & Ecclestone, 2004; Kozhevnikov, 2007; Pashler, McDaniel, Rohrer, & Bjork, 2009; Peterson, Rayner, & Armstrong, 2009), a basic understanding of their concepts allows occupational therapy professionals to further tailor learning experiences to the strengths and abilities of their clients.

Cognitive styles are generally defined as relatively stable ways of processing information from an individual's environment (Kozhevnikov, 2007). They include whether an individual tends to focus holistically or analytically on new information. For example, does a client prefer to discuss the whole occupational therapy process—from evaluation, to intervention, to outcomes—initially, or would the client prefer to focus on just one aspect at a time? Another cognitive style, termed *field (in)dependence*, looks at whether or not a person relies heavily on the environment to interpret information. Someone who relies heavily on environmental cues may benefit from working in a group setting where social cues may enhance the intervention process.

Learning styles and preferences are factors that affect learning behavior specifically. The experiential learning theory (Kolb & Kolb, 2005) describes learning as a process where an experience is grasped through concrete experience or abstract conceptualization and then transformed into new knowledge for an individual through reflective observation or active experimentation. In other words, a client may prefer to consider home modifications to prevent falls by actively practicing these strategies in the clinic or by more abstractly talking through them with an occupational therapy practitioner. Then he or she may prefer to take some time to reflect on these strategies before implementing them, or prefer to experiment with these strategies at home between occupational therapy sessions.

Clients may have preferences for the perceptual mode in which they learn. Some clients may prefer to learn visually with pictures and diagrams, aurally through audio recordings or discussions, visually through reading written text, or kinesthetically through active manipulation of learning materials (Fleming & Bonwell, 2006). Clients may, for example, prefer to complete a home program with a video, written, or audio guide depending on their learning preferences.

## Learner Readiness

After understanding the learning needs and abilities of clients, it is important to assess their readiness. The student or client must see a need to learn what is being taught and be ready to engage in the learning process. Readiness to learn will be affected by a variety of factors both internal and external to the client. Because learning depends on readiness levels in different parts of the brain (National Research Council, 2000), internally the individual's systems, especially sensory systems, need to be functioning at an appropriate level so that information can be both received and processed (Ayres, 1973). Cognitive, emotional, and psychological readiness are also aspects of learner readiness. Clients who are, for example, currently stressed by an acute health problem may find their readiness to learn and their ability to retain information affected (Gustafsson et al., 2010). Externally, it is important to determine whether the context and conditions for working with a client are also ready for the teaching-learning process. If the environment is too noisy or the number of sessions is limited, it is important to consider what learning can be completed in these scenarios with a client who is ready to engage in the teaching-learning process.

## Learner Motivation

Motivation and readiness facilitate the teaching-learning process. When a client is both able to grasp new learning and is motivated to do so, learning will be more successful. Clients may be motivated extrinsically by rewards or consequences; motivation may be intrinsic, in that clients engage in learning for their own satisfaction or self-improvement. Generally, intrinsic motivation is most potent (Radel, Sarrazin, Legrain, & Wild, 2010). If the new learning is personally relevant, functional, utilitarian, or contributes to helping others, it is often more meaningful to the learner. In addition, materials that are neither too hard nor too easy, but instead are at the "just-right challenge" for a client, will avoid frustration or boredom and promote motivation. Motivation can also be contagious; learners often become motivated to learn if they sense genuine excitement and investment in the teaching-learning process by instructors or their peers (Radel et al., 2010). This speaks to the potential power of occupational therapy professionals and peers to motivate learners in a wide variety of contexts including group treatment, continuing education courses, and classrooms.

## Developmental Stages of Learning

Identifying the developmental level at which a client or student functions will help the occupational therapy practitioner or teacher tailor the teaching-learning process appropriately. Development from infancy through old age must be considered (Bastable & Dart, 2011), including typical development, delays in development, and possible regression in the case of an injury or illness such as brain injury or dementia. Psychosocial and cognitive development are commonly considered. In order, Erikson's stages of psychosocial development focus on the development of trust, autonomy, initiative, industry, identity, intimacy, generativity, and ego integrity (Bastable & Dart, 2011). Piaget's stages of cognitive development look at learning from sensorimotor, preoperational, concrete operations, and formal operations perspectives (Piaget, 1954). When working with an infant, the focus may be on developing trust in new movement patterns through exploring toys with the occupational therapy practitioner and caretakers; when working with an adult, more abstract discussion of roles and routines may help a client consider his or her contributions, successes, and areas for modification in his or her occupational plans for the future.

Another perspective on development may be in terms of the four levels of thinking: dualism, multiplicity, contextual relativism, and commitment within relativism (Perry, 1968). A dualistic thinker views knowledge as either correct or incorrect. This type of thinker is challenged by ambiguity and uncertainty and wants and needs structure and concrete examples. The new Level II fieldwork student will likely need structure to know what to do and how to do it. Beginning client expectations would be similar: the need for concrete, real examples and practice within a structured environment to support learning and transfer. A learner at the multiplicity level is learning to think with support from evidence, sees peers as legitimate sources of knowledge, and values independent thought. A student at this level desires evidence to support opinions and may balk at structure, while a client may ask for justification or proof that the approach being used is valid. Those within the contextual relativism level find all knowledge to be contextual, use metacognition, seek out many opinions, and look for connections. They insist on choice and commitment and may seek help from an authority figure. Clinically, this is the client who may combine traditional therapy with complementary approaches. The commitment within relativism stage would be represented by the expert clinician who has made professional commitments. Clinically, it would be represented by a client who has committed to providing education and support to those clients with similar diagnoses. Knowing at which Perry level students or clients are performing provides some of the information needed to design an appropriate learning environment (Figure 11-1).

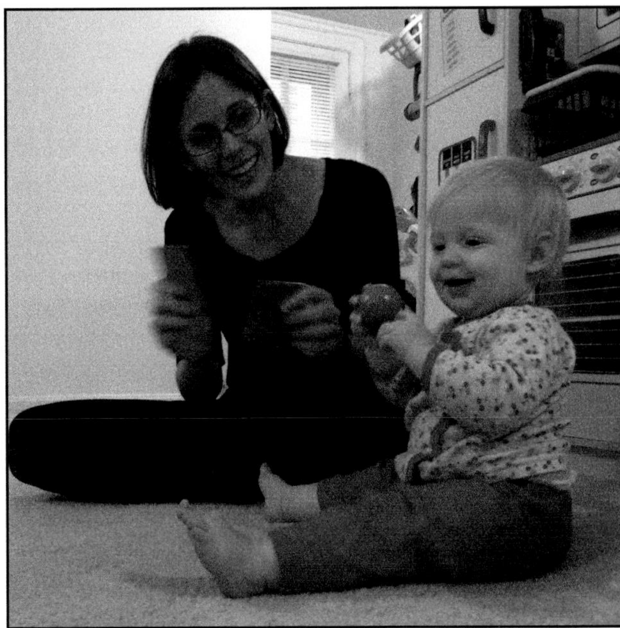

**Figure 11-1.** Working with a child in early developmental stages.

## Literacy Level

Assessing the learning needs of a client includes determining his or her literacy level. This includes gathering information about the primary language of communication, his or her general ability to comprehend spoken and written language, as well as his or her literacy in health information. Smith and Gutman (2011) report that the average American reads at a 6th grade level, much lower than the 10th grade level in which most information is communicated. This indicates a huge gap in what we say or write and what our clients may understand. We have a responsibility to be sure that what we communicate is at the appropriate literacy level so that our clients are able to fully grasp the information we provide to them.

When it comes to health literacy specifically, or the "ability of individuals to gather, interpret, and use information to make suitable health-related decisions" (Pizur-Barnekow & Darragh, 2011, p. 1), approximately half of all Americans have low health literacy. That is, they have "difficulty understanding and acting on health information" (Smith & Gutman, 2011, p. 367). We need to be sure that our services include advancing clients' health literacy, if necessary (Levasseur & Carrier, 2012). For example, if a client with diabetes is unable to read and follow multistep directions to test insulin levels and take medication appropriately, we have a role in improving his or her ability to carry out these health-promoting activities. Just as we complete activity analyses to determine client needs in daily occupations, we can "deconstruct health activities" (Smith & Gutman, 2011, p. 368) and how they interact with clients' unique environments. We can then work to educate clients in the difficult areas of their health activities, thereby increasing intervention effectiveness (Smith & Gutman, 2011) as well as their health literacy and ability to make appropriate and optimal health choices (Pizur-Barnekow & Darragh, 2011).

It is best to assess health literacy confidentially and informally. Formal testing of literacy skills may upset or isolate clients. Instead, a question such as, "How confident are you filling out medical forms by yourself?" (Cornett, 2009, p. 5) may be sufficient for determining that a client could benefit from assistance with health information. Additional behavioral cues (Cornett, 2009) may include patients' avoidance of reading pamphlets or filling out forms while in occupational therapy sessions, stating that they have forgotten their glasses or their eyes are tired, or that they will do this at home. Clients with low literacy may not complete intake forms, or may do so incorrectly. When provided written information, their eyes may wander over but not focus on reading material. Clients with low literacy may miss appointments, and may be anxious, confused, or indifferent about written and health information. By attending to such potential indicators of low literacy, we can choose words and handouts most appropriate to the literacy needs of our clients in our teaching-learning process.

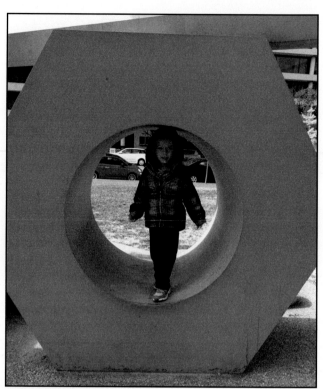

**Figure 11-2.** A child in a playground environment.

## *Context and Culture*

After looking at a client's specific learning characteristics, it is useful to look more broadly at his or her environment, context, and culture. This will help to situate his or her learning needs and appropriately design culturally sensitive teaching approaches. It is important to examine the physical and social environments as well as the cultural, personal, temporal, and virtual contexts of the client (AOTA, 2014) and consider their relation to client education. Understanding whether a company works on a traditional 8-hour day or uses a different temporal rhythm for workers can affect how and when an occupational therapy practitioner provides educational sessions for administration and staff. For example, when working with refugee women from another country, it is important to understand the cultural roles, expectations, and aspirations of the clients. Whether their cultural context is based on a matriarchy or patriarchy can affect how new information is presented and whether it is presented just to the women or also to the men. When working to promote healthy occupational participation for at-risk youth, it is important to note if the physical environment includes safe playgrounds, community centers, or libraries that could promote healthy occupational choices.

In addition to considering the client's context and culture, it is important to be attuned to the context in which the teaching-learning process will occur. Learning environments need to be as authentic as possible, as posited by the situated learning theory (Lave & Wagner, 1991). Social and cultural components of a learning environment also need to be carefully considered. The amount and quality of learning can be helped or hindered by social support, dependent on the individual's perception of the social factors. The opportunity to develop collaborative goals and the freedom to safely err may be among the norms of such an environment and therefore foster learning in a safe place (Figure 11-2).

# Learning Content and Materials

Once the learner profile has been completed, the next step is to design the teaching-learning process and its content. The content is determined largely by the needs of the learner. It often includes client-centered teaching of new occupational skills (Sharry et al., 2002) and should be supported by a strong evidence base.

Greber et al. (2007a, 2007b) formulated the Four-Quadrant Model of Facilitated Learning (4QM) to guide the selection and utilization of specific teaching-learning strategies in occupational therapy practice. This model is grounded in the acquisitional frame of reference, which focuses on developing or acquiring specific skills needed for occupational performance (Greber et al., 2007a). Using a teaching-learning approach based on Vygotsky's social development theory, the occupational therapy practitioner guides the client to learn new skills within an appropriate "zone of proximal development" and by using certain types of teaching-learning strategies (Greber et al., 2007a). The 4QM outlines specific teaching-learning strategies that can be used depending on where the learning opportunity falls along the two continua of (1) facilitator- to learner-initiated and (2) direct to indirect strategy (Greber et al., 2011). Examples of teaching-learning strategies include demonstration (direct, facilitator-initiated), physical prompts (indirect, facilitator-initiated), visual cues (direct, learner-initiated), and self-monitoring (indirect, learner-initiated; Greber et al., 2007b). Preliminary research about the effectiveness of this model has begun and should continue (Greber et al., 2011).

Other research points to the importance of providing information about a client's health conditions and how to manage them as part of client education (Radomski et al., 2009). As summarized by Radomski and colleagues (2009), clients with mild traumatic brain injury who received such education during occupational therapy sessions reported fewer symptoms and shorter symptom duration.

The occupational therapy literature in areas such as stroke rehabilitation (Gustafsson et al., 2010), adult physical disabilities (Sharry et al., 2002), and mild traumatic brain injury (Radomski et al., 2009) emphasizes the importance of providing multisensory and repetitious learning opportunities for clients. That is, clients can benefit from information being presented verbally as well as in written form (Radomski et al., 2009; Sharry et al., 2002), and from demonstration of and active practice or engagement with new learning (Gustafsson et al., 2010). Repetition of the new information may be useful for some learners. Some clients may benefit from teaching opportunities to be provided across occupational therapy sessions, particularly if their cognitive or other learning capacities increase over time or their learning needs change as they progress through various stages of therapy (Gustafsson et al., 2010).

When considering a client at the group or population level, it seems particularly important to provide learning opportunities that target a variety of learning preferences. This will provide a more inclusive learning experience for clients with different learning and cognitive styles within the targeted organization or population.

## Process

In addition to the learning content, it is important to plan how, when, and where the teaching-learning process takes place. Much of this is determined by the information gathered in the learner profile about clients' abilities, readiness, motivation, developmental stage, literacy level, context, and culture. This planning can be done concretely with the client and significant others by setting objectives for the learning in addition to those for the occupational therapy intervention. These objectives may include the amount of time and practice needed for learning, and whether and where transfer of learning should be promoted for the clients we are serving.

In addition to learning objectives, the teaching-learning process is guided by carefully selected pedagogy, educational approaches, and health behavior change theories appropriate to specific clients, their needs, and their characteristics. Just as we select theories and models to guide our occupational therapy interventions, we should choose teaching-learning theories that support our efforts to educate our clients in various areas and topics.

### Learning Objectives

As objectives for occupational therapy intervention are developed with the client, specific objectives for learning new information may be included. It is important to consider not only the content of what the client desires to learn, but also the timing and sequence of the teaching-learning process. For example, the learning objectives may describe when new information will first be presented and how often it will be reinforced in the provision of therapy services (Gustafsson et al., 2010). Learning objectives should include the following:

- Where the learning will take place
- The duration of the teaching-learning process
- What the learner will demonstrate at the end of the teaching-learning process
- How well the learner will perform at the end of the teaching-learning process

Additional considerations for learning objectives might include whether the new knowledge or skill will be transferred to new situations or occupations. The amount of time and the pace of learning should be considered in relation to the complexity or volume of material and the client's learning characteristics. And finally, the amount of practice needed to master new aspects of occupational performance should also be considered when writing learning objectives and carrying out the teaching-learning process.

The revised taxonomy of educational objectives, also called *Bloom's revised taxonomy*, provides one framework for describing "what we expect or intend students [or clients] to learn as a result of instruction" (Krathwohl, 2002, p. 212). According to this framework, learning occurs both in the realm of knowledge and in terms of cognitive processes. For example, we may want clients to learn new factual knowledge, such as details about health concerns or disease processes. Or we may want occupational therapy students to understand new conceptual knowledge, such as specific theories, models, and frameworks in occupational therapy. We may have procedural knowledge objectives for clients, where they learn to do something new, such as how to work with a new piece of adaptive equipment to continue desired occupational engagement in painting, basketball, bathing, dressing, or cooking. Knowledge can also be metacognitive, where students or clients become more aware of how cognition works and what cognitive strategies work best for their own learning to be effective.

Learning objectives may also target the cognitive processes of learning (Krathwohl, 2002). These range from simpler tasks such as remembering knowledge, to understanding, applying, analyzing, and evaluating knowledge. Most complex is the cognitive process of creating, whereby the learner combines knowledge "to form a novel, coherent whole or make an original product" (Krathwohl, 2002, p. 215). For example, we may develop occupational therapy learning objectives where a client both remembers a self-calming strategy as well as learning to apply or implement this strategy in a variety of contexts. Occupational therapy students may search and read the published research literature about a particular area of practice and then work at the highest cognitive levels to analyze the findings, evaluate or critique what is known and what gaps may exist in the literature, and then create a finished product such as a summary of the literature or a sample plan for intervention in the researched area of practice.

## Pedagogy and Andragogy

The teaching-learning process may be approached differently depending on the age of the learner. Typically, a pedagogical approach is selected for children. This is where the teacher instructs by imparting knowledge to the learner. The teacher decides what is to be learned, when it is to be learned, and designs an appropriate environment in which the learning can occur.

When working with adults, a different approach may be useful. Andragogy, or the teaching of adults, is where the teacher assumes the role of a facilitator or a guide in the learning process. In this format, the learner assumes more responsibility for the learning, often choosing what is to be learned. The teacher and learner may be learning together, rather than the traditional transfer of knowledge from expert to novice. In this approach, the teacher may also challenge the learner to progress to higher levels of cognition (Bloom, 1956) and personal development (Cross, 1984).

An awareness of adult learning principles (Knowles, 1980) factors into using andragogy effectively. Hallmarks of adult learners are their need to know and be self-directed. They exhibit a readiness to learn, want to be involved in their learning, and are thus strongly internally motivated. They also want to immediately apply what they have learned, often to solve a problem that spawned their interest in learning. Adult learners bring a host of experiences and often a problem-centered approach to their learning. They assume responsibility for their learning; they desire choices as to how they will learn and, often, what they will learn. They want to voice what they already know, based on their life experience, and build on that knowledge. They value the experience of others, are willing to take risks, and are committed to lifelong learning (Cross, 1984; Knowles, 1980). These concepts may apply to occupational therapy students, participants in continuing education courses, and adult clients who are the experts on their lives and know what they want, but may need help strategizing how to get there (Figure 11-3).

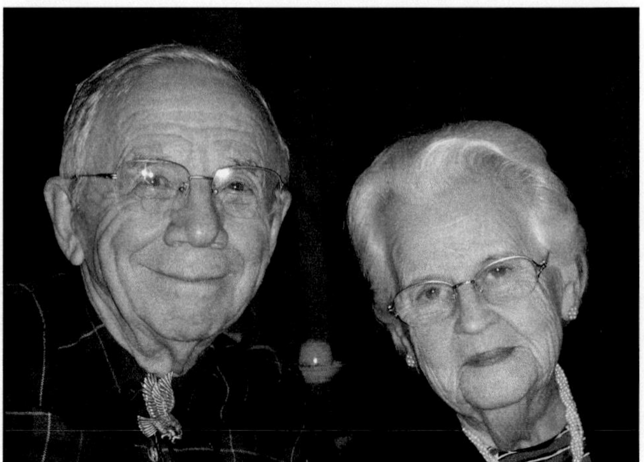

**Figure 11-3.** Adult learners.

The typical role of an occupational therapy practitioner is to facilitate learning during the therapeutic process by clarifying the goal, designing appropriate learning environments, teaching strategies for acquiring learning, providing feedback, and structuring practice opportunities to enhance transfer (Trombly, 1995). In the provision of occupational therapy services, the practitioner may need to make use of both teaching approaches and their varied concepts. Whether pedagogy or andragogy is selected may depend on the client and the progress of therapy. When working with a client or fieldwork student, the occupational therapy professional may find that it is necessary to use a pedagogical approach to structure the environment at the beginning of therapy or a fieldwork placement and, with progress, have the client or student choose which task to work on and self-structure the environment.

## Educational Frames of Reference

Education has a number of teaching and learning theories and embedded frames of reference that need to be understood to design the environment that will best meet the needs of the client or student. Block and Chandler (2005) identify three frames of reference often used in schools: behaviorism, cognitivism, and constructionism. Behaviorism grew out of stimulus-response and classical and operant conditioning theories; it promotes the teacher or occupational therapy practitioner to design the structure of the classroom or clinic and the goals for students or clients. Cognitivists encourage discovery within a less-structured environment. Constructivists believe that learners construct their own meaning and thus create their own learning.

A behaviorist approach may be used with clients who have problems controlling their behavior, such as clients with brain injury and children with emotional problems. Students may need more of this behaviorist approach as they begin to learn about the traits of an occupational therapy professional, with a lessening structure occurring as they progress in their learning. Graduate level occupational therapy education, particularly after clinical experience, would encourage a constructionist approach, providing choices for focused learning goals and the opportunity to reflect on and integrate the resulting learning. A clinical example would be encouraging clients during the last stages of community reintegration to choose a specific occupational performance issue to address and then recount their success or problems in performance.

## *Teaching-Learning Models*

Once the appropriate educational approach—or progression of approaches from behaviorism through constructivism—has been selected, specific models for promoting health behavior changes are used to guide specific learning processes. These models describe how we can work with a client to think about, learn about, and implement behaviors that are health-promoting. Examples of such models include the health belief model, transtheoretical theory, social cognitive theory, diffusion of innovations, and ecological models.

### Health Belief Model

The health belief model describes how the client reacts to a perceived health threat and how he or she determines the benefits and barriers to making a change in the health behavior (Champion & Skinner, 2008). This model also discusses how a client's self-efficacy, or belief in his or her ability to make changes, affects the client's ability to make the needed change. For example, when a client receives a diagnosis of diabetes, he or she is faced with choices as to how to maintain or improve health status. A belief in the ability to be successful with instituting healthy behaviors will allow for a more successful outcome.

### Transtheoretical Theory

Transtheoretical theory (Prochaska et al., 1994) is a model of an individual's readiness to change a health behavior. The model describes five progressive stages of change. In the precontemplation stage, an individual may not be considering a health change even if there is a health problem. In the contemplation stage, the individual considers making a health change to address a health concern. In the preparation phase, the individual prepares and may even begin to implement some elements of a behavior change. In the action phase, the individual makes the identified behavior change and continues with the new behavior short term, such as less than 6 months. In the maintenance phase, the individual continues with the new health-promoting behavior in the long term, or for more than 6 months. In this model, it is the educator's position to match the readiness stage of the client to what is being taught and learned. When working in an organization, providing educational sessions about implementing healthy workplace ergonomics may require a variety of sessions at the various stages of change to target individuals who are at different stages to consider, implement, and sustain healthy ergonomic behaviors.

### Social Cognitive Theory

Social cognitive theory (Bandura, 1977) examines the interdependent relationships of the person, his or her environment, and the psychosocial determinants of his or her health behaviors. This theory takes into account the individual self-efficacy and expectations for health that an individual possesses, and how his or her social environment affects his or her health behaviors. It describes how people can learn from observing others and how environmental influences, such as policies or resources, may influence their behavior. In other words, the individual does not engage in health behaviors in isolation, but is influenced by his or her environment as well as his or her internal determinants to engage in certain health behaviors. For example, the professional behavior of occupational therapy students will be molded not just by their individual capacities and beliefs but also by learning from the behavior of occupational therapy professionals with clients and other colleagues in their fieldwork experiences.

### Diffusion of Innovations

This theory looks at how new ideas, practices, or innovations are spread throughout a community or population. It models the diffusion, or spread, of the innovations in relation to their relative advantage over preexisting innovations, their compatibility with the community, the complexity of the innovation, whether the innovation can be tried before it is adopted, and whether the results of the innovation are easily observable or measurable (Oldenburg & Glanz, 2008). This model is particularly helpful in working with communities or populations to influence behavior change.

### Ecological Models

There are a variety of ecological models that look at health behavior. These models view people as embedded in multiple levels of influence on their health behaviors: environmental, policy, social, and psychological (Sallis,

## Evidence-Based Research Chart

| Topic | Evidence |
|---|---|
| Client education | Greber, Ziviani, & Rodger, 2007a, 2007b, 2011; Gustafsson, Hodge, Robinson, McKenna, & Bower, 2010; Radomski, Davidson, Voydetich, & Erickson, 2009; Sharry, McKenna, & Tooth, 2002 |
| Health literacy | Cornett, 2009; Levasseur & Carrier, 2012; Pizur-Barnekow & Darragh, 2011; Smith & Gutman, 2011; |
| Student education | AOTA, 2007a, 2009; Bondoc, 2005; Crist, Scaffa, & Hooper, 2010; Stern, 2005 |
| Teaching-learning models | Bandura, 1977; Champion & Skinner, 2008; Christiansen, Baum, & Bass-Haugen, 2005; Oldenburg & Glanz, 2008; Prochaska et al., 1994; Sallis, Owen, & Fisher, 2008 |

Owen, & Fisher, 2008). All levels can interact with one another, and interventions that target multiple levels are considered most effective for changes in health behavior. An example might be exploring the multiple levels of influence of older adults in an assisted living facility and targeting environmental, administrative policy, and group and individual attitudes and resources to enhance healthy occupational participation of all residents.

It is important to note that different health behavior change models can be used in combination (Christiansen, Baum, & Bass-Haugen, 2005). A combination allows for factors such as motivation, attitude, self-efficacy, and social support to be addressed simultaneously for the greatest likelihood of success.

## Assessment of Learning

As in all areas of practice, assessment of teaching-learning sessions is as important as the planning and implementation of these sessions. Such assessment is best done by both sides: the occupational therapy practitioner and the client, or the educator and the student. The following questions need to be addressed:

- Were learning objectives met?
- What was the quality of performance?
- How much more practice and variability are needed to guarantee transfer of learning?

Gaining the client's perception of the session provides valuable information for future sessions and encourages self-reflection by the client. Pre-test and post-test assessments may provide valuable information about the teaching-learning process. For example, the Canadian Occupational Performance Measure (Law et al., 1998) can reflect elements of new learning as clients report on whether their satisfaction and performance of prioritized areas of occupational performance have improved. When working with families or significant others, time to absorb the material presented and time for questions become critical for carry-over at home. The same is true for students. They need to be able to consider carefully what has been discussed and pose any queries they may have. Taking such time can facilitate clients and their families and students grasping the critical concepts presented and improve the likelihood of appropriate application. The success of therapy and education hinges on a meaningful understanding of what is being taught and the ability to transfer that knowledge to situations when it is needed.

## Summary

This chapter presented an overview of some of the important issues involved in teaching and learning. These include building a learner profile, understanding a client's health literacy, utilizing evidence-based teaching methods, selecting appropriate teaching-learning theories, and assessing learning. Occupational therapy practitioners need to be aware of these issues, understand them, and incorporate them into their clinical and educational interventions for clients, families, students, colleagues, and the general public. Doing this allows for the development of optimal learning environments, ones that foster successful learning and growth, which are the cornerstones of enhanced independence and understanding.

## Student Self-Assessment

1. Do you view occupational therapy practitioners as educators? Consider examples such as your professors and your fieldwork site supervisors. Why or why not? Has this chapter changed your view, and if so, with what content?

2. Consider your most recent or upcoming fieldwork experience. What elements of the learner profile do you think should be included in the occupational profile of clients in this setting?
3. Describe health literacy in your own words. Do you think it is important to promote the health literacy of your clients? How would you propose doing this with clients in your desired area of practice?

## Acknowledgments

I would like to thank Nancy MacRae, MS, OTR/L, FAOTA, for contributions to this chapter from her "Training, Education, Teaching, and Learning" chapter in the First Edition of this textbook.

## Electronic Resources

American Occupational Therapy Association: www.aota.org

National Institutes of Health Clear Communication Initiative: http://www.nih.gov/clearcommunication/healthliteracy.htm

Occupational Therapy in Health Care: http://www.tandfonline.com/loi/iohc20—This journal periodically publishes research articles advancing occupational therapy education

U.S. Department of Health and Human Services, Health Resources and Services Administration: http://www.hrsa.gov/publichealth/healthliteracy

## References

Accreditation Council for Occupational Therapy Education. (2012). 2011 Accreditation Council for Occupational Therapy Education (ACOTE) standards. *American Journal of Occupational Therapy, 66*, S6-S74. doi:10.5014/ajot.2012.66S6

American Occupational Therapy Association. (2007a). AOTA's Centennial Vision and executive summary. *American Journal of Occupational Therapy, 61*, 613-614.

American Occupational Therapy Association. (2007b). Philosophy of occupational therapy education. *American Journal of Occupational Therapy, 61*, 678.

American Occupational Therapy Association. (2009). Scholarship in occupational therapy. *American Journal of Occupational Therapy, 63*, 790-796.

American Occupational Therapy Association. (2014). Occupational therapy practice framework: Domain and process (3rd ed.). *American Journal of Occupational Therapy, 68*(Suppl. 1), S1-S48. doi:10.5014/ajot.2014.682006

American Occupational Therapy Association. (2015). Occupational therapy code of ethics (2015). *American Journal of Occupational Therapy, 69*(Suppl. 3), 6913410030p1-6913410030p8. doi:10.5014/ajot.2015.696S03

Ayres, A. J. (1973). *Sensory integration and learning disorders*. Los Angeles, CA: Western Psychological Services.

Bandura, A. (1977). Self-efficacy: Toward a unifying theory of behavioral change. *Psychological Review, 84*, 191-215.

Bastable, S. B., & Dart, M. A. (2011). Developmental stages of the learner. In S. B. Bastable, P. Gramet, K. Jacobs, & D. L. Sopczyk (Eds.), *Health professional as educator: Principles of teaching and learning* (pp. 151-197). Sudbury, MA: Jones and Bartlett Learning.

Block, M., & Chandler, B. E. (2005). Understanding the challenge: Occupational therapy and our schools. *OT Practice, 10*(1), CE1-CE8.

Bloom, B. S. (1956). *Taxonomy of educational objectives in the classification of educational goals: Cognitive domain (handbook 1)*. New York, NY: McKay.

Bondoc, S. (2005). Occupational therapy and evidence-based education. *Education Special Interest Section Quarterly, 15*, 1-4.

Carrier, A., Levasseur, M., Bedard, D., & Desrosiers, J. (2012). Clinical reasoning process underlying choice of teaching strategies: A framework to improve occupational therapists' transfer skill interventions. *Australian Occupational Therapy Journal, 59*, 355-366.

Champion, V. L., & Skinner, C. S. (2008). The health belief model. In K. Glanz, B. K. Rimer, & K. Viswanath (Eds.), *Health behavior and health education: Theory, research, and practice* (pp. 45-65). San Francisco, CA: Jossey-Bass.

Christiansen, C. H., Baum, C. M., & Bass-Haugen, J. (2005). *Occupational therapy: Performance, participation and well-being* (3rd ed.). Thorofare, NJ: SLACK Incorporated.

Coffield, F., Moseley, D., Hall, E., & Ecclestone, K. (2004). *Learning styles and pedagogy in post-16 learning: A systematic and critical review.* London, England: Learning and Skills Research Centre.

Cornett, S. (2009). Assessing and addressing health literacy. *Online Journal of Issues in Nursing, 14*, manuscript 2.

Crist, P., Scaffa, M., & Hooper, B. (2010). Occupational therapy education and the Centennial Vision. *Occupational Therapy in Health Care, 24*, 1-6.

Cross, P. K. (1984). *Adult learners: Increasing participation and facilitating learning*. San Francisco, CA: Jossey-Bass.

DeCleene, K. E., & Ridgway, A. J. (2013). Therapists as educators: The importance of client education in occupational therapy. *Open Journal of Occupational Therapy, 1*(4), article 5. doi:10.15453/2168-6408.1050

Fleming, N. D., & Bonwell, C. C. (2006). *VARK questionnaire, version 7.0.* Retrieved from http://www.vark-learn.com/english/page.asp?p=questionnaire

Greber, C., Ziviani, J., & Rodger, S. (2007a). The Four-Quadrant Model of Facilitated Learning (part 1): Using teaching-learning approaches in occupational therapy. *Australian Occupational Therapy Journal, 54*, S31-S39. doi:10.1111/j.1440-1630.2007.00662.x

Greber, C., Ziviani, J., & Rodger, S. (2007b.) The Four-Quadrant Model of Facilitated Learning (part 2): Strategies and applications. *Australian Occupational Therapy Journal, 54*, S40-S48. doi:10.1111/j.1440-1630.2007.00663.x

Greber, C., Ziviani, J., & Rodger, S. (2011). Clinical utility of the Four-Quadrant Model of Facilitated Learning: Perspectives of experienced occupational therapists. *Australian Occupational Therapy Journal, 58*, 187-194. doi:10.1111/j.1440-1630.2010.00901.x

Gustafsson, L., Hodge, A., Robinson, M., McKenna, K., & Bower, K. (2010). Information provision to clients with stroke and their carers: Self-reported practices of occupational therapists. *Australian Occupational Therapy Journal, 57*, 190-196.

Knowles, M. (1980). *The modern practice of adult education*. Chicago, IL: Follett Publishing.

Kolb, A. Y., & Kolb, D. A. (2005). *The Kolb learning style inventory—Version 3.1 2005 technical specifications*. Boston, MA: Hay Resources Direct.

Kozhevnikov, M. (2007). Cognitive styles in the context of modern psychology: Toward an integrated framework of cognitive style. *Psychological Bulletin, 133*, 464-481.

Krathwohl, D. R. (2002). A revision of Bloom's taxonomy: An overview. *Theory Into Practice, 41*(4), 212-218.

Lave, J., & Wagner, E. (1991). *Situated learning: Legitimate peripheral participation*. Cambridge, MA: Cambridge University Press.

Law, M., Baptiste, S., Carswell, A., McColl, M. A., Polatajko, H., & Pollock, N. (1998). *Canadian occupational performance measure* (3rd ed.). Thorofare, NJ: SLACK Incorporated.

Levasseur, M., & Carrier, A. (2012). Integrating health literacy into occupational therapy: Findings from a scoping review. *Scandinavian Journal of Occupational Therapy, 19*, 305-314. doi:10.3109/11038128.2011.588724

National Research Council. (2000). *How people learn: Brain mind, experience and school, expanded edition*. Washington, DC: National Academy Press.

Oldenburg, B., & Glanz, K. (2008). Diffusion of innovations. In K. Glanz, B. K. Rimer, & K. Viswanath (Eds.), *Health behavior and health education: Theory, research, and practice* (pp. 313-333). San Francisco, CA: Jossey-Bass.

Pashler, H., McDaniel, M., Rohrer, D., & Bjork, R. (2009). Learning styles: Concepts and evidence. *Psychological Science in the Public Interest, 9*, 105-119.

Perry, W. G. (1968). *Forms of intellectual and ethical development in the college years: A scheme*. New York, NY: Holt, Rinehart and Winston.

Peterson, E. R., Rayner, S. G., & Armstrong, S. J. (2009). Researching the psychology of cognitive style and learning style: Is there really a future? *Learning and Individual Differences, 19*, 518-523.

Piaget, J. (1954). *The construction of reality in the child*. New York, NY: Psychology Press.

Pizur-Barnekow, K., & Darragh, A. (2011). *AOTA's societal statement on health literacy*. Retrieved from http://www.aota.org/Practitioners/Official/SocietalStmts/Health-Literacy.aspx?FT=.pdf

Prochaska, J. O., Velicer, W. F., Rossi, J. S., Goldstein, M. G., Marcus, B. H., Rakowski, W., et al. (1994). Stages of change and decisional balance for 12 problem behaviors. *Health Psychology, 13*, 39-46.

Radel, R., Sarrazin, P., Legrain, P., & Wild, T. C. (2010). Social contagion of motivation between teacher and student: Analyzing underlying processes. *Journal of Educational Psychology, 102*, 577-587.

Radomski, M. V., Davidson, L., Voydetich, D., & Erickson, M. W. (2009). Occupational therapy for service members with mild traumatic brain injury. *American Journal of Occupational Therapy, 64*, 646-655.

Sallis, J. F., Owen, N., & Fisher, E. B. (2008). Ecological models of health behavior. In K. Glanz, B. K. Rimer, & K. Viswanath (Eds.), *Health behavior and health education: Theory, research, and practice* (pp. 465-485). San Francisco, CA: Jossey-Bass.

Sharry, R., McKenna, K., & Tooth, L. (2002). Brief report—Occupational therapists' use and perceptions of written client education materials. *American Journal of Occupational Therapy, 56*, 573-576.

Smith, D. L., & Gutman, S. A. (2011). Health literacy in occupational therapy practice and research. *American Journal of Occupational Therapy, 65*, 367-369.

Stern, P. (2005). A holistic approach to teaching evidence-based practice. *American Journal of Occupational Therapy, 59*, 157-164.

Trombly, C. A. (1995). *Occupational therapy for physical dysfunction* (4th ed.). Baltimore, MD: Williams and Wilkins.

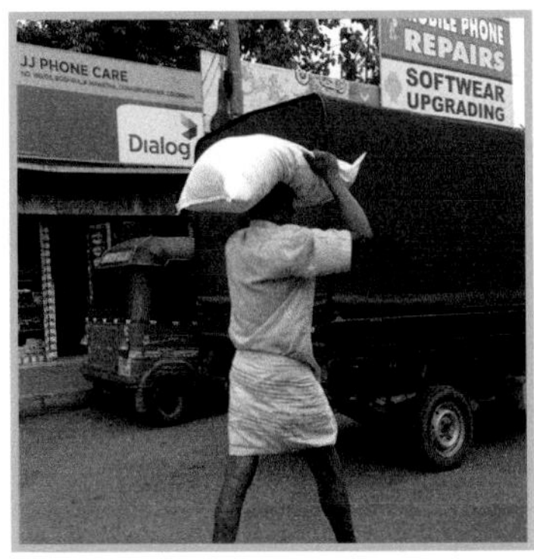


# 12

# Safety and Support

Claudia E. Oakes, OTR/L, PhD

**ACOTE STANDARDS EXPLORED IN THIS CHAPTER**

B.2.8, B.2.9

**KEY VOCABULARY**

- **Safety:** The state of being protected from injury or harm.
- **Support:** To sustain or maintain so that an individual may participate in meaningful occupation.



Jacobs, K., & MacRae, N. (Eds.).
*Occupational Therapy Essentials for Clinical Competence, Third Edition* (pp. 161-174).

This chapter addresses ways in which occupational therapy practitioners and students can take steps to optimize their personal safety and the safety of their clients. It also addresses ways in which practitioners support clients' occupational performance to promote satisfaction and well-being. Practitioners need to think about safety from two points of view. First, how do we, as members of the health care team, work to ensure that all clients receiving care in the health care system are free from harm? Second, how do we, as occupational therapy practitioners, with a unique skill set, help clients to manage/function as safely as possible in their environment?

## Broad Issues in Patient Safety

Issues related to safety in health care came to the forefront when the Institute of Medicine published the report "To Err is Human" in 1999 (Kohn, Corrigan, & Donaldson, 1999). That groundbreaking report estimated that between 48,000 and 96,000 people die every year as a result of medical error. In the immediate aftermath of the report, much of the focus was at the individual level, that is, the careless or reckless mistakes that were made by health care providers that resulted in harm to clients. Over time, however, the emphasis changed to focus on ways in which the broader health care system could create a culture of safety in which everyone recognized his or her role in promoting the safety and well-being of clients (DiCuccio, 2015; Donaldson, 2008). An impressive amount of research related to safety has been published in journals such as *Journal for Healthcare Quality*, *Journal of Patient Safety*, and *Joint Commission Journal of Quality and Safety*. The aim of much of the research is to gather and disseminate evidence on the best practices to promote client safety (National Quality Forum, 2010; Shekelle et al., 2013).

A further outcome of the Institute of Medicine report was the development of General Patient Safety Goals. Initially created by a Patient Safety Advisory Committee, a group of professionals appointed by The Joint Commission in 2003, these broad-ranging goals are updated yearly. The National Patient Safety Goals (The Joint Commission, 2016) are available at http://www.jointcommission.org/standards_information/npsgs.aspx.

Many of the National Patient Safety Goals are applicable to occupational therapy practitioners, including the following:

- Improve accuracy of patient identification
- Improve effectiveness of communication among caregivers
- Improve safety in using medications
- Reduce the risk of health care-associated infections
- Reduce the risk of patient harm resulting from falls
- Prevent health care-associated pressure ulcers
- Identify safety risks inherent in the patient population

It is essential for all occupational therapy practitioners to recognize their vital part in ensuring client safety. Detecting the presence of hazards in the environment, instructing clients and their families on effective techniques to complete activities of daily living, and communicating concerns about a client's need for supervision are a few examples of the skills and training that occupational therapy practitioners can contribute. More broadly, however, we play a part in instructing clients that they need to advocate for themselves with respect to their health care, to ask questions of physicians if they do not understand what was said at an appointment, and to fully comprehend their diagnosis and treatment plan. If, for instance, a client tells a practitioner that she does not plan to take her medication because she does not think she needs it, the occupational therapy practitioner can reinforce the need to speak with the prescribing physician to ensure complete understanding of the risks and benefits of taking—or not taking—the medication.

## Safety in an Occupational Therapy Context

The *Occupational Therapy Practice Framework* from the American Occupational Therapy Association (AOTA) identifies "safety and emergency maintenance" as instrumental activities of daily living that involve "knowing and performing preventive procedures to maintain a safe environment as well as recognizing sudden, unexpected hazardous situations and initiating emergency action to reduce the threat to health and safety" (AOTA, 2014). This definition can be applied to clients who are addressing issues related to functional independence, as well as to practitioners for use in daily practice.

Safety and support, in the context of occupational therapy, are multifaceted concepts encompassing elements of the person, the environment, the activity, and the interactions among them (Holm, Rogers, & James, 1998). The "person" in the context of safety typically refers to the client, and takes into account client factors that may affect performance, such as impaired balance or memory. The "environment" refers to the physical setting in which the person is functioning, and includes other people who live with or support the client. The "activity" refers to the task that the client is completing, for instance bathing, dressing, or cooking. Any activity may fall on a continuum of risk from "not safe at all" to "very safe." However, it is the interactions among the person, the activity, and the environment that largely dictate whether an activity is safe. For example, consider the activity of meal preparation. There is minimal safety risk for a typical college student who is making a simple meal in an uncluttered kitchen using appliances that are in optimal working condition. However, meal preparation does present a safety risk for a person with impaired vision (interaction between the person and the activity) or for a person who is attempting to cook in a cluttered or inadequately lit work space (interaction between the person and the environment).

Practitioners are routinely called upon to make judgments about clients' safety status, often to help with decision making about discharge. For instance, consider a team meeting in which discharge decisions are being made regarding an inpatient in a rehabilitation setting. Determining whether that client will be safe in a different setting (e.g., at home) requires complex problem-solving and analytical skills. Practitioners make judgments about the likelihood that the client will fall after returning home or whether he or she could safely bathe alone. Assessing the risk requires practitioners to incorporate information from the client, family members, and other team members. Because each person may have a different perception about what it means to be "safe," practitioners are called upon to make clear judgments to aid in the team's decision making.

Of concern in the decision-making process is that professionals tend to rely on objective measures when determining potential threats, whereas laypeople may rely on subjective concerns (Oppe, 1988). So, for example, a practitioner will incorporate information about strength, balance, attention, memory, sensation, and visual acuity of a 35-year-old mother who has multiple sclerosis to determine that she has a high likelihood of getting burned while cooking. The client or a family member, meanwhile, may focus on the individual's familiarity with the kitchen environment, her desire to nurture her family, and her love of cooking to determine that the risk of injury is low. Communicating the results of our assessments—and their links to potential hazards—is a key skill that practitioners must demonstrate.

Safety concerns are present across the continuum of settings in which occupational therapy practitioners work. Although the specific types of safety issues that emerge in acute care, rehabilitation, skilled nursing facilities, schools, and home care may differ, practitioners can use a consistent set of clinical reasoning skills across the settings. Assessing client factors, activity demands, contextual cues, and performance skills provides practitioners with important information about each client's ability to function safely. However, it is worth noting that safety is a dynamic construct. A client may be strong and steady when getting out of bed in the morning but need physical assistance to get back into bed when he is fatigued at the end of the day. Likewise, a client may use caution when taking her time to bathe and dress but if rushed may demonstrate riskier behaviors such as walking across the bedroom without her walker. A child may carefully negotiate playground equipment when he is alone with his mother but may impulsively run or jump when other children join in. As practitioners, we cannot anticipate every situation that the client may encounter in the future, but we can use clinical reasoning skills to make our best assessments of the client's safety.

Efforts to support the functional independence of clients must always be balanced with efforts to maintain their safety; these two well-intentioned objectives are at times in conflict with one another (Oakes, 2011). For example, consider an 80-year-old home care client who resides with her daughter. In the practitioner's assessment, impairments in strength, balance, vision, and judgment lead to a recommendation that the client's daughter provide supervision while bathing. The client, however, may value privacy more than safety, and state that she will bathe on her own. This type of conflict is not easily resolved, and requires open and clear communication on all parts.

Although individual health care facilities provide routine training on safety issues, this chapter provides an overview of the basic issues related to safety. It is not intended to serve as a replacement for individualized safety training specific to a particular setting. All practitioners have a responsibility to receive ongoing training and to adhere to institutional policies and procedures related to safety.

## General Safety Principles

When initiating contact with a client, practitioners and students must take steps to ensure that they are working with the correct client. For hospitalized clients, this may include checking wrist bands or confirming the identity with the client, a family member, or staff. Practitioners must have accurate, up-to-date information about our clients. This may involve reading the medical chart or consulting with other staff members in preparation for the therapeutic encounter. If there is a question with respect to a client's status or his or her ability to engage in therapy (e.g., there may be conflicting information in a client's medical chart), clarification must be obtained before initiating contact with the client. Practitioners must be aware of any precautions or contraindications for intervention, such as the following:

- Orthopedic precautions (e.g., do not flex hips greater than 90 degrees)
- Cardiac precautions (e.g., stop activity if heart rate increases more than 20 beats per minute over baseline)
- Positioning precautions (e.g., do not raise head of bed greater than 30 degrees)

- Weight-bearing precautions (e.g., no more than toe-touch weight bearing on left lower extremity)
- Precautions related to feeding status (e.g., fluid restrictions, thickened liquids only)
- Supervision precautions (e.g., do not leave client unattended)
- Infection control precautions (e.g., don mask, gloves, and gown before entering the client's room)

Practitioners must be aware of any procedures that the client may have undergone and whether any follow-up precautions must be observed. For example, clients may be required to remain on bed rest for a set amount of time following an angiography (Gall, Tarique, Natarajan, & Zaman, 2006).

In addition, therapists must be aware of the effects of drugs and associated common side effects that might relate to occupational therapy. Practitioners should know how to interpret common laboratory values with respect to a client's ability to engage in therapy.

Physical hazards in the environment should be reduced to support occupational performance. The space should be visually inspected to ensure that tripping hazards have been eliminated, sharp objects from previous sessions have been stored, and potentially dangerous objects have been removed. Floors should be clear of liquid and debris.

Practitioners are required to make judgments about what is safe for each individual client. Judgments about materials such as sharp-edged scissors, needles, knives, ovens, and stoves need to be made on a case-by-case basis with each client. The dynamic nature of clients' status requires therapists to continually reassess clients' ability to safely engage in a particular occupation on a given day.

Furthermore, to fully support clients in performing their occupational roles and responsibilities, the practitioner must support the cultural, physical, social, personal, spiritual, temporal, and virtual contexts in which the clients are engaged. For example, some clients may need both safety education and social support to explore the Internet. The therapist must use clinical reasoning during the evaluation and intervention of both safety and support to enhance clients' quality of life.

Practitioners must consider the physical, cognitive, and emotional demands of activities to determine whether participation has the potential to compromise the client's safety. Ongoing occupation analysis helps to ensure an appropriate "fit" among the client, the occupation, and the materials that are needed. Adapting an occupation to provide an appropriate challenge is a fundamental step in providing support for clients and in keeping them safe while allowing them to advance their functional status.

Impaired cognition presents serious safety concerns across intervention settings. Practitioners must be aware of clients' awareness of and ability to respond to potentially dangerous situations. To maintain safety, clients must demonstrate adequate attention, memory, judgment, temporal awareness, problem solving, decision making, and the ability to initiate actions in a timely manner. Occupational therapists are often called upon to determine if a client can safely perform an activity independently. Part of that decision making involves determining the client's ability to identify and respond to unsafe conditions in an effective manner and also what supports might be needed to maximize safe performance. Supports may be environmental (e.g., grab bars), social (e.g., "friendly visitors"), or virtual (e.g., daily email contact).

Following interactions with clients, therapists must use judgment when making decisions about how and where to leave clients. For example, some clients may be left alone in their hospital room, whereas others must be supervised at all times. Some will need assistance with transport to another therapy session. It is important to know each client's status with respect to his or her ability to manage independently after a therapy session has been completed.

## Suicide Risk

Because health and rehabilitation workers treat clients with a wide range of diagnoses and stressors, therapists must be alert to the risk of suicide. Practitioners must be able to accurately assess whether clients have made a suicide attempt, the risk of repetition, if suicidal ideation is present, and if the client feels hopelessness or is likely to act impulsively (Bruce & Borg, 2002). If a client makes indirect comments that suggest he or she has considered suicide, ask directly if there is a plan to commit suicide. Any statement about suicide should be taken seriously and shared with other members of the interprofessional team.

A client who appears to be suicidal should not be left unattended. The practitioner should inform the client that he or she has a responsibility to alert the physician immediately. It is critical to document any statement the client has made relative to a suicide threat, as well as any action that has been taken.

## Infection Control

Infection control is a basic component of clinical practice for all practitioners and students regardless of the practice setting. Therapists must be vigilant in our efforts to curb the spread of infection and reduce our personal risk of becoming infected with contaminated materials as well as be aware of the risk of drug-resistant pathogens.

Methicillin-resistant *Staphylococcus aureus*, vancomycin-resistant *Enterococci*, and some gram-negative bacilli are microorganisms that are resistant to one or more classes of antibiotics. Because there are limited intervention options if an infection develops from one of these organisms, it is critical that all health care workers take steps to reduce the spread of infection. The Centers for Disease Control and Prevention (CDC) developed an online campaign to help hospital workers reduce the risk of spreading drug-resistant pathogens (www.cdc.gov/drugresistance/healthcare/default.htm). Guidelines differ for hospitalized adults, adults receiving dialysis, hospitalized children, long-term care clients, and surgical clients.

Therapists should routinely follow standard precautions that include thorough hand washing and the use of workplace procedures to reduce the risk of transmission of infectious agents. Workplace procedures, or the way tasks are performed, can minimize risk. Workplace procedures include proper waste disposal; appropriate laundry handling; and the proper use of personal protective equipment such as gloves, eye protection, face shields, masks, and gowns.

Standard precautions are a combination of universal precautions and body substance isolation. Universal precautions were developed in the 1980s to prevent the transmission of bloodborne pathogens such as HIV (Occupational Safety and Health Administration [OSHA], 2002a, 2011). Body substance isolation precautions were developed to minimize the risk for transmission of pathogens from moist body substances such as infected respiratory secretions or urine. The CDC developed standard precautions based on the assumption that all blood, body fluids, secretions, excretions (other than sweat), non-intact skin, and mucous membranes may contain infectious agents that could be transmitted to other people (Siegel, Rhinehart, Jackson, Chiarello, & Healthcare Infection Control Practices Advisory Committee, 2007). Some standard precautions are detailed in the following section.

## Hand Hygiene

When properly performed, hand washing can be the single most important way to prevent the spread of disease (Potter & Perry, 2004). Hands should be washed before and after contact with every client. In addition, hand washing should be completed after coming into contact with blood, body fluids, secretions, excretions, or any client care equipment. If contact with these substances takes place, practitioners should wash their hands even if gloves were worn. The correct technique involves rubbing the hands together under running water for at least 15 seconds using a mild soap (Boyce, Pittet, Healthcare Infection Control Practices Advisory Committee, & HICPAC/SHEA/APIC/IDSA Hand Hygiene Task Force, 2002). Rub vigorously under the nails, in between the fingers, and on both surfaces of the hands. Rinse thoroughly under running water. Leave the water running while drying hands and use a clean paper towel to turn off the water. Waterless, alcohol-based, antiseptic rubs are acceptable substitutes for routine hand washing when no visible soil is present. Such rubs may be used when running water is not accessible or convenient, although hands should be washed under running water at the earliest opportunity. The CDC (2015) guidelines for hand washing are available online in an interactive video format at http://www.cdc.gov/handhygiene/Basics.html.

## Gloves

Gloves are a critical component of personal protective equipment used to reduce the risk for transmission of infectious agents. Therapists should don gloves before coming into contact with blood, body fluids, secretions, excretions, and contaminated items and before touching mucous membranes or nonintact skin. For occupational therapy practitioners, it is appropriate to don gloves during sessions involving wound care, oral hygiene, or toileting. Remove gloves immediately after use. The proper technique for removing gloves involves pulling the first glove off by grasping the outer surface of the glove to be removed (not the surface touching the skin) and slipping the glove inside out as it is pulled off the hand. To remove the second glove, slip a nongloved finger under the remaining glove and pull it off while turning it inside out. Dispose of both gloves by touching only the inner glove surface. Do not touch noncontaminated items before removing gloves. Hands should be washed immediately after removing gloves (Boyce et al., 2002).

## Masks, Eye Protection, and Face Shields

Masks, eye protection, and face shields may be needed if it is anticipated that blood, body fluids, secretions, or excretions will splash during interaction with the client. These pieces of personal protective equipment protect the practitioner's eyes, nose, and mouth from exposure to sprayed microorganisms.

## Gowns

A nonsterile gown is used for protecting skin and clothing during interactions when splashes are likely to occur. The cuffs of the gown should be tucked into the top of the gloves. After the session, the gown should be untied, held away from the body while being removed, rolled inside out, and then disposed of in an appropriate container. Hands should be washed immediately after the gown and gloves are removed.

## Client Care Equipment

Care must be taken to prevent the spread of microorganisms on equipment that is used by and with clients. Equipment should be cleaned after use with an approved solution according to institutional policy. Mat tables and adaptive equipment should be cleaned according to departmental policy. Single-use items should be discarded appropriately.

## Linens

Practitioners should take steps to minimize skin and mucous membrane exposure to soiled linens. Practitioners may encounter soiled linens when performing activities of daily living with clients. Gloves should be worn to remove soiled linens; then soiled linens should be placed in an appropriate leak-proof container for transport to laundry.

## Other Precautions

Additional practices, including airborne infection isolation rooms, contact precautions, and droplet precautions, are used to prevent transmission of infectious agents spread by direct or indirect contact with a client or the client's environment (CDC, 2004). These practices reflect a higher standard of infection control than standard precautions. Private rooms, negative airflow pressure, and respiratory protection devices add extra levels of infection control for clients placed under these precautions. Appropriate signage will alert practitioners of the need to follow special precautions.

## Respiratory Hygiene/ Coughing Etiquette

This recent addition to standard precautions (Siegel et al., 2007) broadly applies to all people who enter health care settings, including visitors. For example, a client's family member may have a cough and should therefore use coughing etiquette (e.g., covering the mouth, preferably by coughing into a bent elbow) to reduce the spread of an undiagnosed infection. Respiratory hygiene requires people with coughs or respiratory discharge to cover their mouths when coughing, dispose of used tissues, and wash hands as soon as possible after doing so; wear masks if tolerated; and maintain greater than 3 feet distance from others.

## Vaccinations

The hepatitis B virus presents a serious risk of infection for health care workers (CDC, 2011). The hepatitis B virus series reduces the risk of infection and is available, free of charge, to hospital employees who are at risk of exposure (OSHA, 2012). Health care workers may be asked to sign a declination if they choose not to receive the vaccine. The CDC (2011) recommends that health care workers receive annual influenza vaccinations. Health care workers are advised to get the immunization for measles, mumps, and rubella in the absence of laboratory proof of immunity. Health care professionals should not get the varicella vaccination if they have proof from a health care provider that they have either had the illness or can prove through laboratory testing that they are immune (CDC, 2011). In addition, the CDC (2004) recommends periodic skin testing to detect the presence of tuberculosis for health care workers at risk of exposure.

# Basic First Aid

Occupational therapy practitioners and students should demonstrate competence with basic first aid. It is important to keep current with training, as the standards periodically change.

Contact the American Red Cross (www.redcross.org) for the most up-to-date information and for information about training sessions.

## Burns

Therapists should take care to ensure that burns do not occur during the course of splinting, cooking, or bathing with clients. First-degree thermal burns, which result in reddened skin, should be treated by putting the burned area under cool, running water for 5 minutes. The burned area should be covered with a clean or sterile dressing. Creams or ointments should not be applied. Any more serious injury should be immediately reported and treated by other health care professionals (American Red Cross, 2005a).

## Bleeding

In the event of bleeding, therapists should don gloves and then apply pressure with a sterile dressing. Tourniquets should not be used due to the risk of injury to nerves and/or muscles because of problems associated with ischemia. If a client has a laceration, running water should be applied for up to 5 minutes to clear the area of any foreign matter (American Red Cross, 2005a). Professional judgment is necessary to determine if further medical assistance is necessary.

## Allergies

### Latex

Latex allergies emerged as a significant public health issue in the late 1980s and into the early 1990s. During the 1990s, some estimates suggested that 1 in 10 health care workers had latex allergy, but a shift to powder-free, low-protein latex has resulted in a significant decline in the incidence of allergy (Beezhold & Sussman, 2005). However, even with this reduction, practitioners need to be aware of the symptoms of latex allergy, which include redness and itching (typically on hands); difficulty breathing; wheezing; swelling of skin, lips, and tongue; and shortness of breath. If a person exhibits these symptoms after exposure to latex products, emergency medical attention is required. Be aware that some supplies in the occupational therapy department may contain latex, such as gloves and resistance bands. Latex-free versions of many products are available for clients with latex sensitivities.

### Food Allergies and Anaphylaxis

It is estimated that in the United States, food allergies have been diagnosed in three million children younger than the age of 18 (Gupta et al., 2011). It is important for occupational therapy practitioners to be aware of the presence of food allergies in their clients. Allergies should be taken into account when working with feeding, meal preparation, certain craft activities, or when going on food-related outings. Be aware of the symptoms of an allergic reaction: hives, swelling of lips or tongue, vomiting, trouble breathing, or a drop in blood pressure (anaphylaxis; Sicherer, 2006). Should these symptoms develop, emergency medical attention is required. To prevent accidental ingestion of allergens, always read labels when completing meal preparation activities. Avoid cross-contamination when engaging in cooking activities by keeping utensils separate. For example, always use separate utensils for peanut butter and jelly. Be aware of each client's emergency protocol in the event of accidental ingestion. Reactions to food allergies are commonly treated with an auto-injector of epinephrine (Epi-Pen; DEY, L. P.). It is important to know where the Epi-Pen is located and who is trained in its use.

## Orthostatic Hypotension

A client with orthostatic hypotension demonstrates a decrease in blood pressure of more than 20 mm Hg in systolic and of more than 10 mm Hg in diastolic, while also experiencing a 20% increase in heart rate (Goodman, Fuller, & Boissonnault, 2003). A client may experience confusion, dizziness, visual blurring, and possibly fainting when coming to stand. Practitioners must be aware of the potential causes of orthostatic hypotension to prevent its onset. Some common causes include dehydration, venous pooling, side effects of certain medications, and prolonged immobility. To minimize the risk of orthostatic hypotension in a client who is coming to stand from a supine or seated position, instruct the client to rise slowly, flex and extend the ankles, and lift the arms overhead while tightening the abdominal muscles and exhaling through pursed lips. If symptoms develop, help the client into a supine position with the legs elevated, unless contraindicated. Monitor the client's vital signs including pulse, blood pressure, and respiratory rate. This is particularly important in clients with chronic obstructive pulmonary disease who may not tolerate the "legs elevated" position.

Be aware of the risk of fainting for others in the health care environment. Visitors, including students and volunteers, may be at risk of fainting. This is due to emotional stress and the tendency of blood to pool in the lower extremities while standing with knees locked, as is often the case when observing treatment sessions. To prevent fainting, keep legs moving by marching in place or crossing legs. Warn visitors to alert a staff member if they feel lightheaded or dizzy. Provide assurance that visitors should feel free to leave the immediate area if they feel faint.

## Seizures

If a client has a generalized tonic-clonic or grand mal seizure during an occupational therapy session, the practitioner is responsible for ensuring the client is not injured and that an open airway is maintained. These types of seizures generally last approximately 2 minutes and are characterized by a loss of consciousness, rigidity, jerky movements, and shallow breathing. The client should be gently lowered to the ground, mat table, or bed. Do not make any attempt to prevent the client from biting his or her tongue. Loosen clothing around the client's neck to ensure adequate airflow. Do not restrain the client. After the seizure is complete, place the client in the recovery position, lying on his or her side with his or her hand in front. Call for medical assistance (American Red Cross, 2005a). A seizure that lasts for more than 15 minutes, or a series of seizures that lasts for 20 minutes without regaining consciousness in between may suggest status epilepticus. This is a medical emergency and assistance should be sought at once.

## Diabetes Mellitus

When working with clients who have diabetes mellitus, it is important for practitioners to differentiate between signs and symptoms of low blood sugar (hypoglycemia) and high blood sugar (hyperglycemia). Low blood sugar occurs when blood glucose falls below optimal levels and can occur if a client is engaging in physical activity, if there is too much systemic insulin, or if the client has ingested too little food. Some oral medications used to treat diabetes can also cause low blood sugar. Symptoms are variable and may include shakiness, a sense of weakness, a feeling of anxiety and confusion, dizziness, headache, blurred vision, and/or sweating. Practitioners should be aware that therapy sessions may interrupt the usual meal or snack time and therefore result in hypoglycemia. If a client displays symptoms of hypoglycemia, he or she should have a small snack that has a fast-acting source of sugar, such as juice or hard candy. After the snack, the client should check his or her blood sugar level and then contact a nurse or physician if levels are not within the client's acceptable parameters.

High blood sugar may be caused by overeating, poor coordination of eating, medication, infection, or stress. Clients with hyperglycemia may experience fatigue, low energy levels, frequent urination, and/or excessive thirst. High blood sugar may lead to diabetic ketoacidosis, which is a medical emergency. It is caused by inadequate insulin, vast deviation from diet, fever, or infection. The client may have gradual-onset weakness, stomach pain, body aches, labored breathing, fruity breath, dry mouth, nausea, and/or vomiting. If these symptoms occur, contact medical professionals at once, immediately test blood sugar, and provide the client with plain water (Ross, Boucher, & O'Connell, 2005).

### Cardiac Arrest and Choking

Occupational therapy practitioners should maintain cardiopulmonary resuscitation (CPR) certification to treat a person who is choking or who is experiencing cardiac arrest. Local chapters of the American Red Cross or the American Heart Association may be contacted for information about training courses. Protocols are constantly changing as best practices are updated. A thorough description of these procedures is beyond the scope of this chapter.

## Client Care Equipment

Clients may be connected to intravenous lines, arterial lines, central lines, feeding tubes, chest tubes, ventilators, catheters, and/or a variety of monitors (Figure 12-1). It is essential that the occupational therapy practitioner be aware of the purpose of various tubes and monitors. The practitioner should identify all lines and where they connect. In general, it is wise to avoid tugging, pulling, or occluding lines and to ensure adequate slack before moving the client. If any tension is felt, it is recommended that the practitioner stop and check to determine the cause.

Precautions for each tube, line, or monitor must be identified. For example, an arterial line is a catheter that is placed in the radial artery to continually measure blood pressure. Extra caution must be taken to prevent dislodging an arterial line, as dislodging one will cause profuse bleeding (Potter & Perry, 2004). The practitioner must be aware of institutional policies regarding specific equipment and of any particular precautions for an individual client. In addition, it is important that the practitioner is aware of the parameters for any monitors that are providing information about a client's physiologic state.

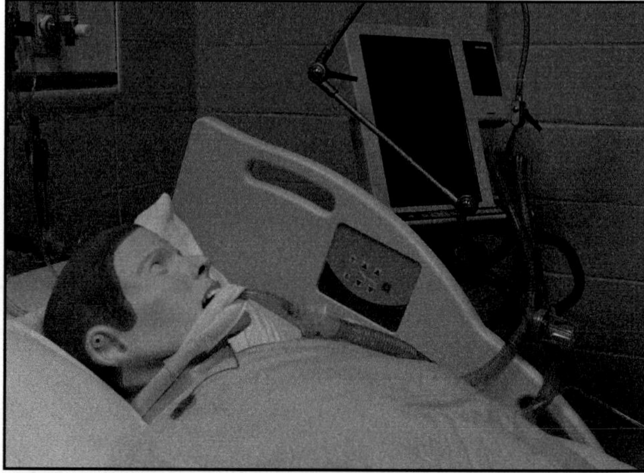

**Figure 12-1.** A patient simulator is an effective way to learn about the purpose and precautions related to client care equipment.

For example, it is generally recommended that activity be stopped if oxygen saturation is below 90%, as measured by a pulse oximeter. The acceptable saturation may be lower in some clients with chronic pulmonary disease (Goodman et al., 2003).

## Hazardous Materials

Therapists should always be aware of the presence of hazardous materials in the occupational therapy department. It is important to know where the material safety data sheets are stored. These sheets are required by OSHA (www.osha.gov). They contain useful information about proper storage of hazards, ways in which products are toxic, information on how to clean a spill, and how to administer first aid if accidental exposure occurs.

## Fire Safety

Therapists should be familiar with the fire safety procedures at their place of employment. This includes knowing the floor map of the facility, the areas for zone evacuation, the location of fire pulls, and the specifics of any emergency plan (OSHA, 2002b). In general, the acronym RACE is helpful to recall in the event of a fire (Potter & Perry, 2004):

- R—Remove all persons who are in immediate danger.
- A—Activate the pull station and call 911.
- C—Close doors to prevent the spread of fire. This includes fire doors, smoke doors, and doors to client rooms.
- E—Extinguish the fire as dictated by department policy.

If a practitioner is called upon to use a fire extinguisher, the acronym PASS guides technique:

- P—Pull the pin to break the glass.
- A—Aim the extinguisher at the base of the fire.
- S—Squeeze the handles together.
- S—Sweep from side to side at the base of the fire.

It is essential that the correct extinguisher is used for the specific type of fire. Labels on extinguishers identify whether they are best used for combustibles, flammable liquids, or electrical fires. More information can be obtained on the OSHA website at www.osha.gov/SLTC/etools/evacuation/portable_use.html.

### *Fire Safety in Clients' Homes*

Practitioners working in home care settings should ensure that clients have smoke detectors in their homes. There should be at least one smoke detector on each level of the home, including the basement. Batteries should be checked at least twice a year. Smoke detectors should be replaced every 8 to 10 years. Therapists should review fire plans with members of the household, which should include the following:

- How to exit the house
- Where to meet outside
- Who is responsible for any person who may need extra help

There should be two methods of egress in every dwelling; this may include a window (U.S. Fire Administration, 2012). It is recommended that people with disabilities notify members of local fire departments to facilitate assistance in the event of an emergency.

## Emergency Preparedness and Disaster Response

Natural and man-made disasters require therapists to respond in an efficient and effective manner to ensure the safety and well-being of clients, family members, and other team members. In the event of a disaster (such as a hurricane) that may limit the ability of health care employees to travel to and from the facility, practitioners may be asked to remain on site to ensure continuity of care. This may involve sleeping at the facility overnight to ensure adequate staffing during the next scheduled shift, or remaining on site to perform other essential functions that are within the scope of practice. This may include transporting clients or assisting with toileting or feeding clients. In the event that the facility needs to be evacuated (perhaps during a flood or power outage), therapists may be needed to assist in moving clients down flights of stairs if the elevators are out of service. It is critical to be aware of the emergency response plan at your place of employment (U.S. Department of Health and Human Services, 2012). For example, in some facilities, the rehabilitation department may be used as a temporary place to hold clients if patient care areas have been damaged.

In addition, occupational therapy practitioners are ideally suited to assist community leaders in preparing for disasters. For example, many towns have plans in place to convert town properties into shelters during mass power outages. Because therapists are aware of the needs of people with a range of disabilities, they can provide useful suggestions about accessibility of shelters, equipment to have available, and ways to assess physical and mental capabilities of residents who occupy the temporary shelter. In the hours and days following disasters, therapists are suited to assist survivors in dealing with stress, maximize safety, and develop routines to facilitate wellness (AOTA, 2011).

When working with clients in their homes, therapists can provide reminders about the importance of preparing an emergency kit that contains first aid supplies, flashlights/batteries, nonperishable food, water, a medication list, and emergency documents. The Red Cross (n.d.) has a complete list of items online, including specific information for older adults, people with disabilities, and children. It is available at http://www.redcross.org/prepare/location/home-family/get-kit.

## Safety During Transfers and Mobility

Therapists should be familiar with the parts of hospital beds, mechanical lifts, and mobility aids before performing transfers or mobility with clients. It is critical to be aware of the procedure for locking bed and wheelchair locks to keep the objects in place. Each client should be positioned in a way that is consistent with precautions specific to his or her condition. Adjusting the height of the bed can ease transfers, requiring less effort for clients and ensuring safety for the practitioner who is assisting.

It is important to have adequate room to work, whether in clients' rooms, in the clinic, or in clients' homes. Practitioners should avoid working in small spaces as much as possible. They should clear unneeded equipment such as bedside tables, extra wheelchairs, or other mobility aids to have adequate room.

Any equipment belonging to an occupational therapy department should be properly maintained. This includes cleaning, ensuring that locks work, and ensuring that all working parts are intact. Routine checks to ensure that every piece of equipment works properly and is stable are important preventive steps to ensure client safety (Kangas, 2002).

The use of proper body mechanics when transferring clients minimizes the risk of injury to practitioners or others who are assisting in the transfer. In general, this involves positioning one's self close to the person being transferred, maintaining a wide base of support, using large muscle groups to move the person, and avoiding twisting movements (Pierson, 1999). In addition, it is important to be aware of any conditions that may affect the client's performance during transfers, such as fragile skin, orthostatic hypotension, amputations, pain, or spasms. Furthermore, it is essential that the practitioner stay current with any precautions or contraindications related to transfers, as these are subject to change. Practitioners must take the time to be aware of best practices regarding injury prevention. For example, research does not support a commonly held belief that back belts reduce injuries caused by lifting (Wassell, Gardner, Landsittel, Johnston, & Johnston, 2001). It is recommended, however, that practitioners use a gait belt with clients when performing transfers or ambulation, unless contraindicated (e.g., after abdominal surgery; Pierson, 1999). A gait belt prevents the practitioner from having to grasp body parts or clothing when providing assistance with mobility. It can also be instrumental in controlling the speed and direction of a fall if the client cannot support his or her own body weight.

Working with clients who are extremely overweight poses potential safety concerns for health care workers and for the clients themselves. Of particular concern is the use of transfer devices and bathroom equipment. Special equipment designed for the bariatric population may be ordered to ensure safety when transferring, bathing, and toileting (Foti & Littrel, 2004). Typically, the weight capacity of durable medical equipment is listed in the ordering information. The practitioner should also consider the distribution of the client's weight, his or her preferred methods of movement, and any anxiety related to mobility.

## Fall Prevention and Restraint Use

Minimizing the incidence of client falls is an important safety consideration for occupational therapy practitioners. This is especially true for older adults and persons with chronic illness who are at an elevated risk. The consequences of a serious fall may include head injury, hip fracture, psychological harm, or death. Falls may be caused by many factors including medications; age-related changes (such as an increased need to urinate at night); visual, balance, strength, or cognitive impairments; or environmental obstacles. Fall prevention efforts are context-specific, but generally include multifaceted interventions such as balance and gait training, medication management, assessment of feet and footwear, environmental modifications, perceived fear of falling, and attention to health concerns such as postural hypotension (American Geriatrics Society, British Geriatrics Society, & American Academy of Orthopedic Surgeons Panel of Falls Prevention, 2011).

The Centers for Medicare and Medicaid Services defines *restraints* as any manual method, physical or manual device, material, or equipment that immobilizes or reduces the ability of a client to move his or her arms, legs, body, or head freely or a drug or medication when it is used as a restriction to manage the client's behavior or restrict the client's freedom of movement and is not a standard intervention or dosage for the client's condition (Centers for Medicare and Medicaid Services, Department of Health and Human Services, 2006).

Historically, restraints were thought to reduce the risk of falling, but research has shown that restraints are ineffective in reducing fall risk. In fact, they can pose serious threats to safety including incontinence, physical injury, and, in some cases, death (Evans & Strumpf, 1990; Miles & Irvine, 1992). Physicians or other licensed independent practitioners are permitted to order physical restraints to treat medical symptoms. The client or surrogate decision makers must consent to their use. Physician's orders must include the circumstances and duration of restraint use, and clients must be carefully monitored while restraints are in use.

Occupational therapy practitioners can play an important part in carefully analyzing a client's fall risk to determine if there are less-restrictive options available. A variety of physical and social supports can minimize reliance on external restraints. In the event that physical restraints are in use, practitioners must ensure that the restraints are applied correctly each time they are fastened to prevent accidental injury. Restraints should be fastened to the frame of the bed or wheelchair rather than to a moveable part, such as a bed rail or arm rest. A strap attached to a bed rail, for example, may tighten when the rail is lifted or lowered, causing injury to the client (Potter & Perry, 2004).

## Home Safety

Working in clients' homes provides an opportunity for the practitioner to make recommendations to enhance safety within the home. Every client presents with different safety needs due to the complex interaction between individual impairments, unique elements of the physical and social environment, and the range of activities performed (Clemson, 1997). When working in clients' homes, practitioners have the ability to observe how activities are performed in their own context, how their social supports influence participation in occupations, and how routines and habits enhance or impede safety.

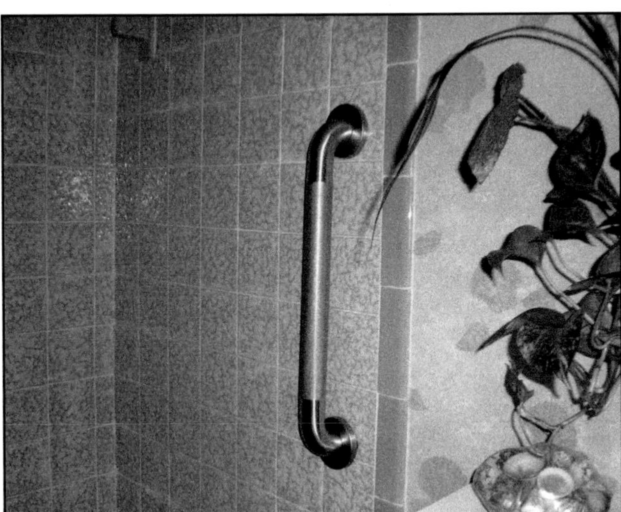

**Figure 12-2.** A grab bar can help a client to safely get in and out of the shower.

The following list is a useful starting point for addressing physical safety in clients' homes:

- Ensure adequate lighting throughout the home; while assessing lighting, also consider blocking light to minimize the effects of glare
- Ensure adequate support during mobility; this may include hand rails on stairs, grab bars in bathrooms, and/or bed mobility aids (Figure 12-2)
- Minimize tripping hazards such as obstacles on floor, unsecured rugs, unfastened door sills or uneven flooring, and electrical cords
- Ensure safe and simple access to commonly used items around the home
- Reduce the risk of scalding injuries by setting the water heater thermostat to no more than 120 degrees
- Prevent electrical injuries by covering outlets, using surge protectors, and keeping electrical cords intact by storing them out of the way of foot traffic

## Personal Safety in Home Care Contexts

Working in clients' homes poses a unique set of safety concerns. Practitioners must take precautions to ensure personal safety when working in the home care environment. It is a safe practice to call before going to a client's home to confirm your arrival. In addition, practitioners should use an escort if there is a perceived threat to personal safety. This is a common service available through many home care agencies. A mobile phone should be readily available (on your person, if possible) in the event of an emergency.

As a means of infection control, it is recommended that practitioners refrain from placing personal items or therapy equipment bags on the ground. Rather, they should be placed over a chair back. Therapy equipment should be appropriately disinfected after each client encounter.

## Areas of Competence

Therapists have a responsibility to "work within their areas of competence" (Reitz et al., 2006, p. 654) and to be aware of their personal limitations in knowledge or expertise. To maintain safe practices, assistance should be sought before performing an evaluation or intervention beyond one's skill set. Additional training, coursework, or education may be needed before working with certain groups of clients. For example, an *American Journal of Occupational Therapy* paper describes the advanced knowledge and skill required for occupational therapy practice in neonatal intensive care units (Vergara et al., 2006). The complexity of this practice setting is compounded by the unique nature of the medical diagnoses, medication regimens, technology, and the family and team dynamics that are present. It is therefore not a recommended practice context for occupational therapy assistants, entry-level occupational therapists, or occupational therapists without prior pediatric experience.

It is imperative for practitioners to allow only authorized personnel to provide intervention. Family members, volunteers, or other unqualified persons should not assist with or carry out interventions they are not capable of completing. When providing caregiver education and training, the practitioner should document his or her competence before allowing the caregiver to complete a task independently. In addition, occupational therapists have a duty to be clear about the roles and responsibilities of the occupational therapy assistant.

Occupational therapy practitioners should report any potentially unsafe practices to a supervisor and work within their means to ensure that the practices are not carried out in the interim. Careful documentation of adverse incidents is necessary. Proper reporting procedures dictated by your institution should be used.

## Summary

Occupational therapy practitioners are instrumental in ensuring that the physical and social environments provide support for client functioning while minimizing the risk of adverse events. Careful attention to the interaction between the person, the environment, and the activity allows practitioners to create situations in which clients can successfully engage in meaningful occupations and enhance their quality of life.

## Evidence-Based Research Chart

| Topic | Evidence |
|---|---|
| Patient safety practices | Shekelle et al., 2013 |
| Safe practices for health care | National Quality Forum, 2010 |
| Hand hygiene | Pittet, Allegranzi, & Boyce, 2009 |
| Home modifications | Stark, Landsbaum, Palmer, Somerville, & Morris, 2009 |
| Fall prevention | American Geriatrics Society, British Geriatrics Society, and American Academy of Orthopedic Surgeons Panel on Falls Prevention, 2011 |

### Case Study

Victor is an 85-year-old single man with a history of polio, necessitating the use of a short-leg brace and a rolling walker. He lives independently in a retirement community. His apartment has a grab bar, handheld showerhead, and tub bench. He was recently hospitalized with pneumonia and is currently in an inpatient rehabilitation facility. He very much wants to return home, but the occupational therapy practitioner has the following concerns. Victor has reduced endurance and cannot tolerate more than 5 to 10 minutes of activity in standing without needing to rest. He has been complaining of left shoulder pain, but the cause is unknown. It is causing minimal difficulty washing and combing his hair. Osteoarthritis makes opening containers difficult, resulting in the occasional need for assistance when preparing meals. While generally cognitively sharp, he demonstrates mild short-term memory loss. Friends help with grocery shopping, and he uses a medication delivery service. He has a call alert button.

**Consider the following questions:**

1. What are the risks to Victor's safety if he returns home alone?
2. What supports may enable him to return home (both existing and potential)?
3. Is ensuring Victor's safety the most important determinant in whether he can return home?
4. To what extent should Victor's wishes factor into the decision making?

Practitioners must engage in lifelong learning to maintain competence in safety-related issues. It is critical to keep current regarding institutional policies and procedures, clients' conditions, and the physical and social environments to optimize safety.

## Student Self-Assessment

1. Assemble a group of at least three people. It may include other students, parents, grandparents, faculty, or friends. Ask each one to state whether he or she thinks the following activities are safe, and why or why not. Discuss how people's perception of the interaction between the person, the environment, and the activity impacts their ideas about the safety of the activity.
   - Walking alone at night
   - Walking down an icy driveway to retrieve the mail from a street-side mailbox
   - Driving overnight to arrive at a destination
   - Changing a tire on the side of a road
   - Standing on a ladder to clean the gutters
   - Changing a lightbulb in a ceiling fixture
   - Renting a room through Airbnb
   - Using Uber for transportation
2. Practice washing your hands according to the CDC standards. Notice how long 15 seconds of scrubbing feels. Practice donning and doffing personal protective equipment.

3. Carefully assess your current living environment to detect the presence of safety hazards. If you locate any hazards, would you consider removing them? Why or why not? What prevents our clients from adhering to our recommendations related to home safety?
4. If you do not already have one, prepare an emergency kit. Use the list provided on the American Red Cross website.

## Electronic Resources

Agency for Healthcare Quality and Research: www.ahrq.gov

American Red Cross: www.redcross.org

Centers for Disease Control and Prevention: www.cdc.gov

The Joint Commission: http://www.jointcommission.org/topics/patient_safety.aspx

National Quality Forum: http://www.qualityforum.org/Home.aspx

## References


American Geriatrics Society, British Geriatrics Society, & American Academy of Orthopedic Surgeons Panel on Falls Prevention. (2011). Summary of the Updated American Geriatrics Society/British Geriatrics Society Clinical Practice Guideline for Prevention of Falls in Older Persons Guidelines for the prevention of falls in older persons. *Journal of the American Geriatrics Society, 59*, 148-157.

American Occupational Therapy Association. (2011). The role of occupational therapy in disaster preparedness, response, and recovery. *American Journal of Occupational Therapy, 65*(Suppl.), S11-S25. doi:10.5014/ajot.2011.65S11

American Occupational Therapy Association. (2014). Occupational therapy practice framework: Domain and process (3rd ed.). *American Journal of Occupational Therapy, 68*(Suppl. 1), S1-S48. doi:10.5014/ajot.2014.682006

American Red Cross. (2005). First aid. *Circulation, 112*(Suppl. I), IV-196–IV-203. Retrieved from http://circ.ahajournals.org/cgi/reprint/112/24_suppl/IV-196

American Red Cross. (n.d.) *Get a kit.* Retrieved from http://www.redcross.org/prepare/location/home-family/get-kit

Beezhold, D., & Sussman, G. (2005). *Lessons learned from latex allergy. Business briefing: global surgery: Future directions 2005.* Retrieved from http://www.touchbriefings.com/pdf/1438/beezhold[1].pdf

Boyce, J. M., Pittet, D., Healthcare Infection Control Practices Advisory Committee, & HICPAC/SHEA/APIC/IDSA Hand Hygiene Task Force. (2002). Guideline for hand hygiene in health-care settings: Recommendations of the Healthcare Infection Control Practices Advisory Committee and the HICPAC/SHEA/APIC/IDSA Hand Hygiene Task Force. *MMWR: Recommendations and Reports, 51*(RR-16), 1-45.

Bruce, M. A. G., & Borg, B. (2002). Suicidal behavior: Critical information for clinical reasoning. In M. A. G. Bruce & B. Borg (Eds.), *Psychosocial frames of reference: Core for occupation-based practice* (3rd ed., pp. 323-324). Thorofare, NJ: SLACK Incorporated.

Centers for Disease Control and Prevention. (2004). Surveillance for tuberculosis infection in health care workers. *Worker Health Chartbook 2004.* NIOSH Publication No. 2004-146. Retrieved from http://www.cdc.gov/niosh/docs/2004-146/appendix/ap-a/ap-a-19.html

Centers for Disease Control and Prevention. (2011). Immunization of health-care personnel: Recommendations of the Advisory Committee on Immunization Practices (ACIP). *MMWR: Recommendations and Reports, 60*(7), 1-48.

Centers for Disease Control and Prevention. (2015). *Hand hygiene in healthcare settings.* Retrieved from http://www.cdc.gov/handhygiene/Basics.html

Centers for Medicare and Medicaid Services, Department of Health and Human Services. (2006). Medicare and Medicaid Programs; Hospital conditions of participation: Patients' rights: Final rule. *Federal Register, 71*(236), 71377-71428.

Clemson, L. (1997). *Home fall hazards: A guide to identifying fall hazards in the homes of elderly people and an accompaniment to the assessment tool, the Westmead Home Safety Assessment.* West Brunswick, Victoria, Australia: Coordinates Publication.

DiCuccio, M. H. (2015). The relationship between patient safety culture and patient safety outcomes: A systematic review. *Journal of Patient Safety, 11*, 135-142.

Donaldson, M. S. (2008). An overview of To Err is Human: Rethinking the message of patient safety. In R. G. Hughes (Ed.), *Patient safety and quality: An evidence-based handbook for nursing.* Rockville, MD: Agency for Healthcare Research and Quality.

Evans, L. K., & Strumpf, N. E. (1990). Myths about elder restraint. *Image: Journal of Nursing Scholarship, 22*(2), 124-128.

Foti, D., & Littrel, E. (2004). Bariatric care: Practical problem solving and interventions. *Physical Disabilities Special Interest Section Quarterly, 27*, 1-3, 6.

Gall, S., Tarique, A., Natarajan, A., & Zaman, A. (2006). Rapid ambulation after coronary angiography via femoral artery access: A prospective study of 1000 patients. *Journal of Invasive Cardiology, 18*, 106-108.

Goodman, C. C., Boissonnault, W. G., & Fuller, K. S. (2003). *Pathology: Implications for the physical therapist* (2nd ed.). Philadelphia, PA: W. B. Saunders Co.

Gupta, R. S., Springston, E. E., Warrier, M. R., Smith, B., Kumar, R., Pongracic, J., & Holl, J. H. (2011). The prevalence, severity, and distribution of childhood food allergy among children in the United States. *Pediatrics, 128*, e9-e17.

Holm, M. B., Rogers, J. C., & James, A. B. (1998). Treatment of occupational performance areas. In M. E. Neidstadt & E. B. Crepeau (Eds.), *Willard & Spackman's occupational therapy* (9th ed., pp. 323-390). Philadelphia, PA: Lippincott Williams and Wilkins.

The Joint Commission. (2016). *National patient safety goals.* Retrieved from http://www.jointcommission.org/standards_information/npsgs.aspx

Kangas, K. M. (2002). Managing transfers and lifting with the complicated patient. *Gerontology Special Interest Section Quarterly, 25*, 1-4.

Kohn L. T., Corrigan J. M., & Donaldson M. (1999). *To err is human: Building a safer health system.* Washington, DC: National Academy Press, Institute of Medicine.

Miles, S. H., & Irvine, P. (1992). Deaths caused by physical restraints. *Gerontologist, 32*(6), 762-766.

National Quality Forum. (2010). *Safe practices for better healthcare: 2010 update: A consensus report.* Washington, DC: National Quality Forum.

Oakes, C. E. (2011). "In their best interest": The challenge of balancing autonomy and beneficence in clinical practice with older adults. *Gerontology Special Interest Section Quarterly, 34*(3), 1-4.

Occupational Safety and Health Administration. (2002a). *Healthcare wise hazards: (Lack of) universal precautions.* Retrieved from http://www.osha.gov/SLTC/etools/hospital/hazards/univprec/univ.html

Occupational Safety and Health Administration. (2002b). *Fact sheet: Fire safety in the workplace.* Retrieved from http://www.osha.gov/OshDoc/data_General_Facts/FireSafetyN.pdf

Occupational Safety and Health Administration. (2011). *Fact sheet: Bloodborne pathogens.* Retrieved from http://www.osha.gov/OshDoc/data_BloodborneFacts/bbfact01.pdf

Occupational Safety and Health Administration. (2012). *Hospital eTool: Bloodborne illnesses: Hepatitis B virus*. Retrieved from http://www.osha.gov/SLTC/etools/hospital/hazards/bbp/bbp.html#HepatitisBVirus

Oppe, S. (1988). The concept of risk: A decision theoretic approach. *Ergonomics, 31*, 435-440.

Pierson, F. M. (1999). *Principles and techniques of patient care* (2nd ed.). Philadelphia, PA: W. B. Saunders Co.

Pittet, D., Allegranzi, B., & Boyce, J. (2009). The World Health Organization guidelines on hand hygiene in health care and their consensus recommendations. *Infection Control and Hospital Epidemiology, 30*, 611-622. doi:10.1086/599166

Potter, P. A., & Perry, A. G. (2004). *Fundamentals of nursing* (6th ed.). St. Louis, MO: Mosby.

Reitz, S. M., Austin, D. J., Brandt, L. C., DeBrakeller, B., Franck, L. G., Homenko, D. F., et al. (2006). Guidelines to the occupational therapy code of ethics. *American Journal of Occupational Therapy, 60*(6), 652-658.

Ross, T. A., Boucher, J. L., & O'Connell, B. S. (Eds.). (2005). *ADA guide to diabetes medical nutrition therapy and education*. Chicago, IL: American Dietetic Association.

Shekelle, P. G., Pronovost, P. J., Scholelles, K., McDonald, K. M., Dy, S. M., Shojania, K., et al. (2013). *Making health care safer II: An updated critical analysis of evidence for patient safety practices*. Rockville, MD: Agency for Healthcare Research and Quality.

Sicherer, S. H. (2006). *Understanding and managing your child's food allergies*. Baltimore, MD: The Johns Hopkins University Press.

Siegel, J. D., Rhinehart, E., Jackson, M., Chiarello, L., & Healthcare Infection Control Practices Advisory Committee. (2007). *2007 guidelines for isolation precautions: Preventing transmission of infectious diseases in healthcare settings*. Atlanta, GA: Centers for Disease Control. Retrieved from http://www.cdc.gov/ncidod/dhqp/pdf/guidelines/Isolation2007.pdf

Stark, S., Landsbaum, A., Palmer, J., Somerville, E. K., & Morris, J. C. (2009). Client-centered home modifications improve daily activity performance in older adults. *Canadian Journal of Occupational Therapy, 76*, 235-245.

U.S. Department of Health and Human Services. (2012). *Healthcare preparedness capabilities: National guidance for healthcare system preparedness*. Retrieved from http://www.phe.gov/preparedness/planning/hpp/reports/documents/capabilities.pdf

U.S. Fire Administration. (2012). *Home fire prevention and safety tips*. Retrieved from http://www.usfa.fema.gov/citizens/home_fire_prev/

Vergara, E., Anzalone, M., Bigsby, R., Gorga, D., Holloway, E., Hunter, J., et al. (2006). Specialized knowledge and skills for occupational therapy practice in the neonatal intensive care unit. *American Journal of Occupational Therapy, 60*(6), 659-668.

Wassell, J. T., Gardner, L. I., Landsittel, D. P., Johnston, J. J., & Johnston, J. M. (2001). A prospective study of back belts for prevention of back pain and injury. *Journal of the American Medical Association, 284*(21), 2727-2732. Retrieved from http://jama.ama-assn.org/cgi/content/abstract/284/21/2727

## Suggested Readings

Galt, K. A., & Paschal, K. A. (2011). *Foundations in patient safety for health professionals*. Sudbury, MA: Jones and Bartlett Publishers.

Gawande, A. (2009). *The checklist manifesto: How to get things right*. New York, NY: Metropolitan Books.

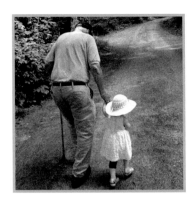

# 13

# Occupational Performance in Natural Environments
## Dynamic Contexts for Participation

*Kathryn M. Loukas, OTD, MS, OTR/L, FAOTA and Hailey C. Davis, MS, OTR/L*

### ACOTE Standards Explored in This Chapter

B.5.17

### Key Vocabulary

- **Context:** The wide array of interrelated variables that influence occupational performance (American Occupational Therapy Association [AOTA], 2014, p. S8).
- **Inclusion:** Full participation in life events and naturally occurring environments for and with people of all abilities.
- **Interdependence:** Functioning with the input from others in a complex and interconnected manner.
- **Least restrictive environment:** The context in which humans participate in daily occupations; the environment that best supports occupational participation.
- **Natural environments:** Contexts that occur in the daily lives of human beings in a society.
- **Nonlinear dynamics:** Complex, open systems that interact in unpredictable flow dynamics versus in a more rigid, linear, cause-effect manner (Champagne, 2008).



Jacobs, K., & MacRae, N. (Eds.).
*Occupational Therapy Essentials for Clinical Competence, Third Edition* (pp. 175-185).

Occupational therapy has evolved in the use of context in intervention planning. Through the history of occupational therapy we have moved from the context of institutional settings that began with the moral treatment paradigm (Letts, Rigby, & Stewart, 2003), to a focus on occupation (Kielhofner, 1992), to practice using the Person-Environment-Occupation Performance Model, which emphasizes natural contexts (Christiansen & Baum, 1991). Early in our history, occupational therapy primarily occurred in the institutional setting. This institutionalization provided a closed system that discouraged individuals from participating in real-life situations in natural settings; it kept our clients and our work invisible to society and inhibited occupational justice and performance (Reed, 2006; Whalley Hammell, 2003). In her landmark Eleanor Clark Slagle lecture, Grady (1995) encouraged occupational therapy practitioners to reach out and build inclusive communities through accessibility, adaptations, hope, and social supports. Our profession continues to move forward toward this ultimate goal.

Today, engagement in purposeful, real-life occupations has become the goal of occupational therapy intervention in most practice settings. The *Occupational Therapy Practice Framework* advocates for occupational therapy practitioners to support participation in occupation in context while considering the multiple factors influencing context, such as performance patterns, client factors, and performance skills (AOTA, 2014a). Occupational therapy has made a paradigm shift from the medical model to the community model to help clients participate in the occupations of "real life" (Scaffa, 2001). Increasing the level of independence is a factor in intervention planning, but not always the ultimate goal. Occupational therapy practitioners need to also recognize and embrace the concept of interdependence. A client who wishes to live in his or her own natural environment may need the assistance of family or caregivers, and that is a worthy goal in achieving occupational life satisfaction. A client who is functioning in the natural rhythm of life, even with assistance, can achieve an individual goal of occupational performance (Hinojosa & Blount, 2000).

Occupational therapy practitioners often use simulation in practice settings to achieve occupation-based goals. A rehabilitation-based occupational therapy practitioner might use the therapy room kitchen to help a client prepare to return home, an occupational therapy practitioner in work reentry therapy might use devices that simulate work tasks such as driving or lifting, a therapist working in early intervention may simulate a play environment in the occupational therapy room to prepare a child to use a playground in the future, and an occupational therapy practitioner in the mental health setting might help a client with functional life skills such as filling out a job application or financial management. Simulations prepare clients for real life, but use of the actual environment is always best for the final goals and discharge planning (Letts et al., 2003). Natural environments are those where the client would actually engage in the occupation in context. These occupations carry with them important social meaning and occupational roles (Pierce, 2003). Typical natural environments include the home, workplace, day care settings, school, places of leisure and recreation, group homes, and the community, including private and public transportation (Hinojosa & Blount, 2000).

Natural contexts for occupational practice include the following (Perr & Bell, 2000):

- The home
- The outdoor environment
- The workplace
- Day care settings, head-start programs, developmental preschools for early intervention
- School-based inclusion in the least restrictive environment
- Community resources for play and leisure, recreation, worship, shopping, dining, and social and community events
- Private and public transportation

As we discuss natural environments in a variety of contexts, the most natural environment of all must not go unmentioned: nature. Interacting with nature benefits people across the lifespan and in various contexts. Nature is a powerful tool that improves self-esteem and mood. Research shows that any amount of "green exercise" is beneficial and that the effects of nature are immediate (Barton & Pretty, 2010). Mood affects all aspects of daily life, such as overall quality of life, motivation, and distress tolerance. Nature is an intervention with only positive side effects, which cannot be said of many medical treatments, such as prescription medications. Occupational therapy practitioners can facilitate client participation in nature as an intervention context when working with clients in various areas of practice, particularly mental health. In addition, accessing nature with older adults, specifically older adults with dementia, improves physical and mental well-being. Interacting with nature can also be a powerful coping strategy for loved ones managing the challenges of caregiving. Affording access to nature provides different ways to stimulate older adults, with or without dementia, and the opportunity to engage in outdoor activities might even help trigger forgotten memories (Clark, 2014).

Today, the positive impacts of nature and playing outdoors are widely known, yet children often have fewer opportunities to engage in outdoor play and access nature (von Benzon, 2010). Evidence suggests that natural environments support children's imaginative play, social skills, and communication, and adds the natural environment as an important place of learning (Dowdell, Gray, &

Malone, 2011). Interacting with nature encourages children to problem solve, exposes them to multiple sensory experiences, and fosters independence and exploration. There is evidence to support the benefits of children with disabilities interacting with nature as well. However, research shows that children with disabilities have even fewer experiences to interact with nature than nondisabled children, which is likely due to society's reaction to their impairment, not their actual disability (von Benzon, 2010). Whenever possible, with safety always at the forefront, occupational therapy practitioners should support and encourage access to nature and the outdoors as a gateway to many functional skills for children.

## Chaos, Complexity, and Nonlinear Dynamics

Chaos theory and the study of nonlinear dynamics is an emerging perspective in the social sciences (Chamberlain & Butz, 1998; Kelso, 1995) and in occupational therapy (Champagne, 2008; Lazzarini, 2004; Royeen, 2003). Dynamic systems theory reflects the importance of the interaction of the complex internal and external systems that make up the whole human being (Case-Smith, 2005; Humphry & Wakeford, 2006; Thelen, 2000). Zoltan (2007) describes the dynamic interactional approach to cognition as "an ongoing production or outcome of the interaction among the individual, the task, and the environment" (p. 16). The environment plays a significant role in the occupations and occupational development of human beings, leading emerging occupational therapy approaches to emphasize contextualism (Humphry & Wakeford, 2006). This contextualism emphasizes the interconnected and inseparable nature of human beings with their environment. According to nonlinear dynamic theory, human beings and behavior are unpredictable, self-organizing systems, each with their own unique initial conditions (Chamberlain & Butz, 1998; Champagne, 2008; Kelso, 1995; Lazzarini, 2004; Royeen, 2003). The person, environment, and occupation are engaged in a transactional relationship, much as the Person-Environment-Occupation Performance Model (Christiansen & Baum, 1991) elucidates, but in a more interactive, holistic, and unpredictable manner. It is essential that occupational therapy practitioners understand the science of chaotic, complex, nonlinear dynamic systems in natural environments. Through this understanding, therapists can facilitate meaningful self-organization of clients in the context of dynamic everyday occupations (Champagne, 2008; Lazzarini, 2004; Royeen, 2003).

## Occupational Therapy Applications

### Play

Play is a primary occupation of childhood. As children play and engage in hands-on activities, they create a strong foundation for learning that gradually builds, preparing them to acquire a myriad of skills including language, social and emotional awareness, problem solving, and self-regulation, among many others (Carlsson-Paige, McLaughlin, & Almon, 2015). Play can take place in a variety of contexts and can be structured or unstructured. In any form, play provides an opportunity for therapists to work with children in their natural environment. Occupational therapists often use play activities as an intervention because play is self-motivating (Case-Smith, 2015). The role of the occupational therapy practitioner may be to adapt a game to include a child with a disability playing with his or her typical peers, to problem solve with a child who has a low frustration tolerance for his or her peers in social situations, or to provide consultation to facilitate greater occupational engagement for a child with a disability.

### Early Intervention

Early intervention programs are designed to enhance the development of children in occupational tasks. The Individuals with Disabilities Education Act (IDEA) mandates these services occur in "natural environments" and in a family-centered context (AOTA, 2006; Stephens & Tauber, 2005). Natural environments in early intervention include kangaroo care of the newborn resting on the parent's abdomen (Figure 13-1); transdisciplinary play environments including play groups, day care centers, preschool, and developmental groups (Loukas, Whiting, Ricci, & Cohen-Konrad, 2012); cultural and religious activities and contexts; and community settings such as shopping or service appointments. The most natural setting occupational therapy could address for a client in the 0- to 3-year-old age range is the family and home environment. Understanding the initial conditions, context, culture, and occupational patterns of the dynamic family system is important and should influence the occupational therapy intervention plan (Figure 13-2). Occupational therapy practitioners working in early intervention take advantage of the natural context in which the occupations and co-occupations of the child and family occur, follow the child's lead, and use natural consequences. Occupational therapists can perform an ecological assessment using the natural environment, whereas the occupational therapy assistant follows through with the intervention plan in the natural context. When children

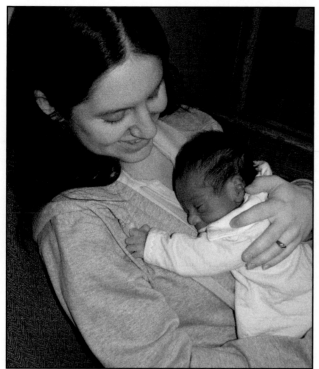

**Figure 13-1.** An early natural environment of kangaroo care is used by a new mother to bond and soothe an infant.

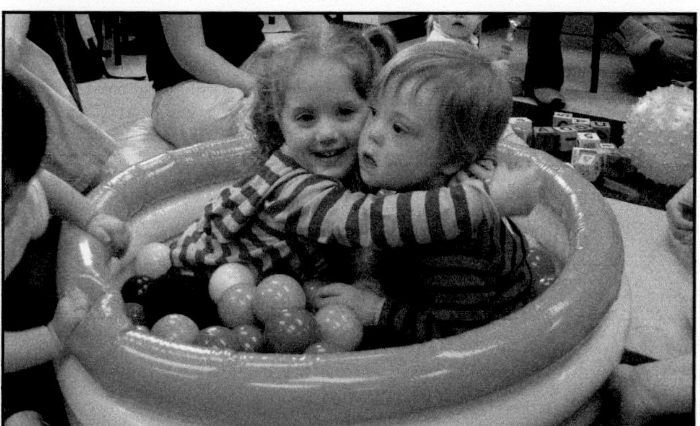

**Figure 13-2.** Early intervention inclusive contexts promote social participation and development.

## Case Example: Lola

Lola is the 9-month-old child of Celeste, a 19-year-old single mother living in a small house with her mother. Lola is a child who is developmentally delayed and just beginning to sit up and roll over. Lola also has some difficulty with eating and feeding and does not sleep well. Samantha, the occupational therapy practitioner, facilitated Celeste to self-organize a routine for the day, including times for feeding, developmental play, and sleep. As a therapeutic activity, Celeste and Samantha worked together to establish a realistic and meaningful routine and put this schedule on the refrigerator with magnets. Samantha's gentle influence regarding the nature of developmental activities facilitated Celeste to find a playgroup for Lola. The dynamic, social, and interactive nature of the playgroup of children and parents began to transform their isolation and improved community participation for both mother and child. The occupational therapy practitioner helped Celeste embed specially selected developmental play activities to enhance motor development into Lola's environment. This served to establish an interconnected bond between mother and child. The context of this play included setting up environments that facilitate development in the living room and outdoors. Sensory modulation input was natural and was included to facilitate Lola's nervous system prior to feeding and to inhibit her system prior to bedtime. As the natural environment of the home became child-development centered, Celeste began to grow in her role as a confident and nurturing mother and Lola began to thrive.

learn skills and develop occupations in the natural environment, it is more likely they will generalize these skills to other areas of their lives (Myers, Case-Smith, & Cason, 2015).

# School-Based Practice

Current IDEA legislation requires that therapy occur in natural environments (Wrights Law, 2013) and for education to occur in the least restrictive environment (AOTA, 2006). The school has many natural environments, all of which are dynamic contexts for occupational performance. These include the classroom, the school bus, the playground, the cafeteria, the gym, the art room, the computer room, and the library. Occupational therapy intervention can occur in all these contexts as direct inclusive therapy or in a consultative approach. The schools have evolved from a model of specialized schools, such as the school for the deaf or the cerebral palsy center, to *mainstreaming*, which put children under the same roof as their typical peers to facilitation of full participation of children in the school environment and routine, which is now termed *inclusion*. Occupational therapy as a profession is dedicated to inclusion and believes all members of society contribute to creating an inclusive community (AOTA, 2009; Dunn et al., 1995b). AOTA asserts that inclusion means all members of society are not only treated equally, but that everyone is provided with the same opportunities to participate in "naturally occurring activities in society" in all contexts (2014b, p. S23), although some may need assistance or adaptations to participate.

To be effective in this complex system, the school-based occupational therapy practitioner must evaluate and affect change in complex and unpredictable ways. This requires facilitating the child, teacher, occupations, and natural environments to support learning and social development in context (Figure 13-3). It is easy to feel overwhelmed with the number of students on an

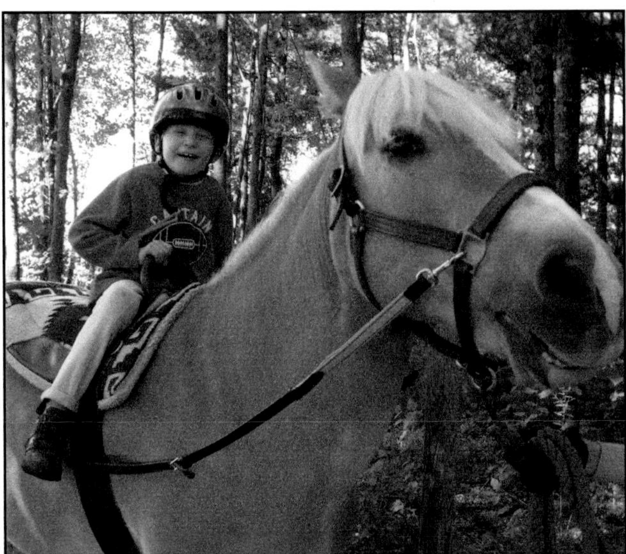

**Figure 13-3.** The outdoor and non-human natural environments facilitate wellness and joy.

**Case Example: Curtis**

Curtis is a child in the second grade. He is full of life and loves to have fun with other children. Curtis is living with cerebral palsy that affects his left side with hemiparesis, but cognitively he is at grade level. Curtis has functional mobility difficulties with negotiating the playground, sitting on the backless benches of the cafeteria, and getting on and off the school bus. He also has fine motor difficulties, which render handwriting and art projects frustrating and very difficult. The occupational therapy practitioners were committed to including Curtis in all activities and settings of the school and adopted an adaptation/compensation contextual approach in his Individualized Education Program (IEP) to enable Curtis to participate successfully in all aspects of the school curriculum. John, the occupational therapy assistant, played with Curtis and his peers on the playground, facilitating Curtis to make good choices in equipment selection and offering ideas on how to safely get on and off the swings and slides. A chair was used at the end of the cafeteria table enabling Curtis to have supportive seating but still eat with his peers. Curtis was given physical assistance on and off the bus for safety reasons. This was facilitated by the occupational therapy practitioners in a manner that was meaningful and social to Curtis, his family, and other children involved. Curtis's classrooms were equipped with a computer with a key guard and elbow supports for school-based written work and some art projects. Dynamic occupational therapy intervention occurred in all school contexts and included the interprofessional team, teachers, parents, and other children in the second grade curriculum for social participation in natural activities of daily living, play, and work contexts.

occupational therapy caseload in school-based practice. Not only is providing the intervention in the natural environment considered best practice, but it is also an effective way to provide interventions to multiple students at one time (e.g., in a fine-motor group at a table in the classroom).

## Instrumental Activities of Daily Living

### *Mental Health*

Occupational therapy has historically played a vital role in promoting mental health through meaningful occupations. While mental health is a specific area of occupational therapy practice, the reality is that mental illness is a reality in all areas of occupational therapy practice across the lifespan including pediatrics, older adults, and rehabilitation, to name a few. It is also important to consider that achieving good mental health is not just the absence of disease or disability but rather the engagement in positive occupations (Barton & Pretty, 2010). As a profession, occupational therapy is well suited to promote mental health from a wellness perspective. It is not uncommon for mental health issues to arise during occupational therapy sessions in the natural environment once the client begins to feel more comfortable with the occupational therapy practitioner. In pediatrics, there is an opportunity for occupational therapy practitioners to teach children in the natural environment how to develop and maintain positive mental health to promote mental health and wellness into adulthood (Bazyk et al., 2015).

Living skills training is a common intervention used in mental health rehabilitation (Tungpunkom & Nicol, 2008). It consists of instrumental activity of daily living skills to support independent living such as financial management, community mobility, meal planning, or establishing child care so that the client can get back to work. Client factors, performance skills, and performance patterns inform the occupational therapy practitioner in choosing the most appropriate intervention. When the natural environment is not available, simulation is effective, although it can be difficult for the client to grasp out of context and it is not as effective as the natural environment. For example, an occupational therapist working in the area of mental health in the context of a hospital may simulate functional life skills for community participation, such as filling out a job application or medication management.

## Work-Based Programs

Transitional return-to-work programs, workplace safety initiatives, ergonomics, sheltered work, employment coaching, volunteer positions, and overall rehabilitation are part of occupational therapy practice and can occur in natural environments (AOTA, 2011). The workplace is where many people spend most weekday hours engaging in productive activities. Occupational therapy practitioners may also consider using a volunteer position as a precursor to the work role. This may serve as a vehicle toward self-actualization and productivity for people with disabling conditions. Clients who are interested in employment may find the natural environment of the workplace to be stimulating and motivating. The occupational therapy practitioner can provide suggestions for how to adapt specific tasks or modify the work environment, complete task analyses of expected activities, and engage the client in the natural positions and conditions necessary for the job. In turn, this provides an opportunity for the occupational therapist to evaluate the client's performance skills, performance patterns, or their readiness to return to work, while the occupational therapy assistant may implement the work-based intervention plan. Transitional work programs typically occur in the clients' natural work environment. Transitional work programs facilitate communication between the client, the employer, and the occupational therapy practitioner to ensure safety and success at work following illness or injury (AOTA, 2012). Although an occupational therapy practitioner's role in work-based programs is typically a result of illness or injury, multiple factors must be considered in the natural environment, such as motor, sensory, perceptual, emotional regulation, or cognition difficulties (AOTA, 2011). Because of time and distance constraints, sometimes occupational therapy practitioners cannot bring their clients to the workplace. If this is the case, the best alternative is to simulate the work situation in physical, temporal, and contextual aspects as closely as possible to maximize the therapeutic impact of intervention.

### Case Example: Ralph

Ralph is a 54-year-old plumber who lost his left (non-dominant) thumb and index finger at the proximal interphalangeal joint in a work-related accident. He is now 2 months post-amputation, participating in outpatient rehabilitation, and has quite a bit of hypersensitivity in the stump areas of his left hand. Ralph is a man who values work at home and the workplace. He is concerned he will not be able to support his family and is anxious to return to his job. Doris, his occupational therapy practitioner, noticed he is not motivated by use of simulations in the outpatient clinic. She tried to set up make-shift plumbing projects, but Ralph insists they are not close to realistic. Doris decides to set up a work-based program on the pipes in Ralph's home. Ralph becomes motivated to use his left hand as a functional assist and the hypersensitivity begins to diminish. As Ralph shows he can still do many plumbing tasks, his wife, Mary, begins to ask about different jobs needed around the house. Ralph complains to her in a good-natured way, but the practitioner can see he is pleased to be back in the role of "Mr. Fix It" in his home. Doris sets up further sessions in the plumbing shop and home environments to facilitate Ralph's return to former performance patterns of work and functional use of the left hand. This dynamic approach to work improves Ralph's relationships, self-image, and mood as his life roles and routines become meaningful again.

## Retirement: Aging in Place

Older adults who wish to age in natural environments, thus "aging in place," may turn to occupational therapy for assistance in that goal (AOTA, 2008; Clark et al., 1997). Occupational therapy is dedicated to developing livable communities where people of all abilities can fully participate (AOTA, 2008). Occupational therapy can occur in this natural environment while facilitating older adults to participate in community programs such as adult day programs, in-home assistance, religious or culturally based activities, and social networks. It is important for older people to stay in their natural environment to maintain the roles, habits, routines, autonomy, and memories associated with their own home and lifestyle. Aging in place allows older adults to maintain their habits, familiar surroundings, and social networks for occupational performance. Changing locations can inhibit an older person, particularly those with cognitive impairments, to regress in their overall functioning and quality of life and may even affect mortality (Edvardsson & Nordvall, 2008). The occupational therapy practitioner, adopting an adaptation/compensation contextual approach, can assist older adults to function in their home through home adaptations, cueing systems, self-organization techniques, and memory enhancement. An emphasis on safety and supported functioning should be established. An occupational therapy practitioner can also train family members or other caretakers on how to best assist older adults with their independent or interdependent functioning (Dunn et al., 1995a; Figure 13-4).

As holistic professionals, occupational therapy practitioners need to also monitor and integrate mental health services as needed when working with older adults (Chippendale, 2014). This is a population in which mental illness, such as depression and anxiety, is prevalent but often overlooked. According to the U.S. Department of Health and Human Services, depression is "common in older adults, but it is not a normal part of aging" (n.d.). Occupational therapy practitioners are in a unique position when working with older adults as they are often

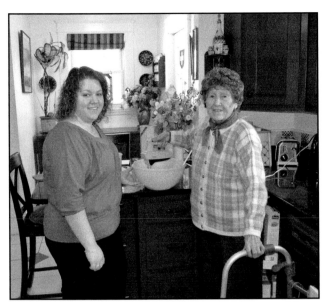

**Figure 13-4.** An occupational therapy practitioner assists an older adult with cooking in the natural environment of the client's home.

### Case Example: Marjorie

Marjorie is a 68-year-old woman in the mid-stage of Alzheimer disease. Her husband, George, age 70, has been very distraught with his wife's behavior and forgetfulness. George works part time as a sales representative and would like to continue his work. The family sought occupational therapy through a center on aging. Nancy, the occupational therapy practitioner at the center, helped the family find resources in the community to assist them. They found an adult day care center for the days George works and through this became involved with a support group for caretakers of people with Alzheimer disease. As George learned more about the importance of taking care of himself, his wife, and his home, he began to self-organize. He hired someone to clean the house, as that had really become a burden for him. In addition, they were able to hire an attendant to sleep over to deal with Marjorie's night wandering and allow George to sleep. Nancy helped George and Marjorie maintain previous routines through a picture calendar for Marjorie. This also helped George effectively engage and interact with his wife in meaningful home tasks that used to be delegated only to her, such as cooking and gardening. While engaging in these occupational tasks, Nancy is able to role-play ways of dealing with Marjorie when she becomes disoriented, belligerent, or confused. These new interactions facilitate George and their children to deal with Marjorie in social and community settings. Due to this occupational therapy intervention, George and Marjorie are able to participate in their home and community in an interdependent manner further in the future.

working on intimate tasks, such as toileting and bathing, which can make the client feel vulnerable. It is not uncommon for signs and symptoms of a mental illness to appear that may be contributing to a decline in occupational performance.

## Best Practice and Safety Considerations in Natural Settings

Because natural settings are not as structured or predictable as those performed in a clinic, they can pose more of a safety risk for clients both physically and psychosocially. It is important to consider a number of recommended practices to ensure positive outcomes. The following recommendations are adapted from Noonan and McCormick (2006) in their work with young children in natural environments:

- Specialize instructional techniques to the client in the natural environment. This can be accomplished by goals that embed meaningful activities in the client's natural environment, making sure that the challenges are not dangerous or too difficult. Task analysis and careful planning are needed for successful therapy in natural environments.
- Ensure that interventions are culturally sensitive and relevant. This may require outside investigation and questions to the client and family members.
- Cultivate team and family involvement. Positive outcomes are more likely to occur with support by the team and the family. Build strong relationships with the therapy team and work collaboratively to support this practice.
- Ecological and contextual assessment. The occupational therapy practitioner should do a thorough ecological assessment for the safety of the client and the therapist. Questions to ask include the following:
    - What are the intervention goals and objectives?
    - Where should the intervention be provided?
    - How should the intervention be provided?
    - When should the intervention be provided?
    - How can the intervention be evaluated? (Noonan & McCormick, 2006, p. 21)
- Positive behavioral support. The occupational therapy practitioner should not provide therapy alone in a natural environment when the behavior of the client/family or safety considerations are questionable. Be sure support is present in any situation that warrants it. Relationship difficulties can also make for difficult or unsafe situations for the client and need to be closely examined prior to the planning of the context of intervention.

## Recommendations for Establishing an Ethical Climate for Privacy and Confidentiality in a Community-Based Practice Setting

- Know and follow the Health Insurance Portability and Accountability Act and Family Educational Rights and Privacy Act regulations, and encourage others to do the same, including notification of privacy procedures to clients and client families.
- Avoid all "hall talk." Establish confidential places to discuss private client matters, and remember casual conversations can quickly turn into conversations with confidential information sharing.
- Make sure your clients understand what is private and what is not, as research indicates many clients do not understand confidentiality (Sankar, Moran, Merz, & Jones, 2003). For our young clients, involve them in decisions using plain language they understand.
- Make all efforts to keep private, professional information confidential. Do not carry confidential reports or files casually. Do not leave them in the bathroom or your open car. Transport confidential items only when absolutely necessary. Keep your computer encrypted or password sensitive for all client-related information.
- Respond "naturally" to questions that occur in typical settings, but be careful not to violate privacy or confidentiality. Make sure paraprofessionals understand their obligations to privacy and do not give more information than is needed.
- Communicate with your clients and their families about what you need to provide best practice as a therapist and what participation in natural environments might entail. Ask about mentioning the disability or educating others; involve them in decisions and discussion. Help clients and parents understand your need for full disclosure of medical information.
- Implicit consent and reasonable expectations of privacy are part of practice when the client and family are involved in a community-based environment. The family and client need to be informed and "agree" to the setting and approach to intervention through an Individualized Education Program, Individual Family Service Plan, or other legal document (J. Boyden, personal communication, July 10, 2006).
- Establish an ethical climate in the community through modeling, educating, and sponsoring workshops with experts. Consider establishment of an ethics program. Use an ethical decision-making model such as the six-step process to assist with difficult decisions (Purtilo & Doherty, 2011; Solum & Schaffer, 2003).

## Summary

Occupational therapy has historically been practiced in a number of contexts from institution, hospital, school, and home. However, emergent best practice indicates the closer we can get our intervention to the natural environment, the more meaningful and effective the occupational performance of our clients will become. This can be accomplished in many settings by finding the best "real-life" context for the occupation in which our client is engaging or wishes to engage. It is important to make sure the safety of the client and therapist are in place through environmental analysis and/or team collaboration. The chaos, complexity, and nonlinear dynamics of interactive systems are essential to consider when using the natural context in intervention planning. Finally, mandatory privacy and confidentiality issues need to be respected in the natural environment. This can be challenging and confusing in the dynamic, unpredictable natural setting, but need to be highly respected for ethical best practice. Occupational participation occurs in the natural occurring contexts and environment of life, not in a contrived clinic environment. The ultimate goal of occupational therapy practice is to facilitate the client to fully participate in all life contexts of individual meaning, interest, and importance.

## Student Self-Assessment

1a. Imagine some of your favorite pastimes and write down three of them. Include the activity and the context in which you like to do that activity.

1b. Describe how your practitioner could best simulate that activity if you ever had occupational therapy.

1c. Describe how an occupational therapy practitioner could modify or assist you to perform that activity in the context you most enjoy it, if you were experiencing:

- ◊ Hemiparesis of your dominant side
- ◊ Severe visual impairment
- ◊ Social anxiety and panic attacks
- ◊ Cognitive impairments including impulsivity and short-term memory deficits

## Evidence-Based Research Chart

| Topic | Intervention | Evidence |
|---|---|---|
| Inclusive preschool | Outdoor play guided by the interdisciplinary Ecology of Human Performance model | Anecdotal and occupational objectives achieved—parent satisfaction (Ideishi et al., 2006) |
| Craft activities in groups at meeting places to support mental health users' everyday occupations | A focused ethnography in which 12 participants engaged in a craft activity in a group facilitated by an occupational therapy practitioner | The craft group facilitated stability and routines that influenced participants' sense of everyday occupation, reduced feelings of helplessness, and provided structure for their lives (Horghagen, Fostvedt, & Alsaker, 2014) |
| Family routines and rituals | Family daily routines, interviews of stories, daily routines and occupation focus on morning activities | Family routines are important for organization and meaning in self-care of children (Segal, 2004) |
| Multicontexts used for brain injury intervention | Single case study incorporating functional tasks in natural environments and contexts of daily life | Brain injury intervention may be enhanced to include the contexts of everyday life (Landa-Gonzalez, 2001) |
| Occupational therapy role in keeping community-based older adults in their homes | Use of assistive devices and focus on safety in functional mobility and overall home-based tasks | Seventeen efficacy studies focusing on decreasing falls, increasing home safety, social participation, and quality of life (Stuetjens et al., 2004) |
| Occupation-based intervention in home-like environments | Single case study demonstrates behavioral, neurological, and qualitative changes in a client with stroke following occupation-based intervention | Study supports use of the occupation-based practice in a home-like environment (Skubik-Peplaski, Carrico, Nicols, Chelette, & Sawaki, 2012) |
| Gardens found to be therapeutic | Access to nature important for healing in an institutional setting | Review of literature supporting therapeutic gardening (Mitrione, 2008) |
| Using pictures of nature as an intervention with older adults | Older adults and college students were shown pictures of nature and pictures of urban images | Results revealed that even images of nature had a positive impact on executive attention in both groups; the urban images did not have the same effect (Gamble, Howard, & Howard, 2014) |

2a. Name some potential safety risks inherent in the following settings:
   - ◊ The kitchen of a client's home
   - ◊ Community mobility with an elder who has Parkinson's disease
   - ◊ The playground
   - ◊ A school field trip to another town
   - ◊ The school bus
   - ◊ The YMCA pool
   - ◊ A summer camp
   - ◊ A group home
   - ◊ A shelter for battered women

2b. Now think critically and problem solve potential precautions to put in place in each of the preceding settings to ensure safety and best practice.

3. Class discussion: Why is privacy and confidentiality more of a concern in natural, "uncontrolled" environments? Please give specific examples.

4. Name three ways that a practitioner can help to achieve an ethical climate of privacy in a natural setting during an activity that promotes real-life social participation.

## References


American Occupational Therapy Association. (2006). *The New IDEA: Summary of the Individuals with Disabilities Education Improvement Act of 2004 (P.L. 108-446)*. Retrieved from www.aota.org

American Occupational Therapy Association. (2008). *AOTA's societal statement on livable communities*. Retrieved from http://www.aota.org/practitioners-Section/Official-Docs.aspx

American Occupational Therapy Association. (2009). *Occupational therapy's commitment to non-discrimination and inclusion*. Retrieved from http://www.aota.org/practitioners-Section/Official-Docs.aspx

American Occupational Therapy Association. (2011). *Occupational therapy services in facilitating work performance*. Retrieved from http://www.aota.org/practitioners-Section/Official-Docs.aspx

American Occupational Therapy Association. (2012). *Occupational therapy services at the workplace: Transitional return-to-work programs [fact sheet]*. Retrieved from http://www.aota.org/-/media/Corporate/Files/AboutOT/Professionals/WhatIsOT/WI/Facts/Transitional.pdf

American Occupational Therapy Association. (2014a). Occupational therapy practice framework: Domain and process (3rd ed.). *American Journal of Occupational Therapy, 68*(Suppl. 1), S1-S48. doi:10.5014/ajot.2014.682006

American Occupational Therapy Association. (2014b). *Occupational therapy's commitment to non-discrimination and inclusion*. Retrieved from http://ajot.aota.org/article.aspx?articleid=1934864&resultClick=3

Barton, J., & Pretty, J. (2010). What is the best dose of nature and green exercise for improving mental health? A multi-study analysis. *Environmental Science and Technology, 44*(10), 3947-3955.

Bazyk, S., Demirjian, L., LaGuardia, T., Thompson-Repas, K., Conway, C., & Michaud, P. (2015). Building capacity of occupational therapy practitioners to address the mental health needs of children and youth: A mixed methods study of knowledge translation. *American Journal of Occupational Therapy, 69*, 6906180060. doi:10.5014/ajot.2015.019182

Carlsson-Paige, N., McLaughlin, G., & Almon, J. (2015). Reading instruction in kindergarten: Little to gain and much to lose. *The Alliance for Childhood and Defending the Early Years*. Retrieved from http://www.allianceforchildhood.org/sites/allianceforchildhood.org/files/file/Reading_Instruction_in_Kindergarten.pdf

Case-Smith, J. (2005). Development of childhood occupations. In J. Case-Smith (Ed.), *Occupational therapy for children* (5th ed., pp. 88-116). St. Louis, MO: Mosby-Elsevier.

Case-Smith, J. (2015). Development of childhood occupations. In J. Case-Smith & J. O'Brien (Eds.), *Occupational therapy for children and adolescents* (7th ed., pp. 65-101). St. Louis, MO: Mosby-Elsevier.

Chamberlain L. L., & Butz, M. R. (1998). *Clinical chaos: A therapist's guide to nonlinear dynamics and therapeutic change*. Philadelphia, PA: Brunner/Mazel.

Champagne, T. (2008). *Sensory modulation and environment: Essential elements of occupation* (3rd ed.). Southampton, MA: Champagne Conferences and Consultation.

Chippendale, T. (2014). Meeting the mental health needs of older adults in all practice settings. *Physical and Occupational Therapy in Geriatrics, 32*(1), 1-9.

Christiansen, C., & Baum, C. M. (1991). *Occupational therapy: Enabling function and well-being*. Thorofare, NJ: SLACK Incorporated.

Clark, F., Azen, S. P., Zemke, R., Jackson, J., Carlson, M., Mandel, D., et al. (1997). Occupational therapy for independent-living older adults. *Journal of the American Medical Association, 278*(16), 1321-1326.

Clark, P. (2014). Nature and the outdoors: Stimulating those with dementia. *Nursing and Residential Care, 16*(6), 336-339.

Dowdell, K., Gray, T., & Malone, K. (2011). Nature and its influence on children's outdoor play. *Australian Journal of Outdoor Education, 15*(2), 24-35. Retrieved from https://une.idm.oclc.org/login?url=http://search.proquest.com.une.idm.oclc.org/docview/1010412777?accountid=12756

Dunn, W., Foto, M., Hinojosa, J., Boyt-Schell, B., Thomson. L., & Hertfelder, S. (1995a). Independence position paper: The American Occupational Therapy Association: Broadening the construct of independence. *American Journal of Occupational Therapy, 49*, 1014.

Dunn, W., Foto, M., Hinojosa, J., Boyt-Schell, B., Thomson. L., & Hertfelder, S. (1995b). Occupational therapy: A profession in support of full inclusion. In *Reference Manual of the Official Documents of the American Occupational Therapy Association, Inc.* Bethesda, MD: AOTA Press.

Edvardsson, D., & Nordvall, K. (2008). Lost in the present but confident of the past: Experiences of being in a psycho-geriatric unit as narrated by persons with dementia. *Journal of Clinical Nursing, 17*(4).

Gamble, K. R., Howard, J. H., & Howard, D. V. (2014). Not just scenery: Viewing nature pictures improves executive attention in older adults. *Experimental Aging Research, 40*(5), 513-530, 18. doi:10.1080/0361073X.2014.956618

Grady, A. P. (1995). Building inclusive community: A challenge for occupational therapy. *American Journal of Occupational Therapy, 49*, 300-310.

Hinojosa, J., & Blount, M. L. (2000). *The texture of life purposeful activities in occupational therapy*. Bethesda, MD: AOTA Press.

Horghagen, S., Fostvedt, B., & Alsaker, S. (2014). Craft activities in groups at meeting places: Supporting mental health users' everyday occupations. *Scandinavian Journal of Occupational Therapy, 21*(2), 145-152. doi:10.3109/11038128.2013.866691

Humphry, R., & Wakeford, L. (2006). An occupation-centered discussion of development and implications for practice. *American Journal of Occupational Therapy, 60*, 258-267.

Ideishi, S. K., Ideishi, R. I., Gandhi, T., & Yuen, L. (2006). Inclusive preschool outdoor play environments. *School System Special Interest Section Quarterly, 13*(2). Bethesda, MD: AOTA Press.

Kelso, J. A. S. (1995). *Dynamic patterns: The self-organization of brain and behavior*. Cambridge, MA: The MIT Press.

Kielhofner, G. (1992). *Conceptual foundations of occupational therapy*. Philadelphia, PA: F. A. Davis Company.

Landa-Gonzalez, B. (2001). Multicontextual occupational therapy intervention: A case study of traumatic brain injury. *Occupational Therapy International, 8*(1), 49.

Lazzarini, I. (2004). Neuro-occupation: The nonlinear dynamics of intention, meaning and perception. *British Journal of Occupational Therapy, 67*(8), 1-11.

Letts, L., Rigby, P., & Stewart, D. (2003). *Using environments to enable occupational performance*. Thorofare, NJ: SLACK Incorporated.

Loukas, K. M., Whiting, A., Ricci, E., & Cohen-Konrad, S. (2012). Transdisciplinary playgroup: Interprofessional opportunities in early intervention practice education. *OT Practice, 17*(3), 8-13.

Mitrione, S. (2008). Therapeutic responses to natural environment using gardens to improve health care. *Minnesota Medicine*. Retrieved from http://www.minnesotamedicine.com/PastIssues/March2008/ClinicalMitrioneMarch2008/tabid/2488/Default.aspx

Myers, C., Case-Smith, J., & Cason, J. (2015). Early intervention. In J. Case-Smith & J. O'Brien (Eds.), *Occupational therapy for children and adolescents* (7th ed., pp. 637-663). St. Louis, MO: Mosby-Elsevier.

Noonan, M. J., & McCormick, L. (2006). *Young children with disabilities in natural environments*. Baltimore, MD: Brookes Publishing Co.

Perr, A., & Bell, P. F. (2000). Moving from simulation to real life. In J. Hinojosa & M. L. Blount (Eds.), *The texture of life purposeful activities in occupational therapy* (pp. 234-257). Bethesda, MD: AOTA Press.

Pierce, D. (2003). *Occupation by design: Building therapeutic power*. Philadelphia, PA: F. A. Davis Company.

Purtilo, R., & Doherty, R. (2011). *Ethical dimensions in the health professions* (5th ed.). St. Louis, MO: Saunders-Elsevier.

Reed, K. L. (2006). Occupational therapy values and beliefs: The formative years: 1904-1929. *OT Practice, April 17*, 21-25.

Royeen, C. B. (2003). Chaotic occupational therapy: Collective wisdom from a complex profession. *American Journal of Occupational Therapy, 57*(6), 609-624.

Sankar, P., Moran, S., Merz, J. F., & Jones, N. L. (2003). Patient perspectives on medical confidentiality. *Journal of General Internal Medicine, 18*(8), 659-669.

Scaffa, M. (2001). *Occupational therapy in community-based settings*. Philadelphia, PA: F. A. Davis Company.

Segal, R. (2004). Family routines and rituals: A context for occupational therapy interventions. *American Journal of Occupational Therapy, 58*, 499-508.

Skubik-Peplaski, C., Carrico, C., Nichols, L., Chelette, K., & Sawaki, L. (2012). Behavioral, neurophysiological, and descriptive changes after occupation-based intervention. *American Journal of Occupational Therapy, 66*, e107-e113. doi:10.5014/ajot.2012.003590

Solum, L. L., & Schaffer, M. A. (2003). Ethical problems experienced by school nurses. *Journal of School Nursing, 19*(6), 330-337.

Stephens, L. C., & Tauber, S. K. (2005). Early intervention. In J. Case-Smith (Ed.), *Occupational therapy for children* (5th ed., pp. 771-793). St. Louis, MO: Mosby-Elsevier.

Stuetjens, E. M., Dekker, J., Bouter, L. M., Jellena, S., Bakker, E. B., & van den Ende, C. H. M. (2004). Occupational therapy for community dwelling elderly people. A systematic review. *Age and Aging, 33*, 453-460.

Thelen, E. (2000). Motor development as foundation and future of developmental psychology. *International Journal of Behavioral Development, 24*(4), 385-397.

Tungpunkom, P., & Nicol, M. (2008). Life skills programmes for chronic mental illnesses. *Cochrane Database of Systematic Reviews, (1)*, doi:10/1002/14651858.CD000381.pub3

U.S. Department of Health and Human Services, National Institute of Mental Health. (n.d.). *Older adults and depression.* Retrieved from http://www.nimh.nih.gov/health/publications/older-adults-and-depression/older-adults-and-depression_141998.pdf

von Benzon, N. (2010). Moving on from ramps? The utility of the social model of disability for facilitating experiences of nature for disabled children. *Disability and Society, 25*(5), 617-625. doi:10.1080/09687599.2010.489313

Whalley Hammell, K. (2003). Changing institutional environments to enable occupation among people with severe physical limitations. In L. Letts, P. Rigby, & D. Stewart (Eds.), *Using environments to enable occupational performance* (pp. 35-53). Thorofare, NJ: SLACK Incorporated.

Wrights Law. (2013). *Special education law.* Retrieved from http://wrightslaw.com/

Zoltan, B. (2007). *Vision, perception, and cognition: A manual for the evaluation and treatment of the adult with acquired brain injury* (4th ed.). Thorofare, NJ: SLACK Incorporated.

## Suggested Readings

Humphrey, R., Gonzalez, S., & Taylor, E. (1993). Family involvement in practice: Issues and attitudes. *American Journal of Occupational Therapy, 47*, 587-593.

Kellegrew, D. H. (2000). Constructing daily routines: A qualitative examination of mothers with young children with disabilities. *American Journal of Occupational Therapy, 54*, 252-259.

Law, M., Cooper, B., Strong, S., Stewart, P., Rigby, P., & Letts, L. (1996). The person-environment-occupation model: A transactive approach to occupational performance. *Canadian Journal of Occupational Therapy, 63*, 9-23.

Ma, H., Trombly, C. A., & Robinson-Podolski, C. (1998). The effect of context on skill acquisition and transfer. *American Journal of Occupational Therapy, 53*, 138-144.

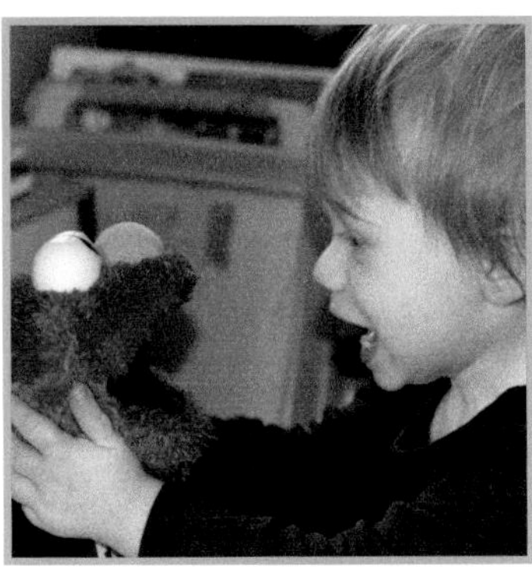

# 14

# Clinical Reasoning

*Mary Elizabeth Patnaude, MS, OTR/L*

**ACOTE STANDARDS EXPLORED IN THIS CHAPTER**

B.2.10, B.2.11

**KEY VOCABULARY**

- **Clinical reasoning:** "The process used by practitioners to plan, direct, perform, and reflect on client care" (Schell & Schell, 2008, p. 443).
- **Experiential learning:** "Involves hands-on experience in a practical setting to test information learned in didactic coursework in an actual practice environment" (Coker, 2010, p. 281).
- **Narrative reasoning:** "The process through which occupational therapy practitioners make sense of people's particular circumstances; prospectively imagine the effect of illness, disability, or occupational performance problems on their daily lives; and create a collaborative story that is enacted with clients and families through intervention" (Schell & Schell, 2008, p. 446).
- **Professional reasoning:** "Cognitive processes used to guide professional actions. Includes the therapy process, as well as reasoning done by supervisors, fieldwork educators, managers, and consultant managers as they conceptualize occupational therapy practice" (Schell, 2009, p. 447).
- **Reflection:** Critical analysis of knowledge and feelings leading to a better understanding of the situation.



Jacobs, K., & MacRae, N. (Eds.).
*Occupational Therapy Essentials for Clinical Competence, Third Edition* (pp. 187-195).

Occupational therapy practitioners include registered occupational therapists and certified occupational therapy assistants. Occupational therapy practitioners therapeutically use everyday activities to enhance participation in meaningful life roles and occupations (American Occupational Therapy Association [AOTA], 2014). To do this effectively, occupational therapy practitioners need to discover the client's story, understand his or her diagnosis or condition, and synthesize all the information into a coherent, evidence-based, client-centered treatment plan. For the intervention process to be effective, occupational therapy practitioners need to use clinical reasoning strategies. Clinical reasoning is "the process used by practitioners to plan, direct, perform, and reflect on client care" (Schell & Schell, 2008, p. 443). Both occupational therapists and occupational therapy assistants are responsible for demonstrating competency in clinical reasoning (AOTA, 2009).

The literature outlines several types of clinical reasoning used by occupational therapy practitioners: narrative, scientific, pragmatic, ethical, and conditional (interactive). Explicit definitions for each of type of clinical reasoning may help occupational therapy students to translate knowledge learned from instructors in didactic coursework to clinical thinking useful for service delivery (Neistadt, 1998). In addition, experiential learning opportunities may also help improve critical thinking and experiential learning, as students delve more deeply into complex issues introduced in didactic coursework and process them through hands-on learning (Coker, 2010; Figure 14-1).

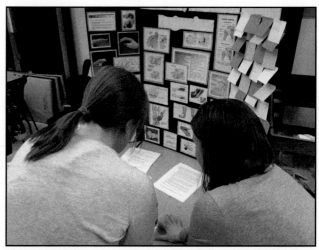

**Figure 14-1.** Entry-level MS occupational therapy students sharpen clinical reasoning skills through an experiential learning opportunity in which they provide an advanced practice seminar.

Occupational therapy practitioners require a high level of skill to successfully use all types of clinical reasoning, due to the complexity involved in the process. To be successful in the occupational therapy process, practitioners must synthesize the knowledge gleaned with each type of clinical reasoning. In the course of intervention treatment planning and delivery, experienced practitioners shift from one type of clinical reasoning to another (Mattingly & Fleming, 1994). Therefore, defining and articulating the type of clinical reasoning being used at any given moment can sometimes be difficult for even the most seasoned occupational therapy practitioner.

## Clinical Reasoning

Clinical reasoning is a multifaceted cognitive process that involves several different layers of thought, evidence, and experience. Because experienced occupational therapy practitioners frequently switch between several types of clinical reasoning during the course of treatment, it may sometimes be difficult for novel practitioners to pinpoint which type of reasoning is being used (Mattingly & Fleming, 1994). Therefore, it might be helpful for the occupational therapy student or entry-level practitioner to analyze evaluation, treatment, and discharge scenarios to help pinpoint the instances of each type of reasoning being used.

In addition, occupational therapy practitioners must use personal experiences, evidence-based practice, and information about the specific client and his or her context to develop clinical reasoning skills. The use of theory can also assist occupational therapy practitioners in developing a high level of clinical reasoning. Hawkins, Elder, and Paul (2010) define clinical reasoning as "thinking through the various aspects of patient care to arrive at a reasonable decision regarding the prevention, diagnosis, or treatment of a clinical problem in a specific patient" (p. 3).

In addition to clinical reasoning, Schell (2009) recommends that occupational therapy practitioners broaden their scope of thought to include professional reasoning. Professional reasoning encompasses a broader scope than clinical reasoning, which traditionally has been applied to medical settings. Professional reasoning includes nonmedical settings, such as homes, schools, and community centers, and the ways in which the outcomes of the reasoning process influence actions and outcomes of service delivery (Figure 14-2).

Both types of reasoning require one to synthesize information to reflect on practice. Therefore, practitioners must understand the various methods of reasoning and the ways in which the outcomes of reasoning direct practice to be successful.

## Case Study

Doug is a 38-year-old single man who works as a computer programmer. He lives alone, and his hobbies include video games, reading, and playing video games and role-playing games with his nephews, who are 16, 13, 11, 9, and 7 years old. He complains of left shoulder, dorsal elbow, and dorsal wrist pain; shoulder weakness; neck pain; left limb paresthesia; and decreased shoulder range of motion.

### Evaluation Procedure

*Interview (Narrative Reasoning)*

- His chief complaint is elbow and wrist pain, which is exacerbated by certain neck and shoulder positions. The pain primarily interferes with sleep because he has difficulty finding a comfortable position at night and driving.
- Interactional reasoning was also used. This client is a family member, and knows me in that context. I had to use my skill as an occupational practitioner to explain (in layperson's language) my rationale for the treatment and intervention I was using. I needed to understand him more thoroughly in his work role (computer programmer).

*Hand Therapy Initial Evaluation (Scientific/Procedural Reasoning)*

- Subjective
  - Forward head posture and decreased use of left upper extremity during functional tasks
  - Elbow and wrist pain (achy) 5 at worst to 0 (at best)
  - Prior level of function: I
  - Current level of function: Mod I
  - Hand dominance: R
  - Work status: Full duty
  - Patient's goals for therapy: To complete activities of daily living (ADLs), instrumental activities of daily living (IADLs), and work tasks with no pain
- Objective (scientific/procedural reasoning)
  - Left shoulder range of motion
    - Flexion 140 degrees
    - Abduction 125 degrees
    - External rotation 75 degrees
    - Supination/pronation 90 degrees
    - Wrist extension 45 degrees
  - Left shoulder strength
    - Flexion/extension 5/5
    - Abduction 4/5
    - External rotation 4/5
  - Special tests (scientific/procedural and conditional reasoning)
    - Cozen's test (to detect lateral epicondylitis): negative
    - Adsen (to detect occlusion of subclavian artery due to thoracic outlet syndrome): negative
    - Spurling (to detect cervical radiculopathy): positive result

### Ethical Reasoning

Nonmaleficence (Schell & Schell, 2008, p 194): Needed to administer special tests with care, to avoid causing more harm to patient, especially with an inflamed nerve root. The reasoning behind choosing the special tests involved conditional reasoning, because I had to think about the whole condition (Fleming, 1991). He complained of seemingly unrelated symptoms: neck, elbow, and wrist pain. Taken alone, dorsal elbow pain can indicate epicondylitis. A negative Cozen's sign ruled this out. The area of pain pointed to radial nerve pathology, which I know originates at the middle trunk of the brachial plexus, at C7. Therefore, I reasoned that his symptoms were originating at the neck. I performed the tests to pinpoint whether it was nerve root or arterial impingement, and determined it to be a nerve root cause.

### Upper Extremity Functional Index (Conditional Reasoning, Looking at Whole Condition and Narrative Reasoning, Trying to Learn More of the Client's Story)

- Scale 0 to 80 (0 = extreme difficulty, 4 = no difficulty)
- 20 items related to work, ADLs, IADLs, etc. (such as lifting, grooming, using tools, etc.)
- The higher the score, the least amount of difficulty
- Doug scored 68/80 (overall moderate difficulty)
  - Moderate difficulty (2): usual work, housework, or school activities
  - A little bit of difficulty in multiple areas: hobbies, lifting items overhead, tying shoes, carrying small items

*(continued)*

## Case Study (continued)

- The results of the upper extremity functional index pointed to the need to perform an ergonomic assessment of his workstation
- A home exercise program was devised (conditional and pragmatic reasoning) that would help ameliorate the symptoms, increase range of motion in affected shoulder, strengthen weak muscles, and be short enough that he would have the time to complete it in his busy daily schedule.

**Assessment (Conditional Reasoning)**

- Decreased range of motion in shoulder abduction and wrist extension (requires the knowledge of normal range of motion)
- Decreased strength in abduction and external rotation
- Pain with overhead activities and lifting moderate amounts of weight
- Forward head posture, which may lead to further impingement of nerve roots

**Plan of Care (Conditional Reasoning)**

- Home exercise program
- Pendulums, external rotation with moderate weight, caudal glides
- Postural retraining: neck range of motion
- Ergonomic assessment (scheduled as soon as possible)
- Manual therapy: to decrease edema and work out trigger points
- ADL retraining

**Summary**

As I was completing this assessment, I really tried to think about each type of clinical reasoning. As I was analyzing it, I found it difficult to pinpoint exactly which type of clinical reasoning I was using. I realized that this is because, as an experienced occupational therapy practitioner, I "used different thinking styles without losing track of some aspects of the problem while (I) shifted attention to another feature of the problem" (Fleming, 1991, pp. 1007-1008.) This exercise emphasized to me that I truly have a multitrack mind when it comes to clinical reasoning.

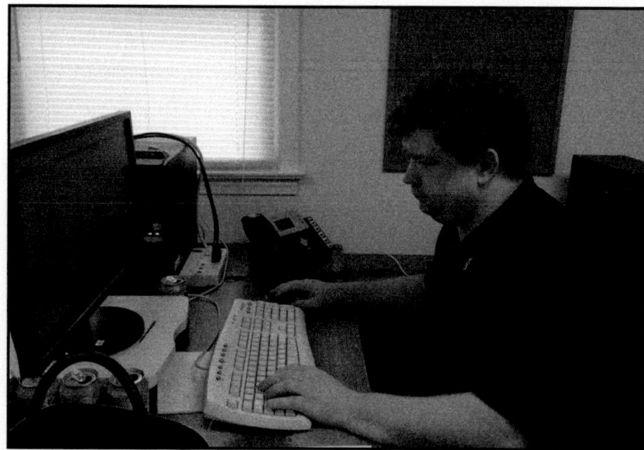

**Figure 14-2.** During a worksite evaluation, an experienced occupational therapy practitioner often switches between several types of clinical reasoning, such as narrative, scientific, and pragmatic.

## *Narrative Reasoning*

Narrative reasoning allows a client to tell a story. The story can be multifaceted, involving his or her life, culture, and illness (Schell & Schell, 2008). It provides information to shape meaningful interventions. The generation of an occupational profile, the first step of the occupational therapy process, is a form of narrative reasoning (Haas, 2014).

"The occupational profile is information that describes the client's occupational history and experience, patterns of daily living, interests, values and needs" (Moyers & Dale, 2007, p. 22). This is important when developing an intervention plan so that the plan is relevant to the client. An occupational therapy practitioner who is skilled at narrative reasoning will synthesize all of this information to devise a client-centered treatment plan. An example of narrative reasoning applied to an upper extremity orthopedic client with a wrist fracture would include the following:

- With whom do you live? This will help the therapist glean whether another individual can help with tasks the client cannot complete at this time.
- For whom are you responsible for care? This will help the therapist know the types of tasks necessary on a daily basis. If a client has an infant or a toddler, there will be much more need for lifting than if the client is retired and lives alone.
- What type of job, if any, do you have? Whether the above client is a stay-at-home mom, with an 8-month-old and a 2-year-old, or a carpenter running his own business, their responsibilities will likely involve tasks that may be contraindicated.
- What do you really want to do that you cannot do now? This is perhaps the most important aspect of narrative reasoning. This gets to the heart of the

client's story. What are his or her hopes and dreams? The client may want nothing more than to cook a big holiday meal or decorate a birthday cake for a grandchild. By keeping this in mind, a skilled occupational therapy practitioner can educate the client on the factors needed to achieve these hopes, and encourage the client if progress in impeded.

When eliciting a client's story, the therapist needs to really listen to the client. This allows the therapist to gauge how things are going, and helps to shape the continuing course of intervention (Schell & Schell, 2008). Therapeutic listening to a client's story really helps form a bond between practitioner and client. This technique of using oneself therapeutically helps the client to feel accepted and comfortable, and allows for an exceptional relationship and trust to be built (Taylor, 2008).

This trust may be further reinforced as a therapist shares some of his or her story as well. Although this is a valuable tool, novice therapists need to be able to forge an effective relationship using narrative while maintaining professional boundaries.

## *Scientific/Procedural Reasoning*

Scientific or procedural reasoning occurs when an occupational therapy practitioner uses foundational knowledge, such as an understanding of human anatomy, biomechanics, physiology, human development, and pathophysiology, to understand the condition with which a client or patient presents. This begins the minute a referral is received. Schell and Schell (2008) define this type of reasoning as "a systematic approach to creating, testing, and using knowledge to make decisions" (p. 92). Because this type of reasoning involves a systematic approach, an occupational therapist completes a systematic process of implementing scientific/procedural reasoning.

The process begins with an evaluation and the development of an occupational profile. The client factors, outlined above, such as injury, illness, disability, and developmental level, are taken into account and used to formulate an intervention plan (Moyers & Dale, 2007). While planning and implementing an intervention plan, occupational therapy practitioners use knowledge of the literature to provide treatments that have the most likely chance of achieving the desired outcome. This process involves the implementation of treatments backed up by evidence or evidence-based treatment (Schell & Schell, 2008).

An example of this type of reasoning applied to wrist fractures involves understanding healing times, the stages of healing, types of fractures, procedures to stabilize fractures, and wrist anatomy. When evaluating and treating a client who has a distal radial fracture, one must keep in mind many factors, a few of which include the time since injury, the age of the client, the type of fracture (displaced vs. nondisplaced), the type of reduction used (closed vs. open), the presence or absence of hardware (internal fixation, external fixation, or none), and precautions (range of motion and weight bearing; Moscony & Shank, 2014).

During the entire process, a practitioner continually evaluates the client and may need to shift gears. This is due to the fact that experienced practitioners often generate several hypotheses and test them frequently (Fleming, 1991). An example of hypothesis shifting in treatment may be when a practitioner uses evidence-based edema reduction techniques, such as active range of motion, and the edema continues to increase. The practitioner may need to shift reasoning to look for another cause, such as an orthotic or cast that is too tight, or another underlying medical cause, such as latent lymphedema.

This type of reasoning requires a solid knowledge of foundational skills, as well as knowledge of the evidence. Students on orthopedic Level II fieldwork rotations and new practitioners need to be mindful of the evidence to ensure the provision of services that will lead to the best outcomes. For instance, the evidence strongly shows that the best way to decrease edema and restore function in the upper extremity is through active range of motion. This can be done through exercise and/or functional activities that require active range of motion of the wrist (e.g., grooming, dressing, and cooking activities). A new practitioner may be tempted to use interventions not supported with strong evidence, such as ultrasound. An occupational therapy practitioner with strong procedural reasoning skills can confidently provide occupation-based interventions that will lead to the best possible outcome for each client.

## *Pragmatic Reasoning*

Occupational therapy practitioners use pragmatic reasoning to understand the practical issues affecting service delivery. Pragmatic reasoning attempts to glean how everyday issues, such as outdated equipment and large caseloads, affect services to clients and family members (Schell & Schell, 2008). This type of reasoning enables occupational therapy practitioners to identify practical strategies for intervention to ensure the highest quality of care. This type of reasoning requires the practitioner to go beyond client factors and consider the context in which the therapeutic intervention takes place, as well as his or her unique attributes and skills (Figures 14-3A and B). Consider the following examples of pragmatic reasoning in various practice settings:

- Children and youth: Would the effectiveness of an intervention to improve fine motor skills be improved if delivered in a quiet room in a private clinic versus in a bustling classroom setting?
- Mental health: How would a client's lack of a safe, consistent living environment help or hinder his or her ability to consistently attend treatment sessions?

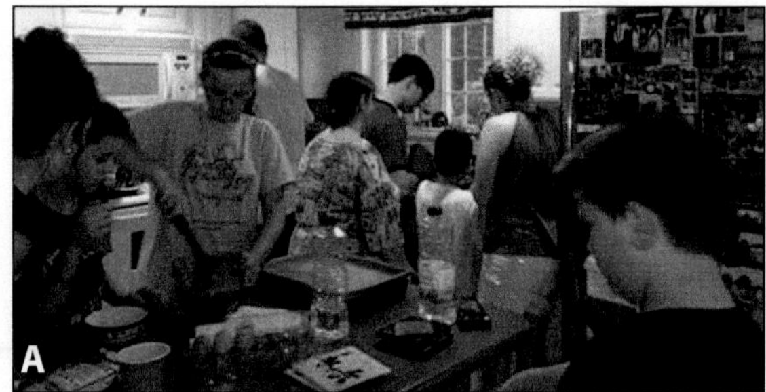


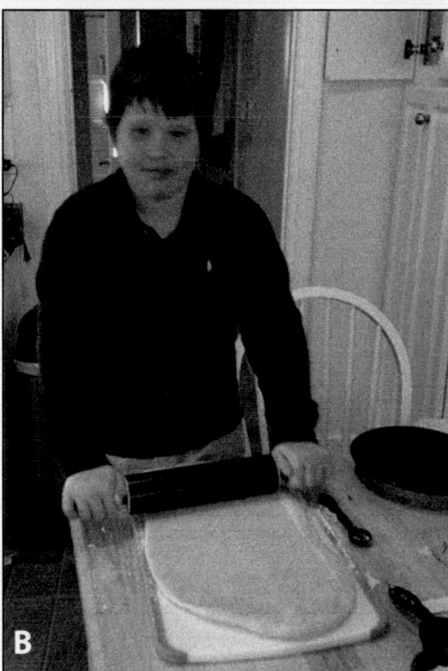


**Figure 14-3.** A meal preparation activity requires a great deal of conditional and pragmatic reasoning (A) when provided in a bustling kitchen with many different people versus (B) when provided in a quiet setting, with 1:1 attention.

- Rehabilitation and disability: How do high productivity demands in acute rehabilitation hospitals influence the types of interventions used by occupational therapy practitioners?
- Health and wellness: What opportunities arise for the occupational therapy practitioner in response to the desire of the "baby boom" population to stay well and independent as they approach and exceed retirement age?
- Productive aging: How do occupational therapy practitioners become more skilled at providing services for individuals who wish to build retirement homes that will allow them to live at home as they age?
- Work and industry: What are the practical differences in providing consultation services to an injured worker's employer versus the worker him- or herself?

## *Ethical Reasoning*

Occupational therapy practitioners use ethical reasoning to drive the intervention process in a way that ensures that all choices made are morally justified. Ethical reasoning introduces the consideration of what "should" be done in the best interest of the person and family. The *Occupational Therapy Code of Ethics* (AOTA, 2015) outlines how the profession is grounded in seven long-standing core values:

1. Altruism
2. Equality
3. Freedom
4. Justice
5. Dignity
6. Truth
7. Prudence

In addition, the *Code of Ethics* outlines enforceable guidelines for professional behavior (AOTA, 2015):

- Beneficence
- Nonmaleficence
- Autonomy
- Justice
- Veracity
- Fidelity

In addition to the *Code of Ethics*, the practitioner must also consider the mission of the facility where the services are provided and/or where the practitioner is employed.

Occupational therapy practitioners with a good understanding and working knowledge of the *Code of Ethics* will be better equipped to navigate moral conflicts. For example, nonmaleficence includes an obligation to not impose the risk of harm to a client (AOTA, 2015). Therefore, an occupational therapy practitioner would abstain from an intervention strategy that he or she knows or suspects may cause harm, even if significant benefits could be gained. Proficiency in ethical reasoning helps one discern situations that truly cause harm from those that may cause a temporary negative effect. An example of this would be temporary pain induced by passive range of motion, which does not cause harm and will likely subside after the treatment is completed.

Ethical reasoning also relates to occupational justice, which "recognizes occupational rights to inclusive participation in everyday occupations for all persons in society, regardless of age, ability, gender, social class, or other differences" (Nilsson & Townsend, 2014, p. 64). Therefore, to be truly ethical, occupational therapy practitioners must demonstrate fairness to all clients with whom they interact. For example, if a client is admitted to an inpatient mental health setting, very dirty and

Table 14-1.

## How Clinical Reasoning Is Applied in Practice

| Therapist/Student Action | Critical Reasoning Used |
|---|---|
| Choice of frame of reference | Ethical |
| Meal preparation intervention for a chef | Narrative |
| Observation of the client's environment | Pragmatic |
| Consultation with family and caregivers | Narrative, conditional |
| Use of the framework to guide decisions | Procedural |
| Choice of intervention approaches | Pragmatic |
| Family/caregiver training activities | Pragmatic |
| Reflection | Conditional |
| Use of evidence-based practice in guiding intervention planning | Scientific, ethical |

Adapted from Haas, K. B. (2014). Clinical reasoning. In K. Jacobs, N. MacRae, & K. Sladyk (Eds.), *Occupational therapy essentials for clinical competence* (2nd ed.). Thorofare, NJ: SLACK Incorporated.

infested with parasites, the occupational therapy practitioner has the obligation to treat him or her regardless of the circumstances. In addition, ethical reasoning can help the novice practitioner tease out fairness and justice from safety. Therefore, despite the obligation to treat all clients with fairness and justice, occupational therapy practitioners should never put themselves in harm's way when providing services.

### Conditional (Interactive) Reasoning

Conditional (or interactive) reasoning combines reasoning about the client (narrative and procedural) with those about the world in which treatment is delivered (ethical and pragmatic). According to Fleming (1991), this type of reasoning includes the ability to really know the client; communicate trust and hope to the client; individualize treatment to the unique goals, abilities, and experiences of each client; and allow for the constant need to adapt treatment in response to successes and failures. For example, an occupational therapy practitioner may have a client who was a professional chef who has sustained brain injury. He expresses the goal to return to a professional kitchen, but exhibits limitations in safety awareness. Although safety is a very big concern, the occupational therapy practitioner must not immediately disregard this goal. Instead, he or she must continually reevaluate it throughout the entire treatment process, making adjustments as the client's condition allows.

## The Use of Reasoning to Improve Clinical Practice

Why do occupational therapy practitioners seek to effectively use clinical and professional reasoning in everyday practice? Schell and Schell (2008) posit that the main reason is to improve practice. Clinical reasoning can be applied to practice to improve outcomes through effective use of research, reflection, and self-direction (Table 14-1).

Consuming research, critically analyzing the research, applying it to practice, and reflecting upon the results are effective tools in improving clinical reasoning (Schell & Schell, 2008). For example, Coker (2010) found that critical thinking and clinical reasoning of students can be improved. This is done with a focus on complex issues in which they are given the opportunity to focus study in depth, with time to process outcomes after the fact. Therefore, it would be beneficial for occupational therapy students to take time to reflect upon experiences received in both the classroom and on fieldwork. Problem-based learning, in which students make connections between clients, generalize from one client to another, and compare treatment approaches, also assists in developing and improving clinical reasoning (Scaffa & Wooster, 2004).

Reflection allows students and occupational therapy practitioners the opportunity to integrate new and previously learned knowledge. It requires that one recall the salient details of a case, critically analyze the information gleaned, synthesize new knowledge with previous knowledge, and evaluate the effectiveness of all this knowledge (Atkins & Murphy, 1993). It also allows practitioners to connect seemingly disparate information in meaningful ways, and enables one to adapt learning from one situation to another as problems arise (Cohn, Coster, & Kramer, 2014).

Expert clinical reasoning requires self-directed learning. Self-directed learning refers to one's ability to take control of one's own learning process (Gibbons et al., 1980). The Professional Development Tool (AOTA, 2003) designed by AOTA, provides a medium for occupational therapists to evaluate current competencies and use critical

## Evidence-Based Research Chart

| Topic | Evidence |
|---|---|
| Clinical reasoning | Carrier, Levasseur, Bedard, & Desrosiers, 2010; Kuipers & Grice, 2009; Mu, Coppard, Bracciano, Doll, & Matthews, 2010; Scaffa & Wooster, 2004; Yancosek & Howell, 2010 |
| Reflection | Bannigan & Moores, 2009; Dunn & Musolino, 2011; Plack & Santasier, 2004 |
| Experiential learning | Coker, 2010; Knecht-Sabres, 2010 |

Adapted from Haas, K. B. (2014). Clinical reasoning. In K. Jacobs, N. MacRae, & K. Sladyk (Eds.), *Occupational therapy essentials for clinical competence* (2nd ed.). Thorofare, NJ: SLACK Incorporated.

reasoning to develop a plan for self-directed learning. This tool is valuable for occupational therapists seeking to stay current utilizing informal learning, as well as those seeking an advanced degree and/or improving critical thinking and clinical reasoning.

## Summary

Occupational therapy practitioners require a high level of skill to successfully use all types of clinical reasoning due to the complexity involved in the process. To be most effective in this process, occupational therapy practitioners must progress through multiple stages of development of clinical reasoning: advanced beginner, competent, proficient, and expert (Neistadt, 1996). In the process, they are transformed from beginners, ruled by exact rules and principles (e.g., exact goniometric measurement of each joint), to experts, able to begin the evaluation process at any point, take cues from clients, and almost effortlessly recognize problems (Neistadt, 1996).

The effective application of clinical reasoning to practice requires the occupational therapy practitioner to understand the type and application of each type (narrative, scientific/procedural, pragmatic, ethical, and conditional) of reasoning. It also requires occupational therapy practitioners use research to evaluate the effectiveness of reasoning and intervention methods. Finally, the occupational therapy practitioner must use reflection and self-direction to synthesize knowledge to assist all consumers of occupational therapy services to fully participate in life through full engagement in meaningful occupations throughout the lifespan (AOTA, 2014).

## Student Self-Assessment

1. How does the use of clinical reasoning strategies lead to an effective intervention process?
2. Compare and contrast the clinical reasoning strategies used by novice occupational therapy practitioners with those used by advanced practitioners.
3. How does the process of reflection fit into the development of advanced clinical reasoning skills?
4. Identify a scenario describing narrative, scientific/procedural, pragmatic, ethical, and conditional reasoning for each of the following practice settings:
   - Children and youth
   - Rehabilitation, disability, and participation
   - Health and wellness
   - Productive aging
   - Work and industry

## Electronic Resources

American Occupational Therapy Association Evidence-Based Practice and Research: http://www.aota.org/practice/researchers.aspx

American Occupational Therapy Association Professional Development Tool: http://www1.aota.org/pdt/p1.htm#

Critically appraised topics related to occupational therapy: www.otcats.com

Evidence-Based Practice Research Group: http://srs-mcmaster.ca/

National Board for Certification in Occupational Therapy (NBCOT), Competency Resources: www.nbcot.org

Occupational Therapy Seeker—evidence-based practice briefs related to occupational therapy: www.otseeker.com

PubMed search engine from the National Library of Medicine and the National Institutes of Health: www.ncbi.nlm.nih.gov/entrez/query.fcgi

# References


American Occupational Therapy Association. (2003, May). *Professional development tool*. Bethesda, MD: Author. Retrieved from http://www.aota.org/pdt

American Occupational Therapy Association. (2009). *Guidelines for supervision, roles, and responsibilities during the delivery of occupational therapy services*. Retrieved from http:// www.aota.org/ Practitioners/ Official/ Guidelines/ 36202.aspx?FT=.pdf

American Occupational Therapy Association. (2014). Occupational therapy practice framework: Domain and process (3rd ed.). *American Journal of Occupational Therapy, 68*(Suppl. 1), S1-S48. doi:10.5014/ajot.2014.682006

American Occupational Therapy Association. (2015). *Occupational therapy code of ethics (2015)*. Retrieved from https://www.aota.org/-/media/corporate/files/practice/ethics/code-of-ethics.pdf

Atkins, S., & Murphy, K. (1993). Reflection: A review of the literature. *Journal of Advanced Nursing, 18*, 1188-1192.

Bannigan, K., & Moores, A. (2009). A model of professional thinking: Integrating reflective practice and evidence based practice. *Canadian Journal of Occupational Therapy, 76*(5), 342-350.

Carrier, A., Levasseur, M., Bedard, D., & Desrosiers, J. (2010). Community occupational therapists' clinical reasoning: Identifying tacit knowledge. *Australian Occupational Therapy Journal, 57*, 356-365. doi:10.1111/j.1440-1630.2010.00875.x

Cohn, E. S., Coster, W. J., & Kramer, J. M. (2014). Conference proceedings—Facilitated learning model to teach habits of evidence-based reasoning across an integrated master of science in occupational therapy curriculum. *American Journal of Occupational Therapy, 68*, S73-S82. doi:10.5014/ajot.2014.685S05

Coker, P. (2010). Effects of an experiential learning program on the clinical reasoning and critical thinking skills of occupational therapy students. *Journal of Allied Health, 39*(4), 280-286.

Dunn, L., & Musolino, G. M. (2011). Assessing reflective thinking and approaches to learning. *Journal of Allied Health, 40*(3), 128-136.

Fleming, M. H. (1991). The therapist with the three-track mind. *American Journal of Occupational Therapy, 45*(11), 1007-1014.

Gibbons, M., Bailey, A., Comeau, P., Schmuck, J., Seymour, S., & Wallace, D. (1980). Toward a theory of self-directed learning: A study of experts without formal training. *Journal of Humanistic Psychology, 20*(2), 41-56.

Haas, K. B. (2014). Clinical reasoning. In K. Jacobs, N. MacRae, & K. Sladyk (Eds.), *Occupational therapy essentials for clinical competence* (2nd ed.). Thorofare, NJ: SLACK Incorporated.

Hawkins, D., Elder, L., & Paul, R. (2010). *The thinker's guide to clinical reasoning*. Dillon Beach, CA: Foundation for Critical Thinking.

Knecht-Sabres, L. J. (2010). The use of experiential learning in an occupational therapy program: Can it foster skills for clinical practice? *Occupational Therapy in Health Care, 24*(4), 320-334. doi:10.3109/07380577.2010.514382

Kuipers, K., & Grice, J. W. (2009). The structure of novice and expert occupational therapists' clinical reasoning before and after exposure to a domain-specific protocol. *Australian Occupational Therapy Journal, 56*, 418-427. doi:10.1111/j.1440-1630.2009.00793.x

Mattingly, C., & Fleming, M. H. (1994). *Clinical reasoning: Forms of inquiry in a therapeutic practice*. Philadelphia, PA: F. A. Davis Company.

Moscony, A. M. B., & Shank, T. (2014). Wrist fractures. In C. Cooper (Ed.), *Fundamentals of hand therapy: Clinical reasoning and treatment guidelines for common diagnoses of the upper extremity* (2nd ed., pp. 312-335). St. Louis, MO: Mosby Elsevier.

Moyers, P. A., & Dale, L. M. (2007). *The guide to occupational therapy practice* (2nd ed.). Bethesda, MD: AOTA Press.

Mu, K., Coppard, B. M., Bracciano, A., Doll, J., & Matthews, A. (2010). Fostering cultural competency, clinical reasoning, and leadership through international outreach. *Occupational Therapy in Health Care, 24*(1), 74-85. doi:10.3109/07380570903329628

Neistadt, M. E. (1998). Teaching clinical reasoning as a thinking frame. *American Journal of Occupational Therapy, 52*(3), 221-229.

Nilsson, I., & Townsend, E. (2014). Occupational justice: Bridging theory and practice. *Scandinavian Journal of Occupational Therapy, 21*, 64-70. doi:10.3109/11038128.2014.952906

Plack, M. M., & Santasier, A. (2004). Reflective practice: A model for facilitating critical thinking skills within an integrative case study classroom experience. *Journal of Physical Therapy Education, 18*, 4-12.

Scaffa, M. E., & Wooster, D. M. (2004). Effects of problem-based learning on clinical reasoning in occupational therapy. *American Journal of Occupational Therapy, 58*(3), 333-336.

Schell, B. A. B. (2009). Professional reasoning in practice. In E. B. Crepeau, E. S. Cohn, & B. A. B. Schell (Eds.), *Willard & Spackman's occupational therapy* (11th ed., pp. 314-327). Philadelphia, PA: Lippincott Williams & Wilkins.

Schell, B. A., & Schell, J. W. (2008). *Clinical and professional reasoning in occupational therapy*. Philadelphia, PA: Lippincott Williams and Wilkins.

Taylor, R. R. (2008). *The intentional relationship: Occupational therapy and use of self*. Philadelphia, PA: F. A. Davis Company.

Yancosek, K. E., & Howell, D. (2010). Integrating the dynamical systems theory, the task-oriented approach, and the practice framework for clinical reasoning. *Occupational Therapy in Health Care, 24*(3), 223-238. doi:10.3109/07380577.2010.496824

# III

# Occupational Therapy Theoretical Perspectives

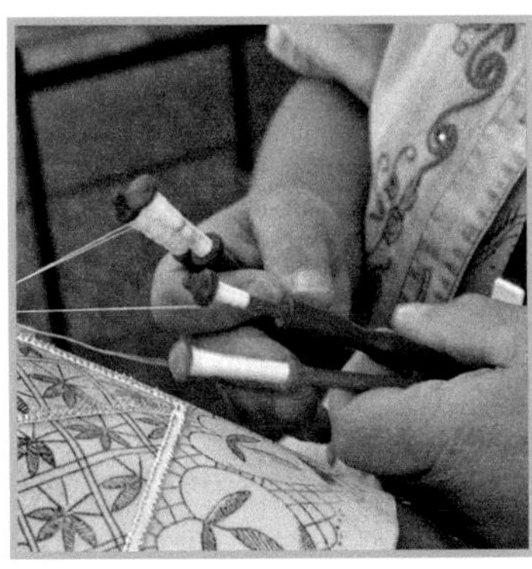

# 15

# Occupational Therapy Theory Development and Organization

Marilyn B. Cole, MS, OTR/L, FAOTA

## ACOTE STANDARDS EXPLORED IN THIS CHAPTER

B.3.1, B.3.2, B.3.4, B.3.6 for master's and doctoral programs
B.3.1, B.3.3 for certified assistant programs

## KEY VOCABULARY

- **Applied theory:** The results of applied research, intended to address problems of practical interest.
- **Basic theory:** Results from basic research addressing general phenomenon.
- **Epistemology:** The dynamics of knowing (Hooper, 2006); how we know what we know.
- **Grounded theory:** The systematic discovery of theory from the data of social research (Glaser & Strauss, 1967; Strauss & Corbin, 1994).
- **Model:** A simplified representation of structure and content that describes or explains complex relationships between concepts (Creek, 2010).
- **Paradigm:** A shared vision encompassing fundamental assumptions and beliefs, which serves as the cultural core of the profession (Kielhofner, 2006).



Jacobs, K., & MacRae, N. (Eds.).
*Occupational Therapy Essentials for Clinical Competence, Third Edition* (pp. 199-216).

Most occupational therapy practitioners and students regard theory as the concern of academia and science, not practice. Although we know that all assessments and interventions have their base in theory, practice focuses on the application of these tools with clients. Theory is elusive, influencing our behaviors, but often without our awareness. Most of us would be surprised at how often we use theory in our daily lives. For decisions as simple as what we eat for breakfast, most of us consider theories about healthy lifestyles. We may feel like eating eggs, bacon, and buttered biscuits, but we may decide on whole grain cereal or yogurt with granola and fresh fruit instead, assuming this to be better for our health long term. Or, we may eat what we want anyway, reasoning that we only live once, so we may as well enjoy it.

Our theories also affect how we react to unexpected situations in life. For example, when Hurricane Sandy headed for the northeastern shores of the United States, news reports used sophisticated weather instruments to predict the trajectory of the storm, estimate its time of arrival, and suggest its likely effect on the people living along the shore. Citizens reacted differently according to their theoretical assumptions. Some assumed that news reports usually exaggerate the situation, and did nothing to prepare. Others dashed out to stores to stock up on supplies. They reasoned that hurricanes generate high winds that knock down power lines and thought about how they might survive without power. They bought foods that do not require cooking or refrigeration, candles, fuel for generators, and batteries to power flashlights, radios, and communication devices. Some even filled bottles and tubs with water for drinking or washing in case the water supply became contaminated. But many people failed to predict the effects of Sandy on the tides, or the volumes of water that high winds could blow into narrow water areas, such as the Hudson River or Long Island Sound. Because people in the northeast do not encounter hurricanes very often, they could not rely on experience. They needed to carry the theory further to imagine the effects of the 12- to 15-foot storm surge that ultimately did most of the damage.

Whenever we make a decision or form an opinion on something, we are using theory in the reasoning process to justify or validate our thoughts and actions. Only through reflection can we become aware of the assumptions we are making—the theories behind our behavior. It is the same with the practice of occupational therapy. In the beginning of the 20th century, occupational therapy practitioners learned techniques and applied them without giving much thought to the theories or assumptions upon which they were based. However, current trends compel us to raise our awareness of frames of reference, to reflect on the outcomes of our tools and techniques, and to read research studies that provide evidence that the theories behind our actions in practice are valid. These are the requirements of evidence-based occupational therapy practice in the 21st century.

In this chapter, we will define theory as it relates to occupational therapy, trace the evolution of theory from occupational therapy's founding in 1917 to the present, and discuss the paradigm shifts in health care within the context of historical events and trends. Finally, we will propose an organizational model for understanding and applying the various levels of theory in occupational therapy practice.

## What Is Theory?

Kerlinger defined theory as "a set of interrelated constructs (variables), definitions, and propositions that presents a systematic view of phenomena by specifying relations among variables, with the purpose of explaining natural phenomena" (1979, p. 64). In occupational therapy, this "scientific" view of theory assumes that knowledge is derived from systematic, controlled, and empirical study of some aspect of human occupational behavior (Table 15-1).

Some well-known theories, such as Newton's gravitational theory and Einstein's theory of relativity, are examples of scientific theories validated through basic research; Skinner's theory of operant conditioning and Bandura's social learning theory (2001) are examples of applied research. This distinction parallels the difference between occupational science and occupational therapy. Occupational science is an academic discipline that is aligned with basic research. Occupational scientists study the form, function, and meaning of occupation without regard to the practical use of the theories generated. Occupational therapy practitioners are mainly concerned with the application of theories in practice. While we may borrow from the theories of occupational science, occupational therapy practitioners look for ways to relate them to our understanding of occupational performance, improvement, enhancement, prevention, health, and wellness (American Occupational Therapy Association [AOTA], 2014), as well as restoration and adaptation, for the clients and populations we serve (see Evidence-Based Research Chart).

Within the existing literature, occupational therapy practitioners can find evidence supporting each of the occupational therapy approaches suggested in the AOTA's *Occupational Therapy Practice Framework: Domain and Process, Third Edition* (2014), with specific populations using a wide range of theories. Occupational therapy practitioners need to develop and test theories that give us evidence about the best ways to enable occupational performance for our clients.

Table 15-1.

## Purposes Served by Theory and Examples

| Purpose | Question Addressed (Theory) | Examples |
|---|---|---|
| Define a concept | What is figure-ground perception? (sensory integration theory) | Ability to recognize shapes of objects in a cluttered line drawing; ability to find two matching black socks in a cluttered drawer |
| Describe | What is good time management? (cognitive behavioral theory) | Ability to plan and execute daily activities to meet one's needs and obligations in an efficient and satisfying manner |
| Correlate | How does exercise relate to successful aging? (biomechanical theory) | Studies show that 30 minutes of moderate exercise each day maintains both mental and physical fitness for older adults |
| Explain why | What causes stress at work? (person-environment-occupation performance model) | Stress is produced when a worker's occupational performance does not match the demands or cultural/social expectations of the workplace |
| Predict | What activities prevent cognitive decline in aging? (cognitive behavioral theory and cognitive theories of aging) | Practicing mentally challenging tasks (e.g., crossword puzzles) and participating socially with others (e.g., playing cards or chess) helps to maintain an aging brain |
| Evaluate | How does volunteering with the homeless help adolescents develop empathy and compassion? (attachment theory and social participation) | Informal personal interactions with persons different from one's self increases the likelihood of finding common ground and developing cultural awareness and sensitivity |

Terminology and definitions adapted from Portney, L. G., & Watkins, M. P. (2009). *Foundations of clinical research: Applications to practice* (3rd ed.). Upper Saddle River, NJ: Prentice-Hall Health.

# How Are Theories Developed?

A theory begins with asking a question. Applied theories represent attempts to solve practical problems. Why do children misbehave in school? What causes people to get stressed out with their jobs? How do some older adults manage to stay healthy and fit well into old age while others do not? The researcher next forms a hypothesis, a possible explanation for something observed. For example, A. Jean Ayres hypothesized that some school children misbehave because they cannot integrate sensory input, resulting in their inability to sit still and pay attention to the teacher. She tested this hypothesis by creating a method to measure the way children process different types of sensory input, mainly vestibular, proprioceptive, and tactile, but also incorporating auditory and visual systems. By evaluating many children, Ayres identified several patterns of sensory dysfunction. When she applied carefully graded sensory input through play activities, she found that some children integrated sensations more effectively, resulting in dramatic improvement of both their classroom behavior and academic learning (Ayres, 1979). Her research resulted in the theory of sensory integration, a frame of reference used widely by occupational therapy practitioners working in school systems today.

## Experimental Research

Experimental research, such as the study just described, uses the scientific method to collect data according to specific criteria, ideally including a random selection of subjects, control of extraneous influences, and some form of manipulation such as an occupational therapy intervention. When a theory has been developed to a certain point, a good way to test the theory is to do an experiment. Two groups of subjects are randomly selected: one group is treated in a designated way (experimental group), while the other group is not (control group). To control for bias or unanticipated influences on the outcome, both groups should be the same in every aspect, except for the intervention being tested. Both groups are evaluated before and after the intervention interval to determine whether the experimental group has changed in a way that is different from the control group. Ayres studied a randomly selected sample of school-age children representative of the normal population, and developed age-equivalent norms for each sensory subtest in her sensory integration battery. This is called a *norm-referenced assessment*, which generated a theory of normal sensory integrative development (Ayres, 1979). Many occupational therapy researchers have tested different parts of Ayres's theory by using specific interventions such as scooter board play and spinning on a tire swing with groups of children who have sensory deficits (Bundy, Lane, & Murray, 2002; Royeen & Luebben, 2009).

When the research subjects are not randomly selected, but are chosen because of their disability status, this type of research is called *quasi-experimental*. Most clinical research falls into this category. The results give occupational therapy practitioners useful evidence about how well certain interventions work with populations with various disabilities.

## Qualitative Research

Qualitative research is the preferred method when a theory is not well developed. Qualitative research begins with a different question, one that is more descriptive rather than cause and effect. For example, a group of occupational therapy practitioners wondered how they could become better time managers. They designed a qualitative study, which involved in-depth interviews with six people they had identified as good time managers—women who successfully juggled marriage, child care, gainful employment, community involvement, and home maintenance. This is called a *purposive sample*. Their interviews included many questions about how the women planned their time, what tools they used, what motivated them, and what made them successful time managers. The results described the nature of good time management and identified some themes that helped us to better understand the concepts involved. Occupational therapy intervention suggestions include the practice of routines, the development of social networks that combine or exchange obligations, and the building of short-term memory and self-management strategies. If taken further, this research could form the basis for a theory of "time mastery" (Cole, 1998).

## Grounded Theory

Grounded theory is a research method that especially reflects the professional trends in occupational therapy today. Like in chaos theory and nonlinear science, developing theory "from the ground up" (Kielhofner, 2006, p. 333) is a self-organizing process. Grounded theory evolves through a form of qualitative research whose purpose is to develop and verify theory, and is one of several types of naturalistic research (DePoy & Gitlin, 2005). This primarily qualitative approach has three phases: (1) It begins with the development of a generative question, (2) followed by identifying a sample of informants for data collection; (3) then the researchers begin a back and forth process of collecting data and analyzing it through a system of identifying categories, themes, and coding, a strategy known as *constant comparative analysis* (Strauss & Corbin, 1994).

This author recently had the opportunity to engage in this exciting process with a colleague, Dr. Karen Macdonald, in a project we called the Productive Aging Study (Cole & Macdonald, 2015). Our research question—"How do retired older adults age productively?"—comes from our observation that some older Americans have discovered the secrets of aging successfully and enjoy continued participation in life, while others have not. Participants were included if in their retirement they remained engaged in at least three productive occupations (self-manager, home manager, caregiver, volunteer, paid worker, and lifelong learner). We interviewed 40 qualified participants, meeting weekly to share and analyze our data. These three themes prevailed in what participants used to age productively:

1. **Self-management:** They managed their own aging process by creating healthy lifestyles, often seeking knowledge and advice from health professionals to manage health conditions and the adverse effects of aging by adapting occupations and environments.
2. **Social connections:** They intentionally made and maintained social relationships, using social support and community resources as necessary to remain engaged in meaningful roles and occupations.
3. **Self-fulfilling activities:** They selected and focused their energy on those occupations that rendered the most meaning, value, and emotional satisfaction—understanding the reality of their own limitations and making the most of their strengths.

To continue the theory development, we then identified some hypothesis-generating statements with the intent of linking the theory to occupational therapy practice. They included occupational therapy roles in client education, consultation, community programs, advocacy, and policy development. Subsequently, an additional level of synthesis occurred that summarized all of the final themes and hypotheses within the original emergent grounded theory of conditional independence. Mosey (1981) stated that postulates of change are the essential parts of any theory that make it useful in practice (p. 37). In this instance, the change we are looking for is what needs to happen so that older adults can age productively, and we determined three postulates:

1. **Situational adaptation:** Looks at all aspects of the environment within which a desired occupation is to be performed, adapting them to overcome barriers or areas of difficulty, and putting appropriate facilitators in place.
2. **Structured performance:** Looks at demands of the tasks to be accomplished within a desired occupation, and adapts these features as necessary to match abilities and accommodate limitations of the performer.
3. **Intentional abilities:** Motivated actions to sustain occupational performance over time, applying knowledge, strengths, skills, and talents, as well as learned strategies that facilitate participation in meaningful social and occupational roles (Macdonald, 2015).

Table 15-2.

**Experimental Versus Qualitative Research in Occupational Therapy**

| Experimental Research | Qualitative Research |
|---|---|
| Includes manipulation, randomization, control | Includes single cases, in-depth interviews, detailed descriptions |
| Theory testing | Theory development |
| Objective reality, correlation, cause and effect, use of quantitative statistics | Subjective reality, personal narratives and perceptions, multiple truths |
| Many subjects | Fewer participants |
| Standardized tests for dependent variables, surveys, controlled observations | Self-reports, attitudes and beliefs, the lived body, the illness experience |

These strategies seem very much like occupational therapy interventions, because they are the conditions under which older adults can remain independent. Conversely, an older adult's continued participation was conditional upon the adaptations he or she made to environments, contexts, and lifestyles and his or her use of available resources, especially sources of social support. In summary, grounded theory can be developed directly from the data collected from clients within occupational therapy practice, using appropriately rigorous research procedures.

In occupational science, qualitative research has been cited as the preferred method for studying the form, function, and meaning of human occupation. When building theories of occupation's role in maintaining and restoring health and functional abilities, qualitative methods have been most useful in determining the outcomes related to client satisfaction and well-being. In general, qualitative methods relate best to theory development, while experimental research works best for theory testing. This description of research has been simplified for clarification purposes. In fact, there are many categories and variations of research not included in this chapter. Table 15-2 compares experimental and qualitative research methods in relation to theory in occupational therapy.

## Evolution of Theory in Science and Occupational Therapy

Occupational therapy theory did not develop in isolation. Historical trends and events have shaped the development of professional theory and practice from the beginning. Some of the trends of the early 1900s included industrialization, economic growth and prosperity, reconstruction after World War I, and a recognition of the need to preserve skilled craftsmanship. Humanism and pragmatism were the predominant philosophical trends influencing the profession's founding and early years. Breines (1987) recognized the predominance of pragmatism at the time of occupational therapy's founding, citing philosophers William James, George Herbert Meade, and John Dewey at the University of Chicago, colleagues of Adolf Meyer and William Dunton (1919), who later applied pragmatic principles to occupational therapy. Pragmatism, based in part on Darwin's theory of evolution, stresses the growth of knowledge and science through adaptation. The Hull House, in association with the University of Chicago, demonstrated pragmatic principles through the practice of arts and crafts and other activities, which served the needs of both individuals and the community. Occupational therapy founder Eleanor Clarke Slagle trained and later taught arts and crafts at the Hull House. Cofounders Susan Tracy and Susan Johnson, both from a nursing background, devoted most of their lives to practicing and teaching the application of occupations such as arts and crafts, work, and self-care tasks to the healing, rehabilitation, and adaptation of persons with disabilities. Although the assumptions of pragmatism were not clearly defined by occupational therapy founders, they were apparent in the focus on learning by doing, mind/body unity, and building health through engagement in occupation. Tracy is the only occupational therapy founder to publish the applied principles of pragmatism in occupational therapy (1918). Most occupational therapy professionals today take a pragmatic approach. Knowledge, ideas, and methods are valued according to their practical usefulness. When we read research studies, we look for ways we can use or apply the results in our own lives and in those of our clients. In doing so, we are using the theory of pragmatism. Perhaps the reason the concept of occupation as therapy has withstood the test

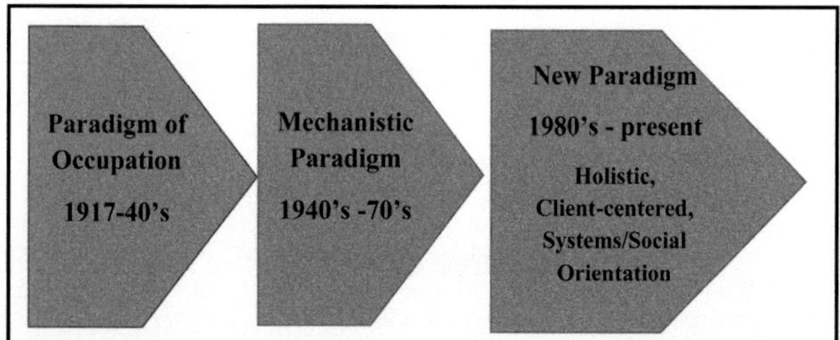


**Figure 15-1.** Paradigm shifts identified by Kielhofner and Burke. (Adapted from Kielhofner, G. [2004]. *Conceptual foundations of occupational therapy* [3rd ed.]. Philadelphia, PA: F. A. Davis Company.)

of time is because of its pragmatic nature. Occupation continues to unify time and space, mind, and body, as well as facilitate the growth and development of individuals and societies.

Kielhofner and Burke (1977) traced the history of epistemological changes that took place in occupational therapy and identified two distinct shifts in occupational therapy's professional paradigm (Figure 15-1). Epistemology is the nature of knowledge and the way it is developed and used. Occupational therapy knowledge through the 1930s was based on humanism and pragmatism. Humanism fueled the profession through its dedication to the betterment of the human condition and the right of each person to respect, dignity, and a meaningful and productive role in society. Professionals learned and collected knowledge about the use of occupations in therapy through extensive apprenticeship and practice of its practical (pragmatic) application with a variety of disabilities: mental illness, long-term infectious diseases such as polio and tuberculosis, and injuries due to industrial accidents or war. Kielhofner and Burke identified this period as the "paradigm of occupation" (1977, p. 679). Paradigms reflect the theoretical base, views of phenomena, range and nature of problems addressed, problem-solving methods, and goals of a scientific discipline (Kuhn, 1970). According to Kuhn, paradigm shifts occur by revolution, not evolution. When new problems that cannot be solved with the old paradigm emerge, a crisis occurs within the discipline, which calls for fundamental and sweeping changes in both theoretical perspectives and methodology.

Paralleling Kuhn's model of theoretical development in basic science, Kielhofner and Burke (1977) identified a crisis period in occupational therapy toward the end of the 1930s when the profession was challenged to become more scientific. Advances in technology and the predominance of the scientific method in basic science, social sciences, and medicine challenged the philosophical validations of morality and social responsibility for the medical and allied medical professions, occupational therapy among them. The scientific method, viewed as the only way to discover basic truths and to substantiate theory, calls for the reduction of the focus of study into its component parts for the purpose of more precise examination and understanding. Reductionism directly opposes the holistic and systems perspective of the original paradigm of occupation. In the mid-20th century, occupational therapy resolved this crisis by becoming more closely aligned with the medical profession. Courses in anatomy and physiology, neurology, psychiatry, and medical conditions were added to the requirements for occupational therapy education. Concurrently, a reductionistic view of illness and disability led to a focus on component parts, the diagnosis of specific problems, and the prescription of specific intervention strategies or methods. This approach views man and the world as machines; when they stop working, the method for restoring them is to locate the part that is broken (diagnosis) and fix or replace it (prescription, intervention). Later, Kielhofner renamed this reductionistic approach the "mechanistic paradigm" (2004, p. 56). According to Kielhofner and Burke (1977), the reductionistic paradigm generated three major theoretical models in occupational therapy: kinesiology (biomechanical, rehabilitative), psychoanalytic (psychodynamic), and sensory integrative (neuroscience, motor control).

Occupational therapy enjoyed a period of stability and growth in the 1950s and 1960s. The discipline benefited from its alliance with medicine, with gains in respectability and status within the medical community; membership on health care teams; and inclusion in legislation, reimbursement, and social policy. For example, the passing of Public Law 94-142 (Education for All Handicapped Children Act) in 1975, requiring children with disabilities to be educated in the least restrictive environment, opened up a whole new area of practice for occupational therapy practitioners treating children in public schools. Many useful assessment and intervention techniques were developed in occupational therapy throughout these decades in collaboration with other scientists and medical professionals (e.g., Bobath's [1990] Neurodevelopmental Treatment [NDT]). However, by the late 1970s, signs of the inadequacy of the mechanistic paradigm became apparent.

In occupational therapy, reductionism had resulted in many extremes of specialization, leading some occupational therapy scholars to view this era as the profession's "identity crisis." The effects of the crisis identified by Kielhofner and Burke in 1977 continue to haunt us in the new millennium, especially in the areas of documentation and reimbursement. The medical profession, which once gave needed recognition to the occupational therapy profession, is itself suffering from cost cutting measures, both public (Medicare Reform and the Omnibus Budget Reconciliation Act [OBRA] of 1987) and private (managed care, malpractice, and health insurance costs; Evanofski, 2003). Although many state licensure laws still require a doctor's prescription for occupational therapy intervention, doctors and other referral sources must choose between several competing service providers (nursing, physical therapy, speech/language therapy, home health aides) for a piece of the ever-shrinking reimbursement pie. Within the profession, the AOTA initiated some remedial measures to resolve the identity crisis, beginning in 1979 with the publication of *Uniform Terminology* (AOTA, 1979), giving the profession a common language and defining the scope of practice. The AOTA further unified the profession by providing standards for the different areas of practice and by establishing the American Occupational Therapy Foundation, which is dedicated to the support of research initiatives. Theory took the form of "frames of reference" in the 1970s (Mosey, 1970), "clinical reasoning" (Mattingly & Fleming, 1994; Rogers, 1983) in the 1980s, and "occupational performance models" in the 1990s (Baum & Christiansen, 2005; Christiansen & Baum, 1997; Dunn, Brown, & McGuigan, 1994; Schkade & Schultz, 1992a, 1992b).

## Professional Trends in the New Millennium

The major trends of the profession may be summarized as holistic, client centered, and systems/socially oriented (Cole & Tufano, 2008). In becoming more holistic, occupational therapy must move away from a reductionistic medical model and instead partner with community organizations in the service of public health. Occupational therapy's method of reimbursement will remain under the umbrella of medicine unless we can demonstrate the value of our services in the broader spectrum of wellness and prevention. The client-centered focus gives occupational therapy a structure for making the transition from clinic to community, with an increased focus on collaborating with clients and establishing stronger therapeutic relationships. From the client-centered perspective, occupational therapy practitioners apply theoretical knowledge and evidence in partnership with clients to assist them in making informed choices, solving occupational problems, and enabling occupational performance. During this decade, client-centered occupational therapy practice has a new focus: enabling occupation (Townsend & Polatajko, 2007). These Canadian authors offer the following updated definition of occupational therapy:

> Occupational therapy is the art and science of enabling engagement in everyday living through occupation; of enabling people to perform the occupations that foster health and well-being; and of enabling a just and inclusive society so that all people may participate to their potential in the daily occupations of life. (p. xxi)

The trend toward a systems/social orientation is evident at many levels. Dynamical systems theories have affected the basic and social sciences; they are evident in the latest revisions of many occupational therapy frames of reference, providing evidence of the importance of environmental and social influences in facilitating or creating barriers to occupational performance. Occupational therapy practitioners need to help clients navigate the vast bureaucracy of the health care system, make use of community resources, and remove barriers to their inclusion in their life occupations. An increased emphasis on social skills in occupational therapy is especially evident in working with children and adolescents. Social reasoning may be defined as "thinking about occupations from a social perspective, including social contexts, expectations, sources of support, and considering the social groups and/or significant relationships within which occupational choices are made and performed" (Cole, 2016, p. 243). On a practice level, the client's social participation—the performance of roles and occupations in social groups such as families, classrooms, work teams, and the community—must become a part of occupational therapy services if we are to enable our clients to find and perform meaningful roles in society (Cole, 2016; Cole & Donohue, 2011). These trends have helped to define the current professional paradigm. The shift away from reductionism has occurred across many disciplines and professions. Evidence of this may be seen in the changes in the systems of health care, both nationally and globally.

## Politics and Health Care

### *Medical Versus Client-Centered Models*

The client-centered model, defined for occupational therapists by the Canadian Occupational Therapy Association in conjunction with Canadian national health care, gained prominence in the United States during the 1990s. For health care professionals, the term *client-centered* refers to the nature of the therapeutic relationship and implies roles for both the professional and the client that are clearly different from those of the medical model (Table 15-3). As occupational therapy moves away from the medical model, the client-centered model serves the purpose of structuring and clarifying our interactions with clients and gives greater importance to our therapeutic use of self. When clients seek occupational therapy services directly or through community agencies rather than being referred by a doctor, their satisfaction with the outcome surpasses the need for precise measurement of functional performance. Ideally, the client's progress in the performance of preferred occupations will lead to greater client satisfaction and will validate the value of occupational therapy in many new areas of practice.

Table 15-3.

**MEDICAL AND CLIENT-CENTERED MODEL COMPARISON**

| Medical Model | Client-Centered Model |
|---|---|
| Patient: Passive recipient of treatment; implies a sick role and a lack of participation or responsibility, requires compliance with doctor's orders | Client: Actively seeks assistance from medical and other professionals or experts; shifts responsibility for solving health problems onto the client |
| Health: Absence of disease; mental and physical fitness and a sense of well-being<br>Disease: Illness or injury affecting ability to perform activities of daily living | Health condition: Any circumstance that interferes with full participation in life |
| Diagnosis: Identification of disease through analysis of signs, symptoms, and syndromes, which allows the doctor to predict the course of illness and to prescribe remedies | Disability: Experienced by the person, sometimes determined by the person's experience of illness; that which prevents the person from participating in life |
| Prescription: Medications or specific techniques or instructions intended to cure disease and/or manage symptoms | Enablement: Sharing expertise, which empowers the client to set reasonable goals and make informed choices regarding interventions to remove barriers to participation in life |
| Objective methods of study, based on experimental research, data gathering, and norms | Subjective methods of study based on qualitative research, looking at each individual's culture, perceptions, and situation |
| Progress is measured by objective measures applied by the medical professional | Outcome includes both objective measures and client satisfaction with results |
| Treatment: Specific medical or surgical procedures prescribed by a doctor or specialist to heal or cure a disease | Intervention: Procedures and strategies created by collaboration between client and professional to overcome barriers to occupational performance |
| Occupational therapy applies expertise to focus on using activities to relieve symptoms, to adapt task demands, or to compensate for disability; rehabilitation ends when the patient has met functional goals established by the occupational therapy practitioner and/or medical treatment team | Occupational therapy practitioner collaborates with client to identify occupational problems and priorities, to set goals, and to enable client participation through supporting skill development, as well as taking preventive actions and/or through adaptation of tasks and environments |

## A Global Perspective of Health

The World Health Organization (WHO) made significant revisions to its classification system that reflect the shift to a holistic and systems perspective of global health care. The *International Classification of Functioning, Disability and Health* (ICF) encompasses all aspects of human health and some health-relevant components of well-being. Its purpose is to be a companion classification system for the 10th Edition of the *International Classification of Disease (ICD-10)*, which classifies all known diseases, both mental and physical. Given the global nature of health care today, the fact that this international guideline confirms the central role of occupation (activity) in health has important implications for occupational therapy. ICF places "activity" at the center of its model and defines the goal of health care efforts as "participation in life" (WHO, 2001).

## Holistic Perspective

The initial publication was entitled *International Classification of Impairments, Disabilities and Handicaps* (WHO, 1980). Each of these terms has been replaced to reflect the shift to a holistic perspective:

- *Handicap* is changed to *participation restriction.*
- *Disability* is changed to *activity limitation.*
- *Impairment* is changed to *health condition*, an umbrella term for not only disease, disorder, injury, and trauma, but also for conditions such as pregnancy, aging, stress, congenital anomaly, and genetic predisposition.

In its 2001 revision, the WHO broadens the horizons of health-related research, service provision, and policy-making beyond the constraints of the medical model. It states, "There is a widely held misunderstanding that ICF is only about people with disability; in fact, it is about all people" (WHO, 2001, p. 7).

## *Systems Orientation*

ICF conceives a person's functioning and/or disability as a "dynamic interaction" between a health condition and contextual factors. Contextual factors are those external factors, "features of the physical, social, and attitudinal world," that facilitate or hinder participation (WHO, 2001, p. 8). Accordingly, ICF is divided into two parts. The first lists the components of human functioning and disability, including body systems and structures, as well as activities and participation, denoting both an individual and a societal perspective. The systems of the human body and the activities represented closely resemble occupational therapy's domain of concern according to the *Framework* (AOTA, 2014).

The second half of ICF lists and classifies contexts in the following categories:

- Products and technology
- Natural and human-made environments
- Support and relationships
- Attitudes
- Services, systems, and policies

The inclusion of so many external or environmental factors reflects the system's view of occupational performance as a product of the interaction between the person, the task, and the environment. The basic language of ICF is compatible with occupational therapy in this regard, stating, "improvement of participation [can be encouraged] by removing or mitigating societal hindrances and encouraging the provision of social supports and facilitators" (WHO, 2001, p. 6). The model of functioning and disability also describes the interaction of ICF components: health conditions, body structures and functions, personal factors, contexts, activities, and participation in life. One can easily see the parallels with the *Framework*, which uses similar terminology and an equally broad perspective of health (AOTA, 2014).

# Interpreting Theoretical Transformations in Occupational Therapy

While the focus on the broader concepts of occupation seems simple and logical in retrospect, its implications for theory development are quite complex. The collective occupational therapy professional community—practitioners, researchers, scholars, and educators who participated in the process of resolving the 1970s crisis—may recognize the fundamental nature of the recent theoretical shifts only through reflection. At first, we thought all that was needed was to articulate our frames of reference. In doing so, we moved from Mosey's three frames of reference to hundreds (Reed & Sanderson, 1999) with no more professional unity than we had before. We failed to recognize the true nature of the Model of Human Occupation (Kielhofner & Burke, 1980) as an occupation-based model, trying instead to define it as one more frame of reference. This worked as well as fitting the proverbial square peg into a round hole.

Then in the 1980s, Joan Rogers (1983) got us thinking about the clinical reasoning process; this approach to unity proved to be a better fit. If occupational therapy practitioners did not all share a common frame of reference, at least they could share a common reasoning process. Mattingly and Fleming (1994) further defined the process of reasoning in occupational therapy, citing three tracks: procedural, interactive, and conditional. Herein lies the beginning of the real transformation—not in the theories of occupational therapy themselves, but in the way we develop these theories. Procedural reasoning applies objective scientific knowledge; interactive reasoning combines objective scientific knowledge with the subjective reality of the individual client's experience (the lived experience); and conditional reasoning considers all of the contexts or systems within which persons exist, live, and perform occupations. Our professional understanding of the process of occupational therapy changed fundamentally as a result of these revelations. We had moved from an exclusively scientific view (procedures such as assessment and intervention) to one that also considered the personal perspective of the client (interactive or client centered) and the contexts (conditional, systems) of occupational performance.

The 1990s focused on two major theoretical trends in occupational therapy: the development of occupation-based models and the movement toward client-centered practice. Occupation-based models moved occupational therapy away from the study of components of occupational performance, which viewed physical, sensory, psychosocial, emotional, and cognitive processes separately. Instead, they refocused our attention on occupation itself. Hooper (2006) explained it as an epistemological transformation, or a shift in the way we define knowledge and in the methods by which we acquire it. The mid-century reductionistic approach led occupational therapy practitioners to develop and research many specific techniques, such as sensory integration for the intervention of children with learning disabilities, biomechanical strategies for the intervention of hand injuries, and cognitive rehabilitation for the intervention of traumatic brain injuries. These applied theories, while useful and valid, represented fragments of occupation developed in isolation of each other. Broader theories of occupation, such as the Model of Human Occupation (Kielhofner & Burke, 1980) and subsequent occupation-based models, served the purpose of defining the interconnections between the fragments or components of occupation. Furthermore, the application of dynamical systems theories influenced the newer occupation-based models in synthesizing much of the specific knowledge developed earlier within the multiple dimensions of occupation (Hooper, 2006).

The move toward client-centered practice represents a similar change in focus—one that questions the nature of reality itself. Creek put it simply as "...the truth is no longer out there" (1997, p. 50), suggesting that truth is not objective, but subjective, and therefore dependent on personal perspectives and specific contexts. The scientific view of truth relies on accurate and objective observations inherent in the scientific method and without regard for human activity. Mosey identifies this view as "rational empiricism," which can serve as a way of thinking about practice, as well as a context for action (1992, p. 42). According to this view of truth, prominent in mid-20th century reductionism, theories are best tested through experimental research, such as the randomized controlled trials typical of medical research. As late as 1999, Holm (2000) referred to the randomized controlled trial as the most valid form of evidence supporting the theories occupational therapy practitioners use in practice. If we compare our research with that of other professions, such as medicine, occupational therapy scholars must recognize that we have a lot of catching up to do.

Citing a postmodernist perspective that is shared with science generally, Creek concluded that "truth is not external, universal, and eternal, but is personal, local, and ephemeral. Occupational therapists, with their concern for the personal experiences of individuals as they live their everyday lives, understand this" (p. 52). Using a subjective view of truth, theories should not be tested using quantitative, experimental research methods; large samples; or statistical analysis. Rather, theories are built through qualitative or ethnographic methodology. While this method has been cited as the least valid from a scientific perspective (Holm, 2000), it has also been viewed as the most relevant method for occupational therapy (Clark, 1993; Zemke, 2004). If we accept this view of reality, using a client-centered approach is more than a new technique. It is the only valid way to build theory in practice. While occupational therapy practitioners may have knowledge of many scientific theories and evidence, they use this expertise differently in client-centered practice, recognizing that the client's perspective is paramount. Theories are only relevant as they relate to specific individuals in specific situations, and the tools and techniques they generate are only valid if they result in positive changes in occupational performance and client satisfaction.

Occupational therapy's "identity crisis" in the 1970s and 1980s precipitated a search for theories to address common threads and unify occupational therapy practice. While many diverse frames of reference in the profession had been identified, we now needed to develop a systematic, theoretical, and scientific basis for occupation itself as intervention. Ironically, this is the same goal proposed by our founders (Dunton, 1919; Quiroga, 1995). By the 1990s, scholars had reflected considerably on the problem of professional identity and had come to understand that the unifying concept for all of the areas of specialization within occupational therapy practice was, quite simply, occupation.

Without this historical background, new students and graduates cannot possibly appreciate the enormity of what has occurred in the occupational therapy profession. Over the past 30 to 35 years, we have witnessed the elevation of occupational therapy from an "allied medical profession" to a profession in its own right, complete with its own body of knowledge and research, its unique theories of occupation, and with a master's degree entry level, the community of scholars needed to continue the quest for prominence as a profession.

## The Current Theoretical Challenge: Standing on the Edge of Chaos

Chaos theory originally came from the fields of mathematics and physics in the 1970s. It has expanded to include a wide range of applications such as the analysis of traffic flow, global weather, group dynamics, health epidemics, and economic trends. For example, in the TV series *Numbers*, character Charlie Epp, a mathematics professor, used chaos theory to help his FBI brother narrow down suspects when solving a crime. The theory has challenged traditional scientific knowledge and methodology at nearly every level. Because of its extreme complexity, chaos theory is not well understood generally, but at the simplest level, it changes the way one views cause and effect, as it renders long-term predictions impossible. A central concept to chaos theory is sensitivity to initial conditions, widely known as the *butterfly effect*. The phrase comes from a presentation given by Edward Lorenz to the American Association for the Advancement of Science in Washington, DC, entitled "Predictability: Does the Flap of a Butterfly's Wings in Brazil Set Off a Tornado in Texas?" (Lorenz, 1972). In other words, even very small changes have the potential to produce large effects, and they do so in ways that are exceedingly complex and unpredictable (Figure 15-2).

Some related terms for chaos are *complexity theory* and *nonlinear science*. The traditional scientific method, implying A + B = C, can be understood as a linear relationship: for example, "if you get a flu shot, you will not get the flu." Proponents of chaos theory believe this type of linear prediction is impossible, because we cannot measure all of the initial conditions; even small mistakes could affect vastly different outcomes. The actual outcome depends on too many factors because human

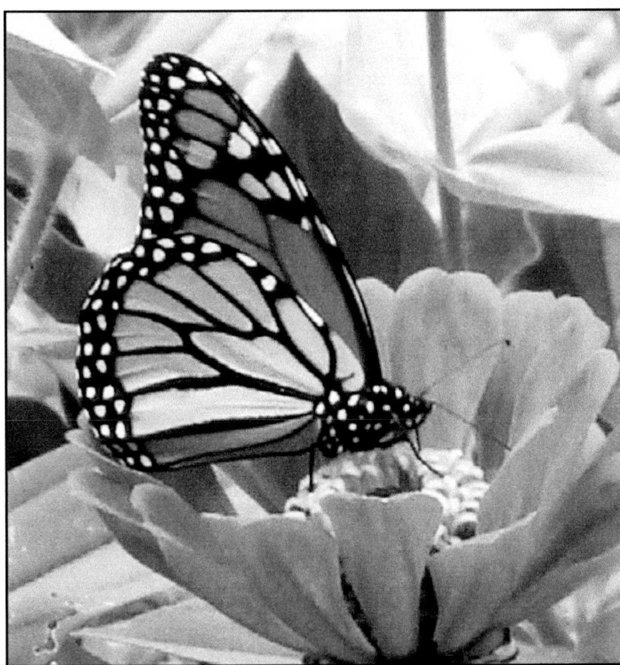

**Figure 15-2.** Lorenz's butterfly effect in chaos theory represents sensitivity to initial conditions contributing to vastly diverse and unpredictable outcomes. (Reprinted with permission from Marilyn B. Cole, 2009.)

systems are extremely complex. The term *chaos* implies a state of disorder, but chaos theory takes us beyond that point—the study of seemingly chaotic systems often leads to self-organization and pattern formation. For this reason, complexity theory might be a more accurate term when applied to human systems.

Occupational therapy practitioners have only begun to understand how complexity theory applies to our profession. Some occupational therapy practitioners have used complexity theory to better understand cognition in the workings of the human brain (Haltiwanger, Lazzarini, & Nazeran, 2007; Lazzarini, 2004, 2005, 2016; Loukas, 2010; Royeen, 2003). Zemke and Clark introduce some similar ideas as dynamical systems theory, a central concept in the study of occupational science (1996). Most of us can accept the idea that the brain is highly influenced by initial conditions, that even small stimuli (called *perturbations* in chaos theory) can produce dramatic and unexpected responses. Lazzarini first used the term *neuro-occupation* to describe more fully how occupation influences and is influenced by brain activity (2005). She believes that the "nonlinear dynamics of brain activity" help us better understand human intention, perception, and meaning in performing occupations, thus providing a link between occupational therapy and occupational science (2016).

In 2017, the AOTA will reach its 100th anniversary. Perhaps we can begin to appreciate occupational therapy as an exceedingly complex intervention that integrates five interactive levels, which Creek (2003) defined as follows:

1. The occupational therapy practitioner as an independent self-organizing system, with all the beliefs, values, skills, tools, knowledge, abilities, and culture that he or she brings to the interaction
2. The client, also as an independent self-organizing system, with all of his or her history, experience at all levels, and contexts, coupled with values, health care beliefs, needs, problems, issues, personal goals, occupations, abilities, skills, attitudes, and interest
3. The context
4. The environment
5. The occupational therapy practitioner's actions

Creek acknowledges the dynamic interactive process that occurs between these levels throughout each treatment session, reflecting the active interchanges that occur within the client-centered partnership, ultimately facilitating new self-organized patterns within the client's occupational life. According to this approach, the real key to positive therapeutic outcomes does not only come from evidence-based practice, nor does it come only from an effective therapeutic relationship, although these remain critical parts of the process. The key lies in finding that place at the edge of chaos, when the system that is the client—surrounded by all the right initial conditions—stands ready to jump in and reorganize itself into a more adaptive being, enabled and empowered to more effectively engage in the occupations that give meaning to life for both the client and the community.

In another attempt to publicly embrace the complex nature of occupation in life and in occupational therapy practice, Florence Clark coined the phrase "high-definition occupational therapy (HDOT)" in her inaugural address as President of the AOTA (Clark, 2010). In a high-definition photograph, one can "zoom in" to read the license plate on a speeding car, or "zoom out" to appreciate the surrounding situations and circumstances. Applying this metaphor to occupational therapy theory, we can zoom in to use biomechanical principles (a reductionistic approach) to help a client strengthen weakened muscles from a stroke and at the same time zoom out to assess and modify the contexts within which the client needs to use those muscles for self-care, mobility, work, and leisure (a holistic perspective). In other words, in the process of occupational therapy treatment, many levels of interactions among variables might be happening simultaneously, with the practitioner intervening at critical points to increase the probability of a positive therapeutic outcome.

Professional reasoning takes occupational therapy into the broader social arenas, expanding the reasoning process to address occupational therapy's position with regard to other disciplines and with health care in general. For example, strategic reasoning (von Bruggen, 2016) was used to establish a network of occupational therapy educators across Europe as a way to share knowledge, standardize curriculums, and generally raise the status of the profession. Collaborative reasoning is used to forge partnerships with community agencies and disability advocacy groups, greatly increasing the level of understanding between occupational therapy service providers and their clients (Birleson, 2016). (See Table 15-4 for updated levels of clinical/professional reasoning.)

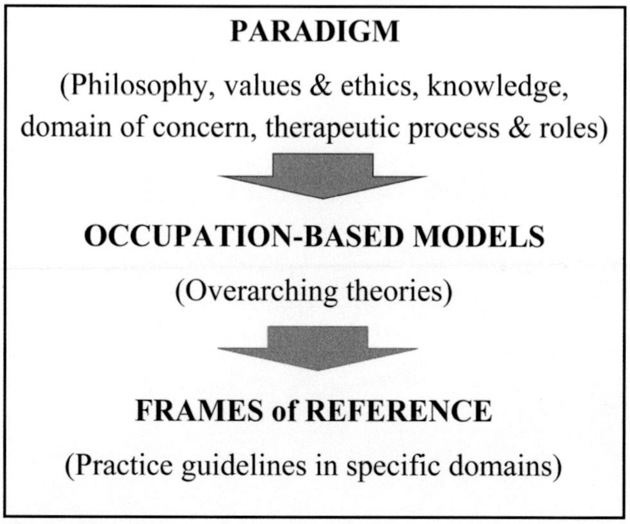

**PARADIGM**

(Philosophy, values & ethics, knowledge, domain of concern, therapeutic process & roles)

**OCCUPATION-BASED MODELS**

(Overarching theories)

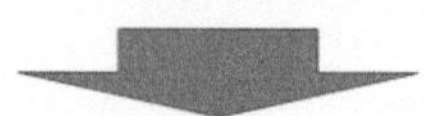

**FRAMES of REFERENCE**

(Practice guidelines in specific domains)

**Figure 15-3.** Proposed taxonomy for the occupational therapy profession. (Adapted from Cole, M. B., & Tufano, R. [2008]. *Applied theories in occupational therapy.* Thorofare, NJ: SLACK Incorporated.)

## Organizing Occupational Therapy Knowledge

Currently, occupational therapy practitioners need both occupation-based models, using a top-down and occupation-first approach (Trombly Latham, 2008), and frames of reference, which address the components of performance using a bottom-up approach. Components such as range of motion or cognition can be targeted for assessment and intervention when these "client factors" are identified as barriers to engagement in occupation. It is comforting to learn that occupation-based models are not going to replace all of the collected wisdom of occupational therapy's more traditional frames of reference. However, as practitioners, occupational therapy practitioners will be expected to use specific techniques within the context of the broader occupation-based models, which requires an understanding of both levels. In fact, occupational therapy students and practitioners need to develop an appreciation of all levels of theory as necessary within our new paradigm of client-centered, holistic, and systems-oriented occupational therapy practice. Mosey (1992) identifies three levels of applied theory in occupational therapy as it had progressed to that point in time:

1. A fundamental body of knowledge including philosophical assumptions, an ethical code, a theoretical foundation of both theories and empirical data, a domain of concern, and legitimate tools. Occupational therapy's professional paradigm and *Framework* fall into this category in our proposed taxonomy because these are common to all practice.
2. An applied body of knowledge that includes sets of guidelines for practice. The occupation-based models addressing the interrelationships of person, environment, and occupation fall into this category in our taxonomy.
3. Practice, which includes action sequences, use of applied knowledge, the clinical reasoning process, and the art of practice. Frames of reference, the most concrete level of theory, fall into this category by providing specific techniques and evidence for specific disabilities.

Taking these distinctions into account, we will clarify some different levels of theory as they currently appear to be understood by our scholars and/or defined by the AOTA. Our proposed organization of theory for occupational therapy appears in Figure 15-3. It includes three levels: occupational therapy paradigm, occupation-based models, and frames of reference. Each of these terms will be defined.

### *Paradigm of Occupational Therapy*

Previously we said that the paradigm in health care has shifted to one that is holistic, client centered, and systems oriented. These broad concepts represent the most general levels of theory. In an attempt to both broaden and unify today's practice, the *Framework* has redefined some of the fundamental concepts of occupational therapy practice and has incorporated many of the concepts from occupation-based models as well. For example, patients are now called *clients*, treatment is redefined as *intervention*, and disease or illness has been replaced by *health condition* (AOTA, 2014). These changes in terminology reflect the shift in focus toward wellness and prevention of disability and imply fundamental changes in the way occupational therapy practitioners will practice in the 21st century.

### *Occupation-Based Models*

The next level includes the occupation-based models, which have been called overarching frames of reference (Dunn, 2000), conceptual models (Reed & Sanderson, 1999), or occupation-based frameworks (Baum & Christiansen, 2005). In occupational therapy, occupation-based models help explain the relationship between the person, the environment, and occupational performance, forming the foundation for the profession's

Table 15-4.

## Expanded Levels of Clinical/Professional Reasoning in Occupational Therapy

| Type of Reasoning | Description | Example |
|---|---|---|
| Scientific | Using logic in systematic ways to make objective decisions | Daily stretching exercise will increase range of motion |
| Procedural | Using evaluation tools and specified intervention strategies | Following hip replacement, the client should not exceed 90 degrees of hip flexion |
| Narrative | Incorporating life history and stories when making occupational choices | As the oldest of four children, Mary has always identified herself as a caregiver |
| Pragmatic | Attending to the practical aspects of service delivery and the best application of one's own skills | When the client expressed extreme fatigue, we did the evaluation seated rather than standing |
| Ethical | Based on beliefs about the right thing to do, acting in the client's best interests | Although Margaret's vision is poor, she wants to continue driving, yet doing so would not be safe for her or others |
| Interactive | Refers to therapist encounters with clients as people, as social beings, and considering their subjective illness and wellness experiences (Mattingly & Fleming, 1994) | Listening to clients, communicating empathy, and gaining their trust |
| Conditional | Applies to the impact of contexts and environments; adaptation to changing circumstances; and clients' life stages, their past, present, and future, and predicting possible client futures (Schell & Schell, 2008) | Using cooking activities as a step toward returning to the role of mother, helping client to envision the process of change |
| Strategic reasoning | A thinking process through which occupational therapy practitioners work out the best course of action to take in a complex situation, or how to position themselves in a constantly changing world (von Bruggen, 2016) | Creating a publicity effort to bring greater recognition to the role of occupational therapy in both health care and health and wellness, targeting community agencies |
| Social reasoning | Thinking about occupations from a social perspective, including social contexts, expectations, sources of support, and considering the social groups and/or significant relationships within which occupational choices are made and performed (Cole, 2016) | Working with nursing home staff to create a social culture that supports resident participation in self-care, activity choices, group decision making, and engagement with community organizations and events outside the facility, including intergenerational interactions |
| Collaborative reasoning | Working in partnership with others, whether with other professionals, the client-practitioner relationship, or practitioners within services collaborating with other organizations to achieve mutual goals (Birleson, 2016) | Occupational therapy providers working in partnership with community advocacy organizations such as an Alzheimer's association |
| Political reasoning | Highlights the need to involve local people in making decisions about public policies and projects that affect them so that development is owned, and therefore more likely to be sustainable (Lorenzo, 2016) | Organizing local seniors to advocate as a group to local governmental agencies to recognize the need for, and to establish and fund, accessible transportation services for elders living independently in the community |
| Development reasoning | Refers to a gradual unfolding or bringing out latent potential in people, their environments, and social systems, including promoting theories and practices for social change (Duncan, 2016) | Occupational therapy programs with traditional Black communities of South Africa to raise funds through production of skilled crafts, and use those funds to educate society about strategies to prevent the spread of AIDS |
| Creative reasoning | People create identities through interaction with their environments, simultaneously inventing solutions for problems with survival and shaping the future directions of mankind | Occupational therapy practitioners encourage creativity in their clients to solve problems with everyday living, simultaneously building on the innovations of those who came before |

Adapted from Schell, B. B., & Schell, J. (2008). *Clinical and professional reasoning in occupational therapy.* Philadelphia, PA: Lippincott Williams and Wilkins and Cole, M. B., & Creek, C. (2016). *Global perspectives in professional reasoning.* Thorofare, NJ: SLACK Incorporated.

focus on occupation. However, they do not provide guidelines for application with specific populations or disability areas. For example, the Canadian Model of Occupational Performance—Enablement (CMOP-E; Townsend & Polatajko, 2007) defines the interactions of person, occupation, and environment, with each of these concepts further defined as the following:

- **Person:** Spirituality as the source of the affective, cognitive, and physical self
- **Occupation:** Consisting of productivity, self-care, and leisure
- **Environment:** Including physical, institutional, cultural, and societal systems

The Canadian model has generated a holistic, client-centered assessment tool, the Canadian Occupational Performance Measure, which can be applied in all areas of occupational therapy practice (Law et al., 2005; Townsend, 1997). This may be understood as a top-down approach, beginning with a client's occupational priorities and goals, and working backward to identify barriers to achieving them.

## Frames of Reference

Theories that explain how therapy works in practice have been called practice models (Kielhofner, 2004; Reed & Sanderson, 1999) or frames of reference (Mosey, 1986, 1992). Frames of reference address specific areas of occupation and help occupational therapists to apply theory with individual clients in specific situations. Most frames of reference were developed to address particular areas of disability. For example, the sensory integration frame of reference was originally developed for the intervention of children with learning disabilities. This frame of reference has produced many specific assessment tools for measuring sensory systems and their motor and cognitive outcomes, as well as tools and techniques for providing specific types of sensory input. The assessment of specific sensory systems and application of remedial strategies demonstrates a bottom-up approach, beginning with foundation skills and working upward toward using these skills during occupational performance. Frames of reference represent the most concrete level of occupational therapy theory.

Certified occupational therapy assistants, as well as master's level occupational therapists, need to have a basic understanding of how the theories used in practice are developed and why. While occupational therapy supervisors may evaluate clients and design appropriate interventions, the certified occupational therapy assistants who carry out intervention plans make many decisions about the details, including the tasks and contexts within which occupational performance takes place. Those everyday decisions need to be consistent with the overall occupation-based models and frames of reference within which the interventions were designed. Since certified occupational therapy assistants spend most of their time working directly with clients, they are the most likely practitioners to be asked to explain why they are doing things a certain way. Theory's role in everyday practice should help all occupational therapy practitioners understand and explain how and why certain interventions will help clients to achieve positive outcomes. Evidence gathered from research studies using the chosen theories will add validity to the strategies being applied in specific situations. For example, a certified occupational therapy assistant working on increasing range of motion in the affected arm of a person who has had a stroke would not choose an activity such as stacking cones if the intervention plan was based on a task-based approach. Asking the client to choose a task such as operating the TV remote or putting away clean flatware in a drawer would be more consistent with a client-centered and task-focused approach.

The knowledge gained from more traditional frames of reference—such as biomechanical, rehabilitative, sensory integrative, or psychodynamic—is still relevant and useful, but using the current professional paradigm, it needs to be applied within occupation-based models of practice. In particular, the client-centered approach has changed the way we perform evaluation and intervention, giving greater importance to therapeutic use of self in the therapeutic relationship. Therapeutic interventions become most meaningful when their relationship to the client's important life roles is outwardly discussed and appreciated by the individuals and groups receiving service.

Chapter 16 reviews some of the more prominent occupation-based models and frames of reference and describes how they are used in practice.

## Summary

Theory development has been addressed in this chapter on two levels—general and specific. Generally, theory begins with a desire to better understand something in our own experience and develop the theory through a continuum of qualitative (ethnographic), descriptive, and quantitative (experimental) research. In occupational therapy specifically, theories have evolved over the history of the profession in response to (or in tandem with) the changing nature of client problems with occupational performance resulting from illness, injury, or another cause, requiring occupational therapy intervention, together with occupational therapy's changing role in the overall system of health care service delivery. From occupational therapy's philosophical roots in humanism and pragmatism, the profession has developed many scientific theories to substantiate its unique focus and methods

## Case Study: Nan

Nan found out about her multiple sclerosis (MS) at the height of her career as the administrator of the recreation therapy department in a large New York City long-term care facility. An active athlete in her younger years, Nan retained her competitive spirit, rejecting disease-based support groups as "whiners" and refusing to allow MS to define her. Instead she embraced rehabilitation, and with the help of occupational therapy adapted her work space so that she could continue a career that she loved. In retirement, Nan and her partner looked for a place with a milder climate where they could engage with others and retain their active lifestyle at a slower pace. They moved to a master planned community with amenities for people of all ages in Denver, Colorado, adapted their home for wheelchair accessibility, and adapted their car with hand controls so Nan could do the driving while her partner navigated. On occasion, Nan used a scooter to navigate public areas. The couple divided household chores, Nan doing the shopping and cleaning while her partner cooked and planned their social and recreational activities. Because fatigue and stress are typical issues with MS, Nan needed to plan for extra time to do certain tasks, and to avoid noise, interruptions, and long waiting times that could cause frustration. On a typical weekday, they spent the morning swimming or volunteering to do work in support of fundraising activities at the Denver Zoo, followed by lunch with friends and an afternoon doing errands and housework or relaxing at home.

However, their challenges didn't end there. Plagued by old athletic injuries, both of Nan's knees required joint replacements, a surgical procedure that was not usually recommended for someone with MS. Again, Nan's competitive spirit kicked in—she won the battle this past August and underwent a double knee replacement. While Nan threw herself into rehabilitation, her partner, a retired occupational therapist, made further adaptations to their home, rearranging their furniture to accommodate a walker; adding grab bars and other supports in the bathroom, bedroom, and kitchen; and organizing storage of needed items. These adaptations helped Nan to return home from rehabilitation to a stress-free environment where she could count on the continued support of a caring partner to ease her continued recovery. Nan was determined to return to the activities she enjoyed: exercising in the pool (Figure 15-4), using her administrative skills to benefit the Denver Zoo, and regularly socializing with friends.

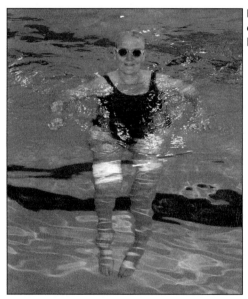

**Figure 15-4.** Nan exercises in the pool several times each week, an especially important routine to maintain strength and flexibility after her double knee replacement surgery.

**Learning activities:** Use the following questions to guide your application of the theory of conditional independence.

1. Situational adaptation: What adaptations were made to the physical and social environments to accommodate Nan's functional issues caused by MS? Give three examples.
2. Structured performance: What were the occupations Nan chose to do? Name three. Discuss how each activity should be structured, and what planning and preparation Nan could do to ensure a better chance of success. As an occupational therapist, what frames of reference might you apply in advising her if needed?
3. Intentional abilities: What were Nan's intentions with regard to occupational participation after her knee surgery? What role did motivation play in her recovery?
4. How did Nan apply self-management, social connections, and self-fulfilling activities to help her overcome barriers to full participation in life?
5. Under what conditions could she engage in her chosen occupations independently? Choose one and explain in detail what you would do as an occupational therapist to assist her with this process.

## Case Study: Jeanette

Jeanette is a 75-year-old woman living alone who had a knee replacement and must learn to use a walker. Her apartment is all one level, but she has a flight of stairs to get from her garage up to her back door. She is able to drive but unable to climb the stairs without assistance. Although her husband died a decade ago and her son and daughter both have families and homes of their own, Jeanette still spends each morning cleaning her three-room apartment and feels frustrated that she cannot continue to do this as before. Jeanette loves to cook but cannot easily reach the items she needs in her cramped kitchenette. Fatigue sets in quickly, preventing her from completing tasks. Although she had participated in several social activities prior to her surgery, she has avoided attending these events following surgery because of her physical issues. She has no problems with toileting or dressing but fears she will fall while getting in and out of the bathtub. Jeanette's daughter and son-in-law live in the next town. Her daughter, Gail, calls several times each day and visits often, even though she works full time. Her grandson, Rob, a college student, has offered to help Jeanette do her shopping on Saturdays.

**Learning activities:**

1. Using the medical model, list five client factors to be addressed in occupational therapy.
2. Using a client-centered approach with Jeanette, write 10 questions you would ask the client or her family members to gain a "holistic" understanding of her occupational problems.
3. Identify three barriers to occupational performance and do an Internet search to learn what theories and applications might be helpful to this case. For example, fear of falling, fatigue, and home adaptation might be relevant areas for Jeanette.

and has broadened into the holistic, client-centered, and systems-oriented practice of the 21st century. Complexity theory (HDOT) compels occupational therapy practitioners to embrace and use all of the collective levels of theory. This includes application of frames of reference, which guide occupational therapy's interventions with specific client occupational issues and priorities within the context of occupation-based models that consider the interrelationships of the client's personal strengths and limitations; the environmental facilitators and barriers to social participation; and the social, cultural, physical, and spiritual nature of human occupation.

## Student Self-Assessment

1. How does theory help therapists make decisions? Give an example.
2. Explain how theory in occupational therapy differs from theory in occupational science.
3. What problems occurred in the occupational therapy profession in the 1930s that caused the paradigm to shift? What problems occurred in the 1970s that caused the professional paradigm to shift again?
4. What are two philosophical schools that influenced the founding of occupational therapy in the early 1900s? Explain each and give an example.
5. What is the purpose of theory? How does it help us with practical problems?
6. Describe two types of research that are used to develop and validate theory.
7. Using the medical model, describe the steps you would follow if you fell and broke your ankle.
8. Using the client-centered model in the broken ankle scenario, what areas of occupational performance would you evaluate to determine what theories should be applied?
9. How does the ICF relate to the professional paradigm of occupational therapy? Name three concepts that are similar.
10. What does the CMOP contribute to occupational therapy's current paradigm in the United States?
11. How is an occupation-based model in occupational therapy different from a frame of reference?
12. What three theoretical trends make up occupational therapy's current paradigm? Describe each briefly.
13. Describe the difference between a "top-down" approach and a "bottom-up" approach to the application of theory in occupational therapy practice.
14. How does a client's social participation affect the occupations that are addressed in therapy, and why is this important to consider?
15. What is complexity theory and how does it change the way occupational therapists apply theoretical principles in practice?
16. What is the meaning of the phrase "standing on the edge of chaos" and how might it apply to the process of occupational therapy practice?

## Evidence-Based Research Chart

| Type of Theory | Examples of Application | Evidence |
|---|---|---|
| Psychological (e.g., Bandura's social cognitive theory, cognitive behavioral theory [2001], or attachment theory) | Influence health practitioners to change their beliefs about consequences if evidence-based practice guidelines are followed<br>Identify barriers to implementing evidence-based practice in practice despite evidence | Michie et al., 2005 |
| Theories of physical and mental health medicine | A mental health quality enhancement research initiative to increase appropriate use of antipsychotic medication among patients with schizophrenia | Sales, Smith, Curren, & Cochevar, 2006 |
| Occupation-based models and frames of reference | Group interventions designed and implemented with use of different theories (both models and frames of reference) across the spectrum of occupational therapy practice | Cole, 2012 |
| Strategic, political, collaborative, creative, social, spiritual, and developmental reasoning approaches | Broadening the spectrum of occupational therapy practice in the larger society, such as establishing social networks, unifying educational standards, forging partnerships with community organizations and initiating efforts that foster needed social change | Cole & Creek, 2016 |

## References


American Occupational Therapy Association. (1979). Uniform terminology for reporting occupational therapy services. *Occupational Therapy News, 35*(11), 1-8.

American Occupational Therapy Association. (2014). Occupational therapy practice framework: Domain and process (3rd ed.). *American Journal of Occupational Therapy, 68*(Suppl. 1), S1-S48. doi:10.5014/ajot.2014.682006

Ayres, A. J. (1979). *Sensory integration and the child.* Los Angeles, CA: Western Psychological Services.

Bandura, A. (2001). Social cognitive theory: An agentic perspective. *Annual Review of Psychology, 52*, 1-26.

Baum, C., & Christiansen, C. (2005). Person-environment-occupation-performance. In C. Christiansen, C. Baum, & J. B. Haugen (Eds.), *Occupational therapy: Performance, participation, and well-being* (3rd ed., pp. 242-267). Thorofare, NJ: SLACK Incorporated.

Birleson, A. (2016). Collaborative reasoning: Working in partnership with third sector organizations. In M. B. Cole & J. Creek (Eds.), *Global perspectives in professional reasoning*. Thorofare, NJ: SLACK Incorporated.

Bobath, B. (1990). *Adult hemiplegia: Evaluation and treatment* (3rd ed.). London, England: Butterworth-Heinemann.

Breines, E. (1987). Pragmatism as a foundation for occupational therapy curricula. *American Journal of Occupational Therapy, 41*(8), 522-525.

Bundy, A., Lane, S., & Murray, E. (2002). *Sensory integration: Theory and practice* (2nd ed.). Philadelphia, PA: F. A. Davis Company.

Christiansen, C., & Baum, C. (1997). Person-environment occupational performance. In C. Christiansen & C. Baum (Eds.), *Occupational therapy: Enabling function and well-being* (2nd ed., pp. 46-71). Thorofare, NJ: SLACK Incorporated.

Clark, F. (1993). Occupation embedded in a real life: Interweaving occupational science and occupational therapy. 1993 Eleanor Clarke Slagle Lecture. *American Journal of Occupational Therapy, 47*(12), 1067-1077.

Clark, F. (2010). High definition occupational therapy: HDOT. *American Journal of Occupational Therapy, 64*, 848-854.

Cole, M. B. (1998). Time mastery in business and occupational therapy. *WORK: A Journal of Prevention, Assessment and Rehabilitation, 10*(2), 119-127.

Cole, M. B. (2012). *Group dynamics in occupational therapy* (4th ed.). Thorofare, NJ: SLACK Incorporated.

Cole, M. B. (2016). Social reasoning in occupational therapy. In M. B. Cole & J. Creek (Eds.), *Global perspectives in professional reasoning.* Thorofare, NJ: SLACK Incorporated.

Cole, M. B., & Creek, J. (2016). *Global perspectives in professional reasoning*. Thorofare, NJ: SLACK Incorporated.

Cole, M. B., & Donohue, M. V. (2011). *Social participation in occupational contexts: In schools, clinics, and communities*. Thorofare, NJ: SLACK Incorporated.

Cole, M. B., & Macdonald, K. (2015). *Productive aging: An occupational perspective*. Thorofare, NJ: SLACK Incorporated.

Cole, M. B., & Tufano, R. (2008). *Applied theories in occupational therapy.* Thorofare, NJ: SLACK Incorporated.

Creek, J. (1997). The truth is no longer out there. *British Journal of Occupational Therapy, 60*(2), 50-52.

Creek, J. (2003). *Occupational therapy defined as a complex intervention.* London, England: College of Occupational Therapists.

Creek, J. (2010). *The core concepts of occupational therapy: A dynamic framework for practice.* London, England: Jessica Kingsley Publishers.

DePoy, E., & Gitlin, L. (2005). *Introduction to research* (3rd ed.). New York, NY: Elsevier.

Duncan, M. (2016). Developmental reasoning in occupational therapy community practice. In M. B. Cole & J. Creek (Eds.), *Global perspectives in professional reasoning*. Thorofare, NJ: SLACK Incorporated.

Dunn, W. (2000). *Best practice occupational therapy: In community service with children and families*. Thorofare, NJ: SLACK Incorporated.

Dunn, W., Brown, C., & McGuigan, A. (1994). The ecology of human performance: A framework for considering the effect of context. *American Journal of Occupational Therapy, 48*(7), 595-607.

Dunton, W. R. (1919). *Reconstruction therapy.* Philadelphia, PA: W. B. Saunders Co.

Evanofski, M. (2003). Occupational therapy reimbursement, regulation, and the evolving scope of practice. In E. B. Crepeau, E. S. Cohn, & B. A. B. Schell (Eds.), *Willard & Spackman's occupational therapy* (10th ed., pp. 887-905). Philadelphia, PA: Lippincott Williams and Wilkins.

Glaser, B., & Strauss, A. (1967). *The discovery of grounded theory: Strategies for qualitative research.* Chicago, IL: Aldine.

Haltiwanger, E., Lazzarini, I., & Nazeran, H. (2007). Application of nonlinear dynamics theory to neuro-occupation: A case study of alcoholism. *British Journal of Occupational Therapy, 70,* 349-357.

Holm, M. B. (2000). The 2000 Eleanor Clarke Slagle Lecture. Our mandate for the new millennium: Evidence-based practice. *American Journal of Occupational Therapy, 54*(6), 575-585.

Hooper, B. (2006). Epistemological transformation in occupational therapy: Educational implications and challenges. *OTJR: Occupation, Participation and Health, 26*(1), 15-24.

Kerlinger, F. N. (1979). *Behavioral research: A conceptual approach.* New York, NY: Holt McDougal.

Kielhofner, G. (2004). *Conceptual foundations of occupational therapy* (3rd ed.). Philadelphia, PA: F. A. Davis Company.

Kielhofner, G. (2006). *Research in occupational therapy.* Philadelphia, PA: F. A. Davis Company.

Kielhofner, G., & Burke, J. P. (1977). Occupational therapy after 60 years: An account of changing identity and knowledge. *American Journal of Occupational Therapy, 31*(10), 675-689.

Kielhofner, G., & Burke, J. P. (1980). A model of human occupation, part 1. Conceptual framework and content. *American Journal of Occupational Therapy, 34*(9), 572-581.

Kuhn, T. S. (1970). *The structure of scientific revolutions* (2nd ed.). Chicago, IL: University of Chicago Press.

Law, M., Baptiste, S., Carswell, A., McColl, M., Polatajko, H., & Pollick, N. (2005). *Canadian occupational performance measure* (4th ed.) Ottawa, Ontario, Canada: CAOT Publications ACE.

Lazzarini, I. (2004). Neuro-occupation: The nonlinear dynamics of intention, meaning and perception. *British Journal of Occupational Therapy, 67,* 342-352.

Lazzarini, I. (2005). A nonlinear approach to cognition: A web of ability and disability. In N. Katz (Ed.), *Cognition and occupation across the life span* (2nd ed., pp. 211-233). Bethesda, MD: AOTA Press.

Lazzarini, I. (2016). Nonlinear reasoning: Restoring the essence of the occupational therapy process. In M. B. Cole & J. Creek (Eds.), *Global perspectives in professional reasoning.* Thorofare, NJ: SLACK Incorporated.

Lorenz, E. (1972). *Predictability: Does the flap of a butterfly's wings in Brazil set off a tornado in Texas?* Retrieved from http://voluntaryboundaries.blogsome.com/2011/02/03/predictability-does-the-flap-of-a-butterflys-wings-in-brazil-set-off-a-tornado-in-texas

Lorenzo, T. (2016). Political reasoning for disability inclusion: Making policies practical. In M. B. Cole & J. Creek (Eds.), *Global perspectives in professional reasoning.* Thorofare, NJ: SLACK Incorporated.

Loukas, K. (2010). Use of the natural environment. In K. Sladyk, K. Jacobs, & N. MacRae (Eds.), *Occupational therapy essentials for clinical competence* (pp. 199-206). Thorofare, NJ: SLACK Incorporated.

Macdonald, K. (2015). A theory of conditional independence. In M. B. Cole & K. C. Macdonald (Eds.), *Productive aging: An occupational perspective* (pp. 231-242). Thorofare, NJ: SLACK Incorporated.

Mattingly, C., & Fleming, M. H. (1994). *Clinical reasoning: Forms of inquiry in a therapeutic practice.* Philadelphia, PA: F. A. Davis Company.

Michie, S., Johnston, M., Abraham, C., Lawton R., Parker, D., Walker, A., on behalf of the Psychological Theory Group. (2005). Making psychological theory useful for implementing evidence based practice: A consensus approach. *Quality and Safety in Health Care, 14,* 26-33.

Mosey, A. C. (1970). *Three frames of reference for mental health.* Thorofare, NJ: SLACK Incorporated.

Mosey, A. C. (1986). *Psychosocial components of occupational therapy.* New York, NY: Raven Press.

Mosey, A. C. (1992). *Applied scientific inquiry in the health professions: An epistemological orientation.* Rockville, MD: AOTA Press.

Portney, L. G. & Watkins, M. P. (2009). *Foundations of clinical research: Applications to practice* (3rd ed.) Upper Saddle River, NJ: Prentice-Hall Health.

Quiroga, V. A. M. (1995). *Occupational therapy: The first 30 years 1900-1930.* Bethesda, MD: AOTA Press.

Reed, K. L., & Sanderson, S. N. (1999). *Concepts of occupational therapy* (4th ed.). Philadelphia, PA: Lippincott Williams and Wilkins.

Rogers, J. C. (1983). The 1983 Eleanor Clarke Slagle Lectureship. Clinical reasoning: The ethics, science, and art. *American Journal of Occupational Therapy, 37*(9), 601-616.

Royeen, C. (2003). Chaotic occupational therapy: Collective wisdom for a complex profession. *American Journal of Occupational Therapy, 57,* 609-624.

Royeen, C., & Luebben, A. (Eds.). (2009). *Sensory integration: A compendium of leading scholarship.* Bethesda, MD: American Occupational Therapy Association.

Sales, A., Smith, J., Curren, G., & Cochevar, L. (2006). Models, strategies, and tools: Theory in implementing evidence-based findings into health care practice. *Journal of General Internal Medicine, 21*(Suppl. 2), S43-S49.

Schkade, J. K., & Schultz, S. (1992a). Occupational adaptation: Toward a holistic approach to contemporary practice, part 1. *American Journal of Occupational Therapy, 46*(9), 829-837.

Schkade, J. K., & Schultz, S. (1992b). Occupational adaptation: Toward a holistic approach to contemporary practice, part 2. *American Journal of Occupational Therapy, 46*(10), 917-925.

Strauss, A., & Corbin, I. (1994). Grounded theory methodology. In N. K. Denzin & Y. S. Lincoln (Eds.), *Handbook of qualitative research* (pp. 217-285). Thousand Oaks, CA: Sage Publishers.

Townsend, E. (1997). *Enabling occupation: An occupational therapy perspective.* Ottawa, Ontario, Canada: Canadian Association of Occupational Therapy Publications.

Townsend, E., & Polatajko, H. (2007). *Enabling occupation II: Advancing an occupational therapy vision for health and well-being, and justice through occupation.* Ottawa, Canada: Canadian Association of Occupational Therapy Publications.

Tracy, S. E. (1918). *Studies in invalid occupation: A manual for nurses and attendants.* Boston, MA: Whitcomb and Barrows.

Trombly Latham, C. A. (2008). Occupation: Philosophy and concepts. In M. V. Radomski & C. A. Trombly Latham (Eds.), *Occupational therapy for physical dysfunction* (6th ed., pp. 339-357). Philadelphia, PA: Lippincott Williams and Wilkins.

von Bruggen, H. (2016). Strategic thinking and reasoning in occupational therapy. In M. B. Cole & J. Creek (Eds.), *Global perspectives in professional reasoning.* Thorofare, NJ: SLACK Incorporated.

World Health Organization. (1980). *International classification of impairments, disabilities, and handicaps.* Geneva, Switzerland: Author.

World Health Organization. (2001). *International classification of functioning, disability and health.* Geneva, Switzerland: Author.

Zemke, R. (2004). The 2004 Eleanor Clarke Slagle Lecture—Time, space, and the kaleidoscopes of occupation. *American Journal of Occupational Therapy, 58*(6), 608-620.

Zemke, R., & Clark, F. (Eds.). (1996). *Occupational science: The evolving discipline.* Philadelphia, PA: F. A. Davis Company.

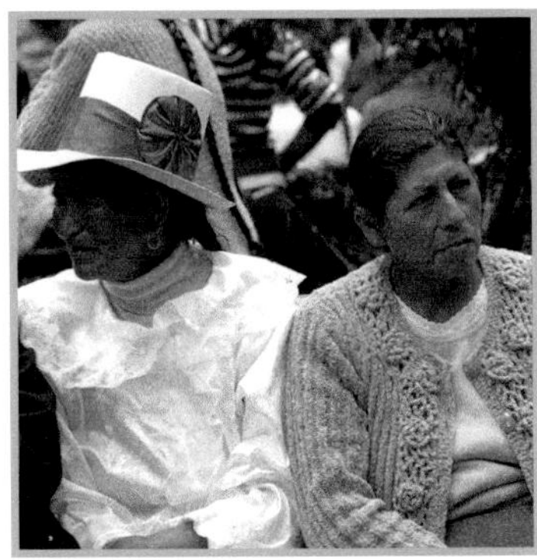

# 16

# Occupational Therapy Theory Use in the Process of Evaluation and Intervention

Roseanna Tufano, LMFT, OTR/L

## ACOTE Standards Explored in This Chapter

B.3.1–B.3.3

## Key Vocabulary

- **Frames of reference:** System of compatible concepts from theory that guides a plan of action within a specific occupational therapy domain of concern (Mosey, 1986).
- **Intervention plan:** A collaborative determination of client-oriented actions meant to enhance occupational performance, including specific targeted outcomes that are based on select models, frames of reference, and evidence.
- **Occupation-based models:** Proposed interaction of person, environment, and occupation that guide the organization of occupational therapy practice (Cole & Tufano, 2008).
- **Occupational profile:** An initial interview process that may be formal or informal. It is meant to reveal the client's personal history, daily living patterns, interests, values, and needs while highlighting problems from the client's perspective concerning the performance of occupations and daily living activities. The client is asked to prioritize goals for intervention.

(continued)



Jacobs, K., & MacRae, N. (Eds.).
*Occupational Therapy Essentials for Clinical Competence, Third Edition* (pp. 217-231).

**KEY VOCABULARY (CONTINUED)**

- **Occupational therapy process:** A multistep clinical reasoning approach conducted by the occupational therapy practitioner. Based on a select model and/or frame(s) of reference, the occupational therapist conducts an occupational profile followed by relevant assessments to formulate an intervention plan. The evaluation and intervention process includes a collaborative client-centered process to determine therapeutic outcomes. An ongoing review of the therapeutic process is necessary to promote best practice outcomes.
- **Theoretical constructs:** Visible and nonvisible ideas and explanations that constitute a concept as parts of a theory.
- **Therapeutic use of self:** A practitioner's intuitive nature that derives from one's personality traits, self-awareness and personal experiences, understanding of human behavior, and observations through the use of the five senses. The practitioner makes conscious use of this nature to engage and affect a therapeutic relationship and foster a meaningful experience for the client.

Occupational therapy is a unique profession with its own specialized therapeutic process. Occupational therapists influence a person's health, well-being, and participation through positive engagement in occupations (American Occupational Therapy Association [AOTA], 2014). While the *Occupational Therapy Practice Framework* document (2014) outlines a linear depiction of the evaluation and intervention process, service delivery is actually more fluid and less predictable in real practice. In essence, practitioners conduct a series of steps in a collaborative manner to seek the best functional outcome for their clients. Occupational therapists respond to the ever-changing data generated by their clients on a daily basis and constantly modify intervention outcomes to ensure best practice.

Beginning with the evaluation phase of service delivery, an occupational therapist's focus is multifaceted. A practitioner's first step in therapy is to complete an occupational profile to learn about a client's wants and needs, problems, and concerns from the person's point of view. Next is an analysis of occupational performance. During this second step, practitioners extrapolate data about a client's performance abilities, patterns, and skills, including supports and barriers within a person's environment and contexts. Practitioners carefully select outcome measures that are used to further assess and gather data for clinical interpretation. An intervention plan is designed collaboratively with the client, highlighting identified outcomes that will enhance occupational performance and overall function. Intervention implementation can now begin with the full understanding that revisions will be made and refined as a client progresses through the therapy process. Occupational therapy practitioners have specialized knowledge and skills to provide a variety of modalities and interventions, all the while monitoring the person's response. Interventions are reevaluated for their effectiveness, and a review of a client's performance will determine if outcomes have been met. Although outcomes are the end result of the occupational therapy process (AOTA, 2014, p. S16), they need to be determined very early in the therapeutic process to guide a practitioner's clinical reasoning. Not only are practitioners responsible to select meaningful outcomes but also to know how to use them to measure progress. The management of effective outcomes includes the refinement of goals and interventions on an ongoing basis. Assessing outcomes data is also needed to make future decisions about the client's life, such as with discharge planning.

It is both hard to describe and learn the complex nature of the evaluation and intervention process in occupational therapy. Basic tenets, derived from theory, guide a practitioner's clinical and professional reasoning in the decision-making process, selection, and delivery of occupational therapy outcomes. In an academic curriculum, students are introduced to the many theories that influence practice. Following graduation, it remains the professional responsibility of every practitioner to keep current with new theories and evidence-based practice approaches as they emerge over time. Understanding the abstract concepts of theory, and subsequently applying theoretical principles to practice, is a required foundational step in the formation of clinical reasoning. As one gains more direct experience and exposure to health care populations and environments, it becomes easier to see the connection between theory and practice.

Our educational standards of practice require that occupational therapy students learn and understand relevant theories, models, and frames of reference as a critical step in their professional development. Next is the ability to apply theoretical approaches to clients across the lifespan and within different practice environments. Joan Rogers was among the first to study clinical reasoning and speak to the complex mind of an occupational therapist (Rogers, 1983). Since her Slagle lecture in the 1980s, many expert practitioners have written about the unique nature of reasoning and thinking that is commonplace to our profession. As we fast forward to our Centennial Vision almost four decades later, we are called upon to become a powerful, widely known, science-driven, and evidence-based profession (AOTA, 2006). This goal can only be reached if we remain a theory-driven profession and conduct evidence-based studies that highlight effective and efficient therapeutic interventions.

In this chapter, the reader will be introduced to common occupational therapy models and frames of reference applicable for practice across the lifespan with different populations. Learning strategies are included to assist the reader to further understand and apply concepts from theory that directly affect practice (see the Evidence-Based Research Chart).

## Understanding Occupation-Based Models and Frames of Reference

How does one begin to learn and understand theories that influence the practice of occupational therapy when there are so many to choose from? This question has been asked by many a student and practitioner. As our occupational therapy scope of practice broadens to include new emerging practice areas and face the complexities of health care, practitioners will need a diverse repertoire of theories, models, and frames of reference from which to base clinical decisions. It serves as an advantage to know about various theories that can complement the changing landscape of populations, settings, and organizational issues within health care practice today.

Clinical reasoning includes the occupational therapist's ability to plan, direct, perform, and reflect on client care (Schell & Schell, 2008, p. 131). The first step in developing clinical reasoning is to study and comprehend the models and frames of reference that are instrumental to best practice. Occupational therapy students and novice practitioners characteristically rely heavily on theory to guide their therapeutic reasoning. Applying a rule-based procedural reasoning approach when making therapeutic decisions can compensate for a practitioner's limited clinical experience (Crepeau & Boyt Schell, 2003).

It is helpful to establish the key terms that organize theoretical knowledge. Understanding the language of theory is necessary to effectively meet the Accreditation Council for Occupational Therapy Education (ACOTE) Standards that are the focus for this chapter. Establishing a common set of definitions or key terms for theory has been one of the profession's greatest challenges. Terms are often used interchangeably in occupational therapy literature. Scholars have agreed to disagree about how to best label concepts that compose our organization of knowledge (Hagedorn, 2001). The terms and definitions included in this chapter are a proposed taxonomy, or classification system, as suggested by Cole and Tufano (2008).

*Theory* describes, explains, and predicts behavior; it helps us to understand the relationship among concepts or events. There are varying degrees and levels of theory. At first, all theories start out as hypothetical guesses. A well-founded theory includes the systematic gathering of data with observation and experimental testing.

*Occupation-based models* are also referred to as *overarching theories* (Dunn, 2000), *conceptual models* (Reed & Sanderson, 1999), or *occupation-based frameworks* (Baum & Christiansen, 2005). These models help to explain the relationship among the person, the environment, and occupational engagement. Occupation-based models help to define the unique role of occupational therapy practitioners and explain how to enhance and promote health and well-being as related to occupational performance and participation. These models also provide the practitioner with guidelines on how to prevent occupational disruptions from occurring across the lifespan.

*Frames of reference*, another type of theory, are based on a system of compatible concepts that guide a plan of action for a specific occupational therapy domain of concern (Mosey, 1986). Frames of reference can be directly applied to address client factors of clinical concern and include whenever possible, the remediation of occupational performance areas, patterns, and skills. This group of theories tends to have more of a disability or problem-based focus. Frames of reference are not suited for all clients and have a limited focus or scope for application that addresses specific body functions and client factors.

Commonly used occupation-based models and frames of reference found in practice will be introduced in this chapter. Continued reading and study will undoubtedly be needed to promote further depth of understanding, analysis, and application to practice.

## Summary of Occupation-Based Models

As discussed in the previous chapter, occupation-based models are designed to focus the attention of practitioners on the nature of occupations and the interdependent relationship that ensues among person, occupation, and environment. Theoretical concepts are often depicted in flow charts that help us to visually see the interactive effect of various components. Common

Table 16-1.

**LIST OF OCCUPATION-BASED MODELS**

| Model | Author | Focus of Concern for Occupational Therapy Practice |
|---|---|---|
| Occupational Behavior | Reilly, 1969 | To prevent and reduce the disruptions and incapacities in occupational behavior that result from injury and illness; health and well-being is represented by a balance of occupational behavior in self-care, work, and leisure/play |
| Model of Human Occupation | Kielhofner & Burke, 1980, 1995, 2002, 2008 | Conceptualized the interactive and cyclical nature of human interaction with one's environment; interplay between person and environment is critical to one's source of motivation, patterns of behavior, and performance |
| Occupational Adaptation | Schkade & Schultz, 1992 | A framework that describes a normal human phenomenon, called adaptation, and its impact on the interactive process between a person and his or her occupational environment |
| Ecology of Human Performance | Dunn, Brown, & McGuigan, 1994 | The interdependent and transactional relationship among a person, his or her context, and the desired task is significant to one's overall performance range within the areas of activities of daily living, work and productive activities, education, leisure/play, and social participation |
| Person-Environment-Occupation Performance | Christiansen & Baum, 1991, 1997, 2005, 2015 | This model views the interdependent and complex relationship among persons and the environment that lead to occupational performance; participation in occupations and personal well-being are enhanced when such factors are optimally congruent to each other |

features among these overarching theories may be summarized in the following ways:

- All are founded by occupational therapists
- All have their roots in broader theories including humanism, holism, general systems, normal development, behavioral and social psychology, and anthropology
- All are client centered
- All provide guidelines for the evaluation and intervention process
- All emphasize the promotion of health and well-being through occupational performance

Table 16-1 represents an inventory of five such models in chronological order. The first occupation-based model was founded by Mary Reilly. She has been credited by many proponents in our profession as the catalyst for the paradigm shift back to occupation during a decade when practice was much more medical-model focused and reductionistic (Kielhofner, 1997). Reilly is famous for her quote: "Man, through the use of his hands as they are energized by his mind and will, can influence the state of his own health" (Reilly, 1962, p. 2). This statement became a consistent premise among all the occupation-based models that soon followed. Reilly also emphasized that the practice of occupational therapy should be guided by theory. She invited practitioners to base their clinical reasoning on organized knowledge (Reilly, 1958). In 1969, Reilly introduced her theory model called *occupational behavior.* This was the first attempt of our profession to promote a general theory for occupational therapy practice. Kielhofner and Burke, originally two students of Mary Reilly, expanded upon the concepts of occupational behavior through further study. These efforts led to the Model of Human Occupation, or MOHO for short.

Kielhofner and his colleagues published MOHO for the first time in 1980 (Kielhofner, 1980a, 1980b; Kielhofner & Burke, 1980; Kielhofner, Burke, & Heard, 1980). MOHO has continued to flourish as a practice model for occupational therapy through the collaborative efforts and substantial studies that have emerged over several decades. Revisions of MOHO occurred in 1995, 2002, and 2008. A randomized survey sent to 1,000 occupational therapists determined that over 80% of therapists use MOHO as their theoretical base for practice (Lee, Taylor, & Kielhofner, 2009). MOHO uniquely proposes a systems view of occupational performance, including the interdependent effect among a person's internal variables and external environmental contexts. This model explains how a person's internal motivation, routines and habits, and performance capacity interact with external feedback from one's physical and social contexts. The external environment affects an individual both positively and negatively, meaning it can facilitate occupational performance or constrain it (Kielhofner, 1997). A person's occupational identity and occupational competency emerges from this complementary relationship among internal and external variables. In summary, MOHO attempts to show the complexities that exist within each person and the role of the environment in shaping one's occupational performance throughout the lifespan. "Through participation in therapeutic occupations, persons transform themselves into more adaptive and healthy beings" (Kielhofner & Barrett, 1997, pp. 204-205).

Mary Reilly also identified another significant construct that influenced the future development of occupation-based models. She believed that as a person is naturally challenged to deal with everyday tasks in life, there is an opportunity to adapt. The adaptation process has had a sustained level of clinical interest among occupational therapists throughout history. Schkade and Schultz first published their Occupational Adaptation model in 1992, describing a comprehensive systems view about the complex nature of the adaptation process as seen in occupational therapy. A central premise to this model is the assumption that as persons become more adaptive, they will become more functional (Schkade & Shultz, 1992). Persons with disrupted or inadequate occupational performance are believed to have a faulty adaptation process at the core. This model focuses on two important phenomena within a complex cycle. Occupational Adaptation begins by labeling the components of adaptation from a normal developmental perspective. Subsequently, the model shows how occupational performance and adaptation are intricately related. Occupational therapists can plan, guide, and implement interventions on various levels to support a person's adaptation while engaging in occupations (Schkade & McClung, 2001). Occupations are a central tool for affecting one's adaptive nature. The Occupational Adaptation model is different from other models in how it defines functional outcomes. Emphasis is on improving adaptation of the individual; a direct change in a person's adaptability will ultimately lead to a change in his or her overall occupational performance.

Dunn, Brown, and McGuigan (1994) identified several issues of professional concern relative to the models of practice that preceded the 1990s. These authors believed that there was not enough attention given to the role of context in occupational therapy practice. Dunn et al. (1994) also drew attention to the benefits of an interdisciplinary relationship among occupational therapy practitioners, educators within school systems, and rehabilitation specialists. As a result, the Ecology of Human Performance (1994) was designed as a model that focused on the interdependent and transactional relationship among a person, his or her context, and the desired task that could be applied not only by occupational therapists but by rehabilitation specialists as well. Tasks are defined as "objective sets of behaviors necessary to accomplish a goal" (Dunn et al., 1994, p. 599). Everyone has a performance range, meaning the number and types of tasks available, that emerges and changes over time. A person's performance range is best understood when observing an individual performing a task within his or her natural context. Healthy functioning includes a high performance range that meets the demands of one's context or environment. Dunn et al. (1994) identified five intervention strategies for occupational therapy application. These strategies were embedded into the *Framework* (AOTA, 2014) and continue to guide the occupational therapy intervention process of today. Here is a listing of the intervention strategies that originated from this model.

1. Create and foster health promotion
2. Establish, remediate, and restore skills or abilities
3. Maintain performance capacities to meet occupational needs
4. Modify contexts and/or activity demands as a form of compensation or adaptation
5. Prevent disability in persons who are at risk for occupational performance problems

The Ecology of Human Performance emerged in a decade that produced the ADA with its focus on social justice at its early stages. Appreciating ecology and advocating for occupational justice are current initiatives in our profession's most recent paradigm shift, namely community integration and practice (Scaffa & Reitz, 2014).

The most current occupation-based model to be published is the Person-Environment-Occupation Performance model. Originating in 1991 by Charles Christiansen and Carolyn Baum, it was updated in 1997, 2005, and most recently 2015. The Person-Environment-Occupation Performance model integrates biomedical science and sociocultural factors from a systems-based perspective. Occupational performance is defined as the doing of meaningful activities, tasks, and roles through complex interactions between the person and environment (Baum, Christiansen, & Bass, 2015). Participation, or active engagement in occupations, results in well-being for individuals and communities alike. Person-Environment-Occupation Performance is considered an ecological, transactional theory meaning that any change in one's capacities, occupational choices, or environmental features could potentially affect outcomes in occupational performance (Baum et al., 2015). Emphasis is placed on client centeredness through a top-down orientation. A client's narrative and occupational history significantly shape the evaluation and intervention process including the identification of problems to be addressed in an intervention plan. Person-Environment-Occupation Performance has been expanded to provide foundational knowledge of interdependent factors that lead to occupational performance as related to individuals, organizations, and population levels (Baum et al., 2015).

## Summary of Frames of Reference

A frame of reference is defined as "a set of interrelated, internally consistent concepts, definitions, and postulates derived from or compatible with empirical data (theory) that provides a systematic description of or prescription for particular designs of the environment for the purpose of facilitating evaluation and effecting change relative to a specified part of the profession's domain of concern" (Mosey, 1986, p. 12). All frames of reference include the following components:

- A clearly defined domain or focus of concern for occupational therapy application
- A listing of compatible concepts derived from broad or meta theories that explain possible causes and/or contributing factors for function and dysfunction patterns
- A definition of how persons demonstrate traits, behaviors, attitudes, and emotions that reflect function and dysfunction according to each theoretical perspective
- A listing of assumptions about how occupational therapy might assist clients in promoting therapeutic change as well as enhancing motivation for engagement in meaningful occupations
- A plan of action meant to guide occupational therapists in the evaluation and intervention process
- Evidence gathered by researchers about the validity of the theoretical concepts outlined and the effectiveness of the techniques used by practitioners according to its guidelines

A brief summary of common frames of reference used in occupational therapy practice is provided next. This list is not all inclusive, as there are many useful and legitimate frames of reference that a practitioner may find relevant for current practice. It is recommended that the reader further explore each of the frames of reference for a more comprehensive understanding by consulting Cole and Tufano (2008), as well as other original publications cited at the end of this chapter.

The psychodynamic frame of reference in occupational therapy encompasses concepts from object relations, ego psychology, humanism, and human spirituality (Bruce & Borg, 2002). Psychodynamic theory has shaped our professional identity, which is based on the humanistic philosophy, as well as provided a theoretical foundation for mental health practice. Since its inception in the early 1900s, occupational therapy has had a long-standing relationship with psychiatry and psychodynamic theories. Eleanor Clarke Slagle's first role as an "occupation therapist" began with persons who had a mental illness. Many occupational therapy scholars have created assessments and intervention groups based on psychodynamic theories. The Azimas (1959) first recognized the therapeutic value of creative activities such as art, music, poetry, drama, dance, and clay/sculpting, also known as *projective techniques*. Gail Fidler (1969), who designed the first task group, emphasized the role of the unconscious in task completion and viewed activities as a means to effectively gratify instinctual needs. Lela Llorens (1966) designed a group program to enhance ego-adaptive skills for children who had experienced trauma. Anne Mosey (1986) founded the analytical frame of reference, which she defined as a "structure for linking psychoanalytic theories, the symbolic potential and reality aspects of activities, and the process of altering intrapsychic content in the direction of providing a more adaptive basis for interaction with the environment." Many facets of psychodynamic theory continue to be currently researched. One example of a modern intervention based on object relations theory is pet therapy. The study of attachment theory continues to be another area of heightened interest in the practice of mental health.

Behavioral frames of reference are represented by a continuum of theories beginning with behavior modification and ending with cognitive behavioral therapy. This group of theories applies the scientific method to human behavior, focusing on the external features of human functioning that can be observed and measured. Significant theorists and contributors to this theory group include Skinner (operant conditioning), Pavlov (classical conditioning), and Bandura (social learning theory). Ann Mosey (1970, 1986) adapted behavioral principles for occupational therapy in her acquisitional frame of reference. The inclusion of behavioral principles are readily found in our practice and often applied for populations with developmental disabilities, school-based populations, autism, various mental disorders, and brain injury. Examples of intervention approaches include applied behavioral analysis, skills training, psychoeducational groups, relaxation training, biofeedback, and systematic desensitization. The common use of reinforcement to increase desired behaviors is a behavioral principle often used in conjunction with other theoretical approaches. Occupational therapy intervention plans include the use of behavioral goals and objectives that are observable and measurable. Royeen and Duncan (1999) have also noted a recent resurgence in behavioral principles to facilitate motor and cognitive skills for children based on Mosey's acquisitional theory.

The biomechanical frame of reference applies the principles of physics to human movement and posture with respect to the forces of gravity. It is a popular theoretical framework for many practitioners who work in rehabilitation and can be applied to both children and adults. It is commonly used with musculoskeletal disorders, cumulative trauma such as back injuries or carpal tunnel syndrome, hand injuries, work hardening, and ergonomics. Intervention focus includes remediation and improvements in strength, range of motion, and endurance. Biomechanical principles guide the design of splints, adaptive seating, and the design and use of prosthetic devices. An example of how this theory can be applied to practice includes positioning of children with motor and postural difficulties to promote engagement in activities and increase occupational functioning (Colangelo, 1999).

Toglia's Dynamic Interactional model to cognitive rehabilitation (2005) has its foundation in neuroscience and its application guidelines within the theory of occupation. Occupational therapists apply this theoretical approach for persons with brain injuries to promote restoration of functional performance. It is based on the central premise that cognitive function is dynamic, context dependent, and modifiable. The Dynamic Interactional model is a complex, systems-based theory with two primary goals for intervention: to remediate skills and to compensate for loss of functioning. Cognitive change depends on the client's ability to learn and generalize information. Enhancing a person's self-awareness about that person's disability and promoting processing strategies are inherent in the therapy process.

Allen's Cognitive Disabilities frame of reference has been updated by Levy (2005) and renamed the Cognitive Disabilities Reconsidered model (Levy, 2005; Levy & Burns, 2006). The six clinically defined cognitive levels and 52 cognitive modes, originally designed by Allen, offer occupational therapists some of the best detailed guidelines for assessing, assisting, and adapting environments for persons with cognitive disabilities. This frame of reference focuses on the role of cognition (a process skill), the role of habits and routines, the effect of physical and social contexts, and the analysis of activity demand. It is often applied for persons with developmental disabilities, dementias, and chronic mental illness such as schizophrenia.

The developmental frames of reference are concerned with establishing or restoring client-chosen, age-appropriate occupations for promotion of meaningful life roles. The occupational therapy profession has continuously been influenced by many developmental theories reflecting childhood (Erikson & Erikson, 1997; Gesell & Armatruda, 1967; Kohlberg, 1973; Piaget, 1972), adulthood (Gilligan, 1982; Levinson, 1978), and aging (Atchley, 1976; Havighurst, 1961; Laslett, 1991). Theories based on neuromaturation include the works of Ayres (1974), King (1974), and the Bobaths (1990), while more generalist views were defined by Llorens (1966) and Mosey (1986). Health conditions and injuries often affect normal development. A practitioner using this approach is concerned with providing a growth-facilitating environment for the stimulation of age-appropriate behavior and skill learning. It is most important to consider the client's view when establishing an intervention plan.

Sensorimotor frames of reference in occupational therapy have been applied to children, adults with mental health conditions, and older adults. Commonly used approaches include Ayres's sensory integration (Bundy, Lane, & Murray, 2002), Dunn's sensory processing (Dunn, 2001), sensory defensiveness (Wilbarger & Wilbarger, 2002), and Ross's five-stage group (Ross & Bachner, 2004). Neuroscientists define sensory integration as the brain's ability to organize sensory information from the body and environment and to produce an adaptive response. Within each of these approaches, interventions are provided by occupational therapists through guided sensory input on a one-on-one or group activity basis.

The next grouping of theories is referred to as motor control and motor learning frames of reference (Cole & Tufano, 2008). Motor control considers one's ability to regulate or direct the mechanisms essential to movement (Shumway-Cook & Woollacott, 2012). Traditional examples of motor control theories include Bobaths' (1990) Neurodevelopmental Treatment, Rood's (1954) sensorimotor approach, Knott and Voss's (1968) Proprioceptive Neuromuscular Facilitation, and Brunnstrom's (1970) movement therapy. Principles of normal neurological development are considered in a reflex-hierarchical or neuromaturational sequence for establishing or restoring functional movement. Motor learning is a process-oriented theory that focuses on repetition, practice, and/or experience in the development of skilled movement (Schmidt & Lee, 2011). Fitts and Posner (1967) defined a three-stage sequential approach to learning that includes cognitive, association, and automatic phases of development. Practitioners strategically provide feedback, in both intrinsic and extrinsic forms, as a critical influence to motor learning. Two types of feedback include knowledge of results and knowledge of performance. Recent models have focused on how movement emerges from the interactive relationship among an individual, the environment, and the task. These client-centered task-oriented frames of reference have an occupation-based focus and incorporate current evidence in neuroscience. Examples include Horak (1991), Carr and Shepherd (1998, 2003), and Bass-Haugen et al. (2008). Motor learning theories currently provide guidelines for restoring functional movement with clients who have a broad range of health conditions. Task accomplishment is the ultimate goal or outcome of therapy. Occupational therapy intervention focuses on assisting clients in developing the optimal motor and cognitive strategies for achieving their functional goals (Cole & Tufano, 2008).

## How to Use Models and Frames of Reference for Occupational Therapy Evaluation and Intervention Process

The process of service delivery is challenging for anyone working in health care today. Most practitioners implement a variety of assessment tools and intervention strategies within their practice. What do theoretical models and frames of reference have to do with the day-to-day delivery of service? Is it OK to rely on more than one theoretical perspective at the same time? While it may appear comfortable for practitioners to rely on familiar therapeutic approaches one may have used over and over again, new research data continue to provide evidence for best-practice approaches. An eclectic practitioner would select "... a method or approach that is composed of elements drawn from various sources" (*Merriam-Webster's Online Dictionary,* n.d.). Imagine if you only had five outfits in your closet to wear every day, regardless of weather conditions in the environment, your internal mood, your external body shape, or the dress occasion. Would you describe your choices as "familiar and comfortable" or "limiting and outdated"? While specializing in one theory approach may seem initially comfortable, like wearing an old pair of shoes, it can also limit the practitioner's ability to be most effective within today's complex health care demands. Not every theory is an appropriate fit for every client; rather, theory should be considered on an individual basis. In like manner, not every theory may be a good match for every occupational therapist. Allowing oneself more choices from a theoretical repertoire, rather than less, in the selection of evaluation and intervention options will increase the likelihood of reaching mutual and desired outcomes. As practitioners, we can look to the *Framework* (AOTA, 2014) for guidance on how to select and apply theory to practice.

The *Framework* (2014) serves as our professional guide, describing how practitioners can integrate theory into the scope of occupational therapy practice. Occupational therapy educational standards of practice emphasize that students must learn how theory serves as the foundation for the evaluation and intervention process. The bridge of applying knowledge to practice is not an easy path of discovery. It must be a deliberate and conscious effort. The following statements represent a summary of suggestions based on both the *Framework* and this author's practical experience for how to use occupation-based models and frames of reference for best-practice outcomes.

Occupation-based models and frames of reference can assist the practitioner in the following ways:

- To understand data and formulate hypotheses about a client's occupational performance issues gathered initially from an occupational profile interview process
- To guide the practitioner in selecting relevant assessments for further data collection
- To create a therapeutic framework for interpreting data and forming initial conclusions about a person's occupational performance within this perspective
- To create collaborative goals with specific outcome measures that are based on sound and rational constructs from theory rather than one's opinion
- To develop an intervention plan for the client utilizing interventions based on best practice and evidence as supported by various models and frames of reference

In summary, the application of theory is a reasoning process that can frame a client's occupational needs and wants as determined from the occupational profile along with the practitioner's analysis of a client's occupational performance (AOTA, 2014). While these two components are significant aspects of a collaborative therapeutic process, there are also other factors that will influence the quality of occupational therapy outcomes. The delivery of occupational therapy services is as much an art as it is a science. It is the practitioner's personality, insights, perceptions, and judgments, also defined as *therapeutic use of self* (AOTA, 2014), that allow the practitioner to form a healthy relationship with clients and affect positive outcomes.

## How to Apply Theoretical Constructs in the Evaluation and Intervention Process

So far, we have identified and introduced five common occupation-based models and eight classifications of frames of reference. As previously noted, the process of integrating theory into practice is a multistep process. Each theory is complex, with intricate levels of related ideas and its own set of terminology. It is common for students to struggle with such abstract concepts; after all, a theory cannot be seen, only understood.

The first step within this clinical reasoning process is to learn each of the models and/or frames of reference individually. A template designed by Cole and Tufano (2008) is provided to assist the reader in gathering key concepts about each model and frame of reference (Table 16-2). The template is based on Mosey's original definition of a frame of reference and how knowledge is organized within this body of knowledge. Categories listed on the left side of the template reflect the various related

Table 16-2.

**TEMPLATE FOR ANALYSIS OF OCCUPATION-BASED MODELS AND FRAMES OF REFERENCE**

| Model or Frame of Reference | Analysis |
|---|---|
| **Focus**<br>Includes the population suited for and domains of practice according to the *Framework* | |
| **Theorists**<br>Includes authors and related theorists who have contributed to this body of knowledge | |
| **Theoretical base**<br>Includes defined compatible constructs that explain possible causes and/or contributing factors for function and dysfunction | |
| **Function**<br>Explains how this theory defines healthy or optimal functioning | |
| **Dysfunction**<br>Explains how this theory defines incapacities or barriers to functioning | |
| **Change**<br>Describes the process for how change is likely to occur according to this theory | |
| **Motivation**<br>Considers the motivating factors that inspire a client to change according to this theory | |
| **Assessment**<br>Identifies both formal and/or informal assessments specifically created or recommended according to this theory | |
| **Intervention guidelines**<br>Describes specific therapeutic techniques or strategies associated with theoretical outcomes based on this theory | |
| **Research**<br>Describes to what extent this theory been validated through research | |

Adapted from Cole, M., & Tufano, R. (2008). *Applied theories in occupational therapy.* Thorofare, NJ: SLACK Incorporated.

parts, or constructs, commonly found in each theory. The student is encouraged to complete this template on each model and/or frame of reference by filling in one section at a time. Further study of references cited at the end of this chapter may be needed to fully complete the template. Students should initially gather and identify the many concepts that compose each theory as identified by each section of the template. A completed template can serve as a study guide and assist the student at a glance to view the overall picture of the theory.

The second learning step is to be able to compare and contrast each model and/or frame of reference to another. The process of distinguishing one theory from another simulates what practitioners do in daily practice. Every practitioner must use clinical judgment in determining best-practice interventions. This reasoning process begins by gathering client data and relying on theoretical explanations to form hypotheses about a client's occupational performance.

Crepeau and Boyt Schell (2003) point out that the major theories in our profession differ in purpose, scope, complexity, extent of development and validation through research, and usefulness in practice (p. 204). In fact, practitioners apply the various levels of theory at different stages of the evaluation, intervention, and outcomes continuum. The occupation-based models help practitioners to develop a perspective on how the client, who engages within a particular environment, is participating in occupations. Constructs from these models relate well to aspects of the *Framework* and the occupational profile because of their holistic and client-centered orientation. Constructs are also rooted in occupational therapy language and theory because each model is authored by an occupational therapist. These models help to identify the range of possibilities when setting collaborative goals for client engagement in occupations as well as identifying barriers to participation. In addition, occupation-based models help us determine ways in which our clients can find meaningful roles in society.

Frames of reference enter the clinical reasoning process as the occupational therapist thinks about problem areas identified by a client. They specifically target select components of the *Framework* such as performance areas, skills patterns, and, most often, client factors. For example, Allen's Cognitive Disability frame of reference specifically addresses the following aspects within the *Framework*: activities of daily living performance areas; process performance skills; the performance patterns of habits, routines, and roles; and client factors defined as mental functions.

Crepeau and Boyt Schell (2003) describe how advanced practitioners tend to incorporate theory into their reasoning process in ways that allow them to use it automatically (i.e., without conscious awareness). Thus, expert occupational therapists may not always be able to articulate the model or frame of reference that they are using. This does not mean that they are not using theory, but rather that its use has become habitual and integrated into their professional reasoning. On the other hand, students who are in the beginning stages of clinical reasoning development may get distracted by their own subjective feelings related to performance anxiety.As novices, it is important to consciously think about procedures and make clinical choices based on objective information deduced from various theoretical approaches (Cole & Tufano, 2008).

Occupational therapy assistants are expected to know about the various occupation-based models and frames of reference used in occupational therapy practice. Understanding these theories will enhance the ability of occupational therapy assistants to have a more comprehensive view of working with a client. As part of their role delineation, occupational therapy assistants are not required to apply the theoretical constructs to practice. Rather, occupational therapy assistants will take direction from the registered occupational therapist on what model and/or frame of reference to employ when providing intervention strategies.

## Summary

The process of understanding relevant occupational therapy theories is often a challenge for students, academicians, and practitioners alike. This chapter attempts to demystify the process for learning about various theories by highlighting common occupation-based models and frames of reference found in current practice. The five occupational therapy models mentioned here represent a holistic, client-centered, and universal application to persons across the lifespan and across all domains of practice. These models support the current health care trend toward prevention of disease and promotion of health, with emphasis on occupational performance. Each model provides a list of guidelines for the occupational therapy practitioner within the evaluation and intervention process. They pose a direct contrast to the frames of reference that are much more prescriptive and specific in nature. Generally speaking, frames of reference are oriented toward restoring, adapting, and/or compensating for the loss of occupational functioning. In their own unique way, these theories are limited in their application scope, each targeting a specific focus of concern within practice. Unlike the occupation-based models, specific assessments, techniques, and strategies are prescribed by each frame of reference for use in the evaluation and intervention process.

As a profession, we look to the *Framework* for guidance on how these models and frames of reference assist the practitioner in the therapeutic process. The art and science of occupational therapy practice includes a two-prong evaluative approach. First, we assess a client's occupational needs while we also consider the practitioner's objective analyses of a client's performance. The delivery of occupational therapy service is an evolving, interactive process affected by both the practitioner's therapeutic use of self and the personality traits of the client. Practitioners need to balance their professional knowledge with the desires and needs of their clients in a collaborative relationship.

It is common for professions such as occupational therapy to develop and consider multiple and often

## Case Example: John

John is a 58-year-old divorced male with two adult children. He is employed at a naval base where he works as a chief engineer. He lives alone in a nearby apartment and reports that his favorite pastime is "hanging out" with his old naval buddies at the local pub. "We look out for each other," John tells the occupational therapy practitioner, who notices missing teeth as he laughs out loud.

The client has been diagnosed with peripheral neuropathy due to chronic alcohol abuse. Recently hospitalized because he reported difficulty walking over a period of 4 months, John thought his "weak legs" were a result of a motorcycle fall that he sustained last year. "I never would have thought that a few beers a day would have given me sea legs!"

John is presently in a rehabilitation center. He is referred to occupational therapy for evaluation of activities of daily living, instrumental activities of daily living, work, rest/sleep, and social/leisure participation. His mood and motivation to recover vary on a daily basis. At times, he expresses sadness and regret about the "many mistakes I made in life." During his initial interview with the occupational therapist, he revealed that he always lived in the moment and hardly thought about the future consequences of his life decisions. "It is time for me to make my peace with my family and with God." Due to the recent health concerns, John has decided to pursue retirement. He wants to return to his second-floor apartment but worries about his ability to climb stairs and care for himself. "What am I going to do all day long?" he questions. John tells the occupational therapy practitioner, "My mind is not as sharp as it used to be. Last week, I left the oven on all night long. If something happens to me in the middle of the night, no one will even know that I am gone."

**Learning Activities**

- After reading the case, fill in as much information as you can gather about John's personal characteristics, his engagement in various occupations, and his social and physical environment. Make a point to identify both supportive factors for change and barriers within each of the three categories.

| Person | Environment | Occupations |
|---|---|---|
| | | |

- Refer to the case of John and identify strengths and concerns by completing the following chart. Consult the *Framework* for the definitions of each category as needed. Based on your knowledge so far about the different theories that serve as foundational knowledge for occupational therapy practice, which models and/or frames of reference would you select for occupational therapy evaluation and intervention for John? Briefly explain your rationale.

| | |
|---|---|
| Occupations (ADLs, IADLs, rest/sleep, education, work, social/leisure participation) | |
| Client factors such as values, beliefs, spirituality; body functions and body structures of concern | |
| Performance skills (motor, process, social interaction) | |
| Performance patterns (habits, routines, rituals, roles) | |
| Contexts and environments (cultural, personal, physical, social, temporal, virtual) | |

## Evidence-Based Research Chart

| Theoretical Foundation | Evaluation and/or Intervention Focus | Evidence |
|---|---|---|
| Occupational performance | Both | Humphry & Wakeford, 2006; Rebeiro, 2001; Rebeiro & Polgar, 1999; Trombly, 1995 |
| Therapeutic use of self | Both | Goulet, Rousseau, & Fortier, 2007; Maitra & Erway, 2006; Polatajko, Davis, & McEwen, 2015; Restall, Ripat, & Stern, 2003; Wilkins, Pollock, Rochon, & Law, 2001 |
| Person-Environment-Occupation Performance model | Both | Letts et al., 1994; Strong et al., 1999 |
| Model of Human Occupation | Both | Boisvert, 2004; Lee et al., 2008 |
| Occupational Adaptation | Both | Schkade & Schultz, 1992; Schultz & Schkade, 1992 |
| Ecology of Human Performance | Both | Dunn, Brown, & McGuigan, 1994; Lund & Nygard, 2004 |
| Frames of reference | Intervention | Capasso, Gorman, & Blick, 2010; Cicerone et al., 2000; Diller, 2005; Hart & Evans, 2006; Henderson, 1999; Jarus & Ratzon, 2005; Johnson & Schkade, 2001; Laatsch et al., 2007; Leichsenring, Hiller, Weissberg, & Leibing, 2006; Mastos, Miller, Eliasson, & Imms, 2007; Roley, Clark, Bissell, & Brayman, 2003; Schaaf & Miller, 2005; Shumway-Cook & Woollacott, 2012; Teasell, Foley, Bhogal, & Speechley, 2003; Watling & Dietz, 2007; Whedon, 2000 |

Reprinted with permission from Cole, M. B., & Tufano, R. (2008). *Applied theories in occupational therapy.* Thorofare, NJ: SLACK Incorporated.

contrasting ideas about practice outcomes. There are many theories from which to choose. For students, academicians, and practitioners inclusively, the process of becoming proficient at understanding and applying the various theoretical constructs for evaluation and intervention purposes takes time and effort. The process begins with learning the basics of each theory and understanding its intended therapeutic purpose. The ability to analyze and select the best theory option for a client requires that a practitioner have a repertoire of models and frames of reference to choose from. This decision-making process encompasses clinical reasoning—a process that is based on knowing what a theory says and how to use it. Understanding theoretical constructs, combined with applying these principles to simulated or real practical experience, fosters the development of clinical synthesis. As stated in our Centennial Vision, we have a professional responsibility to become more science driven. This includes conducting more research studies and basing our clinical decisions on evidence. The integration of theory must drive practice to validate our scope and sustain our unique role as occupational therapy practitioners within the professional world.

## Student Self-Assessment

1. How do today's complex health concerns affect a practitioner's need for theoretical knowledge?
2. How do occupation-based models support the trend toward health promotion and prevention of illness?
3. What are the pros and cons to practicing within a specialty area of occupational therapy versus practicing as a generalist?
4. What is your opinion about the following statements: "theory drives practice" and "practice drives theory"?
5. State some similarities and differences among the two theoretical classifications of practice discussed in this chapter: occupation-based models and frames of reference.
6. How has Mary Reilly influenced the profession of occupational therapy? Consider her quote, "Man, through the use of his hands as they are energized by his mind and will, can influence the state of his own health."
7. When is it appropriate to use more than one theoretical perspective for a given client in occupational therapy practice? Give a specific example.

## References


American Occupational Therapy Association. (2006). *Centennial Vision*. Retrieved from http://www.aota.org/News/Centennial/Background/36516.aspx

American Occupational Therapy Association. (2014). Occupational therapy practice framework: Domain and process (3rd ed.). *American Journal of Occupational Therapy, 68*(Suppl. 1), S1-S48. doi:10.5014/ajot.2014.682006

Atchley, R. C. (1976). *The sociology of retirement*. New York, NY: Halsted.

Ayres, A. J. (1974). *The development of sensory integrative theory and practice*. Dubuque, IA: Kendall Hunt.

Azima, H., & Azima, F. (1959). The therapeutic use of self. *American Journal of Occupational Therapy, 12*, 215-225.

Bass-Haugen, J., Mathiowetz, V., & Flinn, N. (2008). Optimizing motor behavior using the occupational therapy task-oriented approach. In L. Trombly & C. A. Radomski (Eds.), *Occupational therapy for physical dysfunction* (6th ed.). Baltimore, MD: Williams and Wilkins.

Baum, C. M., & Christiansen, C. H. (2005). Person-environment-occupation-performance: An occupation based framework for practice. In C. H. Christiansen, C. M. Baum, & J. Bass-Haugen (Eds.), *Occupational therapy: Performance, participation, and well-being* (3rd ed.). Thorofare, NJ: SLACK Incorporated.

Baum, C. M., Christiansen, C. H., & Bass, J. D. (2015). Person-environment-occupation-performance: An occupation based framework for practice. In C. H. Christiansen, C. M. Baum, & J. Bass-Haugen (Eds.), *Occupational therapy: Performance, participation, and well-being* (4th ed.). Thorofare, NJ: SLACK Incorporated.

Bobath, B. (1990). *Adult hemiplegia: Evaluation and treatment* (3rd ed.). London, England: Heinemann.

Boisvert, R. A. (2004). Enhancing substance dependence intervention. *Occupational Therapy Practice, 9*(10), 11-16.

Bruce, M. G., & Borg, B. (2002). *Psychosocial frames of reference: Core for occupation-based practice* (3rd ed.). Thorofare, NJ: SLACK Incorporated.

Bundy, A. C., Lane, S. J., & Murray, E. A. (2002). *Sensory integration: Theory and practice* (2nd ed.). Philadelphia, PA: F. A. Davis Company.

Capasso, N., Gorman, A., & Blick, C. (2010). Breakfast group in an acute rehabilitation setting: A restorative program for incorporating client's hemiparetic upper extremities for function. *Occupational Therapy Practice, 5*(8), 14-18.

Carr, J., & Shepherd, R. (1998). *Neurological rehabilitation: Optimizing motor performance*. Oxford, United Kingdom: Butterworth Heinemann.

Carr, J., & Shepherd, R. (2003). *Stroke rehabilitation: Guidelines for exercise and training to optimize motor skill*. Edinburgh, Scotland: Butterworth Heinemann.

Christiansen, C. H., & Baum, C. M. (1991). *Occupational therapy: Overcoming human performance deficits*. Thorofare, NJ: SLACK Incorporated.

Christiansen, C. H., & Baum, C. M. (1997). *Occupational therapy: Enabling function and well-being* (2nd ed.). Thorofare, NJ: SLACK Incorporated.

Cicerone, K. D., Dahlberg, C., Kalmar, K., Langenbahn, D. M., Malec, J. F., Bergquist, T. F., & Morse, P. A. (2000). Evidence-based cognitive rehabilitation: Recommendations for clinical practice. *Archives of Physical Medicine Rehabilitation, 81*(12), 159-615.

Colangelo, C. (1999). Biomechanical frame of reference. In P. Kramer & J. Hinojosa (Eds.), *Frames of reference for pediatric occupational therapy* (2nd ed., pp. 377-400). Philadelphia, PA: Lippincott Williams and Wilkins.

Cole, M., & Tufano, R. (2008). *Applied theories in occupational therapy*. Thorofare, NJ: SLACK Incorporated.

Crepeau, E., & Boyt Schell, B. (2003). Theory and practice in occupational therapy. In E. Crepeau, E. Cohn, & B. Schell (Eds.), *Willard and Spackman's occupational therapy* (10th ed.). Philadelphia, PA: Lippincott Williams and Wilkins.

Diller, L. (2005). Pushing the frames of reference in traumatic brain injury rehabilitation. *Archives of Physical Medicine Rehabilitation, 86*(6), 1075-1080.

Dunn, W. (2000). *Best practice occupational therapy: In community service with children and families*. Thorofare, NJ: SLACK Incorporated.

Dunn, W. (2001). The 2001 Eleanor Clarke Slagle lecture: The sensations of everyday life: Empirical, theoretical, and pragmatic considerations. *American Journal of Occupational Therapy, 55*, 608-620.

Dunn, W., Brown, C., & McGuigan, A. (1994). The ecology of human performance: A framework for considering the effect of context. *American Journal of Occupational Therapy, 48*, 595-607.

Eclectic. (n.d.). *Merriam-Webster Online Dictionary*. Retrieved from http://www.merriam-webster.com/dictionary/eclectic

Erikson, E. H., & Erikson, J. M. (1997). *The life cycle completed*. New York, NY: Norton.

Fidler, G. (1969). The task-oriented group as a context for treatment. *American Journal of Occupational Therapy, XXIII*(1), 43-48.

Fitts, P. M., & Posner, M. I. (1967). *Human performance*. Belmont, CA: Brooks/Cole Publishers.

Gesell, A., & Armatruda, C. (1967). *Developmental diagnosis*. New York, NY: Harper and Row.

Gilligan, C. (1982). *A different voice*. Cambridge, MA: Harvard University Press.

Goulet, C., Rousseau, J., & Fortier, P. (2007). A literature review on perception of the providers and clients regarding the use of the client centered approach in psychiatry. *Canadian Journal of Occupational Therapy, 74*(3), 172-182.

Hagedorn, R. (2001). *Foundations for practice in occupational therapy* (3rd ed.). London, England: Churchill Livingstone.

Hart, T., & Evans, J. (2006). Self-regulation and goal theories in brain injury rehabilitation. *Journal of Head Trauma Rehabilitation, 21*(2), 142-155.

Havighurst, R. (1961). Successful aging. *The Gerontologist, 1*, 8-13.

Henderson, S. (1999). Frames of reference utilized in the rehabilitation of individuals with eating disorders. *Canadian Journal of Occupational Therapy, 66*(1), 43-51.

Horak, F. B. (1991). Assumptions underlying motor control for neurologic rehabilitation. In M. J. Lister (Ed.), *Contemporary management of motor control problems: Proceedings of the II STEP conference* (pp. 11-27). Alexandria, VA: Foundation for Physical Therapy.

Humphry, R., & Wakeford, L. (2006). An occupation-centered discussion of development and implications for practice. *American Journal of Occupational Therapy, 60*(3), 258-267.

Jarus, T., & Ratzon, N. Z. (2005). The implementation of motor learning principles in designing prevention programs at work. *WORK: A Journal of Prevention, Assessment and Rehabilitation, 24*, 171-182.

Johnson, J., & Schkade, J. K. (2001). Effects of occupation-based intervention on mobility problems following a cerebral vascular accident. *Journal of Applied Gerontology, 20*(1), 91-110.

Kielhofner, G. (1980a). A model of human occupation, part two. Ontogenesis from the perspective of temporal adaptation. *American Journal of Occupational Therapy, 34*, 657-663.

Kielhofner, G. (1980b). A model of human occupation, part three: Benign and vicious cycles. *American Journal of Occupational Therapy, 34*, 731-737.

Kielhofner, G. (1997). *Conceptual foundations of occupational therapy.* (2nd ed.). Baltimore, MD: Williams and Wilkins.

Kielhofner, G. (2008). *A model of human occupation: Theory and application* (4th ed). Baltimore, MD: Williams and Wilkins.

Kielhofner, G., & Barrett, L. (1997). An overview of occupational behavior. In H. Hopkins & H. Smith (Eds.), *Willard & Spackman's occupational therapy*. Philadelphia, PA: J. B. Lippincott.

Kielhofner, G., & Burke, J. (1980). A model of human occupation, part one: Conceptual framework and content. *American Journal of Occupational Therapy, 34*, 572-581.

Kielhofner, G., Burke, J., & Heard, I. C. (1980). A model of human occupation, part four: Assessment and intervention. *American Journal of Occupational Therapy, 34*, 777-788.

King, L. J. (1974). A sensory integrative approach to schizophrenia. *American Journal of Occupational Therapy, 28*, 529-536.

Knott, M., & Voss, D. E. (1968). *Proprioceptive neuromuscular facilitation* (2nd ed.). New York, NY: Harper & Row.

Kohlberg, L. (1973). Stages and aging in moral development: Some speculations. *The Gerontologist, 1*(3), 497-502.

Laatsch, L., Harrington, D., Hotz, G., Marcantuono, J., Mozzoni, M. P., Walsh, V., & Hersey, K. P. (2007). An evidence based review of cognitive and behavioral rehabilitation treatment studies in children with acquired brain injury. *Journal of Head Trauma Rehabilitation, 22*(4), 248-256.

Laslett, P. (1991). *A fresh map of life: The emergence of the third age*. Cambridge, MA: Harvard University Press.

Lee, S. W., Taylor, R. R., & Kielhofner, G. (2009). Choice, knowledge, and utilization of a practice theory: A national study of occupational therapists who use the Model of Human Occupation. *Occupational Therapy in Health Care, 23*(1), 60-71.

Lee, S. W., Taylor, R., Kielhofner, G. & Fisher, G. (2008). Theory use in practice: A national survey of therapists who use the Model of Human Occupation. *American Journal of Occupational Therapy, 62*(1), 106-117.

Leichsenring, F., Hiller, W., Weissberg, M., & Leibing, E. (2006). Cognitive-behavioral therapy and psychodynamic psychotherapy: Techniques, efficacy, and indications. *American Journal of Psychotherapy, 60*(3), 233-259.

Letts, L., Law, M., Rigby, P., Cooper, B., Stewart, D., & Strong, S. (1994). Person-environment assessments in occupational therapy. *American Journal of Occupational Therapy, 48*(7), 608-618.

Levinson, D. (1978). *The seasons of a man's life*. New York, NY: Ballantine Books.

Levy, L. L. (2005). Cognitive disabilities reconsidered: Rehabilitation of older adults with dementia. In N. Katz (Ed.), *Cognition and occupation across the life span: Models for intervention in occupational therapy*. Bethesda, MD: AOTA Press.

Levy, L. L., & Burns, T. (2006). Neurocognitive practice essentials in dementia: Cognitive disabilities-reconsidered model. *OT Practice, 11*(3), CE1-CE8.

Llorens, L. (1966). Occupational therapy in an ego-oriented milieu. *American Journal of Occupational Therapy, 20*, 178-181.

Lund, M. L., & Nygard, L. (2004). Occupational life in the home environment: The experience of people with disabilities. *Canadian Journal of Occupational Therapy, 71*, 243-252.

Maitra, K. K., & Erway, F. (2006). Perception of client-centered practice in occupational therapists and their clients. *American Journal of Occupational Therapy, 60*, 298-310.

Mastos, M., Miller, K., Eliasson, A. C., & Imms, C. (2007). Goal-directed training: Linking theories of treatment to clinical practice for improved functional activities in daily life. *Clinical Rehabilitation, 21*(1), 47-55.

Mosey, A. (1970). *Three frames of reference for mental health*. Thorofare, NJ: SLACK Incorporated.

Mosey, A. (1986). *Psychosocial components of occupational therapy*. New York, NY: Raven Press.

Piaget, J. (1972). *The psychology of the child*. New York, NY: Basic Books.

Polatajko, H. J., Davis, J. A., & McEwen, S. E. (2015). Therapeutic use of self: A catalyst in the client-therapist alliance for change. In C. H. Christiansen, C. M. Baum, & J. Bass-Haugen (Eds.), *Occupational therapy: Performance, participation, and well-being* (4th ed.). Thorofare, NJ: SLACK Incorporated.

Rebeiro, K. L. (2001). Enabling occupation: The importance of an affirming environment. *Canadian Journal of Occupational Therapy, 68*(2), 80-89.

Rebeiro, K. L., & Polgar, J. M. (1999). Enabling occupational performance: Optimal experiences in therapy. *Canadian Journal of Occupational Therapy, 66*(1), 14-22.

Reed, K. L, & Sanderson, S. N. (1999). *Concepts of occupational therapy* (4th ed.). Philadelphia, PA: Lippincott Williams and Wilkins.

Reilly, M. (1958). An occupational therapy curriculum for 1965. *American Journal of Occupational Therapy, 12*, 293-299.

Reilly, M. (1962). Occupational therapy can be one of the great ideas of 20th century medicine. *American Journal of Occupational Therapy, 16*, 1-9.

Restall, G., Ripat, J., & Stern, M. (2003). A framework of strategies for client-centered practice. *Canadian Journal of Occupational Therapy, 70*(2), 103-112.

Rogers, J. C. (1983). The Eleanor Clarke Slagle lecture: Clinical reasoning: The ethics, science and art. *American Journal of Occupational Therapy, 37*, 601-616.

Roley, S. S., Clark, G. F., Bissell, J., & Brayman, S. J., Commission on Practice. (2003). Applying sensory integration framework in educationally related occupational therapy practice. *American Journal of Occupational Therapy, 57*(6), 652-659.

Ross, M., & Bachner, S. (2004). *Adults with developmental disabilities: Current approaches in occupational therapy* (2nd ed.). Bethesda, MD: AOTA Press.

Royeen, C., & Duncan, M. (1999). Acquisitional frame of reference. In P. Kramer & J. Hinojosa (Eds.), *Frames of reference for pediatric occupational therapy* (2nd ed., pp. 377-400). Philadelphia, PA: Lippincott Williams and Wilkins.

Scaffa, M. E., & Reitz, S. M. (2014). *Occupational therapy in community-based practice settings* (2nd ed.). Philadelphia, PA: F. A. Davis Company.

Schaaf, R. C., & Miller, L. J. (2005). Occupational therapy using a sensory integrative approach for children with developmental disabilities. *American Journal of Occupational Therapy, 11*(2), 143-148.

Schell, B. A., & Schell, J. W. (2008). *Clinical and professional reasoning in occupational therapy*. Baltimore, MD: Lippincott Williams and Wilkins.

Schkade, J. K., & McClung, M. (2001). *Occupational adaptation in practice: Concepts and cases*. Thorofare, NJ: SLACK Incorporated.

Schkade, J. K., & Schultz, S. (1992). Occupational adaptation: Toward a holistic approach to contemporary practice, part 1. *American Journal of Occupational Therapy, 46*, 829-837.

Schmidt, R. A., & Lee, T. D. (2011). *Motor control and learning: A behavioral emphasis* (5th ed.). Champaign, IL: Human Kinetics.

Schultz, S., & Schkade, J. K. (1992). Occupational adaptation: Toward a holistic approach to contemporary practice, part 2. *American Journal of Occupational Therapy, 46*, 917-926.

Shumway-Cook, A., & Woollacott, M. (2012). *Motor control: Translating research into clinical practice* (4th ed.). Baltimore, MD: Lippincott Williams and Wilkins.

Strong, S., Rigby, P., Stewart, D., Law, M., Letts, L., & Cooper, B. (1999). Application of the person-environment-occupation model: A practical tool. *Canadian Journal of Occupational Therapy, 66*(3), 122-133.

Teasell, R. W., Foley, N. C., Bhogal, S. K., & Speechley, M. R. (2003). An evidence-based review of stroke rehabilitation. *Top Stroke Rehabilitation, 10*(1), 29-58.

Toglia, J. (2005). A dynamic interactional approach to cognitive rehabilitation. In N. Katz (Ed.), *Cognition and occupation in rehabilitation: Cognitive models for intervention in occupational therapy*. Bethesda, MD: AOTA Press.

Trombly, C. A. (1995). Occupation: Purposefulness and meaningfulness as therapeutic mechanisms. 1995 Eleanor Clarke Slagle lecture. *American Journal of Occupational Therapy, 49*(10), 960-972.

Watling, R. L., & Dietz, J. (2007). Immediate effect of Ayres's sensory integration-based occupational therapy intervention on children with autism spectrum disorders. *American Journal of Occupational Therapy, 61*(5), 574-583.

Whedon, C. A. (2000). Frames of reference that address the impact of physical environments on occupational performance. *WORK: A Journal of Prevention, Assessment and Rehabilitation, 14*(2), 165-174.

Wilbarger, J., & Wilbarger, P. (2002). The Wilbarger approach to treating sensory defensiveness. In A. Bundy, S. Lane, & E. Murray (Eds.), *Sensory integration: Theory and practice* (2nd ed.). Philadelphia, PA: F. A. Davis Company.

Wilkins, S., Pollock, N., Rochon, S., & Law, M. (2001). Implementing client-centered practice: Why is it so difficult to do? *Canadian Journal of Occupational Therapy, 68*(2), 70-79.

# IV

# Screening, Evaluation, and Referral

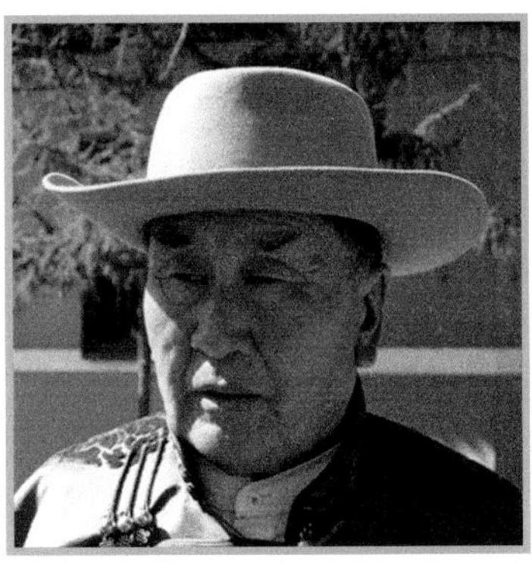

# 17

# SCREENING, EVALUATION, AND REFERRAL

*Jessica J. Bolduc, DrOT, MS, OTR/L*

## ACOTE STANDARDS EXPLORED IN THIS CHAPTER

B.4.1–B.4.3, B.4.5–B.4.10

## KEY VOCABULARY

- **Assessment:** Tools, instruments, procedures, or interactions used during the evaluation process.
- **Client:** The *Occupational Therapy Practice Framework* defines client as persons, groups, including families, caregivers, teachers, employers, and relevant others, and populations. (American Occupational Therapy Association, 2014a).
- **Criterion referenced:** A score from an assessment that can be compared to the skills or performance of a group rather than compared to a normative group (i.e., an assessment designed for children with cerebral palsy about motor performance is criterion referenced when compared to children who also have cerebral palsy rather than the general population of children).
- **Documentation:** A permanent legal record that records the client's occupational therapy service (i.e., evaluation, daily notes, progress notes, discharge).
- **Evaluation:** The process of obtaining and interpreting data necessary to understand the client and initiate treatment.
- **Norm referenced:** A score from an assessment that can be compared to the skills or performance of a "normative" group (e.g., adult grip strength).
- **Referral:** Recommendation for a client to receive occupational therapy; often required to initiate an occupational therapy evaluation.
- **Screening:** The process of gathering information to determine the client's skilled need for occupational therapy.

Jacobs, K., & MacRae, N. (Eds.).
*Occupational Therapy Essentials for Clinical Competence, Third Edition* (pp. 235-248).

The past decade has seen significant changes in the implementation and documentation of occupational therapy services. A variety of factors, both within and outside of our profession, have contributed to these changes. These factors include the view of health and disability in the *International Classification of Functioning, Disability and Health* by the World Health Organization (WHO, 2001), the need for evidence-based practice (American Occupational Therapy Association [AOTA], 2006; Arbesman, Lieberman, & Metzler, 2014), the health care system's mandate for efficiency, the implementation of the electronic medical record, and the publication and implementation of the *Occupational Therapy Practice Framework* (AOTA, 2014a).

With regard to the evaluation process specifically, what is considered to be best practice has led to dramatic improvement in the assessment tools available to practitioners to meet the current responsibilities of an occupational therapy evaluation. In addition to the previously available performance, skill, client-centered, and daily living assessments, the profession now has assessments with focused attention related to occupation, social participation, work, activities of daily living, instrumental activities of daily living, environment/context, educational performance, and play/leisure. This section serves to identify important concepts related to the occupational therapy evaluation process, including information related to each of the aforementioned assessment areas.

## Terms and Definitions

This section is designed to familiarize occupational therapy practitioners with the terms and components of the evaluation process as currently understood within the occupational therapy profession. It is important, however, for practitioners to realize that other professions might use the terms interchangeably or might define them differently. In fact, older occupational therapy texts have offered differing definitions than those described in this chapter because the occupational therapy profession has revised and clarified its understanding of these components over the years. It is important to clarify the occupational therapy perspective during team meetings, when sharing your occupational therapy evaluation results with other professions, or when (as occurs in some instances) preparing a comprehensive evaluation report that includes the work of several disciplines. Screening, assessment, evaluation, and documentation are discussed next.

## Screening

Most often screening will take place at the first occupational therapy encounter. This is a means by which the occupational therapy practitioner determines if further assessment is needed (AOTA, 2010; Sames, 2015). Therefore, intervention planning can never occur with screening information alone. Screening methods can be formal (e.g., a standardized screening instrument or an organization's intake form) or informal (e.g., chart review, interview of a teacher, or the observation of a client). Please refer to A Reason to Screen and to screening examples on the following page.

Although the *Framework* does not specifically discuss the screening process, it is an important component in many institutions. Reasons to complete a screen include the belief that potential problems that could be identified can be addressed by effective and timely occupational therapy interventions (Sames, 2015). Whereas the more experienced practitioner might easily observe a client (informal screen) and determine if additional testing is required, the novice practitioner might need more formalized methods to help determine if a potential difficulty in occupational performance is present. In fact, some might argue that when formalized methods of screening are used, the results factor into the practitioner's clinical decision-making process and form the basis of the occupational therapy evaluation. Screening results are included in the evaluation report as one of the processes used for obtaining information. Occupational therapy assistants can add to the screening information, but only the occupational therapist can determine if further services are needed (Sames, 2015).

## Assessment

Once the need for a comprehensive evaluation is determined, specific assessment tools can be used based on the information deemed necessary and the environment in which the client's occupational performance is limited. If a formalized screening was not completed, the informal methods of chart review and interview (e.g., client profile) would be an appropriate starting point in the evaluation process. Appropriate assessment tools can be identified and implemented by the occupational therapist or the occupational therapy assistant. Although the occupational therapist directs and initiates the evaluation process, the two practitioners can collaboratively determine which assessment(s) can be administered by the occupational therapy assistant based on professional experience, training, establishment of competency, and level of supervision provided. Per the *Guidelines for Supervision, Roles, and Responsibilities During the Delivery of Occupational Therapy Services* (AOTA, 2014b)

## A Reason to Screen

Mrs. Simon, a first-grade elementary school teacher, bumped into Sam, an occupational therapist, in the teachers' lounge. Mrs. Simon and Sam have worked together in the past with previous students. She immediately thought of Mary, a current student who was struggling in class. Mrs. Simon asked if Sam could "just take a look" at Mary. Because the school district had a pre-referral program to assist children within the general education system prior to referral for special education services, Sam asked Mrs. Simon to complete the paperwork that would allow him to review Mary's educational history, observe Mary in the classroom, and send a questionnaire home to Mary's parents.

Upon record review, Mary has been having difficulty since preschool with her fine motor skills and how she organizes educational materials. This was also confirmed via the parent questionnaire. Within the classroom, Mary was observed to sit under her desk with her hands over her ears during morning announcements over the public address system, watch how other children were completing assignments before beginning herself, and rarely finished her workbook assignments within the allotted time. This screening information was sufficient for recommending a complete evaluation to determine Mary's specific difficulties so that an effective occupational therapy intervention plan might be developed. The evaluation report ultimately included these occupational difficulties as examples of the client and contextual factors that interfered with Mary's successful engagement in school-related tasks.

### Sample Screening Tools

| Name | Target |
|---|---|
| The Model of Human Occupation (MOHO) screening tool (Parkinson, Forsyth, & Kielhofner, 2006) | Screen uses MOHO concepts of volition, habituation, skills, and environment to screen the client's occupational functioning |
| Occupational Therapy Adult Perceptual (OT-AP) screening test (Cooke, McKenna, & Fleming, 2005) | Screens adults with agnosia and visual perceptual skills deficits, such as body scheme neglect, apraxia, and acalculia |
| Screening Test for Evaluating Preschoolers (FirstSTEP; Miller, 1993) | Screen detects mild developmental delays in grade school students |

and AOTA's *Standards of Practice* (2010), the occupational therapy assistant can contribute to the "evaluation process by implementing delegated assessments and by providing verbal and written reports of observations and client capacities to the occupational therapist" (p. S19). Although these are professional guidelines, licensure regulations for each state have specific requirements with regard to service providers and supervision, which should be investigated prior to the implementation of service by the occupational therapy assistant. Additionally, relevant principles in the *Occupational Therapy Code of Ethics* (AOTA, 2015) speak to appropriate delegation of tasks and supervision of occupational therapy assistants.

Assessments are the specific tests, tools, or methods used to collect the data needed for a comprehensive evaluation. Appendix B provides information related to commonly used assessment tools. Each assessment manual provides instructions for implementation, application, and interpretation, and it is each practitioner's responsibility to be familiar and competent with each assessment tool that is used as part of his or her practice. Some assessment tools require advanced training and/or certification to implement, whereas some are only applicable to certain populations or age groups. In these cases, it is each practitioner's responsibility to meet the parameters set forth in the manual to ensure ethical implementation in accordance with the test author's guidelines. Novice practitioners can include the acquiring of these skills in their annual professional development plans and request time and financial resources to gain these skills.

There are times when an expert clinical decision is made to implement an assessment outside the boundaries set forth in the manual's implementation guidelines (e.g., not the intended population, procedures modified for language or physical limitations). This practice is frowned upon and should only occur when there are no other means of obtaining data to assist with intervention planning. With regard to reporting the assessment results, however, the data collected in these instances can only be used and reported informally, and scores cannot be reported as they are no longer valid or reliable as reported in the assessment manual. This should be made clear in documentation.

As previously stated, significant changes have occurred in available assessment tools during the past few decades. If, however, a setting requires standardized, client factor-focused assessments, it is the occupational therapist's role to determine how these specific pieces of information integrate with a more comprehensive, occupation-based perspective. For it is only with this clinical process that appropriate and effective interventions can be planned so that occupational engagement, which is part of the continuum of care, will eventually be achieved.

## Standardized Versus Nonstandardized

An assessment is standardized when it is given the same way every time to every client. This enables consistency of testing and scoring. An assessment tool's manual can maximize consistency of professional implementation by outlining a formalized procedure to be followed. The formalized, or standardized, implementation and interpretation methods designed for best practice do not make a tool "standardized." Clinicians need to be clear: A standardized test requires rigorous research and analysis utilizing accepted psychometric procedures.

### Psychometric Properties

- **Reliability, test-retest reliability:** Consistency of a measure; the score obtained reflects a true measure rather than by error
- **Validity:** The assessment measures what it is intended to measure
- **Precision:** Exactness of a measure
- **Sensitivity or responsiveness:** Measure's ability to detect the presence of a problem or condition
- **Clinically important difference:** The smallest change in a test score that is perceived significant by client or therapist
- **Minimal detectable change:** Minimal amount of change that occurs without error that reflects true change in a test score

(Adapted from Kielhofner, 2006; StrokEngine, 2013.)

Standardization guarantees an assessment has psychometric characteristics including a statistical review of reliability and validity, established norms, standard error of measurement, and standardized administration (Cohen, Hinojosa, & Kramer, 2010). Understanding the psychometric properties of each assessment tool that is used allows the practitioners to have confidence in the fairness and consistency of the results. Verifying the assessment tool's reliability (accuracy and stability of the test; getting the same test scores each time the test is given under the same conditions) and validity (measures the constructs, traits, or behaviors it says it will measure) via the test manual and professional literature allows the occupational therapist to speak with authority concerning professional recommendations.

Practitioners sometimes determine that only portions of a standardized assessment are appropriate, or busy practitioners sometimes try to focus on only certain sections of a standardized assessment. This should not be standard practice; when administering a portion of an assessment the scores cannot be reported as valid or reliable. If an assessment tool has several subtests implemented in a particular order or sequence during the standardization process and the practitioner only implements some of those subtests, those scores cannot be fairly compared to the standardized population who completed all subtests in the same sequence. Therefore, if the practitioner has broken the rules of the assessment administration, then the client is denied the full exploration of his or her issues, resulting in a biased assessment of his or her performance.

Among standardized and nonstandardized assessments, there is also a subcategory of assessments encompassing performance-based versus occupation-based assessments. Performance-based assessments, sometimes referred to as *impairment-based*, measure specific units of performance, such as cognition or dexterity (Coster, 2013). This information may be helpful to aid in treatment planning; however, practitioners should be aware that improvement in impairment does not always equate to an improvement in occupation (Hocking, 2001). Occupation-centered assessments help keep practitioners focused on the client and their occupations rather than specific deficits (Hocking, 2001). Some refer to these assessments as *function-based assessments*.

| Performance Based | Occupation Based |
|---|---|
| Nine-Hole Peg Test | Canadian Occupational Performance Measure |
| Range of Motion or Strength Testing | Occupational Self-Assessment |
| Test of Visual Motor Skills | Assessment of Occupational Functioning |

Although one might argue that standardized assessments are preferred given evidence-based practice, this is not necessarily an accurate statement. Occupational therapy leaders have long argued the merits of using a variety of assessment tools to gain the most comprehensive view of client preferences, habits, routines, skills, and occupational performance levels. To improve on the value of obtaining standardized assessment scores, the practitioner's clinical reasoning, professional judgment, and review of evidence-based practice may lead to incorporating nonstandardized alternatives. Hinojosa, Kramer, and Crist (2010) argued that practitioners should question how best to get the needed information rather than what information is needed. Therefore, if nonstandardized methods (e.g., skilled observations, interviews, facility-designed questionnaires, checklists, histories, and/or data collection on the frequency and duration of the identified behavior) are deemed necessary to assessing a client's performance, each practitioner must know his or her own skill level for implementation and interpretation to minimize subjectivity and personal bias.

## Norm Referenced

Most tests are developed using a sample from the "normal" population. As a result, each client's scores can be compared to this "normal population." There are times when a test is developed from a group of persons with similar characteristics (e.g., age, gender, diagnosis). If this "normative" group matches your client's profile, the tool would be appropriate for implementation. Results of a norm-referenced test are often presented in a bell curve with representation of scores or performance as percentages. If an assessment is norm referenced, these data will be available in the assessment manual where you can compare the client's performance to that of group of persons that is similar to him or her (e.g., grip strength testing).

## Criterion Referenced

A criterion-referenced assessment tool outlines a set of objective criteria or skill components used to document what the client is and is not able to master. In this type of assessment, the client's score is then compared to the set of expected criteria rather than to the performance of other people in a normative group. For example, the components of eating with a fork would be the following: (1) visually locates fork on table, (2) reaches for fork, (3) grasps fork, (4) brings fork to plate, (5) scoops or spears food, (6) brings fork to mouth, (7) opens mouth, (8) inserts fork in mouth, (9) closes lips around fork, (10) removes food from fork, and (11) removes fork from mouth. In this scenario, a client's skill level could be documented and future skills requiring intervention can be identified. These tools are particularly helpful for children with physical or mental difficulties where standardized assessment tools that compare a child to a typically developing child's scores are inappropriate or inapplicable.

## Culturally Sensitive Assessments

As previously stated, it is important for the occupational therapy practitioner to use assessment tools in the manner in which they were intended. If the standardization pool used during test development was homogeneous, the results for a client with differing characteristics will be limited and inadequate. For example, if the population sample included 500 men and 52 women, the results would be biased with regard to gender. Although many standardized tests are based on the demographic profile provided by the U.S. Census Bureau and the tool's manual should identify the scope of the population sample used for standardization purposes, it is the clinician's responsibility to interpret the assessment results based on the cultural or ethnic differences of each specific client. For example, if the assessment requires a client to put pictures of his or her bedtime routine in order and he or she places "brush my teeth" after he or she is in bed, this would be clinical data for the practitioner. However, if he did not include the brushing the teeth picture, this might be cultural versus clinical. Similarly, if a client is asked to perform a cooking task as part of an assessment, but in his or her culture it is not his or her role to cook, this may alter the interpretation of the data collected. Taugher (2000) identified this cultural bias in our assessment tools as a primary issue as health care shifts from hospital- or institution-based to community-based, and he posed several scenarios where decreased understanding of a client's cultural patterns might lead to inaccurate assessment of a client's skill level. The following examples could be culturally related or consistent with a diagnostic category:

- Talking fast (as with flight of ideas)
- Slow and laborious talk (as in depression and unable to pull thoughts together)
- Illogical syntax and thought (as in schizophrenia)
- Avoiding eye contact or interactions with others (as in autism)

Lyons (2000) went on to include other examples, such as not sharing during an interview, not following through on home programming, and that clutter in the house yields an unsafe walking environment. Additionally, some cultures have specific gender roles, specific clothing or religious practices, or regard self-care practices in a different light (Black, 2011). A multitude of cultural differences can affect the evaluation process. Wells and Black (2000) defined cultural competency as "lifelong learning designed to foster understanding, acceptance, knowledge, and constructive relations between persons of various cultures and differences" (p. 147). With this definition in mind, it is each practitioner's responsibility to seek out the research information necessary to be efficient, effective, and ethical for the variety of cultural influences on one's specific caseload.

Cultural sensitivity is the last point to be discussed and perhaps the most important. Historically, health care workers have the motto, "Treat the client as I would want to be treated." Salimbene (2000) argued just the opposite in her 10 Tips for Successful Caregiver/Client Interaction. The premise of how "you" want to be treated is based on your cultural background and experiences. If this is not the client's background and you do not recognize that your interactions need to change based on the client's background, then you are not being culturally sensitive. Culturally competent care encompasses understanding the client's "culture and how it impacts health beliefs, health decisions, and activity choices" (Black, 2011, p. 104). With regard to the evaluation process, if you have not educated yourself on the routines, habits, traditions, and practices of a specific client's background, you are not practicing culturally competent care or being culturally sensitive. This is more than simply an insult; this leads to ineffective and inefficient information and inappropriate planning and is professionally unethical (AOTA, 2015).

## Reassessment

In addition to the professional requirements of reassessment for discharge planning purposes, which includes documenting current performance level and planning for additional or follow-up intervention, the documentation of intervention outcomes itself often requires a reassessment. In today's health care environment of accountability, an assessment tool might be used pre- and post-intervention as a mechanism to provide evidence of intervention outcomes, to measure change from the initial evaluation period, request further authorization of therapy visits, and/or to plan for discharge. Additionally, some insurances or payers require reassessment at certain time periods during intervention to support the skilled need of services (Centers for Medicare and Medicaid Services, 2013). Using the same assessment tool would be the easiest method to detect change (i.e., by comparing the reassessment score with the initial assessment score and noting any change in score), but many assessment tools are not designed to be reimplemented (test-retest reliability). For example, if retested with the same standardized tool, the client might know what to expect, be comfortable with the format because he or she has been through it before, or become familiar with the test items from the first implementation. Additionally, different observers, testers, and raters should be factored into the reassessment process (termed *interrater reliability* in the test manual). Each factor would influence the reassessment score. Therefore, familiarity with the assessment tool manual is important for the practitioner to fully understand the strengths and limitations of the assessment tool prior to reimplementation.

Once the assessment tool has been deemed appropriate to readminister, there are additional professional benefits to utilizing a pre- and post-administration of the tool. For example, using pre- and post-assessment data for specific client groups allows the information to be used to compare or evaluate the outcomes for the client group as a whole. It also provides the ability to compare each client's outcomes to the results found in more rigorous research studies completed on the same client group (Mandich, Miller, & Law, 2002).

A point of consideration, however, is the type and purpose of the reassessment. For example, administering a standardized tool before, during, and after intervention might not yield the information needed to alter or redefine a specific client-centered intervention plan. In fact, these tools might miss personal or environmental factors that need to be considered throughout the intervention process. However, ongoing measurements such as rating scales (criterion-referenced tools that identify objectively observable actions or behaviors) or skilled observations related to targeted goal areas would provide immediate feedback. This immediacy allows the practitioner and client to determine if a change in the plan of care is warranted to meet the specific goals for the individual client (Mandich et al., 2002).

## Summary

There is a wide variety of assessment tools available, and picking the appropriate tool for each specific client's profile requires individual consideration. The following list will help the practitioner pick the most appropriate tool while meeting professional standards:

- What is the credibility of the assessment tool, and is it commonly used in the profession?
- Does the occupational therapy literature support the use of this assessment tool as appropriate and applicable to occupational therapy practice?
- Is this tool appropriate, useful, and the best method to obtain the information I need?
- Am I adequately prepared and trained to implement and interpret this assessment?
- Are there any cultural (including education level, English as a first language, etc.) limitations for applicability?
- Does the tool have acceptable psychometric qualities (including reliability, validity, adequate specificity, and sensitivity) for my needs?

After choosing the assessment tool, the practitioner must be prepared to do the following:

- Follow the parameters outlined
- Administer in the manner and for the population which the tool was intended (e.g., if intended for clients with dementia, do not use with clients diagnosed with schizophrenia)
- Interpret as intended and outlined in the manual
- Provide a clinical rationale for any variance in established procedures, and provide a statement indicating that the results were not gained in the manner intended or outlined in the manual
- Use all necessary assessment tools to gather the needed data within the evaluation process to provide the most comprehensive picture of the facilitators of and barriers to participation occupations

# Evaluation

To determine which assessment tools will best yield the necessary information and which pieces of information obtained are most important in understanding the client's needs, one cannot forget that evaluation is a fluid process (see the Eugene example on the following page).

To obtain a comprehensive picture of the client, the evaluation process requires ongoing clinical reasoning and a combination of both standardized and nonstandardized assessment tools (Strickland, 2005). To complete an evaluation, the practitioner must understand

> **Eugene**
>
> After receiving the physician's referral for occupational therapy services, 93-year-old Eugene was assessed for difficulties with feeding. The occupational therapist chose two assessment tools that focused on strength and cognition as areas to focus on based on the referral. Upon seeing the client at the bedside in an acute care setting, the occupational therapist noted that Eugene was unable to sit up in the bed without side and back support. This information prompted the occupational therapist to alter the formal assessment tools originally planned for the evaluation session. Rather, the occupational therapist needed to investigate the client factors and performance skills that affect trunk stability prior to addressing feeding issues.

the strengths and limitations of each assessment tool, identify information that must be obtained outside of standardized or formal methods of the assessment tools previously mentioned, and make effective decisions about how the evaluation needs to be adjusted based on the findings during the evaluation process.

## *Evaluation Factors to Consider*

In preparation for the evaluation process, several underlying issues need to be considered. Specifically, the influence of professional parameters and initiatives (AOTA, 2006, 2010, 2014b, 2015), evidence-based practice mandates (AOTA, 2006; Arbesman et al., 2014), and reimbursement constraints. Additionally, depending on the context in which the evaluation must occur, various factors might be more pertinent than others, while some factors are universal across domains and contexts. This section will discuss considerations that the occupational therapy practitioner must be aware of during the evaluation process.

### Professional

The *Framework* (AOTA, 2014a) provides parameters in which the occupational therapist and occupational therapy assistant must function. Specific information related to the components of this document related to evaluation will be presented in the following section, where the evaluation process is discussed. However, the influence of the *International Classification of Functioning, Disability and Health* (WHO, 2001), from which the *Framework* was created, has greatly changed how the evaluative process is implemented. Specifically, the focus on function, participation, and context have contributed to the development of the *Framework* and are consistent with the long-standing philosophy of occupational therapy to identify the facilitators of and barriers to functional participation in meaningful occupations.

### Evidence-Based Practice

An underlying premise of practice, specifically evaluation, is that decisions need to be made based on evidence. Effective decisions made within the evaluation process yield valuable information that, in turn, leads to appropriate intervention plans and, ultimately, improved outcomes. Muir Gray's (2004) Doing the Right Things Right outline for evidence-based medicine also applies to the occupational therapy evaluation process (Table 17-1). Additionally, evidence-based clinical decision models emphasize clinical expertise and client preference as equally important to research/evidence within the clinical process. This triad allows for the practitioner to use his or her expertise and understanding of client preferences to determine the applicability and appropriateness of the external research evidence. Implementing a client-centered evaluation process, as recommended in occupational therapy literature, fits within this more global model of evidence-based clinical/medical practice. To make these decisions correctly, the occupational therapy practitioner needs to understand the design, rationale, strengths, and limitations of various assessment tools and interface this information with client preferences and clinical reasoning for various client populations.

### Organizational

Whereas the distinct perspective on occupational engagement should always guide evaluative choices, the scope of evaluative responsibilities and procedures is determined by each specific setting. Organizations focusing primarily on client factors or performance skills (e.g., acute rehabilitation, hand therapy) literally set the stage for engagement in meaningful occupations later in the continuum of care. Additionally, each practice setting has its own philosophy, and ensuring a match with the personal philosophy of the practitioner, including values and beliefs, is important because it will factor into the evaluative decisions made. Understanding the scope of practice as defined within a specific organization and ensuring it meets the scope of practice outlined by the professional credentialing body and state licensure laws is imperative prior to the implementation of any occupational therapy service.

The financial constraints of an organization will also influence the evaluative process. The assessment resources available, the time available to complete the evaluation, including implementation, processing information, and documentation, and the requirements of the funding source(s) greatly influence the methods chosen to obtain the necessary information. Therefore, it would be prudent for the practitioner to understand the unique attributes and limitations of the assessment methods within this section, develop a mentoring system to improve clinical reasoning skills related to evaluation implementation, and continually examine personal patterns of performance to meet the demands of current practice.

Table 17-1.

**EVIDENCE-BASED EVALUATION PROCESS**

| Performance | Outcome | Evaluation Implications |
|---|---|---|
| Doing the right things | Increasing effectiveness | • Choose appropriate evaluation methods and procedures to obtain the information critical to intervention planning and referral to others internal and external to the profession<br>• Ask: How can I best obtain the needed information? |
| Doing things right | Efficiency; cost effectiveness | • Adhere to the established professional standards related to the role of the occupational therapist and occupational therapy assistant<br>• Focus on occupational engagement throughout the process<br>• Familiarity with, and knowledge of, specific evaluation methods and procedures yields efficient utilization of time and resources |
| Doing the right things right | Best; quality improvement | • Thorough documentation of the evaluative process results and plan of intervention<br>• Make effective decisions pertaining to the methods necessary to yield the best information for the evaluative purpose and determine the best or most efficient means of obtaining the needed information is both clinically appropriate and fiscally responsible |

### Funding Source and Referral

Understanding the system in which the practitioner works in and having specific knowledge of the funding source(s) or referral options will help to determine the appropriate assessment tool(s) to be used. First, the practitioner needs to be sure of the funding source's evaluation requirements to approve payment can be met. If there are requirements that cannot be completed (e.g., standardized scores are required but there is no tool available given the client's physical limitations), the practitioner needs to contact the funding agency to clearly explain the limitations of the requirements and gain approval to continue in an alternative manner. Second, if the client has expressed concerns during the client profile that do not fall under the domain of the funding agency or the intervention site, this needs to be discussed and alternative or additional arrangements need to be explored with the organization's administration. It may be necessary to refer the client to another discipline or intervention facility.

It is also important to remember that each funding source has rules on who can refer a client to occupational therapy. Typically for third-party payers, it is from a physician. Therefore, if the referral is not generated from the physician, as it is often from another professional, self-initiated by the client, or the client's parent after speaking to others in similar circumstances, having the client contact his or her physician for a prescription for occupational therapy would be necessary to ensure proper and timely payment (see Table 17-1).

## *Evaluation Components*

With regard to an occupational therapy evaluation, the AOTA (2013) emphasizes the need to include client information, reason for referral, an occupational profile, the assessments used, the assessment results, summary and analysis, and recommendations. The first area, client information, will be dependent on the system in which the practitioner works, but it generally includes name, medical record number, age, insurance provider, referring doctor, diagnoses, medical history, medications, precautions, contraindications, and reason for referral (Figure 17-1). There are instances, however, where the client is an organization, population, or community that supports the engagement of individuals in functional activities. In those instances, the client information would include demographics of the group and any other information that would influence the evaluative process necessary to develop an intervention, support, consultation, or education plan for the group. The subsequent components of the evaluation process are as follows with additional information related to specific assessments, assessment results, and assessment analysis presented in the following chapters (Tables 17-2 and 17-3).

### Reason for Referral

First and foremost, it is imperative to understand the reason for referral so that appropriate assessment methods can be identified. Although this may seem to be a basic concept, it is often overlooked. An occupational therapy evaluation referral can come from many sources, with varying levels of information for review and/or with specific outcomes expected. The examples

**Center for Rehabilitation Excellence**
**1 Maine Street, Portland, Maine 04123**
**(888) 207-1234**

**Occupational Therapy Intake/Client Referral**

| Name: | DOB: |
|---|---|
| Address: | Phone: |
| Insurance/ ID Number: | |
| Date of Referral: | Referring Physician: |
| Diagnosis/Code: | |
| Date of Evaluation: | Name of Therapist: |
| Precautions: | |
| Past Medical History: | |
| Reason for Referral: | |
| Employer/Employment: | |
| Goals for Therapy: | |
| Notes: | |

**Figure 17-1.** Sample intake/client profile form.

The hospital in which you work has a standard procedure for a referral to occupational therapy if the admitted client has any injury to the head. In this case, you would have access to files with intake information related to the personal and medical histories, initial medical findings by your organization, reports written by the professionals who have already evaluated the client, and so on. In this scenario, your evaluation would focus on the identification of facilitators of and/or barriers to participation in the client's chosen occupations. In essence, are there occupational performance issues secondary to the diagnostic information warranting occupational therapy services?

A parent calls your clinic to say her neighbor said to call as her baby is colicky and not eating well. In this case, with no other formal documentation available, and the parent potentially not even understanding what occupational therapy can offer, the clinician must obtain as much information as possible to help guide the decision-making process for the evaluation session. Equally important, however, is to remember that the therapeutic relationship begins during this initial conversation.

in the boxes illustrate the diverse nature of referral information. If the referral does not have the required information, it would be the practitioner's responsibility to obtain the required documentation. This lack of information can range from no age on the referral form to the lack of written documentation of medical clearance for the evaluation of a client with a neck injury. Regardless of what information is missing, the importance of complete information is clear.

These types of "systems" referrals often have specific evaluative procedures, outlined via departmental or organizational review, that need to be followed for "eligibility" for occupational therapy services to be determined. Other systems might use this type of procedure, including federal or state programs (e.g., Birth-to-Three and Boards of Education). As a point of clarification, these types of eligibility evaluations were previously termed *diagnostic evaluations* but should not be interpreted to indicate that a simple medical or rehabilitative diagnosis alone would determine eligibility. Rather, identifying the unique, client-specific facilitators of and barriers to functional participation in meaningful activities, which might include a qualifying test/assessment score if mandated, would be the information that determines eligibility (see A Reason for Referral on the following page for an example).

The conversation must be a forum to respond to, respect, and empathize with the parent who is now fearful there is something wrong with his or her child; educate the parent on the types of issues that could be impacting the child's patterns; and provide reassurance that the parent is doing the right thing by investigating any support he or she believes would make his or her child's interactions with the world more calm and joyful. While this may be nonbillable therapeutic time, a full discussion with the parent/client at the time of the intake call would be critical for the process to move forward successfully. In fact, this is the beginning of the therapeutic relationship, and the implications of this concept should not be overlooked. The bottom section of the intake/profile form provided in Figure 17-1 provides a framework for beginning this conversation.

It is important to recognize how these preliminary findings can help form an initial picture of the client. While this assists with designing the approach to the evaluation process, it should not limit the expectations of the client or eliminate the possibility of shifting preliminary plans to accommodate for observations of performance with the distinct perspective of occupation. Additionally, once the client's priorities and preferences are communicated—either by the client or by other significant persons if the client is unable—alternative assessment tools may need to be incorporated.

Table 17-2.

**ENGAGEMENT IN OCCUPATION TO SUPPORT PARTICIPATION IN CONTEXT OR CONTEXTS**

| Performance in Areas of Occupation | Context |
|---|---|
| • Activities of daily living (ADLs)<br>• Instrumental activities of daily living (IADLs)<br>• Education<br>• Work<br>• Play<br>• Leisure<br>• Social participation | • Cultural<br>• Physical<br>• Social<br>• Personal<br>• Spiritual<br>• Temporal<br>• Virtual |
| **Performance Skills** | **Activity Demands** |
| • Motor skills/habits<br>• Process skills/routines<br>• Communication/interaction skills/roles | • Objects used and their properties<br>• Space demands<br>• Social demands<br>• Sequencing and timing<br>• Required actions<br>• Required body functions<br>• Required body structures |
| **Performance Patterns** | **Client Factors** |
| • Habits<br>• Routines<br>• Roles | • Body functions<br>• Body structures |

Adapted from American Occupational Therapy Association. (2014). Occupational therapy practice framework: Domain and process (3rd ed.). *American Journal of Occupational Therapy, 68*(Suppl. 1), S1-S48.

### A Reason for Referral

The local psychologist has been working with an agitated client for the past 3 months. As the agitation has diminished, the psychologist realizes there are underlying difficulties related to home management, life skills, and ongoing issues with holding a job. While you may now have the psychologist's referral and report, which outlines some of the occupational challenges for the client, the underlying reason for these challenges needs to be investigated. This type of evaluation is intended to determine the most appropriate intervention plan rather than eligibility. In this case, the evaluation report might be more descriptive in nature versus simply stating scores from a standardized assessment tool. Stating that a client requires maximum assistance with a task does not delineate specific-enough information; rather, describing the client's function, as with Eugene and self feeding, can facilitate an understanding of barriers and strengths for occupational performance and support the need for continued occupational therapy services.

## Occupational Profile

The occupational profile, defined in the *Framework* as "information that describes the client's occupational history and experiences, patterns of daily living, interests, values, and needs" (AOTA, 2014a, p. S10), identifies and guides understanding of the occupational issues that are important and meaningful to the client. Beginning the evaluation process with an occupational profile also supports the top-down approach to an occupational therapy evaluation as it begins with the client perspective of occupational performance and then works downward to investigate the factors (client specific or contextual) that contribute to occupational limitations.

## Assessments Used and Assessment Analysis

As stated earlier and as illustrated in Appendix B, there are many assessment tools available. Although the following chapters in this section will discuss specific assessment tools that focus on occupational performance components, it is clear that the choice of assessment tool(s) needs to be guided by the occupational profile. Therefore, the occupational therapy evaluation report

Table 17-3.

**Components of an Occupational Therapy Evaluation**

| Category | Description |
|---|---|
| Client profile | For recordkeeping purposes: Name; parent name if appropriate; age; client number if needed; funding identification number; contact information<br>For planning purposes: Pertinent diagnoses; relevant medical history; medications; precautions; limitations; contraindications |
| Reason for referral | Generated by whom; for what reason; what information is being requested and for what purpose; include date of request on documentation |
| Occupational profile | The *Framework* mandates clinicians use a client-centered approach; obtain information that allows the practitioner to understand what is meaningful for the client; client's desired outcomes; past experiences and history contributing to the client's desired outcomes; client priorities and preferences; factors influencing meaningful engagement in occupations |
| Assessments methods/tools used | Per the *Framework*, the evaluation considers performance skills, performance patterns, context, activity demands, and client factors; an evaluation often requires the implementation of multiple assessment tools when possible; minimum expectations are to have sufficient data to plan interventions; document which tools have been used (standardized, norm referenced, criterion referenced, formal, informal, etc.), why implemented, why and how established protocols were not followed if applicable, and how these tools contributed to a full understanding of the client's needs; chosen assessment tools are bias free with regard to cultural (in the broadest sense) issues; practitioners must have required level of skill and knowledge to implement the assessment tool; occupational therapist and occupational therapy assistant mutually determine which tools can be administered by the occupational therapy assistant based on level of expertise, training, supervision, and pertinent regulations |
| Assessment tool(s) results | Score and report all formalized assessment results according to the procedures outlined in the test manual; identify limitations with information obtained if exact testing protocols were unable to be followed; indicate if you believe the assessment results to be accurate or inaccurate for any external reason; make no other assumptions on the data at this time; include skilled clinical observations and other informal findings |
| Analysis and summary | Interpret the assessment findings, summarize strengths and vulnerabilities, and identify the supports and barriers to successful engagement or performance; synthesize the information in a manner consistent with the presenting concerns identified in the referral and the client's life and environment; incorporate information from formal and informal tools, observations, clinical judgment, and how these findings interface with the client's goals, interests, and preferences; do not overinterpret the data—report what you know from your clinical expertise and you can continue to investigate any unsubstantiated hypotheses during the intervention period; provide summary statement of findings |
| Recommendation | Use clinical judgment to determine if services are warranted or additional referrals are necessary; these decisions must relate to the initial referral request, client preferences and priorities, potential intervention approach(es) based on best practice and evidence, and the feasibility of the intervention's success given the evaluative findings; identify the types of service that address the presenting concerns (e.g., education, consultation, direct, monitor); depending on the organization's funding source, this section may include goals, objectives, and specifics about the intervention recommended (e.g., frequency, duration)—otherwise, this information would belong in a plan of care |

needs to identify which tools were used to obtain the data, the rationale for the decision, any alterations to the assessment's procedures required, and how each of these choices contribute to the overarching view of occupation being evaluated. Within the analysis section of the occupational therapy evaluation report, it is important to discuss information from different assessment methods that support the evaluator's analysis as well as information considered to be a contradiction.

## Documentation

Documentation is necessary whenever professional services are provided to a client. Occupational therapists and occupational therapy assistants under the supervision of an occupational therapist determine the appropriate type of documentation and document the services provided with their scope of practice (AOTA, 2013).

Table 17-4.

**DOCUMENTATION REQUIREMENTS**

| | |
|---|---|
| Professional | • Identify and meet agency/organization expectations and ensure these expectations match professional guidelines, licensure, and ethical responsibilities<br>• Write for the reader (target audience)<br>• Differentiate direct observations from opinions regarding the performance (e.g., client stated she is the mother of 13 children vs. client is delusional as she believes she is the mother of 13 children) |
| Legal | • Information for referral to another specialist should be prompt and comprehensive<br>• If using hard copy versus computerized format, documentation should be legible and well organized<br>• Complete required documentation in a timely manner<br>• Remember, every piece of documentation is considered a legal document that can be subpoenaed<br>• All documentation should meet employer, accrediting body, and funding sources requirements<br>• All documentation should be complete and accurate (including dates of service and date of documentation of service if required)<br>• If hard-copy format is used, do not change, remove, or alter your documentation with erasers or correction fluid; simply cross out the error with a single line and initial to indicate it was you who deleted the piece of information; put a line through unused lines or spaces on any forms<br>• Include only first-hand information of what you see or hear versus what the client told you (i.e., client stated he completed the home program once per day versus client completed home program as designed)<br>• Avoid negative statements because, aside from being unprofessional, they can be interpreted as though you disliked the client; then other information would be subject to interpretation<br>• The treating practitioner must sign all documentation, including cosigning as the supervising practitioner as required with name, professional credentials, and date<br>• Client name and identifying information should be on each page of documentation in case pages become separated |

Documentation is an important legal and professional component for all occupational therapy services, and it has an important function within the evaluation process. An evaluation report, which clearly, accurately, and comprehensively outlines the current level of functioning and concerns to be supported by occupational therapy, not only guides entrance into the health care arena, but also offers a framework for communication with the client and other professionals. The evaluation also forms the basis for referral to specialists both internal and external to occupational therapy, establishes the rationale for financial support for services, and provides a mechanism to plan interventions moving forward, which will be compared to this original baseline of performance. Sames (2015) argued that the report of the initial evaluation is the most important document the occupational therapist will write. Components of documentation requirements can be found in Table 17-4, and additional information can be found in Chapter 23.

## *Professional*

As one begins the evaluation report, understanding the target audience or stakeholder will guide the presentation of results. For example, a report for a child's family for program planning purposes might look very different from a report for a third-party payer. Asking who needs the information and why (i.e., funding source, organization, external accrediting agency requirements) will assist the practitioner in producing a report reflective of the practice setting. Despite the nuances, every occupational therapy report should have established components (see Table 17-2).

## *Reimbursement*

Although documentation is important for the continuity of care and therapeutic intervention planning, it is also intricately linked to payment. Regardless of the payment source, documentation is a mechanism to obtain approval for payment through objective client measures. The type and frequency of documentation is generally determined by the payment source (e.g., federal or state programs, third-party payers, grant funding). Thus, to minimize the possibility of claim denial, the practitioner needs to be fully aware of the rules and requirements, including any updates or revisions, prior to report completion. Additionally, effectively communicating this information from the perspective of occupational engagement will help distinguish occupational therapy from other therapeutic services also requesting payment for services, as occupational therapy reports on performance skill deficit and its impact on the client's daily occupations.

## Legal Requirements

Any written communication produced by occupational therapy personnel with regard to a client's care is considered a legal document and should be kept confidential in adherence to professional standards, state laws, and the Health Insurance Portability and Accountability Act (U.S. Department of Health and Human Services, 2002). Not only does the paperwork substantiate that the services were delivered, but it also serves to provide a history of what actually happened on behalf of the client. Even the screening, which led to a full evaluation, should be documented as a client contact in the chart; if it is not documented, it did not happen in the eyes of the law. Therefore, any errors, inconsistencies, or omissions can be used against the practitioner in a court of law. It is imperative for each practitioner to understand the legal requirements of the funding source and the legal implications for the employing agency. Most employers will set the rules of how their staff should perform in terms of documentation, and once the practitioner is aware of the employer's expectations, it is important to be sure the expectations meet professional licensure, guidelines, and ethical expectations. It is the responsibility of the individual practitioner to ensure all of these requirements are met and communicate any disparities to the employer.

Each agency/organization has its own rules on the types of documentation required, as well as its own system of recording the information. If the system is computerized, thorough training for all occupational therapy personnel should be completed, and no other clinician should enter information into the client files of other practitioners. If there are hard-copy files, there may be one formal/official/legal file where all pertinent information needs to be recorded. Thereafter, there may be a clinical file by each clinician for information related to intervention planning, copies of performance measures, and day-to-day information the practitioner needs to monitor and track. Although notes/documents/performance samples are not in the "official" file, they are still considered legal documents, should be kept in a locked file cabinet, and can be subpoenaed in a court of law.

## Summary

The occupational therapy evaluation process is a complicated procedure from a clinical perspective and an administrative process. As the initial evaluation is the entry into occupational therapy services, evaluation from an occupational perspective, competence in administration and interpretation of the assessment tools used, and efficient, accurate, and timely documentation are all necessary. Using the evidence-based medicine model previously discussed (Muir Gray, 2004), Table 17-1 provides a synopsis of this concept with regard to the evaluation process. The remainder of Section IV discusses specific assessment tools and their use in practice.

## Student Self-Assessment

1. From the information provided on Mary's case study in A Reason to Screen, which assessment tools would be appropriate to administer and why? Which frame of reference do the chosen assessments follow? Identify a part of the assessment process an occupational therapy assistant might be able to complete.
2. Complete the Assessment Tool Grid in Appendix B with additional assessment tools from your coursework.
3. Using Appendix B, pick a few assessments from each assessment area and identify if the assessment tool is norm or criterion referenced and why.
4. Identify various state, federal, and private funding sources that might influence the evaluative processes within a given practice setting.
5. Discuss how funding source limitations might influence the documentation of the full scope of your occupational therapy services.
6. Examine your own personal values and beliefs regarding service delivery, and identify how these might influence your approach to an occupational therapy evaluation.
7. Identify the assessment tools appropriate for Eugene's case study given his inability to sit up in bed and its impact on self-feeding.
8. Based on one occupational therapy setting you have observed, create an intake form you believe would be appropriate in that environment.
9. Based on one occupational therapy client you observed this semester, assume the observed session was the evaluation session and complete the information requested in Table 17-2.
10. Referring to Table 17-4, create a list of situations that you have observed throughout your education that might be in conflict with the rules provided. Be prepared to discuss these observations in class.

## Electronic Resources

American Occupational Therapy Association for compliance with Standards of Practice: www.aota.org

Department of Health and Human Services, Centers for Medicare and Medicaid Services: www.cms.hhs.gov

Evidence-Based Practice and Research in Occupational Therapy: http://www.aota.org/practice/researchers.aspx

## REFERENCES


American Occupational Therapy Association. (2006). *AOTA's Centennial Vision*. Retrieved from http://www.aota.org/-/media/Corporate/Files/AboutAOTA/Centennial/Background/Vision1.pdf

American Occupational Therapy Association. (2010). Standards of practice for occupational therapy. *American Journal of Occupational Therapy, 64*(Suppl. 6), S106-S111.

American Occupational Therapy Association. (2013). Guidelines for documentation of occupational therapy. *American Journal of Occupational Therapy, 67*(Suppl. 6), S32-S38.

American Occupational Therapy Association. (2014a). Occupational therapy practice framework: Domain and process (3rd ed.). *American Journal of Occupational Therapy, 68*(Suppl. 1), S1-S48. doi:10.5014/ajot.2014.682006

American Occupational Therapy Association. (2014b). Guidelines for supervision, roles, and responsibilities during the delivery of occupational therapy services. *American Journal of Occupational Therapy, 68*(Suppl. 3), S16-S22.

American Occupational Therapy Association. (2015). Occupational therapy code of ethics. *American Journal of Occupational Therapy, 69*, 1-8.

Arbesman, M., Lieberman, D., & Metzler, C. (2014). Using evidence to promote the distinct value of occupational therapy. *American Journal of Occupational Therapy, 68*, 381-385.

Black, R. M. (2011). Cultural considerations of hand use. *Journal of Hand Therapy, 24*(2), 104-111. doi:10.1016/j.jht.2010.09.067

Centers for Medicare and Medicaid Services. (2013). *Therapy questions and answers*. Retrieved from http://www.cms.gov/Medicare/Medicare-Fee-for-Service-payment/HomeHealthPPS/downloads/therapy_questions_and_answers.pdf

Cohen, M. E., Hinojosa, J., & Kramer, P. (2010). Administration of evaluation and assessments. In J. Hinojosa, P. Kramer, & P. Crist (Eds.), *Evaluation: Obtaining and interpreting data* (3rd ed., pp. 103-122). Bethesda, MD: AOTA Press.

Cooke, D. M., McKenna, K., & Fleming, J. (2005). Development of a standardized occupational therapy screening tool for visual perception in adults. *Scandinavian Journal of Occupational Therapy, 12*(2), 59-71.

Coster, W. J. (2013). Making the best match: Selecting outcome measures for clinical trials and outcome studies. *American Journal of Occupational Therapy, 67*(2), 162-170. doi:10.5014/ajot.2013.006015

Hinojosa, J., Kramer, P., & Crist, P. (Eds.). (2010). *Evaluation: Obtaining and interpreting data*. Bethesda, MD: AOTA Press.

Hocking, C. (2001). Implementing occupation-based assessment. *American Journal of Occupational Therapy, 55*(4), 463-469.

Kielhofner, G. (2006). *Research in occupational therapy: Methods of inquiry for enhancing practice*. Philadelphia, PA: F. A. Davis Company.

Lyons, A. (2000). Cultural competence in occupational therapy practice. *Home and Community Health Special Interest Section Quarterly, 7*, 1-2.

Mandich, A., Miller, L., & Law, M. (2002). Outcomes in evidence-based practice. In M. Law (Ed.), *Evidence-based rehabilitation: A guide to practice* (pp. 49-69). Thorofare, NJ: SLACK Incorporated.

Miller, L. J. (1993). *First STEP screening test for evaluating preschoolers*. San Antonio, TX: Psychological Corp.

Muir Gray, J. A. (2004). *Evidence-based healthcare: How to make health policy and management decisions*. Upper Saddle River, NJ: Pearson Prentice Hall.

Parkinson, S., Forsyth, K., & Kielhofner, G. (2006). *The model of human occupation screening tool*. Retrieved from http://www.uic.edu/depts/moho/assess/mohost.html

Salimbene, S. (2000). *What language does your patient hurt in? A practical guide to culturally competent patient care*. Amherst, MA: Diversity Resources.

Sames, K. M. (2015). *Documenting occupational therapy practice* (3rd ed.). Upper Saddle River, NJ: Pearson Education Inc.

Strickland, L. S. (2005). Evaluation issues in today's practice. In J. Hinojosa, P. Kramer, & P. Crist (Eds.), *Evaluation: Obtaining and interpreting data* (2nd ed., pp. 51-58). Bethesda, MD: AOTA Press.

StrokEngine. (2013). *Glossary of terms*. Retrieved from http://strokengine.ca/assess/definitions-en.html

Taugher, M. (2000). Persons with limited English proficiency: A challenge for home and community practitioners. *Home and Community Health Special Interest Section Quarterly, 7*, 2-4.

U.S. Department of Health and Human Services. (2002). *Standards for privacy of individually identifiable health information*. Retrieved from http://www.hhs.gov/ocr/privacy/hipaa/news/2002/combinedregtext02.pdf

Wells, S. A., & Black, R. M. (2000). *Cultural competency for health professionals*. Bethesda, MD: AOTA Press.

World Health Organization. (2001). *International classification of functioning, disability and health*. Retrieved from http://www.who.int/classifications/icf/icfbeginnersguide.pdf?ua=1

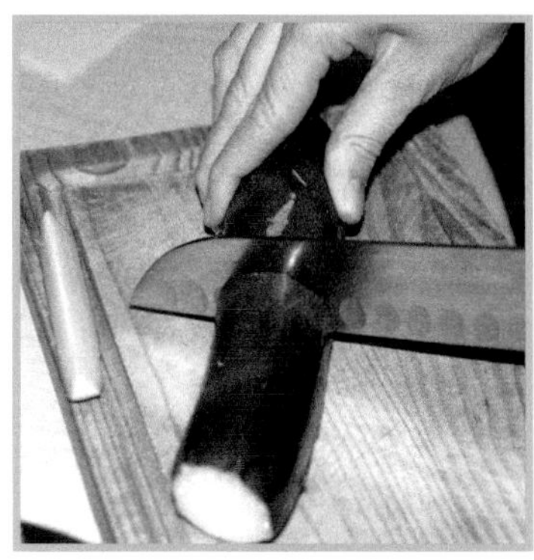

# 18

# Evaluation of Activities of Daily Living and Instrumental Activities of Daily Living

*Lisa Knecht-Sabres, DHS, OTR/L*

**ACOTE STANDARDS EXPLORED IN THIS CHAPTER**

B.2.2, B.4.1, B.4.2, B.4.4, B.4.5

**KEY VOCABULARY**

- **Activities:** "Actions designed and selected to support the development of performance skills and performance patterns to enhance occupational engagement" (American Occupational Therapy Association [AOTA], 2014, p. S41).
- **Activities of daily living (ADLs):** "Activities oriented toward taking care of one's own body. ADLs are also referred to as basic activities of daily living and personal activities of daily living" (AOTA, 2014, p. S19). ADLs consist of bathing, showering, toileting, toilet hygiene, dressing, swallowing, eating, feeding, functional mobility, personal device care, personal hygiene and grooming, and sexual activity (AOTA, 2014).
- **Instrumental activities of daily living (IADLs):** "Activities that support daily life in the home and community that often require more complex interactions than those used in ADLs" (AOTA, 2014, p. S19). IADLs consist of caring for others, caring for pets, child rearing, communication management, driving, community mobility, financial management, health management, health maintenance, home establishment, home management, meal preparation and clean-up, religious and spiritual activities and expression, safety and emergency maintenance, and shopping (AOTA, 2014).

*(continued)*



Jacobs, K., & MacRae, N. (Eds.).
*Occupational Therapy Essentials for Clinical Competence, Third Edition* (pp. 249-264).

**KEY VOCABULARY (CONTINUED)**

- **Occupation:** "Daily activities in which people engage. Occupations occur in context and are influenced by the interplay among client factors, performance skills, and performance patterns. Occupations occur over time; have purpose, meaning, and perceived utility to the client; and can be observed by others (e.g., preparing a meal) or be known only to the person involved (e.g., learning through reading a textbook). Occupations can involve the execution of multiple activities for completion and can result in various outcomes. The *Occupational Therapy Practice Framework* identifies a broad range of occupations; they are categorized as activities of daily living, instrumental activities of daily living, rest and sleep, education, work, play, leisure, and social participation" (AOTA, 2014). "Occupations refer to the everyday activities that people do as individuals, in families, and with communities to occupy time and bring meaning and purpose to life. Occupations include things people need to, want to, and are expected to do" (World Federation of Occupational Therapists, 2012).
- **Occupational profile:** "Summary of a client's occupational history and experiences, patterns of daily living, interests, values, and needs" (AOTA, 2014, p. S13).

Occupational therapy practitioners have a unique perspective of their clients. That is, the expertise of an occupational therapy practitioner lies in his or her ability to appreciate the broad range of human occupations that make up peoples' lives (American Occupational Therapy Association [AOTA], 2014). More specifically, occupational therapy practitioners use occupations for the purpose of enhancing or enabling participation in roles, habits, and routines in the home, school, workplace, community, and other settings (AOTA, 2014). In other words, through engagement of occupation, occupational therapy practitioners attain health and well-being for their clients (AOTA, 2014). The *Occupational Therapy Practice Framework*, hereinafter referred to as the *Framework*, defines occupations as the daily life activities in which people engage. Furthermore, the *Framework* asserts that occupations have significant meaning and value to the client and are central to a client's identity and sense of competence (AOTA, 2014). However, the *Framework* suggests that drawing from multiple classic definitions of occupation described in the occupational therapy literature can add to an understanding of this complex term and concept (AOTA, 2014). For example, the World Federation of Occupational Therapists (2012) defines occupations are "the everyday activities that people do as individuals, in families, and with communities to occupy time and bring meaning and purpose to life…occupations include things people need to, want to, and are expected to do." Whereas, Law, Polatajko, Baptise, and Townsend (1997) define occupations as "activities…of everyday life, named, organized, and given value and meaning by individuals and a culture...occupation is everything people do to occupy themselves, including looking after themselves…enjoying life…and contributing to the social and economic fabric of their communities" (p. 32).

The term *occupation*, as it is used in the *Framework*, and in this chapter, refers to the daily activities in which people engage (AOTA, 2014). According to the *Framework*, occupations are categorized as "activities of daily living, instrumental activities of daily living, rest and sleep, education, work, play, leisure, and social participation" (AOTA, 2014). Thus, since occupational therapy practitioners focus on enabling people to engage or reengage in the everyday occupations and activities that bring meaning and purpose to their lives, the occupational therapy practitioner's evaluation process must include an assessment of relevant, meaningful, and client-centered occupations and daily life activities (Knecht-Sabres, 2014). This chapter will specifically focus on how occupational therapy practitioners should approach the evaluation of activities of daily living (ADLs) and instrumental activities of daily living (IADLs).

The *Framework* defines ADLs as "activities oriented toward taking care of one's own body" and classifies them into the following categories: bathing, showering, toileting, toilet hygiene, dressing, swallowing, eating, feeding, functional mobility, personal device care, personal hygiene and grooming, and sexual activity (AOTA, 2014). ADLs are also referred to as basic activities of daily living and personal activities of daily living (AOTA, 2014). Whereas, according to the *Framework*, instrumental activities of daily living (IADLs) are "activities that support daily life in the home and community that often require more complex interactions than those used in ADLs. IADLs consist of caring for others, caring for pets, child rearing, communication management, driving, community mobility, financial management, health management, health maintenance, home establishment, home management, meal preparation and clean-up, religious and spiritual activities and expression, safety and emergency maintenance, and shopping" (AOTA, 2014).

# Evaluation of ADLs and IADLs

## *Occupational Profile*

The first critical step in any occupational therapy evaluation is to obtain an understanding of the client's occupational profile (AOTA, 2014). As defined in the *Framework*, the occupational profile is "a summary of a client's occupational history and experiences, patterns of daily living, interests, values, and needs" (AOTA, 2014, p. S13). In other words, the occupational profile helps the occupational therapist identify what the client wants or needs to do. To understand the client's perspective regarding his or her individual and unique concerns about occupational performance, it is imperative for the occupational therapist to use a client-centered approach. That is, occupational therapists who commit to taking the time to complete a thorough occupational profile and who truly adopt a client-centered approach to the occupational therapy evaluation and intervention process will be well suited to address each client's individual wants, needs, desires, and priorities regarding the client's occupational performance and meaningful daily life activities. In other words, a comprehensive occupational profile allows the occupational therapist to appreciate what is currently important and meaningful to the client. Gathering information related to the client's occupational profile begins during the initial session with a client; however, a more complete and better understanding of the client's occupational wants, needs, concerns, and priorities typically occurs over time and throughout the entire occupational therapy intervention process. As indicated in the *Framework*, the occupational profile typically includes information related to the client's:

- Concerns relative to occupational performance and daily life activities
- Supports and barriers related to occupational performance
- Occupational history
- Roles, values, and interests
- Occupational patterns and how these patterns have changed over time
- Priorities and desired outcomes related to occupational performance

Therefore, an occupational profile might begin with an open-ended question such as, "Can you please describe to me what a typical day was like for you before you were admitted to the hospital?" and continue with more open-ended and descriptive questions that will paint a complete picture of the client's occupational history, current needs, and priorities. Moreover, as part of a comprehensive occupational profile, a skilled occupational therapist will also be able to begin to appreciate how some of the client factors, performance skills, performance patterns, environmental, as well as contextual factors, may support or inhibit the client's occupational performance (discussed in further detail below). In fact, Shotwell (2014) eloquently describes the occupational therapy evaluation process as similar to the components of dancing. During her analogy, she describes that one of the most difficult parts of the "dance" for the practitioner is knowing what questions to ask and when to ask them. To further develop this analogy, I would assert that a skilled occupational therapist is able to turn the occupational profile into a comfortable conversation and make it look more like a pair of professional dancers, versus someone who is closely following a script or list of questions or looking like someone who is practicing dance moves for the first time.

### Canadian Occupational Performance Measure

Unfortunately, there are very few occupational therapy assessment tools that evaluate occupational performance in a client-centered manner. The Canadian Occupational Performance Measure (COPM; Law et al., 2014) is a personalized, client-centered instrument designed to identify the occupational performance problems as experienced by the client. The COPM is a semi-structured interview that can be used as part of the occupational profile. More specifically, the intent of the COPM is to engage the client in a conversation that focuses on the identification of daily occupations that the client wants to do, needs to do, and/or is expected to do, but is currently unable to accomplish. The COPM focuses on the client's self-perception of his or her occupational performance in the broad categories of the following:

- Self-care, including personal care, functional mobility, and community management
- Productivity, including paid or unpaid work, household management, school, and play
- Leisure, including quiet recreation, active recreation, and socialization (Law et al., 2014)

Because the COPM is intended for use as an outcome measure, it should be administered at the beginning of occupational therapy services, and repeated, as appropriate, to ascertain accomplishment of goals, as identified by the client (Law et al., 2014). There are four main steps related to the COPM interview:

1. The client identifies his or her occupational performance problems
2. The client rates the importance of his or her identified occupational performance problems on a 10-point scale
3. The client chooses up to five of the most important occupational performance problems that he or she wants to address during occupational therapy intervention
4. The client rates his or her own level of performance and satisfaction with performance for each of the top five identified problems (Law et al., 2014)

The COPM can be used with virtually any client regardless of age or diagnosis since this tool can be administered to a family member or caregiver if the client is too young or unable to engage in the interview process (Law et al., 2014). Not only is the COPM an excellent tool to assist the occupational therapist in performing a complete, thorough, and client-centered occupational profile, but, there is also a plethora of research on the COPM, which has repeatedly demonstrated the soundness of this evaluation tool in terms of reliability, validity, and as an effective outcome measure (Colquhoun, Letts, Law, MacDermid, & Missiuna, 2012; Eyssen et al., 2011; Law et al., 2014; McNulty & Beplal, 2008; Richard & Knis-Matthews, 2010).

### Occupational Self-Assessment and the Child Occupational Self-Assessment

The Occupational Self-Assessment (OSA; Baron, Kielhofner, Iyenger, Goldhammer, & Wolenski, 2006) and the Child Occupational Self-Assessment (COSA; Kramer et al., 2014), like the COPM, were developed to capture the client's perceptions of his or her occupational competence. The OSA entails having the client rate his or her level of competence on a variety of items which fall under the three broad categories:

1. Basic tasks of living
2. Managing life and relationships
3. Satisfaction, enjoyment, and actualization

More specifically, the OSA entails having the client respond to a series of statements about his or her occupational competence and is asked to label each area as: (1) I have a lot of problem doing this, (2) I have some difficulty doing this, (3) I do this well, or (4) I do this extremely well. Additionally, the client is asked to rate each statement in terms of how important it is to the client: (1) This is not so important to me, (2) This is important to me, (3) This is more important to me, or (4) This is most important to me. Lastly, the client is asked to identify up to four things that he or she would like to change.

Similarly, the COSA is a client-directed assessment tool and an outcome measure that is designed to capture children's and youth's perceptions regarding their own sense of occupational competence and the importance of everyday activities (Kramer et al., 2014). The COSA consists of a series of statements pertaining to everyday occupational participation, which includes tasks related to ADLs, IADLs, leisure, and performance at school, home, and in the community. The COSA comes in a variety of administrative formats: a rating form with symbols, a rating form without symbols, and a card sort version to be flexible for youth of different ages and abilities. Similar to the OSA, the COSA entails having the child self-rate his or her perception of occupational competence, as well as its level of importance.

## Observation of Occupational Performance

After establishing the client's occupational profile, the next essential step in the evaluation process is to observe the client's occupational performance, ideally within the natural context (AOTA, 2014; Fisher, 2009; Shotwell, 2014). Observation of occupational performance should provide the occupational therapist with vital information concerning supports and barriers to occupational performance (AOTA, 2014), the client's level of independence, as well as the quality of the client's occupational performance, or the degree of physical effort, efficiency, and safety related to the client's performance (Fisher, 2009). Observation of occupational performance is vital to the assessment process, especially because information from an interview alone may be inaccurate. For instance, a client might over- or underestimate his or her performance and/or abilities due to lack of opportunities to perform ADLs and IADLs after an accident, injury, or illness; lack of insight due to cognitive impairments; fear of being admitted to a nursing home; shame, stigma, and/or feelings of self-consciousness; or a myriad of other reasons. Because there are numerous standardized and nonstandardized assessment tools available to assess occupational performance, the shrewd occupational therapist will base his or her decision to use a particular ADL and/or IADL assessment tool on sound clinical reasoning skills (Knecht-Sabres, 2014). In other words, the astute occupational therapist should ask him- or herself a series of questions before selecting a specific assessment tool. For example, the occupational therapist should consider asking him- or herself the following types of questions:

- Which specific ADLs and/or IADLs need to be evaluated for this particular client?
- Which ADL/IADL assessment tools will assess the client's specific occupational needs, wants, and priorities?
- What are the advantages and disadvantages of each ADL and IADL tool under consideration?

- Is there evidence to support the soundness of the ADL/IADL tool(s) under consideration?
- What is the purpose of the evaluation and which assessment tool best addresses the purpose? For instance, is the purpose to determine why the client is having difficulty with occupational performance? Is the purpose to determine if the client is safe and independent with ADL/IADL performance? Is the purpose to provide evidence related to the effectiveness of occupational therapy intervention? Or are there multiple purposes and can one assessment tool meet all of the identified needs of the client and occupational therapist?
- How long does the ADL/IADL assessment tool take to administer, score, and interpret data?
- Is the specific ADL/IADL assessment tool an efficient use of time, and/or feasible given time, financial, and/or environmental constraints (Knecht-Sabres, 2014)?

The therapist who takes time to ensure best practice in every step of the evaluation process is very different from the therapist who decides to use an evaluation tool just because "it's the tool that all of the therapists at the facility use" or because " "I've always done it this way" (Knecht-Sabres, 2014).

After completing the occupational profile, the occupational therapist should have a clear understanding of which specific ADL and/or IADL needs to be observed for each and every individual. As indicated previously, the specific ADL and/or IADL to be assessed should relate directly to the client's unique, needs, wants, goals, and priorities. For example, observation of occupational performance for a client who lives alone, was previously independent in all ADLs and IADLs, does not have social supports, plans on returning to his or her previous environment, and wants and needs to be independent in almost all ADLs and IADLs should be very different from the observation of occupational performance of a client who lives with a spouse, participated in minimal IADLs previously, and has no desire or need to cook, clean, do laundry, or pay the bills. Likewise, the types of ADLs and IADLs to be assessed throughout the lifespan will differ as well. That is, the specific ADLs and/or IADLs that one engages in might be directly influenced by age. For instance, a young child might engage in only some basic ADLs, such as eating, dressing, toileting, and bathing. Whereas an adolescent might engage in all basic ADLs and minimal IADLs such as light housework, light meal preparation, and shopping, while an adult living independently might need and want to perform all ADLs and IADLs, including home maintenance, financial management, care of others, and medication routines.

Because occupational performance involves a transaction between the individual, task, and environment (Law et al., 1996; Metzler & Metz, 2010), it is essential that the occupational therapist not only consider selecting specific assessment tools based on the types of ADLs and IADLs it includes, but also select an assessment tool that provides the practitioner with critical information regarding the individual and the environment. Likewise, the *Framework* also recognizes that the "differences among persons and the occupations they engage in are complex and multidimensional" (AOTA, 2014, p. S6). More specifically, the *Framework* asserts that it is critical to keep in mind that "occupations occur in context and are influenced by the interplay among client factors, performance skills, and performance patterns" (AOTA, 2014, p. S6). To explain further, the *Framework* defines client factors as "the specific capacities, characteristics, or beliefs that reside within the person and influence performance in occupations" (AOTA, 2014, p. S7). For instance, client factors may include, but are not limited to, one's values, beliefs, spirituality, body functions, and body structures. The reader is encouraged to refer to the *Framework* (AOTA, 2014) for a detailed description of many types of client factors. Performance skills, as defined in the Assessment of Motor and Process Skills (AMPS; Fisher & Griswold, 2014), refer to "the smallest observable units of occupational performance" (p. 249) or the goal-directed actions a person carries out as he or she is engaged in naturalistic and relevant daily life task performances. Performance skills are categorized as motor skills, process skills, and social interaction skills (Fisher & Jones, 2012). The reader is encouraged to refer to the *Framework* (AOTA, 2014), Fisher and Griswold (2014), or Fisher and Jones (2012) for a detailed description of performance skills. On the other hand, performance patterns refer to the habits, routines, roles, and rituals used in the process of engaging in occupations or activities that can support or hinder occupational performance (AOTA, 2014, Kielhofner, 2008). The reader is encouraged to refer to the Model of Human Occupation (Kielhofner, 2008), the *Framework* (AOTA, 2014), and *Willard and Spackman's Occupational Therapy* (Boyt Schell, Gillen, & Scaffa, 2014) for a deeper understanding and appreciation of performance patterns.

Thus, when assessing ADLs and IADLs, it is vital to consider the client factors as they will influence the client's wants, needs, abilities, goals, and priorities related to one's ADLs and IADLs; the performance skills, or the motor, process, and social interaction skills, as they underlie the ability to participate in desired occupations and activities; as well as the client's performance patterns to truly understand the frequency and manner in which the ADLs and IADLs are incorporated into a client's life. Likewise, it is as equally as important to consider the physical and social environment, as well as the cultural, personal, temporal, and virtual context related to one's ADLs and IADLs (AOTA, 2014), as these factors may support or hinder occupational performance and will influence the meaningfulness and relevance of one's occupational performance.

Therefore, the most accurate means to assess one's ability to perform his or her ADLs and/or IADLs is to observe the client's performance within its natural context. Not only does the literature suggest that observation of occupational performance within the natural context is a more accurate means of assessment, but researchers have also indicated that it is a better indicator of safety and independence, as well (Linden, Boschian, Eker, Schalen, & Nordstrom, 2005; McNulty & Fisher, 2001). Furthermore, observation of occupational performance in its natural setting and of occupational performance that simultaneously assesses performance skills will provide the skilled occupational therapist with vital information that can be used to determine the primary method of occupational therapy intervention (Fisher & Griswold, 2014). That is, the occupational therapist can use the results of the ADL/IADL assessment to determine if the client's occupational performance can be enhanced by compensation, education, occupational skills training, and/or via enhancing personal factors and body functions (Fisher & Griswold, 2014).

Although there is a surplus of instruments to assess one's ADL/IADL performance, most standardized ADL and IADL evaluation tools have the following limitations:

- They are not designed to be flexible to meet the distinct needs of each individual client
- They do not assess client factors and performance skills in the context of occupational performance
- They do not consider the impact of the environment and context on occupational performance
- They do not provide information as to why the client is having difficulty with his or her ADLs and/or IADLs

These factors have most likely led to the popularity of many "homegrown" and nonstandardized evaluation tools, which, unfortunately, lack evidence to support its use.

The AMPS (Fisher & Jones, 2014) is a client-centered, performance-based, standardized occupational therapy ADL and IADL evaluation tool, which is performed in a familiar environment to the client. The AMPS is unique because the client is able to self-select which ADL and/or IADL item(s) he or she wants to perform, and the client is able to choose from over 15 ADL items and over 100 IADL items (Fisher & Jones, 2014). The AMPS can be used to test any person 2 years and older who has challenges or is at risk of experiencing challenges with ADL and/or IADL task performance (Fisher & Jones, 2014). The AMPS can be administered and scored within 1 hour. Furthermore, because it is computer scored, the results, as well as a computer-generated report, can be ready within minutes. The AMPS can be used to document the client's baseline quality of occupational performance during ADLs and IADLs (Fisher & Jones, 2014). Furthermore, because it is a discreet measure of ADL and IADL performance, it can detect change in ADL ability over time (Fisher & Jones, 2014). In other words, it can be used to demonstrate the effectiveness of occupational therapy interventions. Additionally, it has the advantage that it can provide both a criterion- and norm-referenced perspective of the client's occupational performance (Fisher & Jones, 2014). The AMPS has been standardized on an enormous (~150,000) international sample of persons with and without disabling or medical conditions; however, it requires extensive specialized training to be a reliable and valid rater (Fisher & Jones, 2014). Moreover, because the AMPS directly assesses the motor and process performance skills in the context of occupational performance, the AMPS provides information to the occupational therapist that can aid in the planning of occupational therapy intervention.

The School Function Assessment (SFA; Coster, Deeny, Haltiwanger, & Haley, 1998) is a criterion-referenced assessment that measures a student's ability to participate in a plethora of tasks in a school setting, including ADL performance (e.g., eating and drinking, hygiene, clothing management, functional mobility tasks, and personal care awareness). The SFA is a questionnaire that is designed to measure the student's performance in a wide variety of functional tasks that support the student's participation in the academic and social aspects of elementary education. The SFA contains three scales:

1. Participation
2. Task supports
3. Activity performance

The student's teacher, or any knowledgeable professional within the school environment, can fill out the rating form. Even though the SFA does assess the child's ability to perform ADLs in the school environment, and it considers the environmental modifications and/or lack thereof that may support or hinder performance, unfortunately, it does not formally assess the child's motor, process, and communication-interaction skills, as defined by the AMPS (Fisher & Jones, 2012) and the *Framework* (AOTA, 2014). Furthermore, the SFA does not provide the occupational therapist with any information regarding the student's opinion regarding his or her performance, the student's level of satisfaction related to his or her performance, or which specific activities the student would prefer to address. Thus, if an occupational therapist chooses to administer the SFA, the practitioner will need to use his or her keen observational skills to determine why the client is unable to perform various tasks in the school environment, and perhaps supplement the results of the SFA with information gathered from the occupational profile, or a client-centered assessment, such as the COPM or the School Setting Interview (Hemmingson, Egilson, Hoffman, & Kielhofner, 2005). Regrettably, even though there is a school version of the AMPS, it focuses on school-related tasks, such as cutting, pasting, writing, drawing, and computing, versus performance of ADLs in the school environment (Fisher, Bryze, Hume, & Griswold, 2007).

## Roles of the Occupational Therapist and the Occupational Therapy Assistant During Evaluation of ADLs and IADLs

Even though the occupational therapist and occupational therapy assistant work together in a collaborative partnership, there are distinct differences in the role of the occupational therapist and the occupational therapy assistant. *The Reference Manual of the Official Documents of the American Occupational Association, Inc.* (2012) and the AOTA website (www.aota.org) are excellent resources to identify the most current role delineations for occupational therapists and occupational therapy assistants. This section of this chapter will highlight some of the critical differences for the occupational therapist and occupational therapy assistant when evaluating a client's occupational performance during ADLs and/or IADLs.

It is important to note that the occupational therapist is responsible for directing the evaluation process. Even though the occupational therapy assistant may now contribute to the evaluation process, the occupational therapist is responsible for directing all aspects of the initial contact, including the following:

- Determining the need for service
- Determining the client's goals and priorities
- Defining the problems to be addressed
- Establishing priorities for intervention
- Determining what needs to be assessed and how this should be done
- Determining which specific assessment tasks can be delegated to the occupational therapy assistant
- Interpreting the results of the occupational therapy evaluation

Thus, the occupational therapy assistant can contribute to the evaluation process by implementing delegated assessments, if the occupational therapy assistant has demonstrated service competency in doing so. The occupational therapy assistant is also responsible for providing the occupational therapist with verbal and/or written reports of his or her observations; however, the occupational therapy assistant is not able to interpret the results of observations and/or performance on ADL/IADL assessments (AOTA, 2012).

Furthermore, it is essential that occupational therapy practitioners also familiarize themselves with their state practice act because state regulatory boards include statements related to occupational therapy assistant scope of practice and specific supervision requirements, which can vary from state to state. In addition, it is important to note that Medicare guidelines for rehabilitative services state that occupational therapy practitioners must provide services in accordance with state regulations (www.aota.org).

## Summary

The purpose of this chapter was to introduce the occupational therapy practitioner to the general process of evaluating a person's ability to perform his or her ADLs and IADLs. As previously stated, the first critical step in the evaluation process is to obtain an understanding of the client's occupational history, wants, needs, goals, and priorities (i.e., the occupational profile). After completing the occupational profile, it is vital that the occupational therapist observe the client's occupational performance, ideally in a natural environment, to determine supports and barriers to occupational performance (AOTA, 2014), the client's level of independence, as well as the quality of the client's occupational performance, or the degree of physical effort, efficiency, and safety related to the client's performance (Fisher, 2012). Because occupational performance involves a transaction between the person, task, and environment (Law et al., 1996), it is essential the occupational therapist not only consider selecting a specific ADL/IADL tool based on the activities it evaluates, but he or she also should consider selecting a tool that provides critical information related to the individual and the environment. There is a plethora of ADL and IADL tools available to occupational therapy practitioners. However, best practice entails selecting a specific evaluation tool based on sound clinical reasoning skills and evidence that supports its use. In other words, occupational therapists should be selecting evaluation tools that are occupation-based, client-centered, and have evidence to support the reliability, validity, and utility of the assessment tool. This chapter introduces the reader to a small sampling of ADL and IADL evaluation tools; it is by no means meant to be an exhaustive list! Table 18-1 summarizes a small amount of the ADL and IADL tools available to occupational therapy practitioners and the Evidence-Based Research Chart highlights some of the current evidence to support some of the most researched ADL and IADL tools. Because there is an overabundance of other tools available to the occupational therapy practitioner, the reader is encouraged to refer to books such as *Asher's Assessment Tools: An Annotated Index* (Asher, 2014), *Measuring Occupational Performance: Supporting*

Table 18-1.

## Summary of Selected Activities of Daily Living and Instrumental Activities of Daily Living Evaluation Tools

| Name of Assessment | Areas of Assessment | Type of Client | Format and Specifics of Assessment |
|---|---|---|---|
| Assessment of Motor and Process Skills (AMPS) | Observational evaluation designed to evaluate the quality of a person's performance of ADLs and IADLs, in natural, task-relevant environments | Persons 2 years of age or older<br>Any person who has or is at risk for experiencing challenges with ADL/IADL performance (i.e., any diagnosis or disability)<br>May also be used to assess well persons | Client self-selects ADL/IADL items to perform (occupation based and client centered)<br>There are 17 ADL and more than 100 IADL items<br>Can be administered and scored in 1 hour or less<br>Can be used in any relevant and familiar environment (clinical or community-based)<br>There are 16 motor skill items and 20 process skill items<br>Each motor and process skill item is rated on a 4-point scale<br>4 = competent performance<br>3 = questionable performance<br>2 = ineffective performance<br>1 = unacceptable performance<br>Standardized on ~150,000 persons<br>More than 120 internationally standardized tasks<br>Requires specialized training to be a reliable and valid rater<br>Observation results/scores are inputted into a computer software program and norm-based interpretation is provided, including prediction regarding need for assistance |
| Canadian Occupational Performance Measure (COPM) | Client's self-perception of his or her performance in:<br>(1) self-care (including personal care, functional mobility, and community management);<br>(2) productivity (including paid or unpaid work, household management, school, and play), and<br>(3) leisure (including quiet recreation, active recreation, and socialization productivity) | Any age<br>Any diagnosis or disability<br>Successfully used with children as young as 7 years old; can be used with younger children through parent/caregiver report | Semistructured interview<br>Designed to detect changes in client's self-perception of occupational performance over time<br>Fosters collaboration between client and practitioner<br>Can be used as an initial evaluation and as an outcome measure<br>Can be administered and scored in less than 1 hour<br>Client describes occupations normally performed; client identifies concerns regarding his or her performance during self-care, productivity, and leisure tasks; client evaluates his or her performance and satisfaction regarding occupational performance; client prioritizes his or her problems in occupational performance<br>A 10-point scale is used to indicate client's perception of ability to perform self-care, productivity, and leisure tasks and client's level of satisfaction regarding occupational performance on the five most important occupations to be addressed, as identified by the client |

*(continued)*

Table 18-1 (continued).

## Summary of Selected Activities of Daily Living and Instrumental Activities of Daily Living Evaluation Tools

| Name of Assessment | Areas of Assessment | Type of Client | Format and Specifics of Assessment |
|---|---|---|---|
| Executive Function Performance Test (EFPT) | Utilizes four IADL activities in a naturalistic setting and determines which executive function components are impaired<br>Four tasks: (1) oatmeal preparation;<br>(2) telephone skills;<br>(3) taking medication;<br>(4) paying bills<br>Three components of executive function evaluated are:<br>(1) initiation, (2) execution (organization, sequencing, judgement, and safety); and (3) termination | Adults<br>Diagnoses that may result in executive function deficits (e.g., stroke, traumatic brain injury, multiple sclerosis, schizophrenia) | Top-down performance assessment designed to determine: (1) which executive functions are impacting function; (2) an individual's capacity for independent functioning; and (3) the amount of assistance necessary for task completion<br>Time to administer: 30 to 45 minutes<br>Four tasks:<br>1 = oatmeal preparation<br>2 = telephone skills<br>3 = taking medication<br>4 = paying bills<br>Establishes the amount of assistance necessary for task completion (verbal guidance, direct verbal assistance, physical assistance, and do for the client)<br>Designed to supply the practitioner with information that will help family members understand and support their loved one's performance |
| Performance Assessment of Self-Care Skills (PASS) | Three ADL tasks (oral hygiene, dressing, and trimming toenails)<br>Five functional mobility tasks (bed transfer, stair use, toilet transfer, bathtub and shower transfer, indoor walking)<br>18 IADL tasks (shopping, bill paying by check, checkbook balancing, mailing bills, telephone use, medication management, obtaining critical information from the media [auditory and visual], sweeping, carrying the garbage, changing bed linens, small repairs, home safety, oven use, stovetop use, use of sharp utensils, clean-up after meal, playing bingo<br>Each task has specific directions for set-up and instructions | Adolescents and adults<br>Sample included adults from healthy as well as diagnostic populations<br>Diagnoses include, but are not limited to: arthritis, dementia, cardiopulmonary disease, mental retardation, schizophrenia | A performance-based, criterion-referenced, observational tool that focuses on ADL, IADL, and functional mobility skills<br>26 core tasks (three ADL, five functional mobility, and 18 IADL); patient performance is rated on independence, safety, and adequacy<br>Two versions exist: PASS-Clinic and PASS-Home<br>PASS may be administered in total or selected-items based on client's needs<br>May be used for initial evaluation, intervention planning, assessment of progress, and/or for discharge evaluation/planning<br>Determine amount of change and amount of assistance client requires<br>Helps practitioner understand where the "breakdown" occurs in ability to complete daily living tasks<br>Combines two conceptual foundations of assessment: (1) interactive assessment and (2) graduated prompting<br>Establishes a client's current level of performance without assistance and the type and amount of assistance required for improved performance<br>Incorporates a hierarchy of prompts that are used when there is breakdown in task performance |

*(continued)*

Table 18-1 (continued).

## Summary of Selected Activities of Daily Living and Instrumental Activities of Daily Living Evaluation Tools

| Name of Assessment | Areas of Assessment | Type of Client | Format and Specifics of Assessment |
|---|---|---|---|
| Multiple Errands Test (MET) | The MET evaluates the effect of executive function deficits on everyday functioning through a number of real-world tasks (e.g., purchasing specific items, collecting and writing down specific information, arriving at a stated location)<br>Tasks are performed in a hospital or community setting within the constraints of specified rules<br>The participant is observed performing the test and the number and type of errors (e.g., rule breaks, omissions) are recorded | The MET has been tested on populations with acquired brain injury including stroke<br>The MET should not be used with patients who are confined to bed or participants who require sufficient language skills | Different versions of the MET were developed for use in specific hospitals (MET–Hospital Version and Baycrest MET), a small shopping plaza (MET–Simplified Version), and a virtual reality environment (Virtual MET)<br>For each of these versions, 12 tasks must be performed (e.g., purchasing specific items and collecting specific information) while following several rules<br>The MET-HV was developed for use with a wider range of participants than the original version by adopting more concrete rules and simpler tasks. Clients are provided with an instruction sheet that explicitly directs them to record designated information. Clients must achieve four sets of simple tasks, with a total of 12 separate subtasks. More specifically, for the MET-HV, the client must:<br>Complete six specific errands (purchase three items, use the internal phone, collect an envelope from reception, and send a letter to an external address)<br>Obtain and write down four items of designated information (e.g., the opening time of a shop on Saturday)<br>Meet the assessor outside the hospital reception 20 minutes after the test had begun and state the time<br>Inform the assessor when he or she finishes the test<br>Time taken to complete the assessment is recorded and the total number of errors is calculated |
| Pediatric Evaluation Disability Inventory—Computer Adapted Test (PEDI-CAT) | CAT that measures abilities in three functional domains:<br>1 = daily activities<br>2 = mobility<br>3 = social/cognitive | Can be used across all clinical diagnoses and in community settings<br>Intended for children and youth (birth to 20 years of age)<br>Like the PEDI (pencil version), the PEDI-CAT can be administered by health care professionals, educators, parent report, or other individual familiar with the child | Two versions of PEDI-CAT<br>(1) Speedy or "precision" CAT: Most efficient; administer 10 to 15 items per domain; includes a percentile score, scaled score, and a list of responses to all PEDI-CAT items<br>(2) Content-balanced or "comprehensive" CAT: Administer approximately 30 items per domain; includes a percentile score, scaled score, and an item map showing the location of the response for that domain<br>The PEDI-CAT can be used on multiple occasions (initial, progress, discharge, follow-up) and no minimum is required between assessments<br>The CAT version is intended to provide an accurate and precise assessment while increasing efficiency and reducing respondent burden<br>The PEDI-CAT software uses Item Response Theory statistical models to estimate a child's abilities from a minimum number of the most relevant items or from a set number of items within each domain<br>All respondents begin with the same item in each domain in the middle range of difficulty and the response on that item will determine which item will appear next (a harder or easier item); thus, it avoids irrelevant items<br>Results are displayed instantly with the PEDI-CAT |

## Case Study

Mary is an 80-year-old woman who slipped and fell on ice while attempting to retrieve her morning paper at the end of her driveway. Unfortunately, this fall resulted in the shattering of her right proximal femur and the need for an open reduction internal fixation hip surgery. Because Mary needed to be independent in her ADLs and IADLs to return home, she was admitted to an inpatient rehabilitation facility. Results of the initial occupational profile interview revealed that Mary is widowed and lives alone in a tri-level house. She was completely independent with all her ADLs and IADLs prior to this accident. She is retired, drives a car, and regularly watches her 10-year-old grandson who has a mild disability. Her typical day entailed waking up at approximately 6 a.m.; showering; making her bed; making and eating breakfast, which usually consisted of coffee, juice, and either a muffin, bagel, coffee cake, or cereal; reading the newspaper; doing some light housework, such as laundry, dusting furniture, or ironing; making and eating lunch, which usually consisted of soup, salad, sandwich, and/or leftovers from dinner; bargain shopping; grocery shopping; watching her grandson; making and eating dinner, which usually consisted of chicken or fish, vegetable, salad, and rice or potato; watching TV; reading a book; and going to bed at approximately 10 p.m. Mary stated that she typically sees her adult children on the weekend and gets together with her "lady friends" about once a week for dinner at a restaurant. In terms of Mary's home, it was discovered that she does not have a bathroom on the first floor; her bedroom and master bath are approximately seven steps upstairs (railing on the right side when ascending steps) and her laundry room and powder room are approximately seven steps downstairs (railing on the left side while descending, with a half wall with a sturdy ledge on the right side). Mary typically carried small loads of her laundry to the basement in her hands versus in a bag or basket. Mary has two different ways to access her house; one way is through the garage, but then she has to ascend approximately seven steps to get to her first floor (kitchen area), or she can come in through the front door, which entails walking up a steep incline that often becomes slippery and icy in the winter; furthermore, this entrance also entails ascending two steps without a railing to reach the front door (first floor of house). Through the occupational profile, it became very evident that Mary is very proud of the fact she is a very independent person and that she has been able to remain in her home, even after the passing of her husband about 3 years ago. After obtaining the initial occupational profile, the COPM was administered to gain more specific information regarding Mary's perception of the quality of her performance, her level of satisfaction, and her priorities related to her self-care, productivity, and leisure. The results of the CPOM revealed that Mary's biggest priorities for occupational therapy intervention had do with better performance and satisfaction related to the following ADLs and IADLs: dressing, bathing, cooking, laundry, and being able to get in and out of bed.

### Initial Evaluation

| | COPM Scores for Performance/Satisfaction |
|---|---|
| Dressing: | 4/4 |
| Bathing: | 2/2 |
| Cooking: | 2/2 |
| Laundry: | 0/0 |
| Getting in/out of bed: | 4/4 |

Performance: 1 = Not Able to Do It; 10 = Able to Do It Extremely Well
Satisfaction: 1 = Not Satisfied at All; 10 = Extremely Satisfied

Next, the AMPS was used to assess her performance skills in the context of her performing an ADL task (upper body grooming and total body dressing) and during an IADL task (grilled cheese sandwich and a beverage). Results of the AMPS revealed that, overall, Mary had competent process skills, but had ineffective performance on many of the motor skills, especially with stabilizes, reaches, bends, moves, lifts, walks, transports, and endures. The occupational therapy practitioner determined that the use of compensation, education, and acquisition through occupation skills training would facilitate Mary's ability to regain her safety and independence in her ADLs and IADLs.

*(continued)*

## Case Study (continued)

| Motor Skills | Upper Body Grooming and Total Body Dressing | Grilled Cheese Sandwich and Beverage |
|---|---|---|
| Endures | 2 | 2 |
| Lifts | 4 | 4 |
| Aligns | 2 | 2 |
| Moves | 2 | 2 |
| Transports | 2 | 2 |
| Flows | 2 | 2 |
| Grips | 4 | 4 |
| Reaches | 2 | 2 |
| Bends | 2 | 2 |
| Manipulates | 4 | 4 |
| Walks | 2 | 2 |
| Stabilizes | 2 | 2 |
| Coordinates | 2 | 4 |
| Paces | 2 | 2 |
| Calibrates | 2 | 2 |
| Positions | 2 | 2 |

4 = Competent Performance
3 = Questionable Performance
2 = Ineffective Performance
1 = Unacceptable Performance

| Process Skills | Upper Body Grooming and Total Body Dressing | Grilled Cheese Sandwich and Beverage |
|---|---|---|
| Uses | 4 | 4 |
| Chooses | 4 | 4 |
| Sequences | 4 | 4 |
| Searches/Locates | 4 | 4 |
| Attends | 4 | 4 |
| Inquires | 4 | 4 |
| Gathers | 4 | 4 |
| Heeds | 2 | 4 |
| Terminates | 4 | 4 |
| Navigates | 2 | 2 |
| Handles | 2 | 2 |
| Adjusts | 2 | 2 |
| Continues | 4 | 4 |
| Restores | 4 | 4 |
| Initiates | 2 | 2 |
| Organizes | 3 | 2 |
| Paces | 2 | 2 |
| Notices/Responds | 2 | 2 |
| Benefits | 2 | 2 |
| Accommodates | 2 | 2 |

## Evidence-Based Research Chart

| Topic | Evidence |
|---|---|
| Assessment of Motor and Process Skills | Ayres & Panickacheril, 2015; Fioravanti, Bordignon, Pettit, Woodhouse, & Ansley, 2012; Fisher & Jones, 2012; Gantschnig, Fisher, Page, Meichtry, & Nilsson, 2015; Gantschnig, Page, & Fisher, 2012; Merritt, 2011; Mesa, Heron, Chard, & Rowe, 2014; Rojo-Mota, Pedrero-Perez, Ruiz-Sanchez de Leon, & Page, 2014; Toneman, Brayshaw, Lange, & Trimboli, 2010 |
| Canadian Occupational Performance Measure | Colquhoun, Letts, Law, MacDermid, & Missiuna, 2012; Eyssen et al., 2011; Law et al., 2014; McNulty & Beplal, 2008; Richard & Knis-Matthews, 2010 |
| Executive Function Performance Test | Baum et al., 2008; Cederfeldt, Carlsson, Dahlin-Ivanoff, & Gosman-Hedstrom, 2015; Cederfeldt, Widell, Anderson, Dahlin-Ivanoff, & Gosman-Hedstrom, 2011; Hahn et al., 2014; Katz, Tadmor, Felzen, & Hartman-Maeir, 2007; Raad & Moore, 2012 |
| Performance Assessment of Self-Care Skills | Ciro, Anderson, Hershey, Prodan, & Holm, 2015; Finlayson, Havens, Holm, & Van Denend, 2003; Holm & Rogers, 2008; Rodakowski et al., 2014; Shih, 2008; Skidmore, Rogers, Chandler, & Holm, 2006 |
| Pediatric Evaluation Disability Inventory—Computer Adapted Test | Dumas et al., 2010, 2012; Haley et al., 2010, 2011; Ketelaar & Wassenberg-Severijnen, 2010; Kramer, Coster, Kao, Snow, & Orsmond, 2013; Rich, Rigby, & Wright, 2014; Ying-Chai, Kramer, Liljenquist, & Coster, 2015; Ying-Chai, Kramer, Liljenquist, Feng, & Coster, 2012 |
| Multiple Errands Test | Castiel, Alderman, Jenkins, Knight, & Burgess, 2012; Dawson et al., 2005, 2009; Lanceley, 2015; Maeir, Krauss, & Katz, 2011; Morrison et al., 2013; Pedroli et al., 2013; Poulin, Korner-Bitensky, & Dawson, 2013; Raspelli et al., 2010, 2011 |
| School Function Assessment | Chien, Rodger, Copley, & McLaren, 2014; Daunhauer, Fidler, & Will, 2014; Davies, Soon, Young, & Clausen-Yamaki, 2004; Egilson & Coster, 2004; Gates, Otsuka, Sanders, & McGee, 2008; Liang Hwang, 2005; Liang Hwang & Davies, 2009; Liang Hwang, Davies, Taylor, & Gavin, 2002; Silverman & O'Smith, 2006; West, Dunford, Mayston, & Forsyth, 2014 |
| Child Occupational Self-Assessment | Ayuso & Kramer, 2009; Keller, Kafkes, & Kielhofner, 2005; Keller & Kielhofner, 2005; Kramer, 2008; Kramer, Heckmann, & Bell-Walker, 2012; Kramer, Kielhofner, & Smith, 2010; Ohl, Crook, MacSaveny, & McLaughlin, 2015; ten Velden, Couldrick, Kinébanian, & Sadlo, 2013 |

*Best Practice in Occupational Therapy* (Law, Baum, & Dunn, 2005), and keeping up with the current evidence that supports or does not support use of specific ADL and IADL evaluation tools.

## Student Self-Assessment

1. What is an occupational profile? What type of information should be gathered during an occupational profile?
2. Describe why it is important to observe occupational performance, even after a very thorough occupational profile.
3. In your own words, define ADLs and IADLs. Give at least five examples of each.
4. When selecting an ADL and/or IADL evaluation tool, describe what types of things you should consider before deciding to use a specific ADL/IADL evaluation tool.
5. Search the literature and locate an ADL or IADL tool that you are unfamiliar with. Describe what it assesses, how it goes about the assessment process, what type of clients it should be used with, and summarize the evidence that supports or does not support its usage.
6. Explain how client factors, performance skills, performance patterns, the context, and the environment can influence performance in ADLs and IADLs.
7. In your own words, explain the difference between an activity and an occupation.

8. Compare and contrast the role of the occupational therapist and occupational therapy assistant in the ADL and IADL screening and evaluation process.

# Electronic Resources

American Occupational Therapy Association: www.aota.org

Center for Innovative OT Solutions http://www.innovativeotsolutions.com

Model of Human Occupation Clearinghouse: www.moho.uic.edu

Occupational Therapy: Systematic Evaluation of Evidence: www.otseeker.com

Rehabilitation Measures Database: www.rehabmeasures.org

# References


American Occupational Therapy Association. (2012). *The reference manual of the official documents of the American Occupational Association, Inc.* Bethseda, MD: AOTA Press.

American Occupational Therapy Association. (2014). Occupational therapy practice framework: Domain and process (3rd ed.). *American Journal of Occupational Therapy, 68*(Suppl. 1), S1-S48. doi:10.5014/ajot.2014.682006

Asher, I. (2014). *Asher's occupational therapy assessment tools: An annotated index* (4th ed.). Bethseda, MD: AOTA Press.

Ayres, H., & Panickacheril, A. (2015). The Assessment of Motor and Process Skills as a measure of ADL ability in schizophrenia. *Scandinavian Journal of Occupational Therapy, 22*, 470-477.

Ayuso, D., & Kramer, J. (2009). Using the Spanish Child Occupational Self-Assessment (COSA) with children with ADHD. *Occupational Therapy in Mental Health, 25*, 101-114.

Baron, K., Kielhofner, G., Iyenger, A., Goldhammer, V., & Wolenski, J. (2006). *The Occupational Self-Assessment (OSA) Version 2.2.* Chicago, IL: The Model of Human Occupation Clearinghouse Department of Occupational Therapy, College of Applied Health Sciences, University of Illinois at Chicago.

Baum, C., Tabor Connor, L., Morrison, T., Hahn, M., Dromerick, A., & Edwards, D. (2008). Reliability, validity, and clinical utility of the Executive Function Performance Test: A measure of executive function in a sample of people with stroke. *American Journal of Occupational Therapy, 62*, 446-454.

Boyt Schell, B., Gillen, G., & Scaffa, M. (2014). *Willard and Spackman's occupational therapy* (12th ed.). Philadelphia, PA: Wolters Kluwer/Lippincott Williams and Wilkins.

Castiel, M., Alderman, N., Jenkins, K., Knight, C., & Burgess, P. (2012). Use of the Multiple Errands Test—Simplified version in the assessment of suboptimal effort. *Neuropsychological Rehabilitation, 22*, 734-751.

Cederfeldt, M., Carlsson, G., Dahlin-Ivanoff, S., & Gosman-Hedstrom, G. (2015). Inter-rater reliability and face validity of the Executive Function Performance Test (EFPT). *British Journal of Occupational Therapy, 78*, 563-569.

Cederfeldt, M., Widell, Y., Anderson, E., Dahlin-Ivanoff, S., & Gosman-Hedstrom, G. (2011). Concurrent validity of the Executive Function Performance Test (EFPT) in people with stroke. *British Journal of Occupational Therapy, 74*, 443-449.

Chien, C., Rodger, S., Copley, J., & McLaren, C. (2014). Measures of participation outcomes related to hand use for 2- to 12-year-old children with disabilities: A systematic review. *Child: Care, Health and Development, 40*, 458-471.

Ciro, C., Anderson, M., Hershey, L., Prodan, C., & Holm, M. (2015). Instrumental activities of daily living performance and role satisfaction in people with and without mild cognitive impairment: A pilot project. *American Journal of Occupational Therapy, 69*, 1-10.

Colquhoun, H., Letts, L., Law, M., MacDermid, J., & Missiuna, C. (2012). Administration of the Canadian Occupational Performance Measure: Effect on practice. *Canadian Journal of Occupational Therapy, 79*, 121-128.

Coster, W., Deeny, T., Haltiwanger, J., & Haley, S. (1998). *School Function Assessment (SFA).* San Antonio, TX: The Psychological Corporation.

Daunhauer, L., Fidler, D., & Will, E. (2014). School function in students with Down syndrome. *American Journal of Occupational Therapy, 68*, 167-176.

Davies, P., Soon, P., Young, M., & Clausen-Yamaki, A. (2004). Validity and reliability of the School Function Assessment in elementary school students with disabilities. *Physical and Occupational Therapy in Pediatrics, 24*, 23-43.

Dawson, D., Anderson, N., Burgess, P., Cooper, E., Krpan, K., & Stuss, D. (2009). Further development of the Multiple Errands Test: Standardized scoring, reliability, and ecological validity for the Baycrest version. *Archives of Physical Medicine and Rehabilitation, 90*, S41-S51.

Dawson, D., Anderson, N., Burgess, P., Levine, B., Rewilak, D., Cooper, E., & Stuss, D. (2005). Naturalistic assessment of executive function: The Multiple Errands Test. *Neurorehabiliation and Neural Repair, 19*, 379-380.

Dumas, H., Fragala-Pinkham, M., Haley, S., Coster, W., Kramer J., Kao, Y., & Moed, R. (2010). Item bank development for a revised pediatric evaluation of disability inventory (PEDI). *Physical and Occupational Therapy in Pediatrics, 33*, 332-338.

Dumas, H., Fragala-Pinkham, M., Haley, S., Ni, P., Coster, W., Kramer, J., ... Ludlow, L. (2012). Computer adaptive test performance in children with and without disabilities: prospective field study of the PEDI-CAT. *Disability and Rehabilitation, 34*, 393-401.

Egilson, S., & Coster, W. (2004). School Function Assessment: Performance of Icelandic students with special needs. *Scandinavian Journal of Occupational Therapy, 11*, 163-170.

Eyssen, I., Steultjens, M., Oud, T., Bolt, E., Maasdam, A., & Dekker, J. (2011). Responsivenesss of the Canadian Occupational Performance Measure. *Journal of Rehabilitation Research and Development, 48*, 517-528.

Finlayson, M., Havens, B., Holm, M., & Van Denend, T. (2003). Integrating a performance-based observation measure of functional status into a population-based longitudinal study of aging. *Canadian Journal on Aging, 22*, 185-195. doi:10.1017/S0714980800004505

Fioravanti, A., Bordignon, C., Pettit, S., Woodhouse, L., & Ansley, B. (2012). Comparing responsiveness of the Assessment of Motor and Process Skills and the Functional Independence Measure. *Canadian Journal of Occupational Therapy, 79*, 167-174.

Fisher, A. (2009). *Occupational Therapy Intervention Process Model: A model for planning and implementing top-down, client-centered, and occupation-based interventions.* Fort Collins, CO: Three Star Press.

Fisher, A., Bryze, K., Hume, V., & Griswold, L. (2007). *School AMPS: School Version of the Assessment of Motor and Process Skills* (2nd ed.). Fort Collins, CO: Three Star Press.

Fisher, A., & Griswold, L. (2014). Performance skills: Implementing performance analyses to evaluate quality of occupational performance. In B. Schell, G. Gillen, M. Scaffa, & E. Cohn (Eds.), *Williard and Spackman's occupational therapy* (12th ed.). Philadelphia, PA: Wolters Kluwer/Lippincott Williams and Wilkins.

Fisher, A., & Jones, K. (2012). *Assessment of motor and process skills: Vol. I: Development, standardization, and administration manual* (7th ed.). Fort Collins, CO: Three Star Press.

Fisher, A., & Jones, K. (2014). *Assessment of motor and process skills: Vol. II: User manual* (7th ed.). Fort Collins, CO: Three Star Press.

Gantschnig, B., Fisher, A., Page, J., Meichtry, A., & Nilsson, I. (2015). Differences in activities of daily living (ADL) abilities of children across world regions: A validity study of the Assessment of Motor and Process Skills. *Child: Care, Health, and Development, 41*, 230-238.

Gantschnig, B., Page, J., & Fisher, A. (2012). Cross-regional validity of the Assessment of Motor and Process Skills for use in Middle Europe. *Journal of Rehabilitation Medicine, 44*, 151-157.

Gates, P., Otsuka, N., Sanders, J., & McGee, J. (2008). Relationship between the parental PODCI questionnaire and School Function Assessment in measuring performance in children with CP. *Developmental Medicine and Child Neurology, 50*, 690-695.

Hahn, B., Baum, C., Moore, J., Ehrlich-Jones, L., Spoeri, S., Doherty, M., & Wolf, T. J. (2014). Brief report—Development of additional tasks for the Executive Function Performance Test. *American Journal of Occupational Therapy, 68*, e241–e246.

Haley S., Coster, W., Dumas, H., Fragala-Pinkham, M., Kramer, J., Ni, P., ... Ludlow, L. (2011). Accuracy and precision of the Pediatric Evaluation of Disability Inventory computer-adaptive tests (PEDI-CAT). *Developmental Medicine and Child Neurology, 53*, 1100-1106.

Haley, S., Coster, W., Kao, Y., Dumas, H., Fragala-Pinkham, M., Kramer, J., ... Moed, R. (2010). Lessons from use of the Pediatric Evaluation of Disability Inventory: Where do we go from here? *Pediatric Physical Therapy, 22*, 69-75.

Hemmingsson, H., Egilson, S., Hoffman, O., & Kielhofner, G. (2005). *The School Setting Interview (SSI): Version 3.0*. Chicago, IL: The Model of Human Occupation Clearinghouse Department of Occupational Therapy, College of Applied Health Sciences, University of Illinois at Chicago.

Holm, M., & Rogers, J. (2008). The Performance Self-Care Skills (PASS). In B. Hemphill-Pearson (Ed.), *Assessments in occupational therapy mental health: An integrated approach* (2nd ed., pp. 101-110). Thorofare, NJ: SLACK Incorporated.

Katz, N., Tadmor, I., Felzen, B., & Hartman-Maeir, A. (2007). Validity of the Executive Function Performance Test in individuals with schizophrenia. *OTJR: Occupation, Participation, and Health, 27*, 44-51.

Keller, J., Kafkes, A., & Kielhofner, G. (2005). Psychometric characteristics of the Child Occupational Self-Assessment (COSA), part one: An initial examination of psychometric properties. *Scandinavian Journal of Occupational Therapy, 12*, 118-127.

Keller, J., & Kielhofner, G. (2005). Psychometric characteristics of the Child Occupational Self-Assessment (COSA), part two: Refining the psychometric properties. *Scandinavian Journal of Occupational Therapy, 12*, 147-158.

Ketelaar, M., & Wassenberg-Severijnen, J. (2010). Developments in measuring functional activities: Where do we go with the PEDI-CAT? *Physical and Occupational Therapy in Pediatrics, 30*, 185-189.

Kielhofner, G. (2008). *Model of Human Occupation*. Baltimore, MD: Wolters Kluwer/Lippincott Williams and Wilkins.

Knecht-Sabres, L. (2014). Evaluation of activities of daily living and instrumental activities of daily living. In K. Jacobs, N. MacRae, & K. Sladyk (Eds.), *Occupational therapy essentials for clinical competence* (2nd ed., pp. 215-229). Thorofare, NJ: SLACK Incorporated.

Kramer, J. (2008). A mixed methods approach to building validity evidence: The Child Occupational Self Assessment. Doctoral dissertation, University of Illinois.

Kramer, J., Coster, W., Kao, Y., Snow, A., & Orsmond, G. (2013). A new approach to the measurement of adaptive behavior: Development of the PEDI-CAT for children and youth with autism spectrum disorders. *Physical and Occupational Therapy in Pediatrics, 32*, 34-47.

Kramer, J., Heckmann, S., & Bell-Walker, M. (2012). Accommodations and therapeutic techniques used during the administration of the Child Occupational Self-Assessment. *British Journal of Occupational Therapy, 75*, 495-502.

Kramer, J., Kielhofner, G., & Smith, E. (2010). Validity evidence for the Child Occupational Self-Assessment. *American Journal of Occupational Therapy, 64*, 621-632.

Kramer, J., ten Velden, M., Kafkes, A., Basu, S., Federico, J., & Kielhofner, G. (2014). *Child Occupational Self-Assessment (COSA): Version 2.2*. Chicago, IL: The Model of Human Occupation Clearinghouse Department of Occupational Therapy, College of Applied Health Sciences, University of Illinois at Chicago.

Lanceley, S. (2015). A new approach to the assessment of cognition in drivers: Applying the Multiple Errands Test for use in a simple parking exercise. *British Journal of Occupational Therapy, 78*, 96-99.

Law, M. Baptiste, S., Carswell, A., McColl, M., Polatajko, H., & Pollock, N. (2014). *Canadian Occupational Performance Measure* (5th ed.). Ottawa, Ontario, Canada: CAOT Publications.

Law, M., Baum, C., & Dunn, W. (2005). *Measuring occupational performance: Supporting best practice in occupational therapy*. Thorofare, NJ: SLACK Incorporated.

Law, M., Cooper, B., Strong, S., Stewart, D., Rigby, P., & Letts, L. (1996). The Person-Environment-Occupation Model: A transactive approach to occupational performance. *Canadian Journal of Occupational Therapy, 63*, 9-23.

Law, M., Polatajko, H., Baptise, W., & Townsend, E. (1997). Core concepts of occupational therapy. In E. Townsend (Ed.), *Enabling occupation: An occupational therapy perspective*. Ottawa, Ontario, Canada: Canadian Association of Occupational Therapists.

Liang Hwang, J. (2005). The reliability and validity of the School Function Assessment-Chinese Version. *OTJR: Occupation, Participation, and Health, 25*, 44-54.

Liang Hwang, J., & Davies, P. (2009). Rasch analysis of the School Function Assessment provides additional evidence for the internal validity of the Activity Performance Scales. *American Journal of Occupational Therapy, 63*, 369-373.

Liang Hwang, J., Davies, P., Taylor, M., & Gavin, W. (2002). Validation of School Function Assessment with elementary school children. *OTJR: Occupation, Participation and Health, 22*, 48-58.

Linden, A., Boschian, K., Eker, C., Schalen, W., & Nordstrom, C. (2005). Assessment of Motor and Process Skills reflects brain-injured patients' ability to resume independent living better than neurological tests. *ACTA Neurologica Scandinavica, 111*, 48-53.

Maeir, A., Krauss, S., & Katz, N. (2011). Ecological validity of the Multiple Errands Test (MET) on discharge from neurorehabilitation hospital. *OTJR: Occupation, Participation, and Health, 31*, S38-S46.

McNulty, M., & Beplal, A. (2008). The validity of using the Canadian Occupational Performance Measure with older adults with and without depressive symptoms. *Physical and Occupational Therapy in Geriatrics*, 27, 1-15.

McNulty, M., & Fisher, A. (2001). Validity of using the Assessment of Motor and Process Skills to estimate over-all home safety in persons with psychiatric conditions. *American Journal of Occupational Therapy, 55*, 649-655.

Merritt, B. (2011). Validity of using the Assessment of Motor and Process Skills to determine the need for assistance. *American Journal of Occupational Therapy, 65*, 643-650.

Mesa, S., Heron, P., Chard, G., & Rowe, J. (2014). Using the Assessment of Motor and Process Skills as part of the diagnostic process in an inner-city learning disability service. *British Journal of Occupational Therapy, 77*, 170-173.

Metzler, M., & Metz, G. (2010). Analyzing the barriers and supports of knowledge translation using the PEO model. *Canadian Journal of Occupational Therapy, 77*, 151-158.

Morrison, M., Giles, G., Ryan, J., Baum, C., Dromerick, A., Polatajko, H., & Edwards, D. (2013). Multiple Errands Test-Revised (MET-R): A performance-based measure of executive function in people with mild cerebrovascular accident. *American Journal of Occupational Therapy, 67*, 460-468.

Ohl, A., Crook, E., MacSaveny, D., & McLaughlin, A. (2015). Test–retest reliability of the Child Occupational Self-Assessment (COSA). *American Journal of Occupational Therapy, 69*, 1-4.

Pedroli, E., Cipresso, P., Serino, S., Pallavicini, F., Albani, G., & Giuseppe, R. (2013). Virtual Multiple Errands Test: Reliability, usability and possible applications. *Annual Review of Cybertherapy and Telemedicine, 191*, 38-42.

Poulin, V., Korner-Bitensky, N., & Dawson, D. (2013). Stroke-specific executive function assessment: A literature review of performance-based tools. *Australian Occupational Therapy Journal, 60*, 3-19.

Raad, J., & Moore, J. (2012). Measurement characteristics and clinical utility of the Executive Function Performance Test among individuals with a stroke. *Archives of Physical Medicine and Rehabilitation, 93*, 2139-2140.

Raphael-Greenfield, E. (2012). Assessing executive and community functioning among homeless persons with substance use disorders using the Executive Function Performance Test. *Occupational Therapy International, 19*, 135-143.

Raspelli, S., Carelli, L., Morganti, F., Poletti, B., Corra, B., Silani, V., & Riva, G. (2010). Implementation of the multiple errands test in a NeuroVR-supermarket: A possible approach. *Studies in Health Technology and Informatics, 154*, 115-119.

Raspelli, S., Pallavicini, F., Carelli, L., Morganti, F., Poletti, B., Corra, B., ... Giuseppe, R. (2011). Validation of a neuro-virtual reality-based version of the Multiple Errands Test for the assessment of executive functions. *Annual Review of Cybertherapy and Telemedicine, 167*, 9297.

Rich, D., Rigby, P., & Wright, V. (2014). Mothers' experiences with the Pediatric Evaluation of Disability Inventory (PEDI). *Physical and Occupational Therapy in Pediatrics, 34*, 271-288.

Richard, L., & Knis-Matthews, L. (2010). Are we really client-centered? Using the Canadian Occupational Performance Measure to see how the client's goals connect with the goals of the occupational therapist. *Occupational Therapy in Mental Health, 26*, 51-66.

Rodakowski, J., Skidmore, E., Reynolds, C., Dew, M., Butters, M., Holm, M., ... Rogers, J. (2014). Can performance on daily activities discriminate between older adults with normal cognitive function and those with mild cognitive impairment? *Journal of the American Geriatrics Society, 62*, 1347-1352.

Rojo-Mota, G., Pedrero-Perez, E., Ruiz-Sanchez de Leon, J., & Page, J. (2014). Assessment of the Motor and Process Skills in daily life activities of treated substance addicts. *Scandinavian Journal of Occupational Therapy, 21*, 458-464.

Shih, M. (2008). Multiple perspectives of the functional status of stroke survivors at 3 months post-stroke. Doctoral dissertation, University of Pittsburgh.

Shotwell, M. (2014). Evaluating clients. In B. Schell, G. Gillen, M. Scaffa, & E. Cohn (Eds.), *Williard and Spackman's occupational therapy* (12th ed.). Philadelphia, PA: Wolters Kluwer/Lippincott Williams and Wilkins.

Silverman, M., & O'Smith, R. (2006). Consequential validity of an assistive technology supplement for the School Function Assessment. *Assistive Technology, 18*, 155-165.

Skidmore, E., Rogers, J., Chandler, L., & Holm, M. (2006). Dynamic interactions between impairment and activity after stroke: Examining the utility of decision analysis methods. *Clinical Rehabilitation, 20*, 523-535.

ten Velden, M., Couldrick,L., Kinébanian, A., & Sadlo, G. (2013). Dutch children's perspectives on the constructs of the Child Occupational Self-Assessment (COSA). *OTJR: Occupation, Participation and Health, 33*, 50-58.

Toneman, M., Brayshaw, J., Lange, B., & Trimboli, C. (2010). Examination of the change in Assessment of Motor and Process Skills performance in patients with acquired brain injury between the hospital and home environment. *Australian Occupational Therapy Journal, 57*, 246-252.

West, S., Dunford, C., Mayston, C., & Forsyth, R. (2014). The School Function Assessment: Identifying levels of participation and demonstrating progress for pupils with acquired brain injuries in a residential rehabilitation setting. *Child: Care, Health and Development, 40*, 689-697.

World Federation of Occupational Therapists. (2012). *Definition of occupation*. Retrieved from http://www.wfot.org/aboutus/aboutoccupationaltherapy/definitionofoccupationaltherapy.aspx

Ying-Chai, K., Kramer, J., Liljenquist, K., & Coster, W. (2015). Association between impairment, function, and daily life task management in children and adolescents with autism. *Developmental Medicine and Child Neurology, 57*, 68-74.

Ying-Chai, K, Y., Kramer, J., Liljenquist, K., Feng, T., & Coster, W. (2012). Comparing the functional performance of children and youths with autism, developmental disabilities, and no disability using the Revised Pediatric Evaluation of Disability Inventory Item Banks. *American Journal of Occupational Therapy, 66*, 607-616.

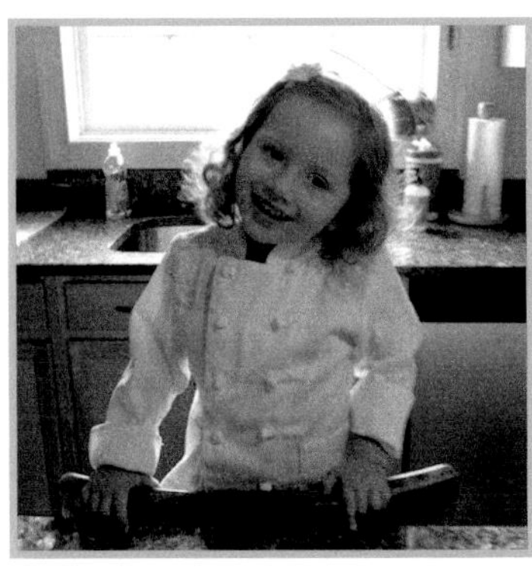

# 19

# Evaluation of Education and Work

Barbara Larson, MA, OTR/L, FAOTA

**ACOTE STANDARDS EXPLORED IN THIS CHAPTER**

B.4.4

**KEY VOCABULARY**

- **Client:** Entity that receives occupational therapy services.
- **Client-centered evaluation:** Focus is on the client's priorities; client is an active participant in the evaluation process.
- **Context:** Conditions that exist in and around the person; may influence the client's performance, and the process of service delivery.
- **Education:** Occupational performance area that includes activities for being a student and participating in learning activities.
- **Environment:** The external factors—physical, social, and attitudinal—that have an effect on how people live their lives.
- **Evaluation:** Includes the occupational profile and the analysis of occupational performance.
- **Occupational performance:** The ability to perform in life activities.
- **Occupational profile:** Information on the client's occupational history and experiences, patterns of daily living, interests, values, and needs.
- **Work:** Occupational performance area that includes activities needed for engaging in paid employment or volunteer activities.



Jacobs, K., & MacRae, N. (Eds.).
*Occupational Therapy Essentials for Clinical Competence, Third Edition* (pp. 265-275).

The health, productivity, and efficiency of persons, groups, or populations can be greatly affected by illness, injury, or incidences that interrupt the ability to engage in meaningful occupational performance. Central to occupational therapy practice is an understanding of the value and use of occupation (American Occupational Therapy Association [AOTA], 2014a, 2014b; Hooper et al., 2015; Mitcham, 2014; Weaver, 2015). This chapter focuses on the components and factors involved in the evaluation of education and work as occupational performance areas. The *Occupational Therapy Practice Framework* (AOTA, 2014b) provides definition to occupational therapy practice and guidance to practitioners in evaluation and as intervention decisions are made. The important task demands and performance factors that may need to be assessed to plan effective interventions will be discussed.

## Education

Education is both a primary therapeutic tool and a primary occupational performance area. When the occupational therapist is planning the educational experiences, education is a primary therapeutic tool. For a child in a classroom or for a college student, education is a primary occupational performance area. In other cases, education might be a more casual experience, such as an adult participating in a continuing education experience or otherwise learning a new skill. In each case, there are relevant barriers to learning.

Education has been described as the work of children (Larson, 2004). The barriers to a child being able to perform as a student may include sensory processing disorder, development delays, and physical disabilities. Psychosocial deficits such as autism, behavioral problems, and those things that interfere with the ability of a child to take advantage of a learning experience are also potential barriers (Case-Smith & Arbesman, 2008; Weaver 2015). To maximize the child's learning experience, it is important for the occupational therapy practitioner to approach the student-instructor relationship from a child's learning perspective (Mitcham, 2014). Occupational therapy practitioners need to establish strategies for collaboration with teachers to make sure the gains made in therapy are transferred to the classroom (Rens & Joosten, 2014). The occupational therapist must determine the most appropriate assessment for the identified problems (AOTA, 2014b, 2015a; de Klerk, Buchanan, & Pretorius, 2015; Schaaf et al., 2015). One example of a highly sophisticated assessment for limitations in sensory integration is the Sensory Integration and Praxis Tests (Bodison & Mailloux, 2006). Another assessment is the Sensory Profile, which measures sensory processing abilities in young children with autism (Brown, Morrison, & Stagnitti, 2010).

Besides carefully selecting the accurate assessment, the occupational therapist must consider the environment and context in which the assessment takes place (AOTA, 2015b). The child's positioning, proximal distal stability (Smith-Zuzovsky & Exner, 2004), as well as the furniture the child sits on related to the testing activity are important and could influence test performance and outcomes (Costigan & Light, 2010; Naider-Steinhart & Katz-Leurer, 2007). In a study of children's work, the author's findings indicated that kindergarten, first, and second graders view handwriting as work. The author thus cautions therapists to view this activity in a work context, "promoting quiet and concentration, setting standards, and encouraging students to achieve them through persistent effort" (Larson, 2004, p. 377). These findings are supported in a study by Wallen, Duff, Goyen and Froude (2013), on assessment and intervention for children with handwriting difficulties, where the results advocated "a shift away from impairment or deficit-oriented approaches to assessment of underlying capacity" (p. 368). The authors stated the assessment should also include "the actual process and output of handwriting generalized under differing conditions" (Wallen et al., 2013, p. 368).

In like manner, there are numerous straightforward sensorimotor, cognitive, and psychosocial deficits (Hildebrand, 2015; Law, Baum, & Dunn, 2005) that can interfere with the adult's occupational performance and, subsequently, the individual's ability to participate in educational experiences. Interviews, observations, a review of medical records, and client history information provide the necessary data to allow the therapist to gain an understanding of the individual's life activities (AOTA, 2014b). The occupational therapist uses standardized or nonstandardized assessments to determine how the occupational performance in those life activities is affected (AOTA, 2014b; Law et al., 2005).

Determining an individual's priorities during the assessment phase allows the occupational therapist to carefully and selectively design education programs that address the needs and wants of the adult (Schepens, Panzer, & Goldberg, 2011). The importance of doing this is illustrated in a study involving the development of a health education program for an elderly population with macular degeneration (Dahlin Ivanoff, Sonn, & Svensson, 2002). The authors concluded that to maintain a sense of security in daily occupations, health education programs should be founded on the needs and problems of the elderly age group (Dahlin Ivanoff et al., 2002). In another study on fall prevention education for older adults, the authors described the importance of using individual assessment information to develop the educational message (Schepens et al., 2011). In a systematic literature review of occupation and activity-based health management and maintenance interventions for adults, Arbesman and Mosley (2012) found increased effectiveness in health education programs that were client centered and needs based.

In selecting assessment tools, the Canadian Occupational Performance Measure can be used to identify client priorities and determine individual needs and wants. The Canadian Occupational Performance Measure assesses self-perception of performance and satisfaction of daily occupations over time (Baptiste, 2010). Problems in occupational performance areas are identified and weighted in terms of importance to the client. The therapist sets client-centered goals for the education program based on those identified priorities (Law et al., 2005; Wolf & Baum, 2011). Along with identifying problems carefully and selecting the appropriate assessment, the occupational therapist must interpret findings accurately and cautiously. It is important to understand the purpose and outcome of each assessment used to plan appropriate interventions. Consideration must be given to each client factor and contexts and environments as they influence performance areas (AOTA, 2014b).

Changing behavior is an important outcome of client education. Whether looking at the occupation of children, the voluntary or educational occupations of adults, or when using learning as a therapeutic approach, there are, as previously discussed, a host of barriers that can interfere with the educational process. These barriers must be evaluated in the context of relevant health behavior and health education theories and models. Health promotion and education programs guided by health behavior theories were shown to positively affect behavior change (Glanz, Rimer, & Viswanath, 2015). The Health Belief Model, the Theories of Planned Behavior and Reasoned Action, and Social Cognitive Theory will be presented next. It should be noted the theory of health behavior and health education is a comprehensive field of study and has been researched extensively (Glanz et al., 2015). The following look at selected models and theories should be viewed as an introduction to further study and investigation.

## The Health Belief Model

The Health Belief Model, which focuses on individual health behavior, supports that, in general, individuals will take action to ward off, screen for, or control ill health under certain circumstances (Rimer & Brewer, 2015; Skinner, Tiro, & Champion, 2015). For behavior change to succeed, people must feel threatened by their current situation and believe that change of a specific kind will be beneficial and result in a valued outcome at an acceptable cost (Rimer & Brewer, 2015; Skinner et al., 2015). People must also feel competent to implement that change. As clients move toward goal attainment, the occupational therapy practitioner should reinforce their successes verbally, while behavior problems should be treated as opportunities to analyze and control the factors that cause the problem.

## Theories of Planned Behavior and Reasoned Action and the Integrated Behavior Model

The theories of Planned Behavior and Reasoned Action focus on the values, beliefs, and motivational factors that influence the likelihood an individual will perform specific behaviors, as well as the perceived control the person has over the behavior (Montaño & Kasprzyk, 2015; Rimer & Berwer, 2015). The Theory of Reasoned Action addresses volitional control, the motivation of the individual, while the Theory of Planned Behavior accounts for the intentions and beliefs effected by factors outside the person's control (Montaño & Kasprzyk, 2015). The Integrated Behavior Model is a combination of the Theories of Reasoned Action and Planned Behavior, as well as constructs from other behavioral theories. In the Integrated Behavior Model, the individual must have the motivation or intention to perform the behavior as well as the knowledge and skill to carry it out. The behavior should be meaningful with few or no environmental constraints that would interfere with performance. Over time, the performance of the behavior should become habitual, lessening the importance of intention, which has been identified as the most important determinant to behavior (Montaño & Kasprzyk, 2015). Understanding these theories can guide the occupational therapist in how to best design educational messages that result in improved health behaviors.

## Social Cognitive Theory

Social Cognitive Theory, formerly known as Social Learning Theory, addresses both the methods of promoting behavior change and the psychosocial dynamics underlying health behavior (Kelder, Hoelscher, & Perry, 2015; Tougas, Hayden, McGrath, Huguet, & Rozario, 2015). Social Learning Theory was renamed Social Cognitive Theory in the 1970s by social psychologist and researcher Albert Bandura. As cited in Kelder et al. (2015), Bandura renamed the theory "in order to emphasize the increasingly important role of observation and cognitive factors in learning, understanding, and predicting behavior" (p. 160). From a cognitive viewpoint, Social Cognitive Theory emphasizes what people think. In Social Cognitive Theory, behavior is influenced by cognitive, behavioral, physical, and environmental factors. Among the cognitive factors is self-efficacy, which equates a person's level of confidence with the ability to control behavior. Self-efficacy has been identified as one of the most important prerequisites for behavior change (Kelder et al., 2015). Self-efficacy is an important factor in not only Social Cognitive Theory, but also within other health behavior theories and models (Kelder et al., 2015; Rimer & Brewer, 2015). While self-efficacy refers to the individual, collective efficacy addresses the issues of groups and can be an important factor to consider when addressing behavior change at the group or population level (Kelder et al., 2015). Understanding how individuals perceive, interpret, and recall information is critical in creating an environment for behavior change (Kelder et al., 2015). In planning educational messages, goals should be set in increments similar to a given behavior, possible to achieve, and meaningful and relevant to the individual or individuals being served.

The factors that influence Social Cognitive Theory—cognitive, behavioral, physical, and environmental—when combined, play a vital role in increasing the success of behavior change (Heaney & Viswanath, 2015; Kelder et al., 2015).

The application of the theories and models support clinical reasoning and help the occupational therapy practitioner build therapeutic relationships with clients and caregivers that are vital to effecting behavior change (Duggan & Street, 2015). Current theorists of client–provider relationships blend social and psychological perspectives and interpersonal influences to explain how the characteristics and behaviors of others affect a person's attitudes, feelings, and behavior. The model of relationship-centered health care builds on the theories of client-centered relationships. Relationship-centered health care focuses on the concepts of autonomy, open shared communication, and consideration of client preferences (Duggan & Street, 2015). A number of factors may interfere with clients' understanding and recall of information in the health care setting. Hunter, Dignan, and Shalash (2012), in a study on health literacy, found the main areas of concern to be with text formatting, vocabulary level, and amount of information in education materials. Jargon and vocabulary that are too complex for the majority of clients are often present in verbal and written information. Situational influences affect a client's ability to attend to and recall information, and the different backgrounds between provider and client often hamper their communication (Hunter et al., 2012).

Communication should be constructed to meet the needs of the audience. In a qualitative study on becoming a health education expert, Svavarsdóttir, Siguróardóttir and Steinbekk (2015) identified several characteristics of expert patient educators, "a thorough up-to-date knowledge of the subject, a holistic view of the patients' situation, and sensitivity to and knowledge about their psychological well-being" (2015, p. 4). The results of the study also showed the importance of communication skills in providing meaningful information that would motivate patients to change their behavior. The authors of the study stated, "the most prominent signs of an expert educator were considered the ability to know when a patient is ready to receive information, being sensitive to the patients' interests and learning needs, and the context of the situation" (Svavarsdóttir et al., 2015, p. 4).

Occupational behavior is influenced by the client's physiological, cognitive, and psychological conditions. These conditions also affect the client's ability to learn (Berkeland & Flinn, 2005). The occupational therapy practitioner needs to create a comfortable, safe environment in which the client can benefit from the educational experience. Client education is important in the practice of occupational therapy. Written materials, while most commonly used in client education, need to reflect the reading level and comprehensibility of the reader to be effective (Friedman, Cosby, Boyko, Hatton-Bauer, & Turnbull, 2011; Griffin, McKenna, & Tooth, 2006).

Teaching and learning provide clients with a way to take action, explore possibilities, and engage in occupation, and they are fundamental to the occupational therapy process (Berkeland & Flinn, 2005). "In designing teaching and learning experiences, practitioners consider models or frameworks for client education, principles of adult learning, and the mechanics of constructing education programs" (Berkeland & Flinn, 2005, p. 421). Client education is a vital link between the occupational therapy practitioner and those individuals under his or her care (AOTA, 2014b; Griffin et al., 2006).

## Work

Work is important socially and economically and it often defines our place in a community. Work has been an integral part of occupational therapy since the early 1900s (Hanson & Walker, 1992). Occupational therapy grew out of the moral treatment movement. Employment, recreation, and self-care came to be important components in the intervention of those with mental illness as the handling of those in asylums became more humane (Hanson & Walker, 1992; Harvey-Krefting, 1985). The development of the veterans hospital in 1922 provided occupational therapy for "therapeutic, economic and diversional reasons" (Hanson & Walker, 1992, p. 57). Work programs were developed to treat those with chronic illnesses and were held in or near sanatoriums. The industrial era of the mid-1930s saw the introduction of curative workshops serving workers who were injured in industrial accidents (Hanson & Walker, 1992). In the 1950s, the focus of the injured worker became return to gainful employment (Harvey-Krefting, 1985). The 1970s brought the first work hardening programs, with the ultimate goal of returning to work (Wyrick, Ogden Niemeyer, Ellexson, Jacobs, & Taylor, 1991). As practice evolves and the needs of those individuals we serve change, assisting individuals to participate in meaningful work roles continues to be the goal of the occupational therapy practitioner in work practice (AOTA, 2011). Work provides a sense of structure, meaning, and economic security in our lives (Matheson, 2001; Rice, 2014). In the event of chronic disease or disability, an individual's ability to work is often compromised. In the rehabilitation process, the evaluation of the worker, development of work skills, and maintaining worker behaviors are an important part of occupational therapy practice (AOTA, 2011, 2014b; Matheson, 2001; Rice, 2014). Deficits in body structures or body functions that interfere with performance skills may limit the ability of the individual to meet the activity and occupational demands work requires (AOTA, 2014b, Steffan & Tosi, 2012; WHO, 2001).

In the evaluation of work, occupational therapists must consider the multiple contexts and activity demands that affect performance (AOTA, 2015b). According to Sandqvist and Henriksson (2004), and supported by Cook and Lukersmith (2010), work function assessment includes participation in work as it relates to society, work performance as it relates to the client, and the client's capacity as it relates to physical and psychological functioning. A client's deficits in the occupational performance area of work may be both physical and psychological (AOTA, 2011, 2014b; Pomake, Franche, Murray, Khushrushahi, & Lampiem, 2012). When work is interrupted, or when the individual is not able to continue working, the public recognition and identity as a worker is missing. The individual may lose the sense of being a productive member of society (Cook & Lukersmith, 2010; Pomake et al., 2012; Rice, 2014). The order and expectations of work can provide the stability an individual needs to move forward with overall life activities.

Understanding the psychosocial aspects of disability is as important as having knowledge of those injuries and illnesses that affect the worker's abilities to perform essential job functions. Psychological events could be triggered by family or work stress. Sociocultural issues such as age discrimination could displace a worker (Abma, Amick, van der Klink, & Bültmann, 2013; Rice, 2014). Neurological, sensory, or other changes related to aging could affect a worker's safety and productivity (Algarni, Gross, Senthilselvan, & Battié, 2015; Rice, 2014). The occupational therapist works with other professionals in addressing issues affecting an individual's ability to work. These professionals may include employers, human resource departments, safety personnel, or case managers (Larson & Ellexson 2015; Rice, 2014). In the past, physical illnesses or injuries have been the primary focus of the employer. There is a definite need in the workplace for occupational therapists to address the performance deficits in those individuals who suffer the effects of mental illness (Larson & Ellexson, 2015; Pomake et al., 2015; Rice, 2014). Competitive work has been shown to be valuable to integrating individuals with schizophrenia into the community. A study in Japan demonstrated how important competitive work, along with clinical support and occupational and vocational rehabilitation services, was in providing individuals with schizophrenia the motivation, income, and stability to move into the community (Oka et al., 2004).

Following a lack of acknowledgment, the recognition of anxiety and depressive disorders in the workplace and the employer costs associated with these illnesses are now being documented (Langlieb & Kahn, 2005; Pomake et al., 2015). "Research, improved treatment options, and a gradual lessening of the stigma associated with mental illness have created an environment in which their importance to the employer community is more apparent" (Langlieb & Kahn, 2005, p. 1099). In the evaluation of work, the ability to analyze job tasks is critical. Identifying the physical job requirements allows the occupational therapy practitioner to determine job adaptations or modifications or to assist an employer to make reasonable accommodations for a qualified individual with a disability (Americans with Disabilities Act [ADA], 1990; ADA Amendments of 2008; Larson & Reineke Lyth, 2011; Rice, 2014). Knowing the physical job requirements is necessary to identify the potential for ergonomic changes, determine options for transitional work, write functional job descriptions, and design post-offer tests. Work injury prevention and management is a specialized field requiring knowledge of specific assessment and intervention strategies, as well as an understanding of the legislation and regulation governing this area of practice (Adam, Strong, & Chipchase, 2014; AOTA, 2011, 2014b; ADA, 1990, 2008; Rice, 2014; Rothmore, Karnon, & Aylward, 2013). Occupational therapists with specialized training and experience would be considered occupational health and safety practitioners (Rothmore et al., 2013).

A comprehensive evaluation looks at the physical requirements of the work, the worker, and the workplace to gain an understanding of factors affecting participation in work. A thorough job analysis should be performed with consideration given to the activity demands of the work such as the forces, angles, weights, distances, and repetitions the job requires; the design or layout of the work area; organization of the work; and the tools and equipment used to perform the job (AOTA, 2011; Larson & Reineke Lyth, 2011; Rice, 2014). Knowledge of gender, age, skill level, and general health of an individual worker or worker population is an important factor in identifying both strengths and limitations in performance skills and patterns (Abma et al., 2013; Larson & Ellexson, 2015; Rice, 2014). Focusing on the physical aspects of the worker and the physical environment of the workplace is important, as is guiding clients toward healthy behavior change. Rothmore, Karnon, and Aylward (2013), in an article on musculoskeletal injury at work, stated, "The structuring of injury prevention advice according to behavior change principles has been proposed by researchers as a means to improve its effectiveness" (Rothmore et al., 2013, p. 344). Understanding health behavior and health behavior change is important in making decisions that are relevant and meaningful to clients and result in healthy behavior changes at the workplace. Functional Capacity Evaluation (FCE), a comprehensive tool used to evaluate an individual's physical capacities related to work abilities, has been around since the 1980s (Isernhagen, 1995; Rice, 2014). FCE provides an objective measure of an individual's physical abilities related to specific work tasks. Cheng and Cheng (2011) studied the predictive ability of the FCE in return to work following a radial wrist fracture. The authors determined that, on the basis of standard testing items in a given FCE protocol, a job-specific FCE could be developed. They determined that a job-specific FCE could have better predictive validity in relation to the work ability status of patients with a specific injury than of patients with a nonspecific injury (Cheng & Cheng, 2011). In a study by Pas et al. (2014), FCE was found to be useful for the assessment of work ability and in making return-to-work recommendations.

The complexities involved in assessing work performance require observing and testing worker skills and abilities in the context of the job and workplace in which the worker intends to work. Based on a review of FCE literature (Gouttebarge, Wind, Kuijer, Sluiter, & Frings-Dressen, 2010), a three-step procedure was proposed to select specific tests from an FCE to address functional limitations in individuals with musculoskeletal complaints:

1. Establishing the medical condition of the worker with musculoskeletal complaints and related functional limitations
2. Assigning the activities limited by the medical condition
3. Selecting the functional tests from the full FCE method measuring the limited activities (Gouttenbarge et al., 2010, p. 113)

Environmental and psychosocial factors must also be considered (AOTA, 2011; Larson & Ellexson, 2015; Rice, 2014). After analyzing the assessment data, the occupational therapist draws conclusions on which to base clinical decisions that will guide workers toward engagement in meaningful, purposeful work activities.

Occupational therapists use education as a therapeutic tool, designing education programs for clients based on the needs and wants identified in the assessment. The programs could include injury prevention, stress management, safety, proper body mechanics, postural awareness, pain management strategies, joint protection, and symptom awareness (AOTA, 2014b).

To be effective in the role of educator, the occupational therapy practitioner must create an environment for learning, becoming aware of the persons or populations being served, understanding the principles of how individuals learn, and selecting the most appropriate teaching approach (Duggan & Street, 2015; Friedman et al., 2011; Svavarsdóttir et al., 2015). As stated earlier, it is important for occupational therapists to be aware of the reading level and comprehensibility of the education materials, as well as the individual client's or population's reading ability and comprehension level. Material should be written at a fifth- to sixth-grade reading level, have a clear purpose, and be meaningful and relevant to the audience (Griffin et al., 2006; Hunter et al., 2012).

A clinical example illustrates this point. A client arrived at an outpatient facility for a scheduled functional capacity assessment. Prior to beginning the test, the client was given medical forms to read and sign. He completed the required paperwork, and the occupational therapist began the assessment. As the test progressed, the client followed directions but appeared frustrated and was not engaged in the process. The therapist decided to stop the test and talk with the client. The client confided that he was upset because of the paperwork he was given to fill out when he came into the clinic. He signed the forms but did not know what he was signing. He said he was a poor reader and embarrassed to ask for assistance. Once the therapist was made aware of the situation, she carefully and thoughtfully reviewed the forms to make sure he understood what he had signed. The client's attitude changed. He was now able to fully participate in the functional assessment.

This issue raised the following concerns. First, the client's uncooperative behavior was a result of his inability to read and understand the forms, not because he did not want to fully participate in the functional assessment. Second, the facility had not created an environment in which the client felt comfortable to ask for assistance. The occupational therapist's ability to recognize and address the needs and wants of the client allowed him to fully participate in and benefit from the functional assessment. The results provided the occupational therapist with vital information in intervention planning. With the engagement of the client in the process, the outcome was directed toward increasing the individual's health and well-being for participation in the occupation of work (AOTA, 2014b; Law, 2002).

The following includes examples of laws and accompanying resources that address the industry as a whole. The Occupational Safety and Health Act of 1970 is a federal law that governs occupational health and safety in the private sector and in the federal government in the United States. Its main goal is to ensure employers provide employees with an environment free from recognized hazards that are causing or are likely to cause physical harm or death. The Act also requires employees to comply with occupational safety and health standards and all rules and regulations covered in the Act. The Occupational Safety and Health Act (1970) established the Occupational Safety and Health Administration and the National Institute for Occupational Safety and Health. Both organizations promote safety and health in the workplace and protection of workers. The Job Accommodation Network is a service provided by the U.S. Department of Labor's Office of Disability Employment Policy. The Job Accommodation Network provides free expert and confidential guidance on workplace accommodation and disability employment issues.

Work injury prevention and management is a specialized field requiring knowledge of specific assessment and intervention strategies, as well as an understanding of the legislation and regulation governing this area of practice (Adam et al., 2014; AOTA, 2011, 2014b; ADA, 1990, 2008; Rice, 2014; Rothmore et al., 2013). Occupational therapy practitioners with specialized training and experience would be well positioned to provide services in the specialized area of occupational health (Rothmore et al., 2013).

## Role of the Occupational Therapy Assistant

The occupational therapy assistant shares a collaborative role with the occupational therapist in the performance areas of work and education. The occupational therapist evaluates, whereas the occupational therapy assistant, working under the supervision of the occupational therapist, assists in the evaluation process by gathering and sharing data (Accreditation Council for Occupational Therapy Education, 2011; AOTA, 2011, 2014c).

The occupational therapist focuses on problem identification, problem analysis, and the planning required for problem solution. The occupational therapy assistant focuses on delivering direct services and documenting client response and progress (AOTA, 2011, 2014c). The occupational therapy assistant collects and reports selected information during the evaluation process. The occupational therapy assistant may be asked to participate in the interview process, assist in the development of an education program, or facilitate education and training sessions.

The occupational therapy assistant, having successfully completed an accredited occupational therapy assistant program, has the knowledge, skills, and abilities required to be part of a work rehabilitation team (Moyers, 1999). Assisting with job analysis, providing continuity in a work-hardening or work-conditioning program, and reporting client physical and behavior changes to the occupational therapist are important occupational therapy assistant roles. Specializing in work allows the occupational therapy assistant to gain a depth of skill and knowledge in this area (James & Kehrhahn, 2005). This valued experience enhances what the occupational therapy assistant brings to the team and benefits the therapeutic process for all occupational therapy practitioners. While it is the responsibility of the occupational therapist to delegate responsibilities to the occupational therapy assistant, service competency is the responsibility of the occupational therapy assistant (AOTA, 2014c, 2015a). The occupational therapist and the occupational therapy assistant demonstrate and document service competency for clinical reasoning and judgment during the service delivery process, as well as for the performance of specific techniques, assessments, and intervention methods used (AOTA, 2015a).

## Summary

To facilitate meaningful participation in the evaluation of education or work, the occupational therapy practitioner needs to create an environment in which clients can focus on and attend to tasks, have a sense of choice or control over the activity, and experience a sense of mastery (AOTA, 2014b, 2015b; Law, 2002). In the evaluation of the performance areas of work and education, identifying both the physical and psychosocial needs of the client is a crucial step in addressing problems manifested by those needs. Whether developing educational materials for persons, groups, or populations, consideration must be given to factors that contribute to health behavior change. In the evaluation of the work, the occupational therapist addresses the complexities involved in both return to work and worker retention. The aging workforce, worker safety and productivity, and accommodation for individuals with disabilities present the occupational therapist with important professional challenges. To be effective requires knowledge of the culture of the workplace, an understanding of the physical and psychological issues related to work illness and injury, and an acute awareness of pertinent laws and regulations governing the industry. The occupational therapy practitioner is well positioned to guide clients toward meaningful participation in the occupations of education and work.

## Student Self-Assessment

1. Locate and review client education materials of your choice. Evaluate the clarity, reading level, and appropriateness for the intended population. Document positive findings as well as any changes you would make to improve the materials for the intended population.
2. Identify what contextual and environmental issues you need to consider when teaching handwriting skills to young children with sensory processing deficits.
3. Review the educational theories and models discussed in the chapter and identify the common themes.
4. Research the ADA website (www.ada.gov) to review cases involving rulings on mental health issues in the workplace.

### Case Example

The client is a 54-year-old woman who works in a light manufacturing industry that specializes in die cutting. Her job responsibilities include the production line and product inspection. The physical demands of her job require frequent use of her upper extremities and include pushing, pulling, overhead reach, and sustained overhead work to change the die in the machine. The client has worked for the company for 15 years. She has been treated for thoracic outlet syndrome and continues to complain of left shoulder and neck pain. She has frequent doctor visits and has been on light duty for several months, stating that she cannot do her regular job. Table 19-1 illustrates both worker and employer issues that, in the past, have impeded the return-to-work process for this individual. The occupational therapist has been asked to evaluate the individual's current functional level related to her essential job functions. The human resources department at the company is working on case resolution and plans to use the functional assessment findings along with vocational data in the company's final placement decision.

The employer, in reviewing the injury logs from the production line, identified several reports of shoulder problems. Based on this information, the employer met with a group of workers to gather data on their concerns about the physical demands of the die cutting production job. Following the meeting, the employer engaged the services of the occupational therapist to do an ergonomic job analysis. As a result of the analysis, the employer was able to determine changes that would increase the safety and productivity of the workers.

Table 19-1.

**Issues Impeding Return to Work**

| Worker Issues | Employer Issues |
|---|---|
| • Bad body schema | • Chronically absent from work |
| • No responsibility for own health and well-being (e.g., poor shoes, footwear)<br>• Multiple physical complaints<br>• Poor work habits | • Employee was not performing the essential job functions on a full-time basis<br>• Employee was frequently late, and needed reminders to keep on task |
| • Various work restrictions<br>• Unhappy with job | • Employee had various work restrictions over the years that were never reevaluated |
| • Personal issues outside of work affecting job satisfaction<br>• Spouse on disability | • Performance issues were never addressed<br>• Employee had heavy use of worker's compensation, medical, and disability systems |

5. List the three components of work function assessment described by Sandqvist and Henriksson (2004).
6. Access the Job Accommodation Network (www.jan.wvu.edu) on the Internet and determine how it can be used to address the client's need for reasonable accommodations.
7. Explain why both physical and psychological issues must be considered when evaluating a client's deficits in the occupational performance area of work.
8. Describe how the principles from the educational theories and models discussed in the chapter are useful in establishing therapeutic relationships.
9. Working with a peer, identify the occupational therapy assistant's role in the evaluation of an individual with deficits affecting work performance.
10. Describe how education is both a primary therapeutic tool and a primary occupational performance area.

## Electronic Resources

Americans with Disabilities Act: www.ada.gov

Job Accommodation Network: https://askjan.org

National Institute on Aging: www.nia.nih.gov

National Institute for Occupational Safety and Health: www.cdc.gov/niosh

Occupational Safety and Health Administration: www.osha.gov

## References

Abma, F. I., Amick, B., C., van der Klink, J. J. I., & Bültmann, U. (2013). Prognostic factors for successful work functioning in the general working population. *Journal of Occupational Rehabilitation, 23*, 162-169. doi:10.1007/s10926-012-9410-0

Accreditation Council for Occupational Therapy Education. (2011). *Accreditation Council for Occupational Therapy Education (ACOTE) Standards and Interpretive Guide (effective July 31, 2013) August 2012 Interpretive Guide Version*. Retrieved from http://www.aota.org/Educate/Accredit/DraftStandards/50146.aspx?FT=.pdf

## Evidence-Based Research Chart

| Topic | Subject/Activity | Evidence |
|---|---|---|
| Educational theories and models | Behavior change; self-efficacy | Kelder, Hoelscher, & Perry, 2015; Montano & Kasprzyl, 2015; Rimer & Brewer, 2015; Skinner, Tiro, & Champion, 2015; Tougas, Hayden, McGrath, Huguet, & Rozario, 2015 |
| Health education | Needs and problems | Arbesman & Mosley, 2012; Dahlin Ivanoff, Sonn, & Svensson, 2002; Glamz, Rimer, & Viswanath, 2015; Schepens, Panzer, & Goldberg, 2011 |
| | Comprehension, reading level; communication | Friedman, Cosby, Boyko, Hatten-Bauer, & Turnbull, 2011; Griffin, McKenna, & Tooth, 2006; Hunter, Dignan, & Shalash, 2012; Svavarsdóttir, Siguróardóttir, & Steinbekk, 2015; Viswanath, Finnegan, & Goullist, 2015 |
| Sensory deficits | Assessments | Bodison & Mailloux, 2006; Brown, Morrison, & Stagnitti, 2010; Case-Smith & Arbesman, 2008; Watling, Deitz, & White, 2001 |
| Handwriting | Positioning | Naider-Steinhart & Katz-Leurer, 2007; Smith-Zuzovsky & Exner, 2004; Wallen, Duff, Goyen, & Frode, 2013 |
| Client centered | Self-perception | Duggan & Street, 2015; Law, 2002; Law, Baum, & Dunn, 2005 |
| Children's work | Education; classroom | Larson, 2004; Mitcham, 2014; Rens & Joosten, 2014 |
| Work | Psychological issues | Abma, Amick, van der Klink, & Bültmann, 2013; Cook & Lukersmith, 2010; Langlieb & Kahn, 2005; Oka et al., 2004; Sandqvist & Henriksson, 2004 |
| | History | Hanson & Walker, 1992; Harvey-Krefting, 1985; Wyrick, Ogden Niemeyer, Ellexson, Jacobs, & Taylor, 1991 |
| Work assessment | Functional Capacity Evaluation | Cheng & Cheng, 2011; Gouttebarge, Wind, Kuijer, Sluiter, & Frings-Dressen, 2010; Isernhagen, 1995; Pas, Kuijer et al., 2014 |
| Essential job functions | Reasonable accommodations | Americans with Disabilities Act, 1990; Americans with Disabilities Act Amendments, 2008; Larson & Reineke Lyth, 2011 |
| Work performance | Measurement | Matheson, 2001; Rice 2014 |


Adam, K., Strong, K., & Chipchase, L. (2014). Readiness for work injury management and prevention: Important attributes for early graduate occupational therapists and physiotherapists. *WORK, 48,* 576-578. doi:10.3233/WOR–141912

Algarni, F. S., Gross, D. P., Senthilselvan, A., & Battié, M. C. (2015). Aging workers with work-related musculoskeletal injuries. *Occupational Medicine, 65*(3), 229-237.

American Occupational Therapy Association. (2011). Occupational therapy services in facilitating work performance. *American Journal of Occupational Therapy, 65*(Suppl.), S55-S64. doi:10.5014/ajot.2011.65S55

American Occupational Therapy Association. (2014a). Scope of practice. *American Journal of Occupational Therapy, 68*(Suppl. 3), S34-S40.

American Occupational Therapy Association. (2014b). Occupational therapy practice framework: Domain and process (3rd ed.). *American Journal of Occupational Therapy, 68*(Suppl. 1), S1-S48. doi:10.5014/ajot.2014.628006

American Occupational Therapy Association. (2014c). Guidelines for supervision, roles, and responsibilities during the delivery of occupational therapy services. *American Journal of Occupational Therapy, 68*(Suppl.), S16-S22.

American Occupational Therapy Association. (2015a). Occupational therapy code of ethics. *American Journal of Occupational Therapy, 69*(Suppl. 3), 6913410030. doi:10.5014/ajot.2015.696S03

American Occupational Therapy Association. (2015b). Occupational therapy's perspective on the use of environments and contexts to facilitate health, well-being, and participation in occupations. *American Journal of Occupational Therapy, 64*(Suppl. 6), S57-S69. doi:10.5014/ajot.2015.696S05

Americans with Disabilities Act of 1990, Pub. L. No. 101-336, §2, 104 Stat. 328 (1991).

Americans with Disabilities Act Amendments of 2008, Pub. L. No. 110-325, 42 USCA § 12101 (2008).

Arbesman, M., & Mosley, L. J. (2012). Systematic review of occupation- and activity-based health management and maintenance interventions for community-dwelling older adults. *American Journal of Occupational Therapy, 66*, 277-283. doi:10.5014/ajot.2012.003327

Baptiste, S. (2010). In M. Curtin, M. Molineux, & J. Supyk-Mellson (Eds.), *Occupational therapy and physical dysfunction: Enabling occupation* (6th ed., pp. 151-160). London, England: Elsevier.

Berkeland, R., & Flinn, N. (2005). Therapy as learning. In C. H. Christiansen, C. M. Baum, & J. Bass Haugen (Eds.), *Occupational therapy: Performance, participation, and well-being* (3rd ed., pp. 420-448.). Thorofare, NJ: SLACK Incorporated.

Bodison, S., & Mailloux, Z. (2006). The Sensory Integration and Praxis Tests: Illuminating struggles and strengths in participation at school. *OT Practice, 11*(17), CE1-CE8.

Brown, T., Morrison, I. C., & Stagnitti, K. (2010). The convergent validity of two sensory processing scales used with school-age children: Comparing the sensory profile and the sensory processing measure. *New Zealand Journal of Occupational Therapy, 57*(2), 56-65.

Case-Smith, J., & Arbesman, M. (2008). Evidence-based review of intervention for autism used in or of relevance to occupational therapy. *American Journal of Occupational Therapy, 62*, 416-429.

Cheng, A. S. K., & Cheng, S. W. C. (2011). Use of job-specific functional capacity evaluation to predict the return to work of patients with a distal radius fracture. *American Journal of Occupational Therapy, 65*, 445-452.

Cook, C., & Lukersmith, C. (2010). Work rehabilitation. In M. C. Curtin, M. Molineux, & J. Supyk-Mellson (Eds.), *Occupational therapy and physical dysfunction: Enabling occupation* (6th ed., pp. 391-408). London, England: Elsevier.

Costigan, F. A., & Light, J. (2010). Effect of seated position on upper-extremity access to augmentative communication for children with cerebral palsy: Preliminary investigation. *American Journal of Occupational Therapy, 64*, 596-604. doi:10.50/ajot.2010.09013

Dahlin Ivanoff, S., Sonn, U., & Svensson, E. (2002). A health education program for elderly persons with visual impairments and perceived security in the performance of daily occupations: A randomized study. *American Journal of Occupational Therapy, 56*(3), 322-330.

de Klerk, S., Buchanan, H., & Pretorius, B. (2015). Occupational therapy had assessment practices: Cause for concern? *South African Journal of Occupational Therapy, 45*(2), 13-19.

Duggan, A., & Street, R. L. (2015). Interpersonal communication in health and illness. In K. Glanz, B. K. Rimer, & K. Viswanath (Eds.), *Health behavior and health education: Theory, research, and practice* (5th ed., pp. 243-268). San Francisco, CA: Jossey Bass.

Friedman, A. J., Cosby, R., Boyko, S., Hatten-Bauer, J., & Turnbull, G. (2011). Effective teaching strategies and methods of delivery for patient education: A systematic review and practice guideline recommendations. *Journal of Canadian Education, 26*, 12-21.

Glanz, K., Rimer, B. K., & Viswanath, K. (2015). The scope of health behaviors. In K. Glanz, B. K. Rimer, & K. Viswanath (Eds.), *Health behavior and health education: Theory, research, and practice* (5th ed., pp. 3-22). San Francisco, CA: Jossey Bass.

Gouttebarge, V., Wind, H., Kuijer, P. P. F. M., Sluiter, J. K., & Frings-Dressen, M. H. W. (2010). How to assess physical work-ability with functional capacity evaluation methods in a more specific and efficient way? *WORK, 37*, 111-115.

Griffin, J., McKenna, K., & Tooth, L. (2006). Discrepancy between older clients' ability to read and comprehend and the reading level of written educational materials used by occupational therapists. *American Journal of Occupational Therapy, 60*(1), 70-80.

Hanson, C. S., & Walker, K. F. (1992). The history of work in physical dysfunction. *American Journal of Occupational Therapy, 46*(1), 56-62.

Harvey-Krefting, L. H. (1985). The concept of work in occupational therapy: A historical review. *American Journal of Occupational Therapy, 39*(5), 301-307.

Heaney, C. A., & Viswanath, K. (2015). In K. Glanz, B. K. Rimer, & K. Viswanath (Eds.), *Health behavior and health education: Theory, research, and practice* (5th ed., pp. 151-158). San Francisco, CA: Jossy-Bass.

Hildebrand, M. W. (2015). Effectiveness of interventions for adults with psychological or emotional impairment after stroke: An evidenced based review. *American Journal of Occupational Therapy, 69*, 6901180050. doi:10.5014/ajot.2015.012054

Hooper, B., Mitcham, D. M., Taff, S. D., Prie P., Krishnagiri, S., & Bilics, A. (2015). The issue is: Energizing occupation as the center of teaching and learning. *American Journal of Occupational Therapy, 69* (Suppl. 2), 6912360010. doi:10.5014/ajot.2015.018242

Hunter, E. G., Dignan, M., & Shalash, S. (2012). Evaluating allied health inpatient rehabilitation educational materials in terms of health literacy. *Journal of Allied Health, 41*(2), e33-e37.

Isernhagen, S. J. (1995). Contemporary issues in functional capacity evaluation. In S. J. Isernhagen (Ed.), *Comprehensive guide to work injury management* (pp. 410-429). Gaithersburg, MD: Aspen.

James A. B., & Kehrhahn, M. T. (2005). Professional development. In S. Ryan & K. Sladyk (Eds.), *Ryan's occupational therapy assistant: Principles, practice issues, and techniques* (4th ed., pp. 560-570). Thorofare, NJ: SLACK Incorporated.

Kelder, S. H., Hoelscher, D., & Perry C. L. (2015). How individuals, environments, and health behaviors interact. In K. Glanz, B. K. Rimer, & K. Viswanath (Eds.), *Health behavior and health education: Theory, research, and practice* (5th ed., pp. 67-74). San Francisco, CA: Jossey-Bass.

Langlieb, A. M., & Kahn, J. P. (2005). How much does quality mental health care profit employers? *Journal of Occupational and Environmental Medicine, 47*(10), 1099-1109.

Larson, B. A., & Ellexson, M. T. (2015). In I. Söderback (Ed.), *International handbook of occupational therapy interventions* (2nd ed., pp. 687-696). Geneva, Switzerland: Springer.

Larson, B., & Reineke Lyth, J. (2011). Writing physical job demands for return-to-work. *Work and Industry Special Interest Section Quarterly, 25*(4), 1-4.

Larson, E. A. (2004). Children's work: The less-considered childhood occupation. *American Journal of Occupational Therapy, 58*(4), 369-379.

Law, M. (2002). Participation in the occupations of everyday life. *American Journal of Occupational Therapy, 56*(6), 640-649.

Law, M., Baum, C. M., & Dunn, W. (2005). Occupational performance assessment. In C. H. Christiansen, C. M. Baum, & J. Bass-Haugen (Eds.), *Occupational therapy: Performance, participation, and well-being* (3rd ed., pp. 338-370). Thorofare, NJ: SLACK Incorporated.

Matheson, L. N. (2001). Measuring work performance from an occupational performance perspective. In M. Law, C. M. Baum, & W. Dunn (Eds.), *Measuring occupational performance: Supporting best practice in occupational therapy* (pp. 103-120). Thorofare, NJ: SLACK Incorporated.

Mitcham, M. D. (2014). Education as engine (Eleanor Clarke Slagle lecture). *American Journal of Occupational Therapy, 68*, 636-648. doi:10.5014/ajot.2014.68001

Montaño, D. E., & Kasprzyk, D. (2015). Theory of reasoned action, theory of planned behavior, and the integrated behavioral model. In K. Glanz, B. K. Rimer, & K. Viswanath (Eds.), *Health behavior and health education: Theory, research, and practice* (5th ed., pp. 95-124). San Francisco, CA: Jossey-Bass.

Moyers, P. A. (1999). The guide to occupational therapy practice. *American Journal of Occupational Therapy, 53*(3), 247-322.

Naider-Steinhart, S., & Katz-Leurer, M. (2007). Analysis of proximal and distal muscle activity during handwriting tasks. *American Journal of Occupational Therapy, 61*(4), 392-398.

Occupational Safety and Health Act of 1970, Pub. L. No. 91-596, 29 U.S.C.§ 651 et seq.

Oka, M., Otsuka, K., Yokoyama, N., Mintz, J., Hoshino, K., Niwa, S., et al. (2004). An evaluation of a hybrid occupational therapy and supported employment program in Japan for persons with schizophrenia. *American Journal of Occupational Therapy, 58*(4), 466-475.

Pas, L. W., Kuijer, P. P. F. M., Wind, H., Sluiter, J. K. Groothorr, J. W., Brouwer, S., & Grings-Dressen, M. H. W. (2014). Clients' and RTW experts' view on the utility of FCE for the assessment of physical work ability, prognosis for work participation and advice on return to work. *International Archives of Occupational and Environmental Health, 87*, 331-338.

Pomake, G., Franche R. L., Murray, E., Khushrushahi, N., & Lampien T. M. (2012). Work-place-based work disability prevention interventions for workers with common mental health conditions: A review of the literature. *Journal of Occupational Rehabilitation, 19*, 260-273.

Rens, L., & Joosten, A. (2014). Investigating the experiences in a school-based paediatric occupational therapy practice. *Australian Journal of Occupational Therapy, 61*, 148-158.

Rice, V. (2014). Restoring competence for the worker role. In M. V. Radomski & C. A. Trombly Latham (Eds.), *Occupational therapy for physical dysfunction* (7th ed., pp. 870-908). Baltimore, MD: Lippincott Williams and Wilkins.

Rimer, B. K., & Brewer, N. T. (2015). Introduction to health behavior theories that focus on individuals. In K. Glanz, B. K. Rimer, & K. Viswanath (Eds.), *Health behavior and health education: Theory, research, and practice* (5th ed., pp. 67-74). San Francisco, CA: Jossey-Bass.

Rothmore, P., Karnon, J., & Aylward, P. (2013). Implementation of interventions to prevent musculoskeletal injury at work: Lost in translation? *Physical Therapy Reviews, 18*(5), 344-349. doi:10.1179/1743288x13Y.0000000092

Sandqvist, J. L., & Henriksson, C. M. (2004). Work functioning: A conceptual framework. *WORK, 23*(2), 147-157.

Schaaf, R. C., Schoen, S. A., May-Benson, T. A., Parham, L. D., Lane, S. J., Smith Roley, S., & Mallioux, Z. (2015). State of the science: A roadmap for research in sensory integration. *American Journal of Occupational Therapy, 69*, 6906360010. doi:10.5014/ajot.2015.019539

Schepens, S. L., Panzer, V., & Goldberg, A. (2011). Randomized controlled trial comparing tailoring methods of multimedia-based fall prevention education for community-dwelling older adults. *American Journal of Occupational Therapy, 65*(6), 702-709.

Skinner, C. S., Tiro, J., & Champion, V. L. (2015). The health belief model. In K. Glanz, B. K. Rimer, & K. Viswanath (Eds.), *Health behavior and health education: Theory, research, and practice* (5th ed., pp. 68-75). San Francisco, CA: Jossey-Bass.

Smith-Zuzovsky, N., & Exner, C. E. (2004). The effect of seated positioning quality on typical 6- and 7-year-old children's object manipulation skills. *American Journal of Occupational Therapy, 58*(4), 380-388.

Steffan, I. T., & Tosi F. (2012). Ergonomics and the design for all work. *WORK, 41*(Suppl. 1), 1374-1380.

Svavarsdóttir, H. M., Siguróardóttir Á. K., & Steinbekk, A. (2015). How to become an expert educator: A qualitative study on the view of health professionals with experience in patient education. *BMC Medical Education, 15*, 87. doi:10.1186/s12909-015-0370-x

Tougas, M. E., Hayden, J. A., McGrath, P. J., Huguet, A., & Rozario, S. (2015). A systematic review exploring the social cognitive theory of self-regulation as a framework for chronic health condition interventions. *PloS ONE, 10*(8), e013977. doi:1.1371/journal.pone.0134977

Viswanath, K., Finnegan, J. R., & Goullist, S. (2015). Communication and health behavior in a changing media environment. In K. Glanz, B. K. Rimer, & K. Viswanath (Eds.), *Health behavior and health education: Theory, research, and practice* (5th ed., pp. 327-348). San Francisco, CA: Jossey-Bass.

Wallen, M., Duff, S., Goyen, T., & Froude, E. (2013). Respecting the evidence: Responsible assessment and effective intervention for children with handwriting difficulties. *Australian Occupational Therapy Journal, 60*, 366-369.

Watling, R. L., Deitz, J., & White, O. (2001). Comparison of sensory profile scores of young children with and without autism spectrum disorders. *American Journal of Occupational Therapy, 55*(4), 416-423.

Weaver, L. L. (2015). Effectiveness of work, activities of daily living, education and sleep interventions for people with autism spectrum disorder: A systematic review. *American Journal of Occupational Therapy, 69*, 690518002. doi:10.5014/ajot.2015.017962

Wolf, T. J., & Baum C. M. (2011). Improving participation and quality of life through occupation. In G. Gillen (Ed.), *Stroke rehabilitation: A function-based approach* (3rd ed., pp. 66-79). St. Louis, MO: Elsevier Mosby.

World Health Organization. (2001). *International classification of functioning, disability and health* (ICF). Geneva, Switzerland: Author.

Wyrick, J. M., Ogden Niemeyer, L., Ellexson, M., Jacobs, K., & Taylor, S. (1991). Occupational therapy work-hardening programs: A demographic study. *American Journal of Occupational Therapy, 45*(2), 109-112.

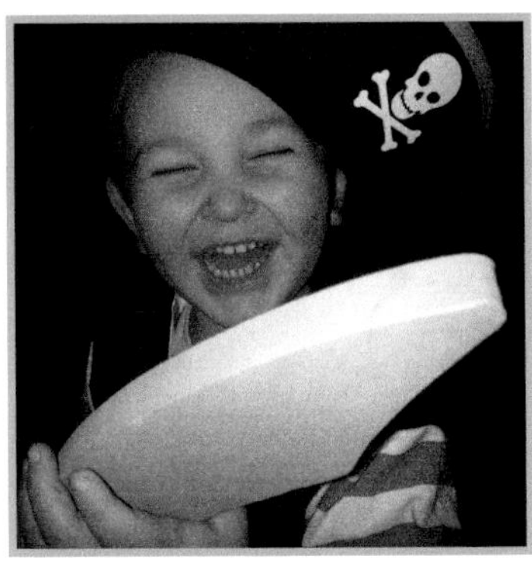

# 20

# Evaluation of Play and Leisure

Lori Vaughn, OTD, OTR/L

**ACOTE STANDARDS EXPLORED IN THIS CHAPTER**

B.4.1, B.4.4, B.4.5

**KEY VOCABULARY**

- **Framing:** Cues that a player offers regarding how he or she wants to be treated (Bateson, 1972).
- **Freedom to suspend reality:** A child's ability to defer the restrictions of realistic play and use his or her imagination to take on new roles and identities and to use objects in a creative way (Bundy, 1997).
- **Internal control:** The individual is the mechanism that drives play. The player is in control of the materials, the play interactions, and some aspects of the outcome (Bundy, 1997; Connor, Williamson, & Siepp, 1978).
- **Intrinsic motivation:** Children are actively engaged in the process of play and are able to continue participation despite barriers and obstacles experienced during the activity (Bundy, 1997; Primeau & Ferguson, 1999).
- **Playfulness:** Describes how an individual approaches any task (not just play or leisure); incorporates intrinsic motivation, internal control, and freedom to suspend reality. It is a characteristic of the person rather than the task (Barnett, 1990; Bundy, 1993).



Jacobs, K., & MacRae, N. (Eds.).
*Occupational Therapy Essentials for Clinical Competence, Third Edition* (pp. 277-298).

## The Occupational Therapy Practitioner's Scope of Practice in the Evaluation of Play and Leisure

According to the American Occupational Therapy Association (AOTA) *Scope of Practice* (2014c), at the core of the values of occupational therapy practice is the understanding and use of occupations. For children and youth, occupations are described as the tasks facilitating learning, enabling the development of important life skills, allowing them to derive pleasure and use creativity, and promoting their ability to thrive. Occupations are also a means and an end, as both a process and a product of intervention (AOTA, 2014b). The domain of occupational therapy is the occupations that people find purposeful and meaningful, enabling individuals to participate in everyday life activities and situations, desired roles, and contexts (AOTA, 2014c). Play activities are defined as "activities pursued for enjoyment and diversion" (AOTA, 2014c, p. S37), and leisure activities are described as "nonobligatory, discretionary, and intrinsically rewarding activities" (AOTA, 2014c, p. S37). In practice, occupational therapy practitioners must consider several factors, including the client's repertoire of occupations, performance skills and patterns used, the influence of contexts on participation, activity demands, and the structures and functions of the client's body (AOTA, 2014c). The AOTA recognizes play and leisure as essential domains of occupational therapy practice for people across the lifespan and the role of practitioners in supporting, enhancing, facilitating, and defending the right of all individuals to engage in this important occupation (Primeau, 2008).

## The Role of the Occupational Therapist and Occupational Therapy Assistant in the Evaluation of Play and Leisure

Occupational therapists have a unique ability to comprehensively, objectively, and quantifiably measure function (Doucet & Gutman, 2013). This ability is essential for measuring progress and for reimbursement purposes, but even more so to ensure the viability and credibility of the profession (Doucet & Gutman, 2013). Evaluations are directed by the occupational therapist and include determination of service need; problem identification and definition; establishment of priorities, goals, and interventions; determination of additional assessment; interpretation of the data; and integration of information. The occupational therapy assistant contributes to the process of evaluation by the implementation of assigned assessments if service competency has been established, provision of verbal and/or written reports based on observations and experience, and dissemination of other pertinent information necessary for the occupational therapist for interpretation and decision making (AOTA, 2014a). Throughout the evaluation process, the occupational therapist develops a client's occupational profile, assesses the client's ability to participate in everyday activities, and works with the client to determine areas of need and priorities for intervention to support engagements in meaningful occupations (AOTA, 2014c, 2015c). Evaluation includes several factors that can affect basic and instrumental activities of daily living, rest and sleep, education, work, play, leisure, and social participation (AOTA, 2014c). Throughout all screening, evaluation, and reevaluation processes, the occupational therapy practitioner must use current and relevant assessment tools and procedures while following established and standardized protocols (AOTA, 2015c). The occupational therapist is responsible for the documentation of evaluation results; however, the occupational therapy assistant can contribute to the documentation process (AOTA, 2015c). The occupational therapist is responsible for determining which specific responsibilities will be delegated to the occupational therapy assistant. The occupational therapy assistant must demonstrate competency, but is also responsible for ensuring that assigned tasks do not extend beyond their scope of practice (AOTA, 2014a).

## The Centennial Vision and the Evaluation of Play and Leisure

In 2007, the AOTA established a vision regarding how the profession would be viewed at its 100th anniversary in 2017. During the intervening decade, AOTA and its members have worked toward becoming a "powerful, widely recognized, science driven, and evidence-based profession with a globally connected and diverse workforce meeting society's occupational needs" (AOTA, 2007, p. 613). Evaluation is an important piece of the vision. Throughout history, occupational therapy practitioners have used a variety of assessment tools, including both standardized and nonstandardized. Both play a role in the evaluation process; however, to continue to move in the direction of the Centennial Vision and become an evidence-based profession, it is important to more fully adopt the use of standardized assessment tools in the evaluation process over homegrown assessments lacking reliability and validity (Hilton, Goloff, Altaras, & Josman, 2013; Radomski & Trombly-Latham, 2008). Assessments focusing on measuring performance in natural environments can both inform practice and increase awareness of innovative practices that are science driven and evidence based with the potential for improved quality of life and client outcomes (Hilton et al., 2013).

## Interprofessional Collaboration in the Evaluation of Play and Leisure

The occupational therapy practitioner is an important member of an interprofessional and collaborative team of health care professionals. Collaboration and consultation with the client, family, and other members of the team is essential to ensure client-centered evaluation and intervention practices (AOTA, 2015b). Mandates for interprofessional collaboration and communication are woven into current Accreditation Council for Occupational Therapy Education (ACOTE) educational standards (2012), and the *Occupational Therapy Code of Ethics* has long included a commitment to fair and respectful treatment of clients and colleagues under the principle of fidelity (AOTA, 2015a, 2015b). In the evaluation of play and leisure, particularly in working with children and youth, it is not unusual for an evaluation to occur "arena" style, in which multiple service professionals are present observing and lending their expertise while one team member conducts the evaluation (Stewart, 2010). This model is presumed to improve the efficiency of service, be more cost effective, be less intrusive to the families, facilitate a more cohesive and collaborative plan of care, and provide a more holistic service delivery model (King et al., 2009). In 2011, domains of competency for collaborative practice were identified by the Interprofessional Education Collaborative Expert Panel (IECE). According to this panel (2011) and Muhlenhaupt, Pizur-Barnekow, Schefkind, Chandler, and Harvison (2015), these competencies include:

- **Values/ethics for interprofessional practice:** These are client-/family-centered values with a focus on the community/population level. This value espouses a commitment to shared purpose, is supportive of the common good, and is committed to the creation of safer and more efficient and effective health care systems.
- **Roles/responsibilities:** This competency relates to the ability to articulate one's professional role and responsibilities to other members of the health care team, to understand the roles and responsibilities of others, and to identify ways for all of the roles and responsibilities to work in concert with each other.
- **Interprofessional communication:** This competency is essential for collaborative practice. It involves the ability to effectively communicate with the recipient of health care services as well as other members of the team in an honest and respectful manner. It also relies on equal contribution and participation from other members of the team.
- **Teams and teamwork:** This competency involves the active participation in client-/family-centered service delivery while minimizing gaps, errors, and redundancy. Other members of the health care team share in the decision-making and problem-solving processes.

## Evaluation of Play

*Children learn as they play.*
*Most importantly, in play children learn how to learn.*

—Dr. O. Fred Donaldson
Author and advocate for play as an alternative to violence and aggression

Play is a concept familiar to everyone. Just the mention of the word can evoke thoughts and emotions. However, the feelings induced are subjective to each individual. A child can be observed while engaged in a variety of play activities, such as playing dress-up or chasing a friend on the playground. An adolescent can be engrossed in playing a video game, or a little leaguer can play baseball. Play is individual to the player and possesses meaning an outside observer can only assume. While the activities can be identified, a clear understanding of a child's intrinsic motivation remains elusive. Contributing to the difficulty with conceptualization are the divergent cultural and societal norms, beliefs, and values associated with play. While play is difficult to understand, it is an inherent part of childhood, how children learn and develop, and how they interact with people and objects in the environment. The first section of this chapter focuses on theories contributing to the concept of play and specific assessment tools used to evaluate play.

### What Is Play?

Despite an inherent personal concept of play subject to individual interpretations, theorists have long struggled to conceive of, develop, and concur on a definitive definition (Parham & Primeau, 1997; Sheridan, Howard, & Alderson, 2011; Takata, 1969). Within the field of occupational therapy, play has been defined as "any spontaneous or organized activity that provides enjoyment, entertainment, amusement, or diversion"

(Parham & Fazio, 2008, p. 448). While the profession has an operational definition of play, there is no denying that the true meaning of play lies within the individual. For example, observers might easily label the previous examples as play; however, the ability to determine what intrinsic value each task holds for the player and what elements of the task constitute a playful experience is much more complex. The challenges in coming to a consensus regarding the definition of play has affected the ability to develop appropriate and culturally relevant assessment tools (Parham & Primeau, 1997), due in part to the inability to find a common language to adequately evaluate and research all of the intricacies of play (Parham & Primeau, 1997) and distinguish it from non-play (Bundy, 1993; Rubin, Fein, & Vandenberg, 1983). Labeling what constitutes play is much more challenging than determining what it is not (Takata, 1969) because it is easy to identify but difficult to define (Johnson, Christie, & Yawkey, 1987; Sheridan et al., 2011). What scholars can agree on is that play is the primary occupation of children (Bundy, 1993; Case-Smith & Kuhaneck, 2008; Heard, 1977; Knox, 1997; Muys, Rodger, & Bundy, 2006; Skard & Bundy, 2008; Welters-Davis & Lawson, 2011), one in which people engage throughout their lifespan (Christiansen, 1991; Kielhofner, 1995; Lautamo & Heikkila, 2011; Primeau, Clark, & Pierce, 1989; Yerxa et al., 1989), and something in which they want to engage, rather than are obliged to engage in (Lautamo & Heikkila, 2011). Children are less concerned with how to define play, but describe their purpose for persistent engagement as "fun" and an escape from "boredom" (Miller & Kuhaneck, 2008). Some of the prevailing operational concepts are found within the constructs of occupational science (Clark et al., 1991), which focus on the study of occupation (Parham & Primeau, 1997). Under this theory, to understand the occupation of play, scholars must study play rather than focus on the performance skills and client factors that can affect play (Parham & Primeau, 1997). In occupational science, play is open ended, limitless, and a completely pleasurable experience (Burke, 1996). Yerxa et al. (1989) stressed the importance of understanding what the process of engagement means to the individual. Another view involves the belief that play is more than a method to achieve a therapeutic end but is an end in and of itself because of its intrinsic value and its ability to promote health. It is inappropriate to view play simply as a therapeutic tool but rather as an entity that should not be reduced to its individual components (Fallon & MacCobb, 2013; Miller & Kuhaneck, 2008). Play has also been linked to the development of creativity, curiosity, humor, imagination, self-efficacy, and communication skills (Caplan & Caplan, 1973; McCune-Nicolich & Bruskin, 1982; Russ, 2003; Saltz & Brodie, 1982; Singer & Singer, 1992) and for the development of physical, cognitive, and social skills, as well as overall quality of life (Kolehmainen et al., 2015; Powrie, Kolehmainen, Turpin, Ziviani, & Copley, 2015; Zwicker, Harris, & Klassen, 2013). While engaged in play, children are at, or close to, their optimal level of development (Vygotsky, 1967, cited in Linder, 1993). It exists for the intrinsic pleasure of the player, and there is no correct or incorrect way to play (Olsen, 1999). Play is also highly dependent on the attitudes and beliefs of the player (Takata, 1974). For this reason, defining play is not the only challenge that is presented—evaluating play may be equally difficult.

## Theories of Play

Occupational therapy practitioners have recognized the value of play as a role and as a method of health promotion. However, not until the work of Mary Reilly (1974) and her students did the profession contribute to the knowledge base of play. Although there is an extensive body of knowledge regarding play theories, much of that knowledge was acquired through other disciplines, especially education and psychology. Still, efforts to develop an occupational therapy theory of play have been limited (Parham & Primeau, 1997). Because much of the knowledge is derived from other disciplines, and because of the unique foci and perspectives of these other disciplines, the ability to develop a comprehensive occupational therapy taxonomy regarding the occupational components of play is challenging (Parham & Primeau, 1997). With the lack of an appropriate taxonomy, practitioners often apply other models of practice to play, which may or may not appropriately address the deficits (Bryze, 1997). Despite the challenges, these disciplines provide a basis on which occupational therapy can build. According to Reilly (1974), an interprofessional explanation is necessary because of the complexity of play.

## Historical Perspectives

History provides several play perspectives. In the research, these theories are typically labeled either classical or modern theories, with World War I as the marker between the two periods (Gilmore, 1971; Mellou, 1994). Classical theories attempted to identify why play existed and define its purpose. These theories were based on philosophical principles rather than scientific research (Ellis, 1973, cited in Parham & Primeau, 1997). Several classical theories have been identified (Gilmore, 1971; Mellou, 1994) and are briefly described in the following examples:

- **Surplus energy theory:** Hypothesized that every organism has a fixed quantity of energy available that must be expended. When the energy is not required for self-preservation, it is manifested in non–goal-directed ways. Because children are typically cared for and do not expend a great deal of energy in these endeavors, they have excess energy and play occurs as a result (Gilmore, 1971; Lieberman, 1977; Mellou, 1994; Parham & Primeau, 1997; Rubin, 1982;

Stagnitti, 2004; Tsao, 2002). Remnants of this theory persist today. Consider parents directing their children to "go outside and play" to burn off some energy.

- **Recreation/relaxation theory:** Proposed that play was a result of a lack of energy and occurred to replenish depleted energy. Because children are always busy learning and acquiring new skills, a great deal of energy is used. Play is relaxing and rejuvenating because there are no cognitive demands (Gilmore, 1971; Lieberman, 1977; Mellou, 1994; Parham & Primeau, 1997; Stagnitti, 2004). Remnants of this theory can be found in the "rejuvenating" outings that occur in the business world and the newfound "energy" a young adult finds after a long day of work when a friend calls to make plans for the evening.
- **Pre-exercise theory (also called the instinct theory):** Hypothesized that play is instinctive and is preparatory for mature adult behavior in the future. As species become increasingly complex on the evolutionary scale, organisms are not born with the required skills to survive in adulthood. For this reason, periods of time during which adaptive skills are acquired are necessary, and play is a method of acquiring these skills. Play is used as rehearsal for adult roles and for the acquisition of skills necessary for survival and adaptation (Parham, 1996; Reilly, 1974; Saracho & Spodek, 1995; Stagnitti, 2004; Tsao, 2002). Remnants of this theory can be found in the preponderance of gender-based toys that are marketed to children to "play house" or to "play pretend" in various life roles.
- **Recapitulation theory:** Postulated that play is part of an evolutionary process. Human development follows an evolutionary path, and the development of play is no exception. For example, children swing and climb trees during an "animal" phase of development (Mellou, 1994; Rubin et al., 1983; Stagnitti, 2004). This theory may also be found in how play behaviors are often described, such as how a person "acts like an animal," and even play equipment, such as the monkey bars.

Modern theories developed after World War I and were based on classical theories. These theorists were more interested in addressing play and how it relates to human development (Parham & Primeau, 1997). Parham and Primeau grouped modern theories into four categories—arousal modulation, psychodynamic, cognitive developmental, and sociocultural theories. These are briefly described as follows:

1. **Arousal modulation theories:** Hypothesized that novelty and uncertainty increase arousal levels, and when aroused, organisms enter an exploratory state. When children are presented with a novel toy or are in a new environment, play is limited because they enter the discovery state, which is cognitively based and requires focused attention. Play is more relaxed as a child experiments with a familiar toy in a known environment (Mellou, 1994; Parham & Primeau, 1997).
2. **Psychodynamic theories:** Based on the works of Freud and Erikson (1959), these theories hypothesized that children develop coping strategies through play. These strategies are "acted out" through play to rehearse for situations that might occur in reality later in life. This allows them to actively mediate stressful events rather than falling prey to anxiety and helplessness (Gilmore, 1971; Parham & Primeau, 1997; Rubin et al., 1983).
3. **Cognitive developmental theories:** Postulated that play is volitional and contributes to the development of cognitive skills, symbolism, adaptation, flexibility, and a repertoire of skills necessary for later life (Bruner, 1972; Mellou, 1994; Parham & Primeau, 1997; Rubin et al., 1983; Sutton-Smith, 1967). These theories further postulate that creativity develops through play. Children also learn the consequences of their actions and self-expression (Gardner, 1982).
4. **Sociocultural theories:** Hypothesized that children learn social and cultural norms and behaviors through play, with both play and culture reciprocally influencing each other. Children also learn the rules of social conduct and the concept of self-identity through playful activities. Empathy and the ability to function as a member of society are learned through game play and games with rules (Mead, 1934, cited in Parham & Primeau, 1997; Roopnarine & Johnson, 1994; Sutton-Smith, 1980).

Whereas many of the classical and modern theories were based in philosophy, psychology, and education, the field of occupational therapy has also been interested in play throughout its history. The early founders stressed the importance of finding a balance between work, rest, play, and sleep (Parham & Primeau, 1997). Play developed as a primary tool when treating children and became synonymous with occupational therapy (Granoff, 1995, as cited in Parham & Primeau, 1997). Economic factors influenced the use of play as a therapeutic tool in the early 20th century. Individuals deemed able to work were placed in work programs, and those unable to work participated in recreational programs (Inch, 1936, cited in Parham & Primeau, 1997). The differentiation between work and play became less defined as practitioners learned that both could exist within a given activity (Parham & Primeau, 1997). Through Mary Reilly's work (1974), play was once again brought to the forefront of occupational therapy and used as a valuable therapeutic and research tool. Reilly recognized the complexity of play, which she described as a "cobweb" through which children learn mastery of their environment and gain the skills and competency required for adulthood. Many of Reilly's students continued her work and have added substantial information to the field, inspiring a new generation of scholars and practitioners.

## Why Evaluate Play?

Researchers have stressed the importance of embracing play as a valid occupational therapy area of practice (Bundy, 1991; Couch, Deitz, & Kanny, 1998; Florey, 1981; Lautamo & Heikkila, 2011). While play is acknowledged as the primary occupation of children (AOTA, 2014b) and one that lasts throughout the lifetime, it is rarely evaluated (Bundy, 1997; Lawlor & Henderson, 1989) and receives less attention in terms of instrument development than other occupations (Brown & Bourke-Taylor, 2014). The reasons for this are varied but are likely related to the lack of assessment tools that truly evaluate play (Bundy, 1993; Bundy, Nelson, Metzger, & Bingaman, 2001; Morrison & Metzger, 2001; Sturgess, 1997). Furthermore, it is acknowledged that observation of a child's play skills in natural environments is important; observation alone does not provide enough objective information with regard to a child's play abilities in the absence of objective, in-depth assessment tools (Bundy, 2005; Sturgess, 1997). Because play and the components that compose play are difficult to define, the ability to quantify and standardize these components can be even more challenging (Kalverboer, 1977), which has traditionally led practitioners to use observations of play behaviors as the primary method of evaluation (Bundy, 2005). However, it is incumbent upon practitioners to use psychometrically sound assessment instruments to inform clinical reasoning and appropriate intervention planning (Brown, 2009; Brown & Bourke-Taylor, 2014). Other constraints diminishing the use of play as a therapeutic tool include negativity regarding play with an emphasis on non–play-based skill development, intervention based on site-specific roles, and reimbursement issues (Couch et al., 1998). Parents with children with disabilities often prefer to focus on physical, rather than play development (Knox, 2008). Assessments exist, but they tend to focus more on play-related skills such as fine motor, gross motor, and cognitive abilities (Bundy, 1997). Although these assessments assist in identifying a child's underlying capabilities and capacity to engage in play, they do not assess play as an occupation (Wallen & Walker, 1995). Current play assessments focusing on skill areas fail to adequately measure alternative concepts of play, such as play through communication or vicarious play, which are often seen in children with disabilities (Graham, Truman, & Holgate, 2015). Assessing the occupation of play provides the practitioner with valuable information regarding developmental levels across several domains, including socialization, pre-academic, motor, communication, and self-awareness (Fewell & Glick, 1993; Florey, 1971; Michelman, 1974; Schaaf, 1990; Takata, 1974), and has been called the "window to development" (Stagnitti, Unsworth, & Rodger, 2000, p. 292). Furthermore, the evaluation of play provides valuable information relative to a child's ability to interact within the environment (Lautamo & Heikkila, 2011).

To effectively evaluate play, it is important to look at the entire occupation of play rather than simply evaluating the related client factors. Play is essential to healthy development as well as a sense of meaning and purpose in life (Kolehmainen et al., 2011). Children who cannot play or who have difficulty engaging in play do not develop the skills necessary for typical development. This difficulty can precipitate lifelong difficulties including decreased participation and satisfaction in occupational roles (Bledsoe & Shepherd, 1982; O'Brien & Shirley, 2001; Stagnitti & Unsworth, 2000), as well as social and emotional well-being (Kolehmainen et al., 2011). Effective assessment of play serves multiple purposes. Play assessments can be used diagnostically to assess development across domains, as well as therapeutically for intervention planning and to determine the effectiveness of intervention (Kelly-Vance & Ryalls, 2005; Miller & Kuhaneck, 2008). Lack of empirically researched assessment tools may also be related to the cultural value that has been placed on play as an occupation. Cultural and societal beliefs have affected the prioritization of areas of focus within the profession, and play has historically been viewed as a volitional rather than compulsory activity such as self-care, work, and education (Bundy, 2005). This lack of tools often leads to the use of informal observation-based evaluation. While this can be a valuable and informative method of obtaining information, there are many factors that can affect the quality of such an evaluation, including the knowledge and experience of the practitioner and his or her ability to adequately interpret the information (Bundy, 2005).

Difficulty evaluating play is further compounded by the lack of culturally appropriate assessment tools. The majority of standardized assessment tools used in pediatric occupational therapy practice were normed on typically developing children from North America and England using items and materials culturally appropriate for those populations, yet they are used to evaluate children from other cultures without consideration of their cultural relevance (Dender & Stagnitti, 2011; Pfeifer, Queiroz, Santos, & Stagnitti, 2011; Richardson, 2015; Thorley & Lim, 2011). This can lead to difficulties in both developing a culturally appropriate intervention plan and an over- or underidentification of children as "delayed" (Dender & Stagnitti, 2011) and place children from other cultures at a disadvantage (Pfeifer et al., 2011). Challenges exist not only in cultural bias that may exist within the tools themselves, but also in the understanding of test-taking procedures and other aspects of the testing, such as time limits (Richardson, 2015). Cultural awareness is essential in evaluating children, particularly in the use of standardized assessments. Use of observation in natural settings is often preferable to use of tools that are culturally inappropriate (Richardson, 2015).

Similar to limited culturally appropriate assessment tools, there is a paucity of tools that adequately measure play in children with disabilities because of the inherent difficulty in determining and measuring participation (Coster & Khetani, 2008; Hoogsteen & Woodgate, 2010; McConachi, Colver, Forsyth, Jarvis, & Parkinson, 2006; Watts, Stagnitti, & Brown, 2014). Despite this, difficulty in play has been identified in children with a variety of diagnoses, including developmental, emotional, learning, and movement/coordination disorders (Cordier, Bundy, Hocking, & Einfeld, 2010; McDonald & Vigen, 2012; Muys et al., 2006; Poulsen, Ziviani, Cuskelly, & Smith, 2007). Because play is central in the lives of children, and practitioners are ethically bound to use a client-centered approach with children and families, it is incumbent on practitioners to evaluate it as an occupation when play is a concern, using culturally and developmentally appropriate assessment tools. Evaluation of play should include the family and caregivers in the process, and whenever possible, it should occur within the child's natural settings of home, school, and community (Townsend, 1997, cited in Primeau, 2003; Richardson, 2015).

Using this top-down, collaborative approach to evaluation, the client and practitioner are able to identify the occupations that children want, need, and have to do and the factors that affect their ability to fully participate in these areas (Coster, 1998; Law et al., 1990; Trombly, 1993). According to Anita Bundy (1997), a comprehensive evaluation of play should include the following five factors:

1. What the player does
2. Why the player enjoys the chosen activity
3. How the player approaches play
4. The player's capacity to play
5. Relative supportiveness of the environment

## What the Player Does

Regardless of the words used to define play, theorists agree that play is activity for its own sake and not one that is based on external factors (Parham & Primeau, 1997; Rubin et al., 1983). In play, it is the process of doing rather than the end product that is rewarding (Rubin et al., 1983). Researchers have identified three factors that comprise play: intrinsic motivation, internal control, and freedom to suspend reality (Bundy, 2002; Morrison, Bundy, & Fisher, 1991; Neuman, 1971). Intrinsic motivation is what drives a child to participate in an activity for pleasure rather than for extrinsic reward (Bundy, 1993). However, it is difficult to assess, as children do not always demonstrate outward expressions of pleasure while engaged in play activities (Morrison et al., 1991). With intrinsic motivation, children are actively engaged in the process of play and are able to continue participation despite barriers and obstacles experienced during the activity (Bundy, 1997; Primeau & Ferguson, 1999). Intrinsic motivation involves pleasure, which differentiates play from work (West, 1990). With internal control, the individual is the mechanism that drives the play. The player is in control of the materials, the play interactions, and some aspects of the outcome (Bundy, 1997; Connor, Williamson, & Siepp, 1978). The child is motivated, is able to modify his or her approach despite challenges, is willing to share materials and equipment, and seeks play opportunities with peers (Bundy, 1997). With the freedom to suspend reality, the child is able to defer the restrictions of realistic play and use his or her imagination to take on new roles and identities and to use objects in a creative way (Bundy, 1997; Rubin et al., 1983). With the ability to suspend reality, the child is able to be mischievous, playful, joking, teasing, and imaginative (Bundy, 1997). This is recognized as important for the acquisition and development of cognitive, social, and language skills (McCune-Nicolich & Fenson, 1984, as cited in Rodger & Ziviani, 1999).

## Why the Player Enjoys the Chosen Activity

As an observer, it can be difficult to understand why an individual chooses a specific activity and what value participation holds for the individual. Theorists have struggled over this concept, attempting to deconstruct the value and purpose ascribed to one activity over another that appears equally enticing (Lawlor, 2003). According to Rubin et al. (1983), play involves self-imposed goals that are subject to change according to the wishes and desires of the player, making it spontaneous. Understanding why a person selects a particular activity and the intrinsic pleasure derived from it is difficult and equally challenging for the player to articulate. Intrinsic motivation is difficult to assess but important to understand if we are to consider play as an important occupation (Bundy, 1997). According to Bruner (1986), it is impossible to understand what an individual is experiencing while engaged in any activity. However, through observation, clues are emitted on which inferences can be drawn. Although motivation is difficult to assess, information can be obtained through the observation of play patterns. Activities in which the child derives pleasure and engages in regularly can provide clues as to the player's motivation (Bundy, 1997). Pleasure is subjective, with each individual deriving something personal from any given activity. Evaluating personal meaning, while difficult, is important if intervention is aimed at building and improving an individual's repertoire of play skills and interests (Bundy, 2001).

## How the Player Approaches Play

It is important to consider not just what a player does, but also how the child approaches play (Bundy, 1993), which has been termed *playfulness* (Barnett, 1990; Bundy, 1993; Lieberman, 1977). Playfulness incorporates intrinsic motivation, internal control, and freedom to suspend reality, but it is not limited to play and may be seen in any activity (Bundy, 1993). In addition to the three factors that comprise play, Bateson (1972) described a fourth factor—framing—that he identified as essential for playfulness. He likened play to a frame through which players offer cues about how they want to be treated. For success, players must be able to give and receive these social cues (Bateson, 1972; Bundy, 1997). With playfulness, the outcome is not as important as the process. It is the individual who determines whether a task is playful, rather than the activity itself (Bryze, 1997; Bundy, 1997). Assessing playfulness may provide practitioners with greater and more valuable information than assessing the play activities themselves (Bundy, 1997). Anita Bundy (1991) recognized the importance of incorporating several factors into the evaluation of play and developed a model of playfulness and a complementary assessment, the Test of Playfulness, which is included in the Evidence-Based Research Chart.

### The Player's Capacity to Play

The player's capacity to play relates to active participation in a play activity (Rubin et al., 1983). Play assessments have historically focused on evaluating the skills necessary to participate in play activities (Bundy, 1997). Fine and gross motor, sensory, and neurological deficits may play a role in play deficits. Although it is important to evaluate these skills to determine how skill performance affects an individual's ability to play, it is not the only area that should be evaluated. The best information will result from an evaluation of these skills within the context of play rather than in isolation (Bundy, 1997). Including a variety of recognizable toys in a familiar environment with minimal intrusion will aid in obtaining the most accurate information of play skills (Rubin et al., 1983).

### The Relative Supportiveness of the Environment

Play represents an interaction of players and the environment in which they play, and a complete evaluation of play must include how the environment supports participation (Bundy, 1997). This environmental assessment should include the caregivers and other individuals, objects, space, safety, comfort, and sensory input relative to their support of play (Bundy, 1997; Olsen, 1999; Parham & Primeau, 1997). A child's daily routines and interactions become incorporated into play experiences and are drawn upon for imagination (Harris, 2000). Children who are deemed "playful" exhibit a decrease in playfulness in a less supportive environment, and conversely, less playful children exhibit an increase in playfulness in a more supportive environment (Bronson & Bundy, 2001; Lieberman, 1977). If environmental factors impede an individual's ability to play, the development of required skills and behaviors may be inhibited (Bryze, 1997; Burke, 1993; Reilly, 1974). Theorists have espoused the benefits of a supportive environment and have advocated the benefits of the reciprocal person–environment interaction, with each influencing the other (Bronson & Bundy, 2001; Kielhofner, 1995; Wicker, 1987). Both physical and social aspects of the environment can influence the development of play skills. The "fit" between the environment and the person is considered positive when the environment is able to meet the individual's needs and when the individual's abilities match the demands imposed by the environment (Pervin, 1968, as cited in Bronson & Bundy, 2001; Rodger & Ziviani, 2006). Boredom or anxiety can exist if the demands of the environment are too low or too high relative to the abilities of the child (Bronson & Bundy, 2001). Play can occur when the child feels comfortable and safe within his or her environment (Hamm, 2006).

## Play Assessments

As indicated earlier in this chapter, play is complex. A thorough evaluation is necessary to determine which factors relate to deficits in this multifaceted occupation. A variety of assessment tools are available; however, they are not inclusive of all potential deficit areas, nor are they wholly occupationally focused. The selection of a play assessment should be carefully considered. Inclusion of the word play in the name of the tool does not necessarily mean that play is being assessed. Therefore, consideration of various tools and options is recommended for an accurate evaluation (Bundy, 1997). Play assessments generally consist of an observation of the child within the context of play to evaluate the child's abilities across all areas when compared to typically developing peers (Kelly-Vance & Ryalls, 2005). These assessments can provide a wealth of information related to a child's areas of strength and areas of need (Fewell, 1991; Kelly-Vance & Ryalls, 2005; Linder, 1993). Neisworth and Bagnato (1988) outlined a continuum of assessment approaches that are typically used by interprofessional assessment teams. Norm-based assessments evaluate a child's developmental level to a similar cohort group. Curriculum-based assessments involve following an individual's achievement along a "developmentally sequenced curriculum" (Neisworth & Bagnato, 1988, p. 27). Adaptive-to-disability assessments allow for altered presentation and response modes and modified responses on test items by a child with sensory impairments to minimize incorrect or false failure on test items. Process assessments examine the changes in a child's reaction to changes in stimuli and can be indicative of a child's cognitive functioning. This includes changes in behavior and can have an effect on the response to the presentation of different stimuli. Judgment-based assessments quantify the impressions and observations of individuals familiar with the child, including parents, caregivers, teachers, and other professionals. This assessment approach is typically used for traits not easily evaluated through other means, including temperament, muscle tone, motivation, and impulse control (Linder, 1993). Ecological assessment examines the child's social, physical, and psychological contexts. Interactive assessment is considered a component of ecological assessment (Linder, 1993) and involves the examination of the social synchronicity of the infant and caregiver. Systematic observation occurs in a child's natural environment of home, school, or community. It may also occur through simulations and/or role-playing and involves measurable, observed aspects of behavior such as frequency, duration, and intensity (Neisworth & Bagnato, 1988). A brief description of play assessments is included in Appendix C to assist the practitioner in selecting the appropriate tool.

## Evaluation of Leisure

*It is in his pleasure that a man really lives; it is from his leisure that he constructs the true fabric of self.*
—Agnes Repplier
American Essayist, 1893

According to Mary Reilly (1974), play possesses both social and biological components. Socially, children learn to interact with both physical and nonphysical aspects of the environment and adapt their responses based on those experiences. Biologically, living things engage in play, which lends to the assumption that, as beings become increasingly complex, the activities in which they engage also become more physically and cognitively complex (Gilfoyle, Grady, & Moore, 1990). As individuals mature beyond childhood, play transforms to leisure, encompassing both social and solitary activities as they continue to refine their understanding of the world and the roles in which they participate (Gilfoyle et al., 1990). While the theoretical beliefs related to leisure have changed throughout history, there is no disputing that, like play, leisure is an important occupation in which we engage and a core concept in the *Occupational Therapy Practice Framework* (AOTA, 2014b).

### What Is Leisure?

Similar to play, theorists have long contemplated the characteristics and value of leisure. The definition of leisure has changed throughout history, adding new elements with each revision. Although each definition added a new dimension to leisure conceptualization, empirical research lagged behind (Esteve, San Martin, & Lopez, 1999). Research indicated that leisure participation, satisfaction, and attitude are positively correlated with satisfaction and quality of life (Bridges & Tancock, 2014; Caldwell & Witt, 2011; Hawkins, 1994; Hawkins, Ardovino, & Hsieh, 1998; Lloyd & Auld, 2002) and has been associated with contributing to promoting and maintaining mental and physical health (Berger, McAteer, Schreier, & Kaldenberg, 2013; Caldwell & Smith, 1988; Coleman & Iso-Ahola, 1993; Passmore, 2003; Tinsley & Tinsley, 1986), as well as positive social functioning (Caldwell & Witt, 2011), decreased mortality (Paganini-Hill, Kawas, & Corrada, 2011), delayed onset of cognitive decline (Källdalen, Marcusson, & Wressle, 2013; Karp et al., 2006), and improved academic performance (Mahoney, 2000). Some research also indicated that leisure affects development by providing opportunities for skill acquisition (Evans & Poole, 1991), social competency, self-awareness, and self-control (Silbereisen, Noack, & Eyferth, 1986, as cited in Passmore, 2003). There have been many terms that have become synonymous with leisure, such as *relaxation, stress-free, freedom from "necessaries,"* and *guilt-free* (Sellar & Boshoff, 2006). Work is often considered obligatory, whereas leisure is the freedom from obligation (Kelly, 1987; Kleiber, 1999; Sellar & Boshoff, 2006). Historically, work has been more highly regarded than leisure, causing the work–leisure dichotomy to exist. Occupational choices were made out of financial necessity and responsibility, creating a barrier to leisure participation and a sense of guilt over what a person can do and what he or she should do (Sellar & Boshoff, 2006). By removing or minimizing the barriers of obligatory tasks, the meaning and experience of leisure is enhanced (Kelly, 1987; Sellar & Boshoff, 2006). Like play in children, leisure has been linked to playfulness (Guitard, Ferland, & Dutil, 2005). The benefits of playfulness in everyday life have been linked to increased creativity, improved ability to heal, increased motivation, and enhanced affect and morale (Auerhahn & Laub, 1987; Etienne, 1982, as cited in Guitard et al., 2005; Lyons, 1987; Tegano, 1990). Despite the benefits, the components of playfulness are different in adults than in children, with adults expressing decreases in spontaneity and tolerance for joy and humor (Guitard et al., 2005; Lieberman, 1977). Guitard et al. (2005) found that playfulness in adults is composed of five components: creativity, curiosity, sense of humor, pleasure, and spontaneity. They further found that playfulness, as defined by the aforementioned components, is helpful in enhancing an individual's occupational performance. Leisure is also similar to play, in that cultural values of leisure time vary. The meaning of "free time" holds different values and beliefs in different societies and cultures (Godbey & Jung, 1991). In English-speaking countries, leisure is equated with free time and can hold a negative value because of its contrast with the concept of work and the value therein (Goodale & Cooper, 1991). There are several factors that affect time use including work beliefs and values, socioeconomic status, politics, gender roles, and weather (Godbey & Jung, 1991). Regardless of the conceptual framework from which leisure is viewed, its intrinsic motivation cannot be denied (Caldwell & Witt, 2011). Occupational therapy practitioners understand the importance of participation in purposeful and meaningful activities with the person at the center of care (Bridges & Tancock, 2014; Njelesani, Teachman, Durocher, Hamdani, & Phelan, 2015). A person-centered approach must address participation in leisure activities across the lifespan.

## Past and Present Theories of Leisure

Theories related to leisure and the use of discretionary time have been in a continuous state of evolution for centuries. It was first defined by Aristotle as being in a state in which an individual was free from the need to toil in laborious tasks and dedicated to more virtuous tasks of self-discovery, self-development, and the pursuit of pleasure (Dare, Welton, & Coe, 1987; Goodale & Cooper, 1991; Sellar & Boshoff, 2006; Veal & Lynch, 2001). These beliefs continued until the period of industrialization and the prevalence of the Protestant work ethic dichotomizing the concepts of work and leisure (Goodale & Cooper, 1991; Primeau, 1996; Sellar & Boshoff, 2006; Veal & Lynch, 2001). Leisure time became that which was left over after domestic and vocational tasks were complete (Veal & Lynch, 2001). It was viewed as a time for consumption, whereas work was a time for production (Goodale & Cooper, 1991). Focus on the concept of leisure as a component of residual time persisted until over 30 years ago, when a shift in thinking occurred. The focus became less of a concept of time and more a concept of the subjective experience of the individual (Primeau, 1996; Suto, 1998; Veal & Lynch, 2001). The perception of the individual became the prevailing determinant in the classification of an activity as leisurely, existing within the individual's consciousness (Kelly, 2000; McDowell, 1984).

## Why Evaluate Leisure?

Like play, leisure is a primary occupation and an important component of well-being (Bridges & Tancock, 2014; Kielhofner, 2008; Turner, Chapman, McSherry, Krishnagiri, & Watts, 2000). Technological advancements, improved health care services, and increased awareness of wellness and prevention have led to an increased number of active, older adults (Stanley, 1995). This number is expected to continue to increase, highlighting the need to ensure that people are able to maintain healthy, active, satisfying existences throughout the lifespan (Sellar & Boshoff, 2006; Stanley, 1995). It is important for health care providers, especially occupational therapy practitioners, to enhance their understanding of the meaning of roles and occupations. Leisure is an important area of practice and is related to improved quality of life, overall health, successful aging, and functional capacity (Charters & Murray, 2006; Easton & Herge, 2011; Law, 2002; Lloyd & Auld, 2002; Sellar & Boshoff, 2006). Like play, leisure can also be viewed as a means to an end and a beneficial area for intervention (Caldwell & Witt, 2011). As such, the necessity to incorporate the evaluation of leisure in occupational therapy is undeniable. However, until recently, the concept of including the subjective experience of the individual in the evaluation was minimal, with a greater focus on more objective factors, including the actual activity and time utilization. This led to the implication that the act of participation was more important than the meaning (Sellar & Boshoff, 2006; Suto, 1998). Understanding the meaning behind participation in certain activities can help practitioners use leisure as a therapeutic activity and enhance the identification of specific barriers that preclude participation (Sellar & Boshoff, 2006; Suto, 1998). To do so effectively, it is important to explore common conceptual factors of leisure, including the temporal, activity, and experiential components. It is also important to consider the role of culture in leisure participation and the concept of leisure as a "flow" experience (Csikszentmihalyi & Kleiber, 1991).

### Leisure as Time

There are certain obligatory activities that everyone engages in to occupy his or her time. Once these activities are completed, certain discretionary time remains. This discretionary time has fluctuated throughout history depending on the prevailing cultural and societal work demands (Csikszentmihalyi & Kleiber, 1991). Despite the existence of this discretionary time, family responsibilities, religious obligations, and personal ambition may drive a person to engage in externally driven projects rather than intrinsically motivating pursuits (Csikszentmihalyi & Kleiber, 1991). The distinction between work and non-work time in defining leisure leads to identifying leisure not as what it is, but rather as what it is not (Henderson et al., 2001). Even when the workday ends, leftover time is not necessarily "free." Long drives are often associated with getting to and from work, and the end of one workday is often the beginning of a second shift of both paid and unpaid labor (Csikszentmihalyi & Kleiber, 1991). Time demands and time use vary from person to person, which is an important consideration in leisure assessment.

### Leisure as Activity

Leisure is identified as activity when engagement occurs for fun and enjoyment, and the activities are categorized according to similar characteristics such as sports, games, outdoor and cultural activities, and socializing (Henderson et al., 2001). Despite the tendency to identify leisure by the activities in which people engage, it is difficult to identify the intrinsic pleasure derived by these activities (Csikszentmihalyi & Kleiber, 1991). This makes it unclear which activities constitute leisure to which individuals. When business executives play golf while discussing business, is this considered work or leisure? Do professional athletes who earn a living playing baseball or football actually work? Is gardening considered work or leisure to a retired person versus a farmer? It is difficult to determine which activities are considered work and which ones are considered leisure and by whom. Researchers tend to identify leisure as those activities that culture identifies as recreational and not engaged in for productive purposes (Csikszentmihalyi & Kleiber, 1991). Csikszentmihalyi (1981) argued that it is more than participation in an activity that constitutes leisure. A single meaningful leisure experience is more significant within a person's life than participation in mundane obligatory experiences over time. For example, participation in a one-time event, such as attendance at a World Series game, may hold greater relevance to an individual than an activity requiring participation over time. However, the frequency of participation in an activity does not determine importance, but perhaps it is the quality of the experience that determines relevance (Csikszentmihalyi & Kleiber, 1991). Participation in meaningful leisure activity can also be impeded by limited opportunities for participation (Kielfhofner, 2009). The activity is less important than the satisfaction derived from engagement (Brown, Frankel, & Fennell, 1991).

### Leisure as Experience

A trend has occurred over the past few decades to shift from the view of leisure as culturally defined, discretionary versus obligatory time, and the subjective experience of the individual (Csikszentmihalyi & Kleiber, 1991). Freedom and intrinsic motivation are essential features of the leisure experience—when an activity is freely selected and engaged in for intrinsic pleasure, it should be considered leisure (Csikszentmihalyi & Kleiber, 1991; Henderson et al., 2001; Neulinger, 1981; Parr & Lashua, 2004). It is a state of mind, and the value of the experience means different things to different people (Estes, 2003; Parr & Lashua, 2005). However, cultural norms and mores cannot be separated from this definition. Some delinquent and vandalistic acts can fall into that definition. Youth gang members who steal and vandalize do so out of free choice and some form of intrinsic pleasure (Csikszentmihalyi & Larson, 1978). Watching television can be considered leisure, but research indicated that it can lead to feelings of apathy and depression (Kubey & Csikszentmihalyi, 1990). To avoid the problem of defining leisure as experience based on these dichotomous viewpoints, two rationalizations can be drawn. First is the admission that leisure can be depressing, tiresome, and even criminal. Second is the idea that an activity cannot be deemed leisure unless it leads to increased positive and culturally accepted experiences in addition to possessing intrinsic motivation and free choice (Csikszentmihalyi & Kleiber, 1991). It is also important to consider the expectations of the occupational therapy practitioners and the clients with regard to what is considered "normal" occupations. For example, participation in leisure activities in later life can be affected by the individual's or the practitioner's perception of what is possible given the process of aging, whether they are applicable to the individual at that time or not. Evidence indicates that these expectations can limit leisure pursuit and participation (Njelesani et al., 2015).

### Leisure as a Construct of Culture

Each society identifies certain activities as work and others as leisure (Henderson et al., 2001). How an individual experiences leisure is often dependent on external factors such as the societal value of work (Parker, 1971, as cited in Henderson et al., 2001). Leisure is encumbered by the influence of social norms, mores, beliefs, and values (Henderson et al., 2001) and cannot occur without consideration of historically conditioned political, economic, and social contexts (Parr & Lashua, 2004). Social influences and peer pressure affect the meaning an individual places on both specific activities as well as the use of discretionary time. Preferences, behaviors, and expectations are dependent, at least in part, on the influence of cultural customs (Henderson et al., 2001).

### Leisure and the Flow Experience

Because of the incongruence of theory related to leisure, the theory of leisure as a "flow experience" was developed and inspired by the work of Abraham Maslow (Csikszentmihalyi & Kleiber, 1991). The research on this theory indicated that when people enjoy what they are doing, the experiential states that they report are similar across cultural, gender, and age boundaries (Csikszentmihalyi, 1990; Csikszentmihalyi & Kleiber, 1991). According to this theory, there is a change in the state of consciousness with the pleasure of the experience. The pleasurable state that is experienced envelops the individual, creating a feeling likened to being engulfed in a current or flow. There is a melding of play and player into a single entity devoid of the "duality of consciousness" typically present in ordinary life—the player becomes the play, able to enjoy new experiences without repercussion (Csikszentmihalyi & Kleiber, 1991, p. 95).

## *Leisure Assessments*

A variety of leisure assessments are available to measure several domains of the leisure experience. Because leisure is subjective, many of the assessments are self-report or interviewer-guided questionnaires (Ben-Arieh & Ofir, 2002; Rosenblum, Sachs, & Schreuer, 2010). Several assessments are described in Appendix C.

## Case Study

Johnny is a 5-year, 2-month-old child with mixed tetraplegic cerebral palsy with bilateral lower extremity and right upper extremity involvement. He also has right homonymous hemianopsia in both eyes. Beth, Johnny's kindergarten teacher, referred him for an evaluation by the XYZ elementary school due to concerns regarding overall academic performance, developmental delays, and limited play skills. With regard to play, she noted concerns with material manipulation, limited construction, decreased attention, limited peer interaction, and apparent lack of interest and participation. Beth also reported concerns with Johnny's limited expressive language and poor motor coordination.

Johnny has attended XYZ school since the age of 3. He attended half-day preschool and is currently attending full-day kindergarten. He has been receiving school-based physical therapy and speech-language services since he began school at the age of 3. He also received physical and occupational therapy through early intervention, beginning at approximately 6 months of age.

He lives at home with both parents, Karen and William; a 12-year old sister, Amanda; and a 9-year old brother, Benjamin. Johnny was the result of a premature birth, occurring at 34 weeks' gestation. He experienced hypoxia at birth and hydrocephalus shortly thereafter. He currently has a ventricular-peritoneal shunt. He spent approximately 1 month in the neonatal intensive care unit. Johnny has been generally healthy. He has typical hearing; however, a reliable visual examination has been difficult to conduct due to his limited expressive language. His limited expressive language has also affected his peer relationships and his participation in classroom, gym, and recess activities.

His parents would like to see Johnny develop improved play skills in an attempt to foster stronger peer relationships. The occupational therapist decided to use the Revised Knox Preschool Play Scale (Knox, 2008) to evaluate Johnny's play. Because the parents were also concerned about his peer relationships, the occupational therapist wanted to use an assessment that evaluated the occupation of play during free play activities. As suggested in the assessment instructions, Johnny was observed for periods of at least 30 minutes in different play situations.

The Revised Knox Preschool Play Scale is administered through observation of the child and designed to provide a description of typical behaviors in play from birth through 6 years of age. The assessment items are grouped into four dimensions: Space Management, Material Management, Pretense-Symbolic, and Participation. Within each domain are several factors. Age ranges are scored for each of the domains. In addition, the child receives an overall play age, which is an average of the age scores in the four domains (Knox, 2008).

Johnny's overall play age was 31 months. In the Space Management domain, Johnny's play age was 21 months. The gross motor section was the most challenging. Because of the cerebral palsy, Johnny requires a walker for ambulation. Even with the walker, he tended to use a wide stance. He was not able to stand unsupported; however, he was able to lower himself to the floor by "plopping." Once down, he was able to sit unsupported, but had limited movement from a seated position, with the exception of scooting. His movement appeared to be a means to an end; Johnny did not appear to explore any new movement patterns. Once in a play center, he remained in that center for the entire free play time. He minimally attempted to incorporate his impaired upper extremity into play activities. Johnny scored in the 38-month range for Material Management. He was able to match and compare, but was unable to effectively and efficiently use tools to copy and trace or for other motor tasks. During the observation, Johnny was able to complete a six-piece inset puzzle and built a simple "castle" out of blocks, using only his unimpaired upper extremity and orienting the blocks and the puzzle pieces by stabilizing them against his body. To visually orient the toys/objects, Johnny held them up to his left side to accommodate for the hemianopsia. Johnny scored in the 48-month range for the Purpose section in this domain because he is just beginning to be interested in completing projects. His lowest score within the Material Management domain was Attention, which was in the 24-month range. He was able to play quietly for 7 minutes and with a single object for 5 minutes; however, he did not demonstrate an intense interest in any single object or task beyond the 5 or 7 minutes. Johnny scored in the 36-month age range for the Pretense-Symbolic domain, with both the Imitation and Dramatization sections scored at that level. He was able to use toys representationally and combined play schemes, such as having the toy puppy do a trick, giving it a treat, and then taking it "outside" for a walk. He also engaged in some imaginative play, such as making the dog treat out of play-dough, cooking it in the block oven, and giving it to the puppy. In the domain of Participation, Johnny scored at the 30-month level, with all sections (Type, Cooperation, Humor, and Language) being scored at that level. Johnny primarily engaged in parallel play. He seemed to enjoy the presence of others, but preferred to play independently. He demonstrated some possessiveness with toys and play objects, including grabbing things away from peers who attempted to join him. He engaged in some conversation with others and used words to communicate his thoughts and ideas. He also used basic language skills to ask questions and comment on his play tasks, such as asking the puppy, "Want go outside?"

*(continued)*

**Case Study (continued)**

Based on the results of the overall team evaluation, including the comprehensive occupational therapy evaluation that included use of the Revised Knox Preschool Play Scale, it was determined that Johnny was a candidate for school-based services. Based upon the results of the Revised Knox Preschool Play Scale and in conjunction with the rest of the educational team, the occupational therapist decided to work on more coordinated movement patterns for engagement in play activities. She also decided to work with the teacher and parents on setting up play environments for Johnny that would promote dynamic movement patterns, both within and between activities. In addition, she recommended arranging play activities to accommodate for Johnny's vision. She believed that his play interests might increase if he was able to independently navigate between centers using a scooter board or some other method of movement once he was down on the floor. In addition, she recommended ongoing projects to promote enhanced interest, such as building more complex puzzles that might not be finished in one sitting, or more complex art tasks, such as papier-mâché, that requires multiple sessions to complete. She also recommended use of visual and verbal prompts for Johnny to incorporate his impaired upper extremity into play activities. The occupational therapist also encouraged the teacher to have Johnny share some of his projects with a peer buddy and have a method of displaying his projects, such as an "Artist of the Week" corner of the classroom. With the team and the parents' input, the practitioner developed fine motor goals to improve Johnny's manipulation skills for improved engagement in play. The team also established a system in the classroom wherein only a certain number of children were allowed in a play center at any given time to encourage other children to engage in centers with Johnny rather than large numbers gathering in other centers. A "Circle of Friends" program was also recommended in coordination with the occupational therapist and the speech-language pathologist to encourage social relationships/skill development.

Theories of play and leisure have changed over time. However, both are valuable occupations in which people engage throughout the lifespan. Benefits have been linked to physical, social, and psychological well-being, as well as improved quality of life, self-esteem, and self-identity. As such, assessment of play and leisure through a variety of standardized and nonstandardized assessment tools, interviews, and observation in a variety of contexts is an essential component to developing a complete occupational profile and developing holistic, client-centered intervention.

## Summary

After our basic needs of food and shelter are addressed, play and leisure become a significant foundation for how we define ourselves as human beings. Play is so important in childhood because of its importance in early learning. Leisure provides adults with healthy outlets to the stresses of a fast-paced life. Even adults with strong and meaningful work relationships know the significance of play and leisure for forming important relationships in life. As play and leisure are so individualized, the occupational therapy practitioner must address the meaning of these activities to the client if the client is to return to a rich and full life.

## Student Self-Assessment

1. Observe a child at play. Take note of the following: What is the child playing with? Is the child intrinsically motivated? What evidence do you have to support your answer? Is the child demonstrating internal control? What evidence do you have to support your answer? Is the child free to suspend reality? What evidence do you have to support your answer?
2. If possible, observe the child playing with a peer. Does the child demonstrate the same level of intrinsic motivation, internal control, and freedom to suspend reality?
3. Attend a child or youth sporting event. Are all of the children demonstrating the same level of playfulness? Why or why not?
4. Interview people at different stages of life, such as a high school or college student, new parents, a still-working baby boomer, and a recent retiree. What differences and similarities do these individuals describe in their leisure pursuits? What about their leisure satisfaction? How does each describe his or her quality of life?
5. After completing the above interview, use the Pleasant Activities List available at https://www.robertjmeyersphd.com/download/Pleasant%20Activities%20List%20(PAL).pdf. Based on the responses, develop a client-centered treatment plan to address leisure participation with the individual.
6. Make a play assessment kit. Pediatric practitioners are often itinerant staff, traveling from site to site. This makes it necessary to travel with all of the items that you need for evaluation and intervention. Because you can only use what you can carry, develop a play assessment kit that you can carry in one bag. What toys/activities would you include? Why would you select these toys? Would you carry different items to assess a preschooler and a second grader?

## Evidence-Based Research Chart

| Play | |
|---|---|
| **Assessment** | **Evidence** |
| Assessment of Preschool Children's Participation | Law, King, Petrenchik, Kertoy, & Anaby, 2012 |
| Child Initiated Pretend Play Assessment | Dender & Stagnitti, 2011; Pfeifer, Pacciulio, Santos, Santos, & Stagnitti, 2011; Pfeifer, Queiroz, Santos, & Stagnitti, 2011; Stagnitti, 2002 as cited in Swindells & Stagnitti, 2006; Stagnitti & Unsworth, 2000, 2004; Stagnitti, Unsworth, & Rodger, 2000; Swindells & Stagnitti, 2006; Uren & Stagnitti, 2009 |
| Child Occupational Self-Assessment | Keller, Kafkes, Basu, Federico, & Kielhofner, 2005; Keller, Kafkes, & Kielhofner, 2005; Keller & Kielhofner, 2005; Kramer, Kielhofner, & Smith, 2010 |
| Children's Playfulness Scale | Barnett, 1990, 1991; Bundy & Clifton, 1998; Muys, Rodger, & Bundy, 2006 |
| Revised Knox Preschool Play Scale | Bundy, 1989; Clifford & Bundy, 1989; Fallon & MacCobb, 2013; Harrison & Kielhofner, 1986; Knox, 1974, 1997; Pacciulio, Pfeifer, & Santos, 2010; Rodger & Ziviani, 1999 |
| McDonald Play Inventory | McDonald & Vigen, 2012 |
| My Child's Play Questionnaire | Schneider & Rosenblum, 2014 |
| Play Assessment for Group Settings | Lautamo & Heikkila, 2011; Lautamo, Kottorp, & Salminen, 2005; Lautamo, Laakso, Aro, Ahonen, & Tormakangas, 2011 |
| Play History | Behnke & Fetkovich, 1984; Rodger & Ziviani, 1999; Stagnitti et al., 2000; Takata, 1969 |
| Play in Early Childhood Evaluation System | Cherney, Kelly-Vance, Gill, Ruane, & Ryalls, 2003; Gill-Glover, McCaslin, Kelly-Vance, & Ryalls, 2001, as cited in Kelly-Vance & Ryalls, 2005; Kelly-Vance & Gill-Glover, 2002, as cited in Kelly-Vance & Ryalls, 2005; Kelly-Vance, Gill, Ruane, Cherney, & Ryalls, 1999, as cited in Kelly-Vance & Ryalls, 2005; Kelly-Vance, Needelman, Troia, & Ryalls, 1999; Kelly-Vance, Gill, Schoneboom, Cherney, Ryan, Cunningham, & Ryalls, 2000, as cited in Kelly-Vance & Ryalls, 2005; Kelly-Vance, Ryalls, & Glover, 2002; King, McCaslin, Kelly-Vance, & Ryalls, 2003, as cited in Kelly-Vance & Ryalls, 2005; McCaslin, King, Kelly-Vance, & Ryalls, 2003, as cited in Kelly-Vance & Ryalls, 2005; Ryalls, Gill, Ruane, Cherney, Schoneboom, Cunningham, & Ryan, 2000, as cited in Kelly-Vance & Ryalls, 2005; Kelly-Vance & Ryalls, 2005 |
| Preschool Play Scale | Bledsoe & Shepherd, 1982; Bundy, 1987, as cited in Bundy et al., 2001; Bundy, 1989; Clifford & Bundy, 1989; Couch, 1996; Harrison & Kielhofner, 1986; Kielhofner, Barris, Bauer, Shoestock, & Walker, 1983; Knox, 1974, 1997; O'Brien et al., 2000; Restall & Magill-Evans, 1994; Shepherd, Brollier, & Dandrow, 1994; Tanta, Deitz, White, & Billingsley, 2005; von Zuben, Crist, & Mayberry, 1991 |
| Symbolic Play Test | Casby, 1997; Cunningham, Glenn, Wilkinson, & Sloper, 1985; Gould, 1986; Lowe & Costello, 1988; Power & Radcliffe, 1989 |
| Test of Playfulness | Bretnall, Bundy, & Kay, 2008; Bronson & Bundy, 2001; Bundy, 1997, 2001, 2003; Cameron et al., 2001; Gaik & Rigby, 1994, as cited in Cameron et al., 2001; Hamm, 2006; Harkness & Bundy, 2001; Hess & Bundy, 2003; Liepold & Bundy, 2000; Muys et al., 2006; O'Brien et al., 2000; O'Brien & Shirley, 2001; Okimoto, Bundy, & Hanzlik, 2000; Reed, Dunbar, & Bundy, 2000; Rodger & Ziviani, 2006; Wilkes-Gillan, Bundy, Cordier, & Lincoln, 2014 |
| Transdisciplinary Play-Based Assessment | Friedli, 1994; Kelly-Vance & Ryalls, 2005; Kelly-Vance et al., 1999; Myers, McBride, & Peterson, 1996; Rodger & Ziviani, 1999 |
| Penn Interactive Peer Play Scale | Castro, Mendez, & Fantuzzo, 2002; Coolahan, Fantuzzo, Mendez, & McDermott, 2000; Fantuzzo, Coolahan, Mendez, McDermott, & Sutton-Smith, 1998; Fantuzzo, Mendez, & Tighe, 1998; Fantuzzo et al., 1995; Mendez, Fantuzzo, & Cicchetti, 2002; Mendez, McDermott, & Fantuzzo, 2002 |

## Evidence-Based Research Chart

| Leisure | |
|---|---|
| **Assessment** | **Evidence** |
| Activity Card Sort | Albert, Bear-Lehman, & Burkhardt, 2009; Chan, Chung, & Packer, 2006 (Hong Kong version); Doney & Packer, 2008; Eriksson et al., 2011; Everard, Lach, Fisher, & Baum, 2000; Hamed et al., 2011 (Arab Heritage version); Hamed & Holm, 2013 (Arab heritage version); Katz, Karpin, Lak, Furman, & Hartman-Maeir, 2003; Laver-Fawcett & Mallinson, 2013 (United Kingdom version); Orellano, 2008 (Spanish version); Packer, Boshoff, & DeJonge, 2008 (Australian version); Packer, Girdler, Boldy, Dhaliwal, & Crowley, 2009; Sachs & Josman, 2003 |
| Children's Assessment of Participation and Enjoyment and Preference for Activities for Children | Bedell & Coster, 2008; Goltz & Brown, 2014; Hochhauser & Engel-Yeger, 2010; King et al., 2003, 2004, 2007; Kolehmainen et al., 2015; Law et al., 2006; McMullan, Chin, Froude, & Imms, 2012; Potvin, Snider, Prelock, Kehayia, & Wood-Dauphinee, 2013; Shikako-Thomas, Majnemer, Law, & Lach, 2008 |
| Children's Leisure Assessment Scale | Rosenblum, Sachs, & Schreuer, 2010 |
| Interest Checklist/Activity Checklist | Katz, 1988; Klyczek, Bauer-Yox, & Fiedler, 1997; Matsutsuyu, 1967, 1969; Nakumara-Thomas & Kyougoku, 2013 (Japanese version); Nakamura-Thomas, Kyougoku, & Forsyth, 2014 (Japanese version); Nakamura-Thomas & Yamada, 2011 (Japanese version); Rogers, Weinstein, & Figone, 1978 |
| Leisure Activity Profile | Mann & Talty, 1991 |
| Leisure Assessment Inventory | Hawkins, 1993, 1994; Hawkins, Ardovino, & Hsieh, 1998; Hawkins & Freeman, 1993 |
| Leisure Attitude Scale | Ragheb & Beard, 1982; Ragheb & Tate, 1993; Siegenthaler & O'Dell, 2000 |
| Leisure Boredom Scale | Gordon & Caltabiano, 1996; Iso-Ahola & Weissinger, 1990; Wegner, Flisher, Muller, & Lombard, 2002 |
| Leisure Competence Measure | Kloseck, Crilly, Ellis, & Lammers, 1996; Kloseck, Crilly, & Hutchinson-Troyer, 2001 |
| Leisure Diagnostic Battery (1) | Beard & Ragheb, 1983; Trottier, Brown, Hobson, & Miller, 2002 |
| Leisure Diagnostic Battery (2) | Chang & Card, 1994; Ellis & Witt, 1986; Peebles, McWilliams, Norris, & Park, 1999; Thomas, 1999; Witt & Ellis, 1984 |
| Leisure Satisfaction Scale | Beard & Ragheb, 1980; DiBona, 2000; Lysyk, Brown, Rodrigues, McNally, & Loo, 2002; Ragheb & Griffith, 1982; Ragheb & Tate, 1993; Raj, Manigandan, & Jacobs, 2006; Siegenthaler & O'Dell, 2000; Trottier et al., 2002 |
| Pediatric Activity Card Sort | Mandich, Polatajko, Miller, & Baum, 2004 |
| Pleasant Activities Checklist | Roozen, Evans, Wiersema, & Meyers, 2009; Roozen et al., 2008 |
| Preferences for Activities of Children | King et al., 2003, 2007 |
| Victoria Longitudinal Study Activity Questionnaire | Jopp & Hertzog, 2010 |

# Electronic Resources

Alliance for Childhood: www.allianceforchildhood.org

Building Healthy Inclusive Communities Through the National Center on Health, Physical Activity, and Disability (NCHPAD): http://www.nchpad.org

Leisure Studies Association: www.leisurestudies.org

National Institute for Play: www.nifplay.org

# References


Accreditation Council for Occupational Therapy Education (2012). 2011 Accreditation Council for Occupational Therapy Education (ACOTE) standards. *American Journal of Occupational Therapy, 66*, S6-S74. doi:20.5014/ajot.2012.66S6

Albert, S. M., Bear-Lehman, J., & Burkhardt, A. (2009). Lifestyle-adjusted function: Variation beyond BADL and IADL competencies. *The Gerontologist, 49*, 767-777.

American Occupational Therapy Association. (2007). AOTA's Centennial Vision and executive summary. *American Journal of Occupational Therapy, 61*, 613-614. doi:10.5014/ajot.61.6.613

American Occupational Therapy Association. (2014a). Guidelines for supervision, roles, and responsibilities during the delivery of occupational therapy services. *American Journal of Occupational Therapy, 68*(Suppl. 3), S16-S22. doi:10.5014/ajot.2014.686S03

American Occupational Therapy Association. (2014b). Occupational therapy practice framework: Domain and process (3rd ed.). *American Journal of Occupational Therapy, 68*(Suppl. 1), S1-S48. doi:10.5014/ajot.2014.682006

American Occupational Therapy Association. (2014c). Scope of practice. *American Journal of Occupational Therapy, 68*(Suppl. 3), S34-S40. doi:10.5014/ajot.2014.686S04

American Occupational Therapy Association. (2015a). Importance of interprofessional education in occupational therapy curricula. *American Journal of Occupational Therapy, 69*(Suppl. 3), 6913410020p1-6913410020p14. doi:10.5014/ajot.2015.696S02

American Occupational Therapy Association. (2015b). Occupational therapy code of ethics. *American Journal of Occupational Therapy, 69*(Suppl. 3), 6913410030p1-6913410030p8. doi:10.5014/ajot.2015.696S03

American Occupational Therapy Association. (2015c). Standards of practice for occupational therapy. *American Journal of Occupational Therapy, 69*(Suppl. 3). 6913410057p1-6913410057p6. doi:10.5014/ajot.2015.696206

Auerhahn, N., & Laub, D. (1987). Play and playfulness in Holocaust survivors. *Psychoanalytic Study of the Child, 42*, 45-58.

Barnett, L. A. (1990). Playfulness: Definition, design, and measurement. *Play and Culture, 3*(4), 319-336.

Barnett, L. A. (1991). The playful child: Measurement of a disposition to play. *Play and Culture, 4*(1), 51-74.

Bateson, G. (1972). Toward a theory of play and fantasy. In G. Bateson (Ed.), *Steps to an ecology of the mind* (pp. 14-20). New York, NY: Bantam.

Beard, J. G., & Ragheb, M. G. (1980). Measuring leisure satisfaction. *Journal of Leisure Research, 12*(1), 20-33.

Beard, J. G., & Ragheb, M. G. (1983). Measuring leisure motivation. *Journal of Leisure Research, 15*(3), 219-228.

Bedell, G. M., & Coster, W. (2008). Measuring participation of school-aged children with traumatic brain injuries: Considerations and approaches. *Journal of Head Trauma Rehabilitation, 23*(4), 220-229.

Behnke, C. J., & Fetkovich, M. M. (1984). Examining the reliability and validity of the play history. *American Journal of Occupational Therapy, 38*(2), 94-100.

Ben-Arieh, A., & Ofir, A. (2002). Time for (more) time-use studies: Studying the daily activities of children. *Childhood, 9*, 225-248. doi:10.1177/0907568202009002805

Berger, S., McAteer, J., Schreier, K., & Kaldenberg, J. (2013). Occupational therapy interventions to improve leisure and social participation for older adults with low vision: A systematic review. *American Journal of Occupational Therapy, 67*(3), 303-311. doi:10.5014/ajot.2013.005447

Bledsoe, N. P., & Shepherd, J. T. (1982). A study of reliability and validity of a preschool play scale. *American Journal of Occupational Therapy, 36*(12), 783-788.

Bretnall, J., Bundy, A. C., & Kay, F. C. S. (2008). The effect of the length of observation on Test of Playfulness scores. *OTJR: Occupation, Participation, and Health, 28*(3), 13-140.

Bridges, L., & Tancock, K. (2014). Activity is a vital component for a healthy and happy environment. *Nursing and Residential Care, 16*(6), 333-335.

Bronson, M. R., & Bundy, A. C. (2001). A correlational study of a test of playfulness and a test of environmental supportiveness for play. *Occupational Therapy Journal of Research, 21*(4), 241-259.

Brown, B. A., Frankel, B. G., & Fennell, M. (1991). Happiness through leisure: The impact of type of leisure activity, age, gender, and leisure satisfaction on psychological well-being. *Journal of Applied Recreation Research, 16*(4), 368-392.

Brown, T. (2009). Assessing occupation: The importance of using valid tests and measures. *British Journal of Occupational Therapy, 72*, 519. doi:10.4276/030802209X12601857794655

Brown, T., & Bourke-Taylor, H. (2014). Children and youth instrument development and testing articles published in the American Journal of Occupational Therapy, 2009-2013: A content, methodology, and instrument design review. *American Journal of Occupational Therapy, 68*(5), e154-e216. doi:10.5014/ajot.2014.012237

Bruner, E. M. (1986). Experience and its expressions. In V. W. Turner & E. M. Bruner (Eds.), *The anthropology of experience* (pp. 3-30). Urbana, IL: University of Illinois.

Bruner, J. S. (1972). Nature and uses of immaturity. *American Psychologist, 27*(8), 687-708.

Bryze, K. (1997). Narrative contributions to the play history. In L. D. Parham & L. S. Fazio (Eds.), *Play in occupational therapy for children* (pp. 23-34). St. Louis, MO: Mosby.

Bundy, A. C. (1989). A comparison of the play skills of normal boys and boys with sensory integrative dysfunction. *Occupational Therapy Journal of Research, 9*, 84-100.

Bundy, A. C. (1991). Play theory and sensory integration. In A. G. Fisher, E. A. Murray, & A. C. Bundy (Eds.), *Sensory integration: Theory and practice* (pp. 46-68). Philadelphia, PA: F. A. Davis Company.

Bundy, A. C. (1993). Assessment of play and leisure: Delineation of the problem. *American Journal of Occupational Therapy, 47*(3), 217-222.

Bundy, A. C. (1997). Play and playfulness: What to look for. In L. D. Parham & L. S. Fazio (Eds.), *Play in occupational therapy for children* (pp. 52-66). St. Louis, MO: Mosby.

Bundy, A. C. (2001). Measuring play performance. In M. Law, C. M. Baum, & W. Dunn (Eds.), *Measuring occupational performance: Supporting best practice in occupational therapy* (pp. 89-102). Thorofare, NJ: SLACK Incorporated.

Bundy, A. C. (2002). Play theory and sensory integration. In A. C. Bundy, S. J. Lane, & E. A. Murray (Eds.), *Sensory integration: Theory and practice* (2nd ed.). Philadelphia, PA: F. A. Davis Company.

Bundy, A. C. (2003). *Test of playfulness (ToP), version 4*. Sydney, Australia: School of Occupation and Leisure Sciences, The University of Sydney.

Bundy, A. C. (2005). Measuring play performance. In M. Law, C. M. Baum, & W. Dunn (Eds.), *Measuring occupational performance: Supporting best practice in occupational therapy* (2nd ed., pp. 128-149). Thorofare, NJ: SLACK Incorporated.

Bundy, A. C., & Clifton, J. (1998). Construct validity of the children's playfulness scale. In M. C. Duncan, G. Chick, & A. Aycock, *Play and culture studies: Volume 1: Diversions and divergences in fields of play* (pp. 37-47). New York, NY: Ablex Publishing.

Bundy, A. C., Nelson, L., Metzger, M., & Bingaman, K. (2001). Validity and reliability of a test of playfulness. *Occupational Therapy Journal of Research, 21*(4), 276-292.

Burke, J. P. (1993). Play: The life role of the infant and young child. In J. Case-Smith (Ed.), *Pediatric occupational therapy and early intervention* (pp. 198-224). Boston, MA: Andover Medical Publishers.

Burke, J. P. (1996). Variations in childhood occupations: Play in the presence of chronic disability. In R. Zemke & F. Clark (Eds.), *Occupational science: The evolving discipline* (pp. 413-418). Philadelphia, PA: F. A. Davis Company.

Caldwell, L. L., & Smith, E. A. (1988). Leisure: An overlooked component of health promotion. *Canadian Journal of Public Health, 79*(2), S44-S48.

Caldwell, L. L., & Witt, P. A. (2011). Leisure, recreation, and play from a developmental context. *New Directions for Youth Development, 130*, 13-27. doi:10.1002/yd.394

Cameron, D., Leslie, M., Teplicky, R., Pollock, N., Steward, D., Toal, C., & Gaik, S. (2001). The clinical utility of the Test of Playfulness. *Canadian Journal of Occupational Therapy, 68*(2), 104-111.

Caplan, F., & Caplan, T. (1973). *The power of play*. New York, NY: Doubleday.

Casby, M. W. (1997). Symbolic play of children with language impairments: A critical review. *Journal of Speech, Language, and Hearing Research, 40*(3), 468-479.

Case-Smith, J., & Kuhaneck, H. M. (2008). Play preferences of typically developing children and children with developmental delays between ages 3 and 7 years. *OTJR: Occupation, Participation and Health, 28*, 19-29.

Castro, M., Mendez, J. L., & Fantuzzo, J. (2002). A validation study of the Penn interactive peer play scale with urban Hispanic and African American preschool children. *School Psychology Quarterly, 17*(2), 109-127.

Chan, V. W. K., Chung, J. C. C., & Packer, T. L. (2006). Validity and reliability of the Activity Card Sort–Hong Kong version. *OTJR: Occupation, Participation, and Health, 26*, 152-158.

Chang, Y. S., & Card, J. A. (1994). The reliability of the Leisure Diagnostic Battery Short Form Version B in assessing healthy, older individuals: A preliminary study. *Therapeutic Recreation Journal, 28*(3), 163-167.

Charters, J., & Murray, S. B. (2006). Design and evaluation of a leisure educational program for caregivers of institutionalized care recipients. *Topics in Geriatric Rehabilitation, 22*, 334-347.

Cherney, I. C., Kelly-Vance, L., Gill, K., Ruane, A., & Ryalls, B. O. (2003). The effects of stereotyped toys and gender on play-based assessment in children aged 18-47 months. *Educational Psychology, 22*(5), 95-106.

Christiansen, C. H. (1991). Occupational therapy: Intervention for life performance. In C. H. Christiansen & C. M. Baum (Eds.), *Occupational therapy: Overcoming human performance deficits* (pp. 4-43). Thorofare, NJ: SLACK Incorporated.

Clark, F. A., Parham, D., Carlson, M. E., Frank, G., Jackson, J., Pierce, D. ... Zemke, R. (1991). Occupational science: Academic innovation in the service of occupational therapy's future. *American Journal of Occupational Therapy, 45*(4), 300-310.

Clifford, J. M., & Bundy, A. C. (1989). Play preference and play performance in normal boys and boys with sensory integrative dysfunction. *Occupational Therapy Journal of Research, 9*(4), 202-217.

Coleman, D., & Iso-Ahola, S. E. (1993). Leisure and health: The role of social support and self-determination. *Journal of Leisure Research, 25*(2), 111-128.

Connor, F. P., Williamson, G. G., & Siepp, J. M. (Eds.). (1978). *Program guide for infants and toddlers with neuromotor and other developmental disabilities*. New York, NY: Teachers College Press.

Coolahan, K., Fantuzzo, J., Mendez, J., & McDermott, P. (2000). Preschool peer interactions and readiness to learn: Relationships between classroom peer play and learning behaviors and conduct. *Journal of Educational Psychology, 92*(3), 458-465.

Cordier, R., Bundy, A., Hocking, C., & Einfeld, S. (2010). Empathy in the play of children with attention deficit hyperactivity disorder. *OTJR: Occupation, Participation, and Health, 30*, 122-132.

Coster, W. (1998). Occupation-centered assessment of children. *American Journal of Occupational Therapy, 52*(5), 337-344.

Coster, W., & Khetani, M. A. (2008). Measuring participation of children with disabilities: Issues and challenges. *Disability and Rehabilitation, 30*(8), 639-648.

Couch, K. J. (1996). The use of the preschool play scale in published research. *Physical and Occupational Therapy in Pediatrics, 16*(4), 77-84.

Couch, K. J., Deitz, J. C., & Kanny, E. M. (1998). The role of play in pediatric occupational therapy. *American Journal of Occupational Therapy, 52*(2), 111-117.

Csikszentmihalyi, M. (1981). Some paradoxes in the definition of play. In A. T. Cheska (Ed.), *Play as context* (pp. 14-26). West Point, NY: Leisure Press.

Csikszentmihalyi, M. (1990). *Beyond boredom and anxiety: The experience of play in work and games*. San Francisco, CA: Jossey-Bass.

Csikszentmihalyi, M., & Kleiber, D. A. (1991). Leisure as self actualization. In P. J. Brown, B. L. Driver, & G. L. Peterson (Eds.), *Benefits of leisure* (pp. 91-102). State College, PA: Venture Publishing.

Csikszentmihalyi, M., & Larson, R. (1978). Intrinsic rewards in school crime. *Crime and Delinquency, 24*(3), 322-335.

Cunningham, C. C., Glenn, S. M., Wilkinson, P., & Sloper, P. (1985). Mental ability, symbolic play and receptive and expressive language of young children with Down's syndrome. *Journal of Child Psychology and Psychiatry and Allied Disciplines, 26*(2), 255-265.

Dare, B., Welton, G., & Coe, W. (1987). *Concepts of leisure in western thought: A critical and historical analysis*. Dubuque, IA: Kendall/Hunt.

Dender, A., & Stagnitti, K. (2011). Development of the indigenous child initiated pretend play assessment: Selection of play materials and administration. *Australian Occupational Therapy Journal, 58*, 34-42.

DiBona, L. (2000). What are the benefits of leisure? An exploration using the leisure satisfaction scale. *British Journal of Occupational Therapy, 63*(2), 50-58.

Donaldson, O. F. (1993). *Playing by heart: The vision and practice of belonging* (3rd ed.). Deerfield Beach, FL: Health Communications, Inc.

Doney, R. M., & Packer, T. L. (2008). Measuring changes in activity participation of older Australians: Validation of the Activity Card Sort-Australia. *Australasian Journal on Ageing, 27*, 33-37.

Doucet, B. M., & Gutman, S. A. (2013). From the desk of the editor and associate editor: Quantifying function: The rest of the measurement story. *American Journal of Occupational Therapy, 67*, 7-9. doi:10.5014/ajot.2013.007096

Easton, L., & Herge, E. A. (2011). Adult day care: Promoting meaningful and purposeful leisure. *OT Practice, 1*, 20-23, 26.

Ellis, G. D., & Witt, P. A. (1986). The leisure diagnostic battery: Past, present, and future. *Therapeutic Recreation Journal, 20*(4), 31-47.

Erikson, E. H. (1959). *Identity and the life cycle*. New York, NY: International Universities Press.

Eriksson, G. M., Chung, J. C. C., Beng, L. H., Hartman-Maeir, A., Yoo, E., Orellano, E. M., Nes, F. V., deJonge, D., & Baum, C. M. (2011). Occupations of older adults: A cross cultural description. *OTJR: Occupation, Participation and Health, 31*, 182-192.

Estes, C. (2003). Knowing something about leisure: Building a bridge between leisure philosophy and recreation practice. *SCHOLE: A Journal of Leisure Studies & Recreation Education, 18*, 51-66.

Esteve, R., San Martin, J., & Lopez, A. E. (1999). Grasping the meaning of leisure: Developing a self-report measurement tool. *Leisure Studies, 18*(2), 79-91.

Evans, G., & Poole, M. E. (1991). *Young adults: Self perceptions and life contexts.* London, England: Falmer Press.

Everard, K. M., Lach, H. W., Fisher, E. B., & Baum, C. M. (2000). Relationship of activity and social support to the functional health of older adults. *The Journals of Gerontology Series B: Psychological Sciences and Social Sciences, 55,* S208-S212.

Fallon, J., & MacCobb, S. (2013). Free play time of children with learning disabilities in a noninclusive preschool setting: An analysis of play and nonplay behaviours. *British Journal of Learning Disabilities, 41,* 212-219.

Fantuzzo, J., Coolahan, K., Mendez, J., McDermott, P., & Sutton-Smith, B. (1998). Contextually relevant validation of peer play constructs with African-American head start children: Penn interactive peer play scale. *Early Childhood Research Quarterly, 13*(3), 411-431.

Fantuzzo, J., Mendez, J., & Tighe, E. (1998). Parental assessment of peer play: Development and validation of the parent version of the Penn interactive peer play scale. *Early Childhood Research Quarterly, 13*(4), 659-676.

Fantuzzo, J., Sutton-Smith, B., Coolahan, K. C., Manz, P. H., Canning, S., & Debnam, D. (1995). Assessment of preschool play interaction behaviors in young low-income children: Penn interactive peer play scale. *Early Childhood Research Quarterly, 10*(1), 105-120.

Fewell, R. R. (1991). Trends in the assessment of infants and toddlers with disabilities. *Exceptional Children, 58*(2), 166-173.

Fewell, R. R., & Glick, M. P. (1993). Observing play: An appropriate process for learning and assessment. *Infants and Young Children, 5*(4), 35-43.

Florey, L. L. (1971). An approach to play and play development. *American Journal of Occupational Therapy, 25*(6), 275-280.

Florey, L. L. (1981). Studies of play: Implications for growth, development, and for clinical practice. *American Journal of Occupational Therapy, 35*(8), 519-524.

Friedli, C. (1994). *Transdisciplinary play-based assessment: A study of reliability and validity.* Unpublished doctoral dissertation, University of Colorado at Boulder.

Gardner, H. (1982). *Art, mind, and brain: A cognitive approach to creativity.* New York, NY: Basic Books.

Gilfoyle, E. M., Grady, A. P., & Moore, J. C. (1990). *Children adapt: A theory of sensorimotor-sensory development* (2nd ed.). Thorofare, NJ: SLACK Incorporated.

Gilmore, J. B. (1971). Play: A special behavior. In R. E. Herron & B. Sutton-Smith (Eds.), *Child's play* (pp. 311-325). New York, NY: John Wiley and Sons.

Godbey, G. C., & Jung, B. (1991). Relations between the development of culture and philosophies of leisure. In B. L. Driver, P. J. Brown, & G. L. Peterson (Eds.), *Benefits of leisure* (pp. 37-45). State College, PA: Venture Publishing.

Goltz, H., & Brown, T. (2014). Are children's psychological self-concepts predictive of their self reported activity preferences and leisure participation? *Australian Occupational Therapy Journal, 61,* 177-186. doi:10.1111/1440-1630.12101

Goodale, T. L., & Cooper, W. (1991). Philosophical perspectives on leisure in English-speaking countries. In B. L. Driver, P. J. Brown, & G. L. Peterson (Eds.), *Benefits of leisure* (pp. 25-35). State College, PA: Venture Publishing.

Gordon, W. R., & Caltabiano, M. L. (1996). Urban-rural differences in adolescent self-esteem, leisure boredom, and sensation-seeking as predictors of leisure-time usage and satisfaction. *Adolescence, 31*(124), 883-901.

Gould, J. (1986). The Lowe and Costello Symbolic Play Test in socially impaired children. *Journal of Autism and Developmental Disorders, 16*(2), 199-213.

Graham, N. E., Truman, J., & Holgate, H. (2015). Parents' understanding of play for children with cerebral palsy. *American Journal of Occupational Therapy, 69*(3), 6903220050p1-6903220050p9

Guitard, P., Ferland, F., & Dutil, E. (2005). Toward a better understanding of playfulness in adults. *OTJR: Occupation, Participation, and Health, 25*(1), 9-22.

Hamed, R., AlHeresh, R., Dahab, S. A., Collins, B., Fryer, J., & Holm, M. B. (2011). Development of Arab Heritage Activity Card Sort. *International Journal of Rehabilitation Research, 34,* 299-306.

Hamed, R., & Holm, M. B. (2013). Psychometric properties of the Arab Heritage Activity Card Sort. *Occupational Therapy International, 20*(1), 23-34.

Hamm, E. M. (2006). Playfulness and the environmental support of play in children with and without developmental disabilities. *OTJR: Occupation, Participation, and Health, 26*(3), 88-96.

Harkness, L., & Bundy, A. C. (2001). The test of playfulness and children with physical disabilities. *OTJR: Occupation, Participation, and Health, 21*(2), 73-89.

Harris, P. L. (2000). *The work of the imagination.* Oxford, United Kingdom: Wiley-Blackwell.

Harrison, H., & Kielhofner, G. (1986). Examining reliability and validity of the preschool play scale with handicapped children. *American Journal of Occupational Therapy, 40*(3), 167-173.

Hawkins, B. A. (1993). An exploratory analysis of leisure and life satisfaction of aging adults with mental retardation. *Therapeutic Recreation Journal, 27*(2), 98-109.

Hawkins, B. A. (1994). Leisure as an adaptive skill area. *AAMR News & Notes, 7*(1), 5-6.

Hawkins, B. A., Ardovino, P., & Hsieh, C. M. (1998). Validity and reliability of the leisure assessment inventory. *Mental Retardation, 36*(4), 303-313.

Hawkins, B. A., & Freeman, P. A. (1993). Correlates of self-reported leisure among adults with mental retardation. *Leisure Sciences, 15,* 131-147.

Heard, C. (1977). Occupational role acquisition: A perspective on the chronically disabled. *American Journal of Occupational Therapy, 31,* 243-247.

Henderson, K. A., Bialeschki, M. D., Hemingway, J. L., Hodges, J. S., Kivel, B. D., & Sessoms, H. D. (2001). *Introduction to recreation and leisure services* (8th ed.). State College, PA: Venture Publishing.

Hess, L. M., & Bundy, A. C. (2003). The association between playfulness and coping in adolescents. *Physical and Occupational Therapy in Pediatrics, 23*(2), 5-17.

Hilton, C. L., Goloff, S. E., Altaras, O., & Josman, N. (2013). Review of instrument development and testing studies for children and youth. *American Journal of Occupational Therapy, 67*(3), 30-54. doi:10.5014/ajot.2013.007831

Hochhauser, M., & Engel-Yeger, B. (2010). Sensory processing abilities and their relation to participation in leisure activities among children with high-functioning autism spectrum disorder (HFASD). *Research in Autism Spectrum Disorders, 4*(4), 746-754.

Hoogsteen, L., & Woodgate, R. L. (2010). Can I play? A concept analysis of participation in children with disabilities. *Physical and Occupational Therapy in Pediatrics, 30*(4), 325-339.

Interprofessional Education Collaborative Expert Panel. (2011). *Core competencies for interprofessional collaborative practice: Report of an expert panel.* Washington, DC: Interprofessional Education Collaborative.

Iso-Ahola, S. E., & Weissinger, E. (1990). Perceptions of boredom in leisure: Conceptualization, reliability, and validity of the Leisure Boredom Scale. *Journal of Leisure Research, 22*(1), 1-17.

Johnson, J. E., Christie, J. F., & Yawkey, T. D. (1987). *Play and early childhood development.* Glenview, IL: Scott Foresman.

Jopp, D. S., & Hertzog, C. (2010). Assessing adult leisure activities: An extension of a self-report activity questionnaire. *Psychological Assessment, 22*(1), 108-120.

Källdalen, A., Marcusson, J., & Wressle, E. (2013). Interests among older people in relation to gender, function, and health-related quality of life. *British Journal of Occupational Therapy, 76*(2), 87-93.

Kalverboer, A. F. (1977). Measurement of play: Clinical application. In B. Tizard & D. Harvey (Eds.), *Biology of play* (pp. 100-122). Philadelphia, PA: J. B. Lippincott.

Karp, A., Paillard-Borg, S., Wang, H. X., Silverstein, M., Winblad, B., & Fratiglioni, L. (2006). Mental, physical and social components in leisure activities equally contribute to decrease dementia risk. *Dementia and Geriatric Cognitive Disorders, 21*, 65-73. doi:10.1159/00089919

Katz, N. (1988). Interest checklist: A factor analytical study. *Occupational Therapy in Mental Health, 8*(1), 45-55.

Katz, N., Karpin, H., Lak, A., Furman, T., & Hartman-Maeir, A. (2003). Participation in occupational performance: Reliability and validity of the activity card sort. *OTJR: Occupation, Participation, and Health, 23*(1), 10-17.

Keller, J., Kafkes, A., Basu, S., Federico, J., & Kielhofner, G. (2005). *The Child Occupational Self Assessment (COSA) (Version 2.1)*. Chicago, IL: University of Illinois, College of Allied Health Sciences, Department of Occupational Therapy, Model of Human Occupation Clearinghouse.

Keller, J., Kafkes, A., & Kielhofner, G. (2005). Psychometric characteristics of Child Occupational Self Assessment (COSA), part one: An initial examination of psychometric properties. *Scandinavian Journal of Occupational Therapy, 12*, 147-158.

Keller, J., & Kielhofner, G. (2005). Psychometric characteristics of the Child Occupational Self Assessment (COSA), part two: Refining the psychometric properties. *Scandinavian Journal of Occupational Therapy, 12*, 147-158. doi:10.1080/11038120510031761

Kelly, J. R. (1987). *Freedom to be: A new sociology of leisure*. New York, NY: Macmillan.

Kelly, J. R. (2000). Leisure, play, and recreation. In J. R. Kelly & V. J. Freysinger (Eds.), *21st century leisure: Current issues* (pp. 14-24). San Francisco, CA: Benjamin-Cummings Publishing Company.

Kelly-Vance, L., Needelman, H., Troia, K., & Ryalls, B. O. (1999). Early childhood assessment: A comparison of the Bayley Scales of Infant Development and a play-based assessment in two-year-old at-risk children. *Developmental Disabilities Bulletin, 27*(1), 1-15.

Kelly-Vance, L., & Ryalls, B. O. (2005). A systematic, reliable approach to play assessment in preschoolers. *School Psychology International, 26*(4), 398-412.

Kelly-Vance, L., Ryalls, B. O., & Glover, K. G. (2002). The use of play assessment to evaluate the cognitive skills of two- and three-year-old children. *School Psychology International, 23*(2), 169-185.

Kielhofner, G. (1995). Environmental influences on occupational behavior. In G. Kielhofner, *A model of human occupation: Theory and application* (pp. 91-111). Baltimore, MD: Lippincott-Raven.

Kielhofner, G. (2008). *A model of human occupation: Theory and application* (4th ed.). Baltimore, MD: Lippincott Williams and Wilkins.

Kielhofner, G. (2009). *Conceptual foundations of occupational therapy practice* (4th ed.). Philadelphia, PA: F. A. Davis Company.

Kielhofner, G., Barris, R., Bauer, D., Shoestock, B., & Walker, L. (1983). A comparison of play behavior in nonhospitalized and hospitalized children. *American Journal of Occupational Therapy, 37*(5), 305-312.

King, G. A., Law, M., King, S., Hurley, P., Hanna, S., Kertoy, M., & Rosenbaum, P. (2007). Measuring children's participation in recreation and leisure activities: Construct validation of the CAPE and PAC. *Child: Care, Health and Development, 33*(1), 28-39.

King, G., Law, M., King, S., Hurley, P., Rosenbaum, S. H., Hanna, S., ... Young, N. (2004). *Children's Assessment of Participation and Enjoyment and Preferences for Activities of Children (CAPE/PAC) manual*. San Antonio, TX: Psychological Corporation.

King, G., Law, M., King, S., Rosenbaum, P., Kertoy, M. K., & Young, N. L. (2003). A conceptual model of the factors affecting the recreation and leisure participation of children with disabilities. *Physical and Occupational Therapy in Pediatrics, 23*(1), 63-90.

King, G., Strachan, D., Tucker, M., Duwyn, B., Desserud, S., & Shillington, M. (2009). The application of a transdisciplinary model for early intervention services. *Infants and Young Children, 22*(3), 21-223.

Kleiber, D. A. (1999). *Leisure experience and human development: A dialectical interpretation*. New York, NY: Basic Books.

Kloseck, M., Crilly, R. G., Ellis, G. D., & Lammers, E. (1996). Leisure competence measure: Development and reliability testing of a scale to measure functional outcomes in therapeutic recreation. *Therapeutic Recreation Journal, 30*(1), 13-26.

Kloseck, M., Crilly, R. G., & Hutchinson-Troyer, L. (2001). Measuring therapeutic recreation outcomes in rehabilitation: Further testing of the leisure competence measure. *Therapeutic Recreation Journal, 35*(1), 31-42.

Klyczek, J. P., Bauer-Yox, N., & Fiedler, R. C. (1997). The interest checklist: A factor analysis. *American Journal of Occupational Therapy, 51*(10), 815-823.

Knox, S. (1974). A play scale. In M. Reilly (Ed.), *Play as exploratory learning: Studies of curiosity behavior* (pp. 247-266). Thousand Oaks, CA: Sage Publications.

Knox, S. (1997). Development and current use of the Knox Preschool Play Scale. In L. D. Parham & L. S. Fazio (Eds.), *Play in occupational therapy for children* (pp. 35-51). St. Louis, MO: Mosby.

Knox, S. (2008). Development and current use of the revised Knox Preschool Play Scale. In L. D. Parham & L. S. Fazio (Eds.), *Play in occupational therapy for children* (2nd ed., pp. 35-51). St. Louis, MO: Mosby.

Kolehmainen, N., Francis, J. J., Ramsay, C. R., Owen, C., McKee, L., Ketelaar, M., & Rosenbaum, P. (2011). Participation in physical play and leisure: Developing a theory and evidence based intervention for children with motor impairments. *BMC Pediatrics, 11*, 100-107.

Kolehmainen, N., Ramsay, C., McKee, L., Missiuna, C., Owen, C., & Francis, J. (2015). Participation in physical play and leisure in children with motor impairments: Mixed methods study to generate evidence for developing an intervention. *Physical Therapy, 95*(10), 1374-1386.

Kramer, J. M., Kielhofner, G., & Smith, E. V., Jr. (2010). Validity evidence for the child occupational self assessment. *American Journal of Occupational Therapy, 64*, 621-632. doi:10.5014/ajot.2010.08142

Kubey, R., & Csikszentmihalyi, M. (1990). *Leisure and the benefits of television*. New Brunswick, NJ: L. Erlbaum.

Lautamo, T., & Heikkila, M. (2011). Inter-rater reliability of the play assessment for group settings. *Scandinavian Journal of Occupational Therapy, 18*, 3-10.

Lautamo, T., Kottorp, A., & Salminen, A. L. (2005). Play assessment for group settings: A pilot study to construct an assessment tool. *Scandinavian Journal of Occupational Therapy, 12*, 136-144.

Lautamo, T., Laakso, M., Aro, T., Ahonen, T., & Tormakangas, K. (2011). Validity of the Play Assessment for Group Settings: An evaluation of differential item functioning between children with specific language impairment and typically developing peers. *Australian Occupational Therapy Journal, 58*, 222-230.

Laver-Fawcett, A. J., & Mallinson, S. H. (2013). Development of the Activity Card Sort–United Kingdom version. *OTJR: Occupation, Participation, and Health, 33*(3), 134-145. doi:10.3928/15394492-20130614-02

Law, M. (2002). Participation in the occupations of everyday life. *American Journal of Occupational Therapy, 56*, 640-649.

Law, M., Baptiste, S., McColl, M., Opzoomer, A., Polatajko, H., & Pollock, N. (1990). The Canadian Occupational Performance Measure: An outcome measure for occupational therapy. *Canadian Journal of Occupational Therapy, 57*(2), 82-87.

Law, M., King, G., King, S., Kertoy, M., Hurley, P., Rosenbaum, P., et al. (2006). Patterns of participation in recreational and leisure activities among children with complex physical disabilities. *Developmental Medicine and Child Neurology, 48*(5), 337-342.

Law, M., King, G., Petrenchik, T., Kertoy, M., & Anaby, D. (2012). The assessment of preschool children's participation: Internal consistency and construct validity. *Physical and Occupational Therapy in Pediatrics, 32*(3), 272-287.

Lawlor, M. C. (2003). The significance of being occupied: The social construction of childhood occupations. *American Journal of Occupational Therapy, 57*(4), 424-434.

Lawlor, M. C., & Henderson, A. (1989). A descriptive study of the clinical practice patterns of occupational therapists working with infants and young children. *American Journal of Occupational Therapy, 43*(11), 755-764.

Lieberman, J. N. (1977). *Playfulness: Its relationship to imagination and creativity*. New York, NY: Academic Press.

Liepold, E. E., & Bundy, A. C. (2000). Playfulness in children with attention deficit hyperactivity disorder. *OTJR: Occupation, Participation, and Health, 20*(1), 61-82.

Linder, T. W. (1993). *Transdisciplinary play-based assessment: A functional approach to working with young children* (2nd ed.). Baltimore, MD: Paul H. Brookes.

Lloyd, K. M., & Auld, C. J. (2002). The role of leisure in determining quality of life: Issues of content and measurement. *Social Indicators Research, 57*(1), 43-71.

Lowe, M., & Costello, A. J. (1988). *Symbolic play test* (2nd ed.). Windsor, Berkshire, England: NFER-Nelson.

Lyons, M. (1987). A taxonomy of playfulness for use in occupational therapy. *Australian Journal of Occupational Therapy, 34*(4), 152-156.

Lysyk, M., Brown, G. T., Rodrigues, E., McNally, J., & Loo, K. (2002). Translation of the Leisure Satisfaction Scale into French: A validation study. *Occupational Therapy International, 9*(1), 76-89.

Mahoney, J. L. (2000). Participation in school extracurricular activities as a moderator in the development of antisocial patterns. *Child Development, 71*, 502-516.

Mandich, A. D., Polatajko, H., Miller, L., & Baum, C. (2004). *Pediatric Activity Card Sort*. Ottawa, Ontario, Canada: CAOT Publication ACE.

Mann, W. C., & Talty, P. (1991). Leisure activity profile: Measuring use of leisure time by persons with alcoholism. *Occupational Therapy in Mental Health, 10*(4), 31-41.

Matsutsuyu, J. S. (1967). The interest checklist. *American Journal of Occupational Therapy, 11*, 179-181.

Matsutsuyu, J. S. (1969). The interest checklist. *American Journal of Occupational Therapy, 23*(4), 323-328.

McConachie, H., Colver, A. F., Forsyth, R. J., Jarvis, S. N., & Parkinson, K. N. (2006). Participation of disabled children: How should it be characterized and measured? *Disability and Rehabilitation, 28*(18), 1157-1164.

McCune-Nicolich, L., & Bruskin, C. (1982). Combinatorial competency in symbolic play and language. In D. J. Pepler & K. H. Rubin (Eds.), *The play of children: Current theory and research* (Vol. 6, pp. 30-45). New York, NY: Karger.

McDonald, A. E., & Vigen, C. (2012). Reliability and validity of the McDonald play inventory. *American Journal of Occupational Therapy, 66*, e52-e60. doi.org/10.5014/ajot.2012.002493

McDowell, C. F. (1984). An evolving theory of leisure consciousness. *Society and Leisure, 7*, 53-87.

McMullan, S., Chin, R., Froude, E., & Imms, C. (2012). Prospective study of the participation patterns of grade 6 and year 8 students in Victoria, Australia in activities outside of school. *Australian Occupational Therapy Journal, 59*(3), 197-208.

Mellou, E. (1994). Play theories: A contemporary review. *Early Child Development and Care, 102*, 91-100.

Mendez, J. L., Fantuzzo, J., & Cicchetti, D. (2002). Profiles of social competence among low-income African American preschool children. *Child Development, 73*(4), 1085-1100.

Mendez, J. L., McDermott, P., & Fantuzzo, J. (2002). Identifying and promoting social competence with African American preschool children: Developmental and contextual considerations. *Psychology in the Schools, 39*(1), 111-123.

Michelman, S. (1974). Play and the deficit child. In M. Reilly (Ed.), *Play as exploratory learning* (pp. 157-207). Thousand Oaks, CA: Sage Publications.

Miller, E., & Kuhaneck, H. (2008). Children's perceptions of lay experiences and play preferences: A qualitative study. *American Journal of Occupational Therapy, 62*(4), 407-415.

Morrison, C. D., Bundy, A. C., & Fisher, A. G. (1991). The contribution of motor skills and playfulness to the play performance of preschoolers. *American Journal of Occupational Therapy, 45*(8), 687-694.

Morrison, C., & Metzger, P. (2001). Play. In J. Case-Smith, A. S. Allen, & P. N. Pratt (Eds.), *Occupational therapy for children* (pp. 528-544). St. Louis, MO: Mosby.

Muhlenhaupt, M., Pizur-Barnekow, K., Schefkind, S., Chandler, B., & Harvison, N. (2015). Occupational therapy contributions in early intervention: Implications for personnel preparation and interprofessional practice. *Infants and Young Children, 28*(2), 123-132.

Muys, V., Rodger, S., & Bundy, A. C. (2006). Assessment of playfulness in children with autistic disorder: A comparison of the children's playfulness scale and the test of playfulness. *OTJR: Occupation, Participation, and Health, 26*(4), 159-170.

Myers, C. L., McBride, S. L., & Peterson, C. (1996). Transdisciplinary, play-based assessment in early childhood special education: An examination of social validity. *Topics in Early Childhood Special Education, 16*, 102-127.

Nakamura-Thomas, H., & Kyougoku, M. (2013). Relationship between interests and health-related quality of life in older people. *British Journal of Occupational Therapy, 76*(4), 162-168.

Nakamura-Thomas, H., Kyougoku, M., & Forsyth, K. (2014). Relationships between interest, current, and future participation in activities: Japanese Interest Checklist for the Elderly. *British Journal of Occupational Therapy, 77*(2), 103-110. doi:10.4276/030802214X13916969447317

Nakamura-Thomas, H., & Yamada, T. (2011). A factor analytic study of the Japanese Interest Checklist for the Elderly. *British Journal of Occupational Therapy, 74*(2), 86-91.

Neisworth, J. T., & Bagnato, S. J. (1988). Assessment in early childhood special education: A typology for independent measures. In S. L. Odom & M. B. Karnes (Eds.), *Early intervention for infants and children with handicaps: An empirical base* (pp. 23-49). Baltimore, MD: Paul H. Brookes Publishing Co.

Neulinger, J. (1981). *To leisure: An introduction*. Boston, MA: Allyn & Bacon.

Neuman, E. A. (1971). *The elements of play*. New York, NY: MSS Information Corporation.

Njelesani, J., Teachman, G., Durocher, E., Hamdani, Y., & Phelan, S. K. (2015). Thinking critically about client-centred practice and occupational possibilities across the life-span. *Scandinavian Journal of Occupational Therapy, 22*(4), 252-259. doi:10.3109/11038128.2015.1049550

O'Brien, J., Coker, P., Lynn, R., Suppinger, R., Pearigen, T., Rabon, S., et al. (2000). The impact of occupational therapy on a child's playfulness. *Occupational Therapy in Health Care, 12*(2), 39-51.

O'Brien, J. C., & Shirley, R. J. (2001). Does playfulness change over time? A preliminary look using the test of playfulness. *Occupational Therapy Journal of Research, 21*(2), 132-139.

Okimoto, A. M., Bundy, A., & Hanzlik, J. (2000). Playfulness in children with and without disability: Measurement and intervention. *American Journal of Occupational Therapy, 54*(1), 73-82.

Olsen, L. J. (1999). Psychosocial frame of reference. In P. Kramer & J. Hinojosa (Eds.), *Frames of reference for pediatric occupational therapy* (2nd ed., pp. 323-375). Baltimore, MD: Lippincott Williams and Wilkins.

Orellano, E. (2008). *Occupational participation of older Puerto Rican adults: Reliability and validity of a Spanish version of the Activity Card Sort*. Unpublished doctoral dissertation, Fort Lauderdale, FL: Nova Southeastern University.

Pacciulio, A. M., Pfeifer, L. I., & Santos, J. L. (2010). Preliminary reliability and repeatability of the Brazilian version of the Revised Knox Preschool Play Scale. *Occupational Therapy International, 17*(2), 74-80. doi:10.1002/oti.289

Packer, T. L., Boshoff, K., & DeJonge, D. (2008). Development of the Activity Card Sort–Australia. *Australian Occupational Therapy Journal, 55*, 199-206.

Packer, T. L., Girdler, S., Boldy, D. P., Dhaliwal, S. S., & Crowley, M. (2009). Vision self-management for older adults: A pilot study. *Disability & Rehabilitation, 31*, 1353-1361.

Paganini-Hill, A., Kawas, C. H., & Corrada, M. M. (2011). Activities and mortality in the elderly: The leisure world cohort study. *Journal of Gerontology, Series A: Biological Sciences and Medical Sciences, 66*, 559-567. doi:10.1093/Gerona/glq237

Parham, L. D. (1996). Perspectives on play. In R. Zemke & F. Clark (Eds.), *Occupational science: The evolving discipline* (pp. 71-80). Philadelphia, PA: F. A. Davis Company.

Parham, D. L., & Fazio, L. S. (2008). *Play in occupational therapy for children* (2nd ed.). St. Louis, MO: Mosby.

Parham, L. D., & Primeau, L. A. (1997). Play and occupational therapy. In L. D. Parham & L. S. Fazio (Eds.), *Play in occupational therapy for children* (pp. 2-21). St. Louis, MO: Mosby.

Parr, M. G., & Lashua, B. D. (2004). What is leisure? The perceptions of recreation practitioners and others. *Leisure Sciences, 26*(1), 1-17.

Parr, M. G., & Lashua, B. D. (2005). Students' perceptions of leisure, leisure professionals and the professional body of knowledge. *Journal of Hospitality, Leisure, Sport, and Tourism Education, 4*(2), 16-26.

Passmore, A. (2003). The occupation of leisure: Three typologies and their influence on mental health in adolescence. *OTJR: Occupation, Participation, and Health, 23*(2), 76-83.

Peebles, J., McWilliams, L., Norris, L. H., & Park, K. (1999). Population-specific norms and reliability of the leisure diagnostic battery in a sample of patients with chronic pain. *Therapeutic Recreation Journal, 33*(3), 135-141.

Pfeifer, L. I., Pacciulio, A. M., Santos, C. A., Santos, J. L., & Stagnitti, K. E. (2011). Pretend play of children with cerebral palsy. *Physical and Occupational Therapy in Pediatrics, 31*(4), 390-402.

Pfeifer, L. I., Queiroz, M. A., Santos, J. L. F., & Stagnitti, K. E. (2011). Cross-cultural adaptation and reliability of child initiated pretend play assessment (ChIPPA). *Canadian Journal of Occupational Therapy, 78*(3), 187-195.

Potvin, M. C., Snider, L., Prelock, P., Kehayia, E., & Wood-Dauphinee, S. (2013). Children's Assessment of Participation and Enjoyment/Preference for Activities of Children: Psychometric properties in a population with high-functioning autism. *American Journal of Occupational Therapy, 67*, 209-217. doi:10.5014/ajot.2013.006288

Poulsen, A. A., Ziviani, J. M., Cuskelly, M., & Smith, R. (2007). Boys with developmental coordination disorder: Loneliness and team sports participation. *American Journal of Occupational Therapy, 61*, 451-462. doi:10.5014/ajot.61.4.451

Power, T. J., & Radcliffe, J. (1989). The relationship of play behavior to cognitive ability in developmentally disabled preschoolers. *Journal of Autism and Developmental Disorders, 19*(1), 97-107.

Powrie, B., Kolehmainen, N., Turpin, M., Ziviani, J., & Copley, J. (2015). The meaning of leisure for children and young people with physical disabilities: A systematic evidence synthesis of qualitative studies. *Developmental Medicine and Child Neurology, 57*(11), 993-1010. doi:10.1111/dmcn.12788

Primeau, L. A. (1996). Work and leisure: Transcending the dichotomy. *American Journal of Occupational Therapy, 50*(7), 569-577.

Primeau, L. (2003). Play and leisure. In E. B. Crepeau, E. S. Cohn, & B. A. Boyt Schell (Eds.), *Willard and Spackman's occupational therapy* (10th ed., pp. 354-363). Philadelphia, PA: Lippincott Williams and Wilkins.

Primeau, L. A. (2008). AOTA's societal statement on play. *American Journal of Occupational Therapy, 62*(6), 707-708.

Primeau, L. A., Clark, F., & Pierce, D. (1989). Occupational therapy alone has looked upon occupation: Future applications of occupational science to pediatric occupational therapy. *Occupational Therapy in Health Care, 6*, 19-32.

Primeau, L. A., & Ferguson, J. F. (1999). Occupational frame of reference. In P. Kramer & J. Hinojosa (Eds.), *Frames of reference for pediatric occupational therapy* (2nd ed., pp. 469-516). Philadelphia, PA: Lippincott Williams and Wilkins.

Radomski, M. V., & Trombly-Latham, K. (Eds.). (2008). *Occupational therapy for physical dysfunction*. Philadelphia, PA: Lippincott Williams and Wilkins.

Ragheb, M. G., & Beard, J. G. (1982). Measuring leisure attitude. *Journal of Leisure Research, 14*(2), 155-167.

Ragheb, M. G., & Griffith, C. A. (1982). The contribution of leisure participation and leisure satisfaction to life satisfaction of older persons. *Journal of Leisure Research, 14*(4), 295-306.

Ragheb, M. G., & Tate, R. L. (1993). A behavioral model of leisure participation, based on leisure attitude, motivation and satisfaction. *Leisure Studies, 12*(1), 61-70.

Raj, J. T., Manigandan, C., & Jacobs, K. S. (2006). Leisure satisfaction and psychiatric morbidity among informal carers of people with spinal cord injury. *Spinal Cord, 44*(11), 676-679.

Reed, C. N., Dunbar, S. B., & Bundy, A. C. (2000). The effects of an inclusive preschool experience on the playfulness of children with and without autism. *Physical and Occupational Therapy in Pediatrics, 19*(3), 73-89.

Reilly, M. (1974). *Play as exploratory learning*. Thousand Oaks, CA: Sage Publications.

Restall, G., & Magill-Evans, J. (1994). Play and preschool children with autism. *American Journal of Occupational Therapy, 48*(2), 113-120.

Richardson, P. K. (2015). Use of standardized tests in pediatric practice. In J. Case-Smith & J. C. O'Brien (Eds.), *Occupational therapy for children and adolescents* (7th ed., pp. 163-191). St. Louis, MO: Elsevier Mosby.

Rodger, S., & Ziviani, J. (1999). Play-based occupational therapy. *International Journal of Disability, Development and Education, 46*(3), 337-365.

Rodger, S., & Ziviani, J. (Eds.). (2006). *Occupational therapy with children: Understanding children's occupations and enabling participation*. Malden, MA: Wiley-Blackwell.

Rogers, J. C., Weinstein, J. M., & Figone, J. J. (1978). The interest check list: An empirical assessment. *American Journal of Occupational Therapy, 32*(10), 628-630.

Roopnarine, J. L., & Johnson, J. E. (1994). The need to look at play in diverse cultural settings. In J. L. Roopnarine, J. E. Johnson, & F. H. Hooper (Eds.), *Children's play in diverse cultures* (pp. 1-8). Albany, NY: State University of New York Press.

Roozen, H. G., Evans, B. E., Wiersema, H., & Meyers, R. J. (2009). The influence of extraversion on preferences and engagement in pleasant activities in patients with substance abuse disorders: One size fits all? *Journal of Behavior Analysis in Health, Sports, Fitness and Medicine, 2*(1), 55-66.

Roozen, H. G., Wiersema, H., Strietman, M., Feij, J. A., Lewinsohn, P. M., Meyers, R. J., Koks, M. & Vingerhoets, J. J. M. (2008). Development and psychometric evaluation of the Pleasant Activities List. *American Journal on Addictions, 17*, 1-14.

Rosenblum, S., Sachs, D., & Schreuer, N. (2010). Reliability and validity of the children's leisure assessment scale. *American Journal of Occupational Therapy, 64*, 633-641. doi:10.5014/ajot.2010.08173

Rubin, K. H. (1982). Early play theories revisited: Contributions to contemporary research and theory. In D. J. Pepler & K. H. Rubin (Eds.), *Play of children: Current theory and research* (Vol. 6, pp. 4-14). New York, NY: Karger.

Rubin, K. H., Fein, G. G., & Vandenberg, B. (1983). Play. In P. Mussen & E. M. Hetherington (Eds.), *Handbook of child psychology, socialization, personality and social development* (Vol. 4, 4th ed., pp. 693-774). New York, NY: Wiley.

Russ, S. W. (2003). Play and creativity: Developmental issues. *Scandinavian Journal of Educational Research, 47*(3), 291-303.

Sachs, D., & Josman, N. (2003). The activity card sort: A factor analysis. *OTJR: Occupation, Participation, and Health, 23*(4), 165-174.

Saltz, E., & Brodie, J. (1982). Pretend play training in childhood: A review and critique. In D. J. Pepler & K. H. Rubin (Eds.), *Play of children: Current theory and research* (Vol. 6, pp. 97-113). New York, NY: Karger.

Saracho, O. N., & Spodek, B. (1995). Children's play and early childhood education: Insights from history and theory. *Journal of Education, 177*(3), 129-148.

Schaaf, R. C. (1990). Play behavior and occupational therapy. *American Journal of Occupational Therapy, 44*(1), 68-75.

Schneider, E., & Rosenblum, S. (2014). Development, reliability, and validity of My Child's Play (MCP) questionnaire. *American Journal of Occupational Therapy, 68*(3), 277-285.

Sellar, B., & Boshoff, K. (2006). Subjective leisure experiences of older Australians. *Australian Occupational Therapy Journal, 53*(3), 211-219.

Shepherd, J., Brollier, C., & Dandrow, R. (1994). Play skills of preschool children with speech and language delays. *Physical and Occupational Therapy in Pediatrics, 14*(2), 1-20.

Sheridan, M. D., Howard, J., & Alderson, D. (2011). *Play in early childhood from birth to six years* (3rd ed.). London, England: Routledge.

Shikako-Thomas, K., Majnemer, A., Law, M., & Lach, L. (2008). Determinants of participation in leisure activities in children and youth with cerebral palsy: A systematic review. *Physical and Occupational Therapy in Pediatrics, 28*(2), 155-169.

Siegenthaler, K. L., & O'Dell, I. (2000). Leisure attitude, leisure satisfaction, and perceived freedom in leisure within family dyads. *Leisure Sciences, 22*(4), 281-296.

Singer, D. G., & Singer, J. L. (1992). *The house of make-believe: Children's play and the developing imagination.* Cambridge, MA: Harvard University Press.

Skard, G., & Bundy, A. (2008). The Test of Playfulness. In L. D. Parham & L. S. Fazio (Eds.), *Play in occupational therapy for children* (2nd ed., pp. 71-94). St. Louis, MO: Mosby.

Stagnitti, K. (2004). Understanding play: The implications for play assessment. *Australian Occupational Therapy Journal, 51*(1), 3-12.

Stagnitti, K., & Unsworth, C. (2000). The importance of pretend play in child development: An occupational therapy perspective. *British Journal of Occupational Therapy, 63*(3), 121-127.

Stagnitti, K., & Unsworth, C. (2004). The test-retest reliability of the child-initiated pretend play assessment. *American Journal of Occupational Therapy, 58*(1), 93-99.

Stagnitti, K., Unsworth, C., & Rodger, S. (2000). Development of an assessment to identify play behaviors that discriminate between the play of typical preschoolers and preschoolers with pre-academic problems. *Canadian Journal of Occupational Therapy, 67*(5), 291-303.

Stanley, M. (1995). An investigation into the relationship between engagement in valued occupations and life satisfaction for elderly South Australians. *Journal of Occupational Science, 2*(3), 100-114.

Stewart, K. B. (2010). Purposes, processes, and methods of evaluation. In J. Case-Smith & J. C. O'Brien (Eds.), *Occupational therapy for children* (6th ed., pp. 193-215). Maryland Heights, MO: Mosby Elsevier.

Sturgess, J. L. (1997). Current trend in assessing children's play. *British Journal of Occupational Therapy, 60*(9), 410-414.

Suto, M. (1998). Leisure in occupational therapy. *Canadian Journal of Occupational Therapy, 65*(5), 271-278.

Sutton-Smith, B. (1967). The role of play in cognitive development. *Young Children, 22*, 361-370.

Sutton-Smith, B. (1980). A sportive theory of play. In H. B. Schwartzman (Ed.), *Play and culture* (pp. 10-19). West Point, NY: Leisure Press.

Swindells, D., & Stagnitti, K. (2006). Pretend play and parents' view of social competence: The construct validity of the Child-Initiated Pretend Play Assessment. *Australian Occupational Therapy Journal, 53*(4), 314-324.

Takata, N. (1969). The play history. *American Journal of Occupational Therapy, 23*(4), 314-318.

Takata, N. (1974). Play as prescription. In M. Reilly (Ed.), *Play as exploratory learning* (pp. 209-246). Thousand Oaks, CA: Sage Publications.

Tanta, K. J., Deitz, J. C., White, O., & Billingsley, F. (2005). The effects of peer-play level on initiations and responses of preschool children with delayed play skills. *American Journal of Occupational Therapy, 59*(4), 437-445.

Tegano, D. W. (1990). Relationship of tolerance ambiguity and playfulness to creativity. *Psychological Reports, 66*, 1047-1056.

Thomas, D. W. (1999). Evaluating the relationship between premorbid leisure preferences and wandering among patients with dementia. *Activities, Adapting and Aging, 23*(4), 33-48.

Thorley, M., & Lim, S. M. (2011). Considerations for occupational therapy assessment for indigenous children in Australia. *Australian Occupational Therapy Journal, 58*, 3-10.

Tinsley, H. A., & Tinsley, D. J. (1986). A theory of attributes, benefits, and causes of the leisure experience. *Leisure Sciences, 8*, 1-45.

Trombly, C. (1993). Anticipating the future: Assessment of occupational function. *American Journal of Occupational Therapy, 47*(3), 253-257.

Trottier, A. N., Brown, G. T., Hobson, S. J., & Miller, W. (2002). Reliability and validity of the leisure satisfaction scale (LSS—Short form) and the adolescent leisure interest profile (ALIP). *Occupational Therapy International, 9*(2), 131-144.

Tsao, L. (2002). How much do we know about the importance of play in child development? Review of research. *Childhood Education, 78*(4), 230-234.

Turner, H., Chapman, S., McSherry, A., Krishnagiri, S., & Watts, J. (2000). Leisure assessment in occupational therapy: An exploratory study. *Occupational Therapy in Health Care, 12*(2/3), 73-85.

Uren, N., & Stagnitti, K. (2009). Pretend play, social competence and involvement in children aged 5-7 years: The concurrent validity of the child initiated pretend play assessment. *Australian Occupational Therapy Journal, 56*, 33-40.

Veal, A. J., & Lynch, R. (2001). *Australian leisure* (2nd ed.). Frenchs Forest, New South Wales, Australia: Longman.

von Zuben, M. V., Crist, P. A., & Mayberry, W. (1991). A pilot study of differences in play behavior between children of low and middle socioeconomic status. *American Journal of Occupational Therapy, 45*(2), 113-118.

Wallen, M., & Walker, R. (1995). Occupational therapy practice with children with perceptual motor dysfunction: Findings of a literature review and survey. *Australian Occupational Therapy Journal, 42*, 15-25.

Watts, T., Stagnitti, K., & Brown, T. (2014). Relationship between play and sensory processing: A systematic review. *American Journal of Occupational Therapy, 68*(2), e37-e46. doi:10.5014/ajot.2014.009787

Wegner, L., Flisher, A. J., Muller, M., & Lombard, C. (2002). Reliability of the leisure boredom scale for use with high school learners in Cape Town, South Africa. *Journal of Leisure Research, 34*(3), 340-351.

Welters-Davis, M., & Lawson, L. M. (2011). The relationship between sensory processing and parent-child play preferences. *Journal of Occupational Therapy, Schools, and Early Intervention, 4*, 108-120.

West, J. (1990). Play, work, and play therapy: Distinctions and definitions. *Adoption and Fostering, 14*(4), 31-37.

Wicker, A. W. (1987). Behavior settings reconsidered: Temporal stages, resources, internal dynamics, context. In D. Stokols & I. Altman (Eds.), *Handbook of environmental psychology* (pp. 613-653). New York, NY: Wiley.

Wilkes-Gillan, S., Bundy, A., Cordier, R., & Lincoln, M. (2014). Evaluation of a pilot parent-delivered play-based intervention for children with attention deficit hyperactivity disorder. *American Journal of Occupational Therapy, 68*(6), 700-709.

Witt, P. A., & Ellis, G. D. (1984). The leisure diagnostic battery: Measuring perceived freedom in leisure. *Society and Leisure, 7*(1), 109-124.

Yerxa, E. J., Clark, F., Jackson, J., Parham, D., Pierce, D., Stein, C., & Zemke, R. (1989). An introduction to occupational science. A foundation for occupational therapy in the 21st century. *Occupational Therapy in Health Care, 6*(4), 1-17.

Zwicker, J., Harris, S., & Klassen, A. (2013). Quality of life domains affected in children with developmental coordination disorder: A systematic review. *Child: Care, Health, and Development, 39*, 562-580.

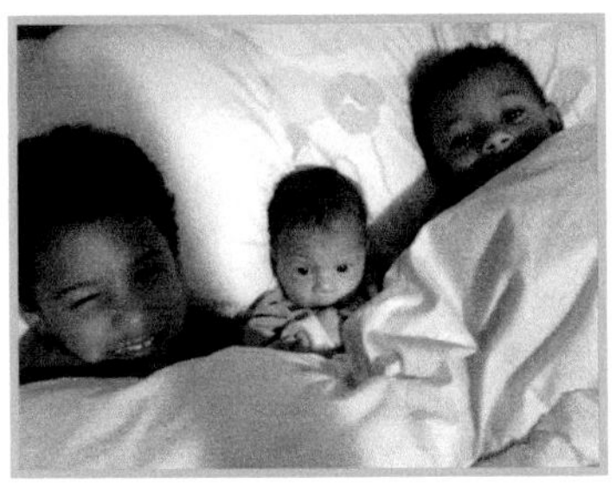

# 21

# Evaluation of Occupational Performance in Rest and Sleep

*Michelle Goulet, MS, OTR/L*

**ACOTE STANDARDS EXPLORED IN THIS CHAPTER**

B.1.4, B.4.1–B.4.4

**KEY VOCABULARY**

- **Central sleep apnea:** A breathing-related sleep disorder caused by the brain's inability to send signals to the diaphragm or other muscles of the respiratory system.
- **Circadian process:** The process within our body that uses environmental cues (light/dark cycle) to train the body to have the ability of knowing when to sleep even if there are no environmental cues present at a given time.
- **Efficiency:** The ratio of total sleep time to time spent in bed.
- **Hypersomnia:** Excessive sleep, usually occurring during the day or at times when sleeping would normally not be considered appropriate.
- **Insomnia:** The inability or great difficulty falling asleep, maintaining sleep, or not feeling refreshed upon waking.
- **Latency:** The duration of time between going to bed and falling asleep.
- **Mental rest:** Freeing one's mind of anything that exhausts or drains the mind while obtaining peace and calmness.
- **Narcolepsy:** Excessive sleepiness accompanying frequent daytime attacks of sleep; there is usually a bilateral loss of muscle tone during these sudden sleep attacks, known as cataplexy, and can be connected with feelings of intense emotion.

*(continued)*



Jacobs, K., & MacRae, N. (Eds.).
*Occupational Therapy Essentials for Clinical Competence, Third Edition* (pp. 299-309).

### KEY VOCABULARY (CONTINUED)

- **Obstructive sleep apnea:** A breathing-related sleep disorder caused by a hindrance in the airway.
- **Periodic limb movements:** Repetitive, twitching leg jerks that occur every 20 to 60 seconds during sleep onset, decreasing as one falls into a deeper sleep.
- **Physical rest:** Cessation of taxing physical activity and relaxing one's body.
- **Rapid eye movement (REM) behavior disorder:** Nerve conduction is not inhibited like normal REM sleep where there is a cease of transmission with muscle activity; persons may violently thrash around during sleep, acting out a dream they are having and potentially causing injury or harm to either themselves or their bed partner.
- **Rest:** A way to restore energy through easy or effortless acts that provide a break from mental and physical activities; there are three components of rest: physical, mental, and spiritual.
- **Restless leg syndrome:** A feeling of discomfort and the desire to move, more commonly the legs, but sometimes also the arms, while falling asleep or waking during the night; the uncomfortable feeling is described as a creeping, crawling, tingling, burning, or itching feeling.
- **Sleep:** A sequence of activities resulting in going to sleep, staying asleep, and maintaining health through participating in sleep.
- **Sleep adequacy:** The feeling of being rested and refreshed after a night of sleep.
- **Sleep debt:** The amount of time an individual is awake. Therefore, the longer an individual stays awake, the more sleep debt he or she accumulates.
- **Sleep diary:** Journals that are kept for a period of a couple weeks to a month or more so that practitioners can identify patterns and discrepancies from what bed partners report and potential reasons why a client may be experiencing sleeping difficulties.
- **Sleep hygiene:** The overall term as to how a client combines aspects of both sleep preparation and sleep participation to create quality and quantity within nighttime sleep.
- **Sleep participation:** The act of engaging in restful sleep.
- **Sleep preparation:** Routines that prepare the client for a comfortable rest.
- **Spiritual rest:** Freeing one's mind of any burdens through relaxation.

One of occupational therapy's original founders, Adolf Meyer, established four occupational performance areas, including work, play, rest, and sleep. Meyer (1922) concluded that a balance must be established between the four performance areas to promote healthy living. Even though our founders emphasized the importance of rest and sleep for a balanced life, the majority of occupational therapy research and practice is still primarily on work, education, play, self-care, and leisure (Nurit & Michal, 2003). Occupational therapy practitioners must remain conscious of the profession's theoretical basis and be sure to establish a balance between all occupational performance areas, including rest and sleep.

This chapter will focus on those frequently neglected areas of occupation, rest and sleep. It will explore what exactly constitutes rest and sleep according to the occupational therapy profession and the medical field. It will touch on improving clients' sleep hygiene as well as the preparation of their sleep. Common sleep disorders across the lifespan will also be identified. Lastly, evaluations and assessments that may be used in the occupational therapy process will be suggested.

## REST

Rest is an area of occupation that was established during the beginning years of the occupational therapy profession and has since been apparent in occupational therapy literature. Meyer (1922) was the first to classify human occupations and established work, play, rest, and sleep as primary performance areas. In addition to establishing the performance areas, Meyer (1922) focused on a balance between the four for healthy living. In later years,

Mosey (1981) supported Meyer's theory by addressing the need for balance between work, play, and rest in his philosophical assumptions. Along with Meyer and Mosey, Llorens (1991) revised her original perception of occupational performance from work, education, play, self-care, and leisure to include rest and relaxation. Many pioneers within the occupational therapy profession have included rest and relaxation as a performance area throughout time. As a result, rest is currently an important part of the *Occupational Therapy Practice Framework* (American Occupational Therapy Association [AOTA], 2014).

Rest is described as "effortless actions that interrupt physical and mental activity resulting in a relaxed state" (AOTA, 2014, p. S20). When individuals engage in a restful activity, they are restoring energy and renewing interest in engagement (AOTA, 2014). Although different for each individual, restful activities can include listening to relaxing music, reading, walking, sitting quietly, or lying down, but not engaging in sleep.

There are three components of rest: physical rest, mental rest, and spiritual rest (Nurit & Michal, 2003). Physical rest includes cessation of taxing physical activity and relaxing one's body. An example of physical rest could be when an individual who is engaging in a tiring game of soccer retreats to the sideline to give his or her body a break from the strenuous physical activity. Mental rest is freeing one's mind of anything that exhausts or drains and obtaining peace and calm. An example of mental rest would be taking a break from studying for an important exam by taking a walk or listening to relaxing music. Spiritual rest includes establishing inner peace, harmony, nirvana, and calm, and is often attained by many people through meditation.

Although physical and mental rest are the two types of rest primarily incorporated throughout daily routines, the idea of "rest" has been tied to spirituality and various religions throughout history. Tibetan Buddhism describes meditation as rest. Meditation is a state of relaxation; its purpose is to free an individual's mind of any burdens. In addition, within the Christian, Jewish, and Muslim religions, specific times and places are dedicated to rest and prayer (Nurit & Michal, 2003). There is a strong link between spirituality and rest and relaxation. There is also a strong link between meaningful occupations and spirituality. There are many ways that an individual can find spirituality through everyday activities. Simple activities such as reading, listening to music, writing, walking, being in nature, and gardening can be turned into meaningful and spiritual activities. Most all of the activities listed are also non-taxing and relaxing. According to Christiansen (1997), "any occupation can be spiritual if attention is given to its style and context" (p. 170). Therefore, similarly to incorporating spirituality into certain activities, most activities have the potential to be restful and relaxing. Spirituality and rest are closely related for some individuals; it is crucial for practitioners to address spirituality within the realm of rest.

A balance between rest and performance areas allows individuals to maintain energy and power to continue with leisure pursuits, work, and play, as well as other activities of daily living. The amount of rest an individual has incorporated into the daily routine will affect that individual's ability to perform daily activities. As an occupational therapy practitioner, it is important to educate clients about incorporating rest into one's routine and establishing a balance between activities and time for rest. In addition, more important than educating individuals about balanced routines and how to include rest, practitioners must demonstrate this practice by allowing clients ample time for rest during therapy. Whether the client needs mental, physical, or spiritual rest, the practitioner should organize therapy in a way that this performance area is included. In addition, when helping a client establish a balance between activities and a time for rest, practitioners must also take into consideration that a balance between performance areas and other activities of daily living is individualized; a balanced routine to one client may not be a balanced routine to another.

## Sleep

Sleep is a sequence of activities resulting in going to sleep, staying asleep, and maintaining health through participating in sleep (AOTA, 2014). Like "rest," sleep was also one of the four major performance areas determined by Meyer (1922). In the English language, rest and sleep are often used interchangeably. Even though it is a common misconception that rest and sleep hold the same meaning, studies show that being asleep and resting are not the same. Resting takes place when one is awake and engages in a calm, relaxing activity. Sleep is a state of unconsciousness with special restorative functions (Nurit & Michal, 2003).

A typical adult falls asleep within 10 minutes and goes through a series of four sleep stages. The stages consist of three non-rapid eye movement stages (NREM) and one rapid eye movement (REM) stage. A typical adult will go through the series of sleep stages three to five times during a night. On average, the sleep cycle repeats every 90 minutes, with REM sleep occupying the majority, of the cycle, about 80% (Tobaldini et al., 2013; Valenza, Rodenstein, & Ferández-de-las-Peñas, 2011). When sleep is recorded via brain waves, eye movements, and muscle movements, the five sleep stages can be identified. During stage one, the eyelids may begin to close and eyes may move laterally, known as slow eye movements, and the pupils become smaller. People describe this stage as being half-awake and half-asleep. When an individual progresses to stage two, short bursts of bilateral parietal area waves, also known as *sleep spindles*, appear. Individuals occasionally exhibit small, jerky muscle movements and one's heart rate and respiratory rate begin to slow. During stage three, which is considered the deeper stage of sleep, there is an increase in high-amplitude delta waves. Muscle tone begins to decrease with the exception of the diaphragm (Izac, 2006; Tobaldini et al., 2013; Valenza et al., 2011; Wilson, 2008). Restorative functions within the body take place during this deep sleep. If woken during the third sleep stage, individuals feel tired for a while after being woken. The last stage is REM sleep, which includes decreased muscle tone, inhibition of postural muscles, twitching seen with distal flexor muscles, and REMs (Izac, 2006). This is the stage during which most dreams occur (Wilson, 2008).

There is no specific number of hours of sleep a person needs per night. The amount of sleep an individual needs for optimal functioning varies from person to person. Even though there is no magic number, sleep duration can be specified to different populations, such as infants, adolescents, and adults, but even within these groups, sleep needs are still individual. According to the National Sleep Foundation (2016b), general recommended sleep durations are:

- Newborns (0 to 3 months): 14 to 17 hours
- Infants (4 to 11 months): 12 to 15 hours
- Toddlers (1 to 2 years): 11 to 14 hours
- Preschoolers (3 to 5 years): 10 to 13 hours
- School-aged children (6 to 13 years): 9 to 11 hours
- Teenagers (14 to 17 years): 8 to 10 hours
- Young adults (18 to 25 years): 7 to 9 hours
- Adults (26 to 64 years): 7 to 9 hours
- Older adults (over 65 years): 7 to 8 hours

Sleep is a homeostatic process. An individual's need to sleep and the amount of sleep required depends on the time elapsed since the last time that individual slept and how many hours of sleep was achieved during that time. While individuals are awake, sleep debt accumulates. The longer an individual stays awake, the more sleep debt he or she accrues. If an individual has a large amount of sleep debt, the body will add extra hours onto future sleep periods or it will engage in short sleep bursts, known as *microsleeps* (for 3 to 30 minutes) until the sleep debt has been restored (Luyster, Strollo, Zee, & Walsh, 2012).

Another process involved in controlling an individual's need to sleep is the circadian process. The circadian process is controlled within the suprachiasmatic nucleus in the hypothalamus and repeats about once every 24 hours. The suprachiasmatic nucleus is responsible for hormone release, regulating body temperature, melatonin, and the sleep–wake cycle. There are three components to the circadian process. The first component is the pathways that correspond with environmental cues, such as the light–dark cycle, that indicate the need for our bodies to sleep. The second component is a circadian pacemaker that is responsible for specific rhythms that cycle through a 24-hour period. The circadian pacemaker helps our body know when sleep is needed when environmental cues, such as the light–dark cycle, are absent. Lastly, the third component is the output pathways controlled by the circadian pacemaker (Luyster et al., 2012).

Sleep is programmed into the human brain for a good reason—it is essential for survival and our bodies require adequate sleep to properly function. Even though no human studies have been conducted, research suggests that sleep deprivation along with longer sleep durations may be associated with cardiovascular disease, diabetes mellitus, and obesity. According to an International Bedroom Poll conducted by the National Sleep Foundation in 2013, 56% of Americans reported "less sleep than needed on workdays" with an average sleep time of 6 hours and 31 minutes. On the contrary, only 44% of Americans reported a "good night's sleep almost every night." It is suggested that adults require 7 to 9 hours of sleep per night (National Sleep Foundation, 2016b). Given this information, more than half of Americans may not be receiving the optimal number of hours of sleep and/or receiving good quality sleep. Optimal sleep has been achieved when an individual wakes feeling rested and energized. Multiple factors contribute to maintaining a consistent and optimal sleep duration as well as good sleep quality on a nightly basis. To engage in healthy sleep routines and habits, there are two components to sleep that must be incorporated. These components are sleep preparation and sleep participation.

## Sleep Preparation

The *Framework* (AOTA, 2014) describes sleep preparation as engaging in routines that prepare the client for a comfortable rest. These routines may include tasks such as grooming, dressing/undressing, calming activities (reading, listening to music, etc.) to help the client fall asleep, spiritual or religious routines, establishing sleep patterns that support growth and health, and preparing the physical environment. Tasks of sleep preparation are often associated with a client's nighttime or sleep routine.

### Nighttime/Sleep Routines

Routines are patterns of behavior that are observable, regular, repetitive, and that provide structure for daily life. Healthy routines play an important role in client's sleep participation because they assist in preparing the client for nighttime and letting the body know that it is time to go to sleep. Each client's routine is different from another and may include many aspects such as engaging in calming activities (reading, yoga, knitting, listening to music), hygiene (brushing teeth, bathing, changing clothes), meditation, prayer, or going to bed at a consistent time (AOTA, 2014). There are also tasks that would be considered unhealthy to include in a client's routine including drinking caffeine or alcohol, which will cause one's body to wake up once metabolized, eating too much or too little, watching television, or viewing information on a computer or cellular phone (Vinson et al., 2010).

Practicing healthy sleep routines reduces sleep loss while improving clients' physical and emotional health (Morin et al., 1999). Therefore, it is important that the clients feel comfortable in their environment where they can practice familiar routines, have the materials needed to complete tasks of routines, and the means to complete routines at a reasonable time and pace set by themselves. As occupational therapy practitioners, it is our domain to assess our clients' nighttime routines and determine factors that may be hindering their sleep. Once the client has been assessed, intervention includes assisting clients to identify healthy patterns/routines for bedtime, recommending strategies or adaptive equipment if needed to improve the quantity/quality of their sleep, and possible referral to specialists or testing if indicated.

### Sleep Participation and Sleep Hygiene

Sleep participation involves taking care of a personal need for sleep, which includes cessation of activities to ensure onset of sleep, napping, sustaining a sleep state without disruption, nighttime care of toileting needs, hydration, etc. (AOTA, 2014). Disruption in a client's sleep routine will have an effect on the client's sleep adequacy and the feeling of being rested and refreshed after a night of sleep. This can be disrupted in three different ways. One is sleep latency, the duration of time between going to bed and falling asleep; another is sleep efficiency, or the ratio of total sleep time to time spent in bed; and last is the client's duration of sleep, which is the total number of minutes spent sleeping (Morin & Espie, 2003). For adequate sleep, a client should fall asleep within 15 minutes of lying down and stay asleep for at least 85% of the time in bed (Sateia, Doghramji, Hauri, & Morin, 2000). Sleep hygiene involves the aspects of both sleep preparation and sleep participation to create quality and quantity within nighttime sleep. Involving poor hygiene in one's nighttime routine may be the cause of sleeplessness, interrupted sleep, or the onset of sleep disorders.

Healthy sleep hygiene practices may include:

- Avoid napping during the day; it can disturb the normal pattern of sleep and wakefulness.
- Avoid stimulants such as caffeine, nicotine, and alcohol too close to bedtime; although alcohol is well known to speed the onset of sleep, it disrupts sleep in the second half as the body begins to metabolize the alcohol, causing arousal.
- Exercise can promote good sleep. Vigorous exercise should be performed in the morning or late afternoon. A relaxing exercise, like yoga, can be done before bed to help initiate a restful night's sleep.
- Food can be disruptive right before sleep; stay away from large meals close to bedtime. Dietary changes can also cause sleep problems; if someone is struggling with a sleep problem, it is not a good time to start experimenting with spicy dishes. And, remember, chocolate has caffeine.
- Ensure adequate exposure to natural light. This is particularly important for older people who may not venture outside as frequently as children and adults. Light exposure helps maintain a healthy sleep–wake cycle.
- Establish a regular relaxing bedtime routine. Try to avoid emotionally upsetting conversations and activities before trying to go to sleep. Do not dwell on or bring your problems to bed.
- Associate your bed with sleep. It is not a good idea to use your bed to watch TV, listen to the radio, or read.
- Make sure the sleep environment is pleasant and relaxing. The mattress and pillows should be comfortable, and the bedroom should be cool (between 60°F and 67°F) and free from noise and light (National Sleep Foundation, 2016a).

## Sleep Disorders

There are many reasons why clients' sleep may be disrupted across the lifespan. More often than not, sleeping difficulties are the result of other underlying medical conditions or the side effects of medications. This is one of the reasons why sleep disorders tend to be more common in older adults. With age also comes an increase in medical conditions or problems that may affect sleep on their own and an increase in the use of medication that may have effects on sleep (Westley, 2004). According to the American Psychiatric Association's (APA) *Diagnostic and Statistical Manual of Mental Disorders* (2000), sleep disorders fall into one of many different categories.

Insomnia affects many people, more so in the older population. It is the inability or great difficulty falling asleep, maintaining sleep (APA, 2000; Rajki, 2011), or not feeling refreshed upon waking (Subramanian & Surani, 2007). The degree to which insomnia affects someone falls into three categories: transient, acute, and chronic. Transient insomnia occurs no more than a few nights a week. Acute insomnia is less than 3 or 4 weeks of sleeping difficulty, and chronic insomnia is when the sleeping difficulty lasts beyond 1 month (Rajki, 2011). Insomnia may also be characterized based on its causes. For instance, when insomnia cannot be linked to a health condition, it is considered *primary insomnia*; when it can be attributed to a particular health problem, it is known as *secondary insomnia* (Subramanian & Surani, 2007).

## Case Study

Jane is a 21-year-old woman who is finishing her last semester in college. Jane is constantly busy with school, writing final papers and studying for exams. On top of completing her schoolwork, Jane plays intramural soccer and is the president of the Sustainability Club. Her involvement in both of these programs, along with attending classes, forces Jane to stay up late at night to complete her schoolwork. Jane reports after she finishes studying or writing papers at 1:00 a.m., she does not feel tired right away and needs to watch television or use her computer for about an hour before she can fall asleep. Jane also reports drinking coffee and taking naps throughout the day. On the weekends, Jane likes to go out with friends and drink socially. Jane reports that drinking usually helps her to fall asleep immediately when she returns home. Jane reports feeling constantly tired and run down.

**Consider the following questions:**

1. What would be the first step in evaluating Jane?
2. Is there a specific assessment you would choose to evaluate Jane?
3. What questions are important to ask during the evaluation?
4. What sleep habits may be interfering with Jane's quality of sleep?
5. Based on the information provided during the evaluation, develop an intervention plan for Jane.

The opposite of insomnia, hypersomnia, is characterized by excessive sleep, usually occurring during the day or at times when sleeping might not be considered appropriate (Westley, 2004). Hypersomnia may cause "clinically significant distress" in functioning for patients within social, occupational, and/or other important areas of daily living (APA, 2000).

Narcolepsy is much less common but can also cause significant distress within patients' lives. It presents as excessive sleepiness accompanying frequent daytime attacks of sleep. There is usually a bilateral loss of muscle tone during these sudden sleep attacks, known as cataplexy, and can be connected with feelings of intense emotion (APA, 2000). The difficulty of performing everyday tasks is not hard to imagine when one must be aware of the risk of falling asleep at any given moment.

Sleep may also be affected by breathing-related sleep disorders, such as obstructive sleep apnea, caused by a hindrance in the airway, or central sleep apnea in which the brain does not send signals to the diaphragm or other muscles of the respiratory system (Rajki, 2011; Westley, 2004). In both cases, clients often complain of increased sleepiness during the day with headaches occurring in the morning and a decrease in functioning during daytime activities. During the night when the client is sleeping, breathing will periodically cease for periods of 10 seconds or greater. The breathing cessation causes the person to wake because the brain recognizes the decrease in oxygen. These episodes of ceased breathing may even occur up to or more than 20 times within one night (Rajki, 2011; Vitiello, 2000; Westley, 2004). Snoring is also a characteristic of obstructive sleep apnea, often more noticed by bed partners than the actual patients themselves (Rajki, 2011). Sleep apnea is more common in men and also more common with older populations (Vitiello, 2000).

Circadian rhythm sleep disorders affect many people regardless of age; these disorders disrupt one's usual sleep–wake cycle. These disruptions in the usual circadian sleep–wake pattern cause excessive sleepiness and sometimes insomnia, both of which have a profound effect on a patient's ability to perform everyday tasks effectively. There are four types: jet lag, shift work, unspecific, and delayed sleep phase, in which one may go to bed late or get up late with an inability to fall asleep or get up at a preferred earlier time (APA, 2000).

Restless leg syndrome presents as discomfort and the desire to move, more commonly the legs, but sometimes also the arms, while falling asleep or waking during the night. The uncomfortable feeling is described as a creeping, crawling, tingling, burning, or itching feeling. Movements of the legs relieve the uncomfortable sensations, but delay falling asleep and often wake the person during the night, both of which lead to daytime sleepiness. This sleep disorder is more common in women and older adults, affecting 10% to 30% of those older than 65 years of age (APA, 2000; Rajki, 2011).

Often occurring hand-in-hand with restless leg syndrome, but more common on its own, is periodic limb movements. These are repetitive, twitching leg jerks that occur every 20 to 60 seconds during sleep onset, decreasing as one falls into a deeper sleep. The limb movements cause affected individuals to wake frequently, but they may not be aware of what actually woke them; bed partners are commonly the ones to provide such information. These frequent awakenings cause increased daytime sleepiness, thus also have a profound effect on the performance of everyday occupations (APA, 2000; Rajki, 2011).

Sleep can also be affected by dreams. Nightmare disorder is characterized by one waking from a deep sleep caused by extremely frightening dreams that commonly involve death or other threats to survival or one's security. Upon waking, one is able to orient oneself to reality, contrary to sleep terror disorder. Sleep terror disorder is related in that it also involves the sleeper waking from a frightening dream. The abrupt waking of the person is usually accompanied by a panicky scream, tachycardia, rapid breathing, and sweating. Although incapable of recalling the dream, the affected individual is unable to be consoled by others and often wakes disoriented and confused (APA, 2000).

During REM sleep, usually there is a cease of transmission with muscle activity. REM behavior disorder is just the opposite, in which nerve conduction is not inhibited. Persons may violently thrash around during sleep, acting out a dream they are having and potentially causing injury or harm to either themselves or their bed partner (APA, 2000; Rajki, 2011). These episodes are more common in males and usually occur later into the sleep cycle, as opposed to sleepwalking disorder, which tends to occur during the beginning third of a sleep cycle. During sleepwalking disorder, individuals may get out of bed and walk around. Their expression is blank and they are unresponsive to others who may attempt to communicate with them. While sleepwalking, arousal is very difficult, and if the person does wake, there is usually no recollection of the episode (APA, 2000).

As mentioned previously, sleep disorders are more commonly caused by an underlying medical condition or can be attributed to a side effect of certain medications. Diagnoses that have an increased chance of affecting sleep are the following (Misra & Malow, 2008):

- Arthritis causes sleep interruption secondary to pain and an increased chance of having restless leg syndrome.
- Gastroesophageal reflux disease has a two-way relationship with sleep because lying down increases the chance of reflux and reflux often results in the person wakening.
- Congestive heart failure has been linked with the inability to maintain sleep, resulting in daytime sleepiness.
- Patients with diabetes mellitus have an increased chance of comorbidities with restless leg syndrome, periodic limb movement disorder, or obstructive sleep apnea.
- Patients with dementia struggle with the ability to regulate sleep and sleep patterns; this is known as *sundowning*. The severity of a client's dementia parallels the severity of sleep disturbance. These changes in sleep often do not cause distress to the client, but instead more so to the caregiver because the client's sleep rhythm does not match up with routine daily activities (Westley, 2004).
- Chronic pain can be a factor in difficulty falling asleep, frequent awakenings during the night, and not having restful sleep. In addition, sleep deprivation can decrease pain tolerance and thus exacerbate pain symptoms (Gooneratne et al., 2011).
- Depression and anxiety often cause an increase in the number of times a person wakes during the night, how early a person may rise, and difficulty falling asleep caused by racing thoughts or too much on one's mind (Rajki, 2011).

Side effects of medications vary greatly; it is not uncommon for medications to disrupt the ability to maintain, begin, or have restful sleep. Specific medications affecting sleep include the following (Misra & Malow, 2008; Rajki, 2011; Subramanian & Surani, 2007):

- Beta blockers disrupt sleep by causing vivid dreams or nightmares, general increased waking during the night, or insomnia.
- Decongestants may contain a specific ingredient that heavily contributes to insomnia, known as *nonselective alpha-adrenoceptor agonists*.
- Antihypertensive drugs can have stimulating effects on clients, disrupting the ability to fall asleep.
- Corticosteroids also contain simulating ingredients affecting one's ability to fall asleep.
- Bronchodilators' stimulating ingredients inhibit the ability to fall asleep.
- Antidepressants, like many other medications, contain ingredients that stimulate a client physically and mentally, making it difficult to fall asleep. These may also exacerbate periodic limb movements or restless leg syndrome.
- Diuretics increase urine output; clients may wake to void more often during the night.
- Beta agonist inhalants and selective serotonin reuptake inhibitors both have been found to affect sleep efficiency, delay the onset of sleep, and increase the amount of times a client wakes during the night.
- Nicotine and alcohol use have been found to decrease a client's sleep continuity throughout the night.

## Evaluation and Assessment

Evaluation and assessment of clients are a crucial part of the occupational therapy process. Often these words are used interchangeably, but they are two different, though related, terms. The evaluation of a client can be thought of as a whole process, whereas the assessment of a client is a piece of the evaluation process (Moyers, 1999).

This process can be thought of as a "top-down" approach (Coster, 1998), in which evaluation begins by focusing on what the client needs and wants to be able to do, as well as what the client can currently do or has done in the past. Lastly, the evaluation identifies the barriers hindering not only the client's performance with occupations but also the client's health in general (AOTA, 2014; Fisher & Short-DeGraff, 1993). This top-down approach supports a more client-centered evaluation versus a disability-centered evaluation. This results in better communication between the practitioner and the client about occupational therapy and ensures that the evaluation process is supporting an occupation-centered intervention (Fisher & Short-DeGraff, 1993). The evaluation process should contain four specific items (Smith, 2006):

1. Personal client information such as name, date of birth, gender, diagnoses, and precautions.
2. Referral information that includes the services requested, by whom they were requested, the client's source of funding, and the length of time that the therapist believes services will be provided.
3. An occupational profile should be obtained and include information about a client's daily activities, values, beliefs, needs, interests, and history. Most important, it should also collect information on the contexts that are causing the most problems and the patient's goals for therapy.
4. Lastly, during the evaluation, assessments should be performed. Assessments are the tools that therapists use to gather information that contribute to the evaluation process. These could be standardized or nonstandardized tests, checklists, or even interviews and skilled observations by the therapist.

## Rest

When performing an occupational profile with a client, it is always important to ask about quiet leisure activities the client performs and considers "restful." In addition, educate the client about the difference between "rest" and "sleep" to gain accurate information in regard to a person's "rest" routines and habits. Asking specific questions surrounding the occupation of rest can give you a good idea about whether clients are providing themselves an adequate amount or too much rest. Examples of these kinds of questions follow:

- Can you describe a typical weekday/weekend day?
- Do you feel like you get enough rest? If not, what do you think stands in the way of you getting enough rest (work, school, family, or illness)?
- What restful activities do you enjoy?
- What helps you relax?
- Do have any difficulty doing the things that help you rest and relax? If so, what do you have difficulty with?

Rest is most commonly evaluated through the use of interviews with a client. However, there are some assessments that specifically ask about rest and relaxation. For instance, the Canadian Occupational Performance Measure (Law et al., 1991) looks at clients' satisfaction with their performance in categories of everyday activities. One of the categories that should be asked about is "quiet recreation," which may include knitting, reading, listening to the radio, and arts and crafts. This category not only provides a practitioner with ideas of what clients enjoy but also gives a clinical picture of how satisfied they are or difficulties they may be having. An Interest Checklist (Katz, 1988; Matsutsuyu, 1969) could also be helpful. This assessment allows a client to individually, or together with a practitioner, check off activities that the client has done in the past year, in the past 10 years, is currently participating in, or would like to pursue in the future. This provides the practitioner with information regarding whether the client has healthy rest/relaxation activities and which ones the client may be experiencing difficulty with. These are only a few examples of assessments available to occupational therapy practitioners.

## Sleep

Typically, sleep is not the reason that clients seek out or are referred to occupational therapy services. Commonly, clients are referred for another reason that may be affecting their sleep or difficulty with sleep is something that is discovered during the evaluation process. During evaluation, it is important to ask about sleep because approximately half of people who experience sleep difficulties do not talk with a health care provider about their sleep complaints (Gooneratne et al., 2011). If a practitioner thinks there may be some underlying issues surrounding sleep, the evaluation may be tailored to provide more focus on these issues. If a spouse or bed partner is available, that individual may also provide key information about the client's sleeping habits because clients are often unaware of what they do when they are sleeping (Rajki, 2011). Some important questions to ask during an evaluation about sleep may include the following (Misra & Malow, 2008; Vitiello, 2000; Westley, 2004):

- What is your normal bedtime routine?
- Do you have difficulties falling or staying asleep? If so:
  - ◊ How long have you been having trouble sleeping?
  - ◊ How long would you say it takes you to fall asleep?
  - ◊ How many times per night do you wake up and for how long?
  - ◊ How does it affect your performance during the day?
  - ◊ Do you feel that you are excessively drowsy during the day?
  - ◊ Do you take naps during the day? If so, for how long and how many naps per day?
  - ◊ What time do you fall asleep at night and get up in the morning? On average, how many hours of sleep do you get per night?
  - ◊ Do you use prescription drugs, over the counter drugs, or alcohol to help you fall asleep?
  - ◊ How much caffeine or alcohol do you consume per day?
  - ◊ Do you exercise? If so, how much do you get per day?

- Also, ask questions about snoring, cessation of breathing, or leg movements and narcoleptic symptoms.

Assessments for the disruption of sleep mainly focus on validating data the practitioner gathered in the extended occupational profile. One of the ways a practitioner can do this is by asking the client to keep a sleep log or sleep diary. The journals are usually kept for a period of 2 weeks to a month or more so that practitioners can identify patterns, discrepancies from what bed partners report, and potential reasons why a client may be experiencing sleeping difficulties (Davidson, Waisberg, Brundage, & Maclean, 2001). Occupational therapy practitioners ask patients to pay special attention to and record information regarding the following (Davidson et al., 2001; Vitiello, Rybarczyk, Von Korff, & Stepanski, 2009):

- How much time clients spent in their bed when they were not sleeping
- If the client took a nap; if so, for how long?
- If the client performed any physical activity that day; if so, for how long and at what time?
- If the client consumed any coffee or alcohol that day; if so, how much and at what time?
- If the client took any medications to aid in falling asleep
- What time the client went to bed and woke up
- The perceived quality of the sleep or how restful the client felt
- If the client woke up during the night; if so, why and for how long? If waking during the night, what did the client do?

The profession of occupational therapy has not adopted or created an assessment that may be used for sleep specifically. However, there are a few sleep assessments created by other professionals within the health care field that occupational therapy practitioners have the clinical knowledge to administer. There are four well-known self-assessments that occupational therapists can either have the patient fill out individually or can fill out with the patient collaboratively.

The Pittsburgh Sleep Quality Index (Buysse, Reynolds, Monk, Berman, & Kupfer, 1989) could be very easily administered by an occupational therapy practitioner, but it is important to know that this assessment requires permission by the creator to be used. It is a 19-item questionnaire that assesses a month-long period of sleep. The assessment has three main focus areas: the client's sleep habits, the effects of the client's sleep disorder, and the potential cause of nighttime sleep disruption (Gooneratne et al., 2011). These focus areas create seven component scores: personal sleep quality, sleep latency, sleep duration, how effective the client's sleep is on a consistent basis, what is causing the sleep disturbance, whether the patient uses sleep medication, and how it affects daytime activities (Misra & Malow, 2008). Scores can range from 0 to 21; anything greater than a score of 5 indicates poor sleep quality (Gooneratne et al., 2011).

There are also more basic assessments that an occupational therapy practitioner would have the clinical knowledge to administer, including the Stanford Sleepiness Scale, the Epworth Sleepiness Scale, and the Sleep Impairment Index. All of these are quick and easy-to-use self-assessments that take a close look at different specific topics (Davidson et al., 2001; Misra & Malow, 2008).

The Stanford Sleepiness Scale is a quick way to test how alert someone is feeling at a given time. The scale ranges from 1 (feeling active, vital, alert, or wide awake) to a 7 (no longer fighting sleep, sleep onset soon, having dream-like thoughts), and after a score of 7, would be sleeping. Assessing a client's degree of alertness throughout the day can give a good idea as to whether the client may not be getting an adequate amount of sleep (Misra & Malow, 2008).

The Epworth Sleepiness Scale assesses the likelihood of a client falling asleep on a 0 (would never doze) to 3 (high chance of dozing) scale during specific given activities. Everyday activities are rated such as sitting and reading, sitting and talking with someone, or being in a car while stopped in traffic. A score of 10 or higher provides reason to check with a health care professional about the possibility of a sleep disorder (Misra & Malow, 2008).

The Sleep Impairment Index asks seven questions that create a score providing information about the severity of a patient's insomnia. Each item is rated on a 5-point scale for a total score between 7 and 35; the higher the score, the more severe the insomnia (Pallesen et al., 2003).

## Student Self-Assessment

1. Name some of your daily activities that are considered "rest."
2. Categorize these activities under the three components of rest: physical rest, mental rest, or spiritual rest.
3. How do these activities help you maintain energy to complete your activities of daily living and instrumental activities of daily living tasks?
4. Are you getting enough quality sleep?
5. What can you do to change your sleep routines, habits, and hygiene?
6. How will improving your sleep duration and/or quality improve your daily functioning?

## Evidence-Based Research Chart

| Topic | Evidence |
|---|---|
| The occupational therapy process | Moyers, 1999 |
| Definition of rest and its components | Christiansen, 1997; Nurit & Michal, 2003 |
| Stages of sleep | Izac, 2006; Valenza, Rodenstein, & Ferández-de-las-Peñas, 2011; Wilson, 2008 |
| Amount of sleep required for specific populations | National Sleep Foundation, 2016b |
| The process of sleep debt and how it affects an individual | Luyster, Strollo, Zee, & Walsh, 2012 |
| Circadian process | Luyster, Strollo, Zee, & Walsh, 2012 |
| Sleep preparation/routines | AOTA, 2014; Morin et al., 1999 |
| Sleep participation/hygiene | Morin & Epsie, 2003; Sateia, Doghramji, Hauri, & Morin, 2000 |
| Sleep disorders | APA, 2000; Rajki, 2011; Subramanian & Surani, 2007; Vitiello, 2000; Westley, 2004 |
| Medical conditions that affect sleep | Gooneratne et al., 2011; Misra & Malow, 2008; Rajki, 2011; Westley, 2004 |
| Medications that affect sleep | Misra & Malow, 2008; Rajki, 2011; Subramanian & Surani, 2007 |

## References


American Occupational Therapy Association. (2014). Occupational therapy practice framework: Domain and process (3rd ed.). *American Journal of Occupational Therapy, 68*(Suppl. 1), S1-S48. doi:10.5014/ajot.2014.682006

American Psychiatric Association. (2000). Sleep disorders. In *Diagnostic and statistical manual of mental disorders* (4th ed.). Washington, DC: Author.

Buysse, D. J., Reynolds, C. F., Monk, T. H., Berman, S. R., & Kupfer, D. J. (1989). The Pittsburgh Sleep Quality Index (PSQI): A new instrument for psychiatric research and practice. *Psychiatry Research, 28*(2), 193-213.

Christiansen, C. (1997). Acknowledging a spiritual dimension in occupational therapy practice. *American Journal of Occupational Therapy, 51*(3), 169-173.

Coster, W. (1998). Occupation-centered assessment of children. *American Journal of Occupational Therapy, 52*(5), 337-344.

Davidson, J. R., Waisberg, J. L., Brundage, M. D., & Maclean, A. W. (2001). Nonpharmacologic group treatment of insomnia: A preliminary study with cancer survivors. *Psycho-Oncology, 10*, 389-397. doi: 10.1002pon.525

Fisher, A. G., & Short-DeGraff, M. (1993). Improving functional assessment in occupational therapy: Recommendations and philosophy for change. *American Journal of Occupational Therapy, 47*(3), 199-201.

Gooneratne, N. S., Tavaria, A., Patel, N., Madhusudan, L., Nadaraja, D., Onen, F., & Richards, K. C. (2011). Perceived effectiveness of diverse sleep treatments in older adults. *Journal of the American Geriatrics Society, 59*(2), 297-303.

Izac, S. M. (2006). Basic anatomy and physiology of sleep. *American Journal of Electroneurodiagnostic Technology, 46*(1), 18-38.

Katz, N. (1988). Interest checklist: A factor analytical study. *Occupational Therapy in Mental Health, 8*(1), 45-55.

Law, M., Baptiste, S., Carswell-Opzoomer, A., McColl, M., Polatajko, H., & Pollock, N. (1991). *Canadian Occupational Performance Measure manual*. Toronto, Ontario, Canada: CAOT Publications.

Llorens, L. (1991). Performance tasks and roles throughout the life span. In C. Christiansen & C. Baum (Eds.), *Occupational therapy: Overcoming human performance deficits* (pp. 45-68). Thorofare, NJ: SLACK Incorporated.

Luyster, F. S., Strollo, P. J., Zee, P. C., & Walsh, J. K. (2012). Sleep: A health imperative. *SLEEP, 35*(6), 727-734.

Matsutsuyu, J. S. (1969). The Interest Checklist. *American Journal of Occupational Therapy, 23*, 323-328.

Meyer, A. (1922). The philosophy of occupational therapy. *Archives of Occupational Therapy, 1*, 1-10.

Misra, S., & Malow, B. A. (2008). Evaluation of sleep disturbances in older adults. *Clinics in Geriatric Medicine, 24*(1), 15-26.

Morin, C., & Espie, C. (2003). *Insomnia: A clinical guide to assessment and treatment*. New York, NY: Kluwer Academic/Plenum Publishers.

Morin, C. M., Hauri, P. J., Espie, C. A., Spielman, A. J., Buysse, D. J., & Bootzin, R. R. (1999). Nonpharmacologic treatment of chronic insomnia. *SLEEP, 22*, 1134-1156.

Mosey, A. C. (1981). *Occupational therapy: Configuration of a profession*. New York, NY: Raven Press.

Moyers, P. A. (1999). The guide to occupational therapy practice. *American Journal of Occupational Therapy, 53*(3), 247-322.

National Sleep Foundation. (2013). *2013 international bedroom poll: Summary of findings*. Retrieved from https://sleepfoundation.org/sites/default/files/RPT195a.pdf

National Sleep Foundation. (2016a). *Healthy sleep tips*. Retrieved from https://sleepfoundation.org/sleep-tools-tips/healthy-sleep-tips

National Sleep Foundation. (2016b). *How much sleep do we really need?* Retrieved from https://sleepfoundation.org/how-sleep-works/how-much-sleep-do-we-really-need

Nurit, W., & Michal, A. (2003). Rest: A qualitative exploration of the phenomenon. *Occupational Therapy International, 10*(4), 227-238.

Pallesen, S., Nordhus, I. H., Kvale, G., Nielsen, G. H., Havik, O. E., Johnsen, B. H., & Skjotskift, S. (2003). Behavioral treatment of insomnia in older adults: An open clinical trial comparing two interventions. *Behaviour Research and Therapy, 41*, 31-48.

Rajki, M. (2011). Sleep problems in older adults. *ADVANCE for Nurse Practitioners and Physician Assistants, 2*(12), 16-22.

Sateia, M. J., Doghramji, K., Hauri, P. J., & Morin, C. M. (2000). Evaluation of chronic insomnia. *American Academy of Sleep Medicine, 23*, 243-308.

Smith, J. (2006). Documentation of occupational therapy services. In H. Pendleton & W. Schultz-Krohn (Eds.), *Pedretti's occupational therapy: Practice skills for physical dysfunction* (6th ed., pp. 110-129). St. Louis, MO: Mosby Elsevier.

Subramanian, S., & Surani, S. (2007). Sleep disorders in the elderly. *Geriatrics, 62*(12), 10-32.

Tobaldini, E., Nobili, L., Strada, S., Casali, K., Braghiroli, A., & Montano, N. (2014). Heart rate variability in normal and pathological sleep. *Frontiers in Physiology, 4*, 294.

Valenza, M. C., Rodenstein, D. O., & Ferández-de-las-Peñas, C. (2011). Consideration of sleep dysfunction in rehabilitation. *Journal of Bodywork and Movement Therapies, 15*, 262-267.

Vinson, D. C., Manning, B. K., Galliber, J. M., Dickinson, L. M., Pace, W. D., & Turner, B. J. (2010). Alcohol and sleep problems in primary care patients: A report from the AAFP National Research Network. *Annals of Family Medicine, 8*(6), 484-492.

Vitiello, M. V. (2000). Effective treatment of sleep disturbances in older adults. *Clinical Cornerstone, 2*(5), 16-24.

Vitiello, M. V., Rybarczyk, B., Von Korff, M., & Stepanski, E. J. (2009). Cognitive behavioral therapy for insomnia improves sleep and decreases pain in older adults with co-morbid insomnia and osteoarthritis. *Journal of Clinical Sleep Medicine, 5*(4), 355-362.

Westley, C. (2004). Sleep: Geriatric self-learning module. *MEDSURG Nursing, 13*(5), 291-295.

Wilson, S. (2008). A good night's sleep, part one: Normal sleep. *Nursing & Residential Care, 10*(11), 543-547.

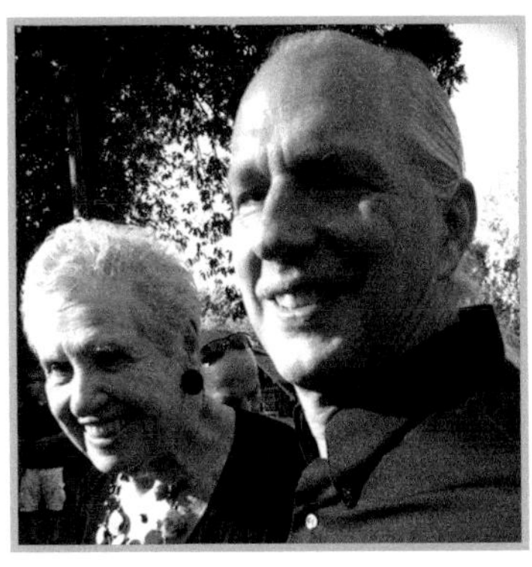

# 22

# Evaluation of Occupational Performance in Social Participation

Danielle J. Cropley, MS, OTR/L and Mary V. Donohue, PhD, OTL, FAOTA

ACOTE STANDARDS EXPLORED IN THIS CHAPTER

B.4.4, B.5.1

KEY VOCABULARY

- **Associative or project participation:** The second most basic level of social participation, in which members of a group briefly work on a task together and incorporate some sharing and competition.
- **Behavioral response:** Ability to express oneself in a social situation using independently generated verbal and nonverbal cues.
- **Cooperative participation (supportive cooperative participation):** Level of engagement in which a group works homogeneously and cooperatively to achieve a task and meet each other's emotional needs while the practitioner or group leader advises rather than participates.
- **Egocentric-cooperative participation (basic cooperative participation):** Engagement in a shared group interest or task with long-term participation aimed at group members meeting the needs of others.
- **Mature participation:** Level of engagement in which group roles and tasks are divided among group members to achieve success, practice flexibility, and develop leaders within the group.
- **Parallel participation:** The most basic level of social participation in which individuals work side by side in a group with little to no interaction.
- **Social cognition:** Ability to analyze, integrate, and plan responses to a continuing social situation.
- **Social participation:** Active engagement in the norms and behaviors of an individual within his or her social system.
- **Social perception:** Ability to receive input from others' social cues.



Jacobs, K., & MacRae, N. (Eds.).
*Occupational Therapy Essentials for Clinical Competence, Third Edition* (pp. 311-323).

The term *social participation* aims to outline the specific norms and behaviors intertwined with other occupations needed for effective engagement with one's family, peers, and community (American Occupational Therapy Association [AOTA], 2014, adapted from Gillen & Boyt Schell, 2014, p. S45). As one of the eight primary areas of occupation, social participation is a fundamental part of a person's occupational identity as it helps to define how a person performs in situations and activities within the social context, as well as the varying levels of dependence one might have with others to fulfill occupational needs (i.e., social interdependence, Magasi & Hammel, 2004). A positive correlation can be drawn between several of the basic tenets of occupational therapy and the principles of interpersonal interactions and relationships needed for useful social participation. Because the AOTA's Accreditation Council for Occupational Therapy Education (ACOTE; 2011) not only identifies two standards on evaluation and intervention for social participation (B.4.4. and B.5.1.), but also requires that occupational therapists "express support for the quality of life, well-being, and occupation of the individual, group, or population to promote physical and mental health and prevention of injury and disease considering the context (e.g., cultural, personal, temporal, virtual and environment)" (B.2.9.), it is essential that occupational therapy practitioners address the complex interrelationship between social participation and well-being.

The *International Classification of Functioning, Disability and Health* (ICF) of the World Health Organization (WHO; 2001) emphasizes the importance of all relationships in its section on activities and participation, as well as the influence occupational therapy can have on improving one's independence in this area. The guidelines provided by the ICF help to outline each level of relationship that is found within an individual's social system from how to relate appropriately to strangers to the complexities of the formal and informal, familial, and intimate relationships one encounters in one's lifetime (WHO, 2001). Each type of relationship and the dynamics found within these relationships can apply to occupational therapy and practitioners' intervention focus on social performance.

Every person's occupational identity is in some way supported and shaped by that person's social system and approach to engaging and interacting with those around them, either in person or through various means of technology and social media. The ACOTE expects occupational therapy practitioners to understand how vital social performance is in relation to occupational balance and one's overall health, wellness, and quality of life. The ACOTE tenets echo the ICF's emphasis on becoming part of an organized social life outside of the family by developing community and civic relationships (WHO, 2001). Appropriate evaluation of social participation is necessary to integrate this area of occupation into therapy successfully, as well as establish therapeutic rapport that meets a client's individual social needs. Therefore, various evaluation processes have been established as a means of preparation for designing interventions for both individual and group interactions.

A social approach, such as the therapeutic use of self, generally provides the most effective means of observing clients' abilities, skills, and behaviors in the area of social participation. These same perceptions developed in observing individuals or groups of clients and in designing interventions prepare the practitioner to consider social aspects of the larger community for an understanding of contextual factors in the management of service delivery. Overall, the evaluation of social participation provides a glimpse into the social supports available to the client before, during, and after therapy, allowing the practitioner to understand each client's strengths and areas for improvement.

## Integration of Social Participation Concepts

Many people perceive the evaluation of social participation as abstract, complex, and subjective in nature. Because the assessment of social cues is not a hard science, this poses a challenge as to how practitioners can accurately evaluate an individual's level of functioning in the social context. Ultimately, practitioners must break down the situational social demands of the environment and context as well as the required actions and performance skills of the client to assess the client's social abilities and desired level of performance (AOTA, 2014).

In occupational therapy, practitioners are most often evaluating clients' functioning during social activity participation, yet this chapter needs to distinguish between the conceptual parts of this term for best understanding. Throughout occupational therapy intervention, activity participation is planned for and incorporated as its basis. In group settings of intervention, the type of participation designed and expected is social activity participation. This distinction is necessary because many mechanical or physical types of intervention may employ activity participation for individuals but not social activity participation (Isaksson, Lexell, & Skär, 2007). Social activity participation is supported by ongoing implementation of social interaction skills (Boyt Schell et al., 2014a, p. S26) consisting of verbal and interpersonal activity interactions. However, further explanation of these general social skills and finer subskills within one-on-one or group interaction is needed. These concepts begin to formulate during young childhood, which is an ideal place to begin exploring the ways in which social participation started being evaluated.

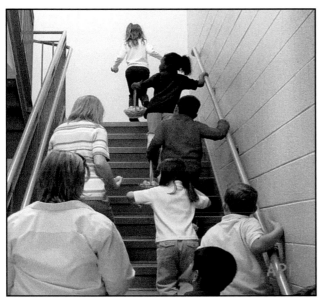

**Figure 22-1.** Parallel level participation. School-aged children transition from one classroom to another, side by side with little to no interaction.

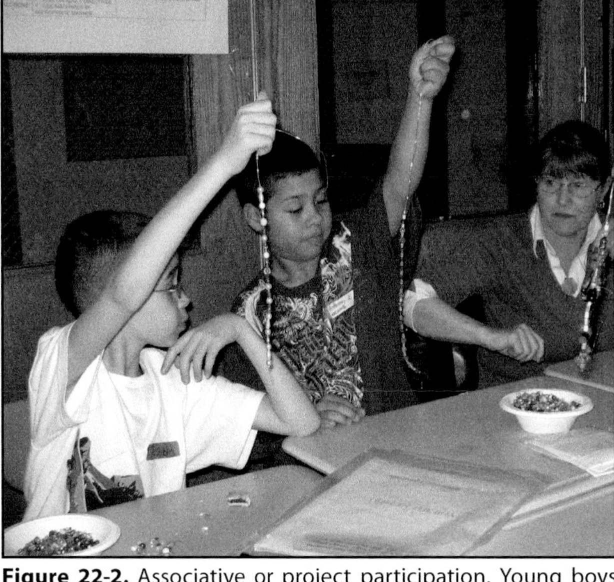

**Figure 22-2.** Associative or project participation. Young boys use crafts as an icebreaker to begin the early stages of interaction.

In her seminal work, Parten (1932) designed a study to evaluate activity group participation of preschool children using the concepts of parallel, associative, and cooperative play. Parten's theoretical base was developmental across children's ages, with the expectation that children would function at higher levels of participation as they advanced in age. She observed 30 children—six children in each of five preschool ages. Collecting 360 data points, Parten reported an association between ages and the three developmental group concept levels. Parten first defined the three levels of social participation as follows:

1. **Parallel participation:** Playing, activities, or working side by side with little to no interaction or sharing. Observable examples include children playing in a sandbox without talking, and older adults doing movement to music at an adult day care program (Figure 22-1).
2. **Associative participation:** Approaching others briefly in verbal or nonverbal interactions as needed. Observable examples include children's games such as Simon Says and Musical Chairs with brief interactions, and young adults using a name game, such as a parachute, to learn each other's names during high school or college orientation (Figure 22-2).
3. **Basic cooperative participation:** Selecting longer activities or tasks for building on mutual self-interest. Observable examples include children dressing up in costumes to role-play and adults choosing to play charades with two teams of people competing against one another.

Parten's concepts have been used most commonly when evaluating the social participation of children; many child psychologists have evaluated children's groups using these concepts. More recently, Parten's schema, or construct of group participation, has been used to evaluate outdoor play, symbolic play, block play, cooperative play, day care centers, and free play programs (Aureli & Colecchia, 1996; Fantuzzo et al., 1996; Field, 1984; Garnier & Latour, 1994; Guralnick, 1990; Howes, 1988; Petrakos & Howe, 1996; Saracho, 1993). All but one study confirmed the association of the children's ages with their level of participation delineated by Parten's three concepts.

Mosey's developmental frame of reference (1968, 1986) took Parten's work a step further by incorporating the original concepts of social participation and added levels of performance for adolescents and adults. Mosey separated Parten's cooperative level into two parts—an egocentric-cooperative level and a cooperative level—and added a mature level. Mosey also included the typical age range when each social skill should emerge as a means of gauging an individual's social abilities in relation to those developing normally. Mosey's modified social participation concepts are as follows, with the parallel group remaining the most basic level (emerging at age 18 months to 2 years):

- **Project participation (similar to Parten's associative participation; emerging at age 2 to 4 years):** Interacting on a task-based level, in which members work individually with some sharing, cooperation, and competition. Observable examples include children in an arts and crafts group and young adults in a cooking class with everyone preparing the same recipe as independently as possible.

**Figure 22-3.** Egocentric-cooperative participation. Group members coordinate a longer, structured task of picnic preparation and eating together.

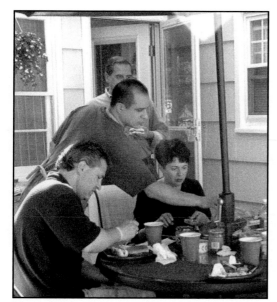

**Figure 22-4.** Cooperative participation. Young boys express emotion in role-playing scenarios in class.

- **Egocentric-cooperative participation (emerging at age 4 to 7 years; presently referred to as *basic cooperative participation*):** Selecting and engaging in a shared interest together on a long-term task that yields group members meeting each other's needs. Observable examples include children in a reading circle and young adults working together on a community art mural (Figure 22-3).
- **Cooperative participation (emerging at age 9 to 12 years; presently referred to as *supportive cooperative participation*):** Fulfilling mutual needs of homogenous and compatible group; the leader or practitioner acts as an advisor rather than a member. Observable examples include adolescents working on leadership or trust exercises and adults in a support group for dealing with grief and loss (Figure 22-4).
- **Mature participation (emerging at age 15 to 18 years):** Varying roles and tasks taken on by members who share leadership and act flexibly when completing tasks and meeting member needs. Observable examples include young adults planning and organizing a group outing and older adults leading their own exercise class (Figure 22-5).

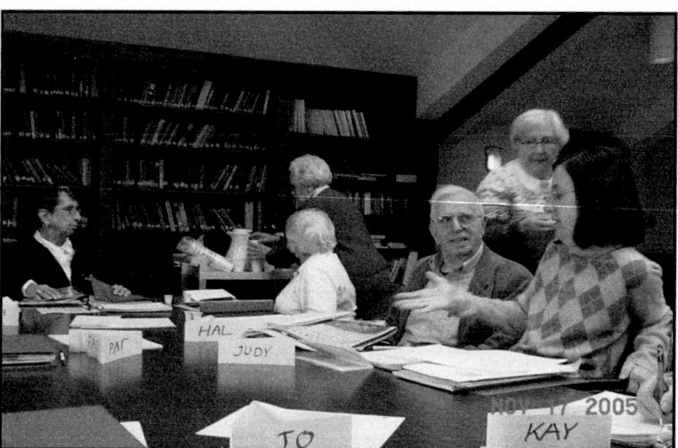

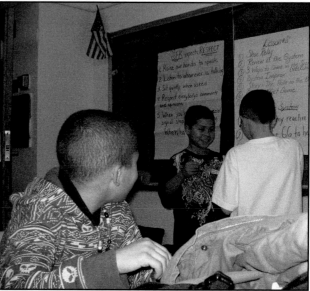


**Figure 22-5.** Mature participation. Members take turns leading a book club, making sure that the task is as important as the group interaction and emotions.

While Mosey's interaction skills appeared to have clinical face validity, they were not tested empirically until recently. However, the concepts of Mosey's five levels of social interactive skills have appealed to many occupational therapy practitioners who continue to publish them in recent textbooks (Cole, 2012; Moyer & O'Brien, 2013; Stoffel & Tomlinson, 2011) and use them in activity group process therapy. The concepts behind these five levels have helped organize the perceptual observations and interventions of occupational therapy practitioners working on social participation in mental health, pediatric, rehabilitation medicine, and geriatric settings.

In conjunction with Parten and Mosey's developmental models, the social skills model provides a basis for understanding the social functions and dysfunctions that practitioners may encounter (Tenhula & Bellack, 2008). Often used with patients diagnosed with schizophrenia, this model breaks down the idea of social competence into three client factors: social perception, social cognition, and behavioral response. Social perception, or one's receiving skills, enable the individual to read both verbal and nonverbal social cues. Building on this, social cognition, or one's processing skills, involves the analysis of the perceived cues, the integration of current and past interactions with an individual, and the planning of an appropriate response to continue participation in a social event. Finally, the behavioral response, or one's expressive skills, allows an individual to provide the social partner with adequate verbal and nonverbal feedback to the previous statement. Ideally, a seamless integration of these three skills is required for functional social participation; failure to achieve one or more of these skills suggests that a social dysfunction is present (Tenhula & Bellack, 2008). To evaluate social participation effectively, identifying the level of some or all of these skills will provide the best understanding of the client's abilities in varying social situations.

## Understanding Observation and Context

Some people are "naturals" at keen observation of others' social participation in terms of verbal and nonverbal cues. Many have acquired expertise through experience working with individuals and groups of people in formal and informal settings. However, others may need guidance or structure to learn what to discern as functional and dysfunctional social skills. For some occupational therapy practitioners, one or more assessment tools can provide the structure needed to guide therapy sessions and develop the necessary observation skills. In whichever of these categories practitioners find themselves, professional development demands that the prospective observer review the available guidelines, manual, or training opportunities before beginning to use a tool.

Some of the methods employed to prepare students and therapists to use the various tools available are training workshops, in-service presentations, seminars, individual coaching, videos, worksheets, and discussion. Of these methods, discussion with others who are knowledgeable about the tool and familiar with the developmental model of social participation has been shown to be most helpful (Smith, 1986). If an observer is at the beginning of the process of developing observation skills, the use of a general observation worksheet during 30 minutes in groups is recommended. Factors such as cooperation, goals, roles, activity involvement, power, attraction, norms, and interaction are valuable to begin with as a focus of interpersonal aspects of function (Borg & Bruce, 1991; Cole, 2005; Howe & Schwartzberg, 2001; Johnson & Johnson, 2000; Posthuma, 2002). Establishing familiarity with these general components of activity group process before undertaking observations with a specific tool for measuring social participation adds to the validity and reliability of the results.

While assessment in the field of occupational therapy is the prerogative of the registered occupational therapist, certified occupational therapy assistants may report and discuss behavioral observations from groups with their occupational therapist supervisor. Therefore, working to establish these skills in all practitioners is just as important as properly administering a social assessment. Table 3 in the *Occupational Therapy Practice Framework* (AOTA, 2014) breaks down the specific social interaction skills that can be observed between two or more individuals in any basic or complex social situation, and these must be reviewed to assist with best practice in social participation evaluation.

Observation within the proper setting and context will also add to the overall quality of the evaluation of one's social participation, as access to and using one's natural environments and contexts during the entire occupational therapy process whenever possible is imperative to best practice. As compared to a clinical setting, observing a client perform socially in environments in which he or she would typically participate will provide a more accurate and thorough understanding of the individual's skills. Depending on the client, an evaluation should combine the right assessment tool with the conditions closest to the natural context to properly assess successful intervention planning that will strengthen and develop the client's current social abilities.

## Social Skill Tools

As identified previously, several tools for assessing occupational performance in social participation and social skills functioning are available for use by occupational therapy practitioners. Each tool addresses various issues related to social interaction and can be used in a variety of settings. Two types of assessments are presented in this chapter: those that were made specifically for occupational therapy practitioners and those found from other fields that are also applicable in occupational therapy (see the Evidence-Based Research Chart). In general, many of these assessments have been found to be particularly useful when working within the mental health population, especially for those living with schizophrenia.

### *Occupational Therapy Assessments for Evaluating Social Participation Performance Patterns and Skills*

Several of the occupational therapy tools that partially or fully address social issues are reviewed here. They are further broken down into those tools that establish performance patterns in the form of an occupational profile and those that look at specific skill sets needed for social participation. The first set of assessments that incorporate the structure of an occupational profile include the Model of Human Occupation Screening Tool (MOHOST), the Occupational Circumstances Assessment Interview and Rating Scale (OCAIRS), and the Role Checklist.

Following these tools is a second section looking at the various skills needed in the context in which a client is required to participate socially. These include the Assessment and Communication of Interaction Skills (ACIS), the Bay Area Functional Performance Evaluation (BaFPE), the Comprehensive Occupational Therapy Evaluation (COTE), the Evaluation of Social Interaction (ESI), the Social Profile, the Role Activity Performance Scale (RAPS), and a Conceptual Framework for Work-Related Social Skills (WSS).

## Tools for Establishing an Occupational Profile

Both the MOHOST (Kielhofner et al., 2009) and the OCAIRS (Forsyth et al., 2005) were developed as tools for gathering an occupational profile under the Model of Human Occupation. The MOHOST includes a section on communication and interaction skills that assesses behavioral categories of nonverbal cues, conversation, vocal expression, and relationships (Kielhofner et al., 2009). In conjunction with this primary section on social functioning, the MOHOST also looks to identify motivation for occupation, patterns of occupation, process skills, and environment—all of which are influenced by social participation. The OCAIRS also looks at one's specific set of communication and interaction skills, as well as the social environment of the client (Forsyth et al., 2005). Furthermore, this tool assesses a variety of areas affected by social functioning, especially with regard to interpreting past experiences and defining long- and short-term goals. Both of these tools have been widely used to structure occupational interviews such that intervention planning and treatment is based on a well-rounded assessment of an individual's strengths and areas of improvement.

The Role Checklist is an additional tool that can be used during an occupational profile, but not as the only basis for evaluation. This tool was developed to be used by an individual independently or with an occupational therapy practitioner to identify major roles in the individual's life (Oakley, Kielhofner, Barris, & Reichler, 1986). Broken down into three parts, the Role Checklist identifies social roles that have been or will be performed in the past, present, and future, as well as the value of each of these roles. This tool is meant to meet the individual needs of each client, specifically identifying the social occupations that have been and will continue to be important. When used in conjunction with an assessment or evaluation, the Role Checklist will help structure intervention planning and rapport building between the client and the occupational therapy practitioner.

## Tools for Identifying Performance Skills

The ACIS (Forsyth, Salamy, Simon, & Kielhofner, 1998) also focuses on individuals and the skills they use to accomplish occupations of daily living. The behavioral categories of the ACIS include an examination of physicality, information exchange, and relations with others. Specifically, as examples, the ACIS looks at gestures, focus of attention, and respect for others as items of assessment. See the Evidence-Based Research Chart for a list of citations of studies used to provide evidence supporting the value of the ACIS.

The BaFPE (Bloomer & Williams, 1979) was developed as a comprehensive tool with two parts: Part A is a Task-Oriented Scale and Part B is called the Social Interaction Scale. This assessment examines people through interviews, at mealtime, and in unstructured and structured oral and activity groups. It examines their verbal communications, psychomotor behaviors, social appropriateness, response to authority, independence, ability to work with others, and participation in groups and programs. The BaFPE evaluates individuals, but not a group as a whole. See the Evidence-Based Research Chart for research carried out to provide evidence of the BaFPE's usefulness. For further research on the BaFPE, refer to Hemphill-Pearson's book on mental health assessment tools (1999).

The COTE is defined as an instrument practitioners use to identify the client factors, performance skills, and patterns of behavior that impede engagement in the occupation of social participation, and is one of the original social skills tools (Brayman, 2008). Originally developed in 1975, the COTE focuses on traditional occupational therapy behaviors (as established by Ayres in 1954) such as punctuality, organization, initiative, responsibility, dependability, attention to detail, neatness, interest, and concentration (Brayman, 2008). The COTE developed into an instrument that uses a checklist format to assess 26 behaviors related to social participation under the categories of general behaviors, interpersonal behaviors, and task behaviors. Various research studies have been established to evaluate the validity and reliability of this tool, yielding evidence to suggest that it is highly effective in structuring the communication skills needed to assess during intervention for both the client and practitioner.

The ESI was initially designed for practitioners to assess an individual's social abilities when engaging in the natural context with client-centered goals and persons the individual would interact with on a regular basis (Fisher & Griswold, 2010). This tool includes an interview to determine the types of social interactions the individual has concerns about participating in, or those skills the client wants or needs to engage in the identified social situations. In total, the ESI has 27 different social interaction items, or skills, that are standardized based on social competency to determine the client's strengths, social dysfunctions, establish a baseline, and plan interventions for improvement (Fisher & Griswold, 2010). Similar to MOHOST, the ESI uses the Rasch measurement model to appropriately assess an individual's quality of social participation and acts as a very sensitive tool. The ESI can also be used for all persons age 2 and older with high rater reliability and person response validity.

The Social Profile was developed in 2009 to empirically evaluate the concepts of social participation as valid and reliable, and then evaluate the level of performance of individuals and group members (Donohue, 2009). A tool of a developmental nature, the Social Profile uses the five levels of social participation concepts (parallel, associative/project, basic cooperative/egocentric-cooperative, supportive cooperative/cooperative, and mature) assembled in an ordinal manner and rated using a Likert scale of 0 to 5. Forty items drawn from various literary sources (Borg & Bruce, 1991; Cole, 2005; Howe & Schwartzberg, 2001; Johnson & Johnson, 2000; Lisina, 1985; Mosey, 1986; Parten, 1932) spread across the five levels were arranged under three topics of activity participation, social interaction, and group membership/roles. These three topics provide an analysis of group participation skill levels designed for practitioners to understand the meaning and dynamics of evaluation for interactive occupation in an appropriate context. Activity participation items evaluate social performance contexts of interaction fostered by the activity. Social interaction items evaluate performance components of a psychosocial nature. Finally, group membership/roles items evaluate performance areas of application to the family and society. Tests of content, construct, and criterion validity were carried out, along with an exploratory factor analysis, to study the validity of the social profile. Item analysis, internal consistency, and interrater reliability statistical analyses were also undertaken (Donohue, 2003, 2005, 2007). Several populations—children, seniors, psychiatric, and drug-abusing adults—were observed by pairs of students and practitioner and student pairs using the Social Profile. The groups were located in inpatient psychiatric services, schools, and senior centers.

The RAPS has an interview-based structure that incorporates a social role component in several of the 12 sections that compose this tool (Good-Ellis, Fine, Spencer, & DiVittis, 1987). Each of the 12 sections aims to address an individual's level of functioning and impact of occupational therapy on individuals with mental illness. Specifically, the RAPS examines varied social relationships and how illness impedes social and role functioning. As social functioning is one of the primary occupations affected by mental illness, the RAPS has been designed to be used in the process of evaluating, intervention planning, and implementing occupational therapy to guide clients back to a functional level of social participation.

The WSS is a conceptual framework of social skills used in psychiatric rehabilitation to delineate the basic skills, core skills, and behaviors needed to guide training for work-related situations (Tsang & Pearson, 1996). This model uses a three-tier hierarchy and showcases several variables seen in the typical workplace environment, such as basic social skills, skills needed to interact with older adults, skills needed to interact with coworkers and subordinates, and skills for handling work-related scenarios. Using this tool will allow practitioners to assess a client's task-related and personal-social competence using this systemic model, although more research is needed in this area for it to be directly applied to the rehabilitation setting (Tsang & Pearson, 1996).

## *Other Relevant Assessments for Evaluating Areas of Performance in Social Participation*

Various other tools developed outside of the field of occupational therapy, but still very relevant, are now examined. These include the Communication Skills Questionnaire (CSQ), the Independent Living Skills Survey (ILSS), the Maryland Assessment of Social Competence (MASC), the Social-Adaptive Functioning Evaluation (SAFE), the Social Functioning Interview (SFI), the Social Functioning Scale (SFS), and the Social Occupational Functioning Scale (SOFS).

### Communication Skills Questionnaire

The CSQ (Takahashi, Tanaka, & Miyaoka, 2006) evaluates the differences within a social skill set when applied to different interpersonal relationships. Because communication skills are essential to other social participation skills, such as social recognition, the CSQ acts as an easy and convenient tool for evaluating interpersonal communication. Unlike other tools discussed that rely on the observations of the occupational therapy practitioner, the CSQ has fewer limitations in that it can be administered by other medical staff, family members of the client, or self-administered. Containing 29 items, the CSQ looks at three categories of cooperative skills, assertive skills, and general communication skills, which include verbal and nonverbal skills. Results of studies of the reliability and validity of the CSQ indicate that this tool could be used as an initial assessment for social skills training for a variety of mental illnesses, although further studies need to be conducted (Takahashi et al., 2006).

### Independent Living Skills Survey

The ILSS was developed as a comprehensive and objective performance measure to assess basic functional living skills, especially for individuals with severe and persistent mental illness (Wallace, Liberman, Tauber, & Wallace, 2000). There are two versions of the ILSS that have been established, one for informants (ILSS-I) and another for self-reporting (ILSS-SR). Each questionnaire aims to establish the view of an individual's community adjustment or the performed tasks needed to live a satisfying, independent life within a community (Wallace et al.,

2000). Both forms of the ILSS address a number of areas of self-care, including appearance and clothing, personal hygiene, care of personal possessions, food preparation and storage, health maintenance, money management, transportation, leisure and community, job seeking, and job maintenance; the ILSS-I also includes sections on eating and social relations. Although the ILSS is not directly related to social participation, addressing the number of times an individual participates in each of these areas enables practitioners to get a better understanding of an individual's strengths for independent living.

### Maryland Assessment of Social Competence

Occupational therapy practitioners and other professionals working with the mental health population, specifically persons with schizophrenia, have found role-playing to be a helpful tool when assessing social abilities. The MASC was a measure designed to evaluate social skills present in simulated social and behavioral situations, as role-playing has been so widely used and recognized as a valid assessment to aid the formation of social skills intervention (Bellack, Brown, & Thomas-Lohrman, 2006). The psychometric properties of the MASC indicate that it is a good tool for measuring social skills abilities, especially between different diagnoses in the chronic psychiatric populations (Bellack et al., 2006). Based on the population being assessed, the MASC uses a number of 3-minute scenes to evaluate general social skills and specific skills needed for interpersonal problem solving. This tool is very sensitive; research shows it works best when the scenarios are planned specifically for the individual or population being examined (Bellack et al., 2006).

### Social-Adaptive Functioning Evaluation

The SAFE (Harvey et al., 1997) was constructed to address the adaptive life functioning deficits faced by older adults living as chronic psychiatric inpatients. This scale is used to measure social-interpersonal, instrumental, and life skills based on the observations of the practitioner, contact with the caregiver, and subject interview, if available. Using a 17-item scale, the SAFE establishes the severity of an individual's impairment concerning the diagnosis, usually schizophrenia, in relation to basic and instrumental activities of daily living, impulse control, and social functions. Overall, the SAFE yields good internal consistency, interrater reliability, and test–retest reliability (Harvey et al., 1997).

### Social Functioning Interview

The SFI is a tool that uses interviewing to gain information on an individual's role functioning, problematic social situations, personal goals, and social skill strengths and weaknesses (Bellack, Mueser, Gingerich, & Agresta, 2004). As a structured social functioning tool, the SFI is a key tool used for interventions such as social skills training, particularly for persons living with schizophrenia. It uses subcategories under each general category that provide guiding questions for discussion to get to know the individual and prevent simple one-word replies (Bellack et al., 2004). The SFI can be used individually or in conjunction with other tools, such as the SFS or MASC.

### Social Functioning Scale

The SFS was constructed to address the areas of social functioning necessary to community maintenance and engagement, particularly for those individuals diagnosed with schizophrenia (Birchwood, Smith, Cochrane, Wetton, & Copestake, 1990). It addresses seven areas of social function, including social engagement and withdrawal, interpersonal behavior, pro-social activities, recreation, independence competence, independence performance, and employment and occupation. Similar to other tools listed previously, the SFS aims to first assess an individual's social strengths and limitations to design a treatment plan with client-centered goals and interventions. Overall, this tool is reliable, valid, and sensitive in measuring an individual's social functioning, specifically impairments, and identifying needs (Birchwood et al., 1990).

### Social Occupational Functioning Scale

The SOFS was also designed to measure the functional status of persons living with schizophrenia. It uses a three-factor structure to address adaptive living skills, social appropriateness, and interpersonal skills with regard to social and occupational functioning (Saraswat, Rao, Subbakrishna, & Gangadhar, 2006). Identified as "simple and easy to administer," the SOFS can be used in inpatient, outpatient, and rehabilitation settings and can be administered by medical practitioners as well as family members (Saraswat et al., 2006). Unlike other tools, the SOFS does not require any formal training and can be used repeatedly throughout treatment.

For further references to assessment tools used in occupational therapy, see *Occupational Therapy Assessment Tools: An Annotated Index*, a comprehensive volume that includes tools from psychology (Asher, 2007). All of these tools examining the dimensions of social participation focus on detailed interaction skills by individuals and groups. Because most treatment of social skills in occupational therapy is carried out in activity groups, it is important to assess the larger issues within levels of interaction in groups and individuals in groups. Therefore, careful selection of the tool(s) used for each client or group of clients is essential for proper evaluation and subsequent intervention.

### Case Study

Allison is a recent occupational therapy graduate who is taking on her first position within a team of clinicians at a community-based facility working with clients who have developmental and psychosocial diagnoses. Allison has been tasked with developing a new task-oriented group for adolescents who have recently been discharged from various hospital or inpatient-based facilities. To help reintegrate these individuals into the community and work force, Allison has decided to structure her group around the development of socially based occupations, and help improve performance to assist her clients with achieving better social appropriateness.

To prepare her group, Allison meets with and evaluates each of her eight group members to establish an occupational profile and baseline of his or her social skills and performance. Given that each of her group members has one or more mental health diagnoses, but no noted developmental delays, Allison selects the COTE to determine what is impeding her clients' social participation, the CSQ to evaluate their interpersonal communication prior to treatment, and the Role Checklist to help assist the group members in building connections with one another. Allison plans to run the group twice a week for a period of 2 months, at which point she will reevaluate each client and measure progress.

Each of the selected tools will guide Allison in making client-centered goals that will target at least two social skills to improve, two social behaviors to modify for appropriate communication, and two coping strategies to ease their difficulty with social anxiety. By developing these skills, Allison will support each client in actively participating in his or her community through becoming an employee or volunteer at a local establishment. The given set of evaluation tools will also allow Allison to make each group tailored to current and future clients, allowing for a sustainable social intervention for her facility.

## Summary

Identifying the skills needed to achieve proper social functioning and participation is imperative to the evaluation of this occupation in overall treatment. Various theories and concepts provide the structure needed to evaluate individual and group social interactions accurately. Research has also been conducted to demonstrate how the evaluation of social participation is an evidence-based practice, further supporting the value and need to address it within the scope of occupational therapy.

Several assessment tools have also been published to include items and sections dedicated to examining the general area of social participation and the various subskills needed for truly successful occupational performance. While some have been developed specifically for occupational therapy practitioners, all are devoted to measuring the varying levels of social functioning around activities and roles that group members assume during group interaction for clinical, educational, and well populations. ACOTE (2006) and AOTA (2014) remind occupational therapy students and practitioners of the importance of social and behavioral foundations of intervention across the lifespan and in each context. There is at least one tool available for each level of social function found in children, adolescents, adults, and older adults.

When emphasizing the need for standardized and nonstandardized screening and assessment tools, ACOTE Standards (2006) provide opportunity for both occupational therapists and assistants to begin with their informal observations of human social behavior in social settings. Occupational therapy assistants can report and discuss their observations of social participation during therapy groups with their occupational therapy supervisors and other team professionals. The occupational therapists may then validate and record these social participation behaviors using occupational therapy assessment tools described in this chapter. Ideally, observations, assessments, and analyses will determine the therapeutic levels used during interventions for the individuals and groups treated.

## Student Self-Assessment

1. Are my observation skills adequate to use a social skills assessment?
2. Do I need training or practice to strengthen my skills of observing group interaction?
3. Would I like to study some aspect of social participation in a research study during my student program in occupational therapy?
4. Should Internet sites, exchanges, or chat room interaction be considered social participation?
5. As a student educated on the different aspects of social participation, am I capable of evaluating my own skills?

# Evidence-Based Research Chart

| Topic | Categories for Observation | Evidence |
|---|---|---|
| Assessment and Communication of Interaction Skills (ACIS; 1998): Individuals<br>Used to accomplish activities of daily living (e.g., gesturing, respecting others, focusing, etc.) | Physicality<br>Information exchange<br>Relations with others | Forsyth, Lai, & Kielhofner, 1999; Helfrich & Aviles, 2001; Keller & Forsyth, 2004 |
| Bay Area Functional Performance Evaluation (BaFPE; 1979): Individuals<br>Part B: Social Interaction Scale (SIS) during interview of the individual, mealtime, unstructured group situation, structured activity group, and structured oral group | Verbal communications<br>Psychomotor behaviors<br>Socially appropriate<br>Response to authority<br>Independence/dependence<br>Ability to work with others<br>Participation in group and program activities | Klyczek, Bloomer, & Fiedler, 1999; Klyczek & Mann, 1990; Mann & Klyczek, 1991 |
| Comprehensive Occupational Therapy Evaluation (COTE; 1975): Individuals<br>Evaluates client factors, performance skills, and behavior patterns affecting occupation | General behaviors (8 subbehaviors)<br>Interpersonal behaviors (6 subbehaviors)<br>Task behaviors (12 subbehaviors) | Brayman, 2008 |
| Communication Skills Questionnaire (CSQ; 2006): Individuals<br>Identifies differences of the same social skill when applied to various relationships | General communication (6 items)<br>Interpersonal communication (23 items) | Takahashi, Tanaka, & Miyaoka, 2006 |
| Evaluation of Social Interaction (ESI; 1992): Individuals<br>Quality of social interaction and desired level of participation in their natural context | Initiation and termination<br>Producing<br>Physical support<br>Shaping content<br>Maintaining flow<br>Verbal support<br>Adaptation | Asplund & Forsberg, 2006; Englund, Bernspång, & Fisher, 1995; Fisher, 2002, 2006; Fisher & Griswold, 2010; Simmons, Griswold, & Berg, 2010 |
| Independent Living Skills Survey (ILSS; 2000): Individuals<br>Basic functional living skills of individuals with severe and persistent mental illness | Community adjustment | Wallace, Liberman, Tauber, & Wallace, 2000 |
| Maryland Assessment of Social Competence (MASC; 1991): Individuals<br>Representative role-playing scenarios that are behaviorally coded | Conversational content<br>Nonverbal content<br>Overall effectiveness | Bellack, Brown, & Thomas-Lohrman, 2006 |
| Model of Human Occupation Screening Tool (MOHOST; 2006): Individuals<br>Section on communication and interaction skills | Nonverbal cues<br>Conversation<br>Vocal expression<br>Relationships | Parkinson, Forsyth, & Kielhofner, 2006; G. Kielhofner, personal communication, November 3, 2006 |
| Role Activity Performance Scale (RAPS; 1987): Individuals<br>Components of social roles | Quality and quantity of social performance | Good-Ellis, Fine, Spencer, & DeVittis, 1987 |
| Social-Adaptive Functioning Evaluation (SAFE; 1997): Individuals<br>Adaptive changes associated with aging and chronic mental illness | Social-interpersonal<br>Instrumental activities of daily living<br>Life skills functioning | Harvey et al., 1997 |

*(continued)*

## Evidence-Based Research Chart (continued)

| Topic | Categories for Observation | Evidence |
|---|---|---|
| Social Functioning Interview (SFI; 2004): Individuals<br>Structured social functioning interview | Role functioning<br>Problematic social situations<br>Personal goals<br>Social skills strengths and weaknesses | Bellack, Mueser, Gingerich, & Agresta, 2004 |
| Social Functioning Scale (SFS; 1990): Groups or Individuals<br>Areas of functioning needed for community maintenance of individuals with schizophrenia | Social engagement/withdrawal<br>Interpersonal behavior<br>Pro-social behaviors<br>Recreation<br>Independence-competence<br>Independence-performance<br>Employment/occupation | Birchwood, Smith, Cochrane, Wetton, & Copestake, 1990 |
| Social Profile (2013): Groups or Individuals<br>Parallel level, associate level, basic cooperative, and supportive cooperative | Activity participation<br>Social interaction<br>Group membership and roles | Bonsaksen, Donohue, & Milligan, 2016; Bonsaksen, Eirum, & Donohue, 2015; Cole & Donohue, 2011; Donohue, 2003, 2005, 2007, 2009, 2013a, 2013b, 2014; Donohue, Hanif, & Wu Berns, 2011 |
| Social Occupational Functioning Scale (SOFS; 2005): Individuals<br>Social functioning and ability to live in a community for persons with schizophrenia | Adaptive living skills<br>Social appropriateness<br>Interpersonal skills | Saraswat, Rao, Subbakrishna, & Gangadhar, 2006 |
| Work-Related Social Skills (WSS; 1996): Groups or Individuals<br>Conceptual framework for work-related skills | Basic social skills<br>Basic social survival skills<br>Job-securing social skills<br>Job-retaining social skills | Tsang & Pearson, 1996 |

## Electronic Resources

American Occupational Therapy Association Special Interest Section—Mental Health: http://www.aota.org/practice/manage/sis/siss/mhsis.aspx

American Speech-Language-Hearing Association: http://www.asha.org (see study on "The Role of Social Participation Intervention")

National Alliance of the Mentally Ill: www.nami.org

National Organization on Disability: www.nod.org

Social Profile: Social-Profile.com

Suicide Prevention: www.save.org

## References


Accreditation Council for Occupational Therapy Education. (2006). *ACOTE standards*. Bethesda, MD: AOTA Press.

Accreditation Council for Occupational Therapy Education. (2011). *Accreditation council for occupational therapy education (ACOTE) standards and interpretive guide (effective July 31, 2013)*. Retrieved from http://www.aota.org/-/media/Corporate/Files/EducationaCareers/Accredit/Draft-Standards/2011%20Standards-and-Interpretive-Guide-August-2013.ashx

American Occupational Therapy Association. (2014). Occupational therapy practice framework: Domain and process (3rd ed.). *American Journal of Occupational Therapy, 68*(Suppl. 1), S1-S48. doi:10.5014/ajot.2014.628006

Asher, I. E. (Ed.). (2007). *Occupational therapy assessment tools. An annotated index* (3rd ed.). Bethesda, MD: AOTA Press.

Asplund, M., & Forsberg, E. (2006). *Bedömning av sociala interaktionsfärdigheter hos personer med generellt god social förmåga – ett steg mot att fastställa användbarheten av BSI-II [Evaluation of social interaction skills of persons with good overall social ability: One step towards establishing the usability of the BSI-II]*. Unpublished bachelor thesis, Department of Occupational Therapy, Umeå University, Umeå, Sweden.

Aureli, T., & Colecchia, N. (1996). Day care experience and free play behavior in preschool children. *Journal of Applied Developmental Psychology, 17*(1), 1-17.

Bellack, A. S., Brown, C. H., & Thomas-Lohrman, S. (2006). Psychometric characteristics of role-play assessments of social skill in schizophrenia. *Behavior Therapy, 37*, 339-352.

Bellack, A. S., Mueser, K. T., Gingerich, S., & Agresta, J. (2004). *Social skills training for schizophrenia: A step-by-step guide* (2nd ed.). New York, NY: Guilford Press.

Birchwood, M., Smith, J., Cochrane, R., Wetton, S., & Copestake, S. (1990). The social functioning scale: The development and validation of a new scale of social adjustment for use in family intervention programmes with schizophrenic patients. *British Journal of Psychiatry, 157*, 853-859.

Bloomer, J., & Williams, S. (1979). *The bay area functional performance evaluation (BaFPE)*. Palo Alto, CA: Consulting Psychologists Press.

Bonsaksen, T., Donohue, M. V., & Milligan, R. M. (2016). Occupational therapy students rating the social profile of their educational group: Do they agree? *Scandinavian Journal of Occupational Therapy, 23*(6), 477-484. doi:10.1080/11038128.2016.1187203

Bonsaksen, T., Eirum, M. N., & Donohue, M. V. (2015). The Social Profile of occupational therapy students' educational groups. *The Open Journal of Occupational Therapy,* 3(3), 4. doi:10.15453/2168-6408.1162

Borg, B., & Bruce, M. A. G. (1991). *The group system: The therapeutic activity group in occupational therapy.* Thorofare, NJ: SLACK Incorporated.

Boyt Schell, B., Gillen, G., & Scaffa, M. (2014). *Willard and Spackman's occupational therapy* (12th ed.). Philadelphia, PA: Wolters Kluwer/ Lippincott Williams and Wilkins.

Brayman, S. J. (2008). The Comprehensive Occupational Therapy Evaluation (COTE). In B. J. Hemphill-Pearson (Ed.), *Assessments in occupational therapy mental health: An integrative approach* (pp. 113-126). Thorofare, NJ: SLACK Incorporated.

Cole, M. B. (2005). *Group dynamics in occupational therapy: The theoretical basis and practice application of group treatment* (3rd ed.). Thorofare, NJ: SLACK Incorporated.

Cole M. B. (2012). *Group dynamics in occupational therapy* (4th ed.). Thorofare, NJ: SLACK Incorporated.

Cole, M. B., & Donohue, M. V. (2011). Social participation in occupational contexts: In schools, clinics and communities. Thorofare, NJ: SLACK Incorporated.

Donohue, M. V. (2003). Group profile studies with children: Validity measures and item analysis. *Occupational Therapy in Mental Health, 19*(1), 1-23.

Donohue, M. V. (2005). Social profile: Assessment of validity and reliability with preschool children. *Canadian Journal of Occupational Therapy, 72*(3), 164-175.

Donohue, M. V. (2007). Interrater reliability of the Social Profile: Assessment of community and psychiatric group participation. *Australian Occupational Therapy Journal, 54*(1), 49-58.

Donohue, M. V. (2009). *Social profile.* Retrieved from http://www.Social-Profile.com

Donohue, M. V. (2013a). *Social Profile. Assessment of social participation in children, adolescents, and adults.* Bethesda, MD: AOTA Press.

Donohue, M. V. (2013b). *The Social Profile for children, adolescents and adults in activities.* Course #1720 Webinar: occupationaltherapy.com

Donohue, M. V. (2014). Social Profile. In I. E. Asher (Ed.), *Asher's occupational therapy assessment tools.* (4th ed., pp. 359-360). Bethesda, MD: AOTA Press.

Donohue, M. V., Hanif, H., & Wu Berns, L. (2011). An exploratory study of social participation in occupational therapy groups. *Mental Health Special Interest Section Quarterly, 34*(4), 1-3.

Englund, B., Bernspång, B., & Fisher, A. G. (1995). Development of an instrument for assessment of social interaction skills in occupational therapy. *Scandinavian Journal of Occupational Therapy, 2,* 17-23.

Fantuzzo, J., Sutton-Smith, B., Atkins, M., Meyers, R., Stevenson, H., Coolahan, K., ... Manz, P. (1996). Community-based resilient peer treatment of withdrawn maltreated preschool children. *Journal of Consulting and Clinical Psychology, 64*(6), 1377-1386.

Field, T. (1984). Play behaviors of handicapped children who have friends. In T. Field, J. L. Roopnarine, & M. Segal (Eds.), *Friendships in normal and handicapped children.* Santa Barbara, CA: Greenwood Publishing Group.

Fisher, A. G. (2002). Cellular identity and lineage choice. *Nature Reviews Immunology, 2,* 977–982.

Fisher, A. G. (2006). Overview of performance skills and client factors. In H. M. Pendleton, & W. Schultz-Krohn (Eds.), *Pedretti's occupational therapy: Practice skills for physical dysfunction* (6th ed., pp. 372-402). St. Louis, MO: Mosby Elsevier.

Fisher, A. G., & Griswold, L. A. (2010). *Evaluation of social interaction (ESI)* (2nd ed.). Fort Collins, CO: Three Star Press.

Forsyth, K., Deshpande, S., Kielhofner, G., Henriksson, C., Haglund, L., Olson, L., ... Kulkarni, S. (2005). *A user's manual for the Occupational Circumstances Assessment Interview and Rating Scale (version 4.0) OCAIRS.* Model of Human Occupation Clearinghouse, Department of Occupational Therapy, College of Applied Health Sciences, University of Illinois at Chicago.

Forsyth, K., Lai, J., & Kielhofner, G. (1999). The assessment of communication and interaction skills (ACIS): Measurement properties. *British Journal of Occupational Therapy, 62*(2), 69-74.

Forsyth, K., Salamy, M., Simon, S., & Kielhofner, G. (1998). *The Assessment of Communication and Interaction Skill (ACIS), version 4.0.* Chicago, IL: MOHO Clearinghouse.

Garnier, C., & Latour, A. (1994). Analysis of group process: Cooperation of preschool children. *Canadian Journal of Behavioural Science, 26*(3), 365-384.

Gillen, G., & Boyt Schell, B. (2014). Introduction to evaluation, intervention, and outcomes for occupations. In B. A. Boyt Schell, G. Gillen, & M. Scaffa (Eds.), *Willard and Spackman's occupational therapy* (12th ed., pp. 606-609). Philadelphia: Lippincott Williams and Wilkins.

Good-Ellis, M. A., Fine, S. B., Spencer, J. H., & DiVittis, A. (1987). Developing a role activity performance scale. *American Journal of Occupational Therapy, 41*(4), 232-241.

Guralnick, M. J. (1990). Peer interactions and the development of handicapped children's social and communicative competence. In H. C. Foot, M. J. Morgan, & R. H. Shute (Eds.), *Children helping children.* London, England: Wiley.

Harvey, P. D., Davidson, M., Mueser, K. T., Parrella, M., White, L., & Powchik, P. (1997). Social-Adaptive Functioning Evaluation (SAFE): A rating scale for geriatric psychiatric patients. *Schizophrenia Bulletin, 23,* 131-145.

Helfrich, C., & Aviles, A. (2001). Occupational therapy's role with victims of domestic violence: Assessment and intervention. *Occupational Therapy in Mental Health, 16*(3/4), 53-70.

Hemphill-Pearson, B. J. (Ed.). (1999). *Assessments in occupational therapy mental health. An integrative approach.* Thorofare, NJ: SLACK Incorporated.

Howe, M. C., & Schwartzberg, S. L. (2001). *A functional approach to group work in occupational therapy* (3rd ed.). Philadelphia, PA: Lippincott Williams and Wilkins.

Howes, C. (1988). Peer interaction of young children. *Monographs of the Society for Research in Child Development, 53*(1), 1-88.

Isaksson, G., Lexell, J., & Skär. (2007). Social support provides motivation and ability to participate in occupation. *OTJR: Occupation, Participation and Health, 27*(1), 23-30.

Johnson, D. W., & Johnson, F. P. (2000). *Joining together: Group theory and group skills* (7th ed.). Upper Saddle River, NJ: Prentice Hall.

Keller, J., & Forsyth, K. (2004). The model of human occupation in practice. *Israel Journal of Occupational Therapy, 13,* E99-E106.

Kielhofner, G., Fogg, L., Braveman, B., Forsyth, K., Kramer, J., & Duncan, E. (2009). A factor analytic study of the model of human occupation screening tool of hypothesized variables. *Occupational Therapy in Mental Health, 25,* 127-137.

Klyczek, J., Bloomer, J., & Fiedler, R. (1999). *Analysis of a shortened BaFPE: Task oriented assessment.* Buffalo, NY: D'Youville College.

Klyczek, J. P., & Mann, W. C. (1990). Concurrent validity of the Task-Oriented Assessment component of the Bay Area Functional Performance Evaluation with the American Association on Mental Deficiency Adaptive Behavior Scale. *American Journal of Occupational Therapy, 44*(10), 907-912.

Lisina, M. I. (1985). *Child-adults-peers: Patterns of communication.* Moscow, Russia: Progress Publishers.

Magasi, S., & Hammel, J. (2004). Social support and social network mobilization in African American woman who have experienced strokes. *Disability Studies Quarterly, 24*(4). Retrieved from http://dsq-sds.org/article/view/878/1053

Mann, W. C., & Klyczek, J. P. (1991). Standard scores for the bay area functional performance evaluation task oriented assessment. *Occupational Therapy in Mental Health, 11*(1), 13-24.

Mosey, A. C. (1968). Recapitulation of ontogenesis: A theory for practice of occupational therapy. *American Journal of Occupational Therapy, 22*(5), 426-438.

Mosey, A. C. (1986). *Psychosocial components of occupational therapy.* New York, NY: Raven Press.

Moyer, E. A., & O'Brien, J. C. (2013). Occupational and group analysis: Adults. In J. C. O'Brien & J. W. Solomon (Eds.), *Occupational analysis and group process.* St. Louis, MO: Elsevier.

Oakley, F., Kielhofner, G., Barris, R., & Reichler, R. K. (1986). The role checklist: Development and empirical assessment of reliability. *Occupational Therapy Journal of Research, 6,* l57-l70.

Parkinson, S., Forsyth, K., & Kielhofner, G. (2006). *The Model of Human Occupation Screening Tool (MOHOST), version 2.0.* Chicago, IL: MOHO Clearinghouse.

Parten, M. B. (1932). Social participation among pre-school children. *Journal of Abnormal and Social Psychology, 27,* 243-269.

Petrakos, H., & Howe, N. (1996). The influence of the physical design of the dramatic play center on children's play. *Early Childhood Research Quarterly, 11*(1), 63-77.

Posthuma, B. W. (2002). *Small groups in counseling and therapy: Process and leadership* (4th ed.). Columbus, OH: Allyn and Bacon.

Saracho, O. N. (1993). A factor analysis of young children's play. *Early Childhood Development and Care, 84*(1), 91-102.

Saraswat, N., Rao, K., Subbakrishna, D. K., & Gangadhar, B. N. (2006). The Social Occupational Functioning Scale (SOFS): A brief measure of functional status in persons with schizophrenia. *Schizophrenia Research, 81,* 301-309.

Simmons, D., Griswold, L. A., & Berg, B. (2010). Evaluation of social interaction during occupational engagement. *Amercian Journal of Occupational Therapy, 64,* 10-17. doi:10.5014/ajot.64.1.10

Smith, D. E. (1986). Training programs for performance appraisal: A review. *Academy of Management Review, 11*(1), 22-40.

Stoffel, V. C., & Tomlinson, J. (2011). Communication and social skills. In C. Brown & V. C. Stossel (Eds.), *Occupational therapy in mental health: A vision for participation* (pp. 298-312). Philadelphia, PA: F. A. Davis Company.

Takahashi, M., Tanaka, K., & Miyaoka, H. (2006). Reliability and validity of communication skills questionnaire (CSQ). *Psychiatry and Clinical Neurosciences, 60,* 211-218.

Tenhula, W. N., & Bellack, A. S. (2008). Social skills training. In K. T. Mueser & D. V. Jeste (Eds.), *Clinical handbook of schizophrenia* (pp. 240-248). New York, NY: Guilford Press.

Tsang, H. W. H., & Pearson, V. (1996). A conceptual framework for work-related social skills in psychiatric rehabilitation. *Journal of Rehabilitation, July/August/September,* 61-66.

Wallace, C. J., Liberman, R. P., Tauber, R., & Wallace, J. (2000). The independent living skills survey: A comprehensive measure of the community functioning of severely and persistently mentally ill individuals. *Schizophrenia Bulletin, 26*(3), 631.

World Health Organization. (2001). *International classification of functioning disability and health (ICF).* Geneva, Switzerland: Author.

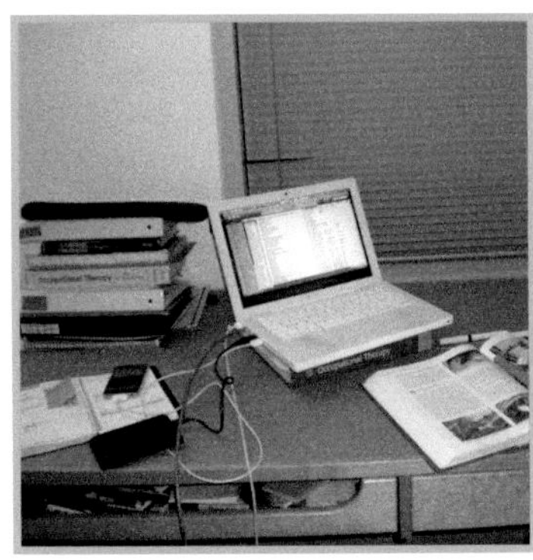

# 23

# Documentation of Occupational Therapy Services

*William R. Croninger, MA, OTR/L and Nancy MacRae, MS, OTR/L, FAOTA*

**ACOTE STANDARDS EXPLORED IN THIS CHAPTER**

B.4.10, B.5.20, B.5.30, B.5.32

**KEY VOCABULARY**

- **DAP:** A documentation format that combines the subjective and objective portions into "D," "A" is the assessment or summary portion, and "P" is for the plan.
- **Discontinuation note:** Documentation that summarizes the course of therapy and makes recommendations.
- **Documentation:** A written account of a therapy session.
- **SOAP note format:** The basic skeletal format for documentation that includes subjective, objective, assessment, and plan portions.



Jacobs, K., & MacRae, N. (Eds.).
*Occupational Therapy Essentials for Clinical Competence, Third Edition* (pp. 325-337).

As occupational therapy practitioners working in a reimbursement-driven health care culture, documentation is an integral part of the process of delivering quality occupational therapy. It affirms our value and uniqueness among health care providers. This is done via the power of everyday life (occupations; Lamb, 2015). Knowing what needs to be included in a clinical note, where it needs to be placed, and how to phrase it are all components of effective and efficient documentation. Reimbursement of occupational therapy services depends heavily on the practitioner demonstrating medical necessity. In this chapter we will introduce you to the framework upon which effective documentation is anchored.

Documentation is a necessary part of the communication process in occupational therapy and serves a number of goals. It is based on the *Occupational Therapy Practice Framework* (American Occupational Therapy Association [AOTA], 2014) and reports on four main areas: screening, evaluation, intervention, and outcomes. This also correlates well with the World Health Organization's *International Classification of Functioning, Disability and Health* (ICF; 2001). The ICF now concentrates on the outcomes of dysfunction, body structures and functions, activities and levels of participation in life, and the environment's effect on performance. A coding system is provided for these factors, which encourages universality of language, thus increasing understanding of professional domains of practice.

Documentation provides a record of interventions and a client's reaction to those interventions. Documentation is an important means to verify that an intervention session has occurred. It is also crucial for stating the goals of intervention, listing baseline data, a description of the plan and the implementation, and a detailing of the outcomes. Complete documentation provides a view of intervention and can be used for retrospective research, comparing the course and outcomes of similar cases.

Documentation promotes communication across the disciplines charged with a single client's care. It notifies the referring physician about the progress of intervention and other disciplines about what goals are being pursued and the specific techniques and media being used. Reinforcement of these can occur in other disciplines' sessions as a way to promote the transfer of learning and the ability to generalize. Documentation can also specify and validate the times an orthosis or adaptive device needs to be worn or used.

Documentation provides a record of care and is thus a legal document that can be and often is used in court. If an intervention session is not documented, it did not occur from the viewpoint of the payer, the administration, and the legal system. If a client becomes involved in a legal case and needs practitioner testimony, documentation is essential for such testimony to be reliable. Because the time span between intervention and a legal case may be long, documentation also provides a memory reference to the testifying practitioner. Documentation is part of the clinical reasoning process. It is represented by a circular diagram (Figure 23-1).

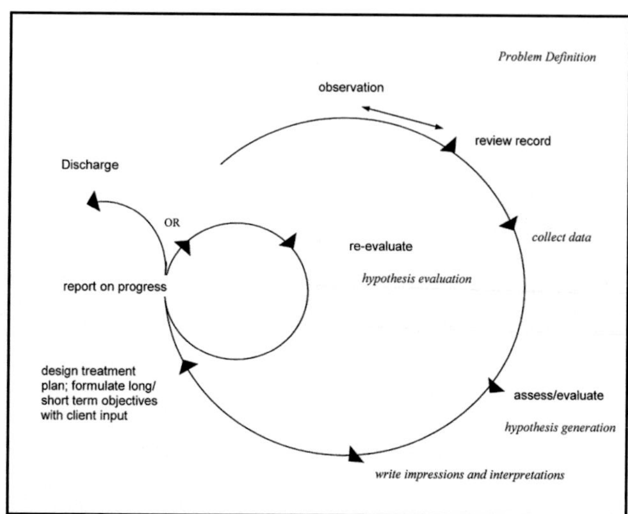


**Figure 23-1.** The occupational therapy process.

Documentation explicates the clinical reasoning process. It can also be fodder for prospective research, providing data for the success or failure of certain intervention approaches. Additionally, it helps the therapist recall what transpired during the last session, can promote reflection on the course of intervention, and can encourage adaptations to sessions. It also reflects our ethical practice. Thus, client notes can be a part of professional growth in improving the clarity of what is written, assessing the intervention's effectiveness, and refining clinical reasoning skills.

During the occupational therapy process, there are various needs for documentation:

- An initial note documents the first meeting and interview of a client.
- An encounter or intervention note is written for each contact with the client.
- The progress note details the continuing and changing status of a client and is generally written every 2 weeks or 10th encounter.
- A discontinuation note summarizes the course of intervention, the types and methods, strategies and activities used, participation of the client, outcomes realized, and recommendations for the future. The latter kind of documentation becomes particularly important to the next practitioner. A discontinuation note needs to provide a history of intervention with the client, detailing what has occurred and providing recommendations for future intervention to make for a smooth transition for continuing therapy.

Documentation can take a number of other forms depending on the setting, such as an educational, business, or industrial setting and area of practice (e.g., industrial rehabilitation and ergonomics). The Individualized Education Program (IEP) is found in an educational setting along with a report written to a parent, teacher, special education administrator, principal, superintendent, etc. In the area of industrial rehabilitation and ergonomics, documentation can take other forms, such as a written job site analysis. In a community setting, it often takes the form of a report of findings to include recommendations. In any context, a commonality is that all documentation, when done properly, promotes and justifies the value of occupational therapy.

One current trend in documentation is called *point of service documentation*. Practitioners are encouraged to address documentation while working with a client. Historically, many practitioners wait until the end of the work day to document interventions. After working with numerous clients over the course of a day, documentation often suffers because the practitioner can easily become confused as to what was done and with whom. Thus accuracy and specificity suffer. Point of service documentation, when performed correctly, allows the practitioner to document within the session and to include client input in each documentation. Some practitioners, however, assign the client a task or exercise and then leave the room to document. This behavior is potentially unsafe as well as defeating the goal of providing an accurate overview of the skilled therapy in a given session (Waite, 2012).

## The Language of Documentation

Formats may vary in different settings and practice areas, but components of good documentation remain the same: documentation needs to be clear, accurate, relevant, and it needs to list exceptions. Additionally, documentation should be succinct, written simply and in an active voice. It also needs to highlight the medical necessity of occupational therapy intervention that connects the need for skilled intervention (Brennan, 2015, p. 9). Functional implications of your interpretation of qualitative and quantitative data need to be made apparent. If intervention is being implemented by a certified occupational therapy assistant, supervisory examples will be necessary. Comorbidities can affect the course and outcome of intervention, so its effect on occupational performance has to be clearly stated. Pain and cognitive dysfunction are examples. Any changes in goals need a careful rationale documented. The writer needs to consider the audience for whom a document is being written. Particularly, when written for nonmedically trained readers, documentation needs to make sense for the designated readers, and it must contain specificity in goals and directions to make it useful. Thus, an official client note in a client chart would likely differ from a progress note sent home to a parent or family member. The content might be similar, but the way it is expressed would differ.

- Example of note in chart: Rose was able to tolerate a 20-minute session in the kitchen. She demonstrated a 15-degree increase in shoulder flexion, allowing her to access items in cabinets above eye level. She was able to gather supplies to make a light lunch.
- Example of note sent to family: Rose is showing improvement in her ability to independently prepare a light lunch for herself.

Another example is a home program written for an outpatient client with deficits in fine motor control of the hand. The program could include suggestions for using everyday activities (e.g., folding clothes, washing and drying dishes) to help improve functional use.

## Process of Documentation

Documentation could be thought of as taking three general forms: initial notes; intervention notes; and discontinuation notes such as discharge, reports, or letters to physicians.

### Basics

Basics need to be included in any client note. Many are common sense, but reminders are needed to ensure inclusion. The basics are presented below.

- Include the following:
  - ◊ Name of client
  - ◊ Date of session
  - ◊ Diagnoses of concern for intervention
  - ◊ How goals have been addressed, with progress or difficulty noted
  - ◊ Any unusual happenings during the session
- Use ink (with appropriate color when designated by site) when writing notes
- Use acceptable terminology and abbreviations (AOTA, 2014)
- Remember to sign name with appropriate initials included
- Most sites do not allow erasures; if you need to correct an error, draw a single line through the mistake and write the correction above and then initial the correction
- Write note as soon after the session as possible
- Be accurate, clear, and relevant
- If extra space remains at the end of the note, draw a line to the end of the section so no one else can add to your documentation

Table 23-1.

**Checklist Sample: Chart Review**

| Criteria | Components |
|---|---|
| Basic information to be retrieved from a chart review | • Date of onset<br>• Admitting diagnosis<br>• Medical history (pertinent medical problems, procedures, preexisting conditions that may affect the evaluation or intervention)<br>• Current medical intervention (medications, procedures, rehabilitation efforts, and progress)<br>• Current medical status (client getting better or deteriorating, intervention plan, discharge plan, results of recent tests, and DNR status; information can be found in nursing and medical notes)<br>• Personal information (age, marital status, family configuration, residence, work history, financial information)<br>• Medication lists (will any medications affect intervention?) |
| Components pertinent to occupational therapy (where you will find the information) | • Medical section (physician notes, pertinent past medical history, general information on social situation, response to intervention, course of intervention, referrals to specialists, upcoming surgeries or procedures, precautions, complications during acute phase that might affect recovery [e.g., infection, hydrocephalus, respiratory distress, seizures])<br>• Nursing section (day-to-day status, response to intervention or disability, often report response to splinting, positioning, activities of daily living, and mobility performances)<br>• Test section (laboratory reports, radiography, computed tomography, magnetic resonance imaging)<br>• Medication lists (sometimes grouped in this section are vital signs, weights, calorie counts)<br>• Professionals section (physical therapy, speech pathology, social work, therapeutic recreation, neuropsychology, vocational rehabilitation evaluations, and progress notes); some institutions have continuous problem-oriented records, and these reports are within the body of the medical section |

Adapted from York, C. D., & MacRae, N. (1993). *Class handout.* Biddeford, ME: Occupational Therapy Department, University of New England.

## Initial Notes

Initial notes are essentially evaluation notes with the specific form varying among entities: general medical, mental health, home health, public education, etc. The initial documentation process can be divided into three stages: actions before meeting the client, the client interview, and actions after the interview.

### Actions Before Meeting the Client

Data collection begins before the client interview. Table 23-1 provides an overview of what and where a therapist working in an acute care physical disabilities setting would look to gather data during an initial assessment from a chart review. If it is possible, the practitioner begins by examining medical records, reports of previous assessments, results of educational testing, and other pertinent documents (Figure 23-2). At this stage, the therapist needs to form a mental "picture" of the client and an idea of what the practitioner is being asked to do. Practitioners should note the following:

- Who is the referral agent (e.g., a physician, a parent, a classroom teacher, another therapist)?
- What is being asked of the therapist (e.g., an orthosis, a safety evaluation, a fine motor writing evaluation)?

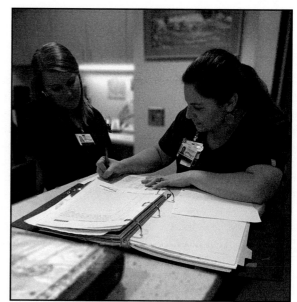

**Figure 23-2.** Chart review.

- If the referral is not clear, then the practitioner needs to follow up with the referring professional to get more information on what outcome is needed.

Using the *Framework* (AOTA, 2014), the practitioner gathers data related to the individual's highest level of performance on each of the following domains: activities of daily living (ADLs) and instrumental activities of daily living (IADLs), education and work, play and leisure, and social participation. If a problem exists, the practitioner then looks for any information on the client's performance skills or performance patterns. The practitioner also looks for information on the client's contexts and any pertinent client factors. He or she continues to review documents, looking for information about diagnoses, any precautions, the client's support systems, and the suspected disposition of the client (e.g., return to home, discharge to skilled nursing facility, or unknown).

An experienced practitioner also looks for information concerning the client's history, interests, and experiences. Although not absolutely necessary, sharing this information with the client often helps build rapport and trust during the next stage.

### The Client Interview

The first meeting with a client sets the tone for future intervention so therapeutic use of self is important. Getting to know the client via an occupational profile helps to collaboratively determine goals and objectives. Knowing how clients feel about their injuries, symptoms, or chronic diseases can facilitate the development of the just-right challenge. The client will also be trying to get to know you, so some self-disclosure may be necessary to show your abilities, as well as your humanity. In reality, two interviews take place during the first meeting. The practitioner is interviewing and assessing the client while the client is conducting a silent interview, determining whether the practitioner is competent and able to be trusted and whether the client can or even wants to work with the practitioner. Not all clients will want to work with you. It may be pain, nausea, fear, or simply a mismatch of personalities. However, in those first few minutes, the weight is on the therapist to demonstrate competency and approachability and to develop trust.

Data collection in the client interview begins at the door, with the therapist noting performance factors such as posture, balance, body symmetry, eye contact, bilateral upper extremity use, and cognition. Following the protocol of the hosting agency, the practitioner records the client's responses to questions and the assessments related to occupational therapy domains and performs an occupational history and profile. Performing the latter can help build rapport and provides points where client and practitioner can connect. Of equal importance is the client's perception of strengths, problems, and his or her goals. Before leaving the client, the practitioner usually discusses findings and any anticipated occupational therapy interventions. In other settings, the practitioner may not discuss the findings with the involved individual because the client may be a disability insurance company, an organization such as a school system, or another professional.

### Actions After the Interview

The therapist now has a clear view of the reasons for referral, the desired outcomes, and the expected outcomes, as well as the client's strengths and problem areas. The therapist must now summarize findings, develop a list of strengths and problem areas, and develop appropriate goals and activities that will help the client achieve those goals and collaboratively determine goals and activities that meet the client's needs. As part of this process, the practitioner also needs to determine the need for skilled intervention, specifically addressing whether an occupational therapist or the certified occupational therapy assistant will deliver the intervention.

## Progress Notes

Usually, each intervention session requires a progress note. It is much shorter than the initial note and commonly details only the date, duration, therapeutic activities used, client reactions, and plan of the next intervention

## Discharge Summary

This type of documentation represents a melding of both the initial and progress note. Providing information that you would like when you work with a client who has had prior occupational therapy is a good guide for what to include. It can include background information that provides an overview of the reason(s) for referral as well as expected outcomes. Next, a thorough synopsis of problem areas and goals, along with progress, is detailed. Client engagement and specific recommendations that are occupation focused provide information that can facilitate a smooth transition to the next occupational therapy practitioner or the rationale for not continuing intervention. It is also informative to include models and methodologies used to inform a subsequent occupational therapy practitioner (Jack & Estes, 2010). The practitioner ends by noting any ongoing problems and recommendations for addressing them. If the client chooses to discontinue services, this also needs to be made clear in the summary (Figure 23-3).

**Occupational Therapy Discharge Summary**

Date of Report: January 15, 2017

Patient: Joyce Smithington, DOB: 4/4/1943, Primary Dx: s/p craniotomy 2° fall
PMH: CVA 6 years prior with R hemiparesis and moderate expressive aphasia
Precautions/contraindications: Ambulates with hemi-walker, patient is a fall risk

Reason for referral to OT: R UE incoordination, decreased ADL participation
Reason for D/C: client has met goals and feels she has received maximum benefit from occupational therapy.

Mrs Smithington has been seen x6 by Home Health Occupational Therapy (HHOT) to increase control of her R UE and maximize independence in ADLS.

Problems/Goals:

Toileting: she reports she is now able to transfer on/off toilet and perform hygiene without assist using her hemi-walker and grab-rails that were recently installed in her bathroom.

Dressing: She is now independent in upper body dressing and needs assist for lower body dressing only for donning shoes and socks. She was not successful using AE: reacher or sock aide.

Meal prep: She is able to independently plan and prepare light meals using AE and a microwave oven.

Home making: she continues to need assistance in home making and has employed an aide x5 weekly.

R UE use: Therapist and patient used a combination of neuro re-education techniques following motor control theories to address R hand in-coordination. The limb is now functional as a gross assist in ADLs.

During her HHOT sessions a home safety evaluation was conducted and her kitchen was organized to make it easier for her to access needed devices and supplies. It was suggested that she have grab rails installed in the bathroom, which she has done.

Recommendations:

1. Continue home health aide to assist with IADLs and monitor for falls as her children all live distantly and her husband recently passed.
2. Encourage enrollment in "Lifeline Monitoring" to allow her access to 24/7 care.
3. The community has a newly formed stroke survivor group which meets biweekly at the YMCA and Mrs. Smithington might enjoy/benefit from participation in their meetings. Transportation can be provided via a local church group.
4. Removal of all scatter rugs.

Thank you for this referral,

Kimberly Golden, MS, OTR/L
Premier Home Health Services
(234) 123-4567

**Figure 23-3.** Discharge summary.

# Documentation Formats

Initial notes, progress notes, and discharge summary are types of documentation, but there are other documentation formats. The types of notes occur across all areas of specialization with formats simply providing different methods of organizing data. Although examples of good documentation can be used during preparation of practitioners for practice, it is recommended that students develop their own style of writing, within the parameters of the basic structure being taught. Developing one's own style makes it easier in the long run because your progress will be smoother and quicker. Having multiple opportunities to practice documenting from real or simulated encounters, or from DVDs, allows for refining efforts, particularly if there is timely feedback given by faculty. Such ungraded practice endeavors allow students to try their hardest but make mistakes of omission or being too detail-oriented, with no consequences but that of learning to appropriately address these in their next notes. After numerous practice efforts, with feedback attempts, then graded assignments can begin, with the goal to write better, not more (Brennan, 2015).

## SOAP

A universally accepted format that organizes findings and provides a firm foundation from which to document from each of the note types is the SOAP or problem-oriented format (Weed, 1969) for the problem-oriented medical record system (Borcherding, 2000). The SOAP format has become the preferred format in many facilities (Sames, 2010). Knowing what needs to be included in each section can guide a practitioner throughout a client session. This format is composed of the following four sections, each with specific areas that need to be addressed and included to have a complete document:

- S, or the subjective portion, includes the reason for referral and any of the following information given to the practitioner by the client or a designated member of the family. It often includes a relevant client quote; a subjective comment can make the note more individual and unique to that client.
    - ◊ History, including prior level of functioning
    - ◊ Lifestyle or home situation
    - ◊ Emotions or attitudes
    - ◊ Client's goals
    - ◊ Client's complaints
    - ◊ Client's response to intervention
    - ◊ Any other information relevant to case or present condition(s)
- O, or the objective portion, includes measurable or observable information.
    - ◊ Objective measurements or observations
    - ◊ Part of intervention already given to client
    - ◊ Relevant client history taken from medical charts (may be setting dependent)
- A, or the assessment portion, includes five sections that together provide the reader with the practitioner's clinical reasoning for goals and intervention. These sections are:
    - ◊ Assets: The strengths of the client and any areas within normal limits. This is an incredibly important section because the identification of the client's strengths facilitates viewing the client as a whole person, not just as one with problems and deficits. Strengths can then be used to assist in intervention.
    - ◊ Problem list: Listing of areas of deficit for occupational performance with a goal to address prioritized problem areas
    - ◊ Long-term goals: Goals that address the functional outcome of the client, worded "To..."
    - ◊ Short-term objectives: Behavioral objectives with a listing of specific methods and activities used
    - ◊ Summary of intervention: Professional summary based on clinical reasoning and experience, with

a succinct correlation between all of the parts. This summary needs to clearly indicate the professional opinion of the practitioner, the course of intervention, and the outcomes attained, as well as prognosis.

- P, or the plan for the future, includes a number of items such as:
  - ◊ Frequency and amount of time a client needs to be seen by the occupational therapist
  - ◊ Location of intervention session
  - ◊ Intervention progression
  - ◊ Client and family education
  - ◊ Equipment needs and equipment ordered/sold to client
  - ◊ Plans for future assessment or reassessment
  - ◊ Plans for discharge
  - ◊ Referral to other services or discharge statement that needs to be carefully phrased ("No need for occupational therapy services at this time," which allows for whatever occupational therapy services may be necessary in the future)

The original SOAP format includes goals in the A section; other authors (Kettenbach, 2009; Sames, 2015) now place goals in the P section.

An example of a pediatric documentation by an occupational therapy student is provided in Figure 23-4. It is longer due to its evaluative nature.

Lauren Zito
2/27/15

**Pediatric documentation:**
**Client:** Max (male) with cerebral palsy; 8 years old

**S:** Max was very interested and engaged in feeding and enjoyed the session

**O:** Client engaged in 25 minute self-feeding activity in his home, with his mother present.

Positioning:
Keekaroo chair with feet on platform, trunk in neutral, chair height slightly inferior to scapula, table height at mid-trunk level.

Client issues:
Feet not flat, weight bearing on balls of feet with R heel at 20° plantar flexion.
Pelvis in slight anterior tilt
Seat cushion not secured properly
Child is leaning laterally to R

While eating, child scoops food into spoon displaying cylindrical grip with L hand on modified spoon, R hand flexed in a fist raised slightly off of table surface. The first 50% of the movement (bowl to mouth) is slow—no food falls off of spoon. The last 50% of the movement speed is increased, child pre-emptively opens his mouth, slightly pronates wrist before the spoon reaches his mouth, causing the spoon to hit his bottom lip before entering mouth—approximately 50% of food falls off of spoon. As child raises L hand to mouth (with spoon) he raises his R hand slightly and extends his thumb. Lips do not close fully around the spoon. Spoon is removed from mouth, lips loosely close and mastication begins. Child purses his lips, protrudes lips and tongue forward, and approximately 50% of food and drool escape (overall) through the middle of his lips.

Slight improvements noted during the second 50% of feeding activity as he maintains approximately 80% of food on spoon. The spoon reaches the inside of his mouth without hitting bottom lip. As child chews, a small amount of food escapes his lips—the child catches some of the escaped food with his spoon, the rest of the food remains on his face. As he fatigues, skills diminish and he misses his mouth at first and hits his cheek with the spoon before reaching his mouth. The child motions with R hand for mom to sit next to him, he then motions with his L hand and smiles. As child releases grip of spoon with L hand, motion is mimicked with R hand (releases his fist). Drooling is observed throughout as well as excess food on his face.

**A:** Based on observation Max displays associate movements with his R hand that indicate hemiplegia, as evidenced by engaging in LUE unilateral feeding. Max exhibited poor lip closure and oral-motor coordination throughout feeding, leading to poor bolus control, food loss from mouth, and excessive drooling. These factors have implications for social participation. He interacted with his mother throughout. Max was moderately successful in feeding himself with the modified spoon and adjusting his posture when verbally cued by his mom. Max improved his coordination with each additional bite, increasing accuracy of spoon to mouth and keeping more food on his spoon, until fatigue set in.

Client issues:
Tongue protrusion causing food to be pushed forward through lips
Potential for embarrassment when eating in social situations.
Fatigue appears to be a challenge
Associated reactions
Positioning

**P:** Max would benefit from OT services to:
improve postural control, oral-motor coordination and control, and increase use of R UE for increased independence and optimal occupational engagement in ADLs, play, and social participation
propose (to family) adjustments to seating by
raising footrest
adding velcro to seat cushion
adding lateral supports to Keekaroo chair for added stability for optimal occupational performance during eating and feeding
OT will include family in future intervention sessions and provide educational support for carryover.
OT will work with SLP to implement eating and feeding interventions.

Adapted from a note written by Lauren Zito
MSOT student

**Figure 23-4.** Pediatric note.

## Description, Assessment, Plan Notes and Findings, Interpretation, and Plan Notes

These other forms vary somewhat from the SOAP version, but they all incorporate the skeletal underpinnings of the SOAP version. The Description, Assessment, Plan (DAP) notes and Findings, Interpretation, and Plan (FIP) notes combine the subjective and objective portions into the D portion, or the description, of the client. The A section is the assessment or summary portion, and the P part is for the plan. A variation of this type of note is the FIP note, standing for findings (both subjective and objective), interpretation (similar to the summary or assessment), and plan.

## Individualized Education Program

The IEP is a standardized format that documents the information determined at an IEP meeting for a specific student. The IEP is a formal process to plan what services and programs are needed for the child to meet educational goals. Guidelines of the Individuals with Disabilities Education Act (U.S. Department of Justice, 2005) establish the format. Elements of an IEP are (Case-Smith, Roger, & Johnson, 2004):

- Present health status
- Present levels of educational performance
- Annual goals and short-term objectives (usually 3 months in length)

Table 23-2.

**SAMPLE CHECKLIST FORMAT**

| Intervention | Date: 9/1 | 9/2 | 9/3 |
|---|---|---|---|
| Minutes taken to complete dressing (upper and lower body) | 30 | 28 | 27 |
| Verbal cues needed to don shoes | 10 | 9 | 8 |

MENTAL HEALTH SOAP NOTE (3 hour OT intervention)

S: "Turn the fire on!" "Wow, this is hard work! We're working hard!"

O: Client seen in the treatment mall kitchen to make an ethnic dish of her choice. Of note is that client has English as a second language and that client is from a different culture than therapist.

Client was not able to list ingredients verbally from memory. Practitioner reassured patient that ingredients readily in kitchen would be procured. Client was able to gather all ingredients, (I) open container and packaging, needing occasional, indirect verbal cues for thoroughness. Patient requested therapist operate equipment and stove.

Client observed to use soiled cup to draw tea from pot. She was cued by practitioner to use a clean cup, initially questioned why but accepted practitioner explanation regarding sanitation. She was able to add ingredients to the main dish but needed maximal verbal cuing for safety when dealing with hot items.

Client declined assist with clean up however failed to remove all food from various items.

A: Client currently operating at ACL 4 but rating may be somewhat influenced by cultural variations between client and practitioner. She demonstrates lack of comfort with various appliances, preferring staff to operate these. She presents with safety risk secondary to this and failure to anticipate items that are hot, such as cooking oil.

P: Pre-plan next activity with client. Continue to work in kitchen to increase comfort with appliances. Monitor meal preparation for unsafe practices.

Adapted from a note written by Amy Walsh

**Figure 23-5.** First mental health note.

MENTAL HEALTH INTERVENTION NOTE (1 hour OT intervention)

SHORT TERM GOAL: Within 14 days client will demonstrate improved thought process as evidenced by safely attending 1 structured group daily and will attend café for meals while maintaining safety 100% of the time.

OT INTERVENTION: OT will provide weekly opportunities to engage in structured and modified activities to promote participation. For example, we will engage in a variety of sensory activities to help her with her alertness.

INTERACTION: When OT arrived and client was in bed. She agreed to meet with her and participate in aromatherapy. Client identified her alertness was "just right". She wanted to make some scented lotion to use after taking a shower. She asked to try something different: sandalwood was offered and the client smelled it and said that she'd like to try it. She said it helped her to feel more relaxed. Client measured out the carrier oil with an indirect verbal cue, the lotion in a separate cup, and the OT put the drops in the oil. Client then poured the scented oil in the lotion and stirred it. She requested OT to make the label for her lotion container and thanked her for assisting her. She later said that she'd return to bed because she felt tired. The possibility of doing some exercise to help increase her alertness next time was discussed and she agreed.

PLAN: Exercise to help increase and extend her alertness. Offer to meet before a group, so she can attend her group right after our alerting intervention.

Adapted from a note written by Amy Walsh

**Figure 23-6.** Second mental health note.

- Special education and related services
- Explanation of nonparticipation
- Participation in assessments
- Dates, frequency, location, and duration of services
- Transition services—begin at age 14 years and annually after that
- Measuring and reporting student progress

Practitioners need to use sound assessment instruments that are nondiscriminatory. Evaluations determine the current ability of the child to perform ADLs and IADLs; his or her ability to access education, work, and play activities; and his or her ability for social participation. Deficit areas are identified, and goals and objectives focus on improving these areas so the child is better able to access the educational process (Sames, 2015). Whereas the Individuals with Disabilities Education Act requires evaluations every 3 years, IEP goals are set annually, usually meeting four times a year to check on the status of the child in reaching outcomes of intervention. An example of an IEP is found in Appendix E.

The Documentation of Occupational Therapy Session during Intervention (DOTSI) has recently been developed and validated for use in pediatrics. It also allows documentation in a unified and professional manner and stimulates clinical reasoning (Bart, Avrech Bar, Rosenberg, Hamudot, & Jarus, 2011).

## Checklists

This format allows for a quick recording of a client's problems and progress using preselected categories. The organization makes it easy for a second therapist to step in if the primary therapist is not available. There are, however, disadvantages in that often there is little room to record observations. Some checklists do not allow the therapist to add problems to the prescribed list (Sames, 2010; Table 23-2).

## Narrative

As implied, this format has data written directly into the client record as soon after the intervention as possible. Narrative notes are commonly free form because there is no universally accepted structure or model for writing them. Although preferred by many therapists, the result is all too often a wordy and poorly organized note. The lack of organization makes it extremely hard for a therapist unfamiliar with the client to step in and provide therapy. It is time consuming and often inefficient to trace back through prior notes in an effort to learn of the client's problems, progress, and clinician's goals. If the organizational sequence provided by the SOAP note structure is used as a guide, this format can be informative and effective. An example of two more narrative type notes, based on SOAP format, for a mental health client are included. They detail a 3-hour intervention and a 1-hour intervention for a client who has been hospitalized for 3 years (Figures 23-5 and 23-6).

## Electronic Health Records

Electronic health records (EHRs), also known as electronic medical records (EMRs), have made slow but steady progress as a means of documentation. As of 2015 they are mandated as part of the Health Information Technology for Economic and Clinical Health Act, a component of the American Recovery and Reinvestment Act of 2009. To encourage hospitals, clinics, and physicians to adopt EHRs, a number of incentives and penalties were set in place (U.S. Department of Health and Human Services for Medicare and Medicaid, Final Rule).

Although the terms *electronic health record* and *electronic medical record* are commonly used interchangeably, they are actually different entities. The EMR is essentially a digital version of an individual's medical record. Think of it as a record that generally stays in-house at the facility where the client is seen or treated. It is not easily shared between entities such as the physician's office and a hospital. The EHR, on the other hand, is meant to be accessible to all entities who have worked with a client. So if you live in Maine, but need to receive medical care in Colorado while on vacation, the EHR would be visible to that physician. The goal here is to have all EMRs from physicians you might have seen in your life accessible to a new physician, researcher, or laboratory.

In a client's EMR, data are generally entered via computer workstations or handheld devices. Individuals involved in a client's care, including medical staff, nursing, and allied health personnel, contribute from evaluations, assessments, and interactions in the respective sections of the document. Data entry is often standardized by being entered via built-in drop-down menus. Narrative can be entered but may be discouraged. The software allows health care workers to examine information entered by other medical personnel; however, data can only be entered into the area of an individual's responsibility. Hospital-based occupational therapy sections often include evaluation, recommendations, and intervention sections. Some systems have a copy forward feature that allows one health care worker to bring data entered by another into an assessment or intervention note. Another feature is that laboratory test values, medical images, and consultation reports are readily available to authorized personnel.

EHRs bring with them both promise and problems. Advocates argue that moving to electronic records will reduce costs and potentially decrease the incidence of medical errors caused by poor handwriting. They should also lead to a standardization of medical terminology as well as abbreviations. Countering potential gains are arguments that EHR systems are often very expensive to implement both in terms of the initial purchase as well as the need to increase information technology staff to maintain the system. At least initially, productivity may decrease as medical and allied health personnel struggle to learn the system. Finally, there is the question of security with EHRs being vulnerable to intrusion both from the outside (hacking) and from within (unauthorized access by medical personnel not involved in a specific client's care).

BRANCH MEDICAL CENTER

Unscheduled Physician's Communication

November 19th, 2015

Patricia Farlow, MD
Superior Orthopedic Surgeons
4321 First Street
Winslow, Maine

Dear Dr. Farlow,
Re: John Smithington, DOB: 4/4/1948, s/p R ARCR

Mr Smithington was seen in outpatient occupational therapy this date per Phase 2 of your Rotator Cuff Repair protocol. He is no longer wearing his sling and has continued to perform his HEP x2 daily.

He reported to clinic this date in obvious discomfort with c/o pain in the R shoulder at 8/10 resting. He states he was playing with his dog yesterday, tripped and fell heavily onto the R shoulder. He heard an audible "pop" in the shoulder and immediately experienced increased pain. The shoulder shows some bruising which had not been present prior to this date. There is no observable edema and he denies alterations in sensation in the limb. No treatment was rendered and I have requested that he restart his sling and contact you immediately.

Sincerely yours,

Kimberly Golden, MS, OTR/L
Staff Occupational Therapist

**Figure 23-7.** First physician letter.

## Professional Letters

Letters are also often required in the occupational therapy process. The practitioner may need to write a letter to a physician, documenting the progress of a client or requesting an extension of a prescription for continued therapy. A letter of referral to a professional colleague may be considered good protocol for getting the kind of information requested. Providing the specifics and detailing concerns help the other professional do a better and more thorough job. A letter may be necessary to a reimbursing agency to document the reasons for a piece of adapted equipment. Photographs of a client with that specified piece of adapted equipment can graphically help demonstrate the difference that piece of equipment will make in the client's life. Another reason for a professional letter may be to ask for a donation or to thank a donor. Two examples of letters to a physician are provided: an encounter note and an unscheduled letter (Figures 23-7 and 23-8).

Letters of reference are requested by new professionals and colleagues who are changing practice sites, jobs, or applying for licensure. Being able to clearly and accurately reflect on a colleague's job performance provides the prospective hiring agency with the information needed to make a good decision. Elements that should be included are the dates you have worked with the colleague

BRANCH MEDICAL CENTER

Therapist's Encounter Note

October 29, 2015

Patricia Farlow, MD
Superior Orthopedic Surgeons
4321 First Street
Winslow, Maine

Dear Dr. Farlow,
Re: John Smithington, DOB: 4/4/1948, s/p R ARCR

Mr Smithington was seen in outpatient occupational therapy this date per Phase I of your Rotator Cuff Repair protocol. He reports to clinic with his surgical arm in sling and resting pain rated at 2/10. Maximal pain is 4/10, described as throbbing. He states he is performing his home exercise program (HEP) x2 daily with minimal discomfort.

Patient received x5 minutes hot pack to the R shoulder concurrent with scapular mobilization by therapist to prepare the joint for PROM. Patient placed in supine with therapist taking surgical shoulder through multiple sets of 5 repetitions each PROM in both ER and GH flexion with a 20 second stretch each repetition. Mr. Smithington continues to meet ROM desired at post op week (POW) 5.

Patient reports he continues to need some assistance from his wife in lower body dressing and bathing. We will progress to POW 6 exercises: pulleys, AAROM in supine and "tabletop" dusting on his following treatment visit.

Sincerely yours,

Kimberly Golden, MS, OTR/L
Staff Occupational Therapist

**Figure 23-8.** Second physician note.

or student, examples of work with clients and team members, personal characteristics, ethical behavior, potential for growth and strengths, and areas in need of improvement in job performance. A grading of your endorsement or lack thereof should end the letter.

## Medical Abbreviations

Knowing how information should be reported in a medical record is as important as knowing what information to include. Historically, health care professionals have used medical abbreviations as a means to shorten the length of time spent writing notes while maintaining thorough client care records. However, there is no universally accepted set of medical abbreviations; therefore, abbreviations accepted at one facility may not be accepted by another. More important, an abbreviation may not have the same meaning at different facilities. In 2001, the Joint Commission on Accreditation of Healthcare Organizations issued an alert related to dangerous medical abbreviations. This was followed in 2005, and most recently in 2012 (Joint Commission, 2012) by the creation of a do not use list. The use of medical abbreviations by health care professionals continues to be both common and controversial. It is, therefore, imperative that practitioners use only the abbreviations accepted at their worksite.

## Goal Writing

Effective goal writing is a vital part of documentation. It is also one of the more difficult skills for new practitioners to perfect. Occupational therapy values a collaborative relationship between the practitioner and client. Therefore, the goals should be developed collaboratively by the client and practitioner. Goals help prioritize intervention, measure the effectiveness of intervention, and assist with keeping health care costs in line.

Goals are composed of a number of components. An easy way to understand the components is by use of an A-B-C-D approach (Kettenbach, 2009, p. 138):

- A represents the who, or the audience; is always client oriented
- B represents the what, or the functional behavior; action words need to be used in this portion of the goal
- C represents the how, with a description of the situation and the circumstances under which the behavior will be accomplished
- D represents some form of measurement, such as percentage, number, or time (i.e., how the outcome will be measured)

An example of each portion of a goal follows:

- Observing hip precautions 100%, the client will don her socks using a sock aid within two intervention sessions.
- Observing hip precautions 100% (measurement), the client (who) will don her socks (what) using a sock aid (how) within two intervention sessions.

Another helpful acronym for effective goal writing is RHUMBA, a goal-writing method developed by the AOTA in the 1970s (Sames, 2010 and modified by the College of St. Catherine in 2001):

- Relevant: Goal must be relevant to the client
- How long: Detail when goal will be met
- Understandable: Goal must be easily understood
- Measurable: Goal must be able to be measured; you must be able to know when and how well the goal has been met
- Behavioral: Goal must be observable
- Achievable: Goal must be able to be accomplished by the client

If these descriptors are used as references by the goal writer, goals have a much better chance of being clear and concise.

Other helpful acronyms that may resonate are:

- RIOT (Wright, 2010) is a form that can assist the school practice occupational therapy practitioner organizing four areas of information. It stands for:
- Review: Do a complete and thorough record review
- Interview: Interview multiple sources, with intent of gathering specific qualitative and quantitative data about supports and barriers to occupational performance (Clark, Cahill, & Ivey, 2015)
- Observe: Collect data as part of problem identification, supporting better understanding of causes of concerns
- Test: Use school-related test and tools

ICEL (Wright, 2010) is another organizing form. It stands for:

- Instruction: How content is delivered
- Curriculum: Identifies the content
- Environment: Context and conditions for learning
- Learner: Unique capacities of the learner

Both of the above are consistent with many of the concepts of the *Framework*.

## Functional Outcomes

Outcomes identify what the client will be able to do functionally because of the intervention. They have resulted from the managed care push for accountability in our health care system, with managed care companies scrutinizing costs to make sure they are receiving value for their expenditures. Outcomes also notify the third-party payer of the functional reason behind the goal formation. More importantly, particularly to reflect the *Framework* (AOTA, 2014), a functional outcome should be seen as contributing to an improved occupational performance that promotes social participation by the client. This exemplifies a shift from focusing on improved strength or range of motion, or components, as the goal of intervention to a more top-down, holistic approach that aims for improved occupational performance. An example of a functional outcome is improved upper extremity functioning to assist in the independence in the ADLs of dressing.

## Administrative Outcomes

Documentation of clients' functional outcomes can also be used to gather administrative outcome data to support research and quality assurance activities of the department.

## Occupational Therapist–Occupational Therapy Assistant Differentiation

Occupational therapy assistants collaborate with occupational therapists throughout the occupational therapy process, from screening and evaluation to discontinuation of services. Assistance is always performed under the supervision of the occupational therapist. The same is true of documentation. Depending on the site, the occupational therapy assistant may contribute to the documentation note or may write the entire note. If the latter is the case, it is most often a progress note, and an occupational therapist's signature is usually required by payers. Because both practitioners contribute to the documentation process, both need to understand what is entailed in the process and how to do it effectively and efficiently. Citing the contributions made by the certified occupational therapy assistant depicts respect for the partnership.

## Summary

For many practitioners, new and experienced, being able to write well-organized and concise documentation is a major challenge, now exemplified by the mantra: write better, not more (Brennan, 2015). Well-crafted assessments and notes help practitioners organize, deliver, assess, and demonstrate occupation-centered intervention, as well as meet the requirements for reimbursement for services. Documentation skill needs to highlight the process of clinical reasoning used within intervention. Effective documentation enhances client care, protects both the practitioner and agency if litigation occurs, demonstrates ethics, and emphasizes the profession's distinct value. Finally, effective documentation allows a trail of thinking and actions that can be later analyzed to demonstrate the efficacy of the profession by research that supports our evidence-based practices. The rewards, therefore, are worth the effort needed to learn this skill. Additionally, letters to others need to reflect not only clinical reasoning, but also the standards of our profession.

## Student Self-Assessment

1. Place the following into its proper location in a SOAP note:
   - ◊ Activities to include AAROM and ADLs concentrating on dressing.
   - ◊ AROM R UE 0 to 150 flexion.

## Evidence-Based Research Chart

| Topic | Evidence |
|---|---|
| Forms of documentation | Bart, Avrech Bar, Rosenberg, Hamudot, & Jarus, 2011; Jack & Estes, 2010 |
| Guidelines for documentation | AOTA Advisory Opinion, 2014; Kettenbach, 2009; Sames, 2015 |

- Using a rolling walker, was close supervision from bed to bathroom and return.
- Nursing reports patient spent a "restless night."
- Client seen x 30 minutes in room to concentrate on lower body dressing.
- Ability to perform dressing independently continues to be decreased secondary to inability to remember sequence.
- "I hate this."
- With distant supervision, client will be able to gather and don all clothing (I) within 20 minutes.
- Client has been seen in occupational therapy x 20 since admission and has met all goals; no further occupational therapy intervention warranted at this time.

2. Reorganize and reformat the following narrative note, shortening it while being concise and thorough. Use approved abbreviations and medical terminology where appropriate.
   - Mr. Jones is a 35-year-old married man who was involved in a motor vehicle accident 24 hours ago. He is complaining of quite a bit of pain in both legs. His car was struck in the driver's side. He broke his left leg and has quite a few bruises and abrasions on the right. He broke his left arm. He has some facial cuts and a concussion. I saw him in his room for about 30 minutes to start the evaluation, but he did not know where he was or what day it was. He does remember his name and what happened to him. I think my goals are to make him independent in dressing by discharge. He should also be independent in mobility during ADLs using the walker that physical therapy provided. He can only put as much pressure on the left leg so as to not break an eggshell at this time. The nurse also said he was in a lot of pain. He rates it as an 8 on a scale of 10. In the memory assessment, he can remember five numbers forward and three numbers backward. I think he will eventually be able to go home, but I'm not sure if he will need rehab first.
3. From the scenario in Question 2, create two properly formatted goals for Mr. Jones.
4. Write a letter to the attending physician, assuming goals have been met and that Mr. Jones is ready for discontinuation from occupational services.

## Electronic Resources

Electronic health records vs. electronic medical records: http://www.healthit.gov/buzz-blog/electronic-health-and-medical-records/emr-vs-ehr-difference/

For further clarification of documentation for occupational therapy, see www.aota.org/pubs/otp/1997-2007/columns/capital briefing/2004/cb-071204.aspx

## References


American Occupational Therapy Association. (2014). Occupational therapy practice framework: Domain and process (3rd ed.). *American Journal of Occupational Therapy, 68*(Suppl. 1), S1-S48. doi:10.5014/ajot.2014.682006

American Occupational Therapy Association Advisory Opinion. (2014). *Ethical considerations for productivity, billing, and reimbursement.* Bethesda, MD: Author.

Bart, O., Avrech Bar, M., Rosenberg, L., Hamudot, V., & Jarus, T. (2011). Development and validation of the Documentation of Occupational Therapy Session during Intervention (D.O.T.S.I.). *Research in Developmental Disabilities, 32*, 719-726.

Borcherding, S. (2000). *Documentation manual for writing SOAP notes in occupational therapy.* Thorofare, NJ: SLACK Incorporated.

Brennan, C. (2015). The do's & don'ts of documentation: Pitfalls to avoid. *OT Practice*, 9-11.

Case-Smith, J., Roger, J., & Johnson, J. (2004). School-based occupational therapy. In J. Case-Smith (Ed.), *Occupational therapy for children* (5th ed., pp. 758-709). St. Louis, MO: Elsevier Mosby.

Clark, G. F., Cahill, S. M., & Ivey, C. (2015). School practice documentation: Documenting and organizing quantitative data. *OT Practice,* 12-15.

Jack, J., & Estes, R. I. (2010). Documenting progress: Hand therapy treatment shift from biomechanical to occupational adaptation. *American Journal of Occupational Therapy, 64*(1), 82-87.

Joint Commission. (2012). *Do not use list.* Retrieved from http://www.jointcommission.org/topics/patient_safety.aspx

Kettenbach, G. (2009). *Writing patient/client notes: Ensuring accuracy on documentation* (4th ed.). Philadelphia, PA: F. A. Davis Company.

Lamb, A. (2015) *AOTA webinar: Demonstrating the distinct value in your daily practice.* Bethesda, MD: AOTA Continuing Education.

Sames, K. (2010). *Documenting occupational therapy practice* (2nd ed.). Boston, MA: Pearson.

Sames, K. M. (2015). *Documenting occupational therapy practice* (3rd ed.). Boston, MA: Pearson.

U.S. Department of Health and Human Services for Medicare & Medicaid Services 42 CFR Parts 4512, 413, 412 et al. *Medicare and Medicaid programs: Electronic health record incentive program: Final rule*. Retrieved from http://www.gpo.gov/fdsys/pkg/FR-2010-07-28/pdf/2010-17207.pdf

U.S. Department of Justice. (2005). *A guide to disability rights laws*. Retrieved from http://www.usdoj.gov/crt/ada/cguide.pdf

Waite, A. (2012). Record time: Point of service documentation strategies help practitioners beat the time crunch. *OT Practice, 17*(1), 9-12.

Weed, L. L. (1969). *Medical records, medical education and patient care: The problem-oriented record as a basic tool*. Cleveland, OH: Case Western Reserve University Press.

World Health Organization. (2001). *International classification of function, disability and health*. Geneva, Switzerland: Author.

Wright, J. (2010). *The RIOT/ICEL matrix: Organizing data to answer questions about student academic performance and behavior*. Retrieved from http://www.interventioncentral. org/sites/default/files/rti_riot_icel_data_collection.pdf

# V

# Intervention Plan
## Formulation and Implementation

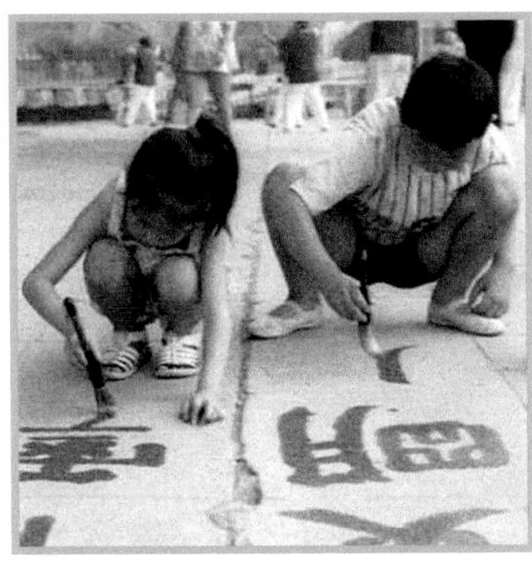

# 24

# INTERVENTION PLANNING AND PROGRAM DEVELOPMENT

*Jane Clifford O'Brien, PhD, OTR/L, FAOTA;*
*Peter DaSilva, MSOT Class 2017; and Jennifer O'Connor, MSOT Class 2017*

**ACOTE STANDARDS EXPLORED IN THIS CHAPTER**

B.5.1–B.5.3, B.7.9

**KEY VOCABULARY**

- **Adapting:** Activities involving changing the actual task. Adapting may involve the use of assistive technology or equipment.
- **Contexts:** The conditions surrounding the client that influence performance, including cultural, physical, social, personal, temporal, and virtual considerations (American Occupational Therapy Association, 2014b).
- **Frames of reference:** Principles, strategies, and specific intervention techniques that guide practice.
- **Grading:** Refers to making activities easier or more difficult for the client.
- **Models of practice:** Overarching philosophy and theories that organize intervention planning (MacRae, 2001).
- **Occupation-based activity:** Involves doing the actual occupation, which provides meaning and is part of one's identity (Fisher, 1998).



Jacobs, K., & MacRae, N. (Eds.).
*Occupational Therapy Essentials for Clinical Competence, Third Edition* (pp. 341-358).

Occupational therapy practitioners work with a variety of clients who have a wide range of abilities and disabilities. A crucial skill in the development of effective intervention planning is the ability to interpret, develop, and use evidence to support practice. Occupational therapy practitioners analyze activity so that they may grade or adapt intervention according to a client's needs. Practitioners also are mindful of safety issues throughout the process and ensure that clients are safe after being discharged from services. Occupational therapy practitioners use activity to help clients return to engagement in the things they find meaningful. This chapter provides an overview of the intervention process by examining how models of practice and frames of reference guide practitioners in their decision making for both intervention and program planning. A description of the role of the occupational therapist and occupational therapy assistant in intervention and program planning is provided.

## Overview of the Intervention Process

Intervention plans provide a map for the occupational therapy process. The occupational therapy practitioner's therapeutic reasoning skills are essential in creating a specific plan for each client. Practitioners use current evidence, knowledge, experiences, and contextual cues to guide and justify the intervention plan. The plan includes the goals of the intervention; who will perform the intervention; and where, when, how often, and how long the intervention will take place. The occupational therapy practitioner provides a rationale for the type of intervention and desired outcomes. Intervention plans clarify the role of the occupational therapy practitioner and specify which team members will collaborate together (Table 24-1).

> Occupational therapy students and novice practitioners learn from carefully describing each part of the intervention plan with a well-developed rationale. As practitioners gain experience, the rationale may not necessarily be written in the plan. However, experienced practitioners should always be able to articulate the rationale for interventions and be aware of current research evidence to support the plan.

The occupational therapist is ultimately responsible for the intervention plan, but he or she receives input from the occupational therapy assistant. Following is further delineation of each practitioner's responsibilities:

- The occupational therapy assistant provides data, updates, observational notes, and information about the client.
- The occupational therapist uses the information provided from the occupational therapy assistant to aid in the development of a plan.
- The occupational therapy assistant and occupational therapist work in collaboration with the client toward the selected goals.
- The occupational therapist provides supervision to the occupational therapy assistant, as needed, depending on the occupational therapy assistant's experience and practice setting requirements.
- Both the occupational therapy assistant and occupational therapist design activities to meet the desired goals (American Occupational Therapy Association [AOTA], 2014a).

## Models of Practice

Occupational therapy is based on the premise that engagement in meaningful activity is beneficial to clients and will help them recover, relearn, or reengage in life's activities (AOTA, 2014b). Because occupational therapy models of practice (as defined by these authors) involve broad theories and a holistic view, they can be used for all clients. The occupational model of practice provides an overview of how to organize one's thinking regarding occupational performance (MacRae, 2001). Occupational therapy models of practice emphasize occupation and describe how factors influence an individual's engagement in occupation.

Occupational therapy models of practice include the Model of Human Occupation (MOHO; Kielhofner, 1985, 2008), Person-Environment-Occupation Performance model (Christiansen & Baum, 1997; Law et al., 1996, 1997), Canadian Model of Occupational Performance and Engagement (Townsend, Brintnell, & Staisey, 1990), and Occupational Adaptation (Schkade & Schultz, 1992). Table 24-2 provides a description of these occupational therapy models of practice. Readers are encouraged to explore these models and choose the one that will be of greatest help to the client. Occupational therapy practitioners use the model of practice to organize their thinking of clients and their abilities (see Chapter 16 for more information on evaluation). Case Study 1 illustrates how a model of practice organizes a practitioner's thinking for intervention planning.

> Some models of practice can also be used as frames of reference, such as the Model of Human Occupation and Occupational Adaptation model.

Table 24-1.

**Outline of Intervention Plan**

| Topic | Description |
|---|---|
| Overview of client's history | Describe the client's occupational performance history, including current situation, medical, social, and environmental |
| Strengths | Include physical, psychosocial, and environmental supports |
| Challenges | Clearly describe what is interfering with client's occupational performance, including client factors, skills, patterns, and contexts |
| Goals and objectives | Goals written in clear, relevant, understandable, measurable, behavioral, and achievable terms |
| Conceptualization of client's situation | Describe your hypothesis regarding what is causing the occupational performance deficits |
| Frame of reference and rationale | Identify a frame of reference to target goals; describe it clearly and state why you chose it for this client |
| Guiding principles of frame of reference | Describe the principles guiding evaluation and intervention; include current research |
| Intervention activities | Outline a variety of activities that fit within the principles and address client's goals |
| Role of practitioner | Determine the role of the practitioner given the frame of reference and client's goals |
| Team members and role | Identify team members and their roles |
| Evaluation and outcome measurements | List evaluation and outcome measurements that address goals, fit the frame of reference, and are congruent with your conceptualization of the client |
| Practical considerations (where, when, frequency, length of program) | A description of where the program will occur, how frequently sessions take place, when sessions occur, and how long they will last |
| Research evidence | Overview of current research as it relates to the specific client needs such as intervention techniques, client factors, contexts, or population characteristics |
| Other considerations | Address safety, medical, physical, and psychological concerns and how they may influence the intervention plan |

## Frame of Reference

The frame of reference provides the occupational therapy practitioner with theory, rationale, strategies, and specific techniques for intervention (Mosey, 1981). Understanding the principles used to develop intervention allows practitioners to identify strategies that are likely to result in expected outcomes based upon research. Table 24-3 provides a description of the features included in a frame of reference.

Commonly used occupational therapy frames of reference include acquisitional (sometimes referred to as developmental), biomechanical, cognitive behavioral, constraint-induced movement therapy, motor control, neurodevelopmental, and sensory integration (Table 24-4). Because frames of reference change as new research becomes available, occupational therapy practitioners are careful consumers of research so they may provide the best care to their clients.

Practitioners continually reevaluate intervention strategies to ensure the frame of reference is effective for the client and the strategies successfully target the client's goals. If the client is not making the desired progress, a closer review of the techniques, principles, and assessment tools described in the frame of reference may provide an alternative plan. A closer inspection of the research and/or protocols associated with the frame of reference may promote success. Alternatively, the occupational therapy practitioner may decide to try another frame of reference altogether. Informed practitioners benefit from the knowledge of many frames of reference. Furthermore, when practitioners understand the principles and theory guiding the frame of reference, they are better able to adapt techniques for clients for whom the frame of reference was not originally intended.

Table 24-2.

## Models of Practice

| Model | Author(s) | Components | Premises |
|---|---|---|---|
| Model of Human Occupation (MOHO) | Kielhofner, 1985, 2008 | Volition<br>Habituation<br>Performance<br>Environment | The human is an open system. The clinician's role is to understand the client in terms of these systems (and subsystems) and intervene to facilitate engagement in occupation. |
| Canadian Occupational Performance Measure (COPM) | Canadian Occupational Therapy Association (Townsend et al., 1990) | Spirituality<br>Occupation<br>Context (institutional included) | The worth of the individual is central to this model. Spirituality is the core of a person. Thus, occupational therapy practitioners must understand the client's spirituality to facilitate engagement in occupations. Performance of occupations takes place within social, physical, and cultural environments. |
| Occupational Adaptation (OA) | Schkade & Schultz, 1992 | Occupations<br>Physical and emotional strengths and weaknesses<br>Examination of available support systems (physical and emotional) | Help people participate in their desired occupations by adapting or modifying the occupation or using other methods to perform the occupation. |
| Person-Environment-Occupation-Performance (PEOP) | Christiansen & Baum, 1997; Law et al., 1996, 1997 | Person<br>Environment<br>Occupation<br>Performance | Occupations are the everyday things people do. PEOP looks at the person in terms of physical, social, and emotional factors. The environment (context) influences the person and occupations. Performance is influenced by person, environment, and occupation factors. The environment includes culture and political institutions. |

Adapted from O'Brien, J. C., & Solomon, J. W. (2006). Scope of practice. In J. W. Solomon & J. C. O'Brien (Eds.), *Pediatric skills for occupational therapy assistants* (2nd ed.). St. Louis, MO: Mosby. Copyright Elsevier Mosby, 2006.

Table 24-3.

## Features of a Frame of Reference

| | |
|---|---|
| Description of theory | The frame of reference begins with a description of the thought process and reasoning for addressing change. The author provides a detailed background of the intentions of the frame of reference based on theory and research evidence. |
| Target population | A description of who will benefit from the strategies provided by the frame of reference, including the rationale for the use with a specific population. |
| Principles used for intervention | The foundation for the intervention includes the specific principles that help practitioners make therapeutic decisions. This section should include research evidence to support each claim. |
| Explanation of client function and dysfunction | A description of the continuum of function and dysfunction as described by the frame of reference helps practitioners understand the scope of the frame of reference. |
| Role of the practitioner | A clear description of the practitioner's role when using this intervention is provided. The frame of reference outlines the strategies and techniques the practitioner uses in therapy. |
| Evaluation and intervention process | The author provides a description of how intervention proceeds using the given techniques. This allows practitioners to observe, assess, and intervene accordingly. |
| Intervention techniques/strategies | Specific intervention techniques and strategies are described so the practitioner is aware of how to proceed in intervention. This section describes the rationale for using the given strategies. |
| Assessment and measurement tools | Assessment tools designed specifically for the frame of reference allow practitioners to operationalize concepts and follow specific guidelines provided. Assessment tools are needed to evaluate clients accordingly. Descriptions of how to measure change are required. |
| Research evidence | Evidence to support the methodology and theoretical premises of the frame of reference. |

## Case Study 1

Evidence exists to support the use of the MOHO (Kielhofner, 2008) in practice (Forsyth, Mann, & Kielhofner, 2005; Lee, Taylor, Kielhofner, & Fisher, 2008). The MOHO provides occupational therapy practitioners with a framework for viewing occupational performance. The following case example provides an overview of how one might use this model for intervention planning.

Mabel is a 75-year-old woman who has diabetes mellitus, heart disease, and arthritis. Recently, Mabel fell and fractured her hip. Mabel has difficulty walking up the stairs and is unable to lift heavy objects. She recently lost her husband and lives on her own in the country. Her daughter lives 1 hour away from her; she is concerned about her mother's ability to live on her own. The occupational therapy practitioner working in acute care received a referral to evaluate and treat Mabel. The therapist frames her thinking and intervention plan using MOHO concepts as illustrated in the following summary.

Volition: Mabel loves to cook and she is known for making delicious fudge. She enjoys watching soap operas and talking to family and friends. Mabel has two dogs. Mabel does not enjoy physical activity but she will go outside to play with the dogs daily. She will periodically go to the mall with a friend. She used to love to do puzzles with her husband; however, she does not do this anymore.

Habituation: Mabel reported that recently she has no desire to watch television or talk to friends. Mabel stated she gets up "whenever," "sort of eats," and takes a shower. Mabel stated she spent her day "hanging out at home." She has a few friends who come to visit, and her daughter visits at least once a week. Mabel sleeps often on the couch. She wakes around 8:00 a.m., cares for dogs, showers, and eats breakfast. Mabel tidies the house, watches television, or visits friends in the afternoon (although not as much lately). She snacks during the day and prepares herself lunch and dinner. Mabel does not follow her diet plan.

Performance: Mabel moved slowly and made little eye contact with the therapist. She followed simple verbal directions and answered questions in complete sentences. Mabel had difficulty moving from her bed to the chair. She has a right hip fracture. Mabel is unable to climb stairs. Mabel sequenced steps to activity, asked questions, and responded to humor.

Environment: Mabel lives in the country. Her daughter visits her weekly. Mabel lives in a two-story house. However, there is a bedroom and bathroom on the first floor. She does not drive, and there is no bus available.

Intervention plan: The occupational therapy practitioner considers Mabel's volition, habituation, performance, and environment when selecting activities and designing the intervention plan. The practitioner is concerned that Mabel's interests (i.e., cooking fudge, watching television, limited physical activity) are contributing to her limited occupational performance. Furthermore, Mabel may be experiencing an inability to adjust to her husband's death. She has not established new habits or routines to support engagement in occupations that will support her physically and emotionally.

The practitioner decides (with Mabel's input) that they will work to help her revisit her joy of cooking. Because the practitioner is working in an acute care setting, the goal of the intervention is to provide Mabel with right hip precautions for healing. The practitioner seeks to determine if Mabel is capable of safely living at home while evaluating her kitchen skills and Mabel's ability to follow hip precautions. Furthermore, the practitioner considers Mabel's environment and works with the physical therapist to be sure that Mabel is safe and mobile in her home. Because winter is approaching, the practitioner meets with the daughter and Mabel to develop strategies for home safety concerning snow shoveling and emergency preparedness in case of power outages. Intervention also includes goals to improve Mabel's habits and routines so that she can reengage in occupations such as cooking, visiting with friends, watching television, and doing puzzles. The plan involves consultation with a dietician and nutritionist so that Mabel learns how to cook healthy foods in consideration of her heart and diabetes mellitus. The practitioner reinforces healthy cooking.

As the practitioner develops a relationship with Mabel, they explore resources in the community that may support Mabel. The daughter decides that once a week they will go to a cooking class together. With Mabel's renewed sense of purpose, she follows hip precautions provided, asks questions, and engages with team members. As Mabel becomes more engaged in her habits and routines, she gains a sense of competency that is required to live independently. Mabel feels empowered to follow the physical activity and nutrition plans (that she helped developed). Together, the practitioner and Mabel develop safety plans. Upon discharge, Mabel and her daughter are comfortable with Mabel living alone with community and family supports.

Table 24-4.

## Frames of Reference

| Frame of Reference | Author(s) | Principles | Treatment Modalities |
|---|---|---|---|
| Biomechanical | Pedretti & Paszuinielli, 1990 | Improve strength, endurance, and range of motion. | Strength: Increase weight of toys or repetitive use of objects.<br>Endurance: Increase time engaged in occupation.<br>Range of motion: Repetitively provide slow, sustained stretch to increase end range. |
| Cognitive-behavioral | Curran, Williams, & Potts, 2009; Turk, Meichenbaum, & Genest, 1983 | Identifying one's thought process and changing how one interprets things. | Identifying negative thought patterns. Developing positive ways to behave by addressing negative thoughts. Challenging one's perceptions and constructing new ways of thinking about behaviors. |
| Constraint-induced movement therapy | Miltner, Bauder, Sommers, Dettmers, & Taub, 1999; Taub et al., 1993 | Intensive intervention to promote the use of the affected upper extremity. | Client's use of unaffected upper extremity is limited, forcing them to use the affected upper extremity. Therapist helps shape (through verbal encouragement and activity selection) client to perform more difficult movements. |
| Developmental (acquisitional) | Llorens, 1976 | Development occurs over time and between skills (e.g., gross and fine motor). Some children experience a gap in their development because of physical, emotional, or social trauma. The occupational therapy practitioner's role is to fill in the gap. | Identify current level of functioning. Work on the next step to achieve the skill. Intervention includes practice, repetition, education, and modeling of skills. |
| Motor control | Shumway-Cook & Woollacott, 2007 | Acquisition of motor skills is based on dynamical systems theory (all systems work on each other for movement to occur, including sensory, motor, and cognitive). | Task-oriented approach: Clients learn motor skills best by repeating the occupations in the most natural setting, varying the requirements. |
| Neurodevelopmental | Bobath, 1975; Schoen & Anderson, 1993, 1999 | Clients learn motor patterns when they feel normal movement patterns. | Clinician uses handling techniques and key points of control to inhibit abnormal muscle tone and facilitate normal movement patterns. |
| Sensory integration | Ayres, 1979 | Children with sensory integration dysfunction have difficulty processing sensory information (vestibular, proprioceptive, tactile). Improvements in sensory processing lead to improved engagement in occupations. | Provide controlled sensory input to improve the child's ability to process sensory stimuli.<br>Use of suspended equipment and the "just-right challenge."<br>Activities are child directed. |

Adapted from Solomon, J. W. & O'Brien, J. C. (2016). The occupational therapy process. In J. W. Solomon & J. C. O'Brien (Eds.), *Pediatric skills for occupational therapy assistants* (4th ed.). St. Louis, MO: Mosby. Copyright Elsevier Mosby, 2016.

Table 24-5.

## Guiding Questions to Consider When Deciding on a Model of Practice or Frame of Reference

| | |
|---|---|
| Setting | Does this model of practice or frame of reference fit within the setting? |
| Population | Does this model of practice or frame of reference address the needs of the population being treated? |
| Basic principles | What is the theory of this model of practice or frame of reference, and does it make sense for the population being treated? Is this model of practice or frame of reference congruent with occupational therapy practice? Is there adequate research to support the theory and principles? |
| Evidence | Has the research supported the use of this model of practice or frame of reference, and if so, with which population? Does this model of practice or frame of reference support cost-effective intervention? Are the assessment tools associated with this model of practice or frame of reference well designed and clinically relevant? Is there documentation that this model of practice or frame of reference can improve the occupations of clients? Is this model of practice or frame of reference congruent with occupational therapy core values and beliefs? |
| Assessment and evaluation | What assessments or tests are compatible with the model of practice or frame of reference? Are the assessments standardized, reliable, and valid? Does the model of practice or frame of reference provide reliable measures for assessment and evaluation? |
| Practical considerations | Does the clinic or site have the equipment necessary to competently use this model of practice or frame of reference? |
| Clinical expertise | Is the practitioner adequately trained to use the associated techniques or assessment tools? How much training is necessary? |

### Case Study 2

The developmental frame of reference (Llorens, 1976) is frequently used to facilitate learning and development in children. This frame of reference relies on identifying the child's level of ability and providing activity to promote the next step. Thus, a developmental approach advocates for practice in a variety of activities. The central principle underlying the developmental approach is that through practice, improved neural synapses occur, resulting in improved performance and improved motor patterns. The following example illustrates the use of the developmental frame of reference to structure intervention.

Trevor is a 2-year-old boy with global developmental delays. Trevor lives at home with his mother, father, and 4-year-old brother in the city. The occupational therapy practitioner begins intervention planning by conducting a developmental assessment to determine the level at which Trevor is functioning in terms of feeding, dressing, bathing, toileting, and play. After completing the Hawaii Early Learning Profile (Warshaw, 2010), a developmental checklist, the practitioner determines a level of functioning for Trevor for gross motor, fine motor, social participation, self-care skills, feeding, dressing, and play. After age levels for these systems are established, the practitioner designs intervention to address the next logical step in development. For example, Trevor will pick up a variety of foods and feed himself (9- to 12-month skill), but he will not bring a spoon to his mouth (12- to 15-month skill) or hold a cup handle (12- to 15.5-month skill). The practitioner works on a variety of developmental skills through play and provides the parents with a home program to reinforce the concepts. This approach emphasizes practice and experience as central to intervention as it improves neural functioning and consequent development.

Practitioners rely on experience, prior knowledge, and research to design and implement effective intervention techniques. Whereas the model of practice provides parameters for viewing and understanding the client, the frame of reference provides a systematic manner by which to conduct intervention. Together, the model of practice and frame of reference help the occupational therapy practitioner define and observe factors influencing occupational performance (Table 24-5).

## Occupation-Based Intervention Plans

Occupations vary from person to person. The occupational therapist collaborates with the client, family, and team members to develop appropriate goals that reflect the client's occupations. Intervention is based on these occupationally based goals developed with the client and family. Therapy goals are designed to create or promote, establish or restore, maintain, modify, and prevent (AOTA, 2014b). The goals are based on helping clients reengage in their occupations, the everyday things we do that provide us with meaning (AOTA, 2014b).

Collaborating with clients and family members on developing goals for occupational therapy services allows the occupational therapist with input from the occupational therapy assistant to understand the client and develop effective intervention plans. Clients who collaborate in goal setting are motivated to participate in therapy and home programs, and they make positive outcomes (Maurer, Smith, & Armetta, 1989; Melchert-McKearnan, Dietz, Engel, & White, 2000; Steinbeck, 1986). Collaborating with clients on goal setting requires skill in interviewing and observation. Interviewing involves asking the client to describe his or her occupational patterns, interests, routines, and performance. It allows the practitioner to better understand the client's narrative story and occupational history.

Occupational therapists use knowledge of the client's narrative, current status, and responses to questions to collaborate on goals for the intervention plan. While many clients can articulate what they would like to gain from therapy, others may not. Until a client is able to define his or her goals verbally, the therapist looks for nonverbal clues that may include investigating past interests, exploring the environment for pictures and objects that express the client's values, or observing facial expressions to determine interests and motivations. The therapist gains information from family members, the client's history, and knowledge of the client's current status. The time taken to understand the client and develop an intervention plan that meets his or her needs makes for a more successful session (Kielhofner, 2008; Law et al., 1996). Therapists use their awareness of the client's narrative, strengths, challenges, occupational desires, and contextual support to develop goals.

Goals are essential features of the intervention plan. Goals are designed to be meaningful and relevant to the person, measurable, achievable, and written clearly. Successful practitioners write goals that the client hopes to achieve. This involves collaboration with the client. Short-term goals are steps toward the long-term goals. The steps are achievable and provide the appropriate challenge, so they serve to motivate the client to continue to achieve. Goals are written so that all who read them can determine how they will be met. Clients are more likely to achieve things that they can see and understand. The mechanics of goal writing are described elsewhere in this book.

Occupation-based intervention plans focus upon enabling the client to achieve a desired occupation. For example, the emphasis of the intervention is to facilitate engagement in dressing, feeding, bathing, self care, instrumental activities of daily living, social participation, education, work, or leisure. The occupational therapy practitioner uses activities that occur within the desired occupation to promote success. Whereas practitioners may provide intervention based on specific components of the occupation with an examination of client factors, they do not lose sight that the purpose is for the client to perform an occupation such as dressing. The therapist and client, together, work to achieve the occupation. The intervention plan may involve remediation (helping the client gain abilities), compensation (completing the occupation despite limited abilities), or adaptation (changing how the occupation is performed). Occupational therapy practitioners focus interventions on occupations by considering the multiple factors that influence one's performance (Gillen, 2013).

## The Influence of Context on Intervention Planning

Intervention plans and strategies depend on the context in which the goal must be achieved. The *Occupational Therapy Practice Framework* (AOTA, 2014b) lists contexts as cultural, physical, social, personal, temporal, and virtual. Table 24-6 illustrates how contexts may influence the intervention plan. Occupational therapy practitioners consider the context in which the occupation occurs when developing the intervention plan because context influences the activity demands and expectations.

## Types of Intervention Activities

### Preparatory Activities

Preparatory activities may include exercise, stretching, range of motion, postural preparation, and positioning (Fisher, 1998). These activities are designed to provide the person with the necessary prerequisite skills. For example, runners stretch before running long distances. In this case, stretching is considered a preparatory activity. Children may participate in hand warm-up exercises or strengthening activities before completing handwriting in school (Figures 24-1A and B). Preparatory activities are required to provide a foundation for occupational performance. After preparatory work is completed, the occupational therapy practitioner may engage the client in purposeful activities.

### Purposeful Activities

Purposeful activities are meaningful to the person or may help the client reach his or her goals (Fisher, 1998). Purposeful activities are chosen by the client, have an end

Table 24-6.

## THE INFLUENCE OF CONTEXT ON INTERVENTION PLANNING

| Context | Considerations for Intervention | Questions | Example |
|---|---|---|---|
| Cultural | Privacy<br>Cultural roles in communication<br>Male and female roles<br>Food<br>Religion<br>Beliefs regarding illness and disease | How does my intervention plan correlate with my client's values?<br>What societal expectations could influence my client's ability to be successful?<br>What is the client's view of functional independence? | Consider privacy issues among cultures when intervening regarding dressing<br>Do not assume everyone celebrates the same religious holidays |
| Physical | Distance for walking<br>Size of space<br>Change terrain<br>Lighting in setting<br>Familiarity of setting<br>Materials for activity (larger or smaller) | Where does the client spend the majority of his or her time?<br>What types of sensory stimuli is the client exposed to?<br>Is the client able to navigate all desirable environments and physical demands?<br>What physical barriers could prevent the client from succeeding?<br>Where will intervention treatment take place? | Consider the physical environment and how to make the activity accessible for client<br>Complete the activity on even terrain<br>Change materials required to complete activity as needed |
| Social | Number of people in the activity<br>Involve familiar or unfamiliar people.<br>Intensity of social exchanges<br>Degrees of structure to the interactions | What type of social interactions does the client participate?<br>What relationships does the client value?<br>Does the client have a supportive social network? | Increase the social demands by inviting unfamiliar people<br>Decrease the social demands by including one close friend and a very structured activity<br>Set clear social rules that do not include intense social interactions<br>Change the social requirements to the activity, such as having the client organize the event versus attend only |
| Personal | Gender<br>Age<br>Generational cohort<br>Socioeconomic status<br>Educational status | How old is the client?<br>To what groups does he or she belong?<br>With what gender does the client identify?<br>Does the client have medical insurance and what kind? | Consider intervention activities that are suitable to the person's gender, age, and generational cohort<br>Increase novelty by selecting less traditional activities |
| Temporal | Time of year<br>Time of day<br>Length of time for the activity<br>Frequency of intervention session<br>Lifespan stage | How long will the intervention sessions take?<br>When can the client engage in therapy?<br>How often can the client engage in therapy?<br>At what point in the lifespan is the client engaging in therapy?<br>At what childhood developmental stage is the client (if applicable)? | Vary the expectations for the time commitment to the intervention activities<br>Keep the time of the activity structured and firm<br>Young adults may be searching for identity through work whereas children engage in play |
| Virtual | Technology<br>Social networks<br>Email<br>Virtual simulations<br>Telecommunication<br>Assistive technology | Does the client have access to electronic devices?<br>Does the client currently partake in electronic communication of any form? If so, what type?<br>Is the client aware of local resources and available educational classes?<br>Would the client benefit from assistive technology?<br>Does the client understand how to use a computer? | Introduce familiar or unfamiliar technology as part of the intervention |

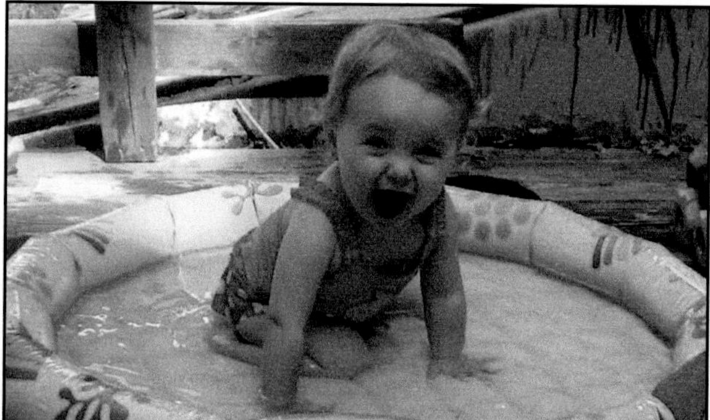

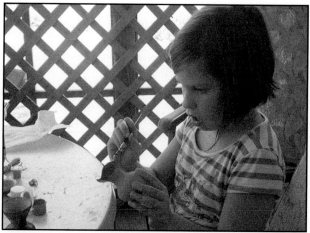

**Figure 24-1A.** Preparatory activity: Weight bearing on both hands builds hand strength for play skills.

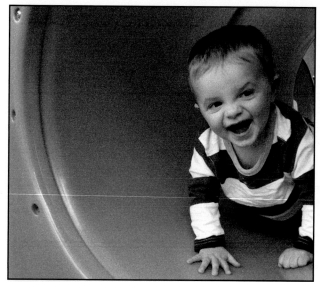

**Figure 24-1B.** Preparatory activity: This young child weight bears on both hands to build up hand strength.

**Figure 24-2A.** Purposeful activity: A child paints a clay vase as a way to improve her hand skills for writing.

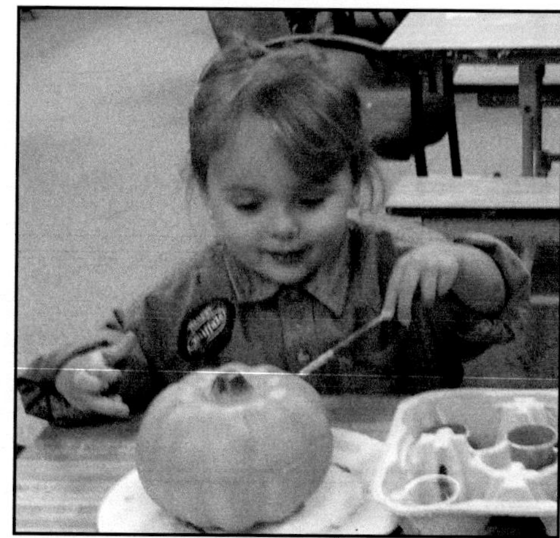

**Figure 24-2B.** Purposeful activity: Painting a pumpkin helps build hand strength for writing.

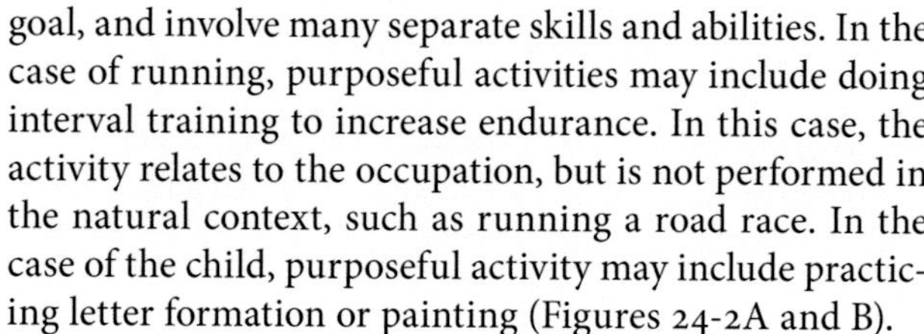

goal, and involve many separate skills and abilities. In the case of running, purposeful activities may include doing interval training to increase endurance. In this case, the activity relates to the occupation, but is not performed in the natural context, such as running a road race. In the case of the child, purposeful activity may include practicing letter formation or painting (Figures 24-2A and B).

## *Occupation-Based Activities*

The goal of occupational therapy intervention is for the client to engage in the chosen occupation. Occupation-based activity involves doing that which provides meaning and is part of one's identity (Fisher, 1998). Using occupation-based activity requires the person use the actual materials and context in which the activity is performed (e.g., a child writing a story in school, a child baking in the kitchen; Figures 24-3A and B). Occupations are personal and thus depend on the client. A skilled occupational therapist takes the time to find out what occupations are most vital to the person's identity and targets intervention accordingly.

A person who enjoys gardening may identify him- or herself as a gardener. This may provide him or her with pleasure, a sense of being, and accomplishment. For this person, returning to gardening is important and a part of his or her identity. For others, gardening may be a task they accomplish every year because it makes the home look better, and for them, being a homemaker is important. In this case, gardening is an activity associated with taking care of the home.

Occupational therapy practitioners use all types of activity in practice. However, intervention should primarily be made up of occupation-based activity (AOTA, 2014b; Fisher, 1998; Gillen, 2013). Engaging in occupations is therapeutic and will lead to larger gains (see Evidence-Based Research Chart). Furthermore, participating in the actual occupation in the natural context promotes adaptation, generalization, and transfer of learning.

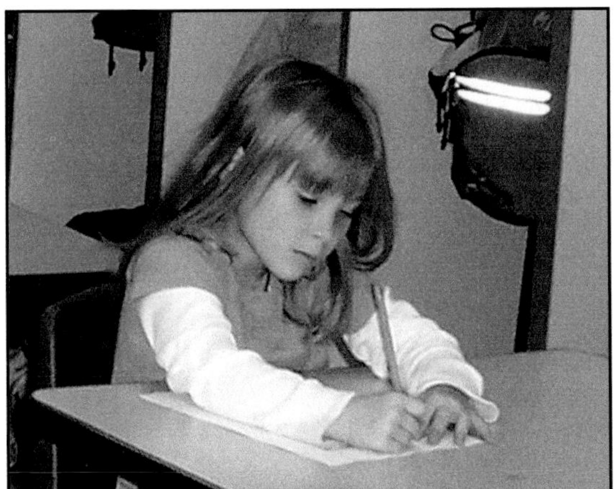

**Figure 24-3A.** Occupation-based activity: A child writes a story about her dog during writing time at school.

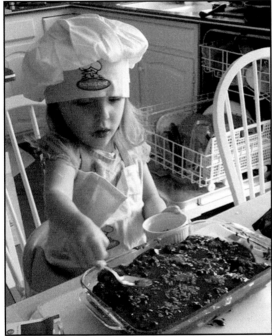

**Figure 24-3B.** Occupation-based activity: A young girl bakes a dessert for the family.

## Activity Analysis

The importance of finding activities that are motivating and purposeful to clients is a key assumption of occupational therapy practice. Occupational therapy practitioners examine individual motivations and desires as essential to the intervention process. After goals and objectives have been established with clients, practitioners design intervention activities to reach these goals.

Practitioners examine the skills and abilities required to achieve the desired goals. They determine body functions and body structures, client factors, contexts, and activity demands. Activity demands include the type of objects used, setting, social demands, movements required, sequencing and timing, costs, and environment in which the activity will occur (AOTA, 2014b). After carefully analyzing these aspects, they design intervention activities to facilitate meaningful engagement in occupation. The detailed analysis provides a thorough description of the activity so that the practitioner is prepared to adjust and modify steps, movements, objects, timing, or the environment as needed. In this way, one activity may work for multiple goals depending upon how the practitioner sets up the activity and the requirements. Table 24-7 provides an example of how one activity can meet multiple goals based upon how the practitioner designs the activity.

## Designing Intervention Activities

Occupational therapy practitioners design intervention activities to target the long- and short-term goals. When developing activities, practitioners consider the client's age, situation, narrative, and contexts. See Table 24-8 for sample intervention activities. Designing creative, novel, meaningful, and culturally relevant activities enhances the effectiveness of therapy sessions and promotes goal attainment. While engaging clients in intervention activities, practitioners use therapeutic use of self to keep clients engaged and enhance the experience. Practitioners facilitate performance and create activities to promote a positive belief in one's skills and abilities.

For example, rather than providing an adult who has lost coordination in the right hand with a fine motor writing worksheet to complete by himself, the practitioner sits with the client. While he engages in the activity, the practitioner observes his position and asks that he sit up more. The practitioner engages in light conversation. The client sighs with frustration and the practitioner empathizes with him. "It is difficult to relearn things." The client becomes tearful and asks if he will ever be able to return to work as a painter. The practitioner, using clinical judgment and knowledge of the client's condition, reassures the client that he will see steady progress over time. The practitioner decides to change the activity so that they work on a simple task involving painting, using a built-up handle paintbrush to help with grip. The client discusses how much he enjoyed painting houses and describes some of the precise aspects of the job. The practitioner asks if he would like to help paint some flower pots that will be used to freshen up the lobby. The client feels valued and closer to achieving his goal to return as a painter.

As illustrated in this example, designing intervention activities involves determining the steps to reach goals, reading the client's cues, listening to the client, and

Table 24-7.

## Using One Activity to Meet Multiple Goals

| Intervention Activity | Occupation Being Addressed | Role of Practitioner | Short-Term Goal |
|---|---|---|---|
| Making a sandwich | Meal preparation | Provide kitchen utensils and lunch supplies. Ask client to make sandwiches as he or she would for family. | Client will independently prepare lunches for a family of four daily for 1 week. |
| | Social participation | In a group setting, require members to share materials, select a menu, and prepare sandwiches. The occupational therapist facilitates social interactions. | Client will spontaneously engage in cooperative social interactions twice during an hour-long group session within 1 week. |
| | Work (fine motor skills) | Provide a variety of spreads, containers to open, different types of utensils to require client to build strength and fine motor coordination. | Client will increase bilateral finger coordination to type 20 words per minute on computer. |

Table 24-8.

## Suggested Activities

| Activity | Description | Goals | Comments |
|---|---|---|---|
| Treasure hunt | Ask a child to follow the written steps to find a treasure. Reinforce the concept of the list. Ask the child to write the steps for an activity to reinforce organization skills. | Increase organization for school | Children will do better if they come up with the system for organizing their work. Be sure to include them in the process and be flexible with the outcome. |
| Lunch group | Have a regular lunch group requiring each client to prepare a part of the meal, depending on his or her ability. When clients are able, require one client to make the entire lunch for the group. Praise the success and have the clients enjoy a lunch break. | Increase ability to prepare meals<br>Increase ability to plan and follow sequential steps<br>Increase hand function | Asking family members, friends, or even other staff members to lunch may help the person feel special and proud of his or her accomplishments. |
| Picture frame | Glue beads on a wooden or cardboard picture frame to decorate it. Place a picture inside the frame upon completion. | Increase hand function<br>Increase activity endurance | Providing a variety of beads, stickers, and paint changes the complexity of the project. |

engaging in therapeutic interactions. Practitioners use creativity and activity analysis to determine intervention activities. Designing intervention activities involves examining multiple factors that influence occupational performance and using therapeutic reasoning to determine the best way to intervene and structure the activity. During the intervention session, practitioners adjust and change (also referred to as *grading and adapting*) activities so that the client is adequately challenged and successful.

## Grading and Adapting

Entry-level occupational therapy practitioners analyze all aspects of activity so that they can design the intervention session to address the client's specific needs and to improve function. Providing clients with the just-right challenge (a challenge that is neither too hard nor too easy) is motivating and therapeutic. If the activity is too difficult or too easy, clients become discouraged or bored and do not want to continue. Therefore, practitioners frequently grade and/or adapt activities so that clients can be successful.

Grading refers to changing the degree of difficulty of an activity so that it is easier or more difficult for the client to complete. Practitioners observe clients as they complete activities and change the degree of difficulty to optimally challenge the client's abilities (Figure 24-4).

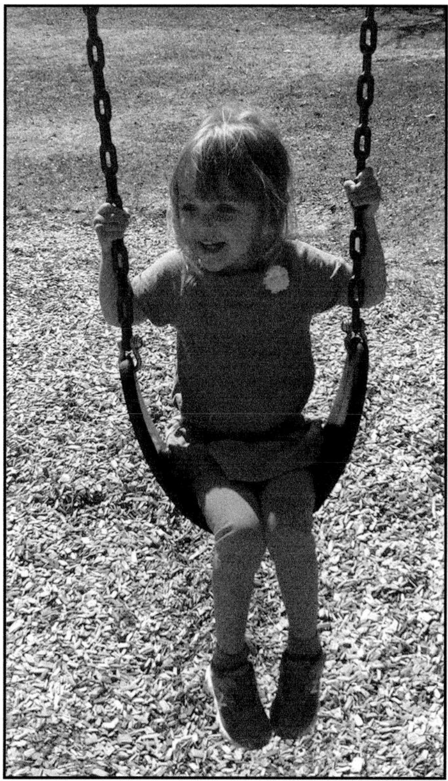

**Figure 24-4.** Grading activity: The young girl swings slowly and low to the ground so she is successful.

Activities may be graded in the following ways:

- Providing more or less direction (consider the type of direction: verbal, demonstrative, written, one-step, two-step)
- Providing more or less physical assistance
- Increasing or decreasing the time requirements
- Adding or subtracting the following:
  - Environmental demands
  - Choices
  - Cognitive or psychological demands
  - Physical demands
  - Social demands
  - Required details

Adapting activities involves changing how the the actual task is completed. Adapting often involves the use of assistive technology, for example, providing clients with a built-up handled spoon to make gripping easier. Other adaptations may include teaching a person to dress using one-hand techniques (Figures 24-5A through C).

Adapting may include the following:

- Technology to change tasks (e.g., cooking food using a microwave instead of an oven)
- Eliminating steps (e.g., buying fruit that has already been cut up) or adding steps
- Performing activities differently (e.g., using food processor instead of cutting vegetables)
- Providing adaptive equipment (e.g., picking things up using a reacher)
- Changing the physical demands of the task (e.g., sitting while dressing)

All activities can be graded or adapted to meet the needs of the client. Practitioners learn to skillfully grade and adapt activities so that the client has success and works toward meeting his or her intervention goals. Occupational therapy practitioners may also address different client factors required to perform by changing the contextual aspects of intervention activities. The goal of therapy is for the client to engage in the occupation in its most natural context. Thus, if the person comes from a large social and/or talkative family, the therapist's job is to help him or her return to this social context. Intervention aimed at having the person return to this environment differs from that in which the client may be returning home with minimal visitors.

## Safety

Throughout the intervention process, the occupational therapy practitioner considers safety issues and addresses the ability of the client to return to occupations

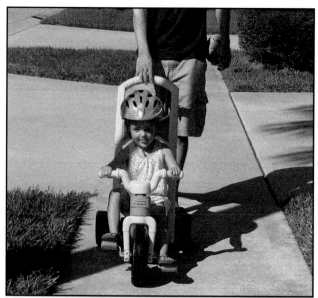

**Figure 24-5A.** Adapting activity: A girl learns to ride a tricycle that has been adapted to make it easier.

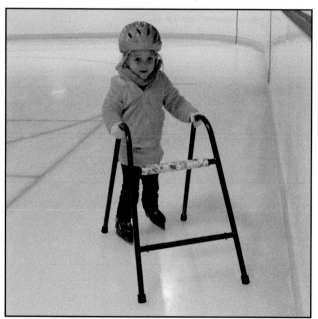

**Figure 24-5B.** Adapting activity: Adapting skating by adding a "walker" for better stability helps this child skate successfully.

in a safe manner. The occupational therapy practitioner carefully watches clients as they perform occupations to determine if judgment, cognition, and physical abilities allow them to be safe. Frequently, the occupational therapist with input from the occupational therapy assistant will perform a home evaluation before discharge to ensure that the environment is safe. The occupational therapy practitioner often adapts and modifies equipment so the client is able to use safety devices (e.g., phone, grab bars). Practitioners use activity analysis skills to evaluate the safety of the environment. They examine how the person performs in the environment and how the environment supports or hinders this performance. The practitioner may also create a safe environment by teaching safety skills (e.g., locking doors).

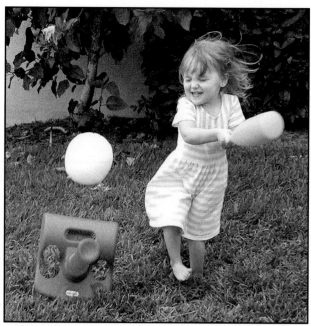

**Figure 24-5C.** Adapting activity: A t-stand adapts softball so that children are more successful.

## Program Development

Occupational therapists with input from occupational therapy assistants may be asked to create programs to meet clients' or groups' needs. Therefore, practitioners benefit from understanding how to develop a sound program. Table 24-9 provides an outline of topics that are included in program development. Like a sound intervention plan, program development begins with a solid understanding of targeted goals. This is best achieved through an understanding of the client population, needs, and setting in which the program will occur, which can be determined through a needs assessment. A needs assessment gathers information from stakeholders, including clients, administrators, and practitioners. Needs assessments provide the practitioner with data on how many people may benefit from the program and what type of program is most beneficial. The data can be obtained through survey, review of existing data, or through a review of literature or existing resources. Once the practitioner understands the need for the program and has collected data to support the program, the practitioner develops activities that address the group's goals while considering the population, setting, and available resources.

Table 24-9.

## Features of Program Development

| Name of Program | Description of Program |
|---|---|
| Purpose | Describes the reason for the program |
| Population (include need) | Outlines the exclusion and inclusion criteria (such as age, gender, developmental level, condition, and diagnoses) |
| Goals and objectives | Clearly identifies the program's goals and objectives |
| Program activities with rationale | Provides an overview of the types of activities and reasoning for the selection |
| Frame of reference or model of practice | Articulates theory and principles guiding therapeutic reasoning |
| Measurements (evaluation and outcomes) | Identifies measurements for evaluation and outcomes and refers to how program and client success will be measured |
| Setting (and space) | Describes physical setting, location, space, and set-up |
| Costs | Explains costs for program to the participant and the agency |
| Equipment and materials | Detailed explanation of materials and equipment required for program |
| Time | Considers time for program, setting up, and cleaning up |
| Number of members of group | Provides a maximum and minimum number of participants for group program |
| Group rules | Details the rules for the program |
| Personnel required | Defines personnel requirements and identifies team members and their roles |
| Procedures, forms, and approvals | Outlines procedures, forms, and approvals needed for program |
| Other | Provides details regarding safety or other considerations for program to run effectively |

Preparation is central to sound program development. Therefore, practitioners examine available literature or research related to the proposed program. Occupational therapy practitioners may use occupational therapy models of practice to develop effective programs. For example, O'Brien et al. (2010) developed the FUN (Fitness, yoU, and Nutrition) program using MOHO as its theoretical model. The FUN program promoted healthy nutritional habits and physical activity in children. Upon reviewing similar programs, practitioners can create goals of the program (Vroman, 2016).

Once the need and goals have been established, the practitioner outlines sample activities, along with timeframe, costs, and setting. Details of the requirements for resources, space, materials, equipment, and transportation are part of program development. It is important to clearly identify personnel needs and associated costs. The practitioner outlines the time, day of week, and nature of the program. A clear description of the rationale for program decisions strengthens the program design. Therefore, practitioners include a review of similar programs with special attention describing how the program will fulfill a unique need.

The program design includes a description of the population for which the program will be created. Practitioners provide information on the population, condition, and intervention strategies and techniques associated with the given population. A review of research evidence adds to this section of the program design. Often times, a description of the theoretical framework underlying the program design is useful and provides practitioners with additional information useful in creating programs.

It is important to develop clear outcome measures when designing a program. These measures provide data to evaluate the effectiveness of the program. When designing a new program, practitioners determine the data they will need to systematically collect for evaluation purposes. For example, practitioners keep records of such things as how many clients benefited from the program, how many clients met their goals, costs, and benefits to the community. Evaluation of outcomes may also include qualitative information from survey or interviews.

## Evidence-Based Research Chart

| Authors | Subjects | Objectives | Definitions | Findings |
|---|---|---|---|---|
| Hetu & Mercier, 2012 | 35 reviewed articles | Provide a review of the literature regarding the influence of object affordance on motor performance, a factor that contributes to the purposefulness of a task. | Three main approaches to increase object affordance relate to number of objects used during task, functional information that the objects convey, and functional goals of the task. | Increasing object affordance produced beneficial effects on motor performance and motor learning. |
| Lee, Lee, & Jung, 2015 | 25 occupational therapy undergraduate students | Investigate the changes from resting of the evoked cortical activity when participants performed three levels of activity. | Adjunctive: activity that focuses on facilitation or inhibiting motion.<br>Enabling: activity that prepares patients for purposeful activity by simulating purposeful activity.<br>Purposeful: activity with a meaningful goal for patient and focus on specific self-care, home management, work, or leisure tasks that are relevant to person.<br>Occupation: activities carried out in the "lived in" environment or community. | Purposeful activity was most complex and generated more brain activity (alpha waves) than adjunctive and enabling. (The authors did not examine occupation.) |
| Orellano, Colon, & Arbesman, 2012 | Systematic review (40 studies) | Examine the effectiveness of occupation and activity-based interventions on community-dwelling older adults' performance of IADLs. | Multicomponent interventions include those provided by more than one discipline. | Evidence that multicomponent interventions improve and maintain IADL performance in community-dwelling older adults is strong. Evidence is moderate for functional task exercise programs and limited for simulated IADL interventions. |
| Wolf, Chuh, Floyd, McInnis, & Williams, 2015 | Systematic review (39 studies) | Examine the evidence supporting the use of occupation-based intervention to improve areas of occupation and social participation post stroke. | Most of the literature targeted ADLs. Interventions included tasks training, repetitive practice, retraining family, Bobath treatment, high intensity dosage of therapy, therapeutic recreation, and high dosage of therapy. | Strong evidence to support use of occupation-based interventions to improve ADL performance in inpatient settings and community settings. |

## Summary

Planning intervention involves determining occupation-based goals, adapting and grading activities, and being mindful of the influence of context on the success of the activity. Intervention planning requires a clear evaluation of the client's strengths and weaknesses and collaboration on occupation-based goals. The occupational therapy practitioner bases intervention on a well-developed frame of reference. The materials, activities, and techniques used vary with clients and goals. Practitioners also develop programs for clients and groups and create clear evaluation guidelines to determine the effectiveness of the programming.

## Student Self-Assessment

1. Develop an activity. Decide on the age, client population, goals, and purpose of the activity. Describe how the activity can be adapted or modified to meet various clients' needs.

2. Analyze the performance skills, client factors, activity demands, and context(s) involved to complete one chosen activity. Provide a detailed description of the steps to complete the activity.
3. Conduct an activity with classmates role-playing different client issues. Discuss how to intervene and change the activity so that each classmate is successful.
4. Interview a person from a culture different from your own. Discuss occupations of importance to him or her and the activities involved. Present the activity to the class, discussing the importance of this to the culture. Provide directions for each class member.
5. Compile a notebook of activities that you may use in clinical settings. Include website references and handouts that may be helpful. Organize the activities so that you can readily find an appropriate one for a client.
6. Examine an occupation prevalent in your area (e.g., lobsterman, basket weaver). What are the skills, client factors, habits, and contextual aspects of this activity? How could you adapt or grade the activity?
7. Find a local resource that may help a client (e.g., recreational center, therapeutic horseback riding center). Find out the cost, benefits, times, and services provided. Share these with your classmates.
8. Develop a program to meet the needs of a population in the community. Identify the goal, activities, space, setting, equipment, and financial resources needed. Determine personnel needs.

## References


American Occupational Therapy Association. (2014a). Guidelines for supervision, roles, and responsibilities during the delivery of occupational therapy services. *American Journal of Occupational Therapy, 68*, S16. doi:10.5014/ajot.2014.686s03

American Occupational Therapy Association. (2014b). Occupational therapy practice framework: Domain and process (3rd ed.). *American Journal of Occupational Therapy, 68*(Suppl. 1), S1-S48. doi:10.5014/ajot.2014.682006

Ayres, A. J. (1979). *Sensory integration and the child.* Los Angeles, CA: Western Psychological Services.

Bobath, B. (1975). Sensorimotor development. *NDT Newsletter, 7*, 1.

Christiansen, C., & Baum, C. M. (1997). Person-environment occupational performance: A conceptual model for practice. In C. Christiansen & C. M. Baum (Eds.), *Occupational therapy: Enabling function and well-being* (2nd ed.). Thorofare, NJ: SLACK Incorporated.

Curran, C., Williams, A. C., & Potts, H. W. (2009). Cognitive-behavioral therapy for persistent pain: Does adherence after treatment affect outcome? *European Journal of Pain, 13*(2), 178-188.

Fisher, A. G. (1998). Uniting practice and theory in an occupational framework. 1998 Eleanor Clarke Slagle lecture. *American Journal of Occupational Therapy, 52*(7), 509-521.

Forsyth, K., Mann, L. S., & Kielhofner, G. (2005). Scholarship of practice: Making occupation-focused, theory-driven, evidence-based practice a reality. *British Journal of Occupational Therapy, 68*(6), 260-268.

Gillen, G. (2013). A fork in the road: An occupational hazard? (Eleanor Clarke Slagle Lecture). *American Journal of Occupational Therapy, 67*, 641-652.

Hetu, S., & Mercier, C. (2012). Using purposeful tasks to improve motor performance: Does object affordance matter? *British Journal of Occupational Therapy, 75*(8), 367-376.

Kielhofner, G. (1985). *A model of human occupation: Theory and application* (3rd ed.). Baltimore, MD: Lippincott Williams and Wilkins.

Kielhofner, G. (2008). *A model of human occupation: Theory and application* (4th ed.). Baltimore, MD: Lippincott Williams and Wilkins.

Law, M., Cooper, B. A., Strong, S., Stewart, D., Rigby, P., & Letts, L. (1996). The person-environment-occupation model: A transactive approach to occupational performance. *Canadian Journal of Occupational Therapy, 63*(1), 9-23.

Law M. L., Cooper, B. A., Strong, S., Stewart, D., Rigby, P., & Letts, L. (1997). Theoretical contexts for practice of occupational therapy. In C. H. Christiansen & C. M. Baum (Eds.), *Occupational therapy: Enabling function and well-being* (2nd ed.). Thorofare, NJ: SLACK Incorporated.

Lee, S. A., Lee, S. H., & Jung, B. K. (2015). Analysis of cortical activation during three types of therapeutic activity. *Journal of Physical Therapy Science, 27*, 1219-1222.

Lee, S. W., Taylor, R., Kielhofner, G., & Fisher, G. (2008). Theory use in practice: A national survey of therapists who use the Model of Human Occupation. *American Journal of Occupational Therapy, 62*(1), 106-117.

Llorens, L. A. (1976). *Application of a developmental theory for health and rehabilitation.* Rockville, MD: AOTA Press.

MacRae, N. (2001). *Unpublished lecture notes: OT 301 foundations of occupational therapy.* Biddeford, ME: University of New England.

Maurer, T., Smith, D., & Armetta, C. (1989). Purposeful activity as exercise. *Occupational Therapy in Mental Health, 9*, 9-20.

Melchert-McKearnan, K., Dietz, J., Engel, J. M., & White, O. (2000). Children with burn injuries: Purposeful activity versus rote exercise. *American Journal of Occupational Therapy, 54*(4), 381-390.

Miltner, W. H., Bauder, H., Sommers, M., Dettmers, C., & Taub, E. (1999). Effects of constraint-induced movement therapy on patients with chronic motor deficits after stroke: A replication. *Stroke, 30*, 586-592.

Mosey, A. C. (1981). *Occupational therapy: Configuration of a profession.* New York, NY: Raven Press.

O'Brien, J., Craib, C., Holmes, L., Keough, K., LePage, L., & O'Brien, E. (2010). *FUN program (Phase I): Development of the Fitness, yoU, and Nutrition (FUN) after school program to improve wellness in elementary school children.* Porland, ME: University of New England.

Orellano, E., Colon, W., & Arbesman, M. (2012). Effect of occupation and activity-based interventions on instrumental activities of daily living performance among community-dwelling older adults: A systematic review. *American Journal of Occupational Therapy, 66*, 292-300.

Pedretti, L. W., & Paszuinielli, S. (1990). A frame of reference for occupational therapy in physical dysfunction. In L. W. Pedretti & B. Zoltan (Eds.), *Occupational therapy: Practice skills for physical dysfunction* (3rd ed., pp. 1-17) St. Louis, MO: Mosby.

Schkade, J. K., & Schultz, S. (1992). Occupational adaptation: Toward a holistic approach in contemporary practice, part I. *American Journal of Occupational Therapy, 46*(9), 829-837.

Schoen, S., & Anderson, J. (1993). Neurodevelopmental treatment frame of reference. In P. Kramer & J. Hinojosa (Eds.), *Frames of reference for pediatric occupational therapy.* Baltimore, MD: Lippincott Williams and Wilkins.

Schoen, S., & Anderson, J. (1999). Neurodevelopmental treatment frame of reference. In P. Kramer & J. Hinojosa (Eds.), *Frames of reference for pediatric occupational therapy* (2nd ed.). Philadelphia, PA: Lippincott Williams and Wilkins.

Shumway-Cook, A., & Woollacott, M. (2007). *Motor control: Theory and practical applications.* Philadelphia, PA: Lippincott Williams and Wilkins.

Solomon, J. W., & O'Brien, J. C. (2016). The occupational therapy process. In J. W. Solomon & J. C. O'Brien (Eds.), *Pediatric skills for occupational therapy assistants* (4th ed., pp. 137-160). St. Louis, MO: Mosby.

Steinbeck, T. M. (1986). Purposeful activity and performance. *American Journal of Occupational Therapy, 40*(8), 529-534.

Taub, E., Miller, N. E., Novack, T. A., Cook, E. W. 3rd., Fleming, W. C., Nepomuceno, C. S., et al. (1993). Technique to improve motor deficit after stroke. *Archives of Physical Medicine and Rehabilitation, 74*, 347-354.

Townsend, E., Brintnell, S., & Staisey, N. (1990). Developing guidelines for client-centered occupational therapy practice. *Canadian Journal of Occupational Therapy, 57*(2), 69-76.

Turk, D. C., Meichenbaum, D., & Genest, M. (1983). *Pain and behavioral medicine: A cognitive behavioral perspective*. New York, NY: Guilford Press.

Vroman, K. (2016). Childhood and adolescent obesity. In J. W. Solomon & J. C. O'Brien (Eds.), *Pediatric skills for occupational therapy assistants* (4th ed.). St. Louis, MO: Mosby.

Warshaw, S. P. (2010). *Hawaii Early Learning Profile (HELP) 0 - 3*. Menlo Park, CA: Vort Corporation.

Wolf, T. J., Chuh, A., Floyd, T., McInnis, K., & Williams, E. (2015). Effectiveness of occupation-based interventions to improve areas of occupation and social participation after stroke: An evidence-based review. *American Journal of Occupational Therapy, 69*, 1-13.

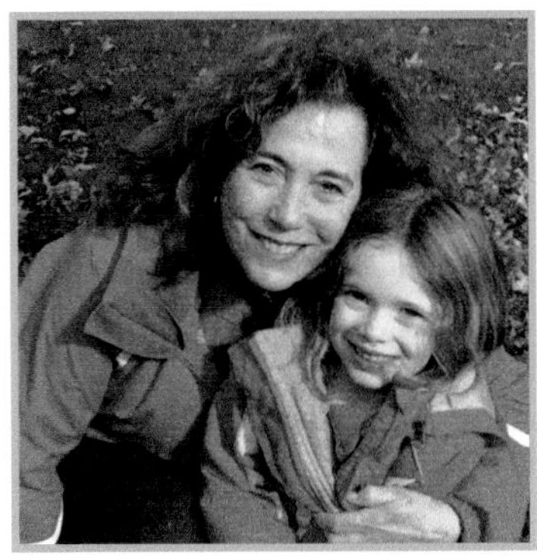

# 25

# Client Factors in Occupational Performance Functioning

Regula H. Robnett, PhD, OTR/L, FAOTA and Jessica J. Bolduc, DrOT, MS, OTR/L

## ACOTE Standards Explored in This Chapter

B.5.6

## Key Vocabulary

- **Anosmia:** Lack of sense of smell.
- **Decubitus ulcers:** Pressure sores due to excessive pressure on or shearing of the skin.
- **Errorless learning:** Learning a skill without making mistakes in performance during the learning process.
- **Executive skills:** Complex cognitive skills (e.g., weighing options, problem solving, multitask planning, and self-monitoring).
- **Ideational apraxia:** Loss of skilled movement patterns that make up task performance, based on the loss of the conceptual idea of performing the task (not on sensorimotor dysfunction).
- **Ideomotor apraxia:** Loss of skilled movement patterns that make up task performance, based on "the loss of access to kinesthetic memory patterns" (Gillen, 2009, p. 112).
- **Isometric contractions:** Muscle contraction during which the muscle maintains a constant muscle length.
- **Isotonic contractions:** Muscle contraction during which the muscle belly shortens while activated.
- **Kinesthesia:** Perception of the direction and movement of one's body and limbs in space.
- **Proprioception:** Perception of a joint's position in space.
- **Task-specific training:** Direct training in tasks without the expectation of generalization of learning.



Jacobs, K., & MacRae, N. (Eds.).
*Occupational Therapy Essentials for Clinical Competence, Third Edition* (pp. 359-382).

Occupational therapy practitioners work with people who have a variety of impairments (and many strengths). The authors acknowledge that these impairments are rarely encountered in isolation. In this chapter, the major categories of impairments are presented in separate sections to more clearly and succinctly explain each one at a fundamental level. During occupational therapy intervention, practitioners use combinations of techniques simultaneously to work holistically on one or more aspects of occupational functioning. This chapter presents a broad overview of occupational therapy interventions focused on providing developmental, remediation, and/or compensatory measures to enhance performance in the realms of physical (including neuromuscular), cognitive (including mental and perceptual), and behavioral skills. Sensory functions (e.g., vision, tactile, auditory, gustatory, olfactory, pain, temperature, pressure, vestibular, proprioception) are also briefly considered. Each section provides a definition and overview of the specific aspect and reviews some of the more common occupational therapy interventions currently in use. Brief overviews of evidence-based practice are included whenever possible.

## Certified Occupational Therapy Assistants

Throughout this chapter, clinicians involved in the intervention process are referred to as occupational therapy practitioners. This is done intentionally because the Accreditation Council for Occupational Therapy Education (ACOTE) Standard on which this chapter is based is exactly the same for both the registered occupational therapist and the certified occupational therapy assistant. Both professionals have the intention of carrying out interventions using clinical reasoning based on occupational therapy principles and evidence-based practice. However, the title occupational therapist is used when referring to the practitioner with a more advanced professional role such as that of an evaluator.

## Intervention Within the *Occupational Therapy Practice Framework*

The occupational therapy process, as described in the *Occupational Therapy Practice Framework* (American Occupational Therapy Association [AOTA], 2014), involves intervention planning, implementation, and follow-up. Although intervention is the core of the occupational therapy process, to be intentionally effective, the intervention phase needs to be based on a comprehensive occupational therapy evaluation appropriate for the setting and the client. The process of intervention planning should incorporate solid theoretical underpinnings and relevant evidence and practice-based research to the extent available. The process, which involves the practitioner working with one or more clients, includes the following types of interventions: creating or promoting, establishing or restoring, maintaining, modifying or compensating, or preventing. The ultimate goal of occupational therapy intervention is "engagement in occupation" or successful participation in those areas of occupation that have personal meaning for the client. Intervention techniques can follow a more functional, real-life "top-down" approach (Trombly, 1993), which includes engagement in occupational tasks as primary aspects of each intervention session, or a "bottom-up" approach, in which therapeutic sessions focus more on the underlying client performance skills or factors (with the intention of transferring these skills to broader occupations outside of the session). Performance skills include motor skills and process skills, whereas client factors include mental functions, sensory functions, neuromuscular and movement-related functions, and bodily functions (AOTA, 2014).

The *Framework* (AOTA, 2014) outlines aspects of performance skills to include motor and praxis, cognitive skills, sensory perceptual, and emotional/behavioral regulation. Each of these skill areas involves actions and behaviors of the client that promote occupational performance. For example, praxis involves planned and sequential motor acts (of any body part that moves) to carry out the motoric aspects of an occupational task. These performance skills are as varied as our occupations and are embedded in all areas of occupation. This chapter includes performance skill areas, but we use the language of the ACOTE Standard.

## Guides for Intervention

Models of practice are outlines used in occupational therapy, based on theory, and are used to conceptualize and guide practice. Models of practice inform decision making to define the evidence-based intervention process, especially in specialized practice areas. This can in turn aid in the justification of reimbursement for occupational therapy services (Miller & Schwartz, 2004).

A frame of reference is "derived from theory and makes use of concepts, definitions, and postulates from a theory or theories…provides principles for action…and can guide the practitioner's decisions" (Ludwig, 2004a, p. 79). Anne Cronin Mosey first started defining frames of reference for practice in the 1970s; she describes frames of reference containing four parts (Ludwig, 2004a, p. 80):

1. Statement of the theoretical basis
2. Delineation of function and dysfunction continua
3. Evaluation
4. Postulates regarding change

The major difference when comparing models of practice and frames of reference is that a model of practice looks to define and guide occupational therapy practice as a whole. A frame of reference links theory to practice in defined areas of occupational therapy practice. Before practitioners can plan interventions for a client, they must reflect on the model of practice and/or frame of reference to be used to guide their clinical reasoning process. Students and recent graduates may have to make more of a conscious effort with this process. Seasoned practitioners tend to evaluate and provide intervention seemingly without considering models of practice and/or frames of reference. With reflection, all practitioners should be able to define what theoretical underpinnings are guiding their practice.

## Intervention Related to Physical Performance

Physical performance generally relies on the supervisory control exerted by the brain. Intact neurological connections within the brain plan and send efferent messages distally to execute the movement in question. The brain provides the control center for motor performance, but the person also needs intact musculature in order to complete movement and manipulation tasks. The aspects of physical performance of primary concern in occupational therapy intervention at the impairment level are range of motion (ROM), strength, balance, coordination, and functional mobility. Successfully completing occupational tasks requires at least minimal levels of ability in these client factors, or the use of adaptations or compensatory measures. The occupational therapist can complete an in-depth activity analysis to determine the specific physical demands of any task under consideration. Ideally, if the task currently exceeds the client's capabilities based on the results of the analysis, the practitioner can then determine how to assist the person by adapting the task or the environment. The physical factors described are applicable for all age groups, but not all people need to be equally capable in all areas to be successful and to feel fulfilled occupationally.

### Biomechanical-Rehabilitation Frame of Reference

As discussed in more detail in other chapters, frames of reference help practitioners guide the way they structure intervention plans. The biomechanical frame of reference is a bottom-up approach to therapy that works well under many different models of practice. The principles that compose this frame of reference, as explained by Cole and Tufano (2008), include ROM, strength, endurance, kinematics, and torque. This frame of reference requires practitioners to look at the underlying musculoskeletal structures when creating the intervention plan for a client. Although this may be a useful tool when trying to understand the biomechanics of a movement, it is a somewhat limited frame of reference in that it does not include the more holistic psychosocial aspects of human motor performance. The rehabilitation frame of reference seeks to enable the highest level of function for occupational performance. Using principles that address underlying musculoskeletal structures to promote recovery, the rehabilitation frame of reference looks to maximize independence through modifying the environment or instructing in the use of adaptive equipment.

### Occupational Adaptation Frame of Reference

Occupational adaptation has been described by Schultz and Schkade over the past two decades as "an internal adaptation process that occurs through engagement in occupation and for successful occupational engagement" using developmental and environmental contexts (Ludwig, 2004b, p. 397). Clients who are able to adapt to their environment are able to function successfully; thus, disability occurs when the client is not able to adapt. Occupational therapy intervention can support the adaptation process to improve occupational performance. This frame of reference spans the life span and all populations.

### Disorders Affecting Physical Performance

When considering physical performance in the scope of biomechanical or rehabilitation frames of reference, common disorders typically are orthopedic in nature, whether elective or accidental. According to the Centers for Disease Control and Prevention (CDC; 2014a), in 2010 there were more than 700,000 elective knee joint replacements, more than 330,000 elective hip joint replacements, and more than 670,000 surgical repairs of fractures. Elective surgeries are increasing in popularity as they can offer pain relief and increase the client's ability to reengage in daily occupations. Hip fractures related to falls account for at least 95% of the 250,000 hospitalizations per year for older adults (CDC, 2015b). Clients undergoing hip surgery from a fall as compared to elective surgeries have a higher level of mortality and complications (LeManach et al., 2015). When occupational therapy services are implemented as soon as possible when medically appropriate, clients are more likely to reach independent levels of occupational performance faster, have shorter hospital stays, and fewer complications (Khan, Ng, Gonzalez, Hale, & Turner-Stokes, 2008). Using intervention approaches utilizing biomechanical or rehabilitation frames of reference can be very beneficial.

Other chronic conditions, such as chronic obstructive pulmonary disease (COPD), congestive heart failure, or chronic renal failure, can also affect a client's endurance and strength and thus occupational performance. In 2009, there were 1.9 million adults with COPD in the United States, with the highest cases in the age range of 75- to 84-year-old adults, with 30,000 adults needing to be hospitalized at some point during the year (Akinbami & Liu, 2011). As of 2010, the CDC reports an average of 400,000 deaths occur annually from COPD, as this lung disease blocks air flow (CDC, 2014b). As for congestive heart failure, when the heart cannot pump enough blood through the body, this condition accounted for 5.8 million adults over the age of 65 and 1 million hospitalizations per year (CDC, 2012). In 2014, 20 million adults in the United States had renal disease with more than 100,000 having end-stage renal disease, which can result in requiring dialysis (mechanical filtering of waste from the blood; CDC, 2014c). These are just a few examples of chronic illnesses that can result in poor health, hospitalization, immobility, and decreased physical ability to perform daily occupations. A practitioner could utilize a biomechanical, rehabilitation, and/or occupational adaptation approach to intervention to maximize physical performance.

## Range of Motion and Strength

As part of a therapeutic evaluation, the occupational therapist needs to at least screen for dysfunction in the realms of ROM and strength. The human body has more than 430 voluntary muscles that move all moveable body parts. For the extremities to be considered "normal" (i.e., within normal limits), people need to be able to move their limbs through full ROM and be able to withstand the application of a maximal amount of resistance during manual muscle testing. Before being able to lift additional weight beyond the weight of the limb or before being able to resist outside pressure, the limb must be able to move through full ROM (unless ROM is compromised by a joint obstruction). As learned through the study of kinesiology, every joint in the human body has a normal or usual ROM. If the joint is compromised in some way through injury, disease, or disuse, then performance in life tasks could be affected, and ROM needs to be addressed as a part of therapeutic intervention. Depending on the cause of the decrease, it may be appropriate to attempt to improve joint mobility through ROM exercises, joint mobilization, and stretching.

When exercises are used in occupational therapy, the use of active ROM is preferred to passive ROM whenever possible. If the client is incapacitated (e.g., if the client is in a coma), active ROM on command is not an option. Those who cannot move limbs on one side of the body (as in hemiparesis secondary to acquired brain injury) may be able to learn to complete a self-ROM program, giving them a degree of control over their movement patterns. Engaging the client in a ROM program (either through exercise or functional activity) is necessary to avoid contractures of the joints caused by immobilization, as well as to provide the person with some degree of normal proprioceptive input, which may enhance personal awareness of the body and the environment.

When ROM is compromised, strength is generally impaired as well. After a client has obtained the maximum ROM for a joint, strength training involving resistance usually begins. "Strength is the capacity of a muscle to exert or endure movement; such as moving a limb, results of complex interactions of neurologic, biomechanical, and cognitive systems" (Hall & Brody, 2005, p. 58). As with ROM, strength can be compromised with the onset of injury, disease, or disuse. Examples include, but are not limited to, spinal cord injury, acquired brain injury, a physical injury to a muscle or joint, or a sedentary lifestyle. Compromised ROM and strength can affect functioning in nearly every occupation. Therefore, physical performance involving ROM and building strength is an important aspect of intervention for many clients.

To increase the strength of a muscle, it needs to contract repeatedly at near maximal capacity. Muscle strengthening involves the utilization of different types of contractions. An isotonic contraction occurs when a muscle shortens in length, such as when a weight is lifted against gravity. An isometric contraction, in comparison, involves holding a muscle contraction at an increased tension point in the muscle. During this type of contraction, the muscle is not shortening while contracting, but rather staying the same length for the duration of the tightening. Exercise groups or individual exercise sessions in occupational therapy often use repeated isotonic contractions with weights and resistance bands. Isometric contractions are used when the limb is immobile, but resisting either an immovable or potentially movable force (e.g., the former may be a wall, while the latter may be a challenging opponent, as in sports). While muscles do need to fatigue to gain strength, overfatiguing muscles can be more damaging than beneficial (Miller Keene, 2003). Soreness can result after one engages in an exercise program, but significant pain should not. Throughout the therapy session, pain should be monitored periodically because it can affect the client's recovery, as well as the client's quality of movement. The practitioner must communicate with the client to ensure that pain is not interfering with overall performance. Pain is considered as an aspect of intervention in a separate section in this chapter.

Making a direct connection between the client's interests, hobbies, or daily activities and the exercise program has shown better adherence rates and outcomes compared to rote exercise alone. This contention is supported by research by Hoppe, Kopp Miller, and Rice (2008) who found that when occupationally embedded exercise is used in comparison to rote exercise, participants experienced better physical and emotional response with regard to level of engagement and motivation. In an interesting aside to usual exercise training, one study compared an exercise program including a virtual reality bicycle exercise tour with a control program just involving the physical exercises. Lee (2015) found the use of virtual reality for exercise in clients post-stroke aided in the improvement of cognitive function, upper extremity motor function, and activities of daily living (ADL) performance. This finding highlights, once again, the interconnectedness of physical and cognitive client factors. Strength training has been shown to decrease resting heart rate, normalize blood pressure, increase cardiac output, and it may lower bad cholesterol levels (Hall & Brody, 2005). Proper diaphragmatic breathing techniques should be incorporated into all strength and ROM exercise programs. Not breathing deeply enough or holding one's breath during exertion can be dangerous, especially for those with compromised cardiac systems (such as when one engages in the Valsalva maneuver).

Resistance training benefits for healthy adults include increased bone strength and muscular fitness. Resistance training, including weight training, can include working with resistance bands, "doing calisthenics that use body weight for resistance (such as push-ups, pull-ups, and sit-ups), carrying heavy loads, and heavy gardening (such as digging or hoeing)" (Office of Disease Prevention and Health Promotion, 2015). The *Physical Activity Guidelines* (Office of Disease Prevention and Health Promotion, 2015) recommend 150 minutes to 300 (5 hours) minutes of moderate-intensity activity a week (or 75 to 150 minutes of vigorous-intensity physical activity a week) for adults 18 to 64 years old. Although discomfort can be acceptable as tolerated, a high level of pain should be avoided, especially if any movement used causes the level of pain to escalate. Any exercise program should be geared to the individual (e.g., physical and health status, personal goals) and can be beneficial even if the recommended parameters for repetitions and frequency cannot be met (Garber et al., 2011).

The sources mentioned previously also recommend strength training for populations who have physical impairments. However, the program would be expected to start at a lower intensity level and the progression would be expected to be slower. Lower intensity level exercise involves activity beyond baseline but fewer than 150 minutes (2 hours and 30 minutes) of moderate-intensity physical activity per week (Office of Disease Prevention and Health Promotion, 2015). Progression to more resistance should occur every week or two if possible, when the person can lift the current weight comfortably a dozen times but still perceives the intensity to be difficult. These guidelines apply to all adult age groups. Sedentary older people, however, may need to start with weights of 2 pounds or even less, take more care in stabilizing at the hip, and may do better on machines not requiring the exerciser to have normal postural control (Feigenbaum, 2001). Few guidelines for specific client populations are available, highlighting the need for further empirical research. Interesting, creative, and occupationally based research projects could involve comparing rote ROM and strength training to the use of repetitive functional tasks such as leisure sports, hobbies, or home management skills.

### Endurance

Endurance as a physical component of occupational therapy intervention is included here only as an adjunct to the other physical aspects of intervention. Decreased endurance manifests itself as an inability to carry through repetitive motions or sustained resistance over time. It results in a decreased ability to complete daily tasks because the person lacks energy. Clients are not likely to be referred to occupational therapy intervention for impaired endurance alone. However, decreased strength is often coupled with lowered endurance. Each contraction of a weakened muscle uses a larger proportion of the overall performance capacity, resulting in the muscle fatiguing more quickly. When aiming to build muscle strength, a high-load regimen with a lower number of repetitions is preferred, but when the focus is on building endurance, a lower amount of resistance or weight over a greater number of repetitions has been determined to be more effective (Breines, 2006).

### Balance/Postural Control

Intact balance or postural control is a prerequisite for safe, ambulatory, functional mobility. Since many daily occupations involve ambulating or moving from one place to another, postural control is an important consideration for the occupational therapy practitioner. This is especially true for practitioners working with those who have sustained acquired brain injuries or who have diagnoses associated with impaired balance such as multiple sclerosis or cerebral palsy. According to Peterson and Clemson (2008), occupational therapy practitioners are well suited to working with elders on fall prevention and rehabilitation due to the profession's in-depth understanding of physical functioning and the contextual and intrinsic factors affecting balance, as well as the practitioner's ability to implement multifactorial, evidence-based interventions. Falls are common among the elderly, with about one-third of community-living elders falling annually (CDC, 2015a). One direct cause of falls is decreased postural control. Balance training can occur in groups, on an individual basis by providing balance exercises and education, or through occupational therapy–related interventions such as virtual reality or Tai Chi courses. In their systematic review, Choi and Hector (2012) determined that fall prevention interventions are often effective in reducing falls by 9%. A number of studies have now been completed on Tai Chi as an intervention to improve balance and strength with overall positive results (e.g., Han et al., 2004; Li et al., 2005; Taylor-Piliae, Haskell, Stotts, & Froehlicher, 2006). An evidence-based review conducted by Nilsen et al. (2015) found that clients post-stroke who participated in repetitive task practice, constraint-induced or modified constraint-induced movement therapy, strengthening and exercise, mental practice, virtual reality, mirror therapy, and action observation (observing with the intent to imitate) can improve upper extremity function, balance and mobility, and/or activity and participation. In two recent studies, both mental practice (Hosseini, Fallahpour, Sayadi, Gharib, & Haghgoo, 2012) and virtual reality balance training (Cho, Lee, & Song, 2012) were shown to improve dynamic balance in older adults post-stroke. A more general community-based course intended to improve balance is called "Stepping On," a 7-week program offered to people 70 years of age and older in Australia. Clemson et al. (2004) reported that the "Stepping On" program resulted in a 31% reduction in falls (p = .025), and that the program was particularly effective for men. A "Matter of Balance," designed by rehabilitation scientists at Boston University, is a similar 8-week program that uses volunteer instructors with occupational therapy and physical therapy consultants or visiting instructors. Chen, Edwards, and Janke (2015) conducted a prospective cohort study and found that the "Matter of Balance" program was effective in reducing falls and reducing the physical risks for falls among older adults.

In a systematic review of 19 randomized controlled trials of interventions to decrease fear of falling, Zijlstra et al. (2007) found overwhelming support for the effectiveness of interventions (including Tai Chi, "Matter of Balance," "Stepping On," and other multifactorial balance programs). Along with a decreased fear of falling, Zijlstra and colleagues also recommended looking at functional outcomes for balance programs (e.g., decreased incidence of falling and increased safe engagement in meaningful activities).

Besides remediating balance through the interventions mentioned, occupational therapy practitioners play a significant role in ensuring safety by helping the client to compensate when balance is impaired. Compensatory safety measures can involve removing clutter from the home and improving organization in the living space. Adaptive equipment such as safety bars, bath seats, and long-handled dustpans can facilitate successful occupational performance in the client's customary daily tasks. Education on fall prevention is a crucial component of occupational therapy in this realm as well. For example, if older people understand the factors affecting balance and the ways to make the environment safer, they are more likely to feel a higher degree of efficacy related to balance and to complete mobility tasks with more awareness of proper body mechanics.

### Case Study 1

Oscar is a 76-year-old single man with chronic emphysema who enjoys hunting, fishing, walking his dogs, and hiking. Recently, Oscar has come down with a cold he cannot seem to get rid of; he has become more sedentary and is not engaging in his normal leisurely occupations. Due to his acute sedentary lifestyle, Oscar has become weaker and has had a fall at home where he was not able to get up. Luckily Oscar does not have any fractures or serious injuries. Oscar was admitted to the hospital with acute exacerbation of his emphysema. During his hospital stay, occupational therapy services were initiated. The occupational therapist completed a thorough evaluation and found that because of Oscar's shortness of breath he has poor endurance for his basic ADLs and his leisurely pursuits. Additionally, Oscar is interested in learning more about strategies for how to manage his chronic condition to be able to complete his ADLs and would like to exercise to regain his lost strength, endurance, and balance.

## Intervention Related to Neuromuscular Disorders

Neuromuscular disorders are a combination of cognitive and physical impairments, often with accompanying sensory dysfunction. This discussion will focus on motor control, which encompasses coordination and movement in general. According to Shumway-Cook and Woollacott (2012), motor control is the brain's ability to regulate the mechanisms required for movement. Movement is the result of neuromuscular interactions involving sensory input to the brain. The central nervous system organizes and interprets this input and then directs subsequent physical actions. When functioning at an adequate level, motor control allows the person to complete essential and optional daily tasks. Intact perceptual and cognitive processes are necessary to carry through purposeful and efficient movement. For example, tossing and catching a ball, feeding oneself, and writing numbers and letters all represent skills that require a high degree of coordination or motor control. The reader should be aware that there are several theories of motor control (reflex, hierarchical, systems, dynamic action, and ecological) and that entire textbooks have been written about this subject. Shumway-Cook and Woollacott (2012) provide a comprehensive resource for those seeking more detail.

## Motor Control Frame of Reference

*Motor control* is the term used to explain how the different body systems interact to perform skilled motor movement. The systems of sensory, motor, and cognition must work with each other to achieve movement (Shumway-Cook & Woollacott, 2012). Through practice or experience, motor control can be improved. Motor learning has occurred when practice or experience has made a positive change in the performance of a motor movement through the use of random and variable practice, decreased amounts of assistance, and through active participation (Mathiowetz, 2011). Although aspects of motor control cover the entire lifespan, the focus for occupational therapy practitioners using motor control models or frames of reference is on initial motor learning in the young and in relearning movement patterns in adults, specifically those with a diagnosis or condition that impairs normal movement.

The ultimate goal of the intervention is to improve occupational performance through the use of the most effective movement patterns possible. While evidence-based practice exists within this realm, it is lacking in its scope. Much has been written in occupational therapy and physical therapy literature about different aspects of motor control intervention, including assessment of motor control, types of learning, types of practice, practice schedules, instructions, and the parameters surrounding feedback. In guiding intervention, Mathiowetz (2011) contends that optimal motor learning is best achieved through occupational therapy intervention that is both individualized and allows for active experimentation, as well as being occupation-based in the client's natural environment.

## Disorders Affecting Motor Control

Cerebral palsy and developmental coordination disorder are two common diagnoses causing movement impairments in children, whereas acquired brain injuries, multiple sclerosis, and Parkinson's disease are common diagnoses interfering with normal movement in adults. Research conducted on motor control and motor learning focuses on the different intervention strategies that occupational therapy practitioners can utilize to improve motor control. More occupation-based research projects in this intervention area, as well in other intervention areas, need to be undertaken. Often in studies examining motor relearning, the Functional Independence Measure is used as an outcome measure, especially to show the gains in motor control in stroke survivors' hemiparetic limbs with the use of constraint-induced movement therapy. In an evidence-based review, Nilson et al. (2011) found evidence for the use of modified constraint-induced movement therapy with clients post-stroke to improve motor control of the hemiparetic limb via 30-minute to 3-hour sessions that range from 2 to 5 days week.

A few research-based articles specifically address the effectiveness of techniques designed to promote the development or relearning of motor skills. They generally compare one type of motor control intervention to another. A study conducted by Hayner, Gibson, and Giles (2010) compared the effectiveness of constraint-induced movement therapy with bilateral treatment of equal intensity for chronic upper extremity dysfunction caused by cerebrovascular accident. "Treatment activities were designed to promote function and active range of motion, were routine and purposeful (e.g., setting the table, washing hands, washing dishes), and were intended to be meaningful, but they were not client-selected occupations (i.e., client-preferred meaningful customary activities)" (Hayner et al., 2010, p. 531). Results suggested that high-intensity occupational therapy using a constraint-induced movement therapy or a bilateral approach can improve upper extremity function in people with chronic upper extremity dysfunction after stroke. In a physiotherapy review that focused on intervention of postural control for those who had sustained a stroke, Pollock, Baer, Pomeroy, and Langhorne (2007) compared orthopedic, neurophysiologic, and motor learning approaches. They determined that one approach was not significantly more effective than the others for improving balance. Since occupational therapy practitioners also work in the realm of postural control, this finding, imprecise as it is, still has meaning for the profession and highlights—once again—the need for more occupation-based research projects in this intervention area and beyond.

## Intervention Involving Functional Activities

While specific types of motor control intervention approaches may not be overwhelmingly better than others based on the research available thus far, a few studies did come to a conclusion that greatly affects the practice of occupational therapy. In a meta-analysis of randomized controlled trials, Park, Maitra, and Martinez (2015) found occupation-based cognitive rehabilitation interventions for clients with traumatic brain injuries have the potential to improve cognitive function and performance of ADLs. Similarly, the systematic review by Orellano, Colon, and Arbesman (2012) found client-centered, occupation-based interventions provide strong evidence in improving and maintaining instrumental ADL performance while exercise and simulated task has only moderate to limited evidence in improvement of performance. To occupational therapy practitioners, the conclusion that occupation-based rather than contrived intervention activity promotes better functioning is self-evident. Yet the need for additional empirical research to substantiate this claim using various daily living tasks that involve motor control remains paramount.

**Case Study 2**

Trudy is an 86-year-old woman with new diagnosis of a transient ischemia attack. She reports to her the emergency room physician that upon awakening this morning she was unable to speak and was unable to move her right arm and leg well when she tried to get out of bed. Initially thinking she was just tired, Trudy went back to sleep. An hour later when she woke up, the symptoms persisted but her speech was slightly better. Trudy was able to notify her husband of her symptoms and emergency services were called. In the ER, physical and occupational therapy are consulted after the physician felt the client was medically stable as her speech was near normal and Trudy was able to move her arm and leg. The question remained if Trudy was safe to return home. The occupational therapist completed a full evaluation including sensory, cognitive, and vision screenings and range of motion, strength, coordination, balance, and functional mobility assessments in the context of the functional task of getting dressed back into the client's personal clothing. Trudy demonstrated safety and independence with all these tasks; Trudy's motor control deficits had seemingly resolved following her transient ischemia attack. Trudy was urged to follow up with her primary care physician to address her risk factors to prevent a more significant stroke that could have more lasting effects on cognition and physical abilities.

# Intervention Related to Mental and Cognitive Skills

Human cognition includes the mental activities associated with thinking, learning, understanding, remembering, (*Merriam-Webster's Online Dictionary*, 2016) and perceiving (e.g., how we interpret sensory information). All purposeful activity is regulated or supervised by one's brain. Therefore, the successful completion of mental activities is based on a foundation of adequate cognition. However, while intact task-specific cognitive functioning is essential, it is not singularly adequate for successful occupational performance. For example, even if a person has the cognitive skills to understand the motions and rules of a specific sport, the individual still may not have the physical performance capacity to carry through the motions to be a successful player. Adequate cognition is crucial, but not necessarily sufficient for competent performance, especially for tasks requiring movement, as most do. Cognitive dysfunction impairing occupational performance can occur at any age due to genetics, developmental delays, trauma, or disease processes such as cerebral palsy, acquired brain injury, mental illness, or dementia (Giles et al., 2013). The *Framework* (AOTA, 2014, p. S22) divides mental functions into the specific mental functions of attention, memory, perception, thought, mental functions of sequencing complex movement, emotional, experience of self and time, and higher level cognitive (functions), including judgment, concept formation, metacognition, executive functions, praxis, cognitive flexibility, and insight. Global mental functions include consciousness, orientation, temperament and personality, energy and drive, and the physiological process of sleep (pp. S22-S23). Performance skill deficits generally affect activities across different areas of occupation. For example, decreases in short-term memory will affect ADLs as well as socialization and work-related tasks.

Occupational therapists evaluate the clients' cognition or mental abilities, especially as these relate to their daily occupational performance. The complex interaction of cognitive capabilities and volition, general behavioral patterns in occupational areas of concern, and the multifactorial contextual factors affecting performance need to be considered because the brain is the executive director of most daily tasks. Based on the outcomes of the cognitive assessment, collaborative client-centered goal setting is vital to ensure meaningful intervention, whether the ensuing intervention is intended to enhance or maintain performance, to provide education, and/or to offer/design compensatory and adaptive measures.

Occupational therapy services in the realm of cognition are often multimodal and fall into the following broad intervention categories (based loosely on AOTA, 2014, p. S33):

- Health promotion (create, promote) to enhance cognitive performance of all people in natural contexts (e.g., brain exercise groups for well elders or community educational groups for those wanting to enhance their knowledge base)
- Remediation or development (habilitation) of cognitive skills and training in specific tasks (e.g., learning new techniques to enhance memory performance [habilitation] or to remediate memory skills that may be declining)
- Maintaining cognitive performance for those who are at risk of losing skills; this may involve using adaptive equipment or adaptive measures such as technological enhancements (e.g., applications for smartphones)
- Compensating for decreased cognitive skills through modification or adaptation (e.g., due to decreased cognitive skills the person may need to simplify meal preparation or the sequence of ADL routines)
- Providing education on cognitive performance in relation to safety, independent living, and/or life quality for the client and the family is often an essential aspect of intervention related to cognitive performance

Table 25-1.

**ALLEN COGNITIVE LEVELS**

| Level | Level of Care/Level of Performance | Milestone Modes |
|---|---|---|
| 0 | Coma | |
| 1 | Awareness | 1.0 Conscious<br>1.4 Swallow<br>1.8 Pivot transfer |
| 2 | Gross body movements | 2.2 Walking<br>2.8 Grab bars |
| 3 | Manual actions | 3.6 Cause and effect |
| 4 | Familiar activity | 4.0 Independent self-care<br>4.2 Discharge to street<br>4.6 Live alone |
| 5 | Learning new activity | 5.0 Intonation in speech<br>5.6 Social bonding<br>Anticipates safety<br>Driving<br>Child care |
| 6 | Planning new activity | 6.0 Premeditated activities |

Adapted from Allen, C. K. (1991). Cognitive disability and reimbursement for rehabilitation and psychiatry. *Journal of Insurance Medicine, 23*(4), 245-247.

The AOTA Commission on Practice *Statement on Cognition, Cognitive Rehabilitation, and Occupational Performance* (2013) spotlights the key features of the models for occupation-based intervention. The approaches include the following (p. S12):

- Global or domain strategy learning and awareness training
- Specific-task training
- Cognitive retraining using functional tasks
- Environmental modification and assistive technology

The Commission on Practice statement (2013) provides valuable case studies further illustrating these approaches.

## Models Related to Cognitive Remediation and Compensation

Both the Commission on Practice *Statement on Cognition, Cognitive Rehabilitation, and Occupational Performance* (2013) and Gillen (2009) list several primary occupation-based cognitive theories in the realm of cognitive rehabilitation. A few of these are briefly described next, but the reader is encouraged to further explore any of interest prior to using them freely in occupational therapy practice.

The Dynamic Interactional model (Toglia, 2005, 2011) emphasizes the dynamic interaction between the person, the activity, and the environment. Performance is likely to vary based on environmental and personal parameters, as well as the demands of the task. For example, the level of personal cognitive processing strategies such as organizing and problem solving may be effective for a specific task but inadequate for another more involved task. Analysis of these interactions, involving both internal and external factors, and the use of cognitive strategies such as developing self-awareness play key roles in this approach, which combines both remediation and compensation.

Allen, Earhart, and Blue (1992) developed the Cognitive Disabilities model, based on Allen's earlier work (1985). In the Cognitive Disabilities Model, the expectation is not that occupational therapy will improve cognition, but rather that intervention will optimize current functioning through the use of environmental cues and adaptations. First, the practitioner must identify the level of functioning through an assessment tool such as the Allen Cognitive Level Screen. The determined cognitive level (1 through 6, with specific modes) guides intervention so that the occupational therapy practitioner can capitalize on the person's cognitive strengths (Levy & Burns, 2005; Table 25-1). For example, someone functioning at a level 4 can pay attention to visual cues and may need set-up and reminders to successfully complete daily tasks. People functioning at this level pose a safety risk because if a hazard is out of sight, they are not likely to attend to it.

The Quadraphonic Approach (Abreu, 1997) is a holistic cognitive rehabilitation approach that considers the client from both the macro- and microlevels, strongly emphasizing the contextual dimensions of intervention to ensure that all of the influential factors on learning are included. This approach, which involves both retraining programs (such as practice drills) and compensatory measures (such as memory aids), was designed specifically for those who exhibit cognitive dysfunction.

Averbuch and Katz (2011) developed the Cognitive Rehabilitation Retraining model for use with adolescents and adults. This model focuses on first assessing general functioning and then enhancing the clients' retained cognitive abilities. Clients build self-awareness (e.g., metacognition) and learn to use alternative cognitive strategies in helping themselves to perceive, process, and act on incoming information. Through improved self-awareness, clients are better able to assess their own capabilities and learn to respond in appropriate ways, thus improving their cognitive functioning related to everyday tasks. For example, a client who needs to improve his or her initiation skills in social situations first builds awareness of the issue and is then guided through occupational therapy intervention about how to approach others through social interaction training (pp. 287-288).

The Cognitive Orientation to Daily Occupational Performance model (CO-OP) was developed by Polatajko and Mandich (2004). It focuses on teaching the cognitive strategy "Goal-Plan-Do-Check" to clients to help them with their everyday cognitive performance. In a series of research projects, McEwen, Polatajko, Huijbregts, and Ryan (2010) used the CO-OP model to determine how well the strategy model improved performance on both trained and untrained tasks, such as cutting with a knife or putting on a coat (p. 551). The practitioner works with the client to learn to use this strategy consistently during engagement in tasks of interest (based on goals and outcomes using the Canadian Occupational Performance Measure). The McEwen et al. (2010) study determined that the CO-OP model held promise to improve motor performance not only in trained tasks, but also to transfer beyond the tasks used during the sessions once the client had learned the general strategic approach.

The Neurofunctional Approach (Giles, 2011) focuses on specific task retraining and compensatory strategies to help people who have sustained severe acquired brain injuries. This approach targets functioning at the occupation level rather than focusing on the impairments themselves. This top-down approach works on skill development through repetitive engagement and practice in tasks that have meaning for the client. Using habits and routines and environmental adaptations, clients enhance their repertoire of appropriate and well-learned behavioral responses.

Maeir et al. (2014) have developed and used an intervention method called The Cog–Fun (Hahn-Markowitz, Manor, & Maeir, 2011), which helps people learn metacognitive executive strategies (stop, recruit effort/persist, check, plan [p. 263]) to overcome barriers to occupational performance. In a cross-over controlled trial, 19 children with attention deficit hyperactivity disorder improved performance and satisfaction scores on the Canadian Occupational Performance Measure and increased executive functioning skills on the BRIEF (Behavior Rating of Executive Function), thus lending support for the use of the Cog–Fun method for children with attention deficit hyperactivity disorder.

## Strategy Learning and Awareness Training

Global strategy learning approaches focus on the strategies to improve general occupational performance, not the remediation of cognitive skills per se. Domain-specific strategy training is designed to manage specific cognitive deficits such as decreased memory or left neglect. Toglia, Rodger, and Polatajko (2012) have developed a detailed framework of cognitive strategy intervention. They describe the use of in-depth strategies to promote improved occupational engagement. Cognitive strategies can be mental or self-verbalization or specific to the task to be accomplished. For example, rehearsal, the use of imagery, and self-coaching are examples of mental cognitive strategies; stimuli reduction, task reorganization, and task simplification are examples of task-specific modification. The authors have also identified the dimensions of cognitive strategies such as source (external or internal), orientation (person or task), purpose, level of visibility, and scope or range (Toglia et al., 2012, p. 229). By helping clients of all ages use cognitive strategies effectively, the occupational therapy practitioner is promoting learning (or relearning) and best possible occupational performance.

An aspect of higher level cognition is self-awareness. Giles et al. (2013) define the self-awareness of one's own cognitive abilities as metacognition. The awareness of self, including the ability to self-monitor and being able to assess one's own strengths and weaknesses, is generally necessary for successful high-level occupational performance. A systematic review of self-awareness training following brain injury conducted by Schmidt, Lannin, Fleming, and Ownsworth (2011) included 12 studies, three of which were randomized controlled studies. The overall consensus was that awareness training tended to have a modest but positive effect on improving self-awareness and a large effect on the participants' level of satisfaction with their performance. Fleming, Lucas, and Lightbody (2006) conducted a pilot study on four adult males with acquired brain injury who demonstrated decreased self-awareness. They determined that an occupation-based program to improve awareness was effective in all four cases, but increased self-awareness was accompanied by increased anxiety across the board. This result highlights the necessity of considering psychosocial aspects of intervention along with the cognitive factors (as well as the physical) at all times. Wales, Hawley, and Sidebotham (2013) reviewed the literature on self-awareness in children who had sustained traumatic brain injury and concluded that self-awareness in children is not the same as that in adults. Therefore when treating children with self-awareness deficits, the developmental nature of this construct must be taken into account. Not surprisingly, more research is advised in the realm of awareness training for both adults and children.

## Cognitive Retraining Using Functional Tasks

Occupational therapy practitioners have a long history of using functional tasks to improve performance, by presenting the just-right challenge for their clients to promote successful engagement. According to the Commision on Practice statement (2013), this approach uses functional activities to improve cognitive performance. The training is context specific, and it is assumed that the learning will be transferred to a new context/task if the task-features are similar enough to support the transition. For example, a near transfer of learning might be represented by learning to use a microwave oven to cook dinner in the clinic and then at home. The appliance and context will be slightly different but usually not so unfamiliar to prevent success in the home environment.

### Specific-Task Training

Specific-task training, as the name implies, involves training of specific meaningful tasks that then get incorporated into the client's daily routines. Repeated engagement in basic ADL routines and other real-world, meaningful tasks for the client are the intervention. Hubbard, Parsons, Neilson, and Carey (2009) suggest that the practitioner "deconstruct" the task to determine the problematic components interfering with performance and then work to have the client "reconstruct" the entire task. Other recommendations include ensuring task variability to generalize learning and using positive reinforcement given in a timely manner to promote learning. Tasks may be taught in a step-by-step, broken-down process, often using errorless learning (not allowing the person to make mistakes along the way), until the entire routine is incorporated into the client's daily repertoire. This training method is described in the Commission on Practice statement (2013) and is based on the work of Giles (Giles, 2011; Giles & Shore, 1989).

## Specific Cognitive Skills

Next we consider specific cognitive skills involved in the habilitation or rehabilitation process. While it is rare for intervention to focus on one skill exclusively without a more global view toward occupational performance in a complex world, the following brief overview is offered to clarify more specific aspects of intervention in the realm of cognition.

The development of cognitive skills often takes place in younger clients who have not been exposed to the cognitive task before, whereas remediation implies that the client was once able to do the task but now cannot due to impairments in brain functioning. Diagnoses and conditions related to cognitive dysfunction are extremely varied and may cause slight, moderate, or severe impairments in just one or many areas of cognition. Even the highest performing individuals cannot be expected to perform at an optimal cognitive level at all times. An important consideration for all populations is how cognitive performance can be optimized by providing both internal and external contexts and environments that promote the highest level of functioning. The *Framework* (AOTA, 2014) includes cultural, personal, temporal, and virtual aspects of context, and both physical and social environments (p. S28). Each of these needs to be considered as performance is context-dependent in the ever-changing world. A few influential factors to consider include comfort level, body positioning, amount and type of environmental stimulation, and physical and mental condition (e.g., nutrition, level of fatigue, pain). The client factors under consideration in this section need to be viewed from this broad multidimensional and interconnected aspects perspective. Remediation of or compensation for decreased cognitive performance generally involves one or more global or specific mental functions such as orientation, attention, memory, and visuospatial perception.

### Orientation

Orientation training involves the repetition of basic orienting information in which the client answers pertinent questions about his or her life situation, such as who, where, what, when, and how. Being able to improve orientation skills is based on the theoretical notion that repetition or practice will help the information stick, especially for those who are expected to make improvements, such as those who have sustained a brain injury and are now in the midst of the healing process. Orientation is related to memory in that it involves remembering key information about aspects of one's life. In a study by Arkin (2000) using 30 biographical items, even those with Alzheimer's disease could improve in basic orientation skills when compared to a control group who had a similar amount of contact but no commensurate orientation training. Carrion, Aymerich, Baillés, and López-Bermejo (2013) included nine randomized controlled trials of orientation training for people with the diagnosis of dementia in a systematic review. The systematic use of reality orientation (in which the client was repeatedly offered personally orientating information) was associated with cognitive improvements, although the progress of the brain disease process was not affected. In addition, addressing orientation, as a component of a hospital-based multimodal delirium prevention program, along with involvement in meaningful tasks and ensuring appropriate sensory stimulation, has been shown to help prevent the onset of delirium (which by its nature includes disorientation) in older adults in an acute hospital setting (Hshieh et al., 2015).

## Attention

Attention, in its various forms, is mediated by the reticular activating system in the brain. Attention is an important aspect of memory in that it is believed that one must be attending to environmental stimulation to remember the information. As might be expected, adequate attention is needed to complete many daily tasks. More difficult tasks such as driving in an unfamiliar city require more focused attention, while automatic tasks such as brushing teeth require less. Attention process training is a common aspect of the cognitive neurorehabilitation techniques developed by Sohlberg and Mateer (2001) and is sometimes undertaken by occupational therapy practitioners. The system is based on practicing bottom-up cognitive exercises to hone in on improving one particular aspect of attention at a time (e.g., sustained, alternating). A Cochrane database of systematic reviews, in an overview of two trials with 56 participants, found attention training following a stroke was generally effective (Lincoln, Majid, & Weyman, 2000). In a randomized controlled trial of 78 stroke patients by Barker-Collo et al. (2009), attention process training was used for the experimental group, compared to those who received standard care. Attention training did seem to have a significant positive effect on decreasing attention deficits following stroke. However, improved attention on retraining exercises may not necessarily correlate with improved functional performance in daily life tasks. Similarly, the participation of 30 children diagnosed with attention deficit disorder in an intense 4-week computerized attention-based neuropsychological treatment regimen resulted in improved attention skills in testing but a lack of definitive generalization to real-life attention tasks (Amonn, Frölich, Breuer, Banaschewski, & Doepfner, 2013). Obviously, more intervention-based research is needed, especially intervention that is focused on improvements that will carry over to daily life skills.

## Memory

Memory has many different facets, including remembering language and common knowledge (both semantic), events (episodic), how to do tasks (procedural), and remembering to actually do specific tasks at a set time in the future (prospective). Memory can also be classified by duration (e.g., immediate, short term, or long term). Working memory tasks are complex in that the person has to temporarily, but simultaneously remember information while engaging in a related or unrelated task (e.g., recalling a phone number while dialing the phone or remembering the rules while playing a game). Not all aspects of memory are amenable to improvement and not all people are candidates for memory training.

Strong empirical evidence supporting the improvement of memory ability after memory practice drills is still lacking for nearly all aspects of memory, although a great deal of memory training research has been conducted. Sohlberg and Mateer (2001) suggested that if improvement does occur, it is more likely due to improvements in the foundational skill of attention (which could improve the process of storing information). A Cochrane review of memory training in older adults (Martin, Clare, Altgassen, Cameron, & Zehnder, 2011) reported inconclusive results regarding the efficacy of memory training but did find some improvements in immediate and delayed verbal recall. Using data from the ACTIVE study involving 629 older adults, Rebok et al. (2013) found that memory training could improve memory performance and that these improvements could potentially be maintained, especially with booster sessions, over a 5-year period. However, the researchers do conclude that memory training does not seem to attenuate the memory decline associated with the aging process.

One technique that has repeatedly been used for people with mild dementia is spaced retrieval training, which is a technique to reinforce memory consolidation by spacing the retrieval of the information to be recalled (e.g., after 1 minute, then 2, then 8, and so on). Oren, Willerton, and Small (2014) conducted a systematic review of spaced retrieval training on semantic memory performance in those with mild dementia. Although initially 454 potential studies were found, only 12 were ultimately included. Although gains in semantic memory were found, additional research needs to be conducted to determine the impact of memory training on general memory performance and overall quality of life. In addition to training to gain memory skills, "memory support systems," used to compensate for decreased memory skills, show promise in improving memory performance in day-to-day tasks. In a randomized controlled group study, Greenaway, Duncan, and Smith (2013) found that memory support systems improved not only functional memory abilities for a group of 40 participants with memory-based mild cognitive impairments, but also their memory self-efficacy and their mood improved. With regard to memory, further research needs to be conducted; for the field of occupational therapy, this research should involve testing the efficacy of functionally based interventions to enhance memory performance related to improvements in functioning in everyday tasks.

## Executive Skills

Levy and Burns (2005) described cognition as based on a hierarchy in which the base is attention and the tip is executive functioning. Executive skills are defined as high-level cognitive skills that involve planning, problem solving, cognitive flexibility, metacognition, and judgment/insight. Monitoring one's own behavior and adapting one's behavior to fit the current situation are also considered executive skills. These high-level skills develop during adolescence and can be easily arrested in their development through common brain injuries involving the frontal and prefrontal lobes. With brain diseases such as Alzheimer's disease, the loss of ability in executive skills happens early in the disease process, while more basic skills are lost later (often in a reverse ontogenetic sequence; Levy & Burns, 2005). A number of approaches for the management of executive dysfunction are detailed in Sohlberg and Mateer (2001). All involve repeated engagement in cognitive activities that challenge the person's level of thinking. Improvement is only expected to occur after rigorous and recurring practice. Unfortunately while training effects are commonly found and often even robust, transfer of learning to daily task performance is often lacking. One recent typical example was a randomized controlled trial using both younger and older adults (N =59). Sandberg, Ronnlund, Nyberg, and Stigsdotter Neely (2014) found that training sessions for basic executive functions such as updating response plans, shifting focus, and inhibiting responses demonstrated gains in executive functioning tasks in all ages of adults, but transfer of training to far transfer (very dissimilar) tasks was not evident in any age group, and only the younger adults had even near transfer success (Sandberg et al., 2014). The lack of consistent real-life performance gains, therefore, remains a concern.

One interesting finding of late has been the influence of physical exercise on cognitive performance including executive skills. For example, a randomized controlled trial of 100 adults by Singh et al. (2014) used both cognitive training and physical training (as well as sham interventions for a control group). They found that not only did the intense physical training improve cognition (including executive functioning), it did so more than the intense cognitive training, though both were found to be more helpful than the control treatments. In a recent pilot study, related results were found. Alloway and Alloway (2015) enrolled 65 middle-aged adults (18 in training group, 27 in a classroom control group, and 20 in a yoga control group). The training group was involved in structured exercises that were "proprioceptively dynamic" (p. 771). The total amount of training was 4.5 hours over two sessions. The experimental group did show improved working memory scores, but once again, it remains inconclusive whether or not the improved scores on working memory tests, actually benefit real life performance, and if so, the duration and intensity of training needed for positive results. Nonetheless, this unique pilot study provides yet one more example of the interconnectedness of physical and cognitive performance.

### Visual Perception

Perceptual skills are higher level, top-of-the-pyramid visual skills (Warren, 1993) that require not only intact visual pathways but also accurate interpretations of the visual information in the right hemispheric occipital and parietal lobes of the brain. Perception also involves the processing and analysis of other types of sensory information in the brain. Due to their complexity, perceptual deficits are some of the most fascinating and difficult problems to treat. They are rarely seen in isolation and are often combined with more general cognitive impairments. Visual perceptual disorders include the inability to recognize common objects (e.g., agnosia), the inability to understand spatial relationships (e.g., figure–ground, right–left, and depth perception impairments), the inability to recognize subtle differences in similar objects and people (e.g., form constancy disorder), the inability to distinguish objects by touch (e.g., astereognosis), and a distortion of body scheme. Included in the realm of perceptual disorders are both ideomotor and ideational apraxias. These are defined as an inability to carry out common motor tasks due to perceptual impairments rather than because of decreased sensation or motor skills. Ideomotor apraxia is less severe because, although the person has lost the "access to kinesthetic memory patterns" (Gillen, 2009, p. 112), the individual may be able to do the task automatically but not be able to simulate the task or do it on command. In the case of ideomotor apraxia, one may display inaccurate, imprecise, uncoordinated, or clumsy movements. Ideational apraxia (or conceptual apraxia) is a loss of the "mental representation" (Gillen, 2009, p. 110) of how to even complete the task (including sequencing the steps of a task). The person does not know how to use objects or understand how the objects needed for a task relate to one another. Difficulty with initiation of the task, due to the more encompassing loss of the concept, and slowed performance is also likely, making ideational apraxia more difficult to remediate. Remediation of perceptual deficits involves repetitive engagement in tasks requiring perceptual skills, starting at the client's level and working up to more complicated tasks as the person is able. Gillen (2009) offers a protocol for instructing and providing assistance and feedback for people with perceptual deficits. These include individualized cueing and assistance based on the client's needs (p. 126).

In a pivotal, classic study involving occupational therapy, Neistadt (1992) compared 45 men in two intervention groups who had perceptual deficits due to brain injuries. One group completed remedial parquetry block assembly and the other worked on functional meal preparation. The results showed that the functional approach was preferable to the remedial approach, although both groups did show improvements in the realm of perception. A more recent study (Vlok, Smit, & Bester, 2011) presented a framework for a visual perceptual training program for young learners between the ages of 7 and 9 years (when perceptual skills are developing). The researchers provided a set protocol and recommended including a set of preparatory eye exercises along with activities to enhance general visual skills and to promote higher level perceptual skills.

Compensation for decreased perceptual skills can involve graded cueing, graded assistance, and giving verbal, physical, or video feedback (Gillen, 2009); simplifying the environment; establishing basic daily routines; and making sure that the environment is safe for someone who has decreased awareness of surroundings. Since supervision may be needed for successful physical completion of basic daily tasks, caregiver training may also be an important aspect of occupational therapy intervention (Gillen, 2009).

Frequently, the research completed on interventions related to perceptual disorders has focused on unilateral neglect, which more often accompanies right-sided lesions of the brain. Cicerone et al. (2004) recommended "relatively intense (i.e., daily)" (p. 1601) visuospatial training, which includes scanning to decrease the level of visual neglect as a practice standard based on the robust evidence of its effectiveness. However, this research group did not recommend the use of isolated computerized exercises as intervention. A Cochrane review of cognitive rehabilitation for spatial neglect following stroke (Bowen, Lincoln, & Dewey, 2007) found that cognitive rehabilitation clearly did result in decreased visual neglect at the impairment level as measured by neuropsychological assessments, but additional research in this area was recommended to ensure that these improvements actually transfer to enhance functioning in day-to-day tasks. A more recent Cochrane systematic review of 23 randomized controlled trials (involving 628 people) was less conclusive. Bowen, Hazelton, Pollock, and Lincoln (2013) determined that there was insufficient evidence to fully support cognitive rehabilitation for the remediation of visual perceptual deficits following stroke. They concluded that more research is still warranted.

Warren (1993), mentioned earlier, described the hierarchical model of visual functioning, and has recommended that occupational therapy practitioners focus on restoring basic visual functioning (visual acuity, visual fields, and oculomotor control) because in doing so, a natural consequence may be the spontaneous recovery of higher level skills.

## Environmental Modification and Assistive Technology

Occupational therapy practitioners consider the global idea of context (AOTA, 2014) throughout the intervention process. Since the environment can both support or hinder occupational performance, it becomes the practitioner's role to modify the environment in such a way as to promote optimal functioning while keeping environmental and other contextual barriers to a minimum. This can be as simple as making sure that lighting is adequate or using high-contrast items. It may also mean ensuring that the client has the most suitable social milieu. In the realm of cognitive rehabilitation, examples are as varied as the creative mind can envision. Basic examples of environmental adaptations to support improved performance may include limiting distractions in the environment, the removal of clutter, the use of labels or signs, or designing the workspace to enhance focused attention.

Current technology can be used freely as tools of the trade. The world has seen the exponential rise in technological advances and options available to the public over the past few decades. The use of technological devices is no longer the exception; most of us incorporate technology into our lives on a daily basis. However, only those devices/applications that fit the client's needs and lifestyle will be helpful. It behooves occupational therapy practitioners to become familiar with the technology related to their realm of practice so that these tools can be incorporated into their interventions as appropriate. By carefully evaluating the desires, needs, skills, and impairments of the client, a clinically reasoned decision can be made regarding the potential usefulness of any device or program. Through task analysis and client evaluation the therapist needs to ensure that the client is both willing and has the capacity to learn to use appropriate available technology. Suitable use of technology (based on skilled evaluation and intervention) can open doors heretofore locked for those with a variety of cognitive impairments.

## Cognitive Performance Remediation or Maintenance

Remediating cognitive performance often involves drills or repeated engagement in tasks with the intended goal being improved skill level in one or more realms of cognition and the ultimate outcome being improved performance in occupations of concern for the client. For example, by improving short-term memory skills, one would likely perform better in classroom testing. Maintaining cognitive performance can also be a goal of occupational therapy rehabilitation, especially for those with neurological conditions expected to worsen over the course of time. Diagnoses such as Alzheimer's disease, Parkinson's disease, and Huntington's chorea are associated with cognitive decline. Therefore, short-term occupational therapy intervention to maintain the current cognitive performance level could be appropriate. The goal of maintaining cognitive skills is forestalling a decline in performance, rather than focusing on improvement. Yet even maintaining function can pose significant challenges when disease processes continue to chip away at functioning. Nussbaum (2003) encouraged those who want to improve or maintain brain health into old age to actively engage the brain through lifestyle choices that encourage new learning. In his list of 10 behaviors to foster optimal brain health, he included healthy eating, not smoking, adequate physical activity, socializing, learning to relax, building strong ties to others, engaging in new and novel learning experiences, and finally, the occupational therapy practitioner's favorite: maintaining valued roles or finding a purpose in life.

## Compensation for Decreased Cognition

When neither improvement nor maintenance of cognitive functioning is the anticipated outcome, therapeutic intervention adjusts its focus to the safe engagement in occupation in spite of persistent cognitive impairments. Compensation for decreased cognition puts the emphasis on changing the actions of others and the context/environment rather than expecting a change in the self (client). This may be true for one aspect of cognition (e.g., memory) even while other cognitive skills could be maintained. For example, if the client has decreased safety awareness, then supervision and/or a more constricted environment may be necessary. Certain complex cognitive activities such as driving no longer would be appropriate, thus other arrangements would need to be made. Environments may need to be more structured and simplified. Establishing routines to capitalize on the use of basic overlearned tasks can help those with significant cognitive deficits maintain ADL skills. Studies by Graff, Vernooij-Dassen, Hoefnagels, Dekker, and de Witte (2003), as well as Hällgren and Kottorp (2005), have demonstrated the effectiveness of occupational therapy in improving ADL performance for those with cognitive impairments. Occupational therapy practitioners, through their keen observation skills, the use of functional cognitive assessments and activity analyses, and their ability to adapt the environment, are often instrumental in assisting the person to continue to live in the least restrictive setting possible. For example, the simple act of removing the stove knobs or putting a safety bar in a strategic location may be what it takes to keep the home safe for the client.

### Case Study 3

Mohammed is a 34-year-old man who sustained a mild traumatic brain injury in a skiing accident. Mohammed was not wearing a helmet while downhill skiing and struck a tree when he lost control on the last run of the day. Mohammed's traumatic brain injury affected his specific and global mental functions of attention, memory, judgment, executive functions, and insight, and global mental functions of orientation and temperament. Mohammed presented in acute rehabilitation with the goal of wanting to return to his home with his wife and two children and to resume his job as an accountant. Upon evaluation, the occupational therapist found Mohammed to have difficulty attending to tasks, was easily distracted, unable to sequence a typical dressing activity such as putting on his clothing for the day, was easily frustrated when he struggled, and was unable to recall the current date and his location in the hospital. While there are many performance deficits to address to enable success in occupational performance, the occupational therapist and occupational therapy assistant collaborated with the client to determine the best and logical place to start. The client wanted to be more independent with self-care tasks. Using cognitive retraining and environmental modification, the client was offered the just-right challenge. In a quiet space with minimal distractors, external cues and simplified clothing were provided to enable the client to attend to task without distractions, and to be able to dress without becoming too frustrated. The occupational therapy practitioners felt that as the client mastered this just-right challenge, they could add additional challenges until the client would be able to sequence a typical dressing activity in his normal household scenario independently.

## Evidence-Based Practice Findings

Cicerone, Mott, Azulay, and Friel (2004) concluded through a nonrandomized controlled intervention study that intensive, holistic cognitive rehabilitation was an effective form of rehabilitation, especially for community reentry for those with traumatic brain injury. An additional positive effect resulted when clients felt satisfied with their level of cognitive functioning. Through a systematic review of the literature from 2003 to 2008, Cicerone et al. (2011) also concluded that there is sufficient evidence to support rehabilitative interventions for attention, memory, social communication skills, and executive functioning for people who have sustained an acquired brain injury. Visuospatial rehabilitation following a lesion to the right brain has been found to be effective, although specific protocols have not been firmly established. Lindsten-McQueen, Weiner, Wang, Josman, and Connor (2014) conducted a systematic review of eight studies involving interventions to manage apraxia. Three treatment approaches were used including errorless learning and gesture and strategy training. While the review determined that the treatment outcomes were clinically significant, transfer to actual improvements in everyday performance was only found in one study. Occupational therapy practitioners certainly can be key players in this team of cognitive rehabilitation experts, especially with their level of expertise in functional and individualized client-centered intervention.

## Intervention Related to Behavioral Skills

Behavioral impairments cannot be entirely separated from cognitive impairments because neurological or cognitive deficits tend to have behavioral manifestations. Behavioral intervention in the *Framework* (AOTA, 2014) is extremely broad and focuses on changing behavior that is inadequate to support successful occupational engagement. Starting at one end of the age spectrum, an example might be a premature infant who has difficulty regulating environmental stimulation and thereby flails, cries, and becomes easily agitated. On the other end of the age spectrum, an older person with Alzheimer's disease may have similar difficulties with related behavioral manifestations. The elder with dementia might lash out and yell instead of cry, but in both cases, the person is not able to respond to the environment appropriately. In these examples, and in a myriad of others involving behavioral dysfunction, occupational therapy intervention may be able to help regulate one's response to the environment.

### *Sensory Integration Frame of Reference*

The foundation of sensory integration took place more than 50 years ago when A. Jean Ayres posited that sensory information from the environment and the body are processed and organized by the central nervous system to enable function (Watling, Koenig, Davies, & Schaaf, 2011). Normal development is supported by intact sensory processing for normal behavior and learning. Intervention is aimed at improving nervous system processing and integration of sensory information to enable optimal occupational performance.

### *Sensory Approach to Practice*

Occupational therapists rely on their client evaluations, knowledge of human performance, and activity analysis to design interventions that will assist people who need to develop skills or need adaptations to function. A common behavioral intervention in the field of pediatric occupational therapy is the use of sensory integration originated by the late Jean Ayres (1979). Sensory integration theory explains the brain's ability to filter, organize, and integrate sensory information to promote learning (Walker, 2004). Ayres believed that sensory input to the human nervous system was necessary for it to evolve. Sensory integration dysfunction is caused by processing problems in the brain, leading to suboptimal functioning (Ayres, 2005). Ayres's theory explained the relationship between the child's ability to interpret sensations from the body and environment and his or her ability to succeed in academic and motor learning (Bundy & Murray, 2002). Sensory integration theory focuses on the role of the tactile, proprioceptive, and vestibular systems. Through observation, Ayres identified the following four areas of dysfunctional sensory processing (Walker, 2004):

1. Visual form and space dysfunction
2. Developmental dyspraxia
3. Deficits in vestibular and bilateral integration
4. Tactile defensiveness

An occupational therapist using sensory integration intervention principles designs individualized programs based on the results of a thorough evaluation. One goal of intervention is to control sensory input so that a child's brain is able to reorganize and adapt (Walker, 2004). Through engagement in play, a child is able to form adaptive responses that will either inhibit or facilitate sensory integration. Intervention is based on normal developmental sequences, posture, and the integration of sensory input. Ayres felt strongly that sensory integration treatment needed to include equipment, such as suspension devices (swings, hammocks), scooter boards, balance boards, therapy balls, and mats that challenge the senses to develop adaptive responses (Walker, 2004). Each child with sensory integration dysfunction will need an individualized plan. When the intervention outcome is successful, the child's behavior no longer interferes with his or her occupational performance.

Related to sensory integration, sensory processing disorder was proposed by Schaaf and Davies (2010). These researchers are turning to neuroscience to explain sensory function/dysfunction into subtypes to enable evidence-based research and the clearer delineation of sensory approaches. Schaaf and Miller (2005) proposed the following three distinct patterns:

1. **Sensory modulation disorder:** Inability to regulate a response to sensory stimulation
2. **Sensory discrimination disorder:** Difficulty interpreting qualities of sensory stimulation
3. **Sensory-based mood disorder:** Poor postural or volitional movement as a result of sensory problems (James, Miller, Schaaf, Nielsene, & Schoen, 2011; Miller, Anzalone, Lane, Cermak, & Osten, 2007)

## *Behavioral Management Strategies*

Behavioral management strategies are often used for children with disruptive behaviors such as aggression, screaming, or self-injurious behaviors that may accompany autism, attention deficit disorder (with or without hyperactivity), as well as sensory integration dysfunction or sensory processing disorder. Strong empirical evidence demonstrating successful interventions is scant, but anecdotal evidence and single-case studies are more abundant. Rosen and Scott (2003) described the behavioral management techniques that can be used with children with autism who appear to be less aware of others in the environment and more focused on their own needs. The occupational therapist can use the analysis and interpretation of ongoing behavior to formulate a plan. The goal is successful occupational engagement in learning activities and at home. Primary techniques include the consistent use of rewards for positive behaviors, redirection or natural consequences for negative behaviors, and environmental restructuring. Rosen and Scott wrote about the use of positive reinforcement, natural consequences, and redirection techniques with a client called Patty (a pseudonym), a 9-year-old with severe self-destructive tendencies. The behavior management strategies allowed Patty to have some choice in selecting tasks, which were introduced slowly with the initial expectation being that she would engage in the task only briefly. The occupational therapy practitioner used edible reinforcements or rewards and picture symbol communication since Patty was initially unable to clearly verbalize her needs. Through a rearrangement of the environment to decrease the level of compulsory stimulation to which Patty was exposed and by providing deep sensory input (e.g., joint compression, bear hugs, and deep massage), occupational therapy intervention was able to help Patty relate to her environment more effectively and to tolerate being in a classroom setting without resorting to maladaptive behaviors. Watling and Schwartz (2004) also described the use of applied behavior analysis for children with developmental disabilities (and later also with grown-ups), specifically positive reinforcement, based on decades of research.

Other aspects of behavior that may be problematic, more often in children, are to be found in those with autism spectrum disorder who tend to have more difficulty than average in social skills, play, and engaging in leisure activities. Those with autism spectrum disorder tend to have both restricted and/or repetitive behaviors both of which can interfere with successful occupational performance in many realms. Tanner, Hand, O'Toole, and Lane (2015) conducted a recent systematic review on the effectiveness of occupational therapy interventions for people diagnosed with autism spectrum disorder. They found strong support for social skills groups and social participation mediated by parents as "therapeutic agents" (p. 5). Also picture-based communications systems and interventions to improve joint attention were found to be helpful, while the evidence for occupational therapy interventions to work on play and leisure participation and decreasing repetitive behaviors was not as strong. Moderate support was found for a few strategies such as water-based exercises and recess interventions to improve social skills. The evidence regarding the use sensorimotor interventions in the realm of improving social skills was found to be inconclusive (Tanner et al., 2015).

### Behavioral Change

When working with adults, behavioral changes are often part of the intervention plan. To promote health and wellness, clients often consider making lifestyle changes. Behavioral changes may be necessary to return to a former level of functioning after an illness or medical event. For example, after having a heart attack, dietary changes may be warranted. Often, behavioral changes are focused on habits that no longer are, or never were, productive or healthy. For example, a few of the common behavioral changes sought by people relate to improving diet, exercising, and giving up unhealthy habits such as smoking or substance abuse. Stress management and working on healthy sleep patterns are also positive outcomes for behavioral change. Occupational therapy practitioners can be helpful in moving people through the stages of change based on the Transtheoretical Model of Behavior Change (precontemplation, contemplation, preparation, action, and maintenance; Prochaska & Velicer, 1997) by collaborating with clients to develop reasonable goals, and by helping them to break down these goals into more distinct and achievable steps or objectives. The role of the occupational therapy practitioner can be to move the client from one stage to the next, always closer to the ultimate goal of an improved and healthier lifestyle. For example, in the precontemplation phase when the person is not yet thinking about making a change in lifestyle, the occupational therapy practitioner can assist the person in making a list of the benefits and drawbacks of a new behavior, such as adopting a diabetic diet for someone with diabetes. Just by acknowledging that there are pros and cons of making a change, the person is beginning to move into the contemplation phase: an acknowledgment that the current diet or situation may not be promoting optimal health.

A supportive intervention technique that relates well to the values of the occupational therapy profession is motivational interviewing, which is used to encourage healthy behavioral changes. Motivational interviewing is a client-centered technique that fits in well with the profession of occupational therapy. Motivational interviewing guides clients through the process of making behavioral changes, if and when they are ready to do so. By using excellent listening skills, affirmations, open-ended questioning, reflections, and summarizing, the occupational therapy practitioner can support and promote healthy changes, while acknowledging that the clients themselves have the expertise and capability to make their own choices and direct their own life course. Miller and Rollnick (2013) provide a helpful, detailed guidebook for motivational interviewing training.

## Summary

With regard to the physical aspects of the client, the evaluation of the client's performance and performance deficits is followed by mutual goal setting. Occupational therapy intervention then takes place to move the client toward the agreed-upon meaningful occupation-centered goals. The process may involve remediation to improve physical performance in one or more physical realms for the purpose of improving occupational performance (e.g., not to just improve movement), compensation (also for improved occupational outcomes), or a combination of both, always depending on the needs and desires of the client. A crucial element of any intervention plan also involves client and/or family education related to safe and effective occupational performance. It should be noted that simple physical outcome goals such as improved strength, ROM, and balance are never sufficient; occupational therapy must always include functional aspects of goals following on the heels of improved physical performance. For example, in occupational therapy, a client may work on improving ROM, but the ultimate goal is improved ability or performance in daily tasks. Occupational therapy sessions often involve providing physically based interventions both in individual and group settings. These interventions may be component- or client factor–based, such as an upper extremity exercise group, balance training, or motor control practice. These would be considered bottom-up sessions. On the other hand, intervention sessions may use either purposeful activities (such as practicing important tasks) or be occupation based, which involves direct engagement in personally meaningful daily tasks (AOTA, 2014).

In the realm of cognitive and perceptual occupational therapy interventions, several theoretical frameworks guide practice. These are varied, sometimes focus on a certain population, and are constantly developing to better inform intervention plans. The Commission on Practice statement (2013) proposes four aspects of intervention in the realm of cognition including the use of global and domain-based strategies or specific-task and awareness training, cognitive retraining using functional tasks, and environmental modification and assistive technology. The chapter also touched upon several components of cognition (attention, memory, executive functioning, and visual perceptual skills) that are often targeted in occupational therapy intervention. The level of functioning in each of these components rarely affects daily performance in an isolated fashion (e.g., influencing just one task), but the factors themselves can be understood more easily when explored individually to gain a basic understanding of their role in enhancing or detracting from successful occupational performance.

Behavioral interventions are briefly touched upon, especially as behavior is influenced by the person's ability to respond to environmental stimulation. Sensory integration developed by Ayres (1979) and more recent theories such as sensory modulation disorder, sensory discrimination disorder, and sensory-based mood disorder, all address the complexity of our human sensory systems and the crucial role that sensory processing plays in occupational performance. Behavioral change, in its many manifestations, is at the core of much of what clients and practitioners seek for positive outcomes, as often clients need to work on making behavioral changes that will improve their lives and promote better performance in the realms of physical, cognitive, emotional, and social performance. Through the use of motivational interviewing and occupational therapy practice skills, practitioners can help to facilitate lifestyle changes and improvement in life satisfaction, as long as the practitioners remain fiercely client centered.

All of the interventions described in this chapter have been condensed for the sake of parsimony in a broad-based text. As stated initially, the impairments—though often described individually—are nonetheless rarely seen in isolation. In addition, although the primary impairment may be cognitive, sensory, behavioral, or physical, these typically have accompanying psychosocial implications. Losses in the realm of client factors and/or performance skills can be traumatic and can result in deep emotional responses in the clients and their significant others. These feelings and accompanying responses can certainly have an influence on the rehabilitation process and should not simply be ignored.

Effective occupational therapy intervention is based on a thorough review of the multifactorial biopsychosocial factors pertinent to the individual client, a full and individualized evaluation, and a strong dose of clinical reasoning to ensure that the subsequent intervention plan is both meaningful to the client and based on the best and most accurate empirical knowledge currently available. The use of appropriate models of practice and frames of reference can help the guide the practitioner to the most client-centered and evidence-based intervention. The preferred method of intervention is to strive toward occupation, since that is the crux of meaning for our profession.

In this chapter, further references are often cited and should be consulted prior to working with clients in the areas described. We need to strive for excellence

## Evidence-Based Research Chart

| Area | Intervention | Evidence |
|---|---|---|
| Physical | Range of motion/strength | Latham, Anderson, Bennett, & Stretton, 2003; Lee, 2015; Lindy et al., 2012; Liu et al., 2011; Mathieux et al., 2009; Mehrholz, Hädrich, Platz, Kugler, & Pohl, 2012; Weiss, Suzuki, Bean, & Fielding, 2000; Xu, Wang, Mai, & He, 2012 |
| | Endurance | Javier & Montagnini, 2011; Singh, Stewart, Franzsen, & MacKay-Lyons, 2011 |
| | Balance/postural control | Chase, Mann, Wasek, & Arbesman, 2012; Clemson et al., 2004; Davison, Bond, Dawson, Steen, & Kenny, 2005; Garcia, Marciniak, McCune, Smith, & Ramsey, 2012; Gillespie et al., 2003; Han et al., 2004; Leland, Elliott, O'Malley, & Murphy, 2012; Li et al., 2005; Taylor-Piliae et al., 2006; Zijlstra et al., 2007 |
| Neuromuscular | Motor control | Chen, Chen, Wu, Wu, & Chang, 2010; Denton, Cope, & Moser, 2006; Dickson, 2002; Foster, Bedekar & Tickle-Degnen, 2014; Pollock, Baer, Pomeroy, & Langhorne, 2007; Whitall, McCombe Waller, Silver, & Macko, 2000 |
| Sensory | Olfactory and gustatory | de Guise, 2015; Gaines, 2010; Heckmann et al., 2005; Neumann et al., 2012; Nordin, Monsch, & Murphy, 1995 |
| | Touch, proprioception, and kinesthesia | Cooper & Canyock, 2013; Imperatore, Reinoso, Chang, & Bodison, 2012; Miller, Chester, & Jerosch-Herold, 2012; Proto, Pella, Hill, & Gouvier, 2009; Winter, Crome, Sim, & Hunter, 2013 |
| | Hearing | Perlmutter, Bhorade, Gordon, Hollingsworth, & Baum, 2010; Sheff, 2010 |
| | Vision | Barstow, Warren, Thaker, Hallman, & Batts, 2015; Gentile, 2005; Perlmutter, Bhorade, Gordon, Hollingsworth, & Baum, 2010; Schoessow, 2010; Smallfield, Clem, & Myers, 2013; Weisser-Pike & Kaldenberg, 2010 |
| | Visual perception | Aki & Kayihan, 2003; Bowen et al., 2007; Cicerone et al., 2011; Lin, Cermak, Kinsbourne, & Trombly, 1996; Vlok, Smit, & Bester, 2011 |
| | Sensory stimulation—coma | Lippert-Grüner, Wedekind, & Klug, 2003; Oh & Seo, 2003 |
| | Pain | Arbesman & Mosley, 2012; Engle, 2011; Stanos, 2012; Szafron, 2011 |
| Cognitive | General cognitive rehabilitation | Cicerone et al., 2011; Gillen et al., 2015; Hayslip, Paggi, Poole, & Pinson, 2009; McHugh & Warren, 2009; Rand, Weiss, & Katz, 2009 |
| | Attention training | Akinwuntan et al., 2010; Loetscher & Lincoln, 2013; Sohlberg & Mateer, 2001 |
| | Memory training | Boman, Stenvall, Hemmingsson, & Bartfai, 2010; Cavallini, Pagnin, & Vecchi, 2003; Cicerone et al., 2011 |
| | Self-awareness | Dirette, 2010; Fleming, Lucas, & Lightbody, 2006; Ownsworth, Fleming, Desbois, Strong, & Kuipers, 2006; Schmidt, Fleming, Ownsworth, Lannin, & Khan, 2012 |
| | Cognitive strategies | Toglia, Rodger, & Polatajko, 2012 |
| Behavioral | Sensory integration/ sensory processing disorder | Arbesman & Lieberman, 2010; Roley et al., 2003; Smith, Press, Koenig, & Kinnealey, 2005 |
| | Behavioral change | Clark, Nigg, Greene, Riebe, & Saunders, 2002; Glasgow, Bull, Gillette, Klesges, & Dzewaltowski, 2002; Hilton, Ackermann, & Smith, 2013 |
| | Motivational interviewing | Miller & Rollnick, 2013 |

in occupational therapy and do the utmost to promote improved quality of life and help clients develop the skills needed to "live life to its fullest," which is, after all, our ultimate goal as professionals within this exhilarating and challenging field.

## Student Self-Assessment

1. Many people have a rather superficial level of understanding of disabilities. We can define them, but we do not truly comprehend what it is like to have impairments. Therefore, a valuable learning tool is to simulate life with a disability. This activity can lend

insight into the difficulties encountered in everyday life. The activity can be completed in a classroom, lab setting, or in the community (although care should be taken not to offend people with disabilities in the community). All of these exercises should be undertaken only under supervision. The following list is just a few examples of how this exercise can work:

- Simulating paralysis of the legs, use a wheelchair to get around. Be sure to go around several buildings, use doors, and roll on graded surfaces.
- Wearing heavy gloves, try to make a peanut butter and crackers snack (or another snack requiring opening containers and using utensils).
- Using just one arm, put on a shirt and shoes, including tying them. You are not allowed to move your "affected" arm.
- Smear lotion on some old sunglasses and put them on. Then try doing a puzzle or playing a game.
- Wearing earplugs and earmuffs, try to write down the words to a song you are listening to on the radio (if there is static on the radio, that's even better).
- Try cleaning a kitchen area or dusting while blindfolded.

2. In small groups of two to four, brainstorm intervention ideas for the impairments listed. Be sure to think of ideas that incorporate remediation and ideas that incorporate compensation or adaptation whenever possible. For example, for decreased sense of smell, although remediation is probably not possible, compensation might involve labeling leftovers with dates, getting a second opinion about perfume (or not wearing any), and making sure that areas are well-ventilated when working with any harmful airborne substances. Remember that the broad list you devise will not be client centered, but it will stimulate your individualized intervention planning when working with people who have the following impairments:
   - Decreased vision
   - Unilateral neglect
   - Ideational/ideomotor apraxia
   - Figure-ground deficit
   - Orientation deficit
   - Decreased attention
   - Decreased short-term memory
   - Decreased endurance
   - Decreased strength
   - Impaired self-awareness

# References


Abreu, B. C. (1997). *The quadraphonic approach*. Galveston, TX: Unpublished course manual.

Aki, E., & Kayihan, H. (2003). The effect of visual perceptual training on reading, writing, and daily living activities in children with low vision. *Fizyoterapi Rehabilitasyon, 14*(3), 95-99.

Akinbami, L. J., & Liu, X. (2011). *Chronic obstructive pulmonary disease among adults aged 18 and over in the United States, 1998–2009*. Retrieved from cdc.gov/nchs/data/databriefs/db63.pdf

Akinwuntan, A. E., Devos, H., Verheyden, G., Baten, G., Kiekens, C., Feys, H., & De Weerdt, W. (2010). Retraining moderately impaired stroke survivors in driving-related visual attention skills. *Topics in Stroke Rehabilitation, 17*(5), 328-336.

Allen, C. K. (1985). *Occupational therapy for psychiatric diseases: Measurement and management of cognitive disabilities*. Boston, MA: Little, Brown, and Company.

Allen, C. K., Earhart, C., & Blue, T. (1992). *Occupational therapy treatment goals for the physically and cognitively disabled*. Rockville, MD: AOTA Press.

Alloway, R. G., & Alloway, T. P. (2015). The working memory benefits of proprioceptively demanding training: A pilot study. *Perceptual and Motor Skills: Learning and Memory, 120*(3), 766-775.

American Occupational Therapy Association. (2014). Occupational therapy practice framework: Domain and process (3rd ed.). *American Journal of Occupational Therapy, 68*(Suppl. 1), S1-S48. doi:10.5014/ajot.2014.682006

Amonn, F., Frölich, J., Breuer, D., Banaschewski, T., & Doepfner, M. (2013). Evaluation of a computer-based neuropsychological training in children with attention-deficit hyperactivity disorder (ADHD). *NeuroRehabilitation, 32*(3), 555-562. doi:10.3233/NRE-130877

Arbesman, M., & Lieberman, D. (2010). Methodology for the systematic reviews of occupational therapy for children and adolescents with difficulty processing and integrating sensory information. *American Journal of Occupational Therapy, 64*(3), 368-374.

Arbesman, M., & Mosley, L. J. (2012). Systematic review of occupation- and activity-based health management and maintenance interventions for community-dwelling older adults. *American Journal of Occupational Therapy, 66*(3), 277-283.

Arkin, S. M. (2000). Alzheimer memory training: Students replicate learning successes. *American Journal of Alzheimer's Disease and Other Dementias, 15*(3), 152-162.

Averbuch, S., & Katz, N. (2011). Cognitive rehabilitation: A retraining model for clients with neurological disabilities. In N. Katz (Ed.), *Cognition, occupation, and participation across the lifespan* (3rd ed., pp. 277-298). Bethesda, MD: AOTA Press.

Ayres, A. J. (1979). *Sensory integration and the child*. Los Angeles, CA: Western Psychological Services.

Ayres, A. J. (2005). *Sensory integration and the child: understanding hidden sensory challenges*. Los Angeles, CA: Western Psychological Services.

Barker-Collo, S. L., Feigin, V. L., Lawes, C. M., Parag, V., Senior, H., & Rodgers, A. (2009). Reducing attention deficits after stroke using attention process training: A randomized controlled trial. *Stroke, 40*(10), 3293-3298.

Barstow, B. A., Warren, M., Thaker, S., Hallman, A., & Batts, P. (2015). Client and therapist perspectives on the influence of low vision and chronic conditions on performance and occupational therapy intervention. *American Journal Of Occupational Therapy, 69*(3), 1-8. doi:10.5014/ajot.2015.014605

Boman, I., Stenvall, C. L., Hemmingsson, H., & Bartfai, A. (2010). A training apartment with a set of electronic memory aids for patients with cognitive problems. *Scandinavian Journal of Occupational Therapy, 17*(2), 140-148.

Bowen, A., Hazelton, C., Pollock, A., & Lincoln, N. B. (2013). Cognitive rehabilitation for spatial neglect following stroke. *Cochrane Database of Systematic Reviews, Jul 1*(7):CD003586. doi:10.1002/14651858.CD003586.pub3

Bowen, A., Lincoln, N. B., & Dewey, M. (2007). Cognitive rehabilitation for spatial neglect following stroke. *Cochrane Database of Systematic Reviews, 2*, CD003586.

Breines, E. B. (2006). Therapeutic occupations and modalities. In H. M. Pendleton & W. Schultz-Krohn (Eds.), *Pedretti's occupational therapy: Practice skills for physical dysfunction* (6th ed.). St. Louis, MO: Mosby Elsevier.

Bundy, A. C., & Murray, E. A. (2002). Sensory integration: A. Jean Ayres' theory revisited. In A. C. Bundy, S. J. Lane, & E. A. Murray (Eds.), *Sensory integration: Theory and practice* (pp. 3-33). Philadelphia, PA: F. A. Davis Company.

Carrion, C., Aymerich, M., Baillés, E., & López-Bermejo, A. (2013). Cognitive psychosocial intervention in dementia: a systematic review. *Dementia and Geriatric Cognitive Disorders, 36*(5-6), 363-375.

Cavallini, E., Pagnin, A., & Vecchi, T. (2003). Aging and everyday memory: the beneficial effect of memory training. *Archives of Gerontology and Geriatrics, 37*(3), 241-257.

Centers for Disease Control and Prevention. (2012). *Hospitalization for congestive heart failure: United States, 2000–2010.* Retrieved from http://www.cdc.gov/nchs/data/databriefs/db108.htm

Centers for Disease Control and Prevention. (2014a). *Inpatient surgery.* Retrieved from http://www.cdc.gov/nchs/fastats/inpatient-surgery.htm

Centers for Disease Control and Prevention. (2014b). *Chronic obstructive pulmonary disease.* Retrieved from http://www.cdc.gov/copd/data2.html

Centers for Disease Control and Prevention. (2014c). *National chronic kidney disease fact sheet, 2014.* Retrieved from http://www.cdc.gov/diabetes/pubs/pdf/kidney_factsheet.pdf

Centers for Disease Control and Prevention. (2015a). *Important facts about falls.* Retrieved from http://www.cdc.gov/homeandrecreationalsafety/falls/adultfalls.html

Centers for Disease Control and Prevention. (2015b). *Hip fractures among older adults.* Retrieved from cdc.gov/homeandrecreationalsafety/falls/adulthipfx.html

Chase, C. A., Mann, K., Wasek, S., & Arbesman, M. (2012). Systematic review of the effect of home modification and fall prevention programs on falls and the performance of community-dwelling older adults. *American Journal of Occupational Therapy, 66*(3), 284-291.

Chen, T., Edwards, J. D., & Janke, M. C. (2015). The effects of the A Matter of Balance program on falls and physical risk of falls, Tampa, Florida, 2013. *Prev Chronic Dis, 12*, 1-10. doi:10.5888/pcd12.150096

Chen, Y., Chen, C., Wu, C., Wu, C., & Chang, Y. (2010). The effects of bilateral arm training on motor control and functional performance in chronic stroke: A randomized controlled study. *Neurorehabilitation and Neural Repair, 24*(1), 42-51.

Cho, K. H., Lee, K. J., & Song, C. H. (2012). Virtual reality balance training with video-game system improves dynamic balance in chronic stroke patients. *Tohoku Journal of Experimental Medicine, 228*, 69-74.

Choi, M., & Hector, M. (2012). Effectiveness of intervention programs in preventing falls: A systematic review of recent 10 years and meta-analysis. *Journal of Post-Acute and Long-Term Care Medicine, 13*(2), 188.e13-188.e21.

Cicerone, K. D., Langenbahn, D. M., Braden, C., Malec, J. F., Kalmar, K., Fraas, M., & Ashman, T. (2011). Evidence-based cognitive rehabilitation: Updated review of the literature from 2003 through 2008. *Archives of Physical Medicine and Rehabilitation, 92*(4), 519-530.

Cicerone, K. D., Mott, T., Azulay, J., & Friel, J. C. (2004). Community integration and satisfaction with functioning after intensive cognitive rehabilitation for traumatic brain injury. *Archives of Physical Medicine and Rehabilitation, 85*(6), 943-950.

Clark, P. G., Nigg, C. R., Greene, G., Riebe, D., & Saunders, S. D. (2002). The study of exercise and nutrition in older Rhode Islanders (SENIOR): Translating theory into research. *Health Education Research, 17*(5), 552-561.

Clemson, L., Cumming, R. G., Kendig, H., Swann, M., Heard, R., & Taylor, K. (2004). The effectiveness of a community-based program for reducing the incidence of falls in the elderly: A randomized trial. *Journal of the American Geriatrics Society, 52*(9), 1487-1494.

Cole, M. B., & Tufano, R. (2008). *Applied theories in occupational therapy: A practical approach.* Thorofare, NJ: SLACK Incorporated.

Commission on Practice. (2013). Statement on cognition, cognitive rehabilitation, and occupational performance. *American Journal of Occupational Therapy, 67*, S9-S31.

Cooper, C., & Canyock, J. D. (2013). Evaluation of sensation and intervention for sensory dysfunction. In H. M. Pendelton & W. Schultz-Krohn (Eds.), *Pedretti's occupational therapy practice skills for physical dysfunction* (7th ed., pp. 575-589). St. Louis, MO: Elsevier Mosby.

Davison, J., Bond, J., Dawson, P., Steen, I. N., & Kenny, R. A. (2005). Patients with recurrent falls attending Accident and Emergency benefit from multifactorial intervention—A randomized controlled trial. *Age and Ageing, 34*(2), 162-168.

de Guise, E., Alturki, A. Y., Laguë-Beauvais, M., LeBlanc, J., Champoux, M. C., Couturier, C., ... Frasnelli, J. (2015).Olfactory and executive dysfunctions following orbito-basal lesions in traumatic brain injury. *Brain Injury, 29*(6), 730-738. doi:10.3109/02699052.2015.1004748

Denton, P. L., Cope, S., & Moser, C. (2006). The effects of sensorimotor-based intervention versus therapeutic practice on improving handwriting performance in 6- to 11-year-old children. *American Journal of Occupational Therapy, 60*(1), 16-27.

Dickson, M. (2002). Rehabilitation of motor control following stroke: Searching the evidence. *British Journal of Occupational Therapy, 65*(6), 269-274.

Dirette, D. (2010). Self-awareness enhancement through learning and function (SELF): A theoretically based guideline for practice. *British Journal of Occupational Therapy, 73*(7), 309-318.

Engle, J. M. (2011). Pain regulation. In C. Brown & V. C. Stoffel (Eds.), *Occupational therapy in mental health: A vision for participation.* Philadelphia, PA: F. A. Davis Company.

Feigenbaum, M. S. (2001). Rationale and review of current guidelines. In J. E. Graves & B. A. Franklin (Eds.), *Resistance training for health and rehabilitation.* Leeds, United Kingdom: Human Kinetics Publishers.

Fleming, J. M., Lucas, S. E., & Lightbody, S. (2006). Using occupation to facilitate self-awareness in people who have acquired brain injury: A pilot study. *Canadian Journal of Occupational Therapy, 73*(1), 44-55.

Foster, E. R., Bedekar, M., & Tickle-Degnen, L. (2014). Systematic review of the effectiveness of occupational therapy: Related interventions for people with Parkinson's disease. *American Journal of Occupational Therapy, 68*, 39-49. doi:10.5014/ajot.2014.008706

Gaines, A. D. (2010). Anosmia and hypnosmia. *Allergy and Asthma Proceedings, 31*, 185-189.

Garber, C. E., Blissmer, B., Deschenes, M. R., Franklin, B. A., Lamonte, M. J., Lee, I. ... Swain, D. P. (2011). Quantity and quality of exercise for developing and maintaining cardiorespiratory, musculoskeletal, and neuromotor fitness in apparently healthy adults: Guidance for prescribing exercise. *Medicine and Science in Sports and Science, 43*(7), 1334-1359.

Garcia, A., Marciniak, D., McCune, L., Smith, E., & Ramsey, R. (2012). Promoting fall self-efficacy and fall risk awareness in older adults. *Physical and Occupational Therapy in Geriatrics, 30*(2), 165-175.

Gentile, M. (2005). *Functional visual behavior in adults: An occupational therapy guide to evaluation and treatment options* (2nd ed.). Bethesda, MD: AOTA Press.

Giles, G. M. (2011). A neurofunctional approach to rehabilitation following brain injury. In N. Katz (Ed.), *Cognition, occupation and participation across the life span* (3rd ed., pp. 351-381). Bethesda, MD: AOTA Press.

Giles, G. M., Radomski, M. V., Champagne, T., Corcoran, M. A., Gillen, G., Kuhaneck, H. M. ... Toglia, J. (2013). Cognition, cognitive rehabilitation, and occupational performance. *American Journal of Occupational Therapy, Nov/Dec*(Suppl.), S9-S31.

Giles, G. M., & Shore, M. (1989). A rapid method for teaching severely brain injured adults how to wash and dress. *Archives of Physical Medicine and Rehabilitation, 70*(2), 156-158.

Gillen, G. (2009). *Cognitive and perceptual rehabilitation: Optimizing function*. St. Louis, MO: Mosby Elsevier.

Gillen, G., Nilsen, D. M., Attridge, J., Banakos, E., Morgan, M., Winterbottom, L., & York, W. (2015). Effectiveness of interventions to improve occupational performance of people with cognitive impairments after stroke: An evidence-based review. *American Journal of Occupational Therapy, 69*(1), 1-13. doi:10.5014/ajot.2015.012138

Gillespie, L. D., Gillespie, W. J., Robertson, M. C., Lamb, S. E., Cumming, R. G., & Rowe, B. H. (2003). Interventions for preventing falls in elderly people. *Cochrane Database of Systematic Reviews, 4*, CD000340.

Glasgow, R. E., Bull, S. S., Gillette, C., Klesges, L. M., & Dzewaltowski, D. A. (2002). Behavior change intervention research in healthcare settings: A review of recent reports with emphasis on external validity. *American Journal of Preventive Medicine, 23*(1), 62-69.

Graff, M. J. L., Vernooij-Dassen, M. J. F. J., Hoefnagels, W. H. L., Dekker, J., & de Witte, L. P. (2003). Occupational therapy at home for older individuals with mild to moderate cognitive impairments and their primary caregivers: A pilot study. *OTJR: Occupation, Participation, and Health, 23*(4), 155-164.

Greenaway, M. C., Duncan, N. L., & Smith, G. E. (2013). The memory support system for mild cognitive impairment: Randomized trial of a cognitive rehabilitation intervention. *International journal of geriatric psychiatry, 28*(4), 402-409.

Hahn-Markowitz, J., Manor, I., & Maeir, A. (2011). Cognitive functional (Cog–Fun) intervention in occupational therapy for children aged 5-10 with ADHD: A pilot study. *American Journal of Occupational Therapy, 65*, 384-392.

Hall, C. M., & Brody, L. T. (2005). Impairment in muscle performance. In C. M. Hall & L. T. Brody (Eds.), *Therapeutic exercise: Moving toward function* (2nd ed.). Philadelphia, PA: Lippincott Williams and Wilkins.

Hällgren, M., & Kottorp, A. (2005). Effects of occupational therapy intervention on activities of daily living and awareness of disability in persons with intellectual disabilities. *Australian Occupational Therapy Journal, 52*(4), 350-359.

Han, A., Robinson, V., Judd, M., Taixiang, W., Wells, G., & Tugwell, P. (2004). Tai Chi for treating rheumatoid arthritis. *Cochrane Database of Systematic Reviews, 3*, CD004849.

Hayner, K., Gibson, G., & Giles, G. M. (2010). Research Scholars Initiative—Comparison of constraint-induced movement therapy and bilateral treatment of equal intensity in people with chronic upper-extremity dysfunction after cerebrovascular accident. *American Journal of Occupational Therapy, 64*(4), 528-539. doi:10.5014/ajot.2010.08027

Hayslip, B., Paggi, K., Poole, M., & Pinson, M. W. (2009). The impact of mental aerobics training on memory impaired older adults. *Clinical Gerontologist, 32*(4), 389-394.

Heckmann, J. G., Stössel, C., Lang, C. J. G., Neundörfer, B., Tomandl, B., & Hummel, T. (2005). Taste disorders in acute stroke: A prospective observational study on taste disorders in 102 stroke patients. *Stroke, 36*(8), 1690-1694.

Hilton, C. L., Ackermann, A. A., & Smith, D. L. (2013). Healthy habit changes in pre-professional college students: Adherence, supports, and barriers. *OTJR: Occupation, Participation and Health, 33*(1), 64-72. doi:10.3928/15394492-20100325-01

Hoppe, K. A., Kopp Miller, D., & Rice, M. (2008). Occupationally embedded exercise versus rote exercise and psychosocial response in college-aged females. *Occupational Therapy in Mental Health, 24*(2), 176-191. doi:10.1080/01642120802055317

Hosseini, S. A., Fallahpour, M., Sayadi, M., Gharib, M., & Haghgoo, H. (2012). The impact of mental practice on stroke patients' postural balance. Journal of Neurological Sciences, 322, 263-267.

Hshieh, T. T., Yue, J., Oh, E., Puelle, M., Dowal, S., Travison, T., & Inouye, S. K. (2015). Effectiveness of multicomponent nonpharmacological delirium interventions: A meta-analysis. *Journal of the American Medical Association Internal Medicine, 175*(4), 512-520.

Hubbard, I. J., Parsons, M. W., Neilson, C., & Carey, L. M. (2009). Task-specific training: Evidence for and translation to clinical practice. *Occupational Therapy International, 16*(3-4), 175-189.

Human cognition. (2016). In *Merriam-Webster's online dictionary* (11th ed.). Retrieved from http://www.merriam-webster.com/dictionary/cognition

Imperatore, B. E., Reinoso, G., Chang, M. C., & Bodison, S. (2012). Proprioceptive processing difficulties among children with autism spectrum disorders and developmental disabilities. *American Journal of Occupational Therapy, 66*(5), 621-624.

James, C., Miller, L. J., Schaaf, R., Nielsene, D. M., & Schoen, S. A. (2011). Phenotypes within sensory modulation dysfunction. *Comprehensive Psychiatry, 52*, 715-724.

Javier, N. S. C., & Montagnini, M. L. (2011). Rehabilitation of the hospice and palliative care patient. *Journal of Palliative Medicine, 14*(5), 638-648.

Khan, F., Ng, L., Gonzalez, S., Hale, T., & Turner-Stokes, L. (2008). Multidisciplinary rehabilitation programmes following joint replacement at the hip and knee in chronic arthropathy. *Cochrane Database of Systematic Reviews, 2*, CD004957. doi:10.1002/14651858.CD004957.pub3

Latham, N., Anderson, C., Bennett, D., & Stretton, C. (2003). Progressive resistance strength training for physical disability in older people. *Cochrane Database of Systematic Reviews, 2*, CD002759.

Lee, K. H. (2015). Effects of virtual reality-based exercise program on functional recovery in stroke patients: Part 1. *Journal of Physical Therapy Science, 27*(6), 1637-1640.

Leland, N. E., Elliott, S. J., O'Malley, L., & Murphy, S. L. (2012). Occupational therapy in fall prevention: Current evidence and future directions. *American Journal of Occupational Therapy, 66*(2), 149-160.

LeManach, Y., Collins, G., Bhandari, M., Bessissiow, A., Boddaert, J., Khiami, F., ... Devereaux, P. J. (2015). Outcomes after hip fracture surgery compared with elective total hip replacement. *Journal of the American Medical Association, 314*(11), 1159-1166. doi:10.1001/jama.2015.10842

Levy, L. L., & Burns, T. (2005). Cognitive disabilities reconsidered. In N. Katz (Ed.), *Cognition and occupation across the lifespan* (2nd ed.). Bethesda, MD: AOTA Press.

Li, F., Harmer, P., Fisher, K. J., McAuley, E., Chaumeton, N., Eckstrom, E., & Wilson, N. L. (2005). Tai Chi and fall reductions in older adults: A randomized controlled trial. *Journals of Gerontology Series A, Biological Sciences and Medical Sciences, 60*(2), 187-194.

Lin, K. C., Cermak, S. A., Kinsbourne, M., & Trombly, C. A. (1996). Effects of left-sided movements on line bisection in unilateral neglect. *Journal of the International Neuropsychological Society, 2*(5), 404-411.

Lincoln, N. B., Majid, M. J., & Weyman, N. (2000). Cognitive rehabilitation for attention deficits following stroke. *Cochrane Database of Systematic Reviews, 4*, CD002842.

Lindsten-McQueen, K., Weiner, N. W., Wang, H.-Y., Josman, N., & Connor, L. T. (2014). Systematic review of apraxia treatments to improve occupational performance outcomes. *OTJR: Occupation, Participation and Health, 34*(4), 183-192.

Lindy, C., Fiatarone, S. M. A., Bundy, A., Cumming, R. G., Manollaras, K., O'Loughlin, P., & Black, D. (2012). Integration of balance and strength training into daily life activity to reduce rate of falls in older people (the LiFE study): Randomised parallel trial. *BMJ, 345*, e4547.

Lippert-Grüner, M., Wedekind, C., & Klug, N. (2003). Outcome of prolonged coma following severe traumatic brain injury. *Brain Injury, 17*(1), 49-54.

Liu, C., Becker, J., Ford, S., Heine, K., Scheidt, E., & Wilson, A. (2011) Effects of upper-extremity progressive resistance strength training in older adults: The missing picture. *Physical and Occupational Therapy in Geriatrics, 29*(4), 255-269.

Loetscher, T. & Lincoln, N. B., (2013). Cognitive rehabilitation for attention deficits following stroke. *Cochrane Database of Systematic Reviews, 5.*

Ludwig, F. M. (2004a). Anne Cronin Mosey. In F. K. Walker & F. M. Ludwig (Eds.), *Perspectives on theory for the practice of occupational therapy* (pp. 69-98). Austin, TX: Pro Ed.

Ludwig, F. M. (2004b). Occupation-based and occupation-centered perspectives. In F. K. Walker & F. M Ludwig (Eds.), *Perspectives on theory for the practice of occupational therapy* (pp. 373-442). Austin, TX: Pro Ed.

Maeir, A., Fisher, O., Bar-Ilan, R. T., Boas, N., Berger, I., & Landau, Y. E. (2014). Effectiveness of cognitive–functional (Cog–Fun) occupational therapy intervention for young children with attention deficit hyperactivity disorder: A controlled study. *American Journal of Occupational Therapy, 68*(3), 260-267.

Martin, M. C., Clare, M., Altgassen, A. M., Cameron, M. H., & Zehnder, F. (2011). Cognition-based interventions for healthy older people and people with mild cognitive impairment. *Cochrane Review, 1,* CD006220.

Mathieux, R., Marotte, H., Battistini, L., Sarrazin, A., Berthier, M., & Miossec, P. (2009). Early occupational therapy programme increases hand grip strength at 3 months: Results from a randomised, blind, controlled study in early rheumatoid arthritis. *Annals of the Rheumatic Diseases, 68*(3), 400-403.

Mathiowetz, V. (2011). Task-oriented approach to stroke rehabilitation. In G. Gillen (Ed.), *Stroke Rehabilitation: A Function-Based Approach* (pp. 80-99). St. Louis, MO: Elsevier.

McEwen, S. E., Polatajko, H. J., Huijbregts, M. P. J., & Ryan, J. D. (2010). Inter-task transfer of meaningful, functional skills following a cognitve-based treatment: Results of three multiple baseline design experiments in adults with chronic stroke. *Neuropsychological Rehabilitation, 20*(4), 541-561.

McHugh, G., & Warren, A. (2009). A report into cognitive intervention strategies with older adults with cognitive impairment: Recommendations for occupational therapy practice. *Irish Journal of Occupational Therapy, 37*(1), 30-37.

Mehrholz, J., Hädrich, A., Platz, T., Kugler, J., & Pohl, M. (2012). Electromechanical and robot-assisted arm training for improving generic activities of daily living, arm function, and arm muscle strength after stroke. *Cochrane Database of Systematic Reviews, 6,* CD006876. doi:10.1002/14651858.CD006876.pub3

Miller, L. J., Anzalone, M. E., Lane, S. J., Cermak, S. A., & Osten, E. T. (2007). Concept evolution in sensory integration: A proposed nosology for diagnosis. *American Journal of Occupational Therapy, 61*(2), 135-140.

Miller, L. K., Chester, R., & Jerosch-Herold, C. (2012). Effects of sensory reeducation programs on functional hand sensibility after median and ulnar repair: A systematic review. *Journal of Hand Therapy, 25*(3), 297-307.

Miller, R. J., & Schwartz, K. (2004). What is theory and why does it matter? In F. K. Walker & F. M Ludwig (Eds.), *Perspectives on theory for the practice of occupational therapy* (pp. 1-26). Austin, TX: Pro Ed.

Miller, W. R., & Rollnick, S. (2013). *Motivational interviewing: Helping people change* (3rd ed.). New York, NY: Guilford Press.

*Miller-Keene Encyclopedia and Dictionary of Medicine, Nursing, and Allied Health* (7th ed.). (2003). Exercise. Retrieved from http://medical-dictionary.thefreedictionary.com/muscle-setting+exercise

Neistadt, M. E. (1992). Occupational therapy treatments for constructional deficits. *American Journal of Occupational Therapy, 46*(2), 141-148.

Neumann, C., Tsioulos, K., Merkomidis, C., Salam, M., Clark, A., & Philpott, C. (2012). Validation study of the "Sniffin' Sticks" olfactory test in a British population: A preliminary communication. *Clinical Otolaryngology, 37*(1), 23-27.

Nilsen, D. M., Gillen, G., Geller, D., Hreha, K., Osei, E., & Saleem, G. T. (2015). Effectiveness of interventions to improve occupational performance of people with motor impairments after stroke: An evidence-based review. *American Journal of Occupational Therapy, 69*(1), 1-9. doi.org/10.5014/ajot.2015.011965

Nordin, S., Monsch, A. U., & Murphy, C. (1995). Unawareness of smell loss in normal aging and Alzheimer's disease: Discrepancy between self-reported and diagnosed smell sensitivity. *Journals of Gerontology Series B. Psychological Sciences and Social Sciences, 50*(4), P187-P192.

Nussbaum, P. (2003). *Brain health and wellness.* Tarentum, PA: Word Association Publishers.

Office of Disease Prevention and Health Promotion. (2015). *Physical activity guidelines for Americans.* Retrieved from http://health.gov/paguidelines/guidelines/

Oh, H., & Seo, W. (2003). Sensory stimulation programme to improve recovery in comatose patients. *Journal of Clinical Nursing, 12*(3), 394-404.

Orellano, E., Colon, W. I. & Arbesman, M. (2012). Effect of occupation- and activity-based interventions on instrumental activities of daily living performance among community-dwelling older adults: A systematic review. *American Journal of Occupational Therapy, 66,* 292-300. doi:10.5014/ajot.2012.003053

Oren, S., Willerton, C., & Small, J. (2014). Effects of spaced retrieval training on semantic memory in Alzheimer's disease: A systematic review. *Journal of Speech, Language, and Hearing Research, 57*(1), 247-270.

Ownsworth, T., Fleming, J., Desbois, J., Strong, J., & Kuipers, P. (2006). A metacognitive contextual intervention to enhance error awareness and functional outcome following traumatic brain injury: A single case experimental design. *Journal of the International Neuropsychological Society, 12*(1), 54-63.

Park, H. Y., Maitra, K., & Martinez, K. M. (2015). The effect of occupation-based cognitive rehabilitation for traumatic brain injury: A meta-analysis of randomized controlled trials. *Occupational Therapy International, 22*(2), 104-116.

Perlmutter, M. S., Bhorade, A., Gordon, M., Hollingsworth, H. H., & Baum, M. C. (2010). Cognitive, visual, auditory, and emotional factors that affect participation in older adults. *American Journal of Occupational Therapy, 64*(4), 570-579.

Peterson, E. W., & Clemson, L. (2008). Understanding the role of occupational therapy in fall prevention for community-dwelling older adults. *OT Practice, 13*(3), CE1-CE8.

Polatajko, H. J., & Mandich, A. (2004). *Enabling occupation in children: The cognitive orientation to daily occupational performance.* Ottawa, Ontario, Canada: CAOT Publications.

Pollock, A., Baer, G., Pomeroy, V., & Langhorne, P. (2007). Physiotherapy treatment approaches for the recovery of postural control and lower limb function following stroke. *Cochrane Database of Systematic Reviews, 1,* CD001920.

Prochaska, J. O., & Velicer, W. F. (1997). The transtheoretical model of health behavioral change. *American Journal of Health Promotion, 12*(1), 38-48.

Proto, D., Pella, R. D., Hill, B. D., & Gouvier, W. D. (2009). Assessment and rehabilitation of acquired visuospatial and proprioceptive deficits associated with visuospatial neglect. *NeuroRehabilitation, 24*(2), 145-157.

Rand, D., Weiss, P. L., & Katz, N. (2009). Training multitasking in a virtual supermarket: A novel intervention after stroke. *American Journal of Occupational Therapy, 63,* 535-542. doi:10.5014/ajot.63.5.535

Rebok, G. W., Langbaum, J. B., Jones, R. N., Gross, A. L., Parisi, J. M., Spira, A. P., ... & Brandt, J. (2013). Memory training in the ACTIVE study: How much is needed and who benefits? *Journal of Aging and Health, 25*(Suppl. 8), 21S-42S.

Roley, S. S., Clark, G. F., Bissell, J., Brayman, S. J., & Commission on Practice. (2003). Applying sensory integration framework in educationally related occupational therapy practice. *American Journal of Occupational Therapy, 57*(6), 652-659.

Rosen, S., & Scott, J. B. (2003). Behavior management strategies for students with autism. *OT Practice, 8*(11), 16-20.

Sandberg, P., Rönnlund, M., Nyberg, L., & Stigsdotter Neely, A. (2014). Executive process training in young and old adults. *Aging, Neuropsychology, and Cognition, 21*(5), 577-605.

Schaaf, R. C., & Davies, P. L. (2010). Evolution of the sensory integration frame of reference. *American Journal of Occupational Therapy, 64*(3), 363-367.

Schaaf, R. C., & Miller, L. J. (2005). Occupational therapy using a sensory integrative approach for children with developmental disabilities. *Mental Retardation and Developmental Disabilities Research Reviews, 11*(2), 143-148.

Schmidt, J., Fleming, J., Ownsworth, T., Lannin, N., & Khan, A. (2012). Feedback interventions for improving self-awareness after brain injury: A protocol for a pragmatic randomised controlled trial. *Australian Occupational Therapy Journal, 59*(2), 138-146.

Schmidt, J., Lannin, N., Fleming, J., & Ownsworth, T. (2011). Feedback interventions for impaired self-awareness following brain injury: A systematic review. *Journal of Rehabilitation Medicine, 43*(8), 673-680.

Schoessow, K. (2010). Shifting from compensation to participation: A model for occupational therapy in low vision. *British Journal of Occupational Therapy, 73*(4),160-169.

Sheff, A. (2010). In the clinic: Meeting the needs of clients with hearing impairments. *OT Practice, 15*(8), 7-8, 21.

Shumway-Cook, A., & Woollacott, M. H. (2012). *Motor control: Translating research into clinical practice* (4th ed.). Philadelphia, PA: Lippincott Williams and Wilkins.

Singh, A., Stewart, A. Franzsen, D., & MacKay-Lyons, M. (2011). Energy expenditures of dressing in patients with stroke. *International Journal of Therapy and Rehabilitation, 18*(12), 683-693.

Singh, M. A. F., Gates, N., Saigal, N., Wilson, G. C., Meiklejohn, J., Brodaty, H., ... Baker, M. K. (2014). The Study of Mental and Resistance Training (SMART) study—Resistance training and/or cognitive training in mild cognitive impairment: A randomized, double-blind, double-sham controlled trial. *Journal of the American Medical Directors Association, 15*(12), 873-880.

Smallfield, S., Clem, K., & Myers, A. (2013). Occupational therapy interventions to improve the reading ability of older adults with low vision: A systematic review. *American Journal of Occupational Therapy, 67*(3), 288-295.

Smith, S. A., Press, B., Koenig, K. P., & Kinnealey, M. (2005). Effect of sensory integration intervention on self-stimulating and self-injurious behaviors. *American Journal of Occupational Therapy, 59*(4), 418-425.

Sohlberg, M. M., & Mateer, C. A. (2001). *Cognitive rehabilitation: An integrative neuropsychological approach*. New York, NY: Guilford Press.

Stanos, S. (2012). Focused review of interdisciplinary pain rehabilitation programs for chronic pain management. *Current Pain and Headache Reports, 16*(2), 147-152.

Szafron, S. H. (2011). Physical, mental, and spiritual approaches to managing pain in older clients. *OT Practice, 16*(3), CE1-CE8.

Tanner, K., Hand, B. N., O'Toole, G., & Lane, A. E. (2015). Effectiveness of interventions to improve social participation,play, leisure, and restricted and repetitive behaviors in people with autism spectrum disorder: A systematic review. *American Journal of Occupational Therapy, 69*, 6905180010. doi:10.5014/ajot.2015.017806

Taylor-Piliae, R. E., Haskell, W. L., Stotts, N. A., & Froehlicher, E. S. (2006). Improvement in balance, strength, and flexibility after 12 weeks of Tai Chi exercise in ethnic Chinese adults with cardiovascular disease risk factors. *Alternative Therapies in Health & Medicine, 12*(2), 50-58.

Toglia, J. P. (2005). A dynamic interactional approach to cognitive rehabilitation. In N. Katz (Ed.), *Cognition and occupation across the life span* (pp. 29-72). Bethesda, MD: AOTA Press.

Toglia, J. P. (2011). A dynamic interactional approach in cognitive rehabilitation. In N. Katz (Ed.), *Cognition, occupation, and participation across the life span* (3rd ed., pp. 161-201). Bethesda, MD: AOTA Press.

Toglia, J. P., Rodger, S. A., & Polatajko, H. J. (2012). Anatomy of cognitive strategies: A therapist's primer for enabling occupational performance. *Canadian Journal of Occupational Therapy, 79*, 225-236.

Trombly, C. (1993). Anticipating the future: Assessment of occupational function. *American Journal of Occupational Therapy, 47*(3), 253-257.

Vlok, E. D., Smit, N, E., & Bester, J. (2011). A developmental approach: A framework for the development of an integrated visual perception program. *South African Journal of Occupational Therapy, 41*(3), 25-33.

Wales, L., Hawley, C., & Sidebotham, P. (2013). How an occupational therapist should conceptualise self-awareness following traumatic brain injury in childhood—a literature review. *British Journal of Occupational Therapy, 76*(7), 325-332.

Walker, K. F. (2004). Jean Ayres. In K. F. Walker & F. M. Ludwig (Eds.), *Perspectives on theory for the practice of occupational therapy* (pp. 145-236). Austin, TX: PRO ED.

Warren, M. (1993). A hierarchical model for evaluation and treatment of visual perception dysfunction in adult acquired brain injury, part 1. *American Journal of Occupational Therapy, 47*(1), 42-54.

Watling, R., Koenig, K. P., Davies, P. L., & Schaaf, R. C. (2011). *Occupational therapy practice guidelines for children and adolescents with challenges in sensory processing and sensory integration*. Bethesda, MD: AOTA Press.

Watling, R., & Schwartz, I. S. (2004). Understanding and implementing positive reinforcement as an intervention strategy for children with disabilities. *American Journal of Occupational Therapy, 58*(1), 113-116.

Weiss, A., Suzuki, T., Bean, J., & Fielding, R. A. (2000). High intensity strength training improves strength and functional performance after stroke. *Archives of Physical Medicine and Rehabilitation, 79*(4), 369-376.

Weisser-Pike, O., & Kaldenberg, J. (2010). Occupational therapy approaches to facilitate productive aging for individuals with low vision. *OT Practice, 15*(3), CE1-CE8.

Whitall, J., McCombe Waller, S., Silver, K. H., & Macko, R. F. (2000). Repetitive bilateral arm training with rhythmic auditory cueing improves motor function in chronic hemiparetic stroke. *Stroke, 31*(10), 2390-2395.

Winter, J. M., Crome, P., Sim, J., & Hunter, S. M. (2013). Effects of mobilization and tactile stimulation on chronic upper-limb sensorimotor dysfunction after stroke. *Archives of Physical Medicine and Rehabilitation, 94*(4), 693-702. doi:10.1016/j.apmr.2012.11.028

Xu, K., Wang, L., Mai, J., & He, L. (2012). Efficacy of constraint-induced movement therapy and electrical stimulation on hand function of children with hemiplegic cerebral palsy: A controlled clinical trial. *Disability and Rehabilitation, 34*(4), 337-346.

Zijlstra, G. A., van Haastregt, J. C., van Rossum, E., van Eijk, J. T., Yardley, L., & Kempen, G. I. (2007). Interventions to reduce the fear of falling in community-living older people: A systematic review. *Journal of the American Geriatrics Society, 55*(4), 603-615.

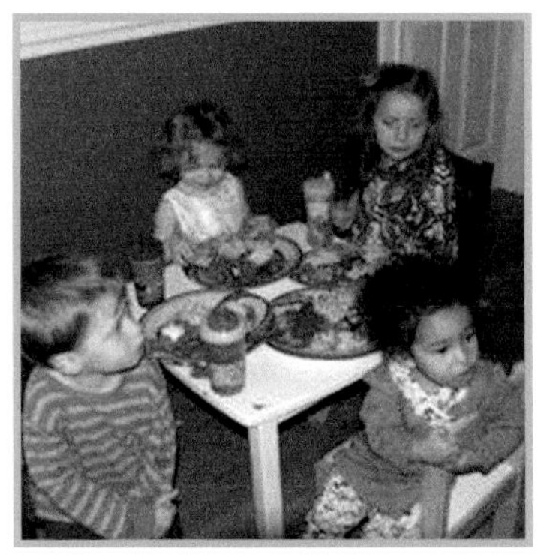

# 26

# Interventions to Enhance Occupational Performance in Activities of Daily Living and Instrumental Activities of Daily Living

*Michael E. Roberts, OTD, OTR/L*

## ACOTE STANDARDS EXPLORED IN THIS CHAPTER

B 5.1–5.6

## KEY VOCABULARY

- **Activities of daily living (ADLs):** Also called basic activities of daily living or personal activities of daily living, activities directed toward caring for one's own body.
- **Adaptation:** Practitioners decrease the demands of the environment and task to meet the client's expected skill level after remediation.
- **Instrumental activities of daily living (IADLs):** Activities that involve interaction with the environment or community, such as pet care, meal preparation, or financial management.
- **Maintenance:** Ensuring continued competency through use of external devices, templates, or skill retraining, despite expectations of potential or eventual declines in occupational performance.
- **Performance context:** Environment in which occupational performance occurs, including the physical environment, available resources, sensory input, temporal and societal influences, or the presence or availability of caregivers.



Jacobs, K., & MacRae, N. (Eds.). *Occupational Therapy Essentials for Clinical Competence, Third Edition* (pp. 383-397).

Occupational performance in activities of daily living (ADLs) and instrumental activities of daily living (IADLs) serve as the foundation for expression of meaning and identity for clients of occupational therapy practitioners (American Occupational Therapy Association [AOTA], 2014; Christiansen, 1999). Evaluation, intervention, and outcomes related to these areas of occupation are of critical importance to effective service delivery. Indeed, this focus on effective self-management of these areas of occupation has served as the defining core of the profession since its earliest days (Meyer, 1922).

## Assessment of ADL and IADL Performance

Evaluation of ADL and IADL performance is comprised of an initial occupational profile and a more focused performance analysis, frequently involving direct observation and standardized assessments (AOTA, 2014). During this first phase of developing and implementing the intervention plan, the frame of reference or model of practice most appropriate for the client is selected, client priorities and perspective are evaluated and incorporated, and the influence of the context of performance is assessed. This process must be ultimately directed by the needs of the client and his or her input. The frame of reference or model of practice must be selected exclusively by an assessment of the client's needs and capacities, not practitioner preference. Evaluation of client priorities drives treatment selection and goal setting. Accurate assessment of client perspective and context are critical to ensuring the durability and applicability of goals and treatment plans throughout the continuum of care.

The occupational profile frequently includes questions like "Tell me about your typical day," "What activities or roles are most important to you?", or "How has your life changed because of your disease/trauma/life change?" These questions allow for identification by the client of the most typical patterns of performance, habits, or roles that comprise their occupational existence. Follow-up questions or active listening techniques can elicit important information about client priorities, perceived obstacles to effective performance, or adaptive/maladaptive strategies for improving performance. Also, occupational history, influence of caregivers or other contextual issues, and client goals may be understood more effectively through effective strategic use of initial interviews with clients. It is important to remember that effective use of the occupational profile and initial interview period must result in specific, occupation-focused priorities to result in an effective intervention plan (AOTA, 2014; Neistadt, 1995). This occupation-directed outcome is important for defining our profession for our clients, and continues as a challenge for practitioners in current practice (McAndrew, McDermott, Vitzakovitch, Warunek, & Holm, 1999; Royeen, 2002).

The next step in the evaluation of ADL and IADL performance is to determine more specifically how to focus the practitioner's efforts through analysis of occupational performance (AOTA, 2014). Informed by the occupational profile, evidence-based practice strategies, and the frame of reference or model of practice most effective for the client, performance is directly observed in the most appropriate context, using standardized assessments where possible (AOTA, 2014). Ideally, tasks such as meal preparation, laundry management, bathing, or dressing are observed and performance assessed in the environment most commonly used by the client. In certain clinical settings or due to particular medical issues, this is not always possible. In these instances, the alternative context must be specifically documented to provide the most complete picture of ADL/IADL performance. Also, observation of performance in a clinical context rather than a client's usual or home context is preferable to relying exclusively on self-report of function (Kempen, Steverink, Ormel, & Deeg, 1996). Research comparing standardized assessments with self-reported IADL status suggests greater accuracy is obtained through performance-based measures (Hilton, Fricke, & Unsworth, 2001), as practitioners may expect.

The order or priority given to assessment of specific performance skills, performance patterns, or client factors depends on the needs and priorities of the client. Utilization of an occupation-focused or "top-down" approach may be effective for certain clients, while a "bottom-up" or component-based approach may be best for other clients (Trombly, 1993, p. 253), and still others receive the most effective treatment through assessment of the client's context and its impact (Weinstock-Zlotnick & Hinojosa, 2004; Wimpenny, Savin-Baden, & Cook, 2014). For example, a client who presents with diabetic peripheral polyneuropathy, an assessment from a top-down approach, may identify decreased client satisfaction with her role as an independent grandparent who cooks brunch for her family every Sunday morning. Her occupational therapy practitioner may determine from the occupational profile to perform a more focused assessment of safety with sharps in the kitchen, foot care as part of her morning self-care routine, and functional mobility assessments in the kitchen during meal preparation to directly identify the roles or occupational priorities most important to this client. A bottom-up approach may also be determined to be the best for this client, including standardized assessments of balance, peripheral sensation, safety awareness, or other foundational skills, which when addressed in the intervention plan are expected to result in resolution of the larger occupational performance issues. The client may benefit most from a contextual assessment first, evaluating the effectiveness of resource utilization, impact of caregivers, and influence of the physical, social, cultural, or temporal environments on the client's performance of her Sunday morning brunch routine. Regardless of the approach, an occupational therapist and occupational therapy assistant can serve as a team in effectively collaborating and prioritizing functional retraining in cases such as this, ensuring comprehensive assessment and intervention with complex cases.

The most effective approach is the one that meets the needs of the client, not the approach with which the practitioners are most comfortable or the one that is routinely used in the setting where assessment occurs. Rather, effectiveness in evaluation depends upon the "fit" of the approach to the client (Weinstock-Zlotnick & Hinojosa, 2004), while maintaining the focus on occupation inherent in occupational therapy practice. This approach should be comprehensive, assessing both performance components and an understanding of limitations in participation for clients, even in more traditionally component-focused practice settings like hand therapy (Weinstock-Zlotnick & Bear-Lehman, 2015).

Nonstandardized assessments of ADL and IADL performance can provide valuable information for intervention plan development, but selection of a frame of reference or model of practice, or an intention of adherence to evidence-based practice, often necessitates the incorporation of standardized assessments of performance of ADLs and IADLs. It is important to note that standardized assessments need not be full self-care assessments to inform intervention planning. Standardized assessments of client factors may prove predictive of self-care performance, such as deficits in categorization and deductive reasoning, logically proving effective predictors of IADL performance (Goverover & Hinojosa, 2002).

The following are a selection of standardized assessments of ADL and IADL performance in current use in occupational therapy clinical practice:

- **Arnadottir OT-ADL Neurobehavioral Evaluation:** Two-part observational assessment with Part 1 focusing on ADL performance in dressing, grooming/hygiene, transfers/mobility, feeding, and communication, and Part 2 correlating 11 areas of impairment with ADL performance to assist the clinicians in identifying the most likely neurological deficit responsible for the observed performance deficits (Arnadottir, 1990).
- **Assessment of Living Skills and Resources:** Interview-based assessment for IADLs that incorporates an appreciation for the impact of available resource utilization as a mitigating or exacerbating factor in determining the true relevance and prioritization of IADL dysfunction (Williams et al., 1991).
- **Assessment of Motor and Process Skills:** Fifty-six tasks typical to IADL routines of children, adolescents, or adults have been deconstructed to allow standardized ratings on specific motor and process skills associated with each task. The occupational therapy practitioner assists the client in identifying several typical tasks from the daily IADL routine for the client. Of these, a small number that are components of the Assessment of Motor and Process Skills are recommended and observed. Competency with performance is assessed and prediction of future IADL function is possible (Fisher, 1999).
- **Barthel Index:** An evaluation of 10 areas of a client's self-care and mobility skills, rated from 0 to 15 (Mahoney & Barthel, 1965). This assessment is typically used to assess functional performance, much like the Functional Independence Measure. Higher scores are associated with greater likelihood of regaining independence after discharge or after completion of rehabilitation services (De Wit et al., 2014).
- **Canadian Occupational Performance Measure:** This semistructured interview is used to identify the client's perception of his or her occupational performance in self-care, productive, and leisure tasks. The five areas identified by the client as most important are rated for performance in addition to satisfaction with performance. A directly client-centered assessment, it can assist the occupational therapy practitioner in tracking perceived effectiveness of the intervention plan (Law et al., 2005).
- **Functional Independence Measure:** Used widely to assess functional performance in physical dysfunction settings, and adapted for use with children as the WeeFIM, the Functional Independence Measure uses a seven-point scale to describe the amount of assistance required for the subject to perform 18 tasks relating to self-care, cognition, and communication. This assessment is multidisciplinary and is part of the Uniform Data System for Medical Rehabilitation (2000).
- **Klein-Bell Activities of Daily Living Scale:** One hundred seventy subtasks of dressing, elimination, mobility, hygiene and bathing, emergency communication, and eating are rated and weighted according to relative importance and difficulty. Observation and scoring results in a score as a percentage of the potential maximum score. This assessment may be used in children and adults (Klein & Bell, 1979).
- **Kohlman Evaluation of Living Skills:** Utilized primarily to determine the likelihood of safe, independent function in the community for clients with psychiatric diagnoses and/or cognitive dysfunction, this assessment combines interview and observation to

determine the number of 18 assessed self-care areas with which a client requires assistance. The assessment covers self-care, safety/health, work and leisure, money management, transportation and telephone use (McGourty, 1979).

- **Minimum Data Set (MDS):** Used for residents in long-term care, and covering a large and comprehensive view of the client's health and function, occupational therapy practitioners are generally contributing to only a few sections, primarily Section G, which relates to mobility and ADL/IADL performance (Nelson & Glass, 1999). Performance of components must be observed, and scores must represent the resident's performance at his or her status of greatest need across all hours within the previous 7 days (Centers for Medicare and Medicaid Services, 2005). Sections of the MDS are also used in determination of placement of cases in Resource Utilization Groups in skilled nursing facilities, which affects reimbursement rates for the facility.
- **Occupational Self-Assessment:** Designed to be used within the Model of Human Occupation, the Occupational Self-Assessment is a self-report assessment that measures client satisfaction with his or her performance of tasks and activities, as well as his or her perceived mastery of his or her environment. These data are then used in collaborative intervention planning sessions to identify client factors, activities, and environmental issues of greatest concern for that particular client. Understandably, this assessment requires a requisite level of insight and cognitive function in the subject to procure useful information (Kielhofner & Forsyth, 2001).
- **Outcome and Assessment Information Set:** Sixteen ADL/IADL performance subtests are included in this very comprehensive home-care assessment. Observation of status is considered best for treatment planning, but assessment strategies are not highly regimented. Questions on this assessment are used to determine reimbursement based on acuity, functional assistance required, complexity, and other factors (Center for Health Services and Policy Research, 1998).
- **Performance Assessment of Self-Care Skills:** This assessment is used with adults to evaluate performance in functional mobility, home management, and basic ADLs, with differing protocols depending upon whether assessment occurs at the client's home or in the clinic of the assessing occupational therapy clinician (Rogers & Holm, 1994). Scoring includes subtask breakdown, a valuable tool in intervention planning.
- **Routine Task Inventory:** For clinicians operating within Allen's cognitive disability model, this assessment relates observed or reported self-care performance to Allen's cognitive levels (Allen, Earhart, & Blue, 1992). The Routine Task Inventory also provides expected performance of tasks correlated to each applicable cognitive level. This assessment provides limited directive instructions on administration, and recommends not using self-report of status with lower functioning clients.
- **Safe at Home:** This assessment is specific to safety and safety awareness of clients in the home environment, involving 12 test items related to typical environmental hazards in the home. The Safe at Home is intended for use with adults (Robnett, Hopkins, & Kimball, 2002).
- **Satisfaction With Performance Scaled Questionnaire:** Subjects for this assessment report the percentage of time in the past 6 months that they were satisfied by their performance in 46 ADL/IADL tasks, differentiated into two subscales: home management and social/community function. Community-dwelling adults can use the information in collaboration with their occupational therapy clinicians to identify and prioritize potential areas of IADL intervention (Yerxa, Burnett-Beaulieu, Stocking, & Azen, 1988).

## Contextual Issues With Assessment

In the current practice environment, there are a number of factors that can affect or influence assessments and outcomes that must be considered in anticipation of developing a treatment plan. A necessary consideration in contemporary practice is reimbursement (see Chapter 41 on reimbursement). Whether discussing the Prospective Payment System, Resource Utilization Groups, Individualized Education Plans, health maintenance organizations, managed care organizations, accountable care organizations, preferred provider options, or any other configuration of reimbursement for occupational therapy services, practitioners must strive for effective outcomes and optimal treatment planning regardless of payer source (AOTA, 20015).

Despite expected adherence to the AOTA *Occupational Therapy Code of Ethics*, some discrepancies have surfaced (see Chapter 50 on ethics). One typical example is research describing functional outcomes for clients with a cerebrovascular accident who receive rehabilitation services. Those who utilized a Medicare health maintenance organization instead of the traditional fee-for-service plans for their treatment received fewer therapy and medical specialist visits, but more home care visits made less progress in functional performance, and were more likely to be living in a nursing home 1 year after their stroke (Kramer et al., 2000). Ideally, practitioners are developing intervention plans as if they were "blind" to reimbursement issues, but incorporating an appreciation of expected utilization limits may help ensure equality of outcomes across payer sources. This must also be accompanied by a renewed focus on demonstrating and communicating the enhanced outcomes uniquely achieved by occupational therapy practitioners (Leland, Crum, Phipps, Roberts, & Gage, 2015).

Practitioners must also be aware of how they are perceived by their clients, and their clients' perceptions of their own function, as these may affect the data collected in assessments and thereby affect intervention planning. Mothers who are engaged in the IADLs of child rearing report that practitioners who present with a more relaxed and friendly demeanor are perceived as having better insight into the daily routine of child rearing and having a greater capacity to "tailor" services to the specific needs of the family (Thompson, 1998). This fact encourages practitioners to be aware of their interactive styles from the development of the intervention plan and to reassess the effectiveness of their therapeutic use of self through the intervention process.

Practitioners may also be affected by their own prejudices regarding settings, populations, and ADL/IADL function. Misguided generalizations may negatively affect the capacity of an intervention plan to most directly and efficiently enhance the functional independence and quality of life for our clients. Research has identified that residents in long-term care facilities perceived themselves to present with significantly higher levels of function than that documented by clinicians (Atwood, Holm, & James, 1994). Dunford, Missiuna, Street, and Sibert (2005) reported that children with a developmental coordination disorder described concerns regarding limitations in performance of self-care and leisure activities, while these deficits were largely not identified by parents or teachers for these children. Additionally, occupational therapy practitioners' reasoning process regarding school readiness for their clients may be influenced by decisions made by parents and teachers, which may be based on a variety of nondevelopmental factors like gender of the client or the client's perceived temperament (McBryde, Ziviani, & Cuskelly, 2004). Awareness regarding preconceptions in assessment of clients becomes a matter of ensuring a professional level of intervention, and this information must be incorporated into the assessment and intervention planning processes.

The environment utilized for assessment and intervention may also affect results of assessment and intervention. As described earlier, assessment in the client's most commonly used performance context is ideal, while observation of performance, regardless of setting, is still preferable to relying solely on self-report of status. Some inpatient facilities invest significant resources into replicating, as closely as possible, contextually appropriate environments for their clients, with the expectation that contextually appropriate settings lead to contextually appropriate carryover. This theory, however, has not been borne out. Richardson, Law, Wishart, and Guyatt (2000) demonstrated that no significant functional performance difference was achieved with the use of contextually appropriate intervention settings. Davis, Hoppes, and Chesbro (2005) reported that there is no substitute for assessment in the clients' home, their most personally relevant context, wherein clients with dementia and IADL dysfunction were found to be largely similar in functional profile except that clients exhibited higher levels of motor skills in their homes. Additional research by Bottari, Dutil, Dassa, and Rainville (2006) found no clear benefit to either home or clinical settings for administration of performance-based assessments.

## Intervention

Once evaluation data are obtained, an intervention plan can be developed, including objectives, expected time frame for goal completion, roles for practitioners, interprofessional collaboration of an occupational therapist/occupational therapy assistant team, and an evidence-based intervention approach within the chosen model of practice or frame of reference (AOTA, 2014). Throughout implementation of the intervention plan, a constant treatment outcomes "feedback loop" informs an evaluation of the plan's efficacy, including not only functional progress with ADLs and IADLs, but also the effectiveness of changes to the available resources, performance context, or therapeutic use of self strategies (AOTA, 2014).

Once the evaluation data have been compiled, and the objectives determined in collaboration with the client and other members of the client's health care team, the most appropriate intervention approach must be selected. The *Occupational Therapy Practice Framework* (AOTA, 2014) describes five approaches: create or promote, establish or restore, maintain, modify, and prevent. Each of these approaches is used in combination with some or all of the others with each client depending upon the client's needs.

### Create or Promote

The create or promote approach, also described as health promotion, involves interventions that facilitate enhancement of health and function in natural contexts of life (AOTA, 2014). This approach may involve utilization of universal design strategies for living spaces or offer cooking classes to enhance nutrition, socialization, and mobility practice in an assisted living facility.

## Establish or Restore

The establish or restore or remediation approach seeks to ensure acquisition and mastery of skills that are absent, lost, or impaired (AOTA, 2014). This approach may include establishing a well-balanced and effective morning ADL routine for a client with a chronic disease, enhancement of activity tolerance in standing for meal preparation or clean-up, or addressing limitations of fine motor control and hand strength to allow return to independence with grooming and oral care after carpal tunnel release surgery.

## Maintain

The maintenance approach, while frowned upon in documentation for rehabilitation settings, is also important for ensuring maximal ADL/IADL performance as its implementation is based on an assumption that without these interventions, occupational performance would decrease (AOTA, 2014). For example, practitioners using this approach may use magnifiers and templates to allow clients with low vision to complete budgeting, check writing, or developing grocery lists. Practitioners may teach the use of timers and pill boxes with clients with chronic mental illness to ensure effective medication management once they are discharged from an inpatient clinical setting. This approach may also be used to train clients with amyotrophic lateral sclerosis in energy conservation and work simplification to delay the outpacing of ADL demands with declining activity tolerance.

## Modify

The modify or adaptation approach (AOTA, 2014) is used quite frequently in rehabilitation settings. In this setting, practitioners use adaptation to decrease the demands of the environment and task to meet the client's expected skill level after remediation. This approach is evident when practitioners teach the use of a sock aid after a client's hip replacement surgery, modify workspaces to maximize ergonomic fit of the client and task, or train clients with chronic obstructive pulmonary disease in the use of tub seats, hand-held showers, and long-handled sponges to decrease trunk flexion and conserve energy during bathing. Given this information, it is important to use adaptive equipment and adaptations judiciously, as too many changes to the home environment, too many new strategies at once, or too great an expenditure of resources to ensure success with adaptations may defeat the initial purpose. The social, developmental, and cultural impact of adaptations and adaptive equipment must be taken into consideration before time and effort are carved out of the intervention plan for their training and use.

## Prevent

Prevention is also utilized as an intervention approach in clients and populations determined to be at-risk. Teaching communication skills to school-aged children to reduce school violence, teaching proper body mechanics during home maintenance and laundry tasks for clients with chronic low back pain, or incorporating effective foot care into the ADL routines of clients with diabetes are all examples of preventative approaches with at-risk clients.

As described earlier, these approaches are not necessarily mutually exclusive, and most effective intervention plans incorporate all of the approaches. For instance, a client with rheumatoid arthritis who presents with pain in both hands with grooming tasks, difficulties with lower body ADLs due to limited joint range of motion and low back pain, and difficulty with food preparation, opening pill bottles, and writing checks due to hand deformities may require all of the approaches to achieve ADL/IADL independence and improved quality of life. This client may require joint protection retraining to prevent future deterioration of joint function. The client may use an occupational therapy selected or fabricated upper extremity splint to prevent further deterioration of joints in his or her hands, as well as maintain range and alignment in the hands at this point. The demands of the client's environment may be modified by introducing adaptive equipment that decreases the demands of tasks to meet the client's current status, such as an adapted built-up toothbrush to decrease the pain and coordination demands of oral care tasks or a dressing stick to reduce the trunk range and low back pain demands of lower body dressing. The practitioner may also assist the client in establishing a new daily routine of ADLs and IADLs to enhance joint protection and energy conservation strategies for daily living tasks that must be completed by the client. Finally, the creation of adaptive equipment or strategies within the client's home environment may reduce dysfunction and pain and may promote greater participation and engagement in occupations that enhance functional independence, such as money management, medication management, laundry and clothing management, or other potentially difficult IADL tasks.

In the previously described example, a number of different "instruments" are utilized by the practitioner in conjunction with the client. These instruments have classifications depending upon their complexity and intention. Preparatory activities are interventions that help a client prepare for functional performance. These may include splinting, modalities, or joint mobilization. In the arthritis example, a practitioner may don or doff a splint for the client, apply moist heat or paraffin to his or her hands, or perform manual joint distraction to enhance joint range of motion and reduce pain. These are not specifically occupation-based activities; however, if they are completed in advance of meal preparation retraining or grooming retraining and the results of the preparatory activities enhance and improve performance, they have been used effectively and appropriately by the practitioner.

Some activities used in occupational therapy are described as purposeful activities, which achieve movement along therapeutic continua through engagement in goal-directed activities (AOTA, 2014). Practice with durable medical equipment for bathroom mobility, such as grab bars, tub seats, or commodes, would qualify as purposeful activities. These practice sessions addressing components of ADLs/IADLs are intended to enhance functional performance, yet have the added benefit of additional focus on the most troublesome components leading to dysfunction, or breaking down occupational performance into manageable "pieces" without losing a focus on ultimate functional independence for the client or his or her caregivers.

Occupation-based activities involve participation in the specific occupations identified by the clients and practitioners as priorities to ensure independence and quality of life. Making a meal in the client's kitchen, training in donning and doffing the client's prosthesis, or practicing wheelchair-level toileting in the client's home bathroom are all examples of occupation-based activities used therapeutically. As expected, progression up the hierarchy of activities to occupation-based activities is often the goal of the intervention plan and an effective strategy for ADL/IADL retraining (Richards et al., 2005; Smallfield & Karges, 2009; Wolf, Chuh, Floyd, McInnis, & Williams, 2015).

These different types of activities are then directed appropriately to address each of the components of the domain of occupational therapy. Client factors are addressed by adaptive equipment use, upper extremity orthosis construction and use, or preparatory methods like joint distraction or modalities. Performance patterns are addressed by joint protection and energy conservation training. Contextual issues are addressed when making environmental changes, using adaptive devices, or addressing temporal issues in training with ADL and IADL routines. Use of upper extremity orthoses, adaptive equipment for lower body dressing, or enhancing body mechanics training may all change activity demands. Teaching joint protection strategies, practicing them, and providing informed feedback to the client would affect and improve performance skills. In this way, all components of the domain of occupational therapy may be addressed (AOTA, 2014). In fact, comprehensive interventions of this type, and of joint protection retraining specifically, have been reported to be effective occupational therapy interventions with clients with rheumatoid arthritis (Niedermann et al., 2012; Steultjens et al., 2006).

It is important to remember that these interventions may address several approaches or aspects of occupational therapy's domain at once, and that the goals of effectively selected occupational tasks address as many components of independence and quality of life as possible. For instance, in the previously described example, an occupational therapist or occupational therapy assistant may address the client's difficulty with check writing through the use of an adapted writing implement and more ergonomically correct writing environment. Addressing this relatively small area of the client's occupational performance may accomplish many objectives at once. Joint degradation may be reduced, pain may be reduced, the client's satisfaction with maintaining financial independence may enhance quality of life and mood, and confidence in the occupational therapy team may improve, therefore enhancing the likelihood of carryover and success of other components of the intervention plan. In this way, an elegantly simple "melody" may enhance the overall effect of the occupational therapy intervention "symphony."

The previous example provides a description of ADL/IADL interventions with a client with a chronic disease. The domain remains the same for acute trauma and disease as well. For example, a client diagnosed with a left hemiparesis and left neglect after a stroke will require a number of different interventions from his or her occupational therapy team members. Given that all of the aspects of the occupational therapy domain will be affected in this clinical situation, a wide variety of interventions are possible. Evidence must be utilized to determine which of the interventions will most likely be of benefit to the client and his or her family. Expected ADL and IADL dysfunctions for a client with left hemiparesis are many. Limited motor function will make bilateral self-care tasks (donning socks, tying shoes) very difficult. All these components of occupational performance may be negatively affected by the onset of the stroke: clothing management during toileting, meal preparation, grooming, medication management, kitchen and bathroom mobility, transfers in the home environment, sexuality, safety with sharps in the kitchen and temperatures in the bathroom, learning use of adaptive equipment or strategies, attention to the left side for functional tasks, balance during functional transfers, and health maintenance of the left side of the body. All of these may have different and changing priorities for the client. All of these may have dozens of different activities that are appropriate for use in intervention by practitioners with this client.

The ADL/IADL retraining process for more acute cases is the same as for chronic cases. The activity selection process depends upon the evidence available, the frame of reference or model of practice, the resources available to the client, the client's priorities, and the impact of other contextual issues, such as service delivery issues or family concerns. For this population in particular, recent research describes the following components critical to successful occupational therapy intervention: use of specific client-identified activities, use of and training with appropriate adaptations, maximizing the familiarity of the context, providing feedback to improve performance, and providing ample practice with the activities (Guidetti & Ytterberg, 2011; Trombly & Ma, 2002).

To illustrate, a number of client characteristics may affect independence in bathing, an important and foundational ADL. The client may highly value the activity and prioritize it for treatment. The client's left hemiparesis, left neglect, and impaired sensation on the left side may negatively affect task completion, safety, and bathroom mobility. Family members may express specific concerns about their ability to use the resources available to them to assist in ensuring the client's independence with this activity. The client may be concerned about the expertise of the occupational therapy team, the efficacy of the bathing retraining plan, or the possibility of institutionalization, all lending expanded meaning to bathing as an occupation-based activity.

The inherent complexity of meaning of the activity within occupational performance for this client in this situation must be seen as an opportunity, not an obstacle by the practitioners with whom this client works. One effective option for the occupational therapy team would be to incorporate the family members in the bathing retraining therapy sessions in as familiar a context as possible, given the clinical situation. If, for instance, the practitioner demonstrates use of adaptations like tub benches, hand-held showers, long-handled sponges, long mirrors, or grab bars to the client and family during a bathing retraining session, a number of objectives are addressed. Primarily, the client's functional performance improves. This activity may also reinforce transfer retraining, skin inspection or other health management strategies, enhancement of activity tolerance, sitting balance, attention to the affected side, problem-solving and scanning retraining, or energy conservation strategies. Demonstrated success with occupational therapy retraining may also enhance self-esteem, build confidence in the occupational therapy team and intervention plan, reduce family concerns about functional outcomes, and enhance carryover of other components of the intervention plan. Utilizing self-care retraining to enhance functional performance directly is also borne out as the most effective strategy for enhancing ADL performance (Walker et al., 2004). With effective application of occupational therapy principles and a specific focus of intervention utilizing ADL retraining, positive results can be achieved with this population with dressing tasks (Christie, Bedford, & McCluskey, 2011) or general self-care and functional mobility (Landi et al., 2006; Sackley et al., 2006). A specific focus on intervention for personal activities of daily living after cerebrovascular accident has even been shown in one review to significantly reduce the incidence of "poor outcomes" described as "death, deterioration, or dependency in personal activities of daily living" in this population (Legg et al., 2007).

Both of these clinical examples demonstrate the richness of ADL and IADL tasks as modalities within the intervention plan, or as melodies within the occupational therapy intervention symphony. Because so many of these tasks are profoundly meaningful, defining, and personal for the clients, even the simplest of ADL or IADL tasks wield significant power to affect many or all aspects of occupational therapy's domain, and therefore are invaluable instruments within the occupational therapy "orchestra" of potential interventions and strategies.

## Therapeutic Outcomes

There are a number of different areas for intervention by practitioners in collaboration with their clients. Practitioners can incorporate movement along an adaptation–gradation continuum to match the demands of the retraining activity to the client's performance level and expected goals. An understanding of the performance skills that are intact may be used to enhance the skills that are lacking. Contexts must be understood and incorporated into treatment planning, especially available resources, influence of caregivers, expected disease or recovery process, and other therapies active with the client. Performance patterns, habits, routines, and roles of the client also may be affected and therefore prioritized for intervention planning (AOTA, 2014). Communication skills, client insight, client goals/priorities, sociocultural and socioeconomic influences, setting, acuity, and developmental level are also important potentially impactful issues to be addressed and utilized in enhancing or focusing the collaboration between clinician and client to maximize the effectiveness of the intervention plan. Currently, new technologies are providing new opportunities for ADL/IADL interventions, including neuroprostheses used with ADL retraining (Hill-Hermann et al., 2008), electronic aids to daily living for clients with acquired brain injuries (Boman, Tham, Granqvist, Bartfai, & Hemmingsson, 2007), mobile and tablet technologies (Weaver, 2015), and virtual reality for community-based shopping tasks (Rand, Weiss, & Katz, 2009).

Each of these potential intervention-maximizing components has an influence on the effectiveness of the practitioner's efforts to improve his or her client's quality of life and move with the client toward functional independence. Not all of the components need to be in effect or be actively addressed at all times in all situations. However, it stands to reason that to treat the whole person, clinicians should be utilizing or manipulating as many of these components at once with each intervention.

One way to envision this strategy is to picture each of the potential intervention components or influences as a musical instrument. Just as there are different kinds of music appropriate for different situations in life, different combinations of these components of ADL/IADL function are addressed in whole or in part depending upon the client and his or her context. For instance, a relatively uncomplicated case, such as an otherwise well client status post an elective orthopedic procedure may require a simpler melody or fewer instruments, say, 1950s-style rock-and-roll. The instruments still need to work together in rhythm, tempo, and key, and be adaptable to the demands of the situation, but can match the complexity of the case more directly.

More complex clinical cases, such as a client who is socioeconomically disadvantaged, diagnosed with a chronic disease, and serves as caregiver to a spouse with a progressive neurological syndrome, will require more intricate interweaving of instruments. A highly skilled clinician "conductor" must ensure all the interventions are of one purpose, directing production of one elegant symphonic masterpiece where the varied, unique, and inherently complex components construct a whole greater than the sum of the parts, more Mozart than Buddy Holly. Regardless of situation, or complexity, recruiting and effectively utilizing as many of the instruments as possible for each client will enhance the holistic, life-changing potential of each intervention plan and thereby ensure the most effective collaboration with clients in their efforts to achieve success in ADL and IADL performance.

## Current Service Delivery Environment

The value of functional independence in self-care is appreciated not only by practitioners and their clients, but also by regulators and purchasers of health care services. More outcome measures related to the efficacy of therapy and health care services in general are focused on function and quality of life, traditional practice domains of practitioners. For example, MDS data are collected on all residents of long-term care facilities that receive Medicare or Medicaid funding. Ninety percent of occupational therapy practitioners responding to a survey reported they were involved in the MDS data collection in the long-term care facilities where they worked, mostly with subsections related to self-care and changes in ADL function (Nelson & Glass, 1999). Given the need for practitioners with this expertise, it is not surprising, therefore, that the change in Medicare reimbursement from a cost-based system to a patient-specific resource utilization system, has been associated with a greater likelihood of receiving occupational therapy services for nonelderly institutional long-term care residents (Wodchis, Fried, & Pollack, 2004).

The value associated with self-care and quality of life is also increasingly appreciated by other clinical professionals with which practitioners frequently collaborate. Multiple research articles describe how the inclusion of occupational therapy and its focus on ADL, self-care, and IADL interventions into interprofessional treatment teams enhances outcomes in function and quality of life (Gitlin et al., 2006; Miyai, 2012; Stark, Landsbaum, Palmer, Somerville, & Morris, 2009; Szanton et al., 2011; Waehrens & Fisher, 2007), reduces caregiver burden (Graff et al., 2006), decreases length of inpatient stays (O'Brien, Bynon, Morarty, & Presnell, 2012), and decreases the use of (and inherent cost of) home health aides for community-dwelling clients (Zingmark & Bernspång, 2011).

This appreciation extends beyond the many interprofessional collaborations, however. Lysaght and Wright (2005) suggested that in work-related practice settings, physical therapy approaches and interventions closely resembled those of occupational therapy practitioners. A psychiatric pilot study described the efficacy of a combined nursing case management and health management skills training program intended to enhance functional independence, independent living, and social functioning, which utilized case workers and nurses, not practitioners (Bartels et al., 2004). In other research, non-occupational therapy psychosocial programs focusing on promoting functional independence, utilizing ADL retraining, client-centered practice, "skill elicitation," and group therapies were lauded as "innovations" in the care of residents with dementia in nursing homes (Haitsma & Ruckdeschel, 2001). Perhaps the most direct example is a description of a 1-week retreat for persons with multiple sclerosis staffed by physical therapists, who assessed participants on self-esteem, quality of life, and ADL self-care (Beatus, O'Neill, Townsend, & Robrecht, 2002). The results of their retreat were described as a significant increase in quality of life related to mental components, but also a lack of significant differences in self-esteem, physical components of quality of life, or functional independence.

These examples are important in that they describe an increased appreciation of professionals with whom practitioners collaborate for the traditional goals of occupational therapy's practice domain; some even attempting to expand their own practice domains to include these traditional occupational therapy goals. Two such examples are physical therapists attempting to expand their scope of practice to include "functional training in self-care and home management (including activities of daily living and instrumental activities of daily living) and functional training in work (job/school/play) and community and leisure integration or reintegration activities (including instrumental activities of daily living, work hardening, and work conditioning)" (American Physical Therapy Association, 2014) and athletic trainers claiming knowledge about implementation of return-to-work programs (Smith, 2006).

This increased appreciation for functional training in other professions is not a substitute, however, for the

### Case Study

Veronica, a 42-year-old married mother of two teenage daughters, and has suffered from intractable right hip joint pain for many months. She had worked in a state government office for about 8 years but was increasingly unable to work because of the pain. Doctors suspected osteoarthritis despite its solitary presentation in her hip. She agreed to an elective total hip replacement and went in for surgery reluctantly. When the surgeons opened up her hip joint for the arthroplasty, they found not arthritic changes, but a stage III osteosarcoma within the joint capsule. She was brought out of the anesthesia and told she instead needed a hemipelvectomy. She underwent the procedure and was admitted to inpatient rehabilitation. She was very tearful and withdrawn for the first 2 weeks of treatment. Later weeks of functional mobility and self-care treatment were hampered by her significant anxiety. She had been assured that it would be very unlikely that the cancer would recur because it was well encapsulated and later scans showed no evidence of recurrence anywhere else in her body.

**Consider the following questions:**

1. What are her priorities for effective functioning at home?
2. Which model of practice and which assessments would you use in intervention planning?
3. What effect will her family have on her recovery?
4. What potential areas of psychosocial dysfunction could limit her function?
5. What would your treatment plan include?
6. Which of Veronica's strengths will you utilize to improve her function?

unique history, tradition, and skill set of occupational therapy practitioners, which has been honed over generations, informed by evidence-based practice, and tempered through a client-centered approach. Current occupational therapy practice has been shown to uniquely enhance occupational functioning in recent research (Alexander, Bugge, & Hagen, 2001; Hagsten, Svensson, & Gardulf, 2004; Hastings, Gowans, & Watson, 2004; Walker et al., 2004). It should be noted, therefore, that appreciation for enhancing quality of life and functional independence among non-occupational therapy clinicians is not a substitute for occupational therapy practitioners' unequalled expertise in addressing ADL and IADL performance.

## Summary

Perhaps the most emblematic interventions utilized by occupational therapists and occupational therapy assistants are those involving ADLs and IADLs. Effective evaluation and treatment of deficits in these occupational performance areas are critical to a client-centered approach, particularly because of their potential for expression of uniquely personal meaning for clients. Successful assessment and interventions related to these areas include standardized evaluations, clinical reasoning within an appropriate model of practice or frame of reference, effective use of proper strategies and approaches, and judicious application of an appreciation for the impact of contextual issues on occupational performance.

## Student Self-Assessment

1. IADL group discussion: Each of these questions can be asked of students in groups, then compiled answers can be presented to the rest of the class and discussed. Discussion can focus on identifying personal stereotypes or assumptions that may impair treatment planning, enhancing understanding of the client perspective, expression of personal values or identity through occupational performance, or the impact of resources on occupational performance, including contextual and caregiver issues.
    - Which IADL tasks are most important to you?
    - Do you believe that there are particular client populations less focused on certain components of self-care?
    - When you are busy or not feeling well, with which ADL and IADL tasks does your performance slip first, either by necessity or choice?
    - If you were working with a client with advanced Parkinson's disease in home care, how would your ADL retraining differ between your work with the client, his or her spouse, and the home health aide?
2. Nontraditional case study: This activity encourages thinking about function and personal values as opposed to rigid diagnosis-based reasoning. Additional information may be added to match recent course content, or role-playing may be used to enhance incorporation of a client-centered approach into treatment planning.

## Evidence-Based Research Chart

| Population | Evidence | References |
|---|---|---|
| Cerebrovascular accident | Client-specific interventions, particularly ADL-specific retraining, enhances independence of function | Christie, Bedford, & McCluskey, 2011; Guidetti & Ytterberg, 2011; Hill-Hermann et al., 2008; Kristensen et al., 2011; Kwan & Sandercock, 2006; Landi et al., 2006; Legg et al., 2007; Rand, Weiss, & Katz, 2009; Richards et al., 2005; Sackley et al., 2006; Trombly & Ma, 2002; Walker et al., 1999, 2004; Wolf et al., 2015 |
| Chronic obstructive pulmonary disease | ADL performance and quality of life improved with simple program | Bendstrup, Ingemann Jensen, Holm, & Bengtsson, 1997 |
| Alzheimer disease/dementia | ADL retraining can improve client quality of life and decrease sense of burden for caregivers | Dooley & Hinojosa, 2004; Graff et al., 2006 |
| Spinal cord injury | Client-centered intervention planning requires a focus on self-care and mobility | Donnelly et al., 2004 |
| Traumatic brain injury | Behavioral observation, task analysis, consistent practice, cue fading, acclimation to electronic aids to daily living are key to success with ADLs/IADLs | Boman et al., 2007; Erikson, Karlsson, Soderstrom, & Tham, 2004; Giles, Ridley, Dill, & Frye, 1997; Waehrens & Fisher, 2007 |
| Multiple sclerosis/ataxia | Combination of contextual changes, adaptations, and orthoses increase ADL function, early intervention improves function and changes sustained through 24 months | Gillen, 2000; Miyai, 2012 |
| Post-traumatic stress disorder, homeless | Role identified for occupational therapy practitioner in addressing IADLs, especially financial management | Davis & Kutter, 1998 |
| Intellectual disabilities | ADL performance hierarchy of difficulty for clients with mild and moderate intellectual disability identified, ADL and IADL performance can be improved even in absence of change in insight | Drysdale, Casey, & Porter-Armstrong, 2008; Hallgren & Kottorp, 2005; Kottorp, Bernspång, & Fisher, 2003 |
| Rheumatoid arthritis | Impact of comprehensive occupational therapy, instruction in joint protection, and splints on functional ability | Niedermann et al., 2012; Steultjens et al., 2006 |
| Orthopedics/hip fracture | Individualized occupational therapy training enhances ADL function, likelihood of independent living, and reduces need for care at home | Hagsten, Svensson, & Gardulf, 2004 |
| Pediatrics/teens/ young adults | Occupational therapy contributes to increased function, cognition, mobility in inpatient setting, increases peer connection, environmental adaptation, independence in 20-day summer program | Chen, Heinemann, Bode, Granger, & Mallinson, 2004; Healy & Rigby, 1999 |
| Cancer/brain tumors | Quality of life improvements may occur later than functional improvements, functional assessments may not sufficiently represent changes in clients | Huang, Wartella, & Kreutzer, 2001; Kasven-Gonzalez, Souverain, & Miale, 2010; Perez de Heredia, Cuadrado, Rodriguez, Lopez, & Miangolarra, 2001 |

*(continued)*

## Evidence-Based Research Chart (continued)

| Population | Evidence | References |
|---|---|---|
| Medical/surgical: Organ transplantation, emergency medicine | Direct correlations between contact with occupational therapy practitioner and greater independence with ADLs and shorter loss of service | Hastings, Gowans, & Watson, 2004; O'Brien, Bynon, Morarty, & Presnell, 2012; Patterson & Williams, 2005 |
| Mental health | Evidence for life skills and IADL training is moderate | Gibson et al., 2011 |
| Mechanical ventilation | Early intervention with occupational therapy practitioner for programs including ADL training are safe and effective from the onset of mechanical ventilation | Pohlman et al., 2010; Schweickert et al., 2009 |
| Community-dwelling elders/ home modification | Daily activity performance and health-related quality of life are enhanced by interdisciplinary programs including occupational therapy and home modification | Gitlin et al., 2006; Stark, Landsbaum, Palmer, Somerville, & Morris, 2009; Szanton et al., 2011; Zingmark & Bernspång, 2011 |

3. Group activity: Nontraditional occupations. This activity can engender discussions about cultural sensitivity, unique challenges to client education or teaching, communication issues, or enhancing the scope of available occupational performance components for use in treatment planning.
   - Have students gain an appreciation for ADL or IADL retraining from the client's perspective by teaching each other how to perform tasks not common to their cultural experience, such as learning to roll sushi, wrap a sari, tie a bowtie, or other tasks with or without simulated impairments/disabilities.
4. Group activity: Stump your classmates. This activity is a lower complexity activity that can be fun as well as educational. Teams of students can either ask other groups to guess the function of a device or present three potential uses for the device and have competing groups guess which potential use is actually correct.
   - Have students dig through catalogs of durable medical equipment and medical suppliers to find obscure adaptive equipment and attempt to "stump" each other in groups as to the purpose and application of the devices.
5. Group activity: Desert island. This can be completed in groups and each group's results discussed and critiqued by their classmates.
   - Each group is given a desert island scenario where they are assigned a disability, impairment, or limitation and an occupational performance context. They are then asked to select the three most important ADLs/IADLs in which to be independent and three most important resources or assistive equipment to have to enhance function and safety (e.g., a married client with total hip replacement precautions in a two-story house, a client with low vision in elderly housing, a married mother of three with hemiplegia and perceptual difficulties in an urban apartment).

## Electronic Resources

Adaptive equipment and durable medical equipment:

www.alimed.com

www.invacare.com

www.sammonspreston.com

## References


Alexander, H., Bugge, C., & Hagen, S. (2001). What is the association between the different components of stroke rehabilitation and health outcomes? *Clinical Rehabilitation, 15*, 207-215.

Allen, C. K., Earhart, C. A., & Blue, T. (1992). *Occupational therapy treatment goals for the physically and cognitively challenged*. Rockville, MD: American Occupational Therapy Association.

American Occupational Therapy Association. (2014). Occupational therapy practice framework: Domain and process (3rd ed.). *American Journal of Occupational Therapy, 68*(Suppl. 1), S1-S48. doi:10.5014/ajot.2014.682006

American Occupational Therapy Association. (2015). Occupational therapy code of *ethics. American Journal of Occupational Therapy, 69*(Suppl. 3).

American Physical Therapy Association. (2014). *Guidelines: Physical therapist scope of practice*. Retrieved from www.apta.org/FuploadedFiles/APTAorg%2FAbout_Us/Policies/Practice/ScopePractice.pdf

Arnadottir, G. (1990). *The brain and behavior: Assessing cortical dysfunction through tasks of daily living*. St. Louis: The C. V. Mosby Co.

Atwood, S. M., Holm, M. B., & James, A. (1994). Activities of daily living capabilities and values of long-term-care facility residents. *American Journal of Occupational Therapy, 48*, 710-716.

Bartels, S. J., Forester, B., Mueser, K., T., Miles, K. M., Dums, A. R., Pratt, S. I., Sengupta, A., Littlefield, C., O'Hurley, S., White, P., & Perkins, L. (2004). Enhanced skills training and health care management for older persons with severe mental illness. *Community Mental Health Journal, 40*, 75-90.

Beatus, J., O'Neill, J. K., Townsend, T., & Robrecht, K. (2002). The effect of a one-week retreat on self-esteem, quality of life, and functional ability for persons with multiple sclerosis. *Neurology Report, 26*(3), 154-159.

Bendstrup, K. E., Ingemann Jensen, J., Holm, S., & Bengtsson, B. (1997). Out-patient rehabilitation improves activities of daily living, quality of life and exercise tolerance in chronic obstructive pulmonary disease. *European Respiratory Journal, 10*, 2801-2806.

Boman, I.-L., Tham, K., Granqvist, A., Bartfai, A., & Hemmingsson, H. (2007). Using electronic aids to daily living after acquired brain injury: A study of the learning process and the usability. *Disability and Rehabilitation: Assistive Technology, 2*(1), 23-33.

Bottari, C., Dutil, E., Dassa, C., & Rainville, C. (2006). Choosing the most appropriate environment to evaluate independence in everyday activities: Home or clinic? *Australian Occupational Therapy Journal, 53*, 98-106. doi:10.1111/j.14401630.2006.00547.x

Center for Health Services and Policy Research. (1998). *Outcome and Assessment Information Set* (OASIS-BI). Denver, CA: Author.

Centers for Medicare and Medicaid Services. (2005). *Minimum Data Set, 2.0*. Washington, DC: U.S. Government Printing Office.

Chen, C. C., Heinemann, A. W., Bode, R. K., Granger, C. V., & Mallinson, T. (2004). Impact of pediatric rehabilitation services on children's functional outcomes. *American Journal of Occupational Therapy, 58*, 44-53.

Christiansen, C. H. (1999). Defining lives: Occupation as identity: An essay on competence, coherence, and the creation of meaning. *American Journal of Occupational Therapy, 53*, 547-558.

Christie, L., Bedford, R., & McCluskey, A. (2011). Task-specific practice of dressing tasks in a hospital setting improved dressing performance post-stroke: A feasibility study. *Australian Occupational Therapy Journal, 58*, 364-369.

Davis, J. & Kutter, C. J. (1998). Independent living skills and posttraumatic stress disorder in women who are homeless: Implications for future practice. *American Journal of Occupational Therapy, 52*, 39-44.

Davis, L. A., Hoppes, S., & Chesbro, S. B. (2005). Cognitive-communicative and independent living skills assessment in individuals with dementia: A pilot study of environmental impact. *Topics in Geriatric Rehabilitation, 21*, 136-143.

De Wit, L., Putman, K., Devos, H., Brinkmann, N., Dejaeger, E., De Weerdt, W., ... Schupp, W. (2014). Long-term prediction of functional outcome after stroke using single items of the Barthel Index at discharge from rehabilitation centre. *Disability and Rehabilitation, 36*(5), 353-358.

Donnelly, C., Eng, J. J., Hall, J., Alford, L., Giachino, R., Norton, K., & Kerr, D. S. (2004). Client-centred assessment and the identification of meaningful treatment goals for individuals with a spinal cord injury. *Spinal Cord, 42*, 302-307.

Dooley, N. R., & Hinojosa, J. (2004). Improving quality of life for persons with Alzheimer's disease and their family caregivers: Brief occupational therapy intervention. *American Journal of Occupational Therapy, 58*, 561-569.

Drysdale, J., Casey, J., & Porter-Armstrong, A. (2008). Effectiveness of training on the community skills of children with intellectual disabilities. *Scandinavian Journal of Occupational Therapy, 15*, 247-255.

Dunford, C., Missiuna, C., Street, E., & Sibert, J. (2005). Childrens' perceptions of the impact of developmental coordination disorder on activities of daily living. *British Journal of Occupational Therapy, 68*, 207-214.

Erikson, A., Karlsson, G., Soderstrom, M., & Tham, K. (2004). A training apartment with electronic aids to daily living: Lived experiences of persons with brain damage. *American Journal of Occupational Therapy, 58*, 261-271.

Fisher, A. G. (1999). *Assessment of motor and process skills* (3rd ed.). Fort Collins, CO: Three Star Press.

Gibson, R. W., D'Amico, M., Jaffe, L., & Arbesman, M. (2011). Occupational therapy interventions for recovery in the areas of community integration and normative life roles for adults with serious mental illness: A systematic review. *American Journal of Occupational Therapy, 65*, 247-256.

Giles, G. M., Ridley, J. E., Dill, A., & Frye, S. (1997). A consecutive series of adults with brain injury treated with a washing and dressing retraining program. *American Journal of Occupational Therapy, 51*, 256-266.

Gillen, G. (2000). Improving activities of daily living performance in an adult with ataxia. *American Journal of Occupational Therapy, 54*, 89-96.

Gitlin, L. N., Winter, L., Dennis, M. P., Corcoran, M., Schinfeld, S., & Hauck, W. W. (2006). A randomized trial of a multicomponent home intervention to reduce functional difficulties in older adults. *Journal of the American Geriatric Society, 54*, 809-816.

Goverover, Y., & Hinojosa, J. (2002). Categorization and deductive reasoning: Predictors of instrumental activities of daily living performance in adults with brain injury. *American Journal of Occupational Therapy, 56*, 509-516.

Graff, M. J. L., Vernooij-Dassen, M. J. M., Thijssen, M., Dekker, J., Hoefnagels, W. H. L., & Olde Rikkert, M. G. M. (2006). Community based occupational therapy for patients with dementia and their care givers: Randomized controlled trial. *British Medical Journal, 333*(7580), 1196.

Guidetti, S., & Ytterberg, C. (2011). A randomized controlled trial of a client-centred self-care intervention after stroke: A longitudinal pilot study. *Disability and Rehabilitation, 33*, 494-503.

Hagsten, B., Svensson, O., & Gardulf, A. (2004). Early individualized post-operative occupational therapy training in 100 patients improves ADL after hip fracture. *Acta Orthopaedics Scandanavia, 75*, 177-183.

Haitsma, K. V., & Ruckdeschel, K. (2001). Special care for dementia in nursing homes: Overview of innovations in programs and activities. *Alzheimer's Care Quarterly, 2*, 49-56.

Hallgren, M., & Kottorp, A. (2005). Effects of occupational therapy intervention on activities of daily living and awareness of disability in persons with intellectual disabilities. *Australian Occupational Therapy Journal, 52*, 350-359.

Hastings, J., Gowans, S., & Watson, D. E. (2004). Effectiveness of occupational therapy following organ transplantation. *Canadian Journal of Occupational Therapy, 71*, 238-242.

Healy, H., & Rigby, P. (1999). Promoting independence for teens and young adults with physical disabilities. *Canadian Journal of Occupational Therapy, 66*, 240-249.

Hill-Hermann, V., Strasser, A., Albers, B., Schofield, K., Dunning, K., Levine, P., & Page, S. J. (2008). Task-specific, patient-driven neuroprosthesis training in chronic stroke: Results of a 3-week clinical study. *American Journal of Occupational Therapy, 61*, 466-472.

Hilton, K., Fricke, J., & Unsworth, C. (2001). A comparison of self-report versus observation of performance using the Assessment of Living Skills and Resources (ALSAR) with an older population. *British Journal of Occupational Therapy, 64*, 135-143.

Huang, M. E., Wartella, J. E., & Kreutzer, J. S. (2001). Functional outcomes and quality of life in patients with brain tumors: A preliminary report. *Archives of Physical Medicine Rehabilitation, 82*, 1540-1546.

Kasven-Gonzalez, N., Souverain, R., & Miale, S. (2010). Improving quality of life through rehabilitation in palliative care: Case report. *Palliative and Supportive Care, 8*, 359-369.

Kempen, G. I., Steverink, N., Ormel, J., & Deeg, D. J. (1996). The assessment of ADL among frail elderly in an interview survey: self-report versus performance-based tests and determinants of discrepancies. *The Journals of Gerontology, Series B, Psychological Sciences and Social Sciences, 51*(5), P254-P260.

Kielhofner, G., & Forsyth, K. (2001). Measurement properties of a client self-report for treatment planning and documenting therapy outcomes. *Scandinavian Journal of Occupational Therapy, 8*, 131-139.

Klein, R. M., & Bell, B. (1979). *The Klein-Bell ADL Scale manual*. Seattle, WA: Educational Resources.

Kottorp, A., Bernspång, B., & Fisher, A. (2003). Activities of daily living in persons with intellectual disability: Strengths and limitations in specific motor and process skills. *Australian Occupational Therapy Journal, 50*, 195-204.

Kramer, A. M., Kowalsky, J. C., Lin, M., Grigsby, J., Hughes, R., & Steiner, J. F. (2000). Outcome and utilization differences for older persons with stroke in HMO and fee-for-service systems. *Journal of the American Geriatrics Society, 48*, 726-724.

Kristensen, H. K., Persson, D., Nygren, C., Boll, M., & Matzen, P. (2011). Evaluation of evidence within occupational therapy in stroke rehabilitation. *Scandinavian Journal of Occupational Therapy, 18*, 11-25.

Kwan, J., & Sandercock, P. (2006). In-hospital care pathways for stroke. *Cochrane Database of Systematic Reviews, 1*, 2006.

Landi, F., Cesari, M., Onder, G., Tafani, A., Zamboni, V., & Cocchi. A. (2006). Effects of an occupational therapy program on functional outcomes in older stroke patients. *Gerontology, 52*, 85-91.

Law, M., Baptiste, S., Carswell, A., McColl, M. A., Polatajko, H. J., & Pollack, N. (2005). *Canadian occupational performance measure* (4th ed.). Ottawa, Ontario, Canada: CAOT Publications ACE.

Leland, N. E., Crum, K., Phipps, S., Roberts, P., & Gage, B. (2015). Health policy perspectives—Advancing the value and quality of occupational therapy in health service delivery. *American Journal of Occupational Therapy, 69*, 6901090010. doi:10.5014/ajot.2015.691001

Legg, L., Drummond, A., Leonardi-Bee, J., Gladman, J. R. F., Corr, S., Donkervoort, M., ... Langhorne, P. (2007). Occupational therapy for patients with problems in personal activities of daily living after stroke: Systematic review of randomized trials. *British Medical Journal, 335*, 922.

Lysaght, R., & Wright, J. (2005). Professional strategies in work-related practice: An exploration of occupational and physical therapy roles and approaches. *American Journal of Occupational Therapy, 59*, 209-217.

Mahoney, F. I., & Barthel, D. W. (1965). Functional evaluation: The Barthel Index. *Maryland State Medical Journal, 14*, 61-65.

McAndrew, E., McDermott, S., Vitzakovitch, S., Warunek, M., & Holm, M. B. (1999). Therapist and patient perceptions of the occupational therapy goal-setting process: A pilot study. *PT and OT in Geriatrics, 17*, 55-63.

McBryde, C., Ziviani, J., & Cuskelly, M. (2004). School readiness and factors that influence decision making. *OT International, 11*(4), 193-208.

McGourty, L. K. (1979). *Kohlman evaluation of living skills*. Seattle, WA: KELS Research.

Meyer, A. (1922). The philosophy of occupational therapy. *Archives of Occupational Therapy, 1*, 11-17.

Miyai, I. (2012). Challenge of neurorehabilitation for cerebellar degenerative diseases. *Cerebellum, 11*, 436-437.

Neistadt, M. E. (1995). Methods of assessing clients' priorities: A survey of adult physical dysfunction settings. *American Journal of Occupational Therapy, 49*, 428-436.

Nelson, D. L., & Glass, L. M. (1999). Occupational therapists' involvement with the Minimum Data Set in skilled nursing and intermediate care facilities. *American Journal of Occupational Therapy, 53*, 348-352.

Niedermann, K., Buchi, S., Ciurea, A., Kubli, R., Steurer-Stey, C., Villiger, P. M., & De Bie, R. A. (2012). Six and 12 months' effects of individual joint protection education in people with rheumatoid arthritis: A randomized controlled trial. *Scandinavian Journal of Occupational Therapy, 19*, 360-369.

O'Brien, L., Bynon, S., Morarty, J., & Presnell, S. (2012). Improving older trauma patients' outcomes through targeted occupational therapy and functional conditioning. *American Journal of Occupational Therapy, 66*, 431-437.

Patterson, S., & Williams, M. (2005). *An occupational therapy consultation provided to older adults presenting to accident and emergency improves ADL functioning and reduces falls and hospital stays*. Retrieved from http://www.otcats.com/topics/CAT-OT&ADLTownsville12Jan2006.html

Perez de Heredia, M., Cuadrado, M. L., Rodriguez, G., Lopez, S., & Miangolarra, J. C. (2001). Eficacia de la Terapia Ocupacional en adolescentes con neoplasias intracraneales: estudio piloto. *Rehabilitacion, 35*(3), 140-145.

Pohlman, M. C., Schweickert, W. D., Pohlman, A. S., Nigos, C., Pawlik, A. J., Esbrook, C. L., ... Kress, J. P. (2010). Feasibility of physical and occupational therapy beginning from initiation of mechanical ventilation. *Critical Care Medicine, 38*, 2089-2094.

Rand, D., Weiss, P. L., & Katz, N. (2009). Training multitasking in a virtual supermarket: A novel intervention after stroke. *American Journal of Occupational Therapy, 63*(5), 535-542.

Richards, L. G., Latham, N. K., Jette, D. U., Rosenberg, L., Smout, R. J., & DeJong, G. (2005). Characterizing occupational therapy practice in stroke rehabilitation. *Archives of Physical Medicine Rehabilitation, 86*, S51-S60.

Richardson, J., Law, M., Wishart, L., & Guyatt, G. (2000). The use of a simulated environment (Easy Street) to retrain independent living skills in elderly persons: A randomized controlled trial. *Journal of Gerontology, 55A*, M578-M584.

Robnett, R. H., Hopkins, V., & Kimball, J. G. (2002). The Safe at Home: A quick home safety assessment. *PT and OT in Geriatrics, 20*, 77-101.

Rogers, J. C., & Holm, M. B. (1994). *Performance assessment of self-care skills (PASS) (Version 3.1)*. Unpublished manuscript, University of Pittsburgh, Pittsburgh, Pennsylvania.

Royeen, C. B. (2002). Occupation reconsidered. *OT International, 9*(2), 111-120.

Sackley, C., Wade, D. T., Mant, D., Atkinson, J. C., Yudkin, P., Cardoso, K., Levin, S., Blanchard Lee, V., & Reel, K. (2006). Cluster randomized pilot controlled trial of an occupational therapy intervention for residents with stroke in UK care homes. *Stroke, 37*, 2336-2341.

Schweickert, W. D., Pohlman, M. C., Pohlman, A. S., Nigos, C., Pawlik, A. J., Esbrook, C. L., ... Kress, J. P. (2009, May 30). Early physical and occupational therapy in mechanically ventilated, critically ill patients: A randomised controlled trial. *Lancet, 373*(9678), 1874-1882. doi:10.1016/S0140-6736(09)60658-9

Smallfield, S., & Karges, J. (2009). Classification of occupational therapy intervention for inpatient stroke rehabilitation. *American Journal of Occupational Therapy, 63*, 408-413.

Smith, K. (2006). Athletic trainers aim to expand scope [electronic version]. *OT Practice, 11*(5), 6.

Stark, S., Landsbaum, A., Palmer, J., Somerville, E. K., & Morris, J. C. (2009). Client-centered home modifications improve daily activity performance of older adults. *Canadian Journal of Occupational Therapy, 76*, 235-245.

Steultjens, E. E. M. J., Bouter, L. L. M., Dekker, J. J., Kuyk, M. M. A. H., Schaardenburg, D. D., & Van den Ende, E. C. H. M. (2006). Occupational therapy for rheumatoid arthritis. *Cochrane Database of Systematic Reviews, 1*.

Szanton, S. L., Thorpe, R. J., Boyd, C., Tanner, E. K., Leff, B., Agree, E., Xue, Q.-L., Allen, J. K., Seplaki, C. L., Weiss, C. O., Guralnik, J. M., & Gitlin, L. N. (2011). Community aging in place, advancing better living for elders: A bio-behavioral environmental intervention to improve function and health-related quality of life in disabled older adults. *Journal of the American Geriatric Society, 59*, 2314-2320.

Thompson, K. M. (1998). Early intervention services in daily family life: Mothers' perceptions of "ideal" versus "actual" service provision. *Occupational Therapy International, 5*, 206-221.

Trombly, C. (1993). Anticipating the future: Assessment of occupational function. *American Journal of Occupational Therapy, 47*, 253-257.

Trombly, C., & Ma, H. (2002). A synthesis of the effects of occupational therapy for persons with stroke, part 1: Restoration of roles, tasks, and activities. *American Journal of Occupational Therapy, 56*, 250-259.

Uniform Data System for Medial Rehabilitation. (2000). *Guide for the Uniform Data Set for Medical Rehabilitation (Including the FIM instrument; version 5.1)*. Buffalo, NY: State University of New York.

Waehrens, E. E., & Fisher, A. G. (2007). Improving quality of ADL performance after rehabilitation among people with acquired brain injury. *Scandinavian Journal of Occupational Therapy, 14*, 250-257. doi:10.1080/11038120601182974

Walker, M. F., Gladman, J. R. F., Lincoln, N. B., Siemonsma, P., & Whitely, T. (1999). Occupational therapy for stroke patients not admitted to hospital: A randomised controlled trial. *Lancet, 354*, 278-280.

Walker, M. F., Leonardi-Bee, J., Bath, P., Langhorne, P., Dewey, M., Corr, S., ... Parker, C. (2004). Individual patient data meta-analysis of randomized controlled trials of community occupational therapy for stroke patients. *Stroke, 35*, 2226-2232.

Weaver, L. L. (2015). Effectiveness of work, activities of daily living, education, and sleep interventions for people with autism spectrum disorder: A systematic review. *American Journal of Occupational Therapy, 69*(5). doi:10.5014/ajot.2015.017962

Weinstock-Zlotnick, G., & Bear-Lehman, J. (2015). Scientific/clinical article: How practitioners specializing in hand therapy evaluate the ability of patients to participate in their daily lives: An exploratory study. *Journal of Hand Therapy, 28*, 261-268. doi:10.1016/j.jht.2014.12.010

Weinstock-Zlotnick, G., & Hinojosa, J. (2004). The issue is: Bottom-up or top-down evaluation: Is one better than the other? *American Journal of Occupational Therapy, 58*, 594-599.

Williams, J. H., Drinka, T. J. K., Greenburg, J. R., Farrel-Holtan, J., Euhardy, R., & Schram, M. (1991). Development and testing of the Assessment of Living Skills and Resources (ALSAR) in elderly community-dwelling veterans. *The Gerontologist, 31*, 84-91.

Wimpenny, K., Savin-Baden, M., & Cook, C. (2014). A qualitative research synthesis examining the effectiveness of interventions used by occupational therapists in mental health. *British Journal of Occupational Therapy, 77*(6), 276-288.

Wodchis, W. P., Fried, B. E., & Pollack, H. (2004). Payer incentives and physical rehabilitation therapy for nonelderly institutional long-term care residents: Evidence from Michigan and Ontario. *Archives of Physical Medicine Rehabilitation, 85*, 210-217.

Wolf, T. J., Chuh, A., Floyd, T., McInnis, K., & Williams, E. (2015). Effectiveness of occupation-based interventions to improve areas of occupation and social participation after stroke: An evidence based review. *American Journal of Occupational Therapy, 69*, 6901180060. doi:10.5014/ajot.2015.012195

Yerxa, E. J., Burnett-Beaulieu, S., Stocking, S., & Azen, S. P. (1988). Development of the satisfaction with scaled performance questionnaire (SPSQ). *American Journal of Occupational Therapy, 42*, 215-222.

Zingmark, M., & Bernspång, B. (2011). Meeting the needs of elderly with bathing disability. *Australian Occupational Therapy Journal, 58*, 164-171.

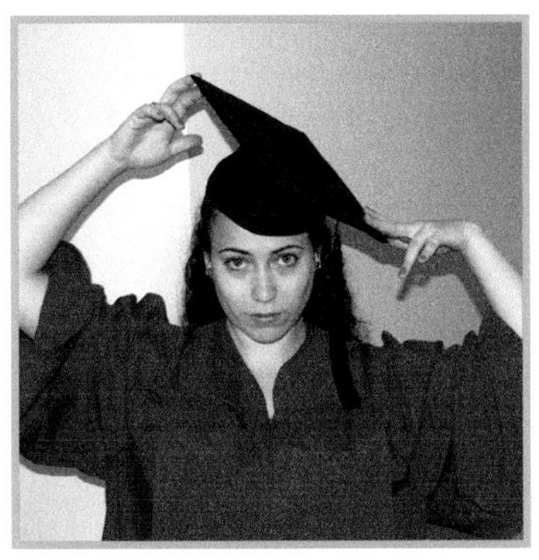

# 27

# Interventions to Enhance Occupational Performance in Education and Work

*Barbara J. Steva, MS, OTR/L*

**ACOTE STANDARDS EXPLORED IN THIS CHAPTER**

B.5.1–B.5.6, B.5.19–B.5.21

**KEY VOCABULARY**

- **Educational activities:** Tasks that facilitate learning, such as reading, writing, and math.
- **Inclusion:** The act of including and providing intervention to students with disabilities in the regular education classroom; adapting the environment for persons with disabilities to be successful in occupations, roles, and activities with others.
- **Individualized Education Program (IEP):** Written legal document developed by the individual education team that incorporates the student's strengths and need areas as well as goals and objectives for intervention.
- **Modification:** A change or alteration.
- **Related service:** Services that may be required for a student to benefit from special education; service providers include, but are not limited to, occupational therapy, physical therapy, social work, and school health services.



Jacobs, K., & MacRae, N. (Eds.).
*Occupational Therapy Essentials for Clinical Competence, Third Edition* (pp. 399-417).

This chapter addresses client identification, evaluation, and intervention within the educational setting, during the process of transition into the work force or post-secondary education, and within the work force. Models of practice are reviewed and discussed as to how they affect practice. Federal laws and regulations are outlined with the outcome of each on occupational therapy practice. The role of the occupational therapist is discussed throughout the chapter.

## Medical and Educational Models of Service Delivery

Occupational therapists must have a clear understanding of the medical and educational service delivery models guiding practice in these areas. Within the medical model, occupational therapy is a primary service provider, and services are provided to promote wellness and independence within the individual's daily occupations. In contrast, occupational therapy within the educational model is a related service in which services supplement the educational program, are provided within the educational setting, and are related to the student's success within that environment. As part of the occupational therapy evaluation, the occupational therapist determines whether or not occupational therapy services are medically necessary or required for successful access to the educational curriculum and setting. Although services may be helpful to the overall function of the student, the therapist evaluates whether the disability or impairment affects the student's ability to access and benefit from the academic instruction before recommending and implementing services. For example, a student diagnosed with cerebral palsy may be referred for an occupational therapy evaluation and found to have challenges with upper extremity function due to limited range of motion and increased muscle tone. This same student is proficient in the use of assistive technology to complete classroom work and independently uses adaptive devices for eating and dressing. It may be determined that although the student may benefit from occupational therapy to address management of muscle tone and range of motion, it is not necessary for the student's ability to access the curriculum or educational setting. Therefore, occupational therapy could be justified within the medical model but not the educational model. Occupational therapists adhere to federal and state mandates by selecting evaluation tools, goals, objectives, and interventions that will address the identified educational needs of the student. Mandates within the Individuals with Disabilities Education Act (IDEA; U.S. Department of Education, n.d.) require that services be provided within the least restrictive environment and support access to the general education or special education curriculum.

## Occupational Therapy in the Educational Setting

Occupational therapy services within the public education setting are provided under federal mandates as outlined in Table 27-1. The Rehabilitation Act was enacted in 1973 (U.S. Department of Education, 2004). This act requires services for all eligible students, enabling them to participate in their regular or special education program. The Education for All Handicapped Children Act (Cengage Learning, n.d.) ensures a free and appropriate public education without discrimination based on disability. This act was amended to become IDEA in 1977, with further amendments made in 1990, 1994, and 2004. Under the original IDEA (1977), students with specific learning disabilities were classified using IQ and individual achievement scores as the primary means of identification. An overidentification of students categorized as having a specific learning disability was suspected when students recognized with specific learning disabilities increased 200% (Vaughn, Linan-Thompson, & Hickman, 2003).

The No Child Left Behind Act of 2001 (U.S. Department of Education, n.d.) reauthorized the Elementary and Secondary Education Act initially enacted in 1965 and impressed the need for all students, including those with disadvantages, to have a fundamental right to access quality education. The Act supported education reform with the proposed outcome being improved individual educational results by establishing standard measurable goals to track student achievement.

The reauthorization of IDEA in 2004 described an additional means of identification, now commonly referred to as Response to Intervention (RtI), to identify students struggling in the classroom. RtI was developed to assist in appropriately recognizing and instructing students before they fail. The role of the occupational therapist within this process varies within states and settings. Occupational therapy consultation and strategies offered to teachers and RtI providers regarding fine motor skill development, visual perception, and sensory processing as it relates to the skills being addressed can be beneficial to the student's success. RtI is a tiered intervention provided within the regular education model that occurs prior to referral to special education. Although models vary in specifics, Berkley, Bender, Peaster, and Saunders (2009) describe a typical model consisting of three tiers. Tier 1 involves large group instruction typically found in a regular education classroom. This may include core instructional interventions provided by the classroom teacher within the context of the regular education classroom. Tier 2 uses small group instruction targeted at specific skill development and guided by evidence-based interventions and close progress monitoring. This instruction is provided in

Table 27-1.

**Public School Laws**

| | |
|---|---|
| Elementary and Secondary Education Act of 1965 | Provided funding to school districts with a high number of students from low-income families |
| The Education for All Handicapped Children Act (P.L. 94-142) | All children, ages 3 to 21, are entitled to a free and appropriate education<br>Parent and student rights and legal recourses are outlined in the event that this right is denied |
| Individuals with Disabilities Education Act (P.L. 108-446) | Services are to be provided to assist the student with a disability to benefit from special education |
| Section 504 of the Rehabilitation Act (P.L. 93-112) | Services are to be provided without discrimination of disability<br>Ensures free and appropriate accommodations and services for eligible students and entitles students with chronic diseases or disabling conditions to modifications that will allow them to participate within the regular or special education program |
| No Child Left Behind Act of 2001 | Reauthorized the Elementary and Secondary Education Act<br>Included Title I services for disadvantaged students |
| Assistive Technology Act of 2004 (P.L. 108-364) | Federally funded program under IDEA that provides access to assistive technology to individuals with disabilities to assist them with access to education, employment, and daily activities |
| Every Student Succeeds Act of 2015 | Reauthorizes the Elementary and Secondary Education Act |

addition to that received within the large group classroom setting. Tier 3, the most intensive tier, provides more concentrated and longer durations of individual instruction with frequent monitoring of progress. If a student progresses through the tiers without meeting specific individualized goals, he or she is referred for a special education evaluation.

In 2009, national and state officials began exploring the need for a standardized set of learning goals that would apply to all students kindergarten through grade 12. The standards were developed as an attempt to ensure that all students who graduate from high school are prepared for entry into college or the work force regardless of their geographical location (Common Core State Standards Initiative, 2016). The standards, addressing English Language Arts/literacy and mathematics, were developed over the course of several years with input from governors, state commissioners of education, and educators. The Common Core State Standards are not mandatory and are adopted by states and territories as they see fit. Currently there are 42 states, District of Columbia, Department of Defense Education Activity, and three U.S. territories that have adopted the Common Core State Standards. School-based practitioners must have an understanding of Common Core State Standards to support the student and educational team by providing appropriate interventions, modifications, and accommodations based on the academic content, expectations, and student need (Carroll, 2014).

In 2015, President Obama's signing of the Every Student Succeeds Act (U.S. Department of Education, n.d.) reauthorized the Elementary and Secondary Education Act and builds on the No Child Left Behind Act's call for expanded support, resources, and outcomes to prepare all students for college and careers.

## Individualized Education Program Team

Occupational therapists collaborate with educational staff and support personnel to ensure that services are available in a timely and appropriate manner. An Individualized Education Program team (IEP team) is formed when a student is not benefiting from academic instruction despite RtI efforts. The team consists of the parent or guardian, the student (when appropriate), at least one regular education teacher, at least one special education teacher, a school administrator, and all other appropriate representatives, such as a psychologist, speech-language therapist, occupational therapist, physical therapist, and social worker. Occupational therapists are related service providers and are included when the team makes a referral stating that the student would benefit from an occupational therapy evaluation.

## Evaluation of the Student

Evaluation in the school setting looks at the primary areas of function and uses a problem-solving approach to identify issues affecting the student's academic progress. Table 27-2 lists skill areas assessed and implications for functional performance within the educational setting. For example, the evaluation assesses sensorimotor

Table 27-2.

## Performance Areas and Functional Implications in the Educational Setting

| Area of Function | Skills Assessed | Potential Impact on Accessing the Educational Curriculum |
|---|---|---|
| Cognitive | Attention | Ability to listen, attend, and benefit from instruction |
| | Problem solving | Ability to use a variety of strategies (increasingly abstract) to solve a problem |
| | Visual perception:<br>• Discrimination | Ability to read and identify safety signs, letters, shapes, or pictures for communication |
| | • Memory | Ability to recall letters, shapes, numbers, and mathematical operations |
| | • Sequential memory | Ability to remember a series of letters or numbers for tasks such as spelling, copying text, remembering phone numbers, and sequencing visual cues within the environment for vocational activities |
| | • Form constancy | Ability to mentally manipulate visual information when some attributes (i.e., size or orientation) have been changed; recognize letters or forms in different contexts such as print to cursive; impacts ability to use mental pictures for tasks such as sequencing the alphabet, using the calendar, telling time, reading maps, and applying mathematical concepts; is an important skill for sewing and construction |
| | • Figure ground | Ability to locate salient information within a busy background such as words, numbers, or mathematical operations on worksheets, text, desk, drawer, bookshelf, or grocery store shelf |
| | • Visual closure/ part or whole relationships | Ability to recognize forms or objects partially hidden or incomplete letters or words; also related to part–whole integration and the ability to see the overall picture of a situation; impacts ability to tell time, perform mathematical skills, and perform mechanical or constructional tasks |
| | • Spatial relationships | Ability to recognize the directionality of letters and numbers (i.e., "b" and "d"); spatial organization of work within lines or on the page; also impacts the ability to use mental pictures to perform tasks such as sequencing the alphabet, using the calendar, telling time, reading maps, and applying mathematical concepts |
| | Visual motor:<br>• Spatial organization | Ability to organize work on a page, space letters and words, set up mathematical operations, complete artwork or projects, conceptualize parts as they relate to the whole |
| | • Directionality | Ability to correctly orient letters, numbers, and shapes; follow instructions of "up, down, right, left" |
| Developmental | Core/postural strength and stability | Ability to maintain an upright, stable, and unsupported position during instruction and tabletop/fine motor work |
| | Fine motor muscle development | Ability to activate the small/intrinsic muscles of the hand with graded controlled force and speed when writing, cutting with scissors, and object manipulation |
| | Bilateral hand coordination | Ability to use both hands together to manipulate objects and participate in physical education, recess, scissor use, writing, and drawing |
| | Eye–hand coordination | Ability to participate in play, physical education, recess, scissor use, writing, and drawing |
| | Motor planning | Ability to navigate obstacles within the classroom, learn new motor tasks such as letter formations, academic games, participation in physical education, recess, and peer interactions |
| Functional | Dressing | Clothing management before/after toileting and outdoor play, fasteners, shoe tying |
| | Mealtime | Utensil use including cutting, spreading, and opening containers |
| | Toileting | Clothing management, navigation of the bathroom environment, hygiene after toilet use |
| | Grooming | Hand washing, wiping face after meals, nose care, general appearance |

skills that may limit access to the physical environment, self-care, or participation in daily tasks expected within the academic setting. Fine motor skills are assessed to ensure adequate appropriate function in tasks requiring manipulation of objects or the use of fine motor tools and manipulatives. Visual motor skills are assessed with a focus on spatial organization, directionality, organization of work on a page, and the ability to control the writing tool for legible writing. Visual perception, inclusive of discrimination, figure ground, form constancy, spatial relationships, part or whole concepts, and memory for one or more forms are important aspects of the evaluation. These areas can affect reading ability; multistep task completion; part or whole concepts; and spatial concepts used in telling time, mathematical operations, and science. Challenges in the area of perceptual skills can also suggest a nonverbal learning disability or assist in excluding this as an identifier if strong perceptual skills are present. Finally, functional self-care skills such as toileting, feeding, grooming, and hygiene are assessed as they relate to the student's ability to participate in the school day (Figure 27-1).

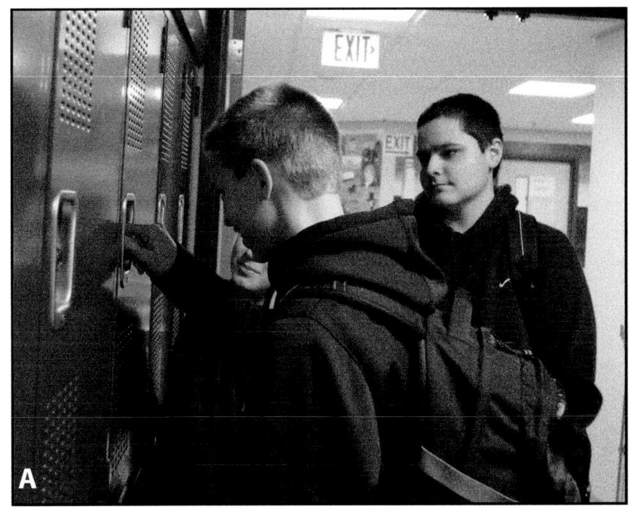


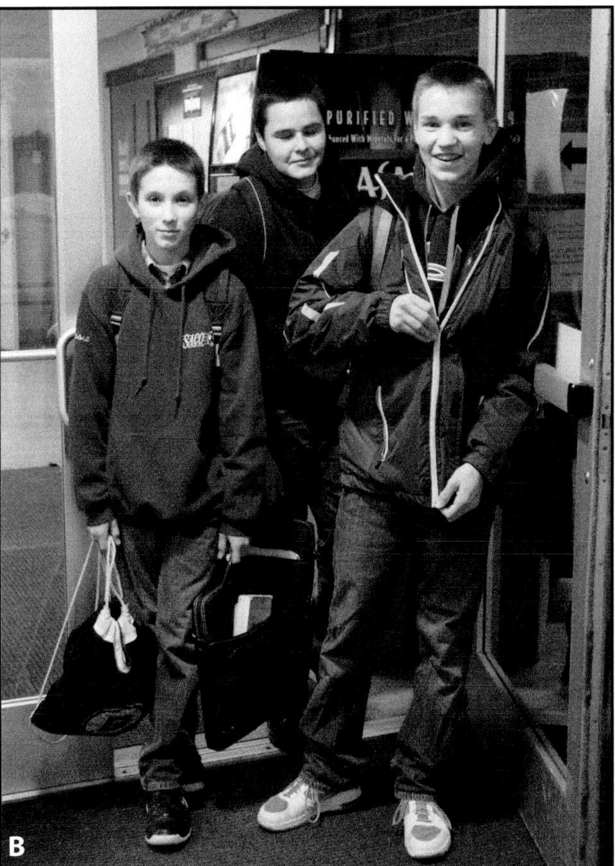


**Figure 27-1.** Daily occupations within the academic setting often require independence with activities involving visual perception and fine motor skill development. (A) Tasks can include opening a combination locker and (B) managing clothing before/after toileting or when entering/leaving the school. Students may require intervention, accommodations, or modifications to assist with these skills.

## Individualized Education Program Development

The team reviews the evaluation/assessment material collected by all disciplines to determine whether the student meets state eligibility requirements for special education. Eligibility is based on exceptional educational need. The team determines whether the information from the evaluations indicates a specific disabling or handicapping condition that prevents the student from participating in and benefiting from academic instruction.

Suchomel (2000) lists the following considerations when determining eligibility for occupational therapy services within the school:

- Does the student have an exceptional educational need that qualifies him or her for special education services, or does he or she qualify for services under Section 504 of the Rehabilitation Act?
- Does the evaluation indicate a need for occupational therapy services by demonstrating a significant delay in one or more areas of occupational performance that is affecting the student's ability to participate in academic tasks?
- Will occupational therapy assist the student in accessing and benefiting from academic instruction?
- Does the student require the skilled service of an occupational therapy practitioner, or can the tasks and interventions be carried out by other personnel?

Table 27-3.

**Representative Goal and Objectives**

| Condition | Behavior | Measurement | Outcome |
|---|---|---|---|
| Under what circumstances you expect the student to perform | What you are expecting the student to do | How you will measure success | Why this area of performance is being addressed |
| "Given..." | "Joey will..." | "...trials, over a 2-week period" "...% of the time during 3 consecutive intervention sessions" | "for use in..." |

**Goal**

Given therapeutic activities, Joey will demonstrate improved strength, endurance, and control in the trunk and upper extremity 70% of the time, as needed for fine motor, visual motor, and academic occupations by December 2017.

**Objectives**

Given therapeutic activities, Joey will demonstrate improved trunk strength and control as seen by the ability to maintain an upright sitting position in a chair or on the floor without external support for 5 minutes (first trimester), 10 minutes (second trimester), and 15 minutes (third trimester), three times per day on 4 of 5 consecutive school days, for use in daily occupations.

Given therapeutic activities, Joey will demonstrate the ability to use bilateral upper extremities at midline for writing, cutting, and playing while in an unsupported sitting position for 3 minutes (first trimester), 5 minutes (second trimester), and 10 minutes (third trimester), three times per day on 4 of 5 consecutive school days, for use in daily occupations.

## Role of the Practitioner in the Evaluation and Development of Individualized Education Program

The occupational therapist establishes the areas and methods that will be used in the evaluation of the student. The occupational therapy assistant collaborates with the occupational therapist by providing observations, collecting data, and administering/scoring assessments within their level of competency. The occupational therapist interprets and reports the information from the assessments. The practitioners collaborate in the development of goals and objectives for intervention. The occupational therapy assistant is a member of the IEP team and can attend the IEP meeting under the direction and supervision of the occupational therapist to report the findings and review goals and objectives (Solomon, 2000).

The occupational therapist provides supervision to the occupational therapy assistant by overseeing service delivery and assisting in his or her professional growth and competence. Frequency of supervision may vary depending on the knowledge and experience of the occupational therapy assistant and his or her ability to ensure safe, effective intervention. The practitioners collaborate to decide on an appropriate amount and method of supervision. Factors to consider include the practice setting, complexity of client needs, requirements of the practice setting, and skills of both the practitioners. Regulations set forth by state and federal agencies must be followed with completion of clear and appropriate documentation of supervision.

## Goals and Objectives

Together, the team determines the student's strength and need areas to develop goals and objectives for the IEP. Occupational therapy goals and objectives are individualized and specific to the student, address educational needs, and are measurable. The goal is overarching and less specific than the objectives. The objectives break the goal into specific tasks or skills required to successfully achieve the goal. Each objective defines the conditions in which you expect to see the student perform well, along with the behavior you wish the student to exhibit, how you are going to measure the behavior, and why you are intervening in this area. The goals and objectives must be directly linked to educational development. Table 27-3 shows a sample goal and objectives.

## Service Delivery Models

The type of practice model that the occupational therapist chooses to employ depends on the educational setting and student needs. Current federal mandates call for instruction to take place in the least restrictive environment. This challenges the occupational therapist to develop an intervention program that can be incorporated into the classroom whenever possible. The model of practice must be determined by carefully examining the classroom environment, the student's needs, and the ability to accomplish the prescribed goals and objectives.

Given the ever-expanding service needs within school-based practice, the workload approach as opposed to caseload approach is gaining acceptance among practitioners and school districts. A caseload approach determines the number of students assigned to a practitioner based on the number of student service hours as determined by the IEP. The workload approach takes all the practitioners work tasks that benefit the student into consideration. In addition to direct and indirect service delivery, a workload approach considers time spent in collaborative efforts with educators, parents, student meetings, and school committees, as well as development and involvement within programs such as response to intervention, travel between school buildings, universal design for learning, and positive behavioral support planning. Based on data collection, the practitioner and administration determine the most appropriate way to implement these services. When developing the workload schedule, practitioners have flexibility to address the needs of all students within the least restrictive environment.

Universal Design for Learning involves curriculum planning that addresses the needs of all students with and without special needs (National Center on Universal Design for Learning, 2012). Universal Design for Learning describes three principles or ways of thinking about learning: the recognition network or "what," strategic network or "how," and the affective network or "why." By posing these questions when designing a learning environment, the educational team is able to use strengths and needs of a student to develop an individualized academic curriculum that best serves each student. The occupational therapist uses his or her observation and assessment skills to recognize patterns of behavior and function that may be influencing the student's ability to participate in the learning environment (Post, 2015). The practitioner can then work with the education staff to develop and provide training, accommodations, and assistive technology for use within the mainstream environment.

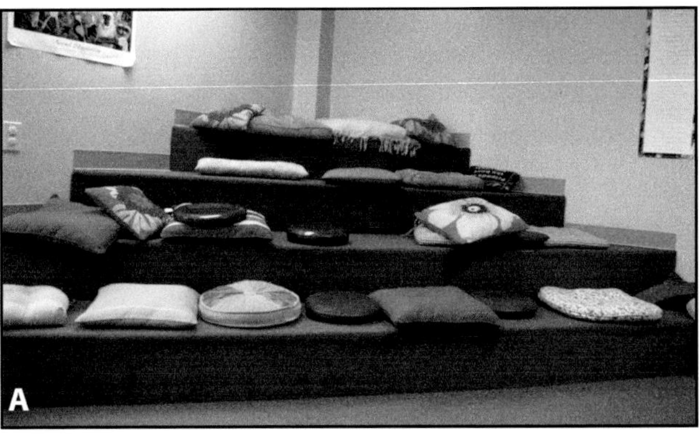

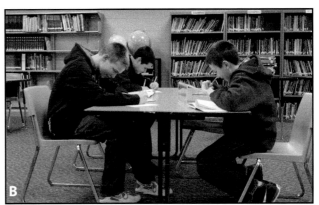

**Figure 27-2.** Through consultation, students can be provided with adaptations and accommodations that promote success. Here, (A) seating options (wiggle seats) and (B) writing strategies (slant board) can be made available to many students within the classroom setting, rather than isolating the student with challenges.

## Direct Service

Direct service occurs individually or in a small group setting. The occupational therapist decides whether this should take place in a setting outside of the classroom, often referred to as "pullout," or in an inclusive setting within the classroom environment. Pullout services involve removal of the student from the classroom for the duration of the therapy session. Inclusive therapy involves the practitioner providing therapy within the classroom environment in a nonintrusive manner. The inclusive model allows the therapist to gain knowledge regarding skills that the student needs to be successful within the classroom and allows the teacher to observe the therapeutic approach, preparing him or her to assist the student during activities when the practitioner is not present. Services are typically provided on a weekly basis for an amount of time discussed and decided on by the IEP team. Inclusion therapy ensures that the intervention supports the educational process and increases the likelihood of generalization of therapeutic techniques throughout the school day. Direct pullout services require ongoing consultation with educational staff outside of the therapy session to ensure carryover of learned tasks. This service delivery is most effective when a student is working on a skill that is significantly below that of peers and intervention within the classroom would be a distraction to other students.

## Consultation

The consultation, or collaboration, model involves the practitioner providing service through direct contact with the teacher or other educational staff working with the student (Figure 27-2). This can be the primary method of service delivery and should always be pursued in addition to the provision of direct services. When providing consultation, the practitioner must have good communication skills and insight to recognize when the tasks being asked of the teaching staff cannot be successfully implemented in the classroom. Teachers provide motivating instruction while implementing modifications and accommodations to students with varying learning styles and speeds. A common mistake of therapists is to overwhelm a teacher with activities, equipment, and specialized programs for one or two children within the classroom. As a result, teachers can become resentful and less receptive to the practitioner's ideas. It is important for the practitioner to be a part of the classroom to which he or she is consulting by observing the environment on an ongoing basis to better understand the inner workings and expectations of the environment and to tailor recommendations to the flow of the classroom schedule.

Dunn (1990) conducted a study of direct service and consultation and the effect of each practice model on student outcomes and adult attitudes. Fourteen preschool- and kindergarten-age children were randomly assigned to either a direct service or a consultation model. Children in both groups achieved nearly 75% of all IEP goals. Teachers in the consultation group, however, reported a 24% greater occupational therapy contribution to goal attainment than the direct service group. Palisano (1989) researched the use of therapist-directed groups and consultation groups. Results revealed statistically higher scores between pre- and post-test scores for the consultation group in the area of motor skills, whereas the therapist-directed group showed clinically higher scores in the area of visual perception. There was no difference in visual motor scores. These findings suggest the need for care in determining the appropriate service delivery model and the need to assess its effectiveness on a regular basis.

## *Termination of Services*

A recommendation to discontinue services is made by the occupational therapist when the established goals and objectives have been achieved. The IEP team is reconvened to review progress and discuss discontinuation of services. The student's disabilities are not necessarily "cured," but he or she is functioning within the academic setting with supports and strategies acquired through occupational therapy intervention. Through effective collaboration with the student's teacher, the occupational therapist can identify and address concerns regarding dismissal. There can be a safety net put in place in the event of regression by developing a measurable goal outlining expected performance. The occupational therapist can step back in to provide more consultation or support to the teacher and student if the goal is not being met. The occupational therapist can help the teacher intervene immediately and support the student when challenged. The therapist does not want to promote a situation in which the student and teacher are unable to function without ongoing intervention by the occupational therapist. The practitioner may slowly withdraw from the immediate environment.

# Alternative Education Settings

Recommendations for an alternative education setting are often made for students at risk for dropping out of school or failing in the public school. Risk factors include the following:

- Truancy
- Low motivation
- Inability to maintain attention
- Low self-esteem
- Behavioral difficulties

These settings incorporate the student's social, emotional, intellectual, physical, spiritual, and moral development with his or her education. Classroom size, teaching styles, and methods are commonly different from those seen in public or traditional school settings. Using questionnaires distributed to educational staff, Dirette and Kolak (2004) studied the needs of students within alternative educational settings. The top three areas of student concern included the following:

- Difficulty with time management
- Lack of participation in healthy play and leisure activities
- Maintenance of healthy lifestyle behaviors

Other areas of concern are as follows:

- Cognitive deficits such as multitasking or the ability to follow multistep instructions
- Higher level thinking skills such as problem solving and retaining/recalling information
- Coping skills
- Anger management
- Poor self-concept

Occupational therapy services are provided within this setting as in a public school setting. These settings are often privately funded and are not obligated by the federal and state mandates guiding special education services. The student's public school district is responsible for evaluating, developing, and implementing an IEP for the student regardless of placement.

## Transition Planning

Legislation guiding the transition from school to the workplace is defined in Section 602(30) of IDEA (U.S. Department of Education, n.d.), which describes "transition services" for students with disabilities beginning at the age of 14 years. By age 16, the IEP should contain a statement regarding services to be provided and designate responsibilities for the student's successful transition into the workplace, higher education, and/or community. Specifically, the mandate is designed as an outcome-oriented process, promoting transition of the student from school to post-school activities. Post-school activities may include post-secondary education, vocational training, supported or unsupported employment, adult services, independent living, or community participation. The transition plan is based on the student's strengths, preferences, and interests. Transition services should include instruction, related services, community experiences, development of employment, post-school adult living objectives, acquisition of daily living skills (as appropriate), and vocational evaluation (U.S. Department of Education, n.d.). The Americans with Disabilities Act (ADA; U.S. Equal Employment Opportunity Commission, n.d.) provides individuals with disabilities an opportunity to fulfill typical roles in the community. The act requires reasonable accommodations for the qualified individual with a disability including accessibility, job restructuring, modifications to equipment and training materials, and provision of qualified readers or interpreters. The intention of the School-to-Work Opportunities Act (Fessler State Board of Education Site, n.d.), jointly managed by the Department of Education and the Department of Labor, is to build partnerships between schools and communities and provide school-to-work programs. This mandate serves to provide opportunities for students to engage in performance-based education and training to prepare them for competitive employment, participation in post-secondary education, and navigation of the workplace. Sanford and colleagues (2011) reported that 55% of individuals with disabilities accessed post-secondary education within 6 years of leaving high school, as compared to 62% of nondisabled peers. Individuals with disabilities were as likely (71%) as their nondisabled counterparts (71%) to be engaged in paid employment outside the home within 6 years of leaving high school.

Occupational therapists can offer knowledgeable and unique perspectives when preparing for education and employment of the student with special needs following high school. It is the occupational therapist's responsibility to understand the current terminology, laws, trends, and interventions that will best serve this population. Depending on the practitioner's role within the school setting and IEP team, advocacy for involvement along with education of school personnel may be needed to promote recognition of the impact and role of occupational therapy in this process.

Occupational therapists contribute to the transition from school to post-secondary education or work by offering skills in the assessment, training, and reinforcement of work skills and behavior. Despite the knowledge and expertise that practitioners have to offer in this area, Kardos and White (2005) found a lack of occupational therapy involvement in transitional planning. Barriers to involvement included transition services being handled by other professionals (special education teachers, guidance or transition coordinators), a lack of understanding of the role of occupational therapy in transition planning, a lack of funding within the school budget to utilize occupational therapy as a transitional team member, a lack of knowledge regarding assessment tools for evaluation in this area, and students being dismissed from occupational therapy prior to age 14 when transition planning is initiated. Asher (2003) described factors that potentially affect successful transition from secondary education to community and areas where practitioners can provide meaningful intervention. These are outlined in Table 27-4.

## Work

Work is one of the primary roles in life that is essential to health and wellness. However, there have been several incomplete definitions. Work has been defined as what people do to earn a living (Brief & Nord, 1990); as an activity done in a specific place and time, on a regular basis (Hearnshaw, 1954); and as employment perceived by individuals as their main occupation, by which they are known, and from which they derive their societal role (Shimmin, 1966). Work may mean different things to different individuals. One may see it as obligatory, whereas another may find it enjoyable regardless of whether there is a monetary value attached to it. The American Occupational Therapy Association's (AOTA) *Occupational Therapy Practice Framework* (2014) describes work as having six components addressed by occupational therapy practice. These are employment interests and pursuits, employment seeking and acquisition, job performance, retirement preparation and adjustment, volunteer exploration, and volunteer participation (Ellexson & Larson, 2011).

Individuals participate in work as a means of financially supporting themselves and their families. After retirement from this role, senior citizens and the elderly often continue to contribute to the workforce through volunteering. This provides a fulfilling experience to individuals who have spent most of their lives in the worker role and may ease their transition to retirement. The terms *work* and *occupation* have evolved to be used synonymously, creating confusion. The *Merriam-Webster Dictionary* defines work as "the labor, task, or duty that

Table 27-4.

**FACTORS FOR SUCCESSFUL SCHOOL/WORK TRANSITION**

| Factor | Evaluation/Assessment Area | Intervention |
|---|---|---|
| Accessibility of the work area | Is adaptive equipment required for positioning or accessibility? | Training in appropriate use of the equipment |
| Student | Sensory, motor, and cognitive-perceptual skills | Development and training in the use of adaptations |
| Task | Analysis of job requirements and components | Preteach the sequence or specific job tasks that may be problematic; develop supports to assist with successful completion of the tasks |
| Skill development | Assessment of job requirements (i.e., standing, finger dexterity) | Develop and implement a program into the school day to work on needed skills |
| Personal care | Independence in self-care | Develop and implement a program involving personal hygiene (i.e., grooming, toileting, eating) into the school day |
| Communication | Evaluation of the need for assistive technology | Develop and implement assistive technology in conjunction with the speech and language clinician as appropriate to enhance communication |
| Job carving | Assessment of the job site to discern any other job possibilities not previously considered | Training in areas required to fulfill other responsibilities within the site |

is one's accustomed means of livelihood," and occupation as "an activity in which one engages" or "the principal business of one's life." Regardless of the reason an individual participates in work-related activities, whether for financial reimbursement or enjoyment, the role of the worker often encompasses the majority of the individual's time each day, making work a primary occupation for him or her.

Before providing any type of intervention within the work environment, a comprehensive evaluation of the worksite and the worker must be completed. A conceptual framework, proposed by Sandqvist and Henriksson (2004), identifies three dimensions for the assessment of work function. These are work participation, work performance, and individual capacity. Work participation refers to the ability of the individual to gain and maintain employment within society. Factors such as public support and the demands on the individual are considered. Work performance refers to the individual's ability to perform the tasks associated with the work activity. Finally, individual capacity refers to the individual's ability to physically and psychologically complete the work activities.

## *Role of the Practitioner in the Evaluation and Intervention Within the Workplace*

Before an individual treatment plan is developed, the occupational therapist conducts a thorough evaluation of the worker's skills and the workplace. The occupational therapist is responsible for all aspects of the evaluation, planning, and intervention process. The occupational therapy assistant works under direct supervision of the occupational therapist to complete this process. Both practitioners work together to ensure the appropriate level of supervision required based on the complexity of client needs; experience of the practitioners; type of practice setting; and state, agency, and other regulatory requirements. The occupational therapist is responsible for conducting the evaluation process, interpreting the results, defining need areas, and developing a treatment plan based on the client's goals and priorities. The occupational therapy assistant participates in the process by implementing tasks deemed appropriate by the occupational therapist. The assistant is responsible for understanding evaluation results and intervention goals. The occupational therapy assistant provides ongoing written and verbal reports to the occupational therapist as the process progresses for effective collaboration in the implementation of the intervention plan and achievement of client goals (AOTA, 2009).

## Intervention

Performance challenges affecting fulfillment of the worker role can be related to motor, sensory, perceptual, and/or emotional skills. In addition, performance patterns, activity demands, or environmental contexts play a part in the successful participation of the worker. Occupational therapy practitioners are skilled in providing services addressing work hardening or conditioning, prework screening, functional capacity assessment and ergonomics, prevocational assessment and training, sheltered or supported employment, and transition from school to work (Ellexson & Larson, 2011).

Intervention is required for those individuals with physical, cognitive, and developmental disabilities, as well as those who become injured as a result of work-related stress or other activities such as carpal tunnel injury, chronic back pain, or brain injury. Interventions may include direct service in the form of job training, training to perform a specific task, muscle strengthening, implementation of task modifications, and accommodations such as ergonomic supports to assist with back pain or repetitive use injuries. Occupational therapists may be used as consultants to the employer to ensure that hiring procedures and job descriptions are nondiscriminatory and the workplace is ergonomically safe for workers and meets ADA regulations (AOTA, 2000). Table 27-5 outlines laws and regulations for services for individuals with disabilities. Social Security or Supplemental Security Income benefits are granted to individuals unable to work due to disability. If and when the individual is ready to explore employment, the Ticket to Work incentive program allows individuals 18 to 64 years of age to receive free employment support services. The program provides incentives to seek or return to work without the threat or fear of losing current health care or cash benefits. Individuals seeking employment have been presented with additional barriers in the areas of employment, vocational rehabilitation, and Ticket to Work knowledge and utilization (Hernandez et al., 2007). Employment barriers include negative employer attitudes to individuals with disabilities, limited transportation options, and limited formal education. Consumers reported vocational rehabilitation to offer only low-paying, temporary, and menial positions in addition to unresponsive and non-collaborative counselors. Consumers' response to their knowledge of the Ticket to Work program revealed poor knowledge of the benefit, fear of losing medical benefits, and limited utilization of the program.

Traditional vocational rehabilitation efforts have focused on "supply-side" training when working with individuals with disabilities who are seeking employment. Supply-side training involves a comprehensive evaluation of the individual's current skills, function, and individual interests for employment. Specific intervention is then provided to teach needed skills for successful participation in the workplace. "Demand-side" training has more recently become a focus in the employment of individuals with disabilities. The demand-side approach looks at the workplace demands and needs (i.e., the employer and workplace involved in hiring and retaining individuals). Chan and colleagues (2010) found barriers to employment of individuals with disabilities to include a lack of the category of disability as part of diversity plans within companies, a lack of resources to recruit and retain persons with disabilities, and inadequate training in the ADA and workplace accommodations.

The practitioner working with individuals with disabilities seeking employment opportunities must work with the clients to develop required physical, cognitive, and social skills. They must also be a resource to potential employers by providing information regarding the needs of the client/worker in addition to providing education and training regarding ADA regulations and accommodations that can be put in place to support both the worker and the employer.

Regardless of the reason for initial referral to occupational therapy, a thorough evaluation of the client's needs and abilities and an analysis of the work task are required before developing an intervention plan (Figure 27-3). Goals and objectives are developed and written in conjunction with the client and with the employer when appropriate. These are objective, task oriented, and measurable to assist in planning for dismissal from occupational therapy services. Knowledge of universal design, construction guidelines, specialized products, and government guidelines is essential in providing guidance to the employer and solutions for the worker within the workplace.

Pohlman, Poosawtsee, Gerndt, and Lindstrom-Hazel (2001) surveyed workers' compensation carriers to assess how occupational therapy programs can best meet the needs of the carriers. Results showed that carriers consider a rehabilitation program successful if the worker is able to return to any job position. The carriers reported that occupational therapy programs are beneficial for returning to work, although it was stated that most carriers did not understand what occupational therapy was or how it could assist in returning an individual to the workforce. This study suggests the need for educating insurance carriers as to the role of the occupational therapist with the worker who has an injury or disability.

## Frames of Reference

A frame of reference and model of practice are used to guide the practitioner's thinking and subsequent intervention plan and activities. The model of practice sets the foundation for the practitioner's thinking while the frame of reference guides the development of critical problem solving and intervention planning. The following section

Table 27-5.

## Workplace Legislation

| Legislation | Provisions |
|---|---|
| Federal Employees Liability (FELA) Act, 1908 (45 U.S.C. 51, et seq.) | • No-fault insurance system<br>• Pays benefits to employees for accidental, work-related injuries and diseases |
| Vocational Rehabilitation Act Amendments of 1943 (P.L. 78-113) | • Amended Vocational Rehabilitation Act of 1920<br>• Includes individuals with physical disabilities, blindness, developmental delays, and psychiatric disabilities<br>• Office of Vocational Rehabilitation established |
| Vocational Rehabilitation Act Amendments (Hill-Burton Act) of 1954 (P.L. 86-565) | • Greater financial support, research and demonstration grants, and professional preparation grants<br>• State agency expansion and improvement grants<br>• Grants to expand rehabilitation facilities |
| Vocational Rehabilitation Act Amendments of 1965 (P.L. 89-333) | • Expanded services to people with disabilities and social handicaps<br>• Money for construction of rehabilitation centers and workshops made available |
| Architectural Barriers Act of 1968 (P.L. 90-48) | • Initiated changes in access for people with disabilities |
| Developmental Disabilities Services and Facilities Construction Act of 1970 (P.L. 91-517) | • States received responsibility for planning and implementing service programs for people with developmental delays, epilepsy, cerebral palsy, and other neurological impairments |
| Occupational Safety and Health Act of 1970 (P.L. 91-596) | • Mandated employers to provide a work environment free of hazards that were likely to cause death or serious harm to workers |
| Rehabilitation Act of 1973 (P.L. 93-112) | • Services expanded to include individuals with more severe disabilities<br>• Provided affirmative action in employment (Section 503) and non-discrimination in facilities (Section 504) by federal contractors and grantees |
| Rehabilitation Act Amendments of 1986 (P.L. 99-506) | • Clarification to include that evaluation of clients must include recreation, employability, and rehabilitation needs |
| Education of the Deaf Act of 1986 (P.L. 99-371) | • Provided technical training and education to prepare people with hearing impairments for employment |
| Omnibus Budget Reconciliation Act of 1987 (P.L. 99-371) | • Allowed states to offer prevocational, educational, and supported employment services to individuals deinstitutionalized prior to the waiver program |
| Americans with Disabilities Act of 1990 (P.L. 101-336) | • Prevented discrimination against people with disabilities<br>• Guaranteed equal protection to individuals with disabilities in employment, public accommodations, transportation, state and local government, and telecommunications |
| Ticket to Work and Work Incentive Improvement Act of 1999 (P.L. 106-170) | • Increased opportunities to recipients of Social Security benefits to obtain employment, vocational rehabilitation, and other support services (from public or private providers, employers, and other organizations) |
| Americans with Disabilities Act Amendments Act of 2008 (P.L. 110-325) | • Focused on discrimination rather than the disability<br>• Made changes in the definition of disability |

Adapted from Ellexson, M., & Larson, B. (2011). Occupational therapy services in facilitating work performance. *American Journal of Occupational Therapy, 65,* s55-s64.

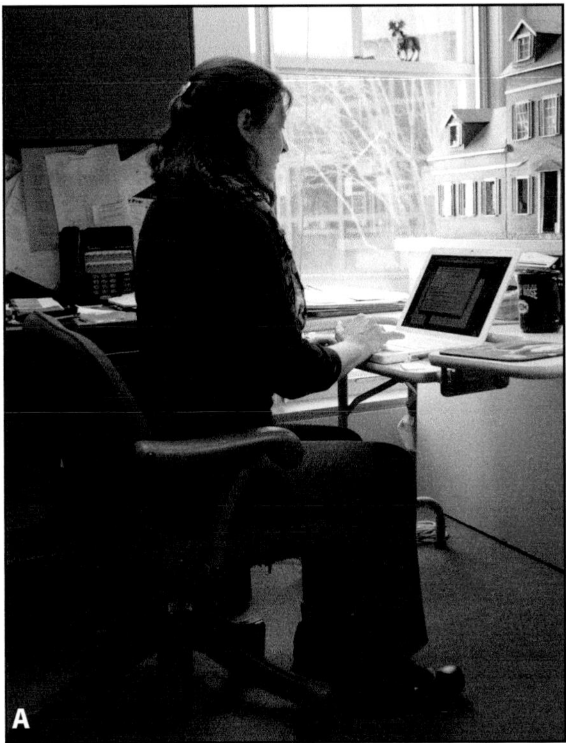

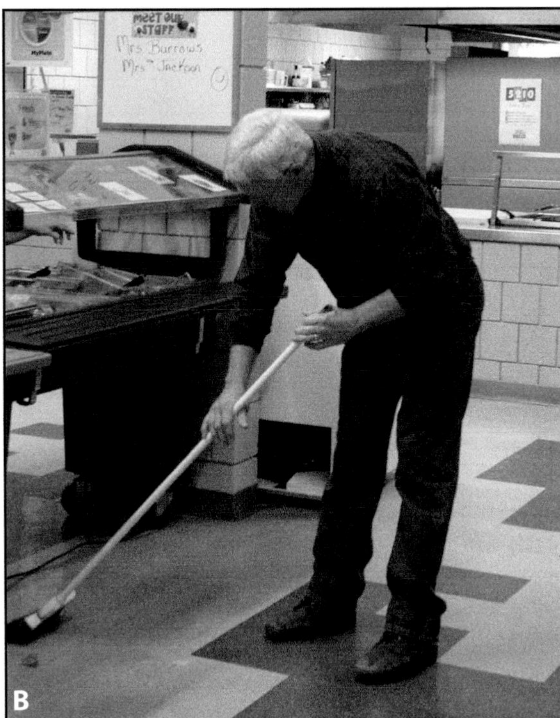

**Figure 27-3.** (A, B) Management and prevention of workplace injuries can involve consultation to employers and staff regarding ergonomics, body mechanics, and work modification.

summarizes a few frames of reference used in school and work intervention. These do not encompass all frames of reference, and the practitioner should be diligent in researching other frames of reference to ensure he or she chooses the appropriate framework in which to plan evaluation and intervention.

## Neurodevelopmental Frame of Reference

The original theories and practice of Neurodevelopmental Treatment (NDT) were developed from the work of Karel and Berta Bobath's intervention of individuals with brain injury. NDT is a sensorimotor approach focusing on motor and postural theories that translate to independence in active tasks (Dunn, 1990). The theories have a strong foundation in normal development and the interpretation of motor responses. These include motor control developing from head to foot, midline to the limbs, and large to small movements. The developmental sequence, integrating primitive reflexes, and achieving developmental milestones are stressed when designing interventions. Mobility is built on stability and progresses outward as the child begins to explore the environment. The trunk is typically where intervention is initiated, progressing to more advanced movements performed away from the trunk. Because NDT focuses on abnormal movement patterns and attempts to extinguish these in favor of more appropriate or typical motor patterns, this theory may not always be effective in treating children with changes in muscle tone, such as cerebral palsy. These children build motor patterns that are successful for them. By changing their motor pattern, they may become dependent in areas or tasks in which they were previously independent.

## Biomechanical Frame of Reference

The biomechanical frame of reference is based in physical science such as kinesiology and physics. A balance between stability and mobility is a primary focus, which takes muscle tone and skeletal alignment into consideration (Dunn, 2000). Muscle tone is the amount of tension in a muscle or muscle group at any given time. Muscle tone is not an exact science and exists along a continuum. Many individuals with high or low muscle tone, relative to "typical," lead functional and productive lives with no detriment to themselves or their lifestyle. An individual with a disorder of the central nervous system may have more severe challenges in regulating the amount of tension present in the muscles during activity or rest. An individual with cerebral palsy may have "high" or "increased" muscle tone resulting from excess tension in the muscles. This leaves the individual at risk for shortened muscle length or contractures due to poor stretch and relaxation. Function is affected due to the decreased ability to relax and tense the muscle as needed for mobility. "Low" or "decreased" muscle tone in an individual is a result of excessive relaxation of the muscles. This leaves the individual at risk for subluxation of joints due to laxity and poor tension in the muscles. Function is affected by a lack of stability. The underlying goal of the biomechanical frame of reference is improved skeletal alignment by developing postural control for use in functional occupations (Dunn, 2000). This can be done through strengthening exercises and activities or the use of positioning devices. Indicators of poor postural control are a decreased ability to maintain an upright position without external support. This is often seen when the individual leans on a table or desk for support or slouches in a chair. These are often seen in school and work settings and can affect an individual's ability to work effectively and efficiently. The biomechanical approach is most commonly used when assessing and providing wheelchairs or splints to improve positioning and function.

## Motor Learning and Motor Control Frame of Reference

The motor learning theory focuses on the process of learning rather than a specific task. Approaches of feedback, feed-forward, and event are described in the literature (Breslin, 1996). The feedback approach relies on information from the environment to provide feedback regarding movement. Arguments to this approach include the closed-loop system, which does not allow for variability in the routine (Gliner, 1985). The feed-forward approach suggests that a motor plan is created prior to carrying out the motor task and is adapted during future use based on feedback from the environment. This is felt to promote variability, although Croce and DePaepe (1989) argued that a separate motor plan for every motor task would be very complex. Gliner (1983) pointed out that these approaches focus on the learner as the primary component and the environment being a secondary factor. The event approach brings both the learner and the environment together and purposeful activity to the forefront. This approach describes the learner as subconsciously choosing the motor plan for a purposeful task from a learned repertoire. The environment provides the learner with feedback regarding the success of the plan, and movements are adjusted at that time or stored for future use. The therapist provides intervention through the use of feedback regarding the success or failure of a movement, structuring the environment or task while the individual engages in a purposeful movement activity (Breslin, 1996). This approach is commonly used within the academic and work settings to address fine motor skill development and skills needed to engage in physical education or playground activities.

## Sensory Integration Frame of Reference

A. Jean Ayres developed Sensory Integration theory in the early 1970s as she attempted to apply neuroscientific knowledge to her practice with children diagnosed with "minimal brain dysfunction," today known as attention deficit hyperactivity disorder. The theory emphasizes the individual's ability to interact with the environment by receiving and organizing sensory information. This information is used to produce an adaptive response and adjust to changes within the environment. Sensory input affects aspects of physical, cognitive, and emotional responses. An individual exhibiting an extreme response to an otherwise benign input such as a gentle tap on the shoulder by a friend would be displaying overresponsivity. Overresponsivity describes the nervous system's state of hyperarousal (fright, fight, or flight), where all input is interpreted as a threat. An individual displaying underresponsivity requires excessive input to register sensory stimulation. This may be the case with the child who loves to spin and purposely crashes to the floor or does not cry when injured. Sensory Integration theory attempts to normalize sensory input to produce an adaptive response that fits the situation at hand.

Sensory Integration theory can be implemented in several ways within the educational or work environment. Many schools and most workplaces do not have the equipment or space to apply optimal intervention using this theory. This approach can be effectively used to develop and implement a sensory diet of activities or strategies to provide individuals with an optimal level of arousal to participate in their academic or work occupations. Table 27-6 reviews the sensory systems and the type of stimulation used to facilitate a calming or alerting response in an individual. These strategies can be used throughout the day to maintain an optimal level of arousal for productive work.

# Summary

The implementation of occupational therapy services within the education and work models requires teamwork and ongoing collaboration with the members of the IEP team or the employers to ensure that individuals are capable of interacting and participating in the tasks being asked of them. The occupational therapist assists in the transition from secondary education into the workforce, independent/supported living, or post-secondary education.

Table 27-6.

**Factors Affecting Sensory Regulation**

| Type of Input | Relaxing/Calming | Alerting |
|---|---|---|
| Vestibular movement of the head through space | • Slow<br>• Rhythmic<br>• Linear—one plane<br>• Movement while on stable ground | • Fast<br>• Jerky<br>• Frequent changes of direction<br>• Angular movement<br>• Suspended equipment |
| Proprioception—compression or stretch of a joint | • Joint compression<br>• Slow stretch<br>• Heavy and sustained resistance | • Quick/unexpected changes<br>• Jarring/jerking<br>• Abrupt stops and starts |
| Tactile—any kind of touch | • Firm/deep pressure<br>• Swaddling<br>• Firm stroking over large areas<br>• Smooth texture<br>• Familiar and predictable<br>• Warmth | • Light touch<br>• Poking<br>• Touch on the face<br>• Rough texture<br>• Unexpected touch<br>• Cold |
| Visual | • Rhythmic<br>• Constant<br>• Blue and green shades<br>• Dim or dark<br>• Familiar and predictable | • Unexpected<br>• Bright colors or lights<br>• Red and yellow shades<br>• Black on white<br>• Changing or moving stimuli |
| Auditory | • Expected<br>• Familiar<br>• Quiet gentle rhythm<br>• Melodic | • Unexpected<br>• Loud<br>• Complex |
| Olfactory | • Familiar—associated with comforting experiences | • All odors |

## Student Self-Assessment

Sam is a 7-year-old boy with cerebral palsy. He is in a regular first-grade classroom with educational support from an educational technician 100% of the day. Sam is independent with ambulation using a rear walker. His upper extremity strength and control are poor, with ataxic movements affecting precision with fine motor tasks. He uses raking finger movements and a lateral pinch to retrieve objects. Release is not always volitional, and he drops many items. Sam is independent in toileting, with the exception of clothing management. At this time, there is a private bathroom within the classroom where Sam's educational technician can assist him as needed. Sam's difficulty in toileting has been an ongoing area of need described by his parents at the IEP meeting. The team agrees that this is an area of need, particularly as he gets older and needs to use one of the public restrooms while at school.

1. Write at least one goal and two objectives to address Sam's independence in self-care while in school.
2. Describe the theoretical model, intervention activities, and potential accommodations or modifications that the occupational therapist may use in Sam's intervention.

Susan, a receptionist, is referred to occupational therapy due to chronic back and shoulder pain resulting from work-related stress. During your evaluation, you find that her computer desk is above elbow level when she is sitting. The computer is set to her right, at an angle to the keyboard, causing Susan to rotate her upper body while working. She schedules appointments and is frequently using the telephone and computer simultaneously, needing to hold the telephone between her ear and shoulder. Susan enjoys her job and does not want to leave in pursuit of other opportunities.

1. Describe the approach most beneficial in the intervention of Susan's pain.

## Evidence-Based Research Chart

| Area Addressed | Topic | Evidence |
|---|---|---|
| Educational settings | Autism | Koenig, Buckley-Reen, & Garg, 2012; Tanner, Hand, O'Toole, & Lane, 2015; Tomchek, Little, & Dunn, 2015 |
| | Handwriting | Alaniz, Galit, Necesito, & Rosario, 2015; Case-Smith, Weaver, & Holland, 2014; Schwellnus et al., 2013 |
| | Evaluation | Pfeiffer et al., 2015 |
| | Attention deficit hypersensitivity disorder | Clince, Connolly, & Nolan, 2016; Lin, Lee, Chang, & Hong, 2014; Maeir et al., 2014 |
| | Mental health | Arbesman, Bazyk, & Nochajski, 2013; Weaver & Darragh, 2015 |
| Workplace | Injuries/illnesses to the back and upper extremities | Amini, 2011; Bohr, 2011; Snodgrass, 2011; Von der Heyde, 2011 |
| | Assistive technology | Banda, Dogoe, & Matuszny, 2011; Burke et al., 2013 |
| | Ergonomics | Esmaeilzadeh, Ozcan, & Capan, 2013; Jaromi, Nemeth, Kranicz, Laczko, & Betlehem, 2012 |
| | Mental health | Arbesman & Logsdon, 2011 |
| Effectiveness | Sensory integration | Urwin & Ballinger, 2005; Vargas & Camilli, 1999; Watling & Hauer, 2015 |
| | Neurodevelopmental intervention | Brown & Burns, 2001; DeGangi, 1994a, 1994b; Jonsdottir, Fetters, & Kluzik, 1997; Kluzik, Fetters, & Coryell, 1990; Lilly & Powell, 1990; Miles Breslin, 1996; Tsorlakis, Evaggelinou, Grouios, & Tsorbatzoudis, 2004 |
| | Motor learning/motor control | Baron & Littleton, 1999; Butler et al., 2001; Miles Breslin, 1996 |
| Alternative education settings | Intervention | Dirette & Kolak, 2004 |

2. Write a care plan for Susan that includes outcome potential, at least one goal, and two objectives.
3. How can the occupational therapist work with Susan's employer to provide accommodations to assist her in working pain free? What are those accommodations?

## Electronic Resources

Education Mandates, Regulations, and Resources: www.ed.gov/index.jhtml

Handwriting Development Standards: http://www.hwtears.com/hwt/why-it-works/handwriting-standards-correlations

Sensory Processing Disorder Foundation Resources: www.spdfoundation.net

Work and School Intervention/Practice Resources: www.aota.org

## References

Alaniz, M. L., Galit, E., Necesito, C. I., & Rosario, E. R. (2015). Hand strength, handwriting, and functional skills in children with autism. *American Journal of Occupational Therapy, 69*, 6904220030.

American Occupational Therapy Association. (2000). Occupational therapy and the Americans with Disabilities Act (ADA). *American Journal of Occupational Therapy, 54*(6), 622-625.

American Occupational Therapy Association. (2009). Guidelines for supervision, roles, and responsibilities during the delivery of occupational therapy services. *American Journal of Occupational Therapy, 63*, 797-803.

American Occupational Therapy Association. (2014). Occupational therapy practice framework: Domain and process (3rd ed.). *American Journal of Occupational Therapy, 68*(Suppl. 1), S1-S48. doi:10.5014/ajot.2014.682006

Amini, D. (2011). Occupational therapy interventions for work-related injuries and conditions of the forearm, wrist, and hand: A systematic review. *American Journal of Occupational Therapy, 65*, 29-36.

Arbesman, M., Bazyk, S., & Nochajski, S. M. (2013). Systematic review of occupational therapy and mental health promotion, prevention, and intervention for children and youth. *American Journal of Occupational Therapy, 67*, e120-e130.

Arbesman, M., & Logsdon, D. W. (2011). Occupational therapy interventions for employment and education for adults with serious mental illness: A systematic review. *American Journal of Occupational Therapy, 65*, 238-246.

Asher, A. (2003). From student to employee: Helping students with disabilities make the transition. *Developmental Disabilities Special Interest Section Quarterly, 26*(4), 1-4.

Assistive Technology Act of 2004, Pub. L. 108-364, 118 Stat. 1707.

Banda, D. R., Dogoe, M. S., & Matuszny, R. M. (2011). Review of video prompting studies with persons with developmental disabilities. *Education and Training in Autism and Developmental Disabilities, 46*, 514-527.

Baron, K. B., & Littleton, M. J. (1999). The model of human occupation: A return to work case study. *WORK, 12*(1), 3-12.

Berkley, S., Bender, W. N., Peaster, L. G., & Saunders, L. (2009). Implementation of Response to Intervention. A snapshot of progress. *Journal of Learning Disabilities, 42*, 85-95.

Bohr, P. C. (2011). Systematic review and analysis for work-related injuries to and conditions of the elbow. *American Journal of Occupational Therapy, 65*, 24-28.

Breslin, D. (1996). Motor learning theory and the neurodevelopmental treatment approach: A comparative analysis. *Occupational Therapy in Health Care, 10*(1), 25-40.

Brief, A. P., & Nord, W. R. (1990). *The meanings of occupational work: A collection of essays*. Lanham, MD: Lexington Books.

Brown, G. T., & Burns, S. A. (2001). The efficacy of neurodevelopmental treatment in paediatrics: A systematic review. *British Journal of Occupational Therapy, 64*(5), 235-244.

Burke, R. V., Allen, K. D., Howard, M. R., Downey, D., Matze, M. G., & Bowen, S. L. (2013). Tablet-based video modeling and prompting in the workplace for individuals with autism. *Journal of Vocational Rehabilitation, 38*, 1-14.

Butler, C., Adams, R., Chambers, H., Abel, M., Damiano, D., Edgar, T., ... McLaughlin, J. (2001), Effects of neurodevelopmental treatment (NDT) for cerebral palsy: An AACPDM evidence report. *Developmental Medicine and Child Neurology, 43*, 778-790.

Carroll, T. C. (2014). *What should the occupational therapy practitioner should know about the Common Core State Standards (CCSS)*. Retrieved from http://www.aota.org/

Case-Smith, J., Weaver, L., & Holland, T. (2014). Effects of a classroom-embedded occupational therapist–teacher handwriting program for first-grade students. *American Journal of Occupational Therapy, 68*, 690-698.

Cengage Learning. (n.d.). *The education for all handicapped children act (PL 94-142) 1975*. Retrieved from http://college.cengage.com/education/resources/res_prof/students/spec_ed/legislation/pl_94-142.html

Chan, F., Strauser, D., Maher, P., Lee, E., Jones, R., & Johnson, E. T. (2010). Demand-side factors related to employment of people with disabilities: A survey of employers in the midwest region of the United States. *Journal of Occupational Rehabilitation, 20*, 412-419.

Clince, M., Connolly, L., & Nolan, C. (2016). Comparing and exploring the sensory processing patterns of higher education students with attention deficit hyperactivity disorder and autism spectrum disorder. *American Journal of Occupational Therapy, 70*, 7002250010.

Common Core State Standards Initiative. (2016). *Common core state standards, development process*. Retrieved from http:// www.corestandards.org/about-the-standards/development-process/

Croce, R., & DePaepe, J. (1989). A critique of therapeutic intervention programming with reference to an alternative approach based on motor learning theory. *Physical and Occupational Therapy in Pediatrics, 9*(3), 5-33.

DeGangi, G. A. (1994a). Examining the efficacy of short-term NDT intervention using a case-study design: Part 1. *Physical and Occupational Therapy in Pediatrics, 14*(1), 71-88.

DeGangi, G. A. (1994b). Examining the efficacy of short-term NDT intervention using a case-study design: Part 2. *Physical and Occupational Therapy in Pediatrics, 14*(2), 21-61.

Dirette, D., & Kolak, L. (2004). Occupational performance needs of adolescents in alternative education programs. *American Journal of Occupational Therapy, 58*(3), 337-341.

Dunn, W. (1990). A comparison of service provision models in school-based occupational therapy services: A pilot study. *Occupational Therapy Journal of Research, 10*(5), 300-320.

Dunn, W. (2000). *Best practice occupational therapy: In community service with children and families*. Thorofare, NJ: SLACK Incorporated.

Ellexson, M., & Larson, B. (2011). Occupational therapy services in facilitating work performance. *American Journal of Occupational Therapy, 65*, s55-s64.

Esmaeilzadeh, S., Ozcan, E., & Capan, M. (2013). Effects of ergonomic intervention on work related upper extremity musculoskeletal disorders among computer workers: A randomized controlled trial. *International Archives of Occupational and Environmental Health, 87*, 73-83.

Fessler State Board of Education Site. (n.d.). *School-to-Work Opportunities Act of 1994*. Retrieved from http://www.fessler.com/SBE/act.htm

Gliner, J. A. (1985). Purposeful activity in motor learning: An event approach to motor skill acquisition. *American Journal of Occupational Therapy, 39*(1), 28-34.

Hearnshaw, L. S. (1954). Attitudes of work. *Occupational Psychology, 28*, 129-139.

Hernandez, B., Cometa, M. J., Velcoff, J., Rosen, J., Schober, D., & Luna, R. D. (2007). Perspectives of people with disabilities on employment, vocational rehabilitation, and the Ticket to Work program. *Journal of Vocational Rehabilitation, 27*, 191-201.

Jaromi, M., Nemeth, A., Kranicz, J., Laczko, T. & Betlehem, J. (2012). Treatment and ergonomics training of work-related lower back pain and body posture problems for nurses. *Journal of Clinical Nursing, 21*(11-12), 1776-1784.

Jonsdottir, J., Fetters, L., & Kluzik, J. (1997). Effects of physical therapy on postural control in children with cerebral palsy. *Pediatric Physical Therapy, 9*(2), 68-75.

Kardos, M., & White, B. P. (2005). The role of the school-based occupational therapist in secondary education transition planning: A pilot survey study. *American Journal of Occupational Therapy, 59*, 173-180.

Kluzik, J., Fetters, L., & Coryell, J. (1990). Quantification of control: A preliminary study of effects of neurodevelopmental treatment on reaching in children with spastic cerebral palsy. *Physical Therapy, 70*(2), 65-76.

Koenig, K. P., Buckley-Reen, A., & Garg, S. (2012). Efficacy of the Get Ready to Learn yoga program among children with autism spectrum disorders: A pretest–posttest control group design. *American Journal of Occupational Therapy, 66*, 538-546.

Lilly, L. A., & Powell, N. J. (1990). Measuring the effects of neurodevelopmental treatment on the daily living skills of 2 children with cerebral palsy. *American Journal of Occupational Therapy, 44*(2), 139-415.

Lin, H.-Y., Lee, P., Chang, W.-D., & Hong, F.-Y. (2014). Effects of weighted vests on attention, impulse control, and on-task behavior in children with attention deficit hyperactivity disorder. *American Journal of Occupational Therapy, 68*, 149-158.

Maeir, A., Fisher, O., Bar-Ilan, R. T., Boas, N., Berger, I., & Landau, Y. E. (2014). Effectiveness of Cognitive–Functional (Cog–Fun) occupational therapy intervention for young children with attention deficit hyperactivity disorder: A controlled study. *American Journal of Occupational Therapy, 68*, 260-267.

Miles Breslin, D. M. (1996). Motor-learning theory and the neurodevelopmental treatment approach: A comparative analysis. *Occupational Therapy in Health Care, 10*(1), 25-40.

National Center on Universal Design for Learning. (2012). *What is universal design for learning*. Retrieved from http://www.udlcenter.org/aboutudl/whatisudl

Palisano, R. J. (1989). Comparison of two methods of service delivery for students with learning disabilities. *Physical and Occupational Therapy in Pediatrics, 9*(3), 79-100.

Pfeiffer, B., Moskowitz, B., Paoletti, A., Brusilovskiy, E., Zylstra, S. E., & Murray, T. (2015). Brief report—Developmental test of visual motor integration (VMI): An effective outcome measure for handwriting interventions for kindergarten, first-grade, and second-grade students? *American Journal of Occupational Therapy, 69*, 6904350010.

Pohlman, J., Poosawtsee, C., Gerndt, K., & Lindstrom-Hazel, D. (2001). Improving work programs' delivery of information and service to workers' compensation carriers. *WORK, 16*(2), 91-100.

Post, K. M. (2015). *Occupational therapy and universal design for learning.* Retrieved from http://wwwaota.org

Sandqvist, J. L., & Henriksson, C. M. (2004). Work functioning: A conceptual framework. *WORK, 23*(2), 147-157.

Sanford, C., Newman, L., Wagner, M., Cameto, R., Knokey, A.-M., & Shaver, D. (2011). *The post-high school outcomes of young adults with disabilities up to 6 years after high school. Key findings from the National Longitudinal Transition Study-2 (NLTS2) (NCSER 2011-3004).* Menlo Park, CA: SRI International.

Schwellnus, H., Carnahan, H., Kushki, A., Polatajko, H., Missiuna, C., & Chau, T. (2013). Writing forces associated with four-pencil grasp patterns in grade 4 children. *American Journal of Occupational Therapy, 67*, 218-227.

Shimmin, S. (1966). Concepts of work. *Occupational Psychology, 40*, 195-201.

Snodgrass, J. (2011). Effective occupational therapy interventions in the rehabilitation of individuals with work-related low back injuries and illnesses: A systematic review. *American Journal of Occupational Therapy, 65*, 37-43.

Solomon, J. W. (2000). *Pediatric skills for occupational therapy assistants.* St. Louis, MO: Mosby.

Suchomel, S. K. (2000). Educational system. In J. W. Solomon (Ed.), *Pediatric skills for occupational therapy assistants.* St. Louis, MO: Mosby.

Tanner, K., Hand, B. N., O'Toole, G., & Lane, A. E. (2015). Effectiveness of interventions to improve social participation, play, leisure, and restricted and repetitive behaviors in people with autism spectrum disorder: A systematic review. *American Journal of Occupational Therapy, 69*, 6905180010.

Tomchek, S. D., Little, L. M., & Dunn, W. (2015). Sensory pattern contributions to developmental performance in children with autism spectrum disorder. *American Journal of Occupational Therapy, 69*, 6905185040.

Tsorlakis, N., Evaggelinou, C., Grouios, G., & Tsorbatzoudis, C. (2004). Effect of intensive neurodevelopmental treatment in gross motor function of children with cerebral palsy. *Developmental Medicine and Child Neurology, 46*(11), 740-745.

U.S. Department of Education. (n.d.). *Building the legacy: IDEA 2004.* Retrieved from http://idea.ed.gov

U.S. Department of Education, (n.d.). *Every Student Succeeds Act.* Retrieved from http://www.ed.gov/essa

U.S. Department of Education, (n.d.). *No Child Left Behind.* Retrieved from http://www2.ed.gov/nclb/landing.jhtml

U.S. Department of Education. (2004). *The Rehabilitation Act.* Retrieved from http://www.ed.gov/policy/speced/reg/narrative.html

U.S. Equal Employment Opportunity Commission. (n.d.). *Americans with Disabilities Act (ADA): 1990–2002.* Retrieved from http://www.eeoc.gov/laws/statutes/ada.cfm

Urwin, R., & Ballinger, C. (2005). The effectiveness of sensory integration therapy to improve functional behaviour in adults with learning disabilities: Five single-case experimental designs. *British Journal of Occupational Therapy, 68*(2), 56-66.

Vargas, S., & Camilli, G. (1999). A meta-analysis of research on Sensory integration treatment. *American Journal of Occupational Therapy, 53*, 189-198.

Vaughn, S., Linan-Thompson, S., & Hickman, P. (2003). Response to Instruction as a means of identifying students with reading/learning disabilities. *Exceptional Children, 69*, 391-409.

Von der Heyde, R. L. (2011). Occupational therapy interventions for shoulder conditions: A systematic review. *American Journal of Occupational Therapy, 65*, 16-23.

Watling, R., & Hauer, S. (2015). Effectiveness of Ayres Sensory Integration and sensory-based interventions for people with autism spectrum disorder: A systematic review. *American Journal of Occupational Therapy, 69*, 6905180030.

Weaver, L. L., & Darragh, A. R. (2015). Systematic review of yoga interventions for anxiety reduction among children and adolescents. *American Journal of Occupational Therapy, 69*, 6906180070.

## Suggested Readings

Baker, N. A., & Jacobs, K. (2003). The nature of working in the United States: An occupational therapy perspective. *WORK, 20*(1), 53-61.

Barris, R., & Kielhofner G. (1985). Generating and using knowledge in occupational therapy: Implications for professional education. *Occupational Therapy Journal of Research, 5*(2), 113-124.

Basu, S., Jacobson, L., & Keller, J. (2004). Child-centered tools: Using the model of human occupation framework. *School System Special Interest Section Quarterly, 11*(2), 1-3.

Berry, J., & Ryan, S. (2002). Frames of reference: Their use in pediatric occupational therapy. *British Journal of Occupational Therapy, 65*(9), 420-427.

Brayman, S. J., Clark, G. F., DeLany, J. V., Garza, E. R., Radomski, M. V., Ramsey, R., et al. (2004). Guidelines for supervision, roles and responsibilities during the delivery of occupational therapy services. *American Journal of Occupational Therapy, 58*(6), 663-667.

Case-Smith, J. (1996). Fine motor outcomes in preschool children who receive occupational therapy services. *American Journal of Occupational Therapy, 50*(1), 52-61.

Clark, G. F., Jackson, L., & Polichino, J. (2011). Occupational therapy services in early childhood and school-based settings. *American Journal of Occupational Therapy, 65*, s46-s54.

Fertel-Daly, D., Bedell, G., & Hinojosa, J. (2001). Effects of a weighted vest on attention to task and self-stimulatory behaviors in preschoolers with pervasive developmental disorders. *American Journal of Occupational Therapy, 55*(6), 629-640.

Fetters, L., & Kluzik, J. (1996). The effects of neurodevelopmental treatment versus practice on the reaching of children with spastic cerebral palsy. *Physical Therapy, 76*(4), 346-358.

Humphries, T., Wright, M., McDougall, B., & Vertes, J. (1990). The efficacy of sensory integration therapy for children with learning disability. *Physical and Occupational Therapy in Pediatrics, 10*(3), 1-17.

Kemmis, B. L., & Dunn, W. (1996). Collaborative consultation: The efficacy of remedial and compensatory interventions in school contexts. *American Journal of Occupational Therapy, 50*(9), 709-717.

King, G. A., McDougall, J., Tucker, M. A., Gritzan, J., Malloy-Miller, T., Alambets, P., et al. (1999). An evaluation of functional, school-based therapy services for children with special needs. *Physical and Occupational Therapy in Pediatrics, 19*(2), 5-29.

Lockhart, J., & Law M. (1994). The effectiveness of a multi-sensory writing programme for improving cursive writing in children with sensorimotor difficulties. *Canadian Journal of Occupational Therapy, 61*(4), 206-214.

Moore, K. M., & Henry, A. D. (2002). Treatment of adult psychiatric patients using the Wilbarger protocol. *Occupational Therapy in Mental Health, 18*(1), 43-63.

Parrott, M. (2001). Further research into specific models of practice. *British Journal of Occupational Therapy, 64*(10), 519.

Scheerer, C. R. (1992). Perspectives on an oral motor activity: The use of rubber tubing as a "chewy." *American Journal of Occupational Therapy, 46*(4), 344-352.

Shamberg, S. (2005). Occupational therapy practitioner role in the implementation of worksite accommodations. *WORK, 24*(2), 185-194.

Soper, G., & Thorley, C. R. (1996). Effectiveness of an occupational therapy program based on sensory integration theory for adults with severe learning disabilities. *British Journal of Occupational Therapy, 59*(10), 475-482.

Storch, B. A., & Eskow, K. G. (1996). Theory application by school-based occupational therapists. *American Journal of Occupational Therapy, 50*(8), 662-668.

VandenBerg, N. L. (2001). The use of a weighted vest to increase on-task behavior in children with attention difficulties. *American Journal of Occupational Therapy, 55*(6), 621-628.

Wilson, B. N., Kaplan, B. J., Fellowes, S., Gruchy, C., & Faris, P. (1992). The efficacy of sensory integration treatment compared to tutoring. *Physical and Occupational Therapy in Pediatrics, 12*(1), 1-36.

World Institute on Disability. (n.d.). *The Ticket to Work and Work Incentives Improvement Act of 1999: Federal fact sheet on Public Law 106-170.* Retrieved from http://www.wid.org/publications/the-ticket-to-work-and-work-incentives-improvement-act-of-1999-federal-fact-sheet-on-public-law-106-170

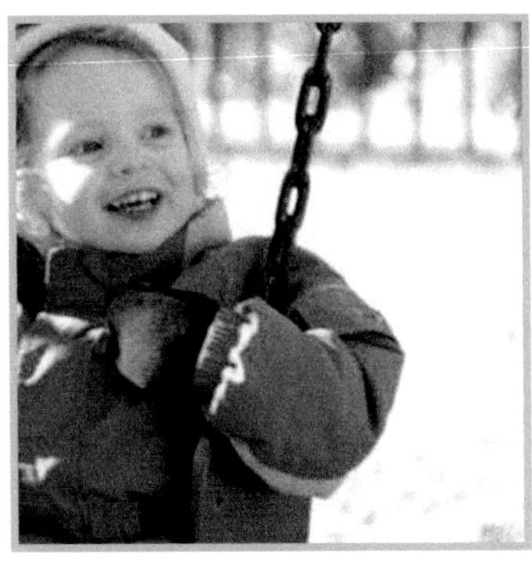

# 28

# Interventions of Play and Leisure

*Bevin Journey, MS, OTR/L and Kathryn M. Loukas, OTD, MS, OTR/L, FAOTA*

**ACOTE STANDARDS EXPLORED IN THIS CHAPTER**

B.5.1–B.5.4

**KEY VOCABULARY**

- **Freedom to suspend reality:** The ability to participate in make-believe activities or pretend play (Bundy, 1997).
- **Fun:** "That which provides mirth and amusement; enjoyment; playfulness" (Parham & Fazio, 1997, p. 250).
- **Internal control:** The extent to which the child is in control of his or her actions and to some aspects of outcome of the activity (Bundy, 1997).
- **Intrinsic motivation:** The self-initiation or drive to action that is rewarded by the activity itself rather than some external reward (Bundy, 1997).
- **Leisure:** "A nonobligatory activity that is intrinsically motivated and engaged in during discretionary time, that is, time not committed to obligatory occupations such as work, self-care, or sleep" (Parham & Fazio, 1997, p. 250).
- **Play:** "Any spontaneous or organized activity that provides enjoyment, entertainment, amusement, or diversion" (Parham & Fazio, 1997, p. 252).
- **Playfulness:** "A behavioral or personality trait characterized by flexibility, manifest joy, and spontaneity" (Parham & Fazio, 1997, p. 252).
- **Recreation:** Adult play or activities whose purpose is to "regenerate energy to support the worker role" (Glantz & Richman, 2001, p. 249).



Jacobs, K., & MacRae, N. (Eds.).
*Occupational Therapy Essentials for Clinical Competence, Third Edition* (pp. 419-431).

Play and leisure activities are one part of the important triad of balance in occupational performance areas: work, play, and self-care across the lifespan (American Occupational Therapy Association [AOTA], 2002; Christiansen, 1991; Kielhofner, 2008). Play has been called "one of the highest achievements of the human species" by one childhood development researcher (Whitebread, Basilio, Kuvalja, & Verma, 2012). In fact, play and leisure participation is such an important part of life, that the ability to access such activities is considered a protected human right by the World Health Organization as part of the United Nations (1948), more recently, these rights specifically include people with disabilities (2008). While engagement in nonwork or self-care activity is valued and supported differently within the cultural context, people around the world and across time have found ways to engage in free-time recreational activities. It is a widely accepted idea that engagement in play and leisure activities contributes to the health of individuals and communities. The pervasive nature of play and leisure occupations throughout the lifespan, across cultures, and in transactive human occupations contributes to the value of occupational therapy practitioners as highly qualified to address engagement in play and leisure as both a process and product of occupational performance. The incorporation of conceptual models of practice enhances the efficacy of occupational therapy practitioners as a holistic health profession. Theory guides critical thinking in occupational therapy by providing a foundation and rationale for practice (Scaffa, 2001), aiding therapists in developing occupation-centered interventions beyond impairment reduction toward meaningful participation in life (Lee, Taylor, Kielhofner, & Fisher, 2008). This chapter focuses on occupational therapy interventions across the lifespan, to plan, implement, and review outcomes of exploration and participation in play and leisure occupations (AOTA, 2014).

## Play and Playfulness

Play is the primary activity, and playfulness is the primary process by which occupational therapy practitioners approach young children and infants (Bundy, 1997). Play facilitates dynamic development within and across domains in physical, cognitive, social, and emotional skills and is the underlying mechanism of learning during the developmental years. Playfulness in childhood, according to Bundy, has three elements: intrinsic motivation, internal control, and the freedom to suspend reality. Suspending reality, or pretend or symbolic play, incorporates an imaginative element that can facilitate a child to develop the skills needed for real life (Bundy, 1993). Writing for the National Institute for Play, Gray (2013) lists the following characteristics of human play: self-chosen and self-directed, intrinsically motivated, guided by rules yet still leaving room for flexibility, imaginative, and conducted in an alert and active frame of mind. To achieve this, occupational therapy practitioners working with young children create a safe environment, ensure activities are fun, make routines part of a game or song, and engage the family or friends in the playful process. During play, a child should feel comfortable, safe, and engaged—the process should be enjoyable for both the client and the therapist.

## Leisure

As humans grow past childhood and take on the roles of adolescence and adulthood, time previously spent in play activities is typically redirected toward leisure participation. The 2003 World Youth Report broadly defines leisure for adolescents as any waking hours not spent at school or work (United Nations, 2003). Recreational leisure activities can consist of components of time, activity, and experience and hold individual meaning to the persons participating. The complex and interconnected process of play and leisure leads contemporary adults to engage in coordinated and complementary leisure. Coordinated leisure activities are those that are work related, such as playing on the company softball team or attending holiday parties at work. Complementary leisure is role related, such as a mother who coaches soccer, a father who works on the set of his children's theater, or partners who accompany an elderly family member on a trip to his or her birthplace (Glantz & Richman, 2001). Extensive research, as documented in the Evidence-Based Research Chart, supports leisure participation as methods of improving overall health and even extending life (Arem et al., 2015).

## Current Influence of Play and Leisure on Occupation

Play and leisure activities increasingly have been tied to national and global current events. The occupations of play and leisure and their relationship to bullying (Stanley, Boshoff, & Dollman, 2012), obesity (Skar & Prellwitz, 2008; Staiano, Abraham, & Calvert, 2013), advancement in STEM curriculum (Zosh, Fisher, Golinkoff, & Hirsh-Pasek, 2013), the healthy aging of Baby Boomers (Koo & Lee, 2013), and feminism and gender issues (Henderson & Gibson, 2013; Stalp, 2015) have all been documented. Despite this, in current occupational therapy practice, play and leisure factors are easily overlooked, perhaps in favor of the more obvious or immediate needs of work and self-care. Another growing factor in addressing play and leisure is examining a client's cultural factors in relation to work and play habits, roles, and routines. Play and leisure have a reciprocal nature when it comes to culture—whereas culture can influence participation in recreational activities, play and leisure can also be a vehicle to access and acquire cultural traits (Holmes, 2013).

## Play and Leisure Deprivation

The importance of play and leisure may best be illustrated through considering the results of occupational deprivation, or factors that preclude participation and occupational engagement in a chosen occupation (Whiteford, 2000). Stuart Brown, the founder of the National Institute of Play, lists "increased prevalence of depression, a tendency to become mired in rigid inflexible perceptions of options available for adaptation, diminished impulse control, less self-regulation, increased addictive predilection, diminished management of aggression, and fragility and shallowness of enduring interpersonal relationships" (2013, p. 30449) as consequences of play deprivation. The lack of productive play and leisure engagement can lead to boredom and unnecessary high-risk behaviors. Miller et al. (2014) found that high school adolescents who self-rated themselves as high in boredom were more likely to engage in high-risk sexual encounters. Children and adults may engage in negative recreational occupations such as self-destructive behavior; addictions such as gambling or substance abuse; compulsions; or aggressive, illegal, or unsafe behaviors during their free time (Moyers, 1999). Clients may also have impoverished habits to be addressed in occupational therapy such as watching too much television and or overeating unhealthy food. It is important for occupational therapy practitioners to find a balance between providing client-centered practice, promoting healthy occupations, and preventing or decreasing unhealthy ones (Table 28-1).

## Evaluation

In-depth evaluation before intervention planning is critical when addressing play and leisure skills to help the practitioner gain a deeper understanding of the complex nature of this area of occupation. See Chapter 20 for more information on assessment of play and leisure skills.

## Intervention Plan

The safety, health, and well-being of the client need to always be the primary focus of the occupational therapy practitioner when addressing play or leisure areas of occupation. Knowing and following precautions may enable a client to feel safe and engaged in a therapeutic play or leisure setting. The intervention planning process follows a comprehensive evaluation by an occupational therapist or the occupational therapist in partnership with the occupational therapy assistant who has demonstrated service competence. The intervention plan is based on the evaluation and interprofessional team input and should encompass the following domains according to the *Occupational Therapy Practice Framework* (AOTA, 2008, 2014).

- **Client factors.** All individual client factors, but especially the areas of values and beliefs, are critical to developing interventions of play and leisure. It is important not to project the therapist's own preconceived personal values onto the client, while maintaining a focus on health-promoting outcomes. Play and leisure skills vary widely across contexts and may have an impact on what activities are considered meaningful. For instance, a family who believes that an infant or child is too fragile for play but would benefit from motor activities could be educated to follow precautions while given specific ideas for interactive play with a medically fragile child.
- **Performance skills.** Posture, mobility, coordination, strength and effort, energy level, cognitive, emotional, sensory, social, and social interaction performance skills are used in the process of play and leisure. Intervention often targets specific areas of performance through interventions that are play or leisure based, creating a fun and engaging therapeutic activity.
- **Performance patterns.** Play and leisure are part of everyday occupations. Play or leisure time routines can be restorative in the balanced lives of human beings. Play, leisure habits, and routines are embedded in roles of individuals, families, and social groups.
- **Contexts and environments.** The dynamic and complex nature of context, environment, and circumstances should be considered, used, and adapted for optimal therapeutic outcomes. Often play and recreational contexts are outdoors or in the community; this can have a very positive therapeutic influence on intervention outcomes. Because the natural environment is less controlled and predictable, safety considerations specific to each client, his or her age, and ability level should always be in place for any therapeutic context.
- **Activity and occupational demands.** Play and leisure choices have unique meaning and relevance to the client. Activity demands are inherent to many properties of play and leisure. Objects and their properties are important in consideration of use of toys, games, sports equipment, etc. Consideration of the space and social demands is an important

Table 28-1.

## Play and Leisure Across the Lifespan

| Age | Description |
|---|---|
| Infancy and preschool | In infancy, play focuses around exploration of surroundings and is sensorimotor based. Infants and young children discover cause-and-effect relationships to develop a purpose to their actions. Play occurs as an interaction between the infant and caregiver and later evolves to include siblings or other children (Knox, 1998). During the preschool years, play becomes more constructive, and symbolic play is refined. Children start to use play to explore social roles. Play often incorporates fine motor activity, refining this skill as well. Play at this stage often occurs at home with parents or siblings (Figure 28-1). |
| School age | School-aged play frequently revolves around rule-governed games, with emphasis on turn taking (Knox, 1998). Play is part of life for school-aged children on the playground at recess, in after-school activities, and during free time. School-aged children also have free leisure time that they need to find positive ways of fulfilling. Middle childhood is a time of engagement with peers in real and important ways. It is a time to make decisions about what occupations are fulfilling and meaningful to them, which can lead to decisions about what leisure activities to pursue in coming years. |
| Adolescence | As children approach adolescence, they begin to engage in more organized or "structured" play and leisure activities such as arts, sports, and other specific individual interests. The main focus of most play and leisure activities in adolescence is socialization. For this age group, it has been found that participation in structured activities can lead to decreased antisocial behavior (Mahoney & Stattin, 2000) and even higher academic grades (Fletcher, Nickerson, & Wright, 2003; Figure 28-2). |
| Adulthood | Time spent pursuing leisure activities varies widely depending on occupational roles and contexts during adulthood. A single man or woman's leisure activities differ greatly from those of new parents, which differ from those of parents of adolescents or a business man or woman, which are again different from those of a retired couple. For parents, leisure activities might be centered around their children's activities. As adults age and children leave the house, more free time emerges for leisure activities such as reading, sewing, ballroom dancing, kayaking, or hiking. Social clubs or religious organizations might become important. Older adults and elders may engage in card groups, restaurant nights, and gardening as an empty nest, retirement, or disability allows more leisure time. |

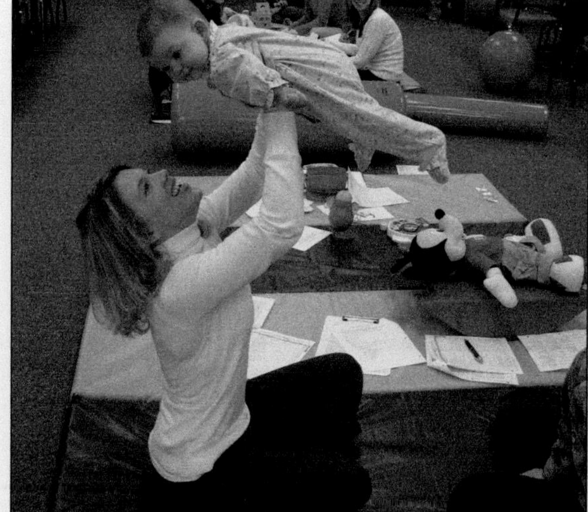

**Figure 28-1.** An occupational therapy student learns occupational development through play.

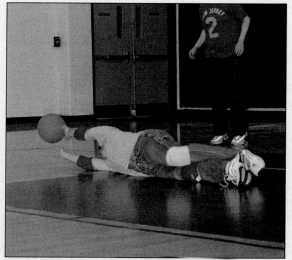

**Figure 28-2.** An athlete plays "Goalball," a sport designed for people who are blind or visually impaired.

part of the decision-making process in intervention. Many sports, games, and play and leisure activities include aspects of sequencing and timing, cognitive demands, social skills, and required body functions and structures, which should be considered by the occupational therapy practitioner.

The occupational therapy intervention plan using play or leisure activities is geared toward the following common approaches (AOTA, 2008; 2014):

- **Create/promote.** Play or leisure programs that target a specific population are examples of occupational therapy intervention that promotes healthy lifestyles. An example is an after-school play and fitness program with recommendations for equipment from an occupational therapy practitioner to promote easy access for all students to promote physical activity and prevent obesity. A Tai Chi program for older adults to promote relaxation and circulation as an effort in fall prevention is another example. Occupational therapy practitioners are always finding more ways to promote health in their communities or workplaces. Many of these programs are play or leisure based.
- **Establish/restore.** Here the play or leisure activity is geared toward factors that are interfering with overall function. The occupational therapy practitioner creatively selects a play or leisure activity that will improve the targeted areas of function through play or leisure activities.
- **Maintain.** A maintenance approach can be used to facilitate preservation of developed skills, habits, etc. For example, this approach might be used to develop an ongoing hiking or basketball group as part of a weight maintenance program or to educate a client about modified cooking equipment to maintain functional independence after being discharged home from an inpatient facility.
- **Modify.** This is an approach to help clients participate in the occupations of their lives by adapting the environment, using adaptive devices, or implementing a compensatory strategy. Adapting toys or games for children with physical disabilities or enlarging text for people with visual impairment to facilitate reading are examples of this approach. Training family members to include their loved one by using adaptations is also under this area of intervention.
- **Prevent.** This area may entail helping people with disabilities engage in activities that require safe and effective movement. Examples are wearing a helmet when using the adaptive bicycle, using a reacher to pick up golf balls, or ensuring that a person with a cognitive impairment understands not to swim alone. People with chronic problems such as back injuries, chronic pain, or mental illness may need an occupational therapist to assist them with a play or leisure program that is healthy and will not exacerbate their disability (AOTA, 2008, 2014).

## Intervention Using Play or Leisure for Occupational Performance

Play and leisure are often used in two ways in occupational therapy practice: play and leisure as a means (process) or play and leisure as an end (product). Play and leisure as a means is described as using these activities as a tool for other goal-oriented outcomes. This can be an important part of occupational therapy intervention and can be used to address many different client factors because clients are more likely to engage and cooperate in fun activities (O'Brien, 2006). Play and leisure as an end, or "outcome," is used when the occupational therapy practitioner is focused on helping the client gain skills and use daily routines in engagement in play or leisure activities (O'Brien, 2006).

Occupational therapy goals are a direct trajectory from the comprehensive evaluation and should lead the intervention planning process for both the occupational therapist and occupational therapy assistant. Goals should be objective, measurable, and client-centered. The following goals presented are broad in scope and are intended to facilitate ideas for intervention planning.

- Play or leisure to improve targeted motor skills or development
    - ◊ James will improve gross and fine motor skills through play with objects and toys in his environment in a variety of developmental positions as measured by improvement to an 18-month developmental level as measured by the Peabody Developmental Motor Scales (Folio & Fewell, 2000).
        - Activity ideas: Creating a supportive context of developmental play incorporating the interdependent contexts of family, play, and child care in the natural environment. Explorative play in positions such as supportive sitting, prone on elbows, or supported standing and interaction with age-appropriate sensorimotor toys should be facilitated.
    - ◊ Through play-based motor activities, Shaniyah will improve trunk control, sitting balance, and upper body control as measured by clinical observation data.
        - Activity ideas: Horseback riding, swimming, playing on a playground.

   - Sharif will engage in selected leisure activities 30 minutes per day to improve overall energy, bilateral arm use, and social participation as measured by self-reported journal entries.
      - Activity ideas: Involvement in an after-school program of choice such as shooting baskets, playing catch with a friend, swimming with a group, playing wiffle ball, or playing volleyball.
- Goals to improve playfulness
   - Layla will engage in make-believe play with her sister with activity set-up as measured by sustaining pretend play activity for three interactions.
      - Activity ideas: Family training and facilitation of make-believe play such as a puppet theater, dress up, or bath-time play.
- Goals to improve psychosocial and behavioral skills
   - Hector will improve emotional control and social interactions when engaging in peer group activities as measured by successful interactions without behavioral outburst three out of four times.
      - Activity ideas: The occupational therapy practitioner can consult with the staff to create contexts that support this goal. Other ideas include board games with one or more peers, "new games," and initiative and cooperative games (possibly done in the physical education class).
   - Mrs. Cooper will actively engage in a leisure activity daily with her husband without outburst for 30 minutes daily as measured by the husband's report.
      - Activity ideas: Consultation with the family and caregivers to create a context of support, safety, and recreation. Simple card games, walking around the block, reading a book to their grandchild, and baking cookies together are ideas that could be incorporated into the intervention plan.
- Goal to improve social interactions and community participation
   - George will interact with peers during recess to negotiate and share equipment three out of four times as measured by educational technician record keeping.
      - Activity ideas: Facilitating play with a group of children along with the client, modeling and scripting communication to share the swings, helping a child wait and then try the slides, engaging a group of children in a four-square game alternating participants.
   - Avery will successfully join the fitness center, interacting with staff as needed as measured by practitioner observation one time per month.
- Goals to add structure and leisure occupations to the daily routine
   - Isabelle will engage in three leisure activities that she will perform independently during free time as measured by group home record keeping.
      - Activity ideas: Explore and engage in leisure activities to add to her list.
   - Terrell will engage in three meaningful leisure-based heavy work activities to effectively transition from home to school daily as measured by sensory diet report card.
      - Activity ideas: Pogo stick, medicine ball, mini trampoline, book deliveries.
- Goals with play or leisure occupations as the outcome
   - As part of the group home program, members will plan and engage in two community recreation activities per month as measured by record keeping and client report.
      - Activity ideas: Choosing and going to a movie or theater event, going to the mall, walking on the high school track, going to an outdoor concert.
   - The Samson family will develop at least five play or leisure activities they can engage in as a family and do one family activity per week as measured by family reporting.
- Goals that use adaptation or compensation for play and leisure involvement
   - Preston will use adaptation in the community, such as his adapted bicycle, for safe and effective play participation with his siblings as measured by family report.
   - Given adaptations for visual deficits, including enlarging the targets, creating tactile boundaries, and adding noise to sports equipment, Ava will fully participate in sports at recreation camp as measured by staff reports, photos, and anecdotal data.
   - Given adaptations such as a card holder, Charlotte will effectively play with her friends on Cards Night for 30 minutes using her hemiplegic left arm as a functional assist as measured by therapist observation and record keeping.
- Goals to prevent disability
   - Virginia will learn and participate in three safe activities to engage in on the playground without injury as measured by inclusive playground therapy record keeping by the occupational therapist.

- ◊ Michael will learn and use safe body mechanics while playing outdoor games such as bocce ball with his friends without pain behaviors as measured by client pain journal data.
- Goals to promote health
    - ◊ The group of people recovering from substance abuse will show increased insight about their addictions and less recidivism after the outdoor adventure program as measured by a 6-week follow-up study.
    - ◊ The older adults in assisted living will show improved balance after the ballroom dance session as measured by improved performance on the Berg Balance Scale.
- Goals to develop positive occupational leisure choices
    - ◊ Jailene will learn three positive leisure activities for physical input that she will engage in instead of reverting to self-abusive behaviors (such as cutting) as measured by staff record keeping.
    - ◊ Joseph will actively participate in a leisure activity of his choice three times a week and refrain from online gambling as measured by reflection journal and anecdotal records.
- Goals to improve self-esteem
    - ◊ Sierah will improve self-confidence and self-esteem through success in community programs such as Special Olympics and choir, as measured by an increase of 10% on scores on the self-esteem checklist.

## Summary

Occupational therapy practitioners enhance contexts and enable performance skills to facilitate play with a purpose for individuals, groups, and populations (AOTA, 2008, 2014). Participation in play and leisure are key areas of occupational therapy intervention. Using models and frames of reference as a guide, play and leisure outcomes should be thoughtfully developed, with interventions planned, implemented, and reviewed as part of the occupational therapy process. Occupational therapy interventions of play and leisure need to be carefully selected and performed with cultural sensitivity and individualized plans. Taking client factors into consideration—such as developmental level, physical and cognitive ability levels, psychosocial skills, and cultural considerations—a wide range of activities can be used in play and leisure interventions. The natural environment of intervention also needs to be considered and modified to facilitate participation of play, leisure, and recreation in context. The outcomes of play and leisure intervention are as dynamic and broad as the occupational therapy spectrum, but they all facilitate occupational performance when they are performed with safety, fun, and enjoyment.

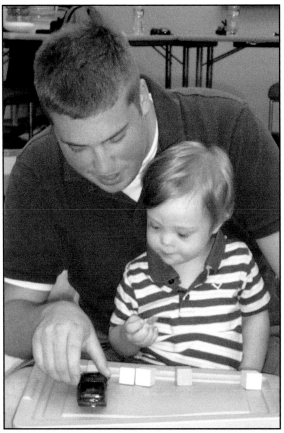

**Figure 28-3.** An occupational therapy practitioner playfully performs a developmental assessment.

## Student Self-Assessment

### *Occupations of Children*

The instructor brings in a variety of toys and games for a wide spectrum of developmental levels and interests. Every student goes to a toy, game, or creative childhood item (Figures 28-3 and 28-4).

1. Answer the following questions:
    - ◊ What thoughts or memories does this item bring back for you?
    - ◊ What ages and gender would most likely use this toy or game?
    - ◊ What skills are necessary to use this toy or game?
    - ◊ What areas of motor development does this toy or game facilitate?
    - ◊ What levels of visual, perceptual, or cognitive development does this toy or game facilitate?
    - ◊ How could this toy or game develop social interaction with other people?
    - ◊ How could this toy or game be modified for a person with physical special needs? For cognitive special needs?

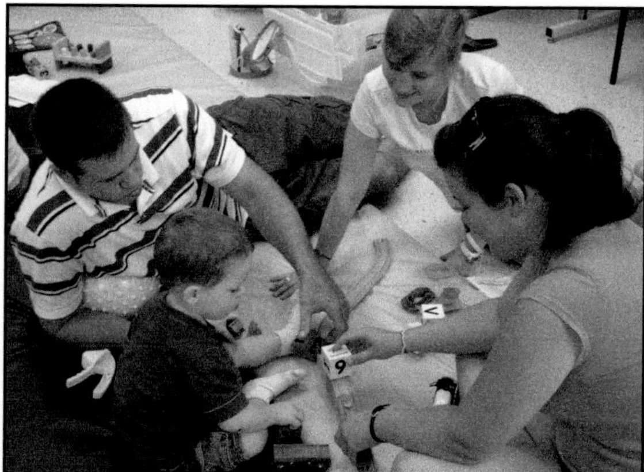

**Figure 28-4.** Occupational therapy students engage a child in play.

- ◊ Is this something that an occupational therapist might use during an intervention? Describe how and with what client and client factors. Include age, diagnosis, and environment.

2. The following is a teaching, learning, and service assignment regarding adaptive equipment, activity, or toy fabrication.
   - ◊ Students are to find a child with special needs through fieldwork or other means and design a piece of play equipment, toy, game, or sport specifically for that individual child or family. The student will then give the child or family the project. Cost limitation: $20. Lab time can be provided for this project.
   - ◊ Criteria
     - * Level of sophistication: Complexity of project
     - * Degree of individualization: Client centered
     - * Safety
     - * Functionality: How well does it work?
     - * Fun factor
     - * Family friendly
     - * Presentation in class
     - * Aesthetics
     - * Level of learning for the student
     - * Creativity
3. Leisure and recreation
   - ◊ The instructor needs to bring in a variety of arts and crafts, games, and sports equipment such as croquet, bocce ball, checkers, Connect Four (Hasbro), Twister (Hasbro), deck of cards, Kings in the Corner, playground ball, table tennis, arts activities such as scrapbooking, etc.
   - ◊ Students are divided into groups. Each group has 5 to 10 minutes to plan and 5 minutes to present or demonstrate one activity. Groups choose a scenario below and an activity to adapt for a successful occupational leisure activity.
     - * The occupational therapy practitioner is working with a middle school child who is significantly visually impaired. The child is participating in a recreational after-school program with typical peers.
     - * The occupational therapy practitioner needs to plan an activity evening for young adult clients with mental retardation and mild obesity who generally like to sit and watch TV and are resistant to physical activity.
     - * The occupational therapy practitioner is working with a client with chronic low back pain and overmedication who is sedentary and depressed. Occupational therapy goals are to promote pain-free movement.
     - * The occupational therapy practitioner is working with a 60-year-old man with significant tremors and balance deficits from Parkinson's disease who wants to participate in activities with his wife.
     - * The occupational therapy practitioner is working with a young man with schizophrenia in a mental health group of four people who have significant difficulties with social interaction.

| Activity | Goals | Adaptations | Expected Outcomes |
|---|---|---|---|
| | | | |
| | | | |
| | | | |

4. Experiential learning: Students who have been involved with work or volunteer work with people in adapted play, leisure, or recreational programming gain valuable insight into the importance and skills involved in adaptive activities. Consider the following experiential activities for students through volunteer experiences, work, or Level I fieldwork:
   - ◊ Therapeutic horseback riding
   - ◊ Adaptive aquatics
   - ◊ Transdisciplinary playgroups (Loukas, Whiting, Ricci, & Cohen-Konrad, 2012)
   - ◊ Camps for children with special needs (e.g., Easter Seals)
   - ◊ Martial arts for people with physical challenges
   - ◊ Special Olympics

# Evidence-Based Research Chart

| Topic | Intervention Description | Evidence |
|---|---|---|
| Playfulness | In a study of 255 adult subjects ages 18 to 67 years, findings include that playfulness was positively correlated with life satisfaction and that engaging in an active lifestyle explained the relationship between playfulness and life satisfaction | Proyer, 2012, 2013 |
| | Playfulness correlated with stress coping skills for 195 university students | Qian & Yarnell, 2011 |
| | Taking information from several questionnaires completed by older adults, this study found that subjects who rated highly "playful" were psychologically upbeat, with traits including being happy, optimistic, cheerful, joyful, positive, relaxed, and enthusiastic | Yarnal & Qian, 2011 |
| | Non–play-specific materials were found to increase playfulness on a school playground with 5- to 7-year-old school children | Bundy et al., 2008 |
| Facilitating the occupation of play (play as an end) | Purposeful "play" activity was more effective than rote exercise in a case study of two children with burn injuries | Melchert-McKearnan, Deitz, Engel, & White, 2000 |
| | Children with autism who had low-registration sensory processing traits participated in fewer leisure activities compared to peers; other sensory processing traits were associated with participation in specific types of leisure tasks | Ismael, Mische Lawson, & Cox, 2015 |
| | Levels of daily physical activity in 83 children ages 6 to 15 years with autism spectrum disorder were examined with only 10 (12%) of participants reporting being physically active; subjects were engaged in solitary play more often than social play activities | Memari et al., 2015 |
| | Praxis deficits, specifically imitative praxis and the domain of ideas and planning, in 32 children with autism spectrum disorder and a mean age of 7.5 greatly affect their ability to successfully participation in play and leisure activities | Bodison, 2015 |
| | By measuring urinary cortisol levels, among 53 pediatric patients ages 7 to 11 years, participating in play activities was an effective method to reduce stress | Potasz, De Varela, De Carvalho, Do Prado, & Do Prado, 2013 |
| | In a small group study (five participants), play interventions improved the social play skills of children with attention deficit hyperactivity disorder as measured at an 18-month follow-up, demonstrating preliminary and long-term effects of a play intervention | Wilkes-Gillan, Bundy, Cordier, & Lincoln, 2014 |
| Play as a means to improve performance skills (play as a means) | Participation in the "Learn to Play" program over 6 months was associated with increased social interaction, connection, and language skills in 19 children with intellectual disabilities | Stagnitti, O'Connor, & Sheppard, 2012 |
| | This study of 128 sixth-grade students found a link from constructive play, to spatial ability, to mathematical word problem solving performance, implying that more frequent engagement in active play could lead to higher performance on ability to solve math word problems | Oostermeijer, Boonen, & Jolles, 2014 |
| | Evidence-based review of interventions used to improve leisure occupations of people with Alzheimer disease shows a positive impact | Letts et al., 2011 |
| | Data collected from the ROOTS study, including 1538 adolescents, showed that subjects with higher perceived family functioning and more friendship qualities or fewer friendship difficulties engaged in more physical activity than peers, and generally demonstrated that family function and friendship are complexly associated with activity level | Atkin et al., 2015 |

*(continued)*

## Evidence-Based Research Chart (continued)

| Topic | Intervention Description | Evidence |
|---|---|---|
| Play as a means to improve performance skills (play as a means) | In data collected from 10,503 adolescents ages 11 to 15 years, a general positive association between physical activity via participation in organized leisure tasks and mental health was found | Badura, Geckova, Sigmundova, van Dijk, & Reijneveld, 2015 |
| | 1,589 adolescents demonstrated that girls 14/15 years of age with low level of leisure time physical activity had increased incidence of poor mental health as 20-/21-year-olds compared to girls with a high level of activity | Poulsen, Biering, & Anderson, 2016 |
| | Researchers found that low level of leisure time in a group of 98 adult patients undergoing hemodialysis for end-stage renal disease was mostly associated with preexisting habits, and recommended promotion of active habits at an early stage of the disease | Rosa et al., 2015 |
| | Children with autism who had low-registration sensory processing traits participated in fewer leisure activities compared to peers; other sensory processing traits were associated with participation in specific types of leisure tasks | Ismael, Mische Lawson, & Cox, 2015 |
| | In 16,642 middle-aged Japanese adults showed that participation in leisure activities including "hobbies or cultural activities" and "exercise or sports" was positively related to mental health status | Takeda, Noguchi, Monmo, & Tamiya, 2015 |
| | Occupation-based life review activity improved symptoms of depression in older adults | Chippendale & Bear-Lehman, 2012 |
| | Longitudinal study of 457 Swedish individuals indicates that late-life participation in both physical and sedentary activities, especially for men, is associated with long-term survival benefits | Agahi, Silverstein, & Parker, 2011 |
| | A cross-sectional study of 237 people with developmental disabilities ages 17 to 65 years living in the community found that leisure participation was primarily solitary and passive, and that subjects desired more engagement in leisure activities with social and physical activity components | Badia, Orgaz, Verdugo, & Ullan, 2013 |
| | Using diary entries over 8 days from 2,022 subjects, it was found that increased leisure time participation significantly reduced the perceived severity of daily stressors the next day, with a stronger effect the more leisure participation occurred | Qian, Yarnal, & Almeida, 2014 |
| Research supporting engagement in leisure activities as a way to improve other performance skills (leisure as a means) | A cross-sectional study of 60 Taiwanese patient-caregiver dyads found that patient with dementia who had intrapersonal barriers to leisure participation was related to depressive symptoms | Chiu et al., 2013 |
| | 942 subjects aged 65 and older demonstrated that increased engagement in hobbies was associated with a decreased risk for dementia | Hughes, Chang, Vander Bilt, & Ganguli, 2010 |
| | 3,209 participants from a pregnancy cohort study investigating relationship between leisure time physical activity and gestational diabetes found that the more pre-pregnancy and early pregnancy active leisure a woman engaged in, the less likely she was to develop gestational diabetes | Badon et al., 2016 |
| | 307 subjects with a mean age of 72 years who participated in cognitive stimulating leisure activities, subjects older than 75 years demonstrated enhanced speed in information processing; subjects younger than 75 years demonstrated less subjective memory decline | Tesky, Thiel, Banzer, & Pantel, 2011 |

(continued)

## Evidence-Based Research Chart (continued)

| Topic | Intervention Description | Evidence |
|---|---|---|
| Research supporting engagement in leisure activities as a way to improve other performance skills (leisure as a means) | Seventy subjects ages 60 to 83 years demonstrated that active musicians had significantly better naming, nonverbal memory recall, visual-motor speed, vasomotor sequencing, and cognitive flexibility | Hanna-Pladdy & MacKay, 2011 |
| | Interventions designed to modify activity demands of leisure were found to be effective for people with Alzheimer's disease | Padilla, 2011 |
| | Leisure activities for older adults with low vision were found effective in occupational therapy using a problem-solving, interdisciplinary approach | Berger, McAteer, Schreier, & Kaldenberg, 2013 |
| Cultural influences | Play is incorporated into work activities with Mayan children | Bazyk et al., 2003 |
| | Sociocultural comparison of Nigerian and American children's games indicate a diversity of styles, values, and approach to play in different cultures | Nwokah & Ikekeonwu, 1998 |
| | In a cross-sectional survey of 19,298 university students from 23 countries, the amount of inactive leisure time varied across cultural and economic development factors | Haase, Steptoe, Sallis, & Wardle, 2004 |
| | Children least likely to have access to recess are those attending school in high-minority, high-poverty, or urban areas | Center for Public Education, 2008 |

- Ski programs for people with physical challenges
- School-based summer recreational programs with inclusion
- Sensory integrative camps
- Developmental preschools

## Electronic Resources

Academy of Leisure Sciences: www.academyofleisuresciences.com

International Play Association: www.ipaworld.org

Play Foundation: www.playfoundation.org

World Leisure Organization: www.worldleisure.org

## References


Agahi, N., Silverstein, M., & Parker, M. G. (2011). Late-life and earlier participation in leisure activities: Their importance for survival among older persons. *Activities, Adaptation and Aging, 35*, 210-222.

American Occupational Therapy Association. (2002). The occupational therapy practice framework: Domain and process. *American Journal of Occupational Therapy, 56*, 609-639.

American Occupational Therapy Association. (2008). The occupational therapy practice framework: Domain and process (2nd ed). *American Journal of Occupational Therapy, 62*(6), 625-683.

American Occupational Therapy Association. (2014). Occupational therapy practice framework: Domain and process (3rd ed.). *American Journal of Occupational Therapy, 68*(Suppl. 1), S1-S48. doi:10.5014/ajot.2014.682006

Arem, H., Moore, S. C., Patel, A., Hartge, P., Berrington de Gonzalez, A., Visvanathan, K., ... Matthews, C. E. (2015). Leisure time physical activity and mortality: A detailed pooled analysis of the dose-response relationship. *JAMA Internal Medicine, 175*(6), 959-967. doi:10.1001/jamainternmed.2015.0533

Atkin, A. J., Corder, K., Goodyer, I., Bamber, D., Ekelund, U., Brage, S, Dunn, V., & van Sluijs, E. M. V. (2015). Perceived family functioning and friendship quality: Cross sectional associations with physical activity and sedentary behaviors. *International Journal of Behavioral Nutrition and Physical Activity, 12*(23). doi:10.1186/s12966-015-0180-x

Badia, M., Orgaz, M. B., Verdugo, M. A., & Ullan, A. M. (2013). Patterns and determinants of leisure participation of youth and adults with developmental disabilities. *Journal of Intellectual Disability Research, 57*(4), 319-332. doi:10.1111/j.1365-2788.2012.01539.x

Badon, S. E., Wartko, P. D., Qiu, C., Sorensen, T. K., Williams, M. A., & Enquobahrie, D. A. (2016). Leisure time physical activity and gestational diabetes mellitus in the omega study. *Medicine and Science in Sports and Exercise,* 48(6), 1044-1052.

Badura, P., Geckova, A. M., Sigmundova, D., van Dijk, J. P., & Reijneveld, S. A. (2015). When children play, they feel better: Organized activity participation and health in adolescents. *BMC Public Health, 15*(1), 1090-1098. doi:10.1186/s12889-015-2427-5

Bazyk, S., Stalnaker, D., Llerena, M., Ekelman, B., & Bazyk, J. (2003). Play in Mayan children. *American Journal of Occupational Therapy, 57*(3), 273-283.

Berger, S., McAteer, J., Schreier, K., & Kaldenberg, J. (2013). Occupational therapy interventions to improve leisure and social participation for older adults with low vision: A systematic review. *American Journal of Occupational Therapy, 67*, 303-311. doi:10.5014/ajot.2013.005447

Bodison, S. C. (2015). Developmental dyspraxia and the play skills of children with autism. *American Journal of Occupational Therapy, 69*(5). doi:10.5014/ajot.2015.017954

Brown, S. L. (2014). Consequence of play deprivation. *Scholarpedia, 9*(5). doi:10.4249/scholarpedia.30449

Bundy, A. C. (1993). Assessment of play and leisure: Delineation of the problem. *American Journal of Occupational Therapy, 47*(3), 217-222.

Bundy, A. C. (1997). Play and playfulness: What to look for. In L. D. Parham & L. S. Fazio (Eds.), *Play in occupational therapy for children* (pp. 52-66). St. Louis, MO: Mosby.

Bundy, A. C., Luckett, T., Naughton, G. A., Tranter, P. J., Wyver, S. R., Ragen, J., ... Spies, G. (2008). Playful interaction: Occupational therapy for all children on the school playground. *American Journal of Occupational Therapy, 62*, 522-527.

Center for Public Education. (2008). *Time out: Is recess in danger?* Retrieved from http://www.centerforpubliceducation.org/Main-Menu/Organizing-a-school/Time-out-Is-recess-in-danger

Chippendale, T., & Bear-Lehman, J. (2012). Effect of life review writing on depressive symptoms in older adults: A randomized controlled trail. *American Journal of Occupational Therapy, 66*(4), 438-446.

Chiu, Y., Huang, C., Kolanowski, A. M., Huang, H., Shyu, Y., Lee, S., ... Hsu, W. (2013). The effects of participation in leisure activities on neuropsychiatric symptoms of persons with cognitive impairment: A cross sectional study. *International Journal of Nursing Studies, 50*, 1314-1325.

Christiansen, C. (1991). Occupational therapy: Intervention for life performance. In C. Christiansen & C. Baum (Eds.), *Occupational therapy: Overcoming human performance deficits*. Thorofare, NJ: SLACK Incorporated.

Fletcher, A. C., Nickerson, P., & Wright, K. L. (2003). Structured leisure activities in middle childhood: Links to well-being. *Journal of Community Psychology, 31*(6), 641-659.

Folio, M. R., & Fewell, R. R. (2000). *Peabody Developmental Motor Scales* (2nd ed). San Antonio, TX: PsychCorp Pearson.

Glantz, C. H., & Richman N. (2001). Leisure activities. In L. W. Pedretti & M. B. Early (Eds.), *Occupational therapy practice skills for physical dysfunction* (5th ed., pp. 249-256). St. Louis, MO: Mosby.

Gray, P. (2013). Definitions of play. *Scholarpedia, 8*(7). doi:10.4249/scholarpedia.30578

Haase, A., Steptoe, A., Sallis, J. F., & Wardle, J. (2004). Leisure-time physical activity in university students from 23 countries: Associations with health beliefs, risk awareness, and national economic development. *Preventative Medicine, 39*.

Hanna-Pladdy, B., & MacKay, A. (2011). The relation between instrumental musical activity and cognitive aging. *Neuropsychology 25*, 378-386.

Henderson, K. A., & Gibson, H. J. (2013). An integrative review of women, gender, and leisure: Increasing complexities. *Journal of Leisure Research, 45*(2), 115-135.

Holmes, R. M. (2013). Children's play and culture. *Scholarpedia, 8*(6). doi:10.4249/scholarpedia.31016

Hughes, T. F., Chang, C. C, Vander Bilt, J., & Ganguli, M. (2010). Engagement in reading and hobbies and risk of incident dementia: The movies project. *American Journal of Alzheimer's Disease, 25*, 432-438.

Ismael, N. T., Mische Lawson, L. A., & Cox, J. A. (2015). The relationship between children's sensory processing patterns and their leisure preferences and participation patterns. *Canadian Journal of Occupational Therapy, 82*(5), 316-324. doi:10.1177/0008417415577421

Kielhofner, G. (Ed.). (2008). *A Model of Human Occupation* (4th ed.). Baltimore, MD: Williams and Wilkins.

Knox, S. H. (1998). Treatment through play and leisure. In M. F. Neistadt & E. B. Crepeau (Eds.), *Willard and Spackman's occupational therapy* (9th ed., pp. 382-390). New York, NY: Lippincott Williams and Wilkins.

Koo, J. E., & Lee, G. U. (2013). The relationship of baby boomers' participation motivation in leisure sports with recovery resilience and life satisfaction. *Journal of Exercise Rehabilitation 9*(2), 263-270. doi: 10.12965/jer.130009

Lee, S. W., Taylor, R., Kielhofner, G., & Fisher, G. (2008). Theory use in practice: A national survey of therapists who use the Model of Human Occupation. *American Journal of Occupational Therapy, 62*, 106-117.

Letts, L., Edwards, M., Berenii, J., Moros, K., O'Neill, C., O'Toole, C., & McGrath, C. (2011). Using occupations to improve quality of life, health and wellness, and client and caregiver satisfaction for people with Alzheimer's disease and related dementias. *American Journal of Occupational Therapy, 64*, 497-504.

Loukas, K. M., Whiting, A., Ricci, E., & Cohen Konrad, S. (2012). Transdisciplinary playgroup: Interprofessional opportunities in early intervention practice education. *OT Practice, 17*(3), 8-13.

Mahoney, J. L., & Stattin, H. (2000). Leisure activities and adolescent antisocial behavior: The role of structure and social context. *Journal of Adolescence, 23*, 113-127.

Melchert-McKearnan, K., Deitz, J., Engel, J. M., & White, O. (2000). Children with burn injuries: Purposeful activity versus rote exercise. *American Journal of Occupational Therapy, 54*(4), 381-390.

Memari, A. H., Panahi, N., Ranjbar, E., Moshayedi, P., Shafiei, M., Kordi, R., & Ziaee, V. (2015). Children with autism spectrum disorder and patterns of participation in daily physical activities and play activities. *Neurology Research International, 2015*. doi:10.1155/2015/531906

Miller, J. A., Caldwell, L. L., Weybright, E. H., Smith, E. A., Vergnani, T., & Wegner, L. (2014) Was Bob Seger right? Relation between boredom in leisure and [risky] sex. *Leisure Sciences, 36*, 52-67. doi:10.1080/01490400.2014.860789

Moyers, P. (1999). The guide to occupational therapy practice. *American Journal of Occupational Therapy, 53*, 246-322.

Nwokah, E. E., & Ikekeonwu, C. (1998). A sociocultural comparison of Nigerian and American children's games. In *Play and Culture Studies* (Vol. 1). London, England: Ablex Publishing.

O'Brien, J. C. (2006). Play and playfulness. In J. W. Solomon & J. C. O'Brien (Eds.), *Pediatric skills for occupational therapy assistants* (pp. 321-342). St. Louis, MO: Mosby.

Oostermeijer, M., Boonen, A. J. H., & Jolles, J. (2014). The relation between children's constructive play activities, spatial ability, and mathematical word problem-solving performance: A mediation analysis in sixth-grade students. *Frontiers in Psychology, 5*, 782. doi:10.3389/fpsyg.2014.00782

Padilla, R. (2011). Effectiveness of interventions designed to modify the activity demands of the occupations of self-care and leisure for people with Alzheimer's disease and related dementias. *American Journal of Occupational Therapy, 65*, 523-531.

Parham, L. D., & Fazio, L. S. (1997). *Play in occupational therapy for children*. St. Louis, MO: Mosby.

Potasz, C., De Varela, M. J. V., De Carvalho, L. C., Do Prado, L. F., & Do Prado, G. F. (2013). Effect of play activities on hospitalized children's stress: A randomized clinical trial. *Scandinavian Journal of Occupational Therapy, 20*, 71-79. doi:10.3109/11038128.2012.729087

Poulsen, P. H., Biering, K., & Anderson, J. H. (2016). The association between leisure time physical activity in adolescence and poor mental health in early adulthood: A prospective cohort study. *BMC Public Health, 16*(3). doi:10.1186/s12889-015-2658-5

Proyer, R. T. (2012). Examining playfulness in adults: Testing its correlates with personality, positive psychological functioning, goal aspirations, and multi-methodically assessed ingenuity. *Psychological Test and Assessment Modeling, 54*(2), 103-127.

Proyer, R. T. (2013). The well-being of playful adults: Adult playfulness, subjective well-being, physical well-being, and the pursuit of enjoyable activities. *European Journal of Humour Research, 1*(1), 84-98.

Qian, X. L., & Yarnal, C. (2011). The role of playfulness in the leisure stress-coping process among emerging adults: An SEM analysis. *Leisure, 35*(2), 191-209.

Qian, X. L., Yarnal, C. M., & Almeida, D. M. (2014) Is leisure time availability associated with more or less severe daily stressors? An examination using eight-day diary data. *Leisure Sciences, 36*, 35-51. doi:10.1080/01490400.2014.860782

Rosa, C. S. C., Bueno, D. R., Souza, G. D., Gobbo, L. A., Freitas, I. F., Sakkas, G. K., & Monteiro, H. L. (2015). Factors associated with leisure-time physical activity among patients undergoing hemodialysis. *BMC Nephrology, 16*, 192. doi:10.1186/s12882-015-0183-5

Scaffa, M. (2001). *Occupational therapy in community-based practice settings*. Philadelphia, PA: F. A. Davis Company.

Skar, L., & Prellwitz, M. (2008). Participation in play activities: A single-case study focusing on a child with obesity experiences. *Scandinavian Journal of Caring Sciences, 22*(2,) 211-219. doi:10.1111/j.1471-6712.2007.00515.x

Stagnitti, K., O'Connor, C., & Sheppard, L. (2012). Impact of the Learn to Play program on play, social competence, and language for children aged 5-8 years who attend a specialist school. *Australian Occupational Therapy Journal, 59*, 302-311.

Staiano, A. E., Abraham, A. A., & Calvert, S. L. (2013). Adolescent exergame play for weight loss and psychosocial improvement: A controlled physical activity intervention. *Obesity, 21*(3). doi:10.1002/oby.20282

Stalp, M. C. (2015). Girls just want to have fun (too): Complicating the study of femininity and women's leisure. *Sociology Compass, 9*(4), 261-271. doi:10.1111/soc4.12260

Stanley, R. M., Boshoff, K., & Dollman, J. (2012). Voices in the playground: A qualitative exploration of the barriers and facilitators to lunchtime play. *Journal of Science and Medicine in Sport, 15*(1), 44-51. doi:10.1016/j.jsams.2011.08.002

Takeda, F., Noguchi, H., Monmo, T., & Tamiya, N. (2015). How possibly do leisure and social activities impact mental health of middle-aged adults in Japan? Evidence from a national longitudinal survey. *PLoS ONE, 10*(10). doi:10.1371/journal.pone.0139777

Tesky, V. A., Thiel, C., Banzer, W., & Pantel, J. (2011) Effects of a group program to increase cognitive performance through cognitively stimulating leisure activities in healthy older subjects. *GeroPsych, 24*, 83-92.

United Nations. (1948). *Universal declaration of human rights*. Retrieved from http://www.un.org/en/universal-declaration-human-rights/

United Nations. (2003). *World youth report: The global situation of young people*. Retrieved from http://www.un.org/esa/socdev/unyin/documents/worldyouthreport.pdf

United Nations. (2008). *Convention on the rights of persons with disabilities*. Retrieved from http://www.un.org/disabilities/documents/convention/convoptprot-e.pdf

Whitebread, D., Basilio, M., Kuvalja, M. & Verma, M. (2012). *The importance of play: A report on the value of children's play with a series of policy recommendations*. Brussels, Belgium: Toys Industries for Europe.

Whiteford, G. (2000). Occupational deprivation: Global challenge in the new millennium. *British Journal of Occupational Therapy, 63*, 200-204.

Wilkes-Gillan, S., Bundy, A., Cordier, R., & Lincoln. M. (2014). Eighteen-month follow-up of a play-based intervention to improve the social play skills of children with attention deficit hyperactivity disorder. *Australian Occupational Therapy Journal, 61*(5), 299-307.

Yarnal, C., & Qian, X. (2011). Older-adult playfulness: An innovative construct and measurement for healthy aging research. *American Journal of Play, 4*(1), 52-79.

Zosh, J. M., Fisher, K., Golinkoff, R. M., & Hirsh-Pasek, K. (2013). The ultimate block party: Bridging the science of learning and the importance of play. In M. Honey & D. E. Kanter (Eds.), *Design, make, play: Growing the next generation of STEM innovators* (pp. 95-118). New York, NY: Routledge.

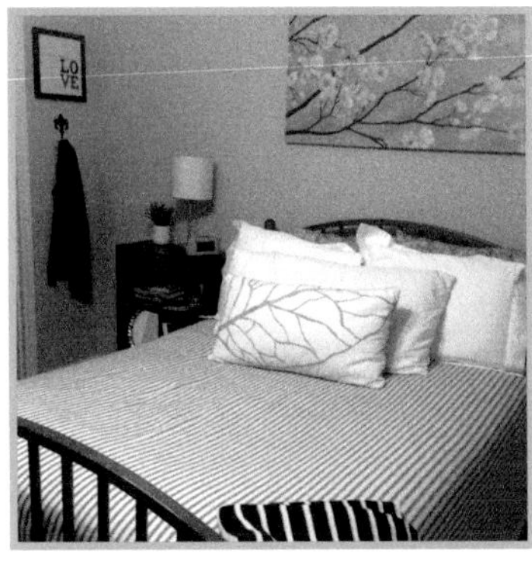

# 29

# Interventions to Enhance Occupational Performance in Rest and Sleep

*Courtney Shufelt, MS, OTR/L*

**ACOTE STANDARDS EXPLORED IN THIS CHAPTER**

B.5.1–B.5.4, B.5.8

**KEY VOCABULARY**

- **Cognitive behavioral therapy:** Is used when a practitioner is aiming to change the way a client thinks about something; this is done using the assumption that the way in which we think about a situation controls how we feel and in turn controls our actions and the consequences to those actions.
- **Health promotion:** Focuses on lifestyle redesign and the balance between one's body, self, and environment to engage in purposeful and meaningful occupations.
- **Primary disability prevention:** Addresses society as a whole, including those who do not have limitations or impairments.
- **Secondary disability prevention:** Focuses on a group or population that is considered at risk for a disease or disability.
- **Tertiary disability prevention:** Meant to increase function and decrease the effects of an illness or injury in those who already have or currently are experiencing its effects.



Jacobs, K., & MacRae, N. (Eds.).
*Occupational Therapy Essentials for Clinical Competence, Third Edition* (pp. 433-440).

Continuing with the occupations of rest and sleep, this chapter discusses how occupational therapists may help to enhance these occupations. The effects of sleep deprivation on our clients' activities of daily living (ADL) and instrumental activities of daily living (IADL) performance are discussed for a general knowledge of what to expect. General and specific intervention guidelines as well as ideas are provided.

## How Lack of Sleep Affects the Human Body

Sleep is important for restoring energy, repairing the physical body, regulating temperature, normalizing emotions, and recharging cognitive function (Luyster, Strollo, Zee, & Walsh, 2012; Ohlmann & O'Sullivan, 2009). Sleep allows the brain to form new neural pathways and synapses (Church, 2012). Healthy sleep habits and routines that promote optimal sleep duration and quality of sleep have a positive impact on ADL and IADL performance. An individual wakes feeling energized and prepared to accomplish mental and physical tasks. On the other hand, when an individual does not receive the amount of sleep his or her body requires, sleep deprivation can occur, and this can affect many aspects of the client's life. Sleep deprivation can affect an individual's functional capabilities by increasing his or her likelihood of accidents, decreasing productivity, increasing fatigue, and increasing health problems (Ohlmann & O'Sullivan, 2009).

Sleep deprivation can be acute or chronic. In acute sleep deprivation, individuals are awake for 24- to 72-hour periods. In chronic sleep deprivation, individuals experience a cumulative sleep loss over several consecutive nights (Kravitz, 2012). Multiple factors can contribute to sleep deprivation, including sleep disorders such as insomnia, sleep apnea, restless leg syndrome, anxiety, depression, certain medications, and other health problems (Wells & Vaughn, 2012). Environmental factors and an individual's lifestyle or routine may also contribute to his or her sleep deprivation.

Researchers have found that sleep deprivation and sleep apnea are linked to cardiovascular disease. During sleep, the body repairs cardiovascular tissues. If deep sleep is interrupted, the body does not have adequate time to repair these tissues, and damage to vital organs can occur (Ohlmann & O'Sullivan, 2009). Sleep deprivation has also been shown to increase heart rate and blood pressure and has been linked to an increase in the incidence of cardiac-related death (Valenza, Rodenstein, & Ferández-de-las-Peñas, 2011). Although damage to vital cardiovascular organs may not be directly apparent to the client or practitioner, it is important for clients and practitioners to remain mindful that sleep is imperative for cardiovascular health, and a client's cardiovascular health affects his or her ability to perform daily activities and tasks.

In addition to cardiovascular health, sleep is also important for maintaining insulin levels within the body. Research has found that after 3 consecutive nights of sleep loss, an individual's insulin sensitivity decreases by 25%. According to Ohlmann and O'Sullivan (2009), sleep deprivation has the potential to decrease glucose tolerance and compromise insulin sensitivity because sympathetic nervous system activity increases, which raises evening cortisol levels and decreases the use of glucose. Cardiovascular health and diabetes mellitus type 2 are two of the most common physical health problems associated with sleep in current research. Other health problems that have the potential to arise from or are made worse by sleep deprivation include obesity (Kravitz, 2012), certain types of cancers (Church, 2012; Luyster et al., 2012; Ohlmann & O'Sullivan, 2009), and digestive problems (Ohlmann & O'Sullivan, 2009).

Many aspects of cognitive functioning have the potential to be influenced by a lack of sleep such as memory, perception, reaction time, attention, and processing. If cognitive processes are not restored during sleep, an individual's ability to engage in tasks that require higher level cognitive functioning will be greatly affected. Specifically, sleep is essential for adequate memory processing. Sleep transforms the information we learn while we are awake into a more concrete memory within different parts of the brain. Researchers believe that during sleep, memories are allocated to other parts of the brain to be stored. This is the brain's way of sorting through important information. Research also suggests that engaging in rapid eye movement and non–rapid eye movement sleep after engaging in a learning activity increases one's ability to retain the information he or she learned during the activity and results in improved performance with the activity the next day (Church, 2012; Dang-Vu et al., 2010). Therefore, sleep is important for the rehabilitation process, specifically the carryover of learned information from one day to another.

Almost all ADL and IADL tasks require some form of cognitive functioning; however, one IADL task that is heavily influenced by sleep deprivation is driving. Driving requires many cognitive skills such as reaction time, memory, attention, sequencing, and processing. When a person is tired and the brain has not received an adequate amount or quality of sleep, these cognitive functions will be impaired. The National Highway Traffic Safety Administration estimates that there are approximately 100,000 police-reported accidents, 1,550 deaths, and 71,000 injuries each year caused by sleep-deprived drivers (Wells & Vaughn, 2012). Because sleep plays an important role in cognitive functioning, not only for success of the task at hand, but also for gains to be made during occupational therapy interventions, the practitioner and client need to make sure adequate sleep is being achieved for the client to retain new information during therapy.

Sleep deprivation affects emotional memories and has been linked to mood disorders as well as the ability to deal with criticism and painful experiences (Church, 2012). How we interpret our personal experiences affects our relationships and ability to survive. It is crucial for individuals to be able to interpret experiences as either rewarding or dangerous. If one's emotional judgment is being affected by sleep deprivation, this can cause dysfunctional emotional processing. Decision making is a large part of the occupational therapy process, and intervention often includes a great amount of emotional involvement from the client, caregivers, family, and occupational therapist. Therefore, if any individual involved in the intervention process is sleep deprived, emotions can be affected and may influence the therapy process, resulting in decreased effectiveness of occupational therapy services.

Although it is hard to see the direct impact of sleep deprivation on an individual's physical health, research supports links between sleep and physical health, psychological and neurological dysfunction, and mood (Valenza et al., 2011). Sleep does play an important role in restoring the health of the body's organs and physiological systems. Regardless of whether a client already has physical, mental, or emotional impairments, a practitioner must encourage healthy sleep habits and routines to maintain optimal overall health. Even though sleep deprivation does not necessarily have immediate physical effects on the body, it does have the potential to cause life-threatening damage over the course of time. Therefore, an occupational therapist should think about the end goals of interventions and treatments, the client's sleep habits and routines, and how they will affect the client's goals and future (Figure 29-1).

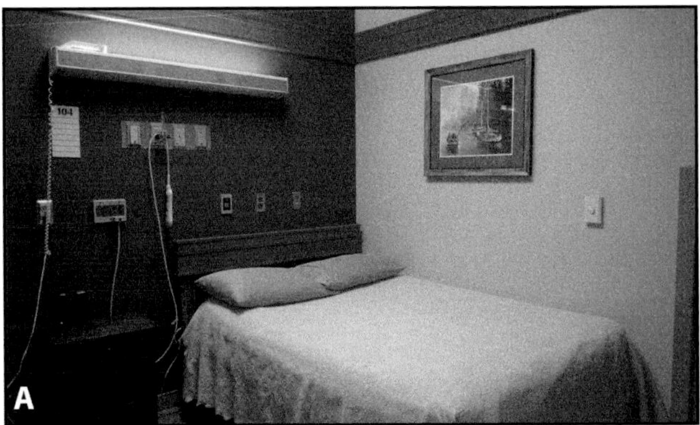


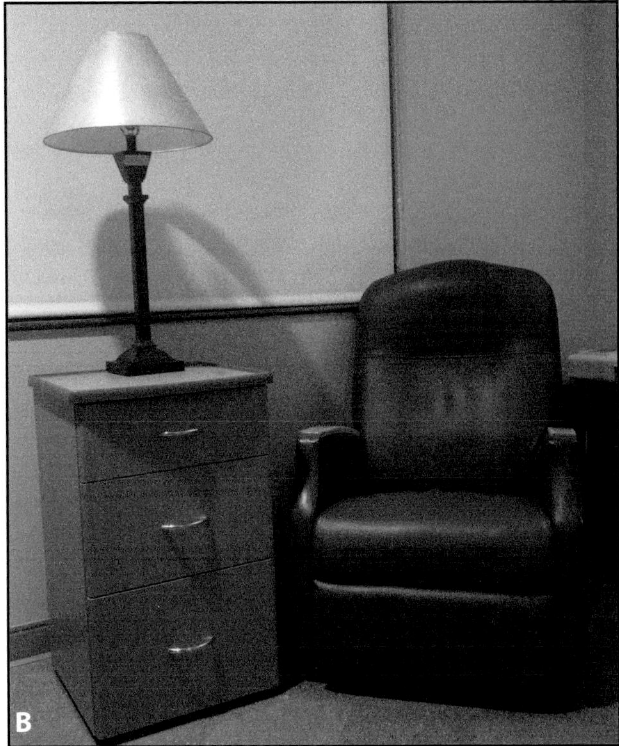


**Figure 29-1.** (A, B) At this particular hospital, the sleep study room is set up to feel more "home-like," with a regular bed versus a hospital bed, as well as a reading area where a patient can participate in a relaxing activity before bed. This is done to produce the most accurate results reflecting what might occur at the client's home.

## Intervention Planning

Before an intervention can begin, an occupational therapist must create a comprehensive intervention plan for the client. This is developed in conjunction with not only the client and other health care professionals such as the occupational therapy assistant, but also the family and caregivers whenever possible. The major parts of an intervention plan include measurable goals; the possible intervention procedures to be used; the amount, frequency, duration, and type of therapy sessions; and any further recommendations and referrals to other health care professionals (Moyers & Dale, 2007). An intervention plan must have the ability to be flexible. There is no guarantee that everything mentioned in the intervention plan will be achieved or even addressed during treatment. Good practice strives to include everything listed because the items were included for particular reasons; however, unforeseen circumstances could affect this. For instance, the client may succeed much quicker than anticipated or may require increased time to reach short-term goals and thus the intervention plan may need to be altered.

When attending to the topic of sleep disturbances, clients are more often than not referred to occupational therapy for other reasons and sleep disturbances are discovered during evaluation. It may come to an occupational therapist's attention during evaluation that a client's sleep disturbances may require a referral to a physician who specializes in sleep. Physicians who specialize in sleep should be contacted when a person has not been diagnosed with a sleep disorder; if the occupational therapist suspects sleep apnea, a nocturnal seizure disorder, or periodic limb movement disorder; if a formal sleep study is needed; or if there is suspicion that medication may need to be reviewed or altered (Westley, 2004). Whether a client ends up seeing a physician who specializes in sleep or if their treatment diagnosis is not specifically stated as a sleep disturbance, occupational therapists can still include improving sleep in the intervention plan. For instance, a patient who is being seen in an outpatient setting for lateral epicondylitis may have difficulty sleeping at night secondary to pain. A goal could be set for reported decreased pain during the night or even a reported full night sleep versus waking up from pain with possible intervention strategies providing a resting hand splint for more functional/protective positioning during sleep to decrease night pain and stiffness upon waking.

According to Moyers and Dale (2007), the intervention process can be classified into five common approaches, which are used individually or in an integrated fashion.

1. **Remediation/restoration** focuses on the components of one's performance including physiological, psychological, neurologic, and biologic processes. It may require the occupational therapist to provide education on techniques and the review of techniques to enable the client to institute new skills, habits, and behaviors within those components that are required for successful performance. An intervention within this category would be providing education on what to do and what not to do to promote adequate sleep or to provide behavioral treatment interventions. When addressing rest with a client who enjoys reading books but has difficulty reading the print, an intervention that falls into this category would be introducing the use of either large-print books, an electronic reader with which font size can be changed accordingly, or audio books depending on the need of the client.
2. **Compensation/adaptation** attends to the possibility of changing the task itself, such as its necessities, the objects it uses, or how the task is accomplished. An occupational therapy practitioner may also decide to change the task environment under this approach. A client who loves to watch his or her favorite television show as relaxation but has difficulty seeing the remote may benefit from a remote control for vision-impaired individuals or a voice activated home system, including the television. A client who experiences sleep difficulties may benefit from a home visit with an occupational therapist to change his or her sleeping environment to make it more conducive for a restful night's sleep or recommending a sleeping wedge for a client who has gastroesophageal reflux disease to decrease the likelihood of increased acid reflux while lying flat (Figure 29-2).

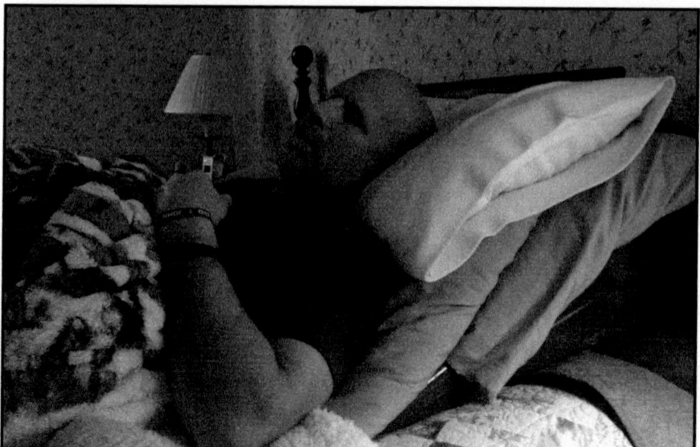

**Figure 29-2.** Using a sleeping wedge can decrease the likelihood that gastroesophageal reflux disease will affect how well you sleep because it prevents the acid reflux that might normally occur if you were lying flat.

3. **Disability prevention** is split up into three different types: primary, secondary, and tertiary.
   - Primary prevention of disability is meant to address society as a whole, including those who do not have limitations or impairments. Providing education throughout the lifespan to all clients about the importance of maintaining good sleep habits and taking time out for rest is a great example of this.
   - Secondary prevention is focused on a group or population that is considered at risk. Providing information about how specific conditions may affect sleep is a good example of protecting those with a higher chance of sleep disturbances.
   - Tertiary prevention seeks to increase function and decrease the effects of an illness or injury in those who already have or currently are experiencing its effects. Providing a group for elders who experience sleeping difficulty on how to improve their sleep, and thus their everyday functioning, displays this type of prevention.
4. **Health promotion** focuses on lifestyle redesign and the balance between one's body, self, and environment to engage in purposeful and meaningful occupations. Current research has even found evidence of decreased amounts of sleep positively affecting weight gain in all age groups, but particularly in those younger than 18 years (Patel & Hu, 2008; Vorona et al., 2005). When discussing the possibilities of sleep disruptions with clients, it is important to educate them on being able to regulate a healthy daily routine juggling rest, work, play, and leisure and how it can affect our mood, relationships, and performance.
5. **Maintenance** of a client's current abilities includes not only tools needed to perform the task but also maintaining the physical ability of the client to per-

form those tasks. With clients who have low vision but enjoy reading, adequate lighting is a simple way to ensure maintenance of this restful activity. For clients who are recovering from surgery, providing a home exercise program not only helps to increase strength and endurance, but also aids in maintaining what strength they do have or have gained back since surgery.

Two specific types of intervention are very helpful when working with clients who experience sleeping difficulties. Both types of interventions have been used separately and in conjunction, resulting in success within groups and on an individual basis. Studies have shown that using cognitive and behavioral treatment approaches are safe and effective alternatives to some medication (Davidson, Waisberg, Brundage, & Maclean, 2001). These two intervention approaches are different; however, they share many of the same qualities and beliefs, making them easy to use in combination with one another.

Cognitive behavioral therapy (CBT) is a therapy approach that is used when a practitioner is aiming to change the way a client thinks about something. The main assumption of CBT is that the way we think about a situation controls how we feel and, in turn, controls our actions and the consequences of those actions. The goal of using CBT with clients who have sleep difficulties is to change the way they think and act in relation to their sleep. Logging the client's sleep is usually the first step, as well as receiving general education about sleep and clients' personal sleep hygiene. Next, occupational therapists work with clients to cognitively restructure their dysfunctional beliefs about sleep, highlighting unrealistic thoughts and irrational fears (Jernelov et al., 2012; Vitiello, 2000; Vitiello, Rybarczyk, Von Korff, & Stepanski, 2009). Eliminating behaviors in the bed or bedroom that are not conducive to sleep is a CBT guideline for sleep intervention. This is done to foster the thinking that the bed and bedroom are meant only for sleep, sex, and activities that help one sleep. Sticking to a sleep–wake schedule and avoiding naps during the day will train a client that there are only certain times when he or she should be sleeping. If a person does not sleep during that time, then he or she should wait until the next sleep-appropriate time (Jernelov et al., 2012; Vitiello, 2000).

Behavioral treatment focuses on the behaviors that one performs surrounding sleep and how changing them can improve the quality of sleep. The aim is to positively affect the emotional connection one has between sleeping and his or her bedroom, rather than the association to the bedroom with his or her difficulty sleeping. There are three main treatment areas used: relaxation techniques, temporal control therapy, and sleep restriction therapy.

Different from CBT, behavioral treatments focus on relaxation techniques, allowing the client to let go of the emotional stressors attached to his or her sleeping difficulties by integrating biofeedback, meditation, and guided imagery as part of his or her sleep routine (Rajki, 2011; Subramanian & Surani, 2007). These strategies, in turn, reduce cognitive and physiologic arousal at bedtime (Vitiello et al., 2009). Similar to a CBT approach are temporal control therapy and sleep restriction therapy of behavioral intervention. Maintaining a consistent sleep/wake cycle and avoiding daytime napping are included with the temporal control aspect; this is accomplished by getting in and out of bed at the same time each day regardless of how the client's sleep went the previous night. Sleep restriction allows a sleep debt to accumulate based on the theory that it will enhance the tendency to sleep at the appropriate time (Subramanian & Surani, 2007).

## Intervention Strategies for Sleep

Once the occupational therapist and occupational therapy assistant understand what intervention plan he or she is going to incorporate into the client's session, then the more specific strategies will be chosen. An occupational therapy assistant has the education and ability to carry out an intervention plan once established by the occupational therapist and can make changes to an intervention plan based on the needs of the client once the occupational therapist has been notified, the changes have been discussed, and the occupational therapist consents. There are three main areas of improving sleep that current research has focused on or has been found to be of importance by opinion including the environment of the bedroom, the client's nutritional habits, and a healthy sleep routine.

The environment of the client's bedroom has many aspects to consider. Interventions that could be used might include a home/bedroom evaluation and education about how to make a bedroom more ideal for sleep. Considering the temperature of the room during sleep can be a huge factor in why a client may have sleep difficulties because sleep quality decreases with increased temperature in the bedroom. Comfortableness of the sheets and of the mattress are well known as to their overall effect on sleep; however, less considered is how the fabric of the sheets and mattress might affect the client's body temperature—more breathable fabrics may allow for increased sleep quality (National Sleep Foundation, 2012-2015b). Similarly, discussing with clients what they wear to bed might provide further information as to sleep disturbances, such as clothing being the reason for overheating, as well as restriction of natural movement during sleep from clothing being too small or large. The amount of light that the body is exposed to, both before bed and during sleep, can have immense implications of the client's quality of sleep. Using electronics or watching

## General Sleep Interventions: The Do's and Don'ts

**Do**

- Eat a healthy, small snack before bed if you prefer
- Go to bed and wake up at the same time each day
- Use a consistent bedtime routine
- Use relaxation techniques to reduce anxiety before bedtime
- Take a nap for 20 minutes or less if you must take one
- Contact your doctor if you suspect a sleep disorder
- Decrease noise and light in your bedroom
- Maintain a consistent exercise program
- Get natural sunlight during the day, especially toward the end of the day

**Don't**

- Drink alcohol or caffeine near bedtime
- Take naps during the day, especially after 2 p.m.
- Use your bed for anything other than sleep, activities that encourage sleep, or sex
- Watch television close to bedtime
- Exercise 2 hours before going to bed
- Eat a big meal before going to bed or go to bed on a full stomach
- Drink liquids close to bedtime if you have urinary urgency
- Keep your bedroom too hot or cold; neutral temperatures are better
- Go to bed unless you feel sleepy
- Stay in bed if you cannot fall asleep

Adapted from Rajki, 2011; Subramanian & Surani, 2007; Vitiello, 2000; and Westley, 2004.

television prior to going to bed disrupts the body's natural circadian rhythm as does having too much light in the room when actually asleep. The darker the room, the more the body will anticipate sleep and stay asleep (Dijk & Archer 2009). Naturally, what you hear in your room also can have a negative or positive effect on sleep. If a client reports having difficulty sleeping because of outside noise, it might be a good idea to recommend that the client use a sound conditioning machine or simply a fan to decrease the amount of noise heard but also to increase the likelihood that the client will sleep through an unexpected noise if it occurs. Smells are not often thought as a consideration when assessing and providing intervention for sleep disturbances; however, strong and abrasive scents can decrease the quality of sleep whereas lavender has been found to elicit relaxing feelings and therefore can encourage sleep. It might be important to note what is next to the client's bed or what is smelled as you walk into the room. Strong scented air fresheners, dirty laundry, or even a smelly gym bag could all have a negative effect on someone's sleep (National Sleep Foundation, 2012-2015b).

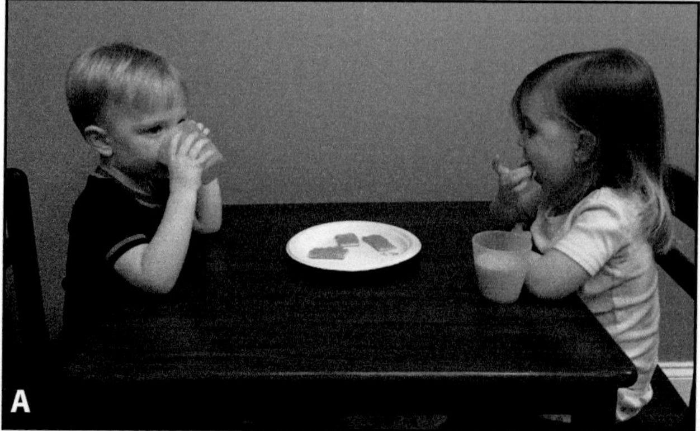

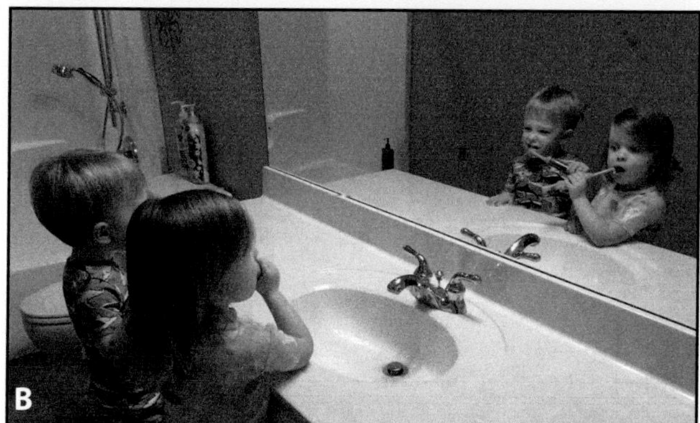

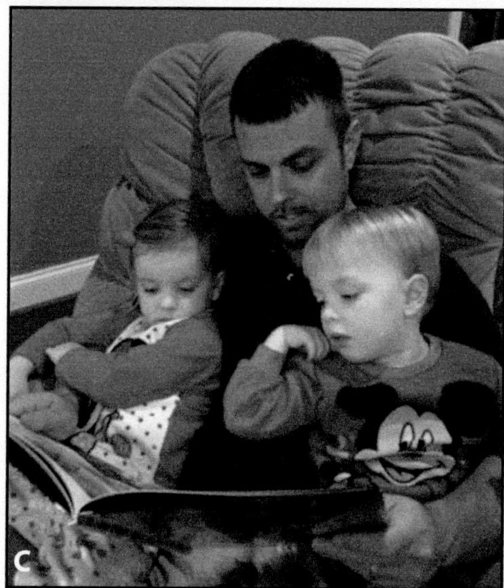

**Figure 29-3.** (A-C) Skyler and Logan always eat a bedtime snack before brushing their teeth and reading a bedtime story with Mom or Dad. A healthy bedtime routine helps these two little ones know that it is almost time for bed.

The overall atmosphere of a client's bedroom is one that should encourage relaxation; if it does not, then making environmental changes might be a quick and easy fix for someone whose everyday activities are being affected by lack of sleep (Figure 29-3).

It is important to watch your nutritional intake throughout the day, but for someone with difficulty

**Case Study**

Margaret is a married 55-year-old woman who works as an elementary school gym teacher and recently underwent a right total knee replacement. She lives with her husband and is currently on summer vacation and has been receiving physical therapy outpatient services for her knee rehabilitation. Two weeks before her knee replacement, lateral epicondylitis was diagnosed and she now presents for outpatient occupational therapy services as well. Throughout evaluation and the first couple treatment sessions, Margaret complains of increased fatigue during the day, difficulty sleeping at night, and admits that she doesn't perform her home exercise program as often as she is supposed to because it "slips her mind." She states she has had difficulty at home adjusting to being "laid up" and often feels bored but is also concerned that she may not be able to do her job secondary to this new onset of "sluggish" behavior.

**Consider the following questions:**

1. What do you suspect is causing Margaret's "sluggish" behavior?
2. What are some aspects of Margaret's life about which you might want to inquire?
3. What type of education would you provide Margaret with and how would you encourage her to incorporate it into her life?
4. What intervention strategies would you use to help Margaret?

sleeping, it could be imperative that changes be made to pre-bedtime food and drink intake, including dinner and bedtime snacks. Studies have shown that in general, diets that have high fat and carbohydrate intake as well as diets that significantly decrease caloric intake either shorten sleep durations or decrease the quality of sleep received (Halson, 2014). Alcoholic beverages are used at night by many to bring on sleepiness, and in the short term, can make one feel sleepy or help one fall asleep. Unfortunately, it also prevents the body from entering the deep stages of sleep and, in general, can decrease the quality of the sleep during the night, leaving the person still feeling lethargic in the morning. If a client complains of sleepiness during the daytime hours, it may be useful to inquire about energy drink intake because the ingredients cause a short-term alertness followed by a longer period of increased fatigue (Davila, 2009). It is a well-known fact that tryptophan can cause drowsiness but is less known that the intake of carbohydrates makes tryptophan more easily absorbed by the brain, which is why carbohydrates can make you feel sleepy as well. Protein intake can increase sleep quality because it creates the building blocks for tryptophan. Thus, a good bedtime snack is one that contains a small amount of protein, carbohydrates, or foods directly rich in tryptophan. Some examples of a good bedtime snack include nuts, such as pumpkin seeds that are rich in tryptophan, cereal with milk, peanut butter with toast, or cheese with crackers (Davila, 2009; Halson, 2014). Interventions focusing on how nutrition plays a role in sleep might include deconstructing a client's eating habits, education for healthy eating and alternative choices, and shopping and/or cooking tasks reintegrating newly learned healthy eating education.

Occupational therapists specialize in the ability to break down and create healthy routines for increased success with ADLs and IADLs. A healthy bedtime routine might include changing your clothes, eating a light snack, grooming tasks, and engaging in a relaxing activity such as reading just before sleep. Most important is maintaining a similar sleep/wake time each day to allow the body to anticipate sleep at night or anticipate waking in the morning, preventing oversleeping and thus difficulty falling asleep the next night (Rajki, 2011). Educating clients about replacing mattresses and pillows is also an intervention incorporating routines that a client should consider to improve his or her sleep; it is recommended that mattresses should be replaced every 8 years or possibly sooner than that if you are older because your body may be more sensitive to degenerative changes in the mattress. Pillows are recommended to be replaced every 2 years or when they do no provided adequate support to maintain the client's head and neck in a neutral position. Making the bed in the morning as well as maintaining clean sheets can also affect your sleep later that night because the majority of people find a clean and neat bedroom and bed lead to better sleep (National Sleep Foundation, 2012-2015a).

## Summary

Sleep and rest are important to client health because it allows the body to rejuvenate so it can have the required energy and concentration for the tasks ahead during the next day. Beyond the fact of needing to be productive for success with ADL and IADL tasks, as mentioned, there are also physiological effects of depriving the body of sleep. Occupational therapists are perfectly placed to provide intervention for sleep disturbances because they look at the person in a multifaceted approach, including not only the person and those around them, but also the environment in which they thrive. Intervention for sleep and rest might include education for lifestyles changes, environmental changes, establishing healthy routines, and ruling out physiological diagnoses. Considering the effects of sleep disturbances during treatment may also assist in success of intervention and healing of other diagnoses because sleep is such an integrated part of overall health and wellness.

## Evidence-Based Research Chart

| Topic | Evidence |
|---|---|
| Occupational therapy process | Moyers & Dale, 2007 |
| Cognitive behavioral therapy used with sleep | Jernelov et al., 2012, Vitiello, 2000; Vitiello, Rybarczyk, Von Korff, & Stepanski, 2009 |
| Behavioral treatment techniques used with sleep | Rajki, 2011; Subramanian & Surani, 2007; Vitiello, Rybarczyk, Von Korff, & Stepanski, 2009 |
| Acute and chronic sleep deprivation and its effects on the body | Kravitz, 2012; Wells & Vaughn, 2012 |
| Sleep deprivation and how it affects an individual's physical health | Ohlmann & O'Sullivan, 2009 |
| Sleep deprivation and how it affects an individual's cognitive functioning | Church, 2012; Dang-Vu et al., 2010 |
| Sleep deprivation and how it affects an individual's emotional processing | Church, 2012 |

## Student Self-Assessment

1. Describe how you feel and what effects you notice when you do not get adequate sleep.
2. Log your sleep for 2 weeks including items that you think would be most important. At the end of the 2 weeks, ask yourself: What did I discover? Is there anything you did not log that might have been helpful to know? If you have sleep disturbances, what do you think causes them? How can you make changes to better your sleep?
3. Describe your perfect sleeping environment. How might it differ from someone else's?

## References

Church, E. J. (2012). Imaging sleep and sleep disorders. *Radiologic Technology, 83*(6), 585-605.

Dang-Vu, T. T., Schabus, M., Desseilles, M., Sterpenich, V., Bonjean, M., & Maquet, P. (2010). Functional neuroimaging insights into the physiology of human sleep. *Sleep, 33*(12), 1589-1603.

Davidson, J. R., Waisberg, J. L., Brundage, M. D., & Maclean, A. W. (2001). Nonpharmacologic group treatment of insomnia: A preliminary study with cancer survivors. *Psycho-Oncology, 10*, 389-397.

Davila, D. (Ed.). (2009, December). *Food and sleep*. Retrieved from https://sleepfoundation.org/sleep-topics/food-and-sleep

Dijk, D., & Archer, S. (2009). Light, sleep, and circadian rhythms: Together again. *PLoS Biology, 7*(6), 1-4.

Halson, S. (2014). Sleep in elite athletes and nutritional interventions to enhance sleep. *Sports Medicine, 44*(1), S13-S23. doi:10.1007/s04279-014-0147-0

Jernelov, S., Lekander, M., Blom, K., Rydh, S., Ljótsson, B., Axelsson, J., & Kaldo, V. (2012). Efficacy of a behavioral self-help treatment with or without therapist guidance for co-morbid and primary insomnia—A randomized controlled trial. *BMC Psychiatry, 12*(1), 5.

Kravitz, L. (2012). Sleep deprivation: Cognitive function and health consequences. *IDEA Fitness Journal*, 18-21.

Luyster, F. S., Strollo, P. J., Zee, P. C., & Walsh, J. K. (2012). Sleep: A health imperative. *Sleep, 35*(6), 727-734.

Moyers, P. A., & Dale, L. M. (2007). The guide to occupational therapy practice (2nd ed.). *American Journal of Occupational Therapy*. Bethesda, MD: AOTA Press.

National Sleep Foundation. (2012-2015a). *Bedroom poll: Summary of findings*. Retrieved from https://sleepfoundation.org/sites/default/files/bedroompoll/NSF_Bedroom_Poll_Report.pdf

National Sleep Foundation. (2012-2015b). *Inside your bedroom: Use your senses!* Retrieved from https://sleepfoundation.org/bedroom/

Ohlmann, K. K., & O'Sullivan, M. I. (2009). The costs of short sleep. *AAOHN Journal, 57*(9), 381-385.

Patel, S. R., & Hu, F. B. (2008). Short sleep duration and weight gain: A systematic review. *Obesity, 16*(3), 643-653.

Rajki, M. (2011). Sleep problems in older adults. *ADVANCE for Nurse Practitioners and Physician Assistants, 2*(12), 16-22.

Subramanian, S., & Surani, S. (2007). Sleep disorders in the elderly. *Geriatrics, 62*(12), 10-32.

Valenza, M. C., Rodenstein, D. O., & Ferández-de-las-Peñas, C. (2011). Consideration of sleep dysfunction in rehabilitation. *Journal of Bodywork and Movement Therapies, 15*, 262-267.

Vitiello, M. V. (2000). Effective treatment of sleep disturbances in older adults. *Clinical Cornerstone, 2*(5), 16-24.

Vitiello, M. V., Rybarczyk, B., Von Korff, M., & Stepanski, E. J. (2009). Cognitive behavioral therapy for insomnia improves sleep and decreases pain in older adults with co-morbid insomnia and osteoarthritis. *Journal of Clinical Sleep Medicine, 5*(4), 355-362.

Vorona, R. D., Winn, M. P., Babineau, T. W., Eng, B. P., Feldman, H. R., & Ware, J. C. (2005). Overweight and obese patients in a primary care population report less sleep than patients with a normal body mass index. *Archives of Internal Medicine, 165*, 25-30.

Wells, M. E., & Vaughn, B. V. (2012). Poor sleep challenging the health of a nation. *Neurodiagnostic Journal, 52*(3), 233-249.

Westley, C. (2004). Sleep: Geriatric self-learning module. *MEDSURG Nursing, 13*(5), 291-295.

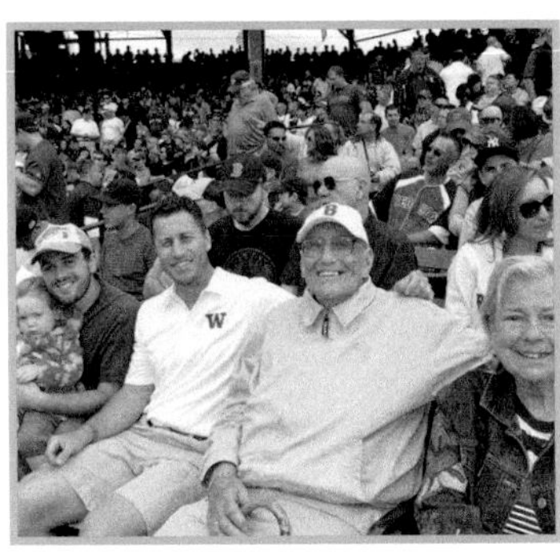

# 30

# Interventions to Enhance Occupational Performance in Social Participation

*Jane Clifford O'Brien, PhD, OTR/L, FAOTA;*
*Meghan McNierney, MSOT Class 2017; and Megha Panchal, MSOT Class 2017*

**ACOTE STANDARDS EXPLORED IN THIS CHAPTER**

B.5.1–B.5.6

**KEY VOCABULARY**

- **Compensation:** Refers to making changes to the activity so that the client can perform despite limitations.
- **Occupation-based activity:** Involves doing the actual occupation, which provides meaning and is part of one's identity (Fisher, 1998).
- **Preparatory activity:** Enables clients to better engage in intervention and may include range of motion, relaxation techniques, sensory-based activities, role-playing, or discussion.
- **Remediation:** The act or process of correcting a fault or deficiency (American Heritage Dictionaries, 2009).



Jacobs, K., & MacRae, N. (Eds.).
*Occupational Therapy Essentials for Clinical Competence, Third Edition* (pp. 441-453).

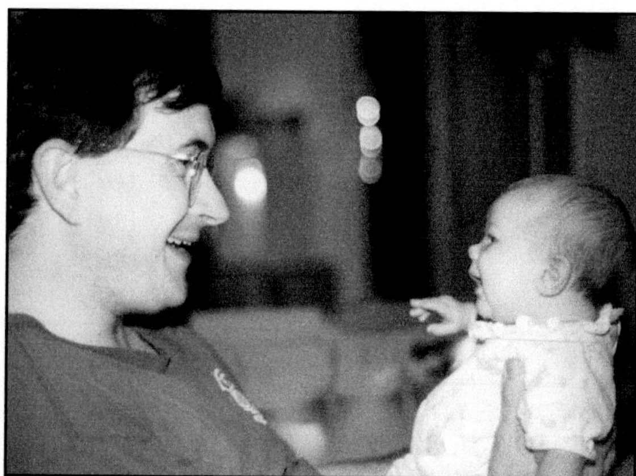

**Figure 30-1.** Face-to-face interaction between father and daughter is central to this social relationship.

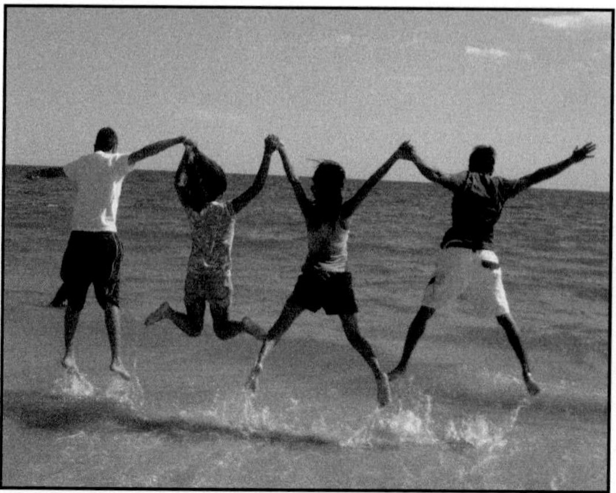

**Figure 30-2.** Jumping is an observable motor skill.

This chapter introduces readers to therapeutic use of occupations and activities for helping clients engage in social participation. The authors introduce techniques practitioners use to facilitate a client's development, remediation, or compensation for social behaviors. Examples are provided of how to grade and adapt the environment, tools, materials, occupations, and interventions to reflect the client's social participation needs. The roles of the occupational therapist and occupational therapy assistant in intervention of social participation are differentiated throughout the chapter.

## Social Participation

Social participation involves the numerous activities and occupations that aid in participation among community, family, and peers (adapted from Gillen & Boyt Schell, 2014). Social participation can occur in face-to-face interactions or through the use of technology such as a telephone call, computer interaction, and video conferencing (American Occupational Therapy Association [AOTA], 2014b; Figure 30-1).

The first step in planning intervention to improve engagement in social participation is to understand the client's needs. This involves collaboration with clients, family members, and significant others. The occupational therapy practitioner designs intervention based on the client's goals, values, beliefs and occupational needs, as well as the health and well-being of the client. While the occupational therapist is ultimately responsible for the intervention plan, the occupational therapy assistant may provide input and data to the process and may be responsible for designing the activities to carry out the established plan (AOTA, 2014a).

In addition to collaborating with clients, the occupational therapy practitioner analyzes the performance skills, client factors, activity demands, and context(s) required for successful social participation. Performance skills are observable elements of action (AOTA, 2014b) and include motor, process, and social interaction skills (Figure 30-2). The occupational therapist evaluates performance skills required for social participation through observation, interviews, and assessments. The following paragraphs provide a description of performance skills and examples of how the skills relate to social participation.

### *Motor Skills*

Occupational therapy practitioners evaluate motor skills that are needed to engage in social events, such as mealtime socializing, outings with friends, community events, theater, and recreational activities. The occupational therapist is ultimately responsible for the evaluation and intervention plan (AOTA, 2014a).

#### Case Study 1

Meena is a 75-year-old women who had a stroke resulting in right-sided weakness. Meena lives alone and can no longer drive, although she enjoys engaging with peers and "lights up" when she speaks with others her age. Meena's occupational therapy practitioner is concerned that once she is discharged, she will no longer have opportunities for social participation. Meena's occupational therapy practitioner and social worker have set up weekly transportation and connected her with a support group for people who have had a stroke in hopes of encouraging her to engage socially after discharge. Prior to discharge, the occupational therapy practitioner further evaluates the motor skills required to interact at the recreational center and in the support group.

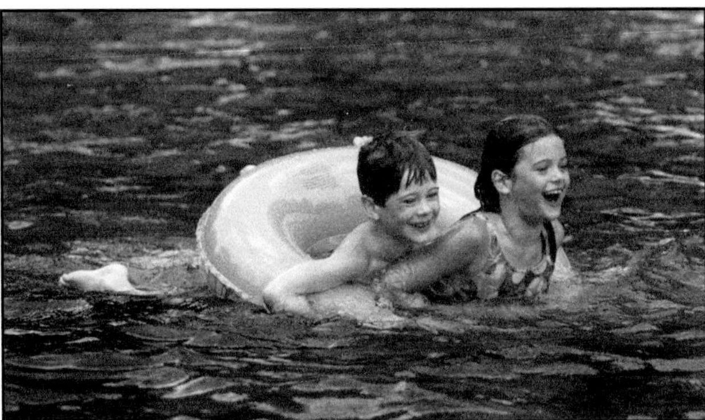

**Figure 30-3.** Children participate in social activities through play.

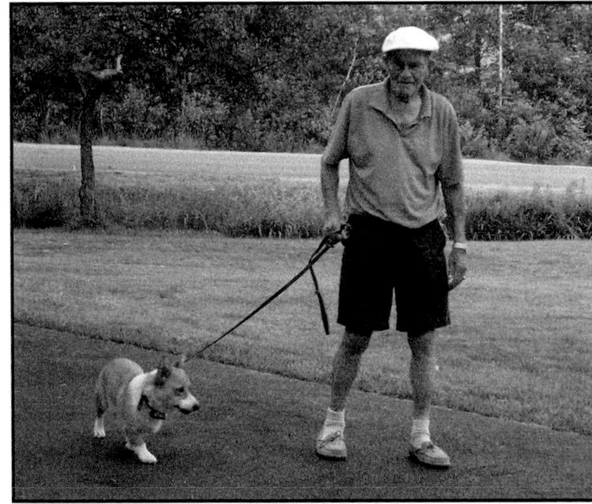

**Figure 30-4.** Gordon walking his dog as part of his daily routine.

In Case Study 1, the occupational therapy assistant provides data to inform Meena's evaluation and plan. The occupational therapy assistant may complete parts of the evaluation once service competency has been established (AOTA, 2014a). The occupational therapist and occupational therapy assistant both develop activities to carry out the intervention plan. As illustrated by Meena's case, social participation may involve transportation, ambulation, sitting, and standing. Meena needs to develop adequate sitting and standing posture, walk to and from the center entrance, and sit for extended periods at the center. She must get up out of the car and chair, use fine motor skills for activities, maintain prolonged periods of attention to activity, and eat a light meal. Social participation involves interacting with others by responding or initiating conversations. People also nod, gesture, and move during social participation. Furthermore, motor skills are required to produce speech. These motor skills are considered when facilitating social participation (Figure 30-3).

### Processing Skills

Social participation involves reciprocal conversation, which requires the person to hear words, read cues, and understand the context of the situation before responding. The processing skills required in Meena's case include initiating, choosing words, inquiring, and sequencing conversation, which have become more difficult for her since the stroke. Meena must also attend, pace, and terminate dialogue. Processing skills that are delayed may cause awkward silences and interfere with socialization. Furthermore, clients who have difficulty with the context of the situation may respond inappropriately.

### Social Interaction Skills

Social interaction skills are essential aspects of engagement in events and activities. Many occupations require social interactions, which can range from asking directions to engaging in detailed personal conversations. In Meena's case, the occupational therapy practitioner observed the following social interaction strengths: looks (makes eye contact), thanks, and takes turns. However, Meena experiences difficulty with producing speech, speaking fluently, placing self, regulating, replying, and expressing emotion. In the rehabilitation setting, Meena easily engages one on one with the practitioner to work on achieving her intervention goals.

## Performance Pattern

The pattern of engagement in social activities provides direction for occupational therapy intervention. The practitioner determines whether the social activity is part of the client's established routines, roles, habits, or rituals. Routines are defined as activities performed on a regular basis to provide structure to the client's daily life (AOTA, 2014b). Consider Gordon, a 78-year-old grandfather who enjoys walking (Figure 30-4). As part of his routine, he walks to the store for the paper each morning, converses with others, and returns home to report. Generally, clients wish to return to engage in their meaningful routines. Gordon would be distressed if he could not partake in this routine because it has become part of his role as a social being. Roles are "a set of behaviors that have some socially agreed upon function for which there is an accepted code of norms" (e.g., mother, father, student, and worker; Christiansen & Baum, 1997, p. 603). As part of his grandfather role, Gordon frequently brings back "treats" for his grandchildren.

Habits are automatic behaviors performed repeatedly (Boyt Schell, Gillen, & Scaffa, 2014, p. 1234). Clients may possess performance patterns that foster engagement in social participation (useful habits) or patterns of performance considered limitations (impoverished habits). As observed with Kenny, a 58-year-old client with traumatic brain injury, who hopes to return to "hanging out" with a group of work friends but has trouble remembering to bathe or groom himself. His habits around hygiene are

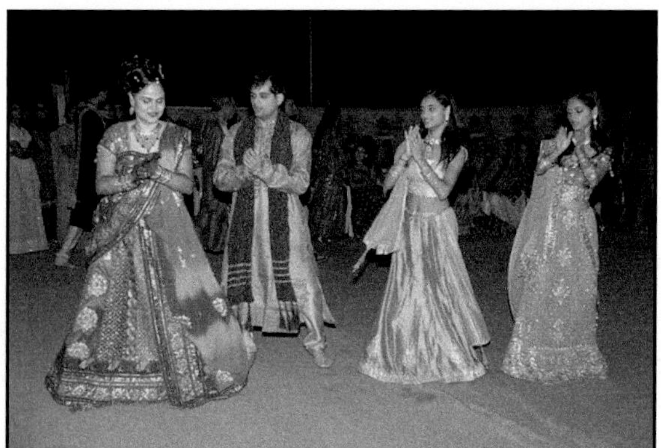

**Figure 30-5.** Indian family engaged in cultural dancing.

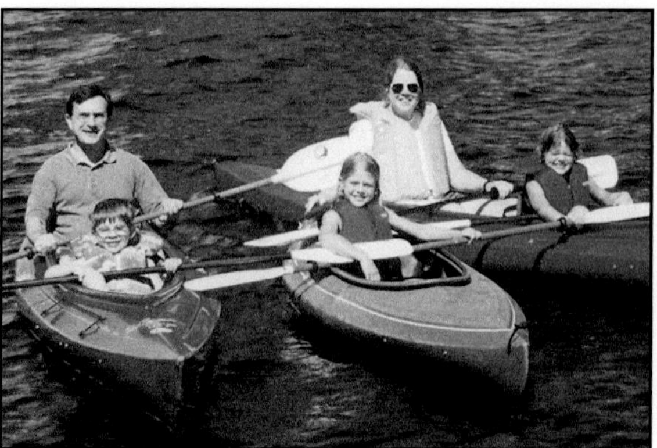

**Figure 30-6.** The lake provides a beautiful outdoor environment to kayak with family.

impoverished because he has no routine or pattern of performance. Although Kenny has many useful habits (e.g., he takes public transportation), his impoverished pattern and dominating habits (e.g., head banging, hand biting) interfere with successful participation.

# Contexts

After the practitioner has an understanding of the client's performance skills and patterns, further evaluation of the context in which the social interaction takes place is considered. The *Occupational Therapy Practice Framework* (AOTA, 2014b) lists cultural, physical, social, personal, virtual, and temporal contexts as important to consider when developing occupation-based intervention. A description of how each context may be considered in terms of social participation is presented along with examples.

## Cultural

Cultures hold different expectations for social participation. The occupational therapy practitioner evaluates cultural expectations for things such as proximity, eye contact, and physical contact (e.g., touch). The expectations of participation in social events vary among cultures and subsequently influence the goals for occupational therapy (Figure 30-5). It is the occupational therapy practitioner's responsibility to be aware of cultural complexities as they relate to social expectations and participation.

Cultural differences are also observed within families. For example, Tonya expressed concern that her 3-year-old son with autism could not play with his cousin at family gatherings every Sunday. The occupational therapy practitioner realized the cultural value of this to the family and worked on play skills with the child, encouraging the mom to bring in his cousin on occasion. Being sensitive to the family's values enabled the practitioner to design client-centered intervention that made a difference to the child and family.

## Physical

The physical space in which social interaction occurs becomes important when examining the activity demands (Figure 30-6). Physical space includes the building, location, surroundings, objects, and set-up of the event. Small intimate gatherings require different social skills than large public events. Activities that occur outside on uneven or hilly terrain may not be accessible to some clients. Background noise or even certain smells may be bothersome to some clients, especially older adults or children with olfactory sensitivity.

## Social

Social situations require different behaviors and may become the source of occupational therapy intervention. Social manners may need to be addressed to help clients participate in specific events. Helping clients address others properly, make conversation, and interact with others are all part of occupational therapy intervention. Others' expectations affect the skills necessary to participate in social events. For example, the training and standards for success differ between formal and informal events and between familiar persons and strangers (Figure 30-7). Clients are expected to behave differently with peers or loved ones than with strangers in public settings. Social activities differ in the type and amount of personal disclosure required.

Occupational therapy practitioners analyze the requirements to prepare clients for social outings, as in the case of Max, a 20-year-old man with muscular dystrophy who freely (and inappropriately) discusses personal issues. Before the actual outing, the occupational therapy practitioner reviewed social expectations for attending the art museum and led clients in a role-play activity to illustrate social behaviors appropriate for the art museum. Max and the occupational therapy practitioner developed a system to remind him when his behavior was not appropriate. After the outing, they discussed Max's

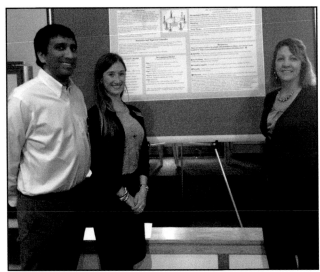

**Figure 30-7.** Peers engage in professional social behaviors as they present research.

performance to reinforce what he did well and to discuss areas for improvement.

## Personal

Social participation requirements vary depending on one's age, gender, educational level, or socioeconomic status. Although the occupational therapy practitioner is not able to change personal context, it must be considered when designing intervention. As commonly understood, adults interact and express themselves differently than children.

Occupational therapy practitioners consider the client's chronological and developmental age when selecting appropriate social activities. For example, an occupational therapy practitioner would not give a rattle to a 12-year-old girl who still mouths objects because this is not considered socially appropriate.

## Virtual

In today's society, heavy emphasis is placed on virtual communication and social media. Communication via computers or technologies may provide a social outlet for some clients. Occupational therapy practitioners may help clients to physically access and use such technology. Practitioners also help clients understand the social expectations and guidelines to protect themselves while using social media sources.

## Temporal

The demands for social participation vary across the lifespan as is illustrated next.

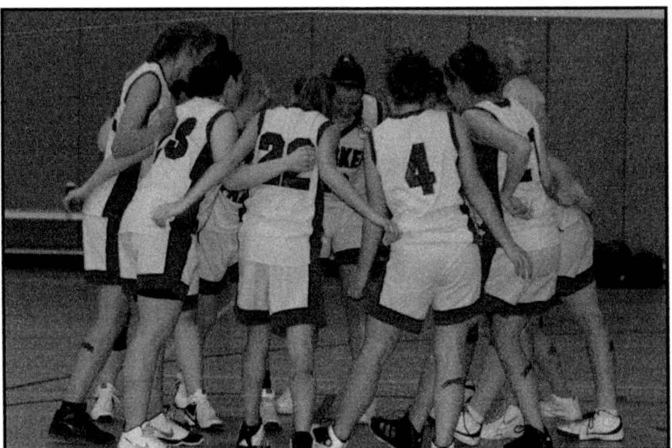

**Figure 30-8.** Adolescents enjoy being part of a team as these high school basketball players.

### Children and Youth

Children and youth may experience difficulty socializing for a variety of reasons, including sensory, behavioral, cognitive, physical, or emotional status. They may struggle with playing with others, reading others' cues, and understanding social expectations. Occupational therapy intervention may be designed to increase the child's ability through role-playing, practice, and coaching. Occupational therapy intervention works to identify and eliminate socially inappropriate behaviors, while developing effective social skills.

### Adolescents

Social groups are important to adolescents, who are beginning to develop their identity. Adolescent peer groups conform to certain rules and expectations. For example, adolescents dress alike, use certain slang phrases, and collectively take up similar mannerisms (Figure 30-8). Adolescents may also have to develop social skills for work. Adolescents need to learn to get along in groups, be heard, negotiate, stand up for themselves, and resist negative influences.

Occupational therapy practitioners work with adolescents who have experienced disease, trauma, or an event that has altered their development (Llorens, 1976). In terms of social participation, adolescents may exhibit a host of problems including inappropriate affect, difficulty initiating or sustaining conversation, and difficulty with boundaries, articulation, or poor judgment. The occupational therapy practitioner may target foundational skills, such as making eye contact, greeting people, and social manners in activities. Occupational therapy interventions work to develop skills such as confidence, assertiveness, flexibility, and understanding of social cues for successful participation in a variety of events.

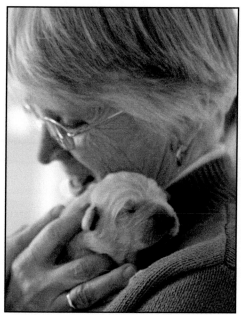

**Figure 30-9.** This older adult establishes a new social avenue by volunteering to spend time caring for pets.

### Adults

Social participation related to intimate and work relationships are key elements of adulthood. Intimate relationships require trust, collaboration, sharing, communication, and reciprocal physical behaviors. Conversely, work relationships require leadership, assertiveness, professional communication, and behavior. Adults are expected to take the lead and participate in community and family activities, as well as model behaviors for children.

### Older Adults

Older adults experience role change as they transition into retirement. As the social activities provided through work decline, they may need to establish new social avenues (Figure 30-9). Older adults may try to refer back to previous occupations that held social meaning, but may experience difficulty due to age-related physical changes. Some older adults may experience a loss of a spouse or loved one, which results in a change of habits, roles, routines, and social support to which they were accustomed.

## Family, Community, Peers, and Friends

Social participation occurs with family, community, peers, and friends. It can occur in person or through the use of technology. Many social rules exist to describe the relationship boundaries and associated interactions. People are expected to behave differently in community settings (e.g., a public fair) than with family (e.g., at home). Thus, social training differs for community versus family activities. Occupational therapy practitioners evaluate the activity demands for socializing with family, community, peers, or friends. By understanding the expectations, roles, rules, and interaction requirements, the practitioner can prepare clients for social events.

**Case Study 2**

Susan is a 35-year-old small business owner, who was in a motor vehicle accident and lost both her lower legs. She is embarrassed by her appearance and that she uses a wheelchair. Socialization is an important aspect of her work setting; however, her fears and embarrassment are preventing her from returning to work. The occupational therapist, with information provided by the occupational therapy assistant, develops an intervention plan to help Susan return to work that also focuses on socialization. The occupational therapist and occupational therapy assistant designed activities to promote social participation. Together, they developed a variety of experiences to help Susan gain skills. The occupational therapist was ultimately responsible for the intervention plan but valued the input provided by the occupational therapy assistant. On several occasions, the occupational therapy assistant provided information so the intervention plan could be modified to more accurately meet Susan's needs. Specifically, they used role-playing, practice, and cognitive awareness of social behaviors to facilitate confidence and positive experiences. Susan is supported as she engages in short successful structured social events with unfamiliar people. As she begins to feel comfortable socializing with her new identity, the practitioner invites work "friends" to social sessions and they begin to help her transition to return to work. Eventually Susan establishes new friendships with others who she meets in rehabilitation and she reestablishes friendships at work prior to returning.

## Occupation and Activities

### *Preparatory Methods*

Clients may experience stress or discomfort interfering with their ability to engage in social activities. Preparatory activities help clients get ready for such interactions. Preparatory methods include relaxation techniques, sensory-based activities, role-playing, discussion, breathing techniques, mental rehearsal, and reviewing the schedule of events. Reviewing rules and expectations may ease anxiety and promote success.

Children or adults who experience tactile defensiveness may find crowds, being touched, or noises difficult to tolerate. They may become anxious, agitated, or distressed in social situations. The occupational therapy practitioner may engage the client in preparatory activities aimed at preparing the nervous system for the interaction. These activities may be used by the client on a regular basis to "calm" the system so that the client is not anxious and ready to engage.

## Purposeful Activity

Occupational therapy practitioners may help clients learn specific social participation skills through engagement in purposeful activity. Purposeful activity is goal-directed activity with an end product (Fisher, 1998). Purposeful activity closely resembles the actual occupation, but it is designed to target specific client factors or performance. The occupational therapy practitioner designs the activity to target the client's needs and challenge the client to develop skills and abilities in the desired area.

For example, the client may show poor social interaction skills by sharing inappropriate personal information with strangers. Using purposeful activity, the occupational therapy practitioner may address this weakness during a role-playing activity or group game involving discussion with a small group of supportive peers before requiring the client perform the social activity in a crowd.

Another occupational therapy intervention example may be sharing craft supplies as one way to increase the ability to ask and communicate with others. Working on group projects or playing on a sports team may be purposeful and assist clients in selected areas of social participation. Clients may work in small groups on expressing frustration making eye contact, engaging in conversations, demonstrating body language, and relating to others through group activities, with the hope that these skills will be generalized to the client's meaningful occupations.

Frequently, the occupational therapy practitioner sets up scenarios for clients to role-play so they may practice the skills before the actual event. The occupational therapy practitioner may support the client by accompanying him or her to social events. Price, Stephenson, Krantz, and Ward (2011) found that clients with spinal cord injury appreciated it when the practitioners engaged in the social activity with them (as a partner) and when they involved family and friends.

## Occupation-Based Activity

The goal of occupational therapy intervention is for clients to perform in the natural setting. For example, helping children get along with others on the playground at the school or day care they attend is the preferred activity, compared to requiring they play in the clinic. Working with siblings so they may play and socialize together at home or taking clients to a public event such as the swimming pool and encouraging them to use socially appropriate behaviors are both occupation-based activities (Figure 30-10). Coaching adults about socially appropriate behaviors and interaction skills by engaging them in community events is an occupation-based activity.

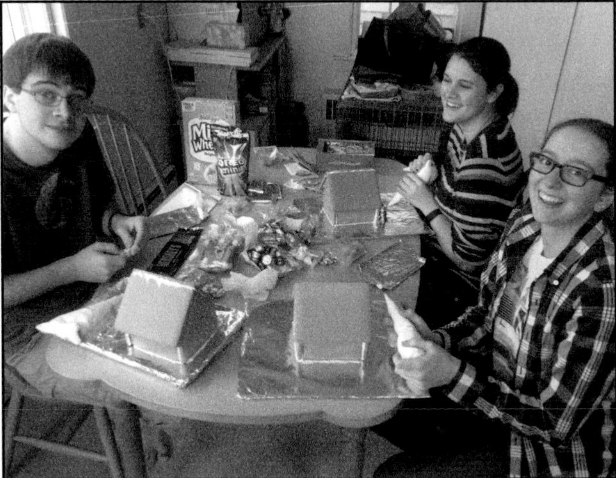

**Figure 30-10.** Siblings make gingerbread houses together at home.

Occupation-based activity requires clients integrate a variety of skills and abilities within the context in which they will perform. Occupation-based activity results in improved generalization and transfer of learning. By doing the actual occupation, clients continue to develop skills, abilities, and their identity.

# Advocacy

Consulting requires clear communication and negotiation skills. Consulting is most frequently conducted by an occupational therapist. The occupational therapy practitioner may decide to serve as a consultant to improve social participation. In this case, the role of the occupational therapist is to help the client identify the problem, try some solutions, and alter them as necessary (AOTA, 2014a). The occupational therapy practitioner does not do the activity with the client but instead recommends activities to enhance the client's functioning. For example, the occupational therapy practitioner may suggest that an adolescent join the Special Olympics or an adult join a social group. Consultation may require the occupational therapist to visit the site and make suggestions to the group leader, coach, client, or family member.

Consultation for social participation may include identifying social groups that the client would enjoy and making specific recommendations to the client or family. The occupational therapist may serve as a consultant on an as-needed basis to help the client problem solve situations as they arise. When consulting, the occupational therapy practitioner is not directly responsible for the outcome (AOTA, 2014a). Consultation may occur to increase social behaviors of clients in group homes, schools, or community setting. The occupational therapy practitioner provides information on the client's abilities and disabilities along with suggestions to help the client be successful. Implementation is overseen by others, and responsibilities for outcomes lie with the client.

## Education and Training

Occupational therapy practitioners frequently educate others about occupations and the impact a disorder, disease, or trauma may have on a client's functioning. Imparting knowledge or educating others about the occupation is part of the intervention process (AOTA, 2014b). The occupational therapy practitioner may educate family members or caregivers on social expectations consistent with a client's diagnosis. Family members may need education on how to best approach and communicate with clients who do not use traditional methods (e.g., computer systems, communication boards). Family members, caregivers, or significant others may also need education on the prognosis of the client to help develop realistic expectations, which is not to be confused with giving up hope. Occupational therapy practitioners also teach others what to expect developmentally from the client. They educate family members and clients about how to grade and adapt activities so the client is successful and how to create effective social interactions for clients with all abilities and disabilities. They also provide education on the legal rights clients have to participate completely in their occupations (e.g., access, billing) and the possibilities for engagement in occupations.

Occupational therapy practitioners are resources to those with disabilities since they often know which programs adapt to clients with special needs. Other resources available to clients allow them to engage in social activities such as transportation systems, adapted sailing programs, hypnotherapy programs, or aquatic programs.

## Occupational Therapy Intervention Approaches

Occupational therapy interventions aimed to increase social participation have been reported to have positive results (Berger, McAteer, Schreier, & Kaldenberg, 2013; Carter et al., 2004; Dumont, Gervais, Fougeyrollas, & Bertrand, 2005; Gol & Jarus, 2005; Krupa, Woodside, & Pocock, 2010; Tanner, Hand, O'Toole, & Lane, 2015; Wolf, Chuh, Floyd, McInnis, & Williams, 2015). See the Evidence-Based Research Chart at the end of the chapter for an overview of research evidence regarding social participation. The AOTA (2014b) defines five occupational therapy intervention approaches: create, establish, maintain, modify, and prevent. The following describes each approach and how occupational therapy practitioners apply the approach to enhance social participation:

- **Create, promote (health promotion):** This approach develops experiences for everyone, not just those with disabilities. Occupational therapy practitioners use this approach to create social experiences for all persons and promote healthy social activities. Examples are as varied as clients, but include developing after school programs for children or creating appropriate social opportunities, such as a tea party or dance. An occupational therapy practitioner using this type of approach sets up the scenario under the premise that the clients have the abilities but need the opportunity to engage in social activity.
- **Establish, restore (remediation, restoration):** This intervention approach works on establishing abilities that have not developed or restoring those that may have been lost (AOTA, 2014b). Developing a client's social skills through role-playing and coaching techniques is one way to establish abilities. This approach requires restoring the underlying factors interfering with the occupation. Helping a client who has had a stroke interact with loved ones is an example of attempting to restore social skills. Many of the behavioral frames of reference work on establishing appropriate social skills through reinforcement methods. Clients are rewarded when their behavior meets the appropriate social standards. Motor control or biomechanical approaches work to increase physical skills that may be interfering with social participation.
- **Maintain:** Occupational therapy practitioners may help clients keep the skills and abilities they currently possess so they do not decline in function. This type of approach may be readily used with deteriorating conditions in which maintaining function is difficult. In this case, the client is expected to keep the skills he or she has without losing function. Thus, the practitioner provides strategies so the client does not lose social skills and develops strategies so the client may participate in desired social activities as long as possible. For example, the occupational therapy practitioner may work with the client to attend a weekly yoga class. The occupational therapy practitioner may work to help the client communicate with others despite decreased functioning. Maintaining social

networks may require educating others involved or helping the client overcome fears.

- **Modify (compensation, adaptation):** This intervention approach requires the occupational therapy practitioner to make changes to the activity or the way in which the client performs the activity. In this case, the expectation is not that the client improves his or her abilities but rather learns to perform the activity differently. Compensation is used to help clients engage in occupations without trying to change the degree of disability. Clients may need to compensate in social activities for poor verbal skills by using assistive technology. More subtle but equally important compensations may be required when a client experiences psychological difficulties interfering with social participation. For example, clients who are anxious in new social systems may be encouraged to seek out a familiar person with whom to attend social activities. The compensation strategy may be that the client only attends those functions for short periods of time, or the client is encouraged to participate in activities with a few familiar peers.
- **Prevent (disability prevention):** Some occupational therapy practitioners develop programs to help those who may be at risk for disability such as programs targeting backpack awareness, healthy computing, childhood obesity, well elderly, work simplification, and fall prevention. The goal of this type of intervention is to prevent future impairments. Social participation programs such as Big Brother Big Sister, peer mentoring groups, day intervention, and adult recreational leagues are designed to increase socialization, friendships, and a sense of belonging. Structured groups provide resources to individuals. These groups may prevent antisocial behaviors or psychosocial disorders (e.g., depression and loneliness) caused by a lack of social interactions. The occupational therapy practitioner may develop a specific group around preventing disability or help a client participate in an existing group. Clients may be involved in book clubs, dance classes, school programs, craft classes, parenting classes, and exercise groups. Clients may form support groups with persons with similar diagnoses. These support groups provide resources and are a source of social participation. Therefore, they help the client meet his or her social needs and identify with others.

## Grading and Adapting Intervention for Social Participation

Grading and adapting activities to address social participation first involves a thorough analysis of the behaviors and expectations required of the activity. Table 30-1 provides a list of factors to consider when grading and adapting social activity. These areas can be modified to make the activity more or less challenging for the client. The occupational therapy practitioner designs intervention to challenge a client while promoting success. For example, the rules and expectations of the social activity may be formal or informal, flexible or inflexible, and explicit or implicit. Requiring a client to engage in a formal event with inflexible rules and as high expectations as might be expected when presenting at a conference increases the social demands and requirements. Conversely, attending an informal gathering with one close friend at a coffee shop may allow the client to be successful.

The practitioner considers if the social activity is new versus old or active versus passive. The number of people involved in the activity and the relationships of group members play an important role in the complexity of the social interactions required. Generally, small task-oriented groups are the least stressful socially. Pairing clients with others who have similar issues may be helpful. The diversity of group members and the content of the activity change the degree of difficulty. Adapting and grading activities require that the practitioner consider the client's strengths and weaknesses when deciding on the type of social activity and how to change the activity so the client will be successful. Working one on one with the client to establish a rapport before a social event may prove useful. Discussing the social rules, boundaries, and consequences before the activity promotes success. Setting firm limits and helping clients work through and socially adapt to different situations is necessary before performing the actual occupation. The occupational therapy practitioner uses his or her skill at analyzing activities to determine the best social intervention activity.

Table 30-2 summarizes a variety of group interventions targeting social participation. Group interventions provide a venue to facilitate social participation.

Table 30-1.

## Factors to Consider When Grading and Adapting Social Participation Activities

| Client's Goal for Activity | Can the Goals Be Facilitated in the Session? |
|---|---|
| Purpose of interactions | Project<br>Goals of group<br>Goals of clients |
| Size of group | Is it adequate to facilitate interactions? |
| Location | Familiar versus unfamiliar<br>Transportation |
| Physical space | Outdoors versus indoors<br>Small versus large<br>Quiet versus noisy<br>Public versus private<br>Formal versus informal |
| Structure | Expectations<br>Expectations of others<br>Roles<br>Degree of investment required<br>Time commitment<br>Degree of supervision |
| Experience | Novelty<br>Frequency of social interaction<br>Risk |
| Behavioral expectations | Rules<br>Complexity of interactions<br>Interaction of members |
| Cultural expectations | Past experiences with activity<br>Meaning ascribed to activity |
| Performance expectations | Degree of difficulty<br>Mobility requirements<br>Social requirements |
| Conclusion | Degree of follow-up available |
| Other | Cost |
| Suitability for client | |
| Modifications needed | |

Table 30-2.

**GROUP INTERVENTIONS**

| Intervention | Description | Application Examples |
|---|---|---|
| Peer support system | A structured relationship to encourage social involvement | Reclaiming Joy Peer Support Intervention: A program where a volunteer and participant are paired together to encourage health and well-being through social interaction and support (Chapin et al., 2013)<br>Social Internet-Based Activities: A therapy session using a coaching method to help older adults explore and use the Internet for socialization (Larsson, Nilsson, & Larsson Lund, 2013) |
| Peer-mediated approach | The process of educating peers to initiate, prompt, and reinforce social interaction, therefore encouraging improvements in the social behaviors | Integrated Play Group: Structuring the play environment with typically developing peers and adult guidance to promote mutually enjoyable social interaction, communication, play, and imagination experiences with children with autism (Wolfberg & Schuler, 1993) |
| Group therapy | Allows the practitioner to meet the needs of several clients at once through careful planning and selection of group members based on their goals | Combined-Strategy Group Intervention: The use of social stories, video modeling, visual cues, positive reinforcement, and parent involvement to educate clients of appropriate social behaviors in a group therapy session (Kroeger, Schultz, & Newsom, 2007; Theimann & Goldstein, 2001) |
| Community-based support | A community environment designed to support the client's independence in various occupations and foster supportive roles | "Village" Model: Designed to support older adults with dementia to maintain their independence and reduce social isolation (Graham, Scharlach, & Wolf, 2014). |

The organization and structure of groups allow participants to be comfortable so that they can work on increasing aspects of social participation, such as initiating conversation, body language, sharing, responding, pacing, and cooperating. The occupational therapy practitioner is aware of the participants' needs and facilitates groups that will encourage clients to practice and repeat skills within the groups so that they may be successful. This will allow clients to learn skills within a safe setting so that they may engage in occupations requiring social participation in their own community and family.

## SUMMARY

Humans are social beings, and as such, social participation is an important occupation for clients of all ages and abilities. Occupational therapy practitioners evaluate the social skills required, considering the contexts of the activity, including the setting in which the activity occurs.

Occupational therapy practitioners help prepare clients for the social interactions by providing them with many opportunities to practice the prerequisite skills, consulting with them and team members, and educating clients on appropriate social behaviors. In this way, the goal of improved social participation can be reached.

## STUDENT SELF-ASSESSMENT

1. Describe the social behaviors required to participate in one social activity. Describe the context in which this activity takes place.
   - Change the context of the aforementioned activity
   - Compare and contrast the differences
2. Describe the aspects of a specific activity requiring social participation, such as going to the coffee shop with friends, using the *Framework* (client factors, activity demands, contexts) as a guide.
3. Make a list of social activities in which you participate.
   - Describe the motor, processing, and social interaction factors involved in three of them.
4. Develop a notebook of social activities and resources for children, adolescents, adults, and elderly persons.
5. Summarize three research articles describing social participation in a given population.

## Evidence-Based Research Chart

| Author/Year | Population | Measurement | Intervention | Results |
|---|---|---|---|---|
| Berger, McAteer, Schreier, & Kaldenberg, 2013 | Adults with low vision | Systematic review (13 articles) | Problem-solving approach<br>Combination of services<br>Social skills training<br>Home and environmental modifications | The strongest evidence supports using a problem-solving approach to improve leisure and social participation in adults with low vision |
| Carter et al., 2004 | Children with Asperger syndrome ages 8 to 15 (n = 12) | Lifestyle Performance Profile Interview | Friendship Club: An afterschool program for children | Positive results per report from children and parents |
| Dumont, Gervais, Fougeyrollas, & Bertrand, 2005 | 53 adults with traumatic brain injury | Self-Efficacy and Social Participation questionnaire | | Perceived self-efficacy explained 40% variance of social participation |
| Gol & Jarus, 2005 | Children with ADHD (n = 27) and without ADHD (n = 24) | Assessment of Motor Processing | Social skills training through meaningful occupations (e.g., art, games, cooking) in groups | AMPS for children with ADHD improved from first to second evaluation (P = .008) |
| Krupa, Woodside, & Pocock, 2010 | 25 participants who had experienced a first episode of psychosis in the previous 5 years | Grounded theory; data from family, friends, participants, personal records, documents | Description of experiences | Individuals are at high risk for disengagement from important and meaningful activity and social participation<br>Conceptualizing critical tasks can provide a useful framework for occupational therapy services |
| Paul-Ward, Kielhofner, Braveman, & Levin, 2005 | Staff members (n = 21) and clients with AIDS (n = 16) | Focus groups | | Staff identified systematic and personal barriers; clients identified only systemic barriers as impacting participation |
| Tanner, Hand, O'Toole, & Lane, 2015 | Autism spectrum disorder | Systematic review (35 articles: 24 Level I, 4 Level II, and 7 Level III) | Examination of a variety of interventions: Virtual reality video modeling)<br>Picture Exchange Communication System<br>Group-based social skills training<br>Parent-mediated<br>Naturalistic behavioral | Strong evidence was found that social skills groups, the PECS, joint attention interventions, and parent-mediated strategies can improve social participation |
| Wolf, Chuh, Floyd, McInnis, & Williams, 2015 | Persons with stroke | Systematic review (3 Level I studies) | Occupation-based interventions to increase social participation<br>Cognitive Orientation to Daily Occupational Performance<br>Chronic Disease Self-Management Program | Moderate evidence from one study for the CO-OP strategy-based intervention<br>Limited evidence to support the use of occupation-based interventions to address social participation goals for people with stroke |

## References


American Heritage Dictionaries (Ed.). (2009). *The American heritage dictionary of the English language* (4th ed.). Boston, MA: Houghton Mifflin Company.

American Occupational Therapy Association. (2014a). Guidelines for supervision, roles, and responsibilities during the delivery of occupational therapy services. *American Journal of Occupational Therapy, 68*(Suppl. 3), S16-S22. doi:10.5014/ajot.2014.686S03

American Occupational Therapy Association. (2014b). Occupational therapy practice framework: Domain and process (3rd ed.). *American Journal of Occupational Therapy, 68*(Suppl. 1), S1-S48. doi:10.5014/ajot.2014.682006

Berger, S., McAteer, J., Schreier, K., & Kaldenberg, J. (2013). Occupational therapy interventions to improve leisure and social participation in older adults with low vision: A systematic review. *American Journal of Occupational Therapy, 67*, 303-311.

Boyt Schell, B. A., Gillen, G., & Scaffa, M. (2014). Glossary. In B. A. Boyt Schell, G. Gillen, & M. Scaffa (Eds.), *Willard and Spackman's occupational therapy* (12th ed., pp. 1229-1243). Philadelphia, PA: Lippincott Williams and Wilkins.

Carter, C., Meckes, L., Pritchard, L., Swensen, S., Wittman, P. P., & Velde, B. (2004). The friendship club: An after-school program for children with Asperger syndrome. *Family and Community Health, 27*(2), 143-150.

Chapin, R. K., Sergeant, J. F., Landry, S., Leedahl, S. N., Rachlin, R., Koenig, T., & Graham, A. (2013). Reclaiming joy: Pilot evaluation of a mental health peer support program for older adults who receive Medicaid. *The Gerontologist, 53*(2), 345-352.

Christiansen, C., & Baum, C. (1997). Person-environment occupational performance: A conceptual model for practice. In C. Christiansen & C. Baum (Eds.), *Occupational therapy: Enabling function and well-being* (2nd ed.). Thorofare, NJ: SLACK Incorporated.

Dumont, C., Gervais, M., Fougeyrollas, P., & Bertrand, R. (2005). Perceived self-efficacy is associated with social participation in adults with traumatic brain injury. *Canadian Journal of Occupational Therapy, 72*(4), 222-233.

Fisher, A. G. (1998). Uniting practice and theory in an occupational framework. 1998 Eleanor Clarke Slagle lecture. *American Journal of Occupational Therapy, 52*(7), 509-521.

Gillen, G. & Boyt Schell, B. (2014). Introduction to evaluation, interpretation, and outcomes for occupations. In B. A. Boyt Schell, G. Gillen, & M. Scaffa (Eds.). *Willard and Spackman's occupational therapy* (12th ed. pp. 606-609). Philadelphia, PA: Lippincott Williams and Wilkins.

Gol, D., & Jarus, T. (2005). Effect of a social skills training group on everyday activities of children with attention-deficit-hyperactivity disorder. *Developmental Medicine and Child Neurology, 47*(8), 539-545.

Graham, C., Scharlach, A., & Wolf, J. (2014). The impact of the "village" model on health, well-being, service access, and social engagement of older adults. *Health, Education and Behavior, 41*(1S). Retrieved from http://heb.sagepub.com.une.idm.oclc.org/content/41/1_suppl/91S.full.pdf+html

Kroeger, K. A., Schultz, J. R., & Newsom, C. (2007). A comparison of two groups delivered social skills programs for young children with autism. *Journal of Autism and Developmental Disorders, 37*, 808-817.

Krupa, T., Woodside, H., & Pocock, K. (2010). Activity and social participation in the period following a first episode of psychosis and implications for occupational therapy. *British Journal of Occupational Therapy, 73*(1), 13-20.

Larsson, E., Nilsson, I., & Larsson Lund, M. (2013). Participation in social internet-based activities: Five seniors' intervention processes. *Scandinavian Journal of Occupational Therapy, 20*(6), 471-480. doi:10.3109/11038128.2013.839001

Llorens, L. A. (1976). *Application of a developmental theory for health and rehabilitation*. Rockville, MD: AOTA Press.

Paul-Ward, A., Kielhofner, G., Braveman, B., & Levin, M. (2005). Resident and staff perceptions of barriers to independence and employment in supportive living settings for persons with AIDS. *American Journal of Occupational Therapy, 59*(5), 540-545.

Price, P., Stephenson, S., Krantz, L., & Ward, K. (2011). Beyond my front door: The occupational and social participation of adults with spinal cord injury. *OTJR: Occupation, Participation and Health, 31*(2), 81-88.

Tanner, K., Hand, B. N., O'Toole, G., & Lane, A. E. (2015). Effectiveness of interventions to improve social participation, play, leisure, and restricted and repetitive behaviors in people with autism spectrum disorder: A systematic review. *American Journal of Occupational Therapy, 69*, 6905180010. doi:10.5014/ajot.2015.017806

Theimann, K. S., & Goldstein, H. (2001). Social stories, written text cues, and video feedback: Effects on social communication of children with autism. *Journal of Applied Behavior Analysis, 34*, 425-446.

Wolf, T. J., Chuh, A., Floyd, T., McInnis, K., & Williams, E. (2015). Effectiveness of occupation-based interventions to improve areas of occupation and social participation after stroke: An evidence-based review. *American Journal of Occupational Therapy, 69*, 6901180060. doi:10.5014/ajot.2015.012195

Wolfberg, P. J., & Schuler, A. L. (1993). Integrated play groups: A model for promoting the social and cognitive dimensions of play in children with autism. *Journal of Autism and Developmental Disorders, 23*, 467-489.

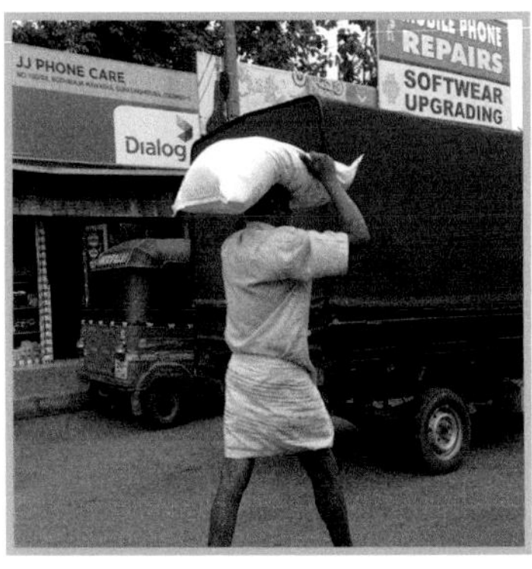


# 31

# Environmental Adaptation and Ergonomics

Linda Miller, OT (C), OTD, CPE

## ACOTE Standards Explored in This Chapter

B.5.9, B.5.23, B.5.24

## Key Vocabulary

- **AbleData:** A web-accessed database that houses unbiased information on products, solutions, and resources to improve productivity and ease of tasks. AbleData is funded by the National Institute on Disability and Rehabilitation through the Office of Special Education and Rehabilitative Services.
- **Americans with Disabilities Act:** Signed into law by Congress in 1990, this Act seeks to prevent discrimination in employment, public buildings and transportation, public accommodations, and telecommunications based solely on disability.
- **Ergonomics/human factors:** A scientific discipline that addresses the interaction between humans and other elements of a system. Through the use of theory, principles, data, and methods, professionals optimize design to support well-being and overall system performance (International Ergonomics Association, 2016).
- **Primary and secondary prevention:** Primary prevention encompasses initiatives to prevent the occurrence of injury or illness. This may include modification of the environment or task. Secondary prevention through modification or adaptation of the environment, tools, or tasks for workers after injury to prevent further decline or reinjury (Bell et al., 1995).

*(continued)*

Jacobs, K., & MacRae, N. (Eds.).
*Occupational Therapy Essentials for Clinical Competence, Third Edition* (pp. 455-465).

**KEY VOCABULARY (CONTINUED)**

- **Tertiary prevention:** Managing medical conditions to prevent further or accelerated deterioration which may result in premature exit from the workforce (Bell et al., 1995).
- **Universal design:** The design of products and environments to the greatest extent possible to support ease of use by everyone regardless of age or ability.

Occupational therapy practitioners consider the client's occupational performance within the environment in which it is performed. Environmental adaptation has the primary goal of modifying the client's environment to maximize participation in his or her occupational roles. It is an attempt to modify the environment to match the client's abilities rather than expecting an individual to meet the demands of the environment.

In this chapter, we will provide a brief overview of the Americans with Disabilities Act (ADA) and its influence on environmental adaptation, the process for determining the appropriate environmental adaptations, and how both ergonomics and universal design can be used by the practitioner to assist with determining effective environmental modifications to meet a client's needs.

## The Environment

When considering environmental adaptation—in the home, at work, school, or in the community—one should consider the following tasks and related environments:

- Travel to a site (e.g., private or public transportation)
- Entry to structures or areas (e.g., parking, entering and exiting a building)
- Movement within the common areas (e.g., lobby, hallway, cafeteria, elevator, bathroom)
- Tasks performed within specific areas (e.g., bathing, dressing, computer work, shopping, playing)

It is important to remember that an environment can be designed appropriately, but the actions, processes, procedures, and training within a task can lead to injury or illness.

### *Transportation*

#### Public Transportation

The ADA of 1990, updated in 2010 and revised in 2012, prohibits discrimination against individuals with disabilities. The goal is to allow access and safe transportation for all individuals with a disability. Public transportation includes modes such as buses, subways, airplanes, and public taxis. It is important to note that access may not always mean immediate access without prior planning, especially when the individual is considering air travel. The client may have to prearrange access so that arrangements can be made to accommodate their needs.

#### Private Transportation

Private transportation is access to and the operation of, either by self or a driver, motor vehicles. Private transportation can be much more challenging than public transportation since the individual may be expected to also be the vehicle operator. The client must be able to access and egress from the vehicle unassisted, access and store mobility aids efficiently, and safely operate the vehicle.

A standard-sized vehicle may be sufficient when the client can transfer to and from the vehicle unassisted. Vehicles with sufficient room behind the front seat can be appropriate when a client has the strength and balance to store a walker, cane, or other device there independently. The client may still require an aid such as a swivel seat or support aid to get in and out of the vehicle. When the weight and size of the mobility aid becomes too difficult for client to handle, power lifts can be utilized. When independent transfers are impossible or not appropriate, a van can become a viable option. Vans may need to be modified to allow entrance and exit via a power lift or ramp. Some are factory made for accessibility while others may be a custom modification made after the vehicle has been purchased. If an existing vehicle needs to be modified to accommodate the client's abilities, it is important to work in conjunction with a vendor to select the correct modification to meet the requirements of the client and ensure safe vehicle adaptation.

Independent operation of the vehicle by the client will require the ability to access controls such as the ignition and accelerator, to control the direction of travel, and to be able to stop. Modifications may entail mechanical assists to lessen the force needed to use and manipulate traditional controls such as a steering wheel, accelerator, and brake (Figure 31-1). For individuals who are short, it is also possible to adapt accelerator and brake controls through the use of commercial extenders.

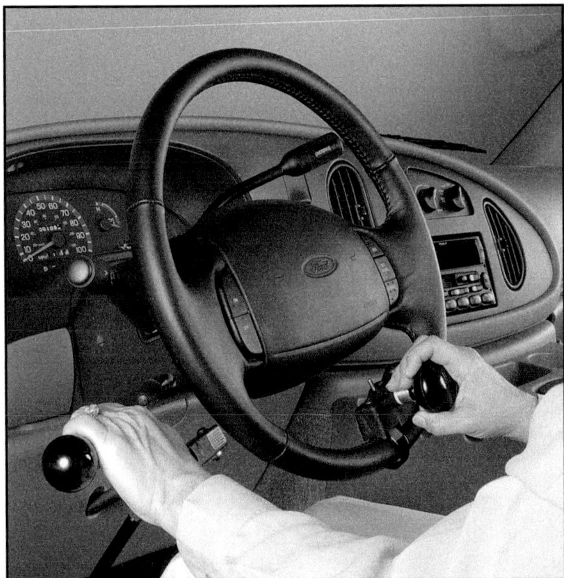

**Figure 31-1.** MPD (Mobility Products & Design) 3500 Push Right Angle hand control with Knob Grip and Offset handle. (Reprinted with permission from Veigel North America dba Mobility Products & Design.)

## Site Accessibility

### Parking Lots/Parkades

When the client arrives at the destination, access to the structure or destination can be a challenge. If the client is using private transportation, he or she will require a parking space to safely access and egress the vehicle, followed by the ability to safely move from the parking area through common areas to access entrances.

### Parking Places and Size

The ADA specifies the number and size of parking spaces that must be accessible. Additionally, regulations specify the number and size of spaces that need to accommodate access for a van.

### Walkways/Passageways

The ADA requires at least one "accessible route" be provided that allows individuals access to and between all accessible areas.

### Entry Doors

The ADA specifies that doors must be 32 inches in width and require no greater than 5 pounds of force to open the door (Figure 31-2). The handles should be lever style, such that it can be operated with the push of a closed fist. It is important to note that the ADA specifies the minimum requirements to meet to regulation.

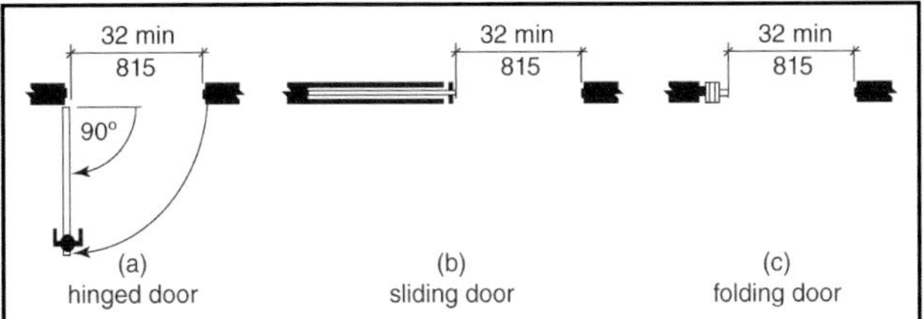


**Figure 31-2.** Door entry. (Reprinted from U.S. Department of Justice. [2010]. *2010 ADA Standards for Accessible Design*. Retrieved from https://www.ada.gov/regs2010/2010ADAStandards/2010ADAStandards_prt.pdf)

### Ramps

One common means of providing access to a private or public facility is via a ramp. A ramp for a public building must meet state and local codes. Ramps for a private residence may or may not be covered by a local code.

The most common specification used for determining how long to make a ramp is the ratio of 1:12, which translates to 12 inches in length for every 1 inch of rise. Ramps must be a minimum of 36 inches between handrails. (Note: The ratio is the maximum angle allowed.) When possible, it is desirable to make the ramp longer to place less stress on the person propelling the wheelchair, whether it is the client or caregiver.

Ramps should be built and positioned over concrete columns. The columns must extend deep enough to go below the normal frost lines of the area to avoid distortion of the ramp through the freeze/thaw cycle. Specification of size and depth for columns will often be covered under local building codes. Construction of a ramp can be very costly. Alternatives exist that are also feasible for private residences (refer to AbleData for potential ideas and options). Information about ramps and the accompanying loan and grant programs can be found at state independent living centers.

## Common Area Access

Common areas can be thought of as within a structure that a client will need to navigate or use. This may include hallways, foyers, cafeterias, and bathrooms, as well as utilization of devices, such as drinking fountains. Guidance for each of these areas can be found under Electronic Resources.

## Task Areas

Task areas can be considered those spaces in which primary occupation takes place. Examples of tasks as they relate to occupation and task are presented in Table 31-1. Occupational therapy practitioners are uniquely positioned to use their skills of activity analysis to examine task areas to meet the client's needs and goals in primary occupational performance areas.

Table 31-1.

**EXAMPLE TASK AREAS WHERE PRIMARY OCCUPATIONS TAKE PLACE**

| Environment | Task Areas |
|---|---|
| Home | Kitchen, bathroom, laundry room, bedroom |
| School | Classroom, gym, library, art room |
| Work | Workspace, storeroom, cafeteria |
| Community | Stores, library, restaurants, banks, theaters |

# THE PROCESS

Collaboration between the practitioner and the client is central to service delivery (American Occupational Therapy Association [AOTA], 2014). When considering environmental adaptation, context is critical to understanding. Depending upon the environment, the therapist may have to also collaborate with other key stakeholders to fully define the demands of the environment and activities. In the following section, strategies to better understand contexts will be outlined for educational, home, work, and community settings.

## Educational Setting

Watson and Wilson (2003) stressed the importance of "participation and engagement" by modifying the classroom and its demands to support all students to participate. Participation in learning activities is argued to be more effective than simply providing a piece of assistive technology, which aids participation, but does not fully allow for engagement. It is important that the school-based therapist works with the teachers and caregivers to fully understand the contexts of the classroom as well as performance skills and activity demands before suggesting alterations in the space or activities.

## Home Setting

For the home care therapist to aid environmental adaptation, he or she will need to meet the client, but may also need to meet with caregivers or family members to explore feasibility of suggestions for the space or activities. For example, to aid use of a mobility aid in a home environment, the therapist may suggest to decrease clutter throughout the house. This may require participation of the family or caregiver to help support implementation and also help determine strategies to ensure pathways are clear and uncluttered.

### Case Study 1

Dorothy was diagnosed with Parkinson disease shortly after her husband died. Her family started to notice she was having difficulty remembering if she had taken her medication and often became extremely anxious. To compensate, Dorothy frequently called her children for guidance to remember to take her medication. During a visit with the family doctor, she asked if she may have mild dementia. An assessment by the psychiatrist returned a diagnosed of Parkinson-related dementia.

An occupational therapist assisted the family by using the *Framework* (AOTA, 2014) to define Dorothy's goals, the requirements of her environment, and to determine her ability to meet those requirements. With the assistance of the family, the therapist was able to determine that Dorothy wished to remain in her own home with assistance from a paid caregiver, participate in social activities at her church, and continue to drive in and around her neighborhood to get groceries. In the areas of independent living and driving, the therapist was able to establish "thresholds events" that would require her to give up her license or move into an assisted living facility. Using the Context and Activity Demands portions of the *Framework*, the therapist identified the performance skills and client factors needed to be successful in the context and activity demands of Dorothy's environment. The therapist asked the family to use a common activities of daily living checklist to identify both performance skills and performance patterns they observed in their mother. The therapist stressed the importance of change over time. Finally, using the assessment reports provided by the psychiatrist, Dorothy, her children, and the therapist were able to develop a plan that included environmental adaptations along with daily visits by a paid caregiver.

## Work Setting

To allow for successful environmental adaptation in the workplace, the therapist will need to conduct a worksite assessment. Prior to performing the assessment, it is important that the therapist contact the employer to prepare for the site visit. The therapist will need to determine if he or she will require specific personal protective equipment such as steel toe boots, safety glasses, or hearing protection to access the site. In some instances, the therapist may also require specialized training such as the Workplace Hazardous Materials Information System or a safety orientation to enter the site. Once onsite, the therapist will need to work with employer representatives to determine both activity and environmental demands. Prior to suggesting site changes in the environment or activities, the therapist should consider the impact changes may have on other workers and the organization so that suggested changes will be adopted and supported.

## Community Setting

Interview the client to determine goals and preexisting performance patterns. Performance skills and client factors can be assessed using standardized or nonstandardized means to understand observed or potential issues related to the client's ability to successfully and safely function in the environment.

# Overview of Ergonomics and Human Factors Engineering

In the preceding pages of this chapter, areas for consideration have been highlighted as well as the process for assessing an environment before determining what modifications might be needed. In this section, an overview of ergonomics and human factors will be provided and their link to modifications associated with the environment, tools, equipment, organizations, and activities.

Ergonomics provides a very useful body of knowledge that will assist practitioners in understanding the activity demands of the task areas (AOTA, 2014), particularly those found in work settings. The application of ergonomic principles can be applied to other contexts, such as learning environment (e.g., schools, libraries).

Jacobs (1999) traced the understanding of the importance of ergonomics back to the earliest tools created by humanoids as they shaped stone implements to fit their own hands and abilities. The International Ergonomics Association (2016) defines ergonomics/human factors as a discipline that addresses the interaction between humans and other elements of a system (Figure 31-3). Ergonomics/human factors is considered "human-centered" design. The primary goal in ergonomics is to design and evaluate products, jobs, tasks, environments, and the organization

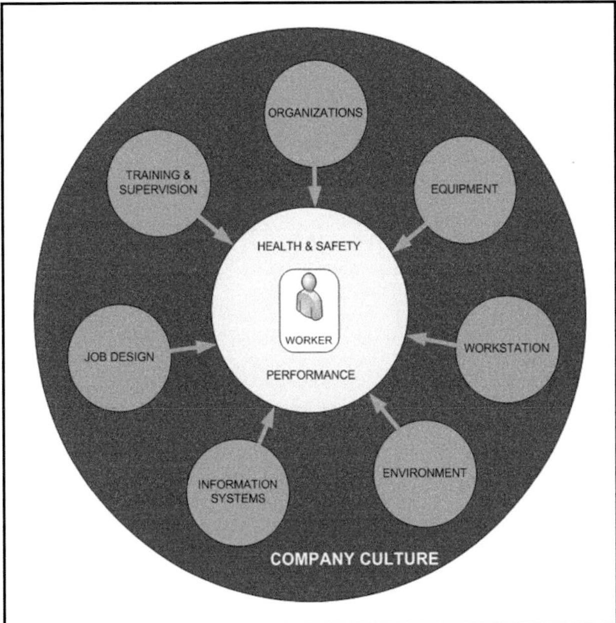


**Figure 31-3.** Ergonomics.

so that they are compatible with the needs, abilities, and limitations of people (International Ergonomics Association, 2016). Today, ergonomics is used in computer workstation set-up, equipment/tool design, and the organization of work in factories.

# Environmental Adaptation and Ergonomics

Ergonomics requires knowledge in a wide range of topics (Table 31-2). For practitioners, ergonomics holds considerable promise. Use of ergonomic techniques can allow the practitioner to gain a full understanding of the contexts and performance skills required to complete a task in its environment. Understanding the demands of the task and its environment can better aid the practitioner's design and adapt the environment to support client independence.

Ergonomics can be used by the occupational therapy practitioner to support primary, secondary, and tertiary prevention initiatives. For example, the practitioner working in primary prevention can analyze the work environment and tasks to determine injury risks. The practitioner can then utilize the ergonomic principles to design strategies to either modify or eliminate concerns to prevent future injury. In the field of ergonomics, there are a number of well-established assessment tools/checklists available through the Occupational Health and Safety Administration (OSHA) and the Washington State Department of Labor and Industries (see Electronic Resources).

Table 31-2.

**FIELDS CONTRIBUTING TO KNOWLEDGE OF ERGONOMICS**

| Subject | Operational Definition | Example |
|---|---|---|
| Physiology | Sensory information: Visual, auditory, olfactory, touch, taste | What color would make a shut-off switch most visible in an emergency situation? |
| Skills | What is the skill set required to operate a piece of equipment? | What is the longest password that the average person can remember? |
| Performance | What are the factors that influence an operator's ability to perform an operation? | How long can a long-distance truck driver safely operate his or her vehicle on the highway? |
| Anthropometrics | Study of human body dimensions; examines both averages and extremes | How far can the average person reach into a refrigerator? |
| Biomedical factors | Effects of environment on workers: Sound levels, temperature, vibration, altitude, humidity, odor, etc. | What effect does temperature have on a worker's ability to perform fine adjustments on a piece of equipment? |
| Safety factors | What could go wrong? What are the consequences of making a wrong choice? | What are the consequences of a distracted vehicle operator shifting the transmission into "park" while moving? |
| Training | How long should a training program be? | What is the minimal amount of time a driver education program needs to significantly reduce the accident rate among new drivers? |
| Manning implications | What is the minimum number of workers we need? | How many craftspeople should be on a team that manufacturers custom-made stairways onsite? |

Adapted from Headquarters, Department of the Army. (1983). *Man-material systems: Human factors engineering program.* AR 602-1, Washington, DC: Author.

## UNIVERSAL DESIGN

Closely aligned with ergonomics is the concept of universal design, "the design of products and environments to be usable by all people, to the greatest extent possible, without the need for adaptation or specialized design" (Mace, 1997, para. 1). Table 31-3 outlines the principles, definitions, and an example of each of the seven principles that guide universal design (The Centre for Universal Design, 1997). Figure 31-4 is an example of one of the principles of equitable use, and Figure 31-5 is an example of low effort.

Universal design can be thought of as an attempt to "get it right from the start." Architects and designers that use universal design principles anticipate that individuals have different abilities by building in "tolerances" so different abilities can be accommodated. In Case Study 2, note how the practitioner analyzed the activity demands of the task. Using ergonomics/human factors principles, the practitioner recognized potential sources of hazards for the workers. The suggested intervention demonstrates a low-tech, cost-effective strategy for reducing worker risk.

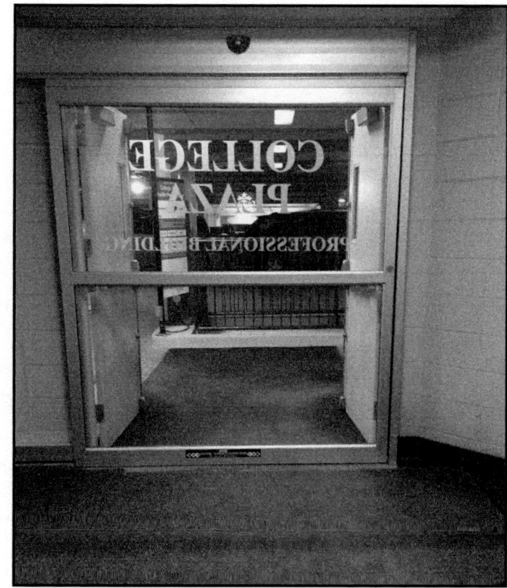

**Figure 31-4.** Equitable use.

Table 31-3.

**Universal Design Principles, Description, and Examples**

| Principle | Description | Example |
|---|---|---|
| Equitable use | Is useful for people of diverse abilities | Smartphone can be adapted to accommodate for low vision by altering the display size and colors |
| Flexibility in use | The design allows for wide range of user abilities | In a public art exhibition, the individual can either select to listen or read relevant information |
| Simple and intuitive | The design or product is easy to understand; understanding does not depend on the user's experience, knowledge, language skills, or current concentration levels | The entrance door is easy to locate |
| Perceptible information | Regardless of ambient conditions or the user's sensory abilities, the design communicates necessary information to the user | In a noisy train station, important information is displayed on signage so that it can still be viewed |
| Tolerance for error | The design minimizes hazards and the adverse consequences of accidental or unintended actions | A software program that asks the user prior to deleting an item if he or she is sure they wish to complete the action |
| Low effort | Designs that require minimal effort to perform the tasks | A sliding automatic door to a building provides access, no effort to push or pull the door open |
| Size and space for approach and use | A space that is designed that does not limit access, reach, manipulation, and use; the user's posture, size, mobility, and/or handedness does not limit access or use | A fully adjustable computer workstation that allows an individual to work while sitting or standing |

Adapted from Burgstahler, S. (2015). *Universal design: processes, principles, and applications.* Retrieved from https://www.washington.edu/doit/sites/default/files/atoms/files/Universal_Design%20Process%20Principles%20and%20Applications.pdf

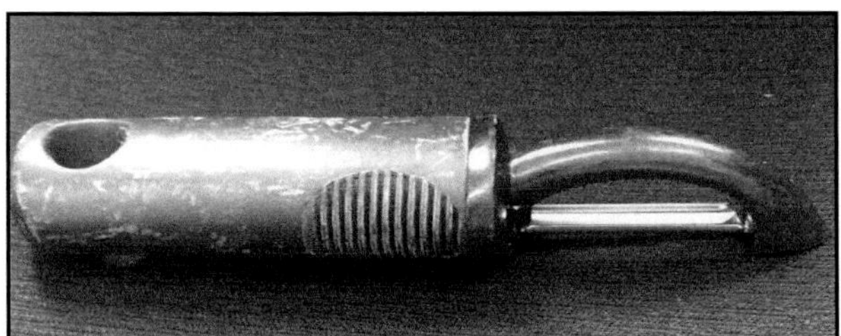

**Figure 31-5.** Low effort.

## Overview of Ergonomics and Process Modification

Controls used to reduce the risk of injury fall into one of the five categories: elimination, substitution, engineering, administrative, or personal protective equipment. Figure 31-6 outlines the hierarchy of controls and their effectiveness (Canadian Centre for Occupational Health and Safety, 2016).

Table 31-4 defines each control and provides an example. A number of resources exist through OSHA (see Electronic Resources).

## Roles and Teams in Environmental Adaptation

The occupational therapy assistant may work with an occupational therapist in the provision of services in environmental adaptation. The standard, however, makes it clear that the occupational therapy assistant may also work independently to modify, adapt, and teach after service competency has been demonstrated. Service competency is a method by which both the occupational therapy assistant and the occupational therapist determine that the clinical skills of each are appropriate and by which the occupational therapist verifies that the occupational therapy assistant is functioning to the ethical, safety, and practice standards of the profession. This is most often achieved by regularly coassessing and cotreating clients and comparing results and treatment methodologies.

As the occupational therapy practitioner and the client explore possible environmental adaptations, it is important that they work with architects and builders (when applicable), vendors, and all key stakeholders that may be affected by the implementation. Key stakeholders

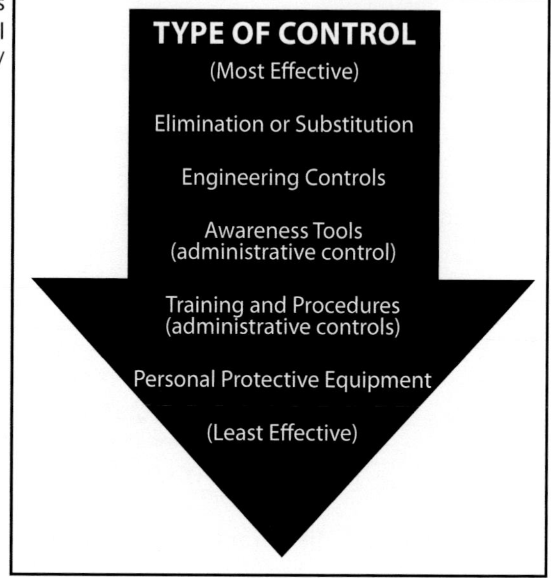


**Figure 31-6.** Hierarchy of controls and effectiveness. (Adapted from Centers for Disease Control and Protection—National Institute for Occupational Safety and Health. [2015]. *Hierarchy.* Retrieved from http://www.cdc.gov/niosh/topics/hierarchy/)

## Case Study 2

A local meat processing facility had an increase in the number of workers reporting hand and wrist discomfort. Individuals' work included cutting sections of meat repetitively to achieve a specific cut. The supervisor of the facility contacted a therapist to come in to provide him with some possible reasons for the increase in worker reported discomfort as well as suggestions to help reduce concerns. The therapist scheduled a worksite visit. She completed a series of interviews with the affected employees and the supervisor. Once she completed her interviews, she went out to the production floor and observed the task. To help the therapist classify the level of risk, she selected a validated assessment tool—the Rapid Upper Limb Assessment.

Upon completion of the Rapid Upper Limb Assessment checklist, it was apparent that the task was characterized by highly repetitive awkward movements of the wrist and high force gripping when handling the knife (Figure 31-7). Upon return to the clinic, the therapist examined the literature and identified that regular sharpening of the knife has resulted in effective outcomes to reduce force.

The therapist returned to the facility and spoke with the supervisor regarding their knife-sharpening protocol. It was determined that many of the new workers were inconsistently sharpening their knives. Working with the plant, the organization implemented a standard knife-sharpening protocol and provided ongoing training to front-line employees on proper sharpening technique. Along with additional education provided by the therapist on injury prevention, the organization realized a drop in discomfort reports.

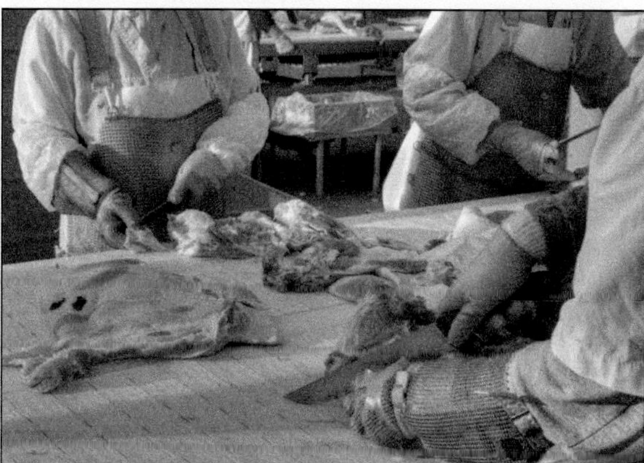

**Figure 31-7.** Meat cutting.

Table 31-4.

**HIERARCHY OF CONTROLS: DEFINITION AND EXAMPLES**

| Level of Control | Description | Example |
|---|---|---|
| Elimination | Physically removing the hazard | This may be achieved through reengineering the design or process—tend to be inexpensive if a project is in a design stage; if the project has already been built can be often very costly |
| Substitution | Replacing the hazard | |
| Engineering | Removing a hazard condition or placing a barrier between a worker and the hazard | Installation of a ceiling lift to assist with patient transfers in a patient care setting |
| Administrative | Change the way individuals perform their work | Providing the client with education and training on safe body mechanics when performing a work task |
| Personal protective equipment | Protecting the worker from the hazard with personal protective equipment | Hard hat, safety shoes, and/or eye protection |

Adapted from the Centers for Disease Control and Prevention—National Institute for Occupational Safety and Health. (2015). *Hierarchy of controls*. Retrieved from http://www.cdc.gov/niosh/topics/hierarchy/

may include a family member or a caregiver in a home environment, supervisors/engineers/human resources in a work environment, and building managers/facility managers in a community setting.

## SUMMARY

Environmental adaptation and ergonomics present occupational therapy practitioners with an important professional challenge. To be effective, the practitioner must be familiar with the client, environment and tasks involved. In this chapter, a process along with resources has been presented for addressing each of these areas.

## STUDENT SELF-ASSESSMENT

1. Assess your computer workstation or that of a friend using the evaluation tool from OSHA-Computer Workstation e-tool. (https://www.osha.gov/SLTC/etools/computerworkstations/checklist_evaluation.html). Once you have completed the detailed report, specify how the workstation should be altered to meet OSHA guidelines (see Electronic Resources).
2. Using a diagnosis provided by your facility, perform a home evaluation on your residence, your parents' home, or a relative's home. How should the site be modified to allow the "client" to remain in the home at a maximal level of independence?
3. Specify a ramp for a residence you live in or one nearby. Your work should be specific enough that a contractor could fabricate it without additional questions. You should include the length of ramp, width, height of handrails, and wheelchair rails. If you need "switchback," you should also state the dimensions for the platform that ties the sections together. Use any of the websites listed in the Electronic Resources.
4. Take some time and go into your local community or at your college/university and locate an example to represent each one of the universal design principles. If you have difficulty identifying an example for each principle's problem, solve a concern you have identified in the environment, and see how you could reengineer the space or product to meet the principle.

## ACKNOWLEDGMENTS

Thanks to Betsy DeBrakeleer, COTA/L, ROH; William R. Croninger, MA, OTR/L; and John E. Lane, Jr., OTR/L, for their work on this chapter in the Second Edition.

## ELECTRONIC RESOURCES

AbleData: http://www.abledata.com

North Carolina State University, Center for Universal Design: https://www.ncsu.edu/ncsu/design/cud/

U.S. Department of Justice, Americans with Disabilities Act: http://www.ada.gov/2010ADAstandards_index.htm

U.S. Department of Labor, Occupational Safety & Health Administration: https://www.osha.gov/SLTC/ergonomics/

Washington State Department of Labor and Industries: http://www.lni.wa.gov/safety/SprainsStrains/

## Evidence-Based Research Chart

| Intervention | Keywords | Evidence |
|---|---|---|
| Americans with Disabilities Act (ADA) | Mixed results in the workplace; limited to negative results in employment; unclear expectations on what constitutes appropriate accommodations making it difficult for employment prospects; people with disabilities per student expenditures; interior designers mainly view ADA as legalistic and punitive; preliminary findings suggested improvements in transportation and accessibility of public buildings; ADA yet to reach potential in designing the built environment | Bell & Heitmueller, 2009; Frieden, 2005; Gius, 2005; Karger & Rose, 2010; Sherman & Sherman, 2012; Wells, 2001 |
| Ergonomics, human factors engineering (HFE) | Mixed results of workstation adjustment on effectiveness to prevent musculoskeletal injuries; return to work; cost effectiveness of ergonomics improvements; parents rank repetitive stress injury low on concerns for children using computers at home; interventions; aircraft cockpit design and HFE | Anema et al., 2004; Helander & Burri, 1995; Kimmerly & Odell, 2009; Schmelzer, n.d.; Steffens et al., 2016; van Eerd et al., 2016; van Holland, Soer, de Boer, Reneman, & Brouwer, 2015 |
| Universal design | Changes still exist with education for interior designers and architects as it relates to universal design and its application; rehabilitation professionals advantageous to assist with application of universal design principles in design projects; designing instructional materials for all learners; designing computer interface (email) for seniors; potential role for physiological anthropologists in improving independence of elders; downloadable booklet: principles, history, case studies in universal design | Crews & Zavotka, 2006; Hawthorn, 2003; Lid, 2014; Olgunturk & Demirkan, 2009; Pisha & Coyne, 2001; Story, Mueller, & Mace, 1998 |
| Environmental adaptation | Architecture and technology used to promote improved quality of life for military with traumatic brain injury; positive and negative aspects of adapting homes for children with disabilities; poor housing related to poor health; justifying occupational therapy at home; effectiveness of home adaptation decreases as client limitations increase in elderly adults | Donald, 2009; Mathieson, Kronenfeld, & Keith, 2002; Pasquina, Pasquina, Anderson-Barnes, Giuggio, & Cooper, 2010; Richards, 2003; Roy, Rousseau, Allard, Feldman, & Majnemer, 2008 |

## References


American Occupational Therapy Association. (2014). Occupational therapy practice framework: Domain and process (3rd ed.). *American Journal of Occupational Therapy, 68*(Suppl. 1), S1-S48. doi:10.5014/ajot.2014.682006

Anema, J., Cuelenaere, B., van der Beek, A., Knol, D., de Vet, H., & van Mechelen, W. (2004). The effectiveness of ergonomic interventions on return-to-work after low back pain; a prospective two-year cohort study in six countries on low back pain patients sick-listed for 3-4 months. *Occupational and Environmental Medicine, 61*, 289-294.

Bell, D., & Heitmueller, A. (2009). The Disability Discrimination Act in the UK: Helping or hindering employment among the disabled? *Journal of Health Economics, 28*(2), 465-480.

Bell, J. G., Bishop, C., Gann, M., Gilbert, M. J., Howe, W., Lamb, C. T., & Turner, M. (1995). A systematic approach to health surveillance in the workplace. *Occupational Medicine*, 305-310. doi:10.1093/occmed/45.6305

Canadian Centre for Occupational Health and Safety. (2016). *Hazard control*. Retrieved from http://www.ccohs.ca/oshanswers/hsprograms/hazard_control.html

Crews, D., & Zavotka, S. (2006). Aging, disability, and frailty: Implications for universal design. *Journal of Physiological Anthropology, 25*, 113-118.

Donald, I. (2009). Housing and health care for older people. *Age and Ageing, 38*(4), 364-367.

Frieden, L. (2005). *NCD and the Americans with Disabilities Act: 15 years of progress*. Retrieved from http://www.ncd.gov/newsroom/publications/2005/15yearprogress.htm

Gius, M. (2005). The effect of the American with Disabilities Act on public education expenditures. *Journal of Social Sciences, 1*(3), 162 165.

Hawthorn, D. (2003). *How universal is good design for older users?* Proceedings of the 2003 conference on universal usability, November 1-11, 2003. Vancouver, British Columbia, Canada. doi:10.1145/957205.957213

Helander, M., & Burri, G. (1995). Cost effectiveness of ergonomics and quality improvements in electronics manufacturing. *Journal of Industrial Ergonomics, 15*(2), 137-151.

International Ergonomics Association. (2016). *Definitions and domains of ergonomics*. Retrieved from http://www.iea.cc/whats/index.html

Jacobs, K. (Ed.). (1999). *Ergonomics for therapists* (2nd ed.). Newton, MA: Butterworth Heinemann.

Karger, H., & Rose, S. R. (2010). Revisiting the Americans with Disabilities Act after two decades. *Journal of Social Work in Disability and Rehabilitation, 9*, 73-86. doi:10.1080/1536710X.2010.493468

Kimmerly, L., & Odell, D. (2009). Children and computer use in the home: Workstations, behaviors and parental attitudes. *WORK, 32*(3), 299-310.

Lid, I. (2014). Universal design and disability: An interdisciplinary perspective. *Disability and Rehabilitation, 36*(16), 1344-1349. doi:10.3109/09638288.2014.931472

Mace, R. (1997). *Universal design*. Retrieved from http://www.design.ncsu.edu/cud/univ_design/ud.htm

Mathieson, K., Kronenfeld, J., & Keith, V. (2002). Maintaining functional independence in elderly adults: The roles of health status and financial resources in predicting home modifications and use of mobility equipment. *The Gerontologist, 42*(1), 24-31.

McAtamney, L., & Corlett, E. N. (1993) RULA: A survey method for the investigation of work-related upper limb disorders. *Applied Ergonomics, 24*(2) 91-99.

Olgunturk, N., & Demirkan, H. (2009). Ergonomics and universal design in interior architecture education. *METU Journal of the Faculty of Architecture, 26*(2), 123-138. doi:10.4305/METU.JFA.2009.2.7

Pasquina, P. F., Pasquina, L. F., Anderson-Barnes, V. C., Giuggio, J. S., & Cooper, R. A. (2010). Using architecture and technology to promote improved quality of life for military services members with traumatic brain injury. *Physical Medicine and Rehabilitation Clinics of North America, 21*, 207-220. doi:10.1016/j.pmr.2009.08.001

Pisha, B., & Coyne, P. (2001). Smart from the start: The promise of universal design for learning. *Remedial and Special Education, 22*(4), 197-203.

Richards, S. (2003). *People leave hospital stable, but not necessarily able: We must help them*. Retrieved from http://0-proquest.umi.com.lilac.une.edu:80/pqdweb?did=351348661&sid=14&Fmt=3&clientId=8421&RQT=309&VName=PQD

Roy, L., Rousseau, J., Allard, H., Feldman, D., & Majnemer, A. (2008). Parental experience of home adaptation for children with motor disabilities. *Physical and Occupational Therapy in Pediatrics, 28*(4), 353-368.

Schmelzer, R. (n.d.). *Human interaction with aircraft cockpit displays*. Retrieved from http://www.eas.asu.edu/~humanfac/ringo.html

Sherman, S., & Sherman, J. (2012). Design professionals and the built environment: Encountering boundaries 20 years after the Americans with Disabilties Act. *Disability and Society*, 51-64. doi:10.1080/09687599.2012.631797

Steffens, D., Maher, C. G., Pereira, L. S., Stevens, M. L., Oliveira, V. C., Chapple, M., ... Hancock, M. J. (2016). Prevention of low back pain: A systematic review and meta-analysis. *JAMA Internal Medicine, 176*, 199-208. doi:10.1001/jamainternmed.2015.7431

Story, M., Mueller, J.. & Mace, R. (1998). *The universal design file: Designing for people of all ages and abilities*. Retrieved from http://eric.ed.gov:80/ERICDocs/data/ericdocs2sql/content_storage_01/0000019b/80/19/ac/11.pdf

van Eerd, D. M. (2016). Effectiveness of workplace interventions in the prevention of upper extremity musculoskeletal disorders and symptoms: An update of the evidence. *Occupational Environmental Medicine, 73*, 62-70. doi:10.1136/oemed-2015-102992

van Holland, B. Soer, R., de Boer, M., Reneman, M., & Brouwer, S. (2015). Preventive occupational health interventions in the meat processing industry in upper-middle and high-income countries: A systematic review on their effectiveness. *International Archives of Occupational and Environmental Health, 88*, 389-402.

Watson, D., & Wilson, S. (2003). *Task analysis: An individual and population approach*. Baltimore, MD: AOTA Press.

Wells, S. (2001). *Is the ADA working—Americans with Disabilities Act*. Retrieved from http://findarticles.com/p/articles/mi_m3495/is_4_46/ai_73848278

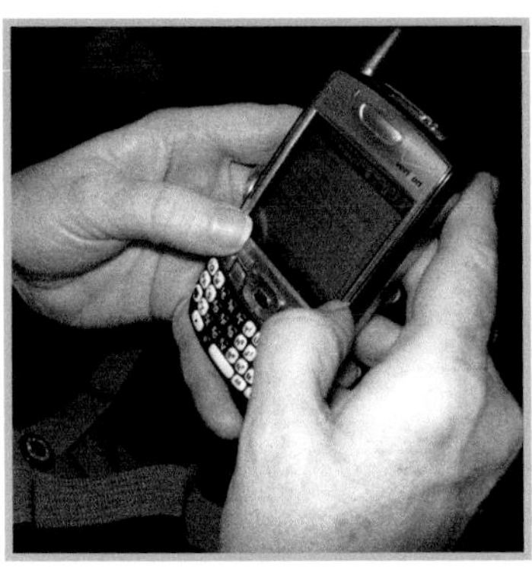

# 32

# Assistive Technology

*Laura Crossley-Marra, MS, OTR/L;*
*Betsy DeBrakeleer, COTA/L, ROH; and William R. Croninger, MA, OTR/L*

## ACOTE Standards Explored in This Chapter

B.5.11

## Key Vocabulary

- **Assistive technology:** Defined by Public Law 100-407, any item, piece of equipment, or product system, whether acquired commercially off the shelf, modified, or customized, that is used to increase, maintain, or improve functional capabilities of individuals with disabilities.
- **Assistive technology service:** Any service that directly assists an individual with a disability in the selection, acquisition, or use of an assistive technology device.
- **High-tech assistive technology:** Items or devices that are expensive, difficult to make, or difficult to find and purchase.
- **Low-tech assistive technology:** Inexpensive items or devices that are simple to make or easy to find and purchase.



Jacobs, K., & MacRae, N. (Eds.).
*Occupational Therapy Essentials for Clinical Competence, Third Edition* (pp. 467-477).

Over the years, assistive technologies have provided essential tools to increase one's independence. As advancements in technology are ever changing, especially in recent years, it is imperative as an occupational therapy practitioner to understand the tools and resources available to clients, to keep up with this fast-paced industry. The 2004 Assistive Technology Act defines assistive technology devices as "any item, piece of equipment, or product system, whether acquired commercially, modified, or customized, that is used to increase, maintain, or improve functional capabilities of individuals with disabilities." Assistive technology devices encompasses a broad spectrum of devices from a simple buttonhook to a complex robotic. Assistive technology service includes "any service that directly assists an individual with a disability in the selection, acquisition, or use of an assistive technology device" (P.L. 108-364.118). The assessment, evaluation, designing, or training individuals in utilizing the assistive technology device are encompassed within assistive technology service (Individuals with Disabilities Education Improvement Act, 2004). Assistive technology service can be delivered by occupational therapy practitioners across practice settings, including acute care, rehabilitation centers, skilled nursing facilities, outpatient facilities, home health agencies, schools, worksites, as well as other community sites. Occupational therapy practitioners provide a unique perspective within the interdisciplinary team to identify, create, and apply assistive technology devices, through understanding clients' individual occupational needs, contexts, and task analysis. When an individual has difficulty or is unable to engage in occupations that are purposeful and meaningful to him or her, assistive technology may provide the means necessary for individuals to complete these occupations, maximizing one's functional independence (AOTA, 2004).

Assistive technology can be classified as low tech or high tech. Low tech is defined as devices that are inexpensive, simplistic, and easily obtained (Cook & Hussey, 1995, p. 7). Examples of low-tech devices include pencil grips, built-up handles, long-handled sponges, and dressing sticks. High-tech devices are more complex and expensive. High-tech devices include robotics, augmented speaking devices, and power wheelchairs. Through technological advances, devices can fluctuate between low-tech and high-tech devices. The first step in determining the appropriate assistive technology device is the evaluation process.

## Evaluation

The American Occupational Therapy Association (AOTA) *Occupational Therapy Practice Framework* (2014) delineates the evaluation process through a thorough analysis of an occupational profile and an analysis of occupational performance. During this process, activity and occupational demands should be examined. Common activities, such as those found in activities of daily living (ADLs), will likely be familiar to the practitioner. Activities that are unfamiliar, such as those found in school, work, or leisure, require additional consultation. In work settings, a job description is helpful, and team members, coworkers, and supervisors may also be able to deepen the practitioner's understanding of the demands and skills necessary. Coworkers or peers who might be affected by the device also need to be considered. To be successful, the practitioner needs a firm grasp of all of the activity components.

Simultaneously, the practitioner should gather information for an occupational profile to identify meaningful activities, impressions of their roles, demands, and skills required to engage in these activities. At this time, it is also appropriate to work with the client to understand performance patterns. What are the habits and routines historically used by the client? Were they successful in the past? What parts of the routine or habit does the client value and seek to maintain? Finally, what limitations does the client place on the nature of any intervention or tool?

The practitioner then assesses the skills required by the activity through completing a comprehensive assessment utilizing valid and reliable formal, nonformal, standardized, and nonstandardized assessments (AOTA, 2014). When a client's performance skills and contextual factors of the activity do not match, and cannot be altered by environmental or process changes, assistive technology devices may be appropriate.

## Assistive Devices

There are a variety of methods for classifying assistive technologies. Angelo (1997) looked at mobility, methods of access, switch types, and the level of technology. Mann and Lane (1991) presented a system that sorts devices by disability: physical, sensory, speech, and cognition. Cook and Hussey (1995) arranged their work by activity area: communication, mobility, sensation, manipulation, and control. All of these ordering systems would seem to be appropriate. A look at assistive technology using a combination of the preceding classification systems follows.

## Occupational Therapy's Role in Assistive Technology Provision

Mann and Lane (1991) noted that the occupational therapy practitioners may work independently in some situations, as when training a client to use a sock aid after a total hip arthroplasty. When the complexity of

**Case Study**

We met Maryanne when she was in her mid-70s. Despite severe arthritis, she had continued to live independently in her own home after the death of her husband. Maryanne had been referred for occupational therapy after replacement of the metacarpophalangeal joints of her left hand. During therapy, she related that she was experiencing significant issues centered on ADLs and home management. Permission for a home evaluation was obtained from her attending physician.

Maryanne escorted us through her home, pointing out problem areas and detailing strategies she had used with various degrees of success. In coming up with a set of possible interventions, we paid attention to her impressions of the task demands, the contexts in which the tasks took place, and her habits and routines. We tried each task to get a feel of the performance skills required. Our understanding of her "space" was then compared with the formal assessments we had on her range of motion, strength, endurance, and information from the physician relative to the expected progress of both her therapy and the disease.

We then met again with Maryanne to present our list of solutions and to get her feedback on her willingness to accept changes to habit and routine. Financial considerations related to the final choice of assistive devices were also discussed. One major issue was that her limited range of motion made opening doors with traditional knobs almost impossible. We selected a commercially available device that clamps over the doorknob and features a lever she could easily use. A second issue related to controlling the faucets in her kitchen. Replacing the controls was not a financial option. However, she was able to use the controls when we attached wooden clothespins to them. These adaptations allowed her to use her closed fist to turn the water on and off. The pins initially slid off the controls quickly, but this was rectified by a small bolt with a nut running through the open portion of the pin.

A final problem of great aggravation to her was her inability to open the windows in her living area on hot days. She was able to close windows with her fists but could not grasp the window hardware to open it. Maryanne had shown us, with great pride, how she used a back scratcher to remove her winter coat. Because she always left her windows open a small amount, we devised a plan where we attached small blocks to each of the windowsills. We then fabricated a slightly stronger "scratcher" that allowed her to use the block as a fulcrum to lever the windows up on warm days. She now had a combination scratcher–lever. A few weeks later, she demonstrated, with great pride, how she could also use the device to open her refrigerator by inserting it into the door handle and pushing against it with her chest.

All tools were decidedly "low-tech" interventions, and only the door handles entailed any cost for Maryanne. She took a considerable amount of pride in helping "her" practitioners. One unintended consequence was that she also became one of the strongest advocates in our community for occupational therapy.

the task(s) requires a team approach, they argued that the occupational therapy practitioner is the individual best prepared to act as its leader.

Angelo (1997) stated that the occupational therapy practitioner frequently serves as the "interface specialist" (p. 8). In this role, the responsibility of the occupational therapist is to assess the client's performance skills and client factors to determine the body part or motion over which the client demonstrates the greatest and most consistent control. Working with other team members, the specific method of access, the switch, and its mounting location can then be selected.

All authors are in agreement that one primary role for the occupational therapy practitioner and other team members is in positioning and seating. Effective, consistent control will not be possible until the client is positioned correctly.

## Augmenting or Adding Mobility

Problems with mobility have a wide variety of potential causes, which may include problems with balance, muscle strength, joint range, control, or sensation. Finally, a limb may not be present in whole or part.

- **Low-tech examples:** Canes, walkers, crutches, lower extremity orthoses, manual wheelchairs. Low-tech mobility devices such as canes, walkers, and crutches are commonly prescribed by the physical therapist, who performs the initial selection, set-up, and training. Thereafter, all team members frequently work to improve a client's functional mobility as during ADLs.
  - ◊ Lower extremity orthoses: Lower extremity orthoses can take many forms and can affect the body at the ankle, knee, hip, or any combination of these. They are frequently used to stabilize the lower extremity, correct deformity, or slow the progression of deformity. In addition to stability functions, they are used to assist in mobility by correcting problems in gait. They are generally fabricated and fitted by an orthotist.

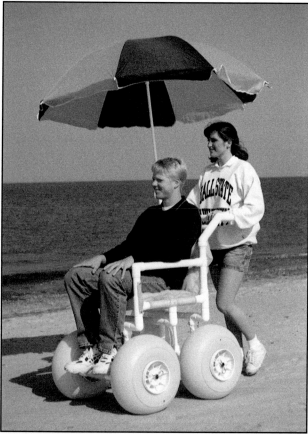


**Figure 32-1.** All-terrain chair. (Reprinted with permission from Assistive Technology, Inc.)

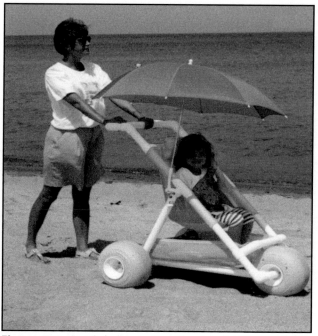

**Figure 32-2.** Beach baby stroller. (Reprinted with permission from Assistive Technology, Inc.)

- ◊ Manual wheelchairs: These are generally coprescribed by attending physical and occupational therapy practitioners.

- **High-tech examples:** Power wheelchairs, personal mobility devices, lower extremity prostheses, robotic and exoskeleton walkers.
  - ◊ Power wheelchairs: These items change dramatically every year. The practitioner should know the products and have a good working relationships with equipment vendors to ensure that the client receives the most appropriate equipment.
  - ◊ Personal mobility devices: A wide range of devices fall into this category (Figures 32-1 and 32-2), from three-wheeled scooters to electric carts to high-tech two-wheeled devices such as the Segway personal transportation device.
  - ◊ Lower extremity prostheses: Although a lower extremity orthosis is used to augment an existing body part, the prosthesis functions to replace a missing body part (Bodeau, 2002). Assessment and prescription require the interprofessional team to look at a diverse set of criteria that includes the cognitive status, function, environment in which the device will be used, client goals, client financial situation, and the level of amputation.
  - ◊ Robotic walker: The robotic walker is a hybrid system under development that adds global positioning, obstacle avoidance, and speech recognition to a rolling walker. Researchers envision this device as a means to allow individuals with cognitive and balance deficits to ambulate more safely.
  - ◊ Exoskeleton walker: Considerable research is being conducted in this area. Unlike the robot walker, the exoskeleton attaches to or is donned by the user. Current devices are aimed at augmenting or enhancing an individual's ability to walk or carry heavy loads over a variety of terrain types.

## Assistive Technology for Upper Extremity Augmentation

The upper extremities are frequently affected by a number of conditions, both congenital and acquired. This classification looks at assistive technology for situations requiring the augmentation or extension of gross motor upper extremity functions including range of motion, strength, sensation, and control.

- **Low-tech devices:** Dressing sticks, reachers, long-handled shoe horns, long-handled bath sponges, sock aids, button hooks, nosey cups, lipped plates, plate guards, built-up utensils, card holders, mouth sticks, pointing devices, and static splints (Figures 32-3 through 32-6).

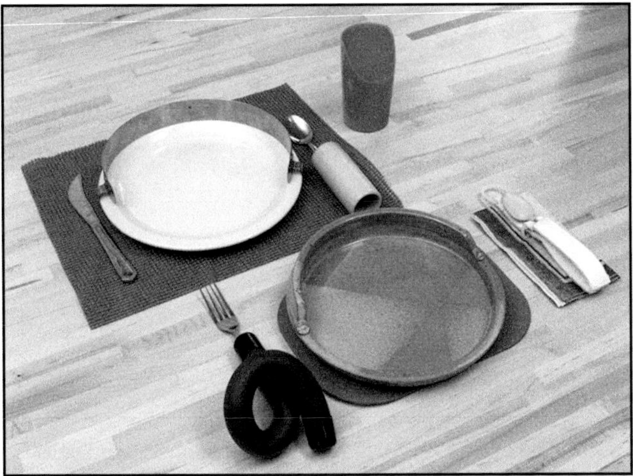

**Figure 32-3.** Low-tech assists for eating. (Reprinted with permission from William R. Croninger.)

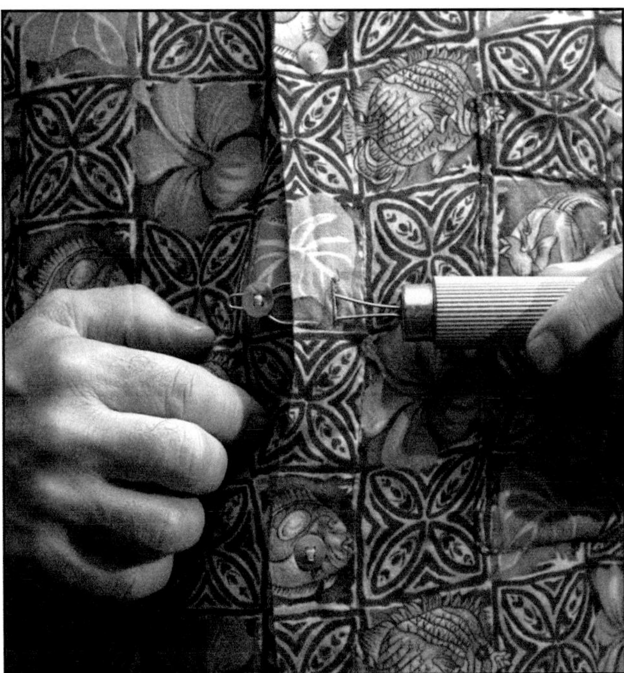

**Figure 32-4.** Low-tech assist for buttoning. (Reprinted with permission from William R. Croninger.)

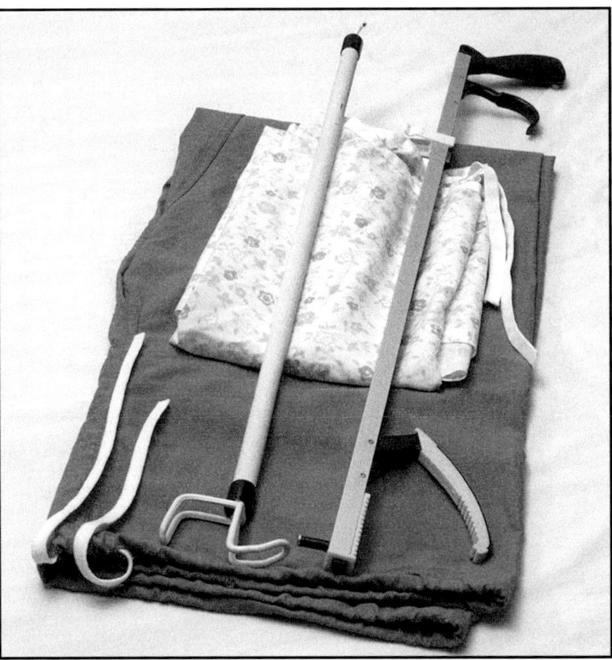

**Figure 32-5.** Low-tech dressing assists. (Reprinted with permission from William R. Croninger.)

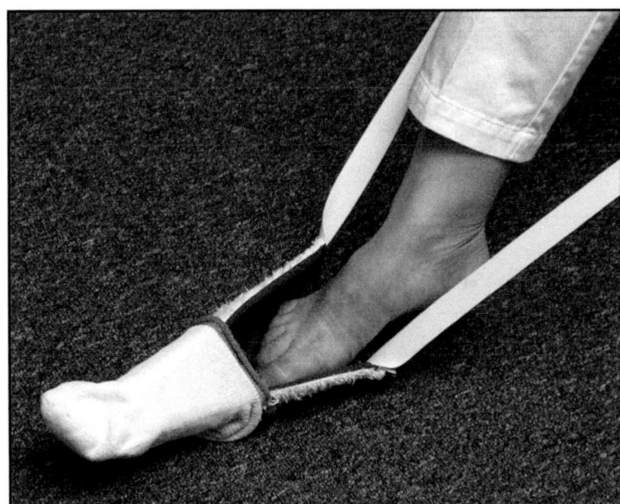

**Figure 32-6.** Low-tech assist for sock donning. (Reprinted with permission from William R. Croninger.)

- **High-tech devices:** Environmental controls, upper extremity prosthetic, robotics, and dynamic splints.

## Assistive Technology for Fine Motor Augmentation

Most of the devices discussed in this chapter allow a user to approach or participate in a task. The fine motor assistive technology is commonly some type of switch. It is critically important because it is the point of interface between user and device. AbleData is again an excellent resource to begin to understand the large variety and types of switches available. Most critical is that the switch be accessible and appropriate for the client. Because it is the most heavily used portion of the intervention, it is also the most common point of failure. Practitioners should always consider the effect of switch failure, both on the client's ability to access the device and on the effect on client safety if a switch fails while the device is being used. The following are two types of switches:

- **Latched:** Latched switches turn a device on or off. After being activated, the device stays in that mode until the switch is reactivated. Examples include light switches, on/off knobs on appliances, and tools that require two-handed operation (Figures 32-7 and 32-8).

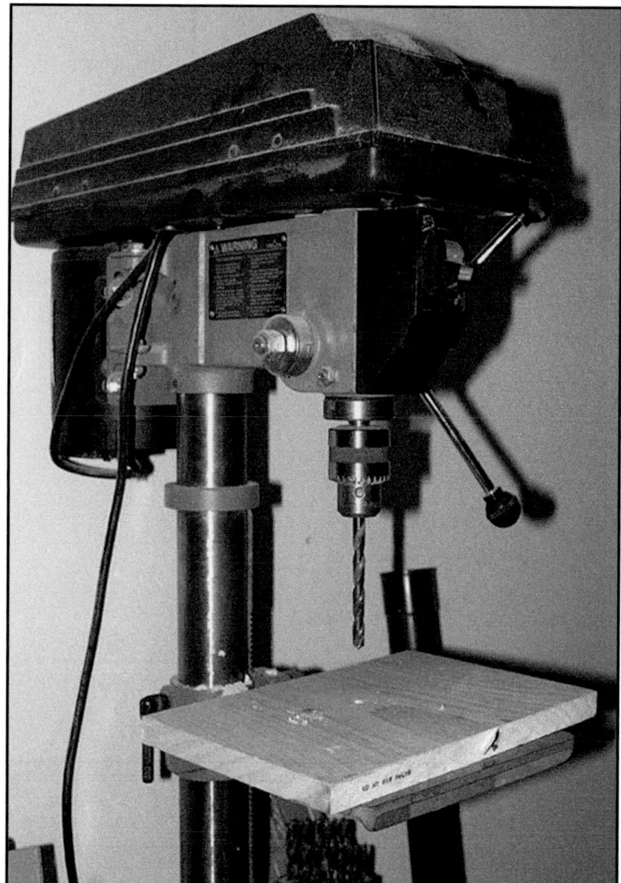

Figure 32-7. Example of tool with a latched switch. (Reprinted with permission from William R. Croninger.)

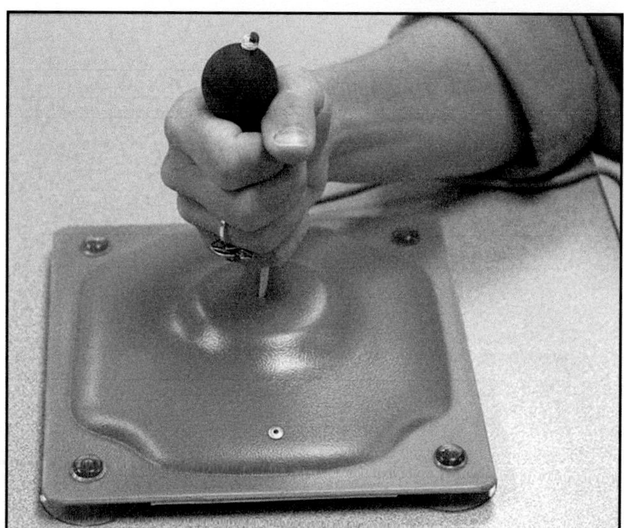

Figure 32-8. Example of a latched switch. (Reprinted with permission from William R. Croninger.)

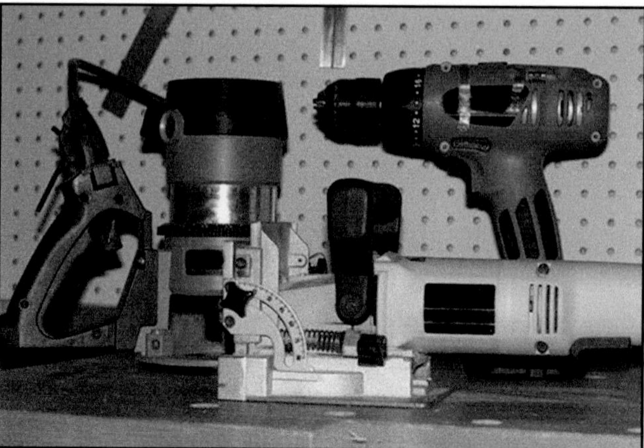

Figure 32-9. Tools with momentary switches. (Reprinted with permission from William R. Croninger.)

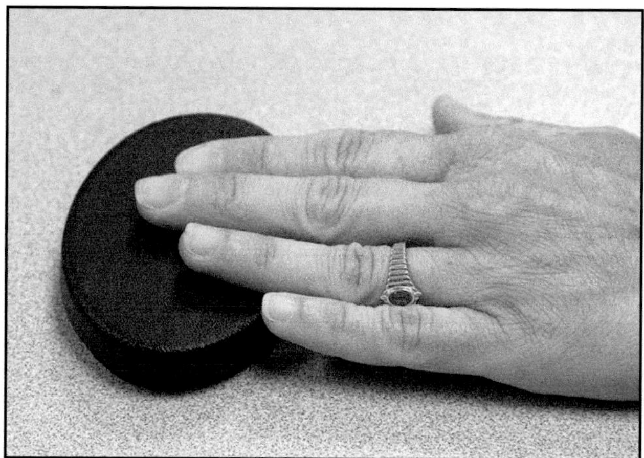

Figure 32-10. Example of a momentary switch. (Reprinted with permission from William R. Croninger.)

- **Momentary:** Momentary switches require constant input or attention to operate. Examples include automobile accelerators and the "triggers" on tools that require fine adjustments while operating (Figures 32-9 and 32-10).

## Assistive Technology for Sensory Augmentation

This assistive technology area is generally thought of as including deficits in vision and hearing. To this, however, should be added technology for individuals who experience altered sensation, whether it is the epicritic or protopathic (informational vs. safety) pathway.

## Hearing

- **Environmental adaptations:** Include modifications to environment to reduce background noise and "auditory clutter."
  - ◊ Low-tech examples: These include sound-deadening materials, amplification, or choice or positioning of furniture. These also include modifications speakers make, such as not standing in front of bright light sources and trimming of mustaches or beards to allow a listener who lip reads a clear view of the speaker's lips.
  - ◊ High-tech examples: In some situations, selective amplification, as in assisted listening devices, is more appropriate. The assisted listening devices involve a microphone (speaker), transmitter, receiver, and earphone (listener) system that allows an individual with diminished hearing to adjust the sound levels produced at the earphones. In this way, an audience can be made up of those who do and do not need amplification.
- **Hearing aids (generally all high tech):** Falling into this category are devices that alert or augment hearing. Buzzers, strobes, flashing lights, and vibratory devices can signal an individual that he or she needs to attend to some event or situation. Hearing aids are classified by the National Institute of Health (National Institute on Deafness and Other Communications Disorders, 2002) using a number of categories:
  - ◊ By style: An in-the-ear hearing aid fits into the outer ear; a behind-the-ear hearing aid is located behind the ear with the earpiece located within the canal; canal aids fit completely within the ear canal; body aids are large devices carried external to the ear and located on the wearer's clothing.
  - ◊ By circuitry: The analog adjustable type is built for a specific client to augment a specific level of hearing loss. The analog programmable type is fabricated to an individual's specific needs—the user can often select a variety of settings depending on the environment he or she is in. The digital programmable type contains a microchip that increases the ability of the device to adjust to the acoustics of varying environments.
- **Cochlear implants:** This assistive technology involves implantation of a device implanted behind the ear. The device bypasses damaged or nonfunctioning parts of the user's ear, sending information directly to the brain.

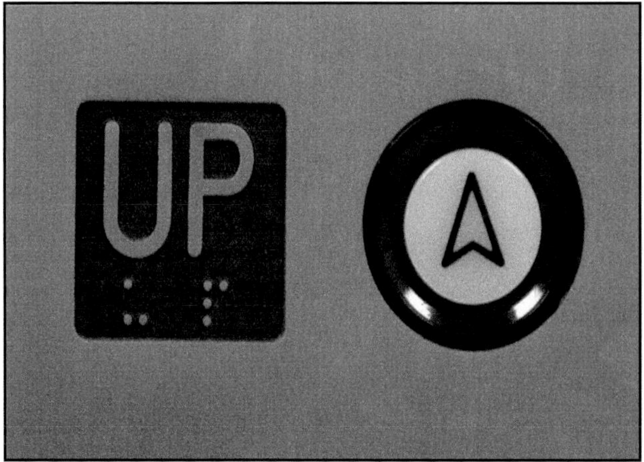


**Figure 32-11.** Low-tech vision assists. (Reprinted with permission from William R. Croninger.)

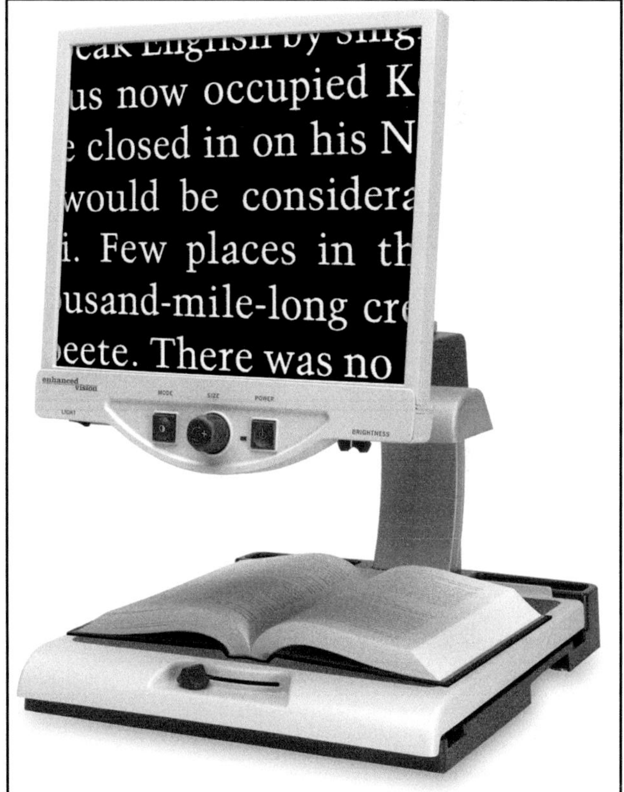


**Figure 32-12.** Merlin: LCD. (Reprinted with permission from Enhanced Vision.)

## Vision

- **Low-tech examples:** Glasses, a magnifying glass, large print, large fonts, alterations to light levels, contrast enhancement, reduction of glare, books and signage in Braille, walking cane (Figure 32-11).
- **High-tech examples:** Scanning or large display device, character enhancement via computer, Braille talkers or typers, digital e-books, tablet computers (Figure 32-12).

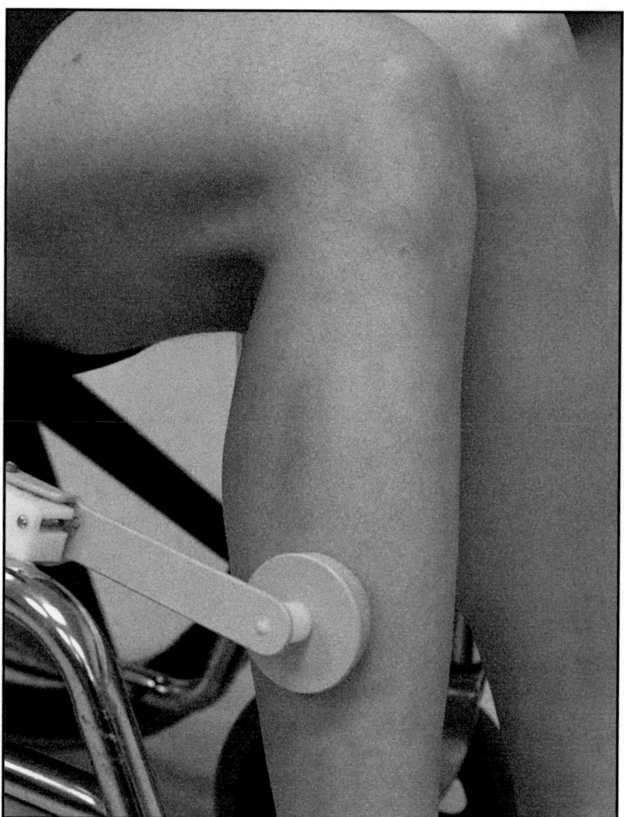

**Figure 32-13.** Locate the switch where the user has the greatest amount of control. (Reprinted with permission from William R. Croninger.)

- ◊ Scanning or large display devices: A large number of devices allow a user to scan print on a page and display it on a screen in real time.
- ◊ Character enhancement: Adds a computer that can enlarge fonts or "speak" words on a page.
- ◊ Braille talkers or typers: Braille typers use a scanner that is moved over a printed page. The device converts the text input to Braille and raises the correct pins under the reader's fingers. Another strategy again uses a scanner to convert text to Braille, but the output is in Braille via a specialized printer.

## Touch

Altered sensation, particularly tactile and pain, has the potential to impose a significant affect on a client's life and well-being. Because the hands are the most common means by which we interact with our environment, loss of tactile sensation makes it more difficult to choose effective assistive technology for other existing conditions. Practitioners need to remember that switches need not always be activated by hand. The key is that the switch be positioned where motor ability allows consistent and accurate access (Figure 32-13).

Loss of sensation in the protopathic pathways (sharp–dull and hot–cold) brings a safety issue into the equation. Clients may not recognize they have come into contact with an object that is sharp or sufficiently cold or hot enough to cause tissue damage. Individuals with decreased peripheral sensation, such as is found after trauma or with diabetes, may not recognize that their fingers, toes, or a complete limb is too cold or hot.

The first strategy could be deemed to be "no tech," in that clients should be trained to attend visually to affected body parts. When the body part cannot be readily visualized, it can often be viewed using a hand mirror or mirror fitted with a universal cuff. Clients should always use thermometers when extremes of temperature may be encountered.

# Assistive Technology for Communications Augmentation

A wide variety of conditions can lead to a decreased ability to communicate. Problems may be congenital, as in a child with dysarthria acquired after a cerebrovascular accident, or progressive, as seen in amyotrophic lateral sclerosis. Strategies involve a wide range of low- and high-tech interventions.

- **No-tech examples:** Gestures, grimaces, "mouthing," eye gaze.
- **Low-tech examples:** Paper and pencil, picture boards, symbol boards, touch talkers, and speech recognition software. Speech recognition and touch talkers were originally considered high-tech interventions. However, both have now become much more commonly available to the general public.
- **High-tech examples:** Tablet computers now have downloadable apps that are used as assistive technology. Some examples, such as the Smarty Ears app, assist in teaching pronunciation skills, articulation, stuttering, and language skills. There are also apps that provide icons, phrases, and videos to assist or supplement speech (Lingraphica). Dedicated software and computer systems use variable strategies for word selection or prediction. Mann and Lane (1991) grouped electronic communication devices into three types by method of access, each with its own advantages and drawbacks.
    - ◊ Direct: Here, the user touches or uses a form of fine motor augmentation to select the response from among a group. The fine motor augmentation could be a mouth stick or one of the many head-mounted electronic pointers that use lasers, infrared, or radio waves.

> **Paying for Assistive Technology**
>
> Technology can be expensive, especially high-tech items. Devices can be paid for out-of-pocket by the consumer; by private health insurances; or by public resources such as Medicare, Medicaid, vocational rehabilitation, and education. Most health insurance companies have a cap, or a limit, to how much they will pay for assistive technology. This makes it imperative that the occupational therapy practitioner do a careful and thoughtful assessment of the client's needs and make only necessary recommendations and document proof of need or medical necessity. Proof of medical necessity often requires a physician's prescription for the assistive technology. Other options for funding include low-interest loans designed specifically for assistive technology and modifications, such as the MPower loan, provided by the state of Maine. Most states have a similar program.
>
> The Assistive Technology Act funds a statewide assistive technology program in each of the 50 states and six territories, and the majority of these programs support assistive technology device reuse or recycle activities. The following website will direct you to those programs: http://www.resnaprojects.org/allcontacts/statewidecontacts.html
>
> Programs such as ALLTECH (http://www.alltech-tsi.org/) and Alpha One (http://alphaonenow.org/classifed_ads.htm) in Maine have online lists of assistive technology, adaptive equipment, and durable medical equipment. Get AT Stuff (http://alphaonenow.org/classifed_ads.htm) is an assistive technology exchange that covers the New England states.
>
> Other options for gently used assistive technology include online resources such as craigslist.com and Uncle Henry's. These types of sites often do not list assistive technology and adaptive equipment as such, but you can search for specific items or look in the "Senior Selections" area for items such as wheelchairs and other devices. An Internet search will produce many links to online options.
>
> There are also local non-online community resources. The Lions Clubs, Kiwanis Clubs, Easter Seals, and local churches are just a few examples.

- Scanning: In this strategy, the device moves through the available choices in a prearranged pattern at a preset pace. When the desired choice is available, often signaled by a light-emitting diode near the choice, the user responds. This method requires less user action but is slower than direct selection.
- Encoding: Symbols, numbers, colors, or letters are used for the desired words or phrases. This requires the least action on the part of the client in exchange for the client learning a new system of symbolizing.

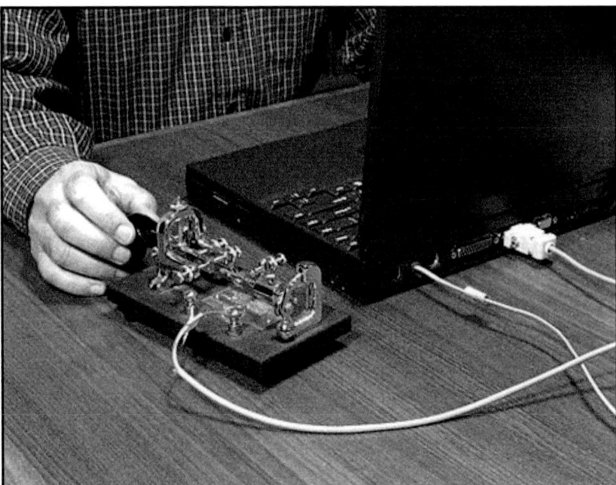

**Figure 32-14.** Example of a Morse code keyer (N7RZ). (Reprinted with permission from Les Kerr.)

## Occupational Therapy Assistant in Assistive Technology

The occupational therapy assistant may work with an occupational therapist in the provision of services in assistive technology provision. The Accreditation Council for Occupational Therapy Education Standard, however, makes it clear that the occupational therapy assistant may also work independently to modify, adapt, and teach after service competency has been demonstrated. Service competency is a method by which both the occupational therapy assistant and the occupational therapist determine that the clinical skills of each are appropriate and by which the occupational therapist verifies the occupational therapy assistant is functioning to the ethical, safety, and practice standards of the profession. This is most often achieved by regularly coassessing and cotreating clients, comparing results and treatment methodologies.

## Morse Code

Morse code is an example of an encoding strategy. In this system, combinations of short and long tones stand for letters, numbers, and abbreviations. With modern equipment, very small hand movements are needed to generate the tonal sequences, which could then be displayed on a computer screen as letters. The computer would add the ability to have a short letter combination, such as "az," stand for an entire phrase just as in when a word processor is used to create a "macro" (Figure 32-14).

## Evidence-Based Research Chart

| Intervention | Keywords | Evidence |
|---|---|---|
| Pediatric | Improve writing, verbal communication | Lancioni et al., 2007; Mihailidis, Tam, McLean, & Lee, 2005; Watson, Ito, Smith, & Andersen, 2010 |
| | Caregiver reasons for use versus non-use (mobility, augmentative communications) | Benedict, Lee, Marrujo, & Farel, 1999 |
| Cognitive | Memory loss, conversation skills | Bourgeois & Mason, 1996; Van Hulle & Hux, 2006 |
| Functional mobility, communication, ADLs | Improved independence | Dahlin Ivanoff & Sonn, 2005; Eriksrud & Bohannon, 2005; Hoenig, Taylor, & Sloan, 2003; Nordenskiöld, 1997; Uustal & Minkel, 2004 |
| | Reasons for use versus non-use | Agree & Freedman, 2003; Arthanat, Nochajski, Lenker, Bauer, & Wu, 2009; Sonn, 1996 |

## Summary

Assistive technology, whether it is a low-tech reacher or high-tech communication device, has the potential to greatly enhance the ability of occupational therapy clients to engage in occupations. Careful use of the *Framework* (AOTA, 2014) greatly enhances the potential interventions that use these technologies will increase clients' independence. The practitioner, however, should pay particular attention to the sources cited in the Evidence-Based Research Chart, which documents why and when assistive technology interventions have not been successful. It is not enough to provide assistive technology devices for our clients. Practitioners must be certain that what is provided is the proper tool, adequate training has been completed, and that there is ongoing support after discontinuation of services is provided.

## Student Self-Assessment

1. Write a definition of assistive technology you could use to explain an assistive technology intervention to the partner of a client.
2. Review Maryanne's story. What other assistive technologies could have been used to assist her in her dressing, cooking, and home management activities?
3. Pick one of your instructors and imagine he or she has lost the use of his or her right upper extremity. Analyze the tasks required by his or her environment and roles. What assistive technology interventions might assist him or her in maintaining his or her occupations? How would you assist him or her with assistive technology if the problem were decreased memory? Decreased mobility?

## Electronic Resources

AbleData, sponsored by the U.S. Department of Education: http://www.abledata.com

American Foundation for the Blind: http://www.afb.org/Section.asp?SectionID=3&TopicID=135&DocumentID=2424

American Speech-Language-Hearing Association: www.asha.org

Communication Disorders (NIDCD)—Cochlear implants: http://www.nidcd.nih.gov/health/hearing/coch.asp

Gallaudet University: http://www.gallaudet.edu

Hearing Loss Association of America: http://www.shhh.org

International Society for Augmentative and Alternate Communication: https://www.isaac-online.org/english/home/

Job Accommodation Network: http://www.jan.wvu.edu

National Institute on Deafness and Other Communication Disorders (NIDCD)—Hearing aids: http://www.nidcd.nih.gov/health/hearing/hearingaid.asp

Rehabilitation Engineering and Assistive Technology Society of North America: http://www.resna.org/

## References

Agree, E., & Freedman, V. (2003). A comparison of assistive technology and personal care in alleviating disability and unmet need. *The Gerontologist, 43*(3), 142-151.

American Occupational Therapy Association. (2004). Assistive technology within occupational therapy practice. *American Journal of Occupational Therapy, 58*, 678-680.

American Occupational Therapy Association. (2014). Occupational therapy practice framework: Domain and process (3rd ed.). *American Journal of Occupational Therapy, 68*(Suppl. 1), S1-S48. doi:10.5014/ajot.2014.682006

Angelo, J. (1997). *Assistive technology for rehabilitation therapies*. Philadelphia, PA: F. A. Davis Company.

Arthanat, S., Nochajski, S. M., Lenker, J. A., Bauer, S. B., & Wu, Y. W. B. (2009). Measuring usability of assistive technology from a multicontextual perspective: The case of power wheelchairs. *American Journal of Occupational Therapy, 63*, 751-764.

Assistive Technology Act of 2004. Pub. L. 108–364.

Benedict, R. E., Lee, J. P., Marrujo, S. K., & Farel, A. M. (1999). Assistive devices as an early childhood intervention: Evaluating outcomes. *Technology and Disability, 11*(1/2), 79-90.

Bodeau, V. (2002). Lower limb prosthetics. *EMedicine from WebMD*. Retrieved from http://www.emedicine.com/pmr/topic175.htm

Bourgeois, M., & Mason, L. A. (1996). Memory wallet intervention in an adult day-care setting. *Behavioral Interventions: Theory and Practice in Residential and Community-Based Clinical Programs, 11*(1), 3-18.

Cook, A. M., & Hussey, S. (1995). *Assistive technologies: Principles and practice*. St. Louis, MO: Mosby.

Dahlin Ivanoff, S., & Sonn, U. (2005). Assistive devices in activities of daily living used by persons with age-related macular degeneration: A population study of 85-year-olds living at home. *Scandinavian Journal of Occupational Therapy, 12*(1), 10-17.

Eriksrud, O., & Bohannon, R. (2005). Effectiveness of the easy-up handle in acute rehabilitation. *Clinical Rehabilitation, 19*(4), 381-386.

Individuals with Disabilities Education Improvement Act of 2004, Pub. L. 108–446, 20 U.S.C. § 1400 et seq.

Hoenig, H., Taylor, D. H., Jr., & Sloan, F. A. (2003). Does assistive technology substitute for personal assistance among the disabled elderly? *American Journal of Public Health, 93*(2), 330-337.

Lancioni, G. E., Singh, N. N., O'Reilly, M. F., Sigafoos, J., Olivia, D., & Baccani, S. (2007). Enabling students with multiple disabilities to request and choose among environmental stimuli through microswitch and computer technology. *Research in Developmental Disabilities: A Multidisciplinary Journal, 28*(1), 50-58.

Mann, W. C., & Lane, J. P. (1991). *Assistive technology for persons with disabilities: The role of occupational therapy*. Bethesda, MD: AOTA Press.

Mihailidis, A., Tam, T., McLean, M. & Lee, T. (2005). An intelligent health monitoring and emergency response system. In S. Giroux & H. Pigot (Eds.), *From smart homes to smart care* (pp. 272-281). Amsterdam, The Netherlands: IOSPress.

National Institute on Deafness and Other Communications Disorders. (2002). *Hearing aids*. Retrieved from http://www.nidcd.nih.gov/health/hearing/hearingaid.asp

Nordenskiöld, U. (1997). Daily activities in women with rheumatoid arthritis. Aspects of patient education, assistive devices and methods for disability and impairment assessment. *Scandinavian Journal of Rehabilitation Medicine Supplement, 37*, 1-72.

Sonn, U. (1996). Longitudinal studies of dependence in daily life activities among elderly persons. *Scandinavian Journal of Rehabilitation Medicine Supplement, 34*, 1-35.

Uustal, H., & Minkel, J. (2004). Study of the Independence IBOT 3000 Mobility System: An innovative power mobility device, during use in community environments. *Archives of Physical Medicine and Rehabilitation, 85*(12), 2002-2010.

Van Hulle, A., & Hux, K. (2006). Improvement patterns among survivors of brain injury: Three case examples documenting the effectiveness of memory compensation strategies. *Brain Injury, 20*(1), 101-109.

Watson, H. A., Ito, M., Smith, O. R., & Andersen, T. L. (2010). Effect of assistive technology in a public school setting. *American Journal of Occupational Therapy, 64*(1), 18-29.

## Suggested Readings

Bellis, M. (n.d.). *Martin Cooper—History of cell phone: Martin Cooper talks about the first cell phone call*. Retrieved from http://inventors.about.com/cs/inventorsalphabet/a/martin_cooper.htm

Office of the Federal Register, National Archives and Records Service, General Services Administration. (2000). Electronic and information technology accessibility standards. *The Federal Register, 65*(246), 80499-80528.

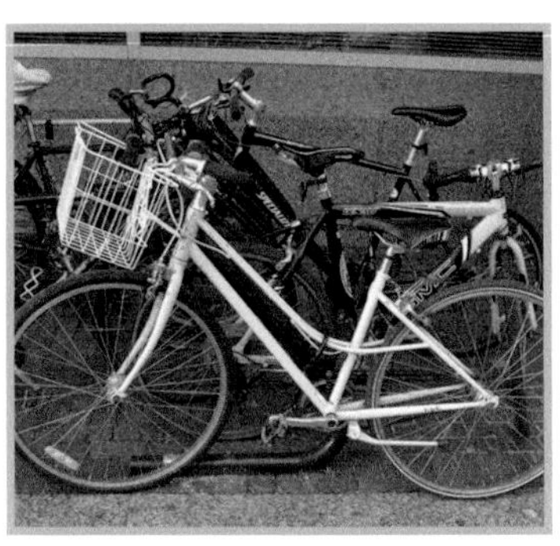

# 33

# Occupation-Centered Functional and Community Mobility

Scott D. McNeil, OTD, MS, OTR/L and Kathryn M. Loukas, OTD, MS, OTR/L, FAOTA

**ACOTE STANDARDS EXPLORED IN THIS CHAPTER**

B.5.12, B.5.13

**KEY VOCABULARY**

- **Bed mobility:** Safely and effectively moving in bed for comfort, skin integrity, and function.
- **Body mechanics:** The utilization of appropriate muscles and positions to complete heavy work safely and efficiently (Brookside Associates, 2007).
- **Community mobility:** Engaging in mobility resulting in successful participation in the community (American Occupational Therapy Association [AOTA], 2014a).
- **Driver recommendations:** The process of making suggestions regarding the safe and efficient ability to engage in the occupation of driving.
- **Driver rehabilitation:** A specialized form of therapy that focuses on evaluation and intervention in the occupation of driving a vehicle.
- **Functional mobility:** "Moving from one position to another during performance of every day activities" (AOTA, 2014a, p. S19).
- **Mobility device care:** The use and care of ambulatory devices to participate in everyday occupations.
- **Positioning and seating systems:** Selection and utilization of a comfortable, supportive wheelchair or chair seat that encourages symmetry, skin integrity, and occupational performance.

*(continued)*



Jacobs, K., & MacRae, N. (Eds.).
*Occupational Therapy Essentials for Clinical Competence, Third Edition* (pp. 479-499).

KEY VOCABULARY (CONTINUED)

- **Transfers:** A specific process of moving effectively from one surface to another to participate in life activities.
- **Wheelchair management:** Selection, utilization, and functional mobility of a wheelchair.
- **Wheelchair selection and accessories:** A client-centered process that generates a product to maximize health and functional independence in wheeled mobility.

Occupational engagement and participation in activities of life require people to move about their environment. Social participation is greatly enhanced when people can freely travel with purpose in their homes, communities, and gathering places. *Functional mobility intervention* is the term occupational therapy practitioners most often use to describe the therapeutic tenets of bringing a client from bed mobility through transfers and finally to community mobility and driving. Safe and effective participation in occupational performance is the goal of such intervention. Functional mobility is defined in the *Occupational Therapy Practice Framework* (American Occupational Therapy Association [AOTA], 2014a) as "Moving from one position or place to another (during performance of everyday activities), such as in-bed mobility, wheelchair mobility, and transfers (e.g., wheelchair, bed, car, shower, tub, toilet, chair, floor). Includes functional ambulation and transportation of objects" (p. S19). It is usually an interprofessional intervention because the occupational therapy practitioner must work closely with the physical therapist, who addresses gait training and functional ambulation, as well as physicians and durable medical equipment vendors involved in wheeled mobility. The occupational therapy practitioner must be fully informed of important factors involved in functional mobility through evaluation of overall important client factors including strength, range of motion, balance, coordination, cognitive processing, perceptual understanding, and visual skills (Bolding, Adler, Tipton-Burton, & Verran, 2013).

Pierce (2002) proposed a basic hierarchy of mobility to address the order in which these skills should be addressed. This adapted pyramid forms the stability, positioning, and mobility necessary to participate in meaningful occupations. The pyramid of skills goes from the foundation or base and moves to the top (Figure 33-1).

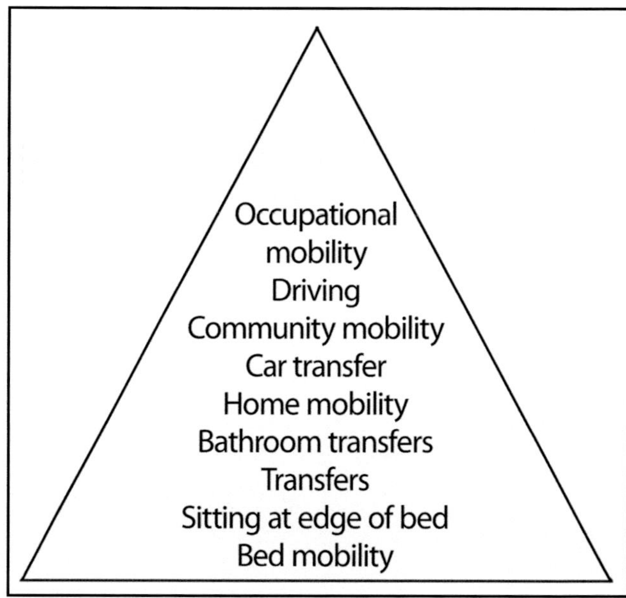


**Figure 33-1.** The occupation-based mobility pyramid. (Adapted from Pierce, S. [2002]. Restoring competence in mobility. In C. A. Trombly & M. V. Radomski [Eds.], *Occupational therapy for physical dysfunction* [5th ed., p. 667]. Philadelphia, PA: Lippincott Williams and Wilkins.)

The occupational therapy practitioner must keep in mind that every client is unique in his or her abilities and approach to mobility in occupation. Prerequisites to functional mobility training include critical thinking of the occupational therapy practitioner regarding client factors and performance patterns, including primary and secondary medical conditions, age, medications, family unit, and lifestyle, and how these factors might affect the client's functioning now and in the future (AOTA, 2014a). Context and environmental opportunities and obstacles are also important to incorporate and adapt if necessary. It is imperative that occupational therapy practitioners learn and use proper body mechanics to safely move, position, and transfer clients.

Functional mobility and community mobility skills must be included in academic programs for both the occupational therapist and occupational therapy assistant (AOTA, 2015). The evaluation of these areas is directed by the occupational therapist, yet the provision of intervention for these occupations may be provided by any occupational therapy practitioner if in accordance with local state regulations (AOTA, 2014b). With this in mind, the following content in this chapter is essential for both levels of occupational therapy practitioner.

## Basic Principles of Body Mechanics

Use of proper body mechanics is essential for the safety of both the occupational therapy practitioner and the client. Alnaser (2007) found in a literature review that patient handling was the most common occupational factor involved in work-based injuries. In addition, occupational therapy practitioners may teach caretakers or instruct clients to facilitate the proper body mechanics of handling and lifting in the home or community.

Principles and techniques to use during handling or lifting include the following (Bolding et al., 2013; Brookside Associates, 2007):

- Assess the context to ensure that you are capable of handling the situation; if not, seek assistance
- Communicate with the person you are handling or lifting and facilitate involvement or independence as much as possible
- Maintain a wide base of support and a stable center of gravity
- Maintain proper body alignment, keeping a square orientation to the client
- Bend at the hips and knees using the larger, stronger muscles, such as the legs, for lifting
- Lift in one smooth motion, keeping your heels down
- Stay as close as possible to the person you are lifting or handling
- Avoid twisting or overstretching by moving your feet in the direction of movement

## Bed Positioning and Mobility

Movement in the bed is usually the first physical task involved in the recovery of occupational performance. The occupational therapy practitioner is often involved with the interprofessional team in assisting the client to position or move in the bed. It is important that the team collaborate and communicate the best positioning movement techniques for each individual client. All team members should facilitate the positioning and movement of the client in the same manner to help the client move in an independent or interdependent manner.

### *Goals of Bed Positioning*

The goals of bed positioning are as follows (Wilson, Lange, & Mandac, 2006):

- Provision of support, comfort, and pain relief
- Normalization of muscle tone
- Promotion of symmetrical positioning
- Improved awareness of affected side and safety of limbs
- Prevention of positions of deformity and pressure sores
- Facilitation of occupational mobility and meaningful activities
- Optimization of occupational performance

### *Precautions*

The occupational therapy practitioner should be aware of her or his own physical capabilities as well as the medical and psychosocial needs and attributes of the client when preparing for occupational mobility. Common client precautions include the following (Bolding et al., 2013):

- Absent or impaired sensation
- Pressure points and length of positioning
- Awareness of skin integrity as friction during movement may cause shearing, particularly over bony prominences
- Deep vein thrombosis from lack of circulation in the legs
- Abnormal muscle tone (hypertonia or hypotonia) with impaired sensation
- Proper positioning of client in bed to prevent foot entrapment
- Orthostatic hypotension caused by a sudden drop in blood pressure when moving from supine to upright positions following long periods of bed rest, resulting in dizziness, nausea, or possible loss of consciousness
- Cognitive challenges

## General Bed Mobility Skills

The occupational therapy practitioner can facilitate the basic movements needed in the occupational performance task of bed mobility. Breaking these tasks into manageable steps can be an effective way to facilitate bed mobility. The occupational therapy practitioner should work with the interprofessional team to develop an individualized approach to bed mobility based on the evaluation of individual client factors, performance patterns, and contexts. Practicing can help the client gain skills and confidence to begin to combine movements for occupational performance. The occupational therapy practitioner needs to then facilitate the use of these skills in independent or interdependent performance patterns and daily routines. Skills needed for effective bed mobility include the following:

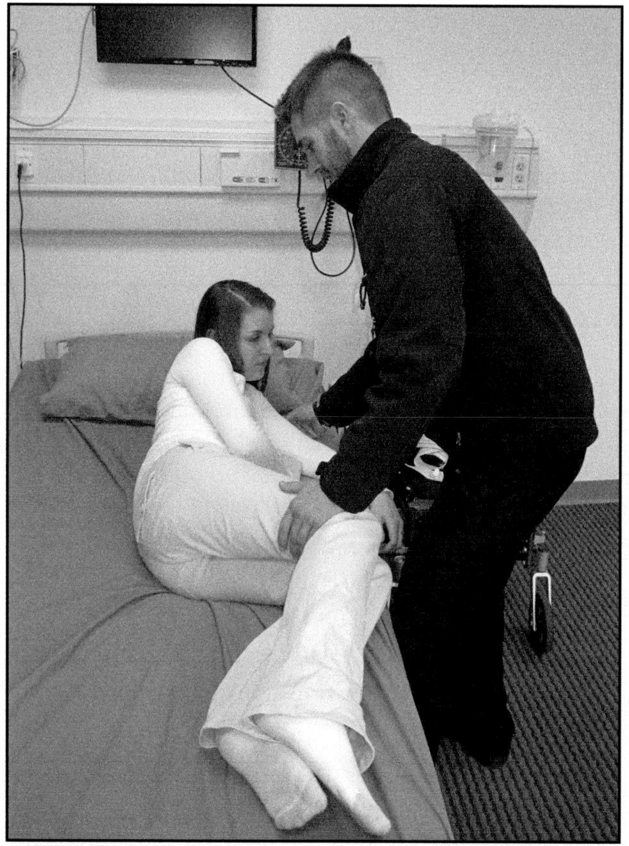

**Figure 33-2.** The occupational therapy practitioner assists the client to safely roll to the side of the bed.

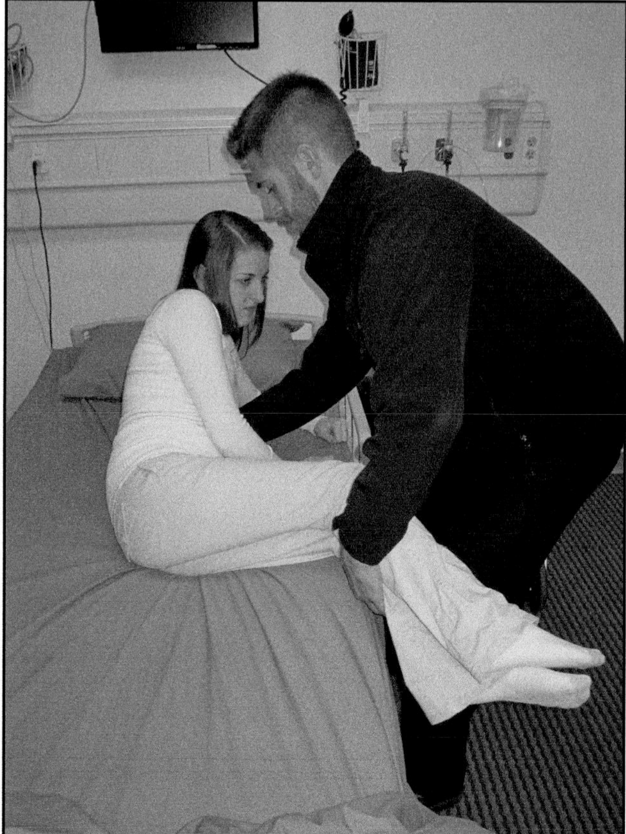

**Figure 33-3.** The occupational therapy practitioner facilitates the transition from side-lying to sitting.

- Rolling (to either side)
- Bridging (pulling the hips up in supine while supporting the pelvis from the legs)
- Scooting up in bed (necessary to reposition one's self in bed)
- Supine, to side lying, to sit
- Moving to either side of the bed

## Adaptive Devices for Bed Mobility

Adaptive equipment may assist a client to move effectively in bed. The occupational therapy practitioner works with the interprofessional team to facilitate independent or interdependent bed mobility individualized to each client. Devices that can facilitate bed mobility in the medical setting or home include the following:

- Bed ladder pull-up
- Leg lifter
- Overhead trapeze bar
- Bed rail assist
- Transfer pole

A draw sheet or positioning sheet can be placed perpendicular to the client under the trunk and hips for dependent bed mobility with two people on either side of the bed (Pierce, 2002).

## Therapeutic Bed Mobility

Bed mobility can be used as the occupational product of therapy, such as when a client is given adaptations for independence, or as an occupational process (Royeen, 2002), such as when the occupational therapy practitioner is facilitating movement, cognitive processing, or perceptual awareness through the occupation of bed mobility. Some examples of performance skills that can be incorporated into bed mobility include the following:

- Awareness of affected side (hemiparesis) or affected extremities (spinal cord injury)
- Upper extremity movement, including scapular mobility
- Weight shift and weight bearing
- Trunk stability and postural control
- Management of affected extremities
- Safe movement and cognitive awareness

Figures 33-2 through 33-4 demonstrate steps of bed mobility.

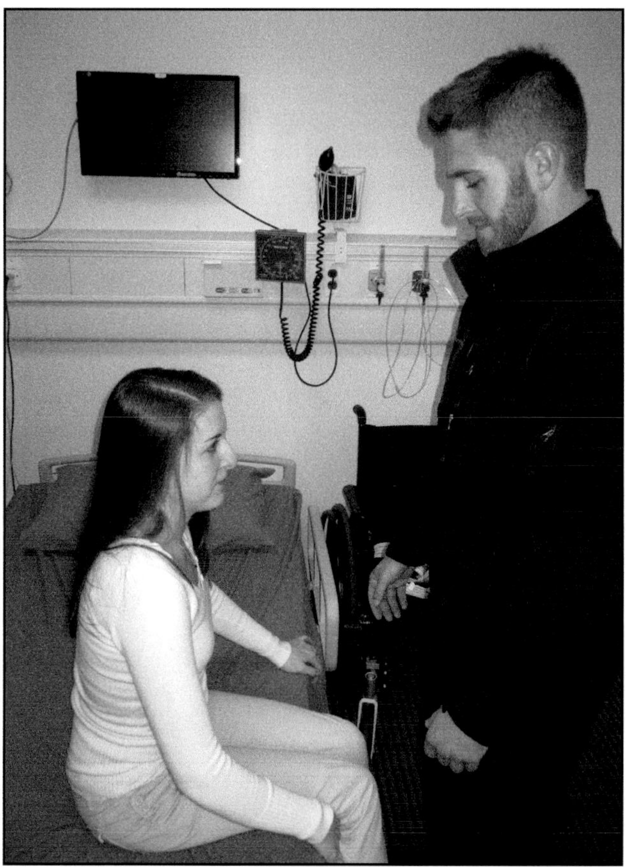

**Figure 33-4.** The client has transferred to the edge of the bed.

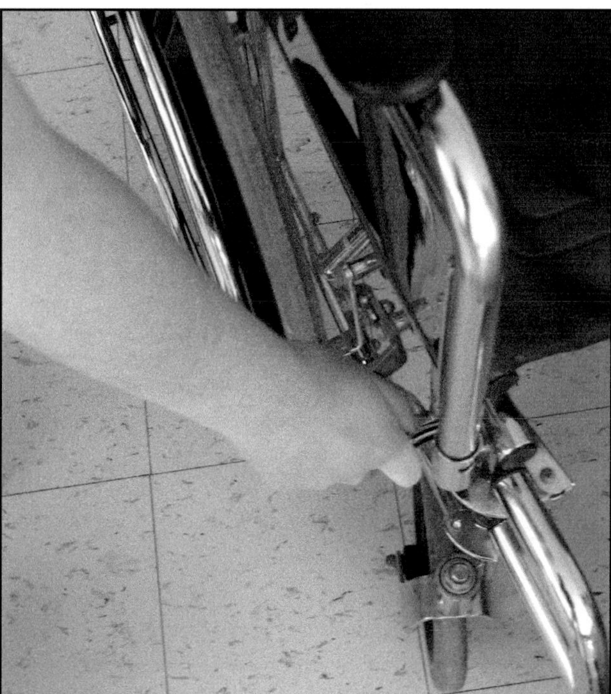

**Figure 33-5.** Properly position the chair ensuring that the wheelchair brakes are locked.

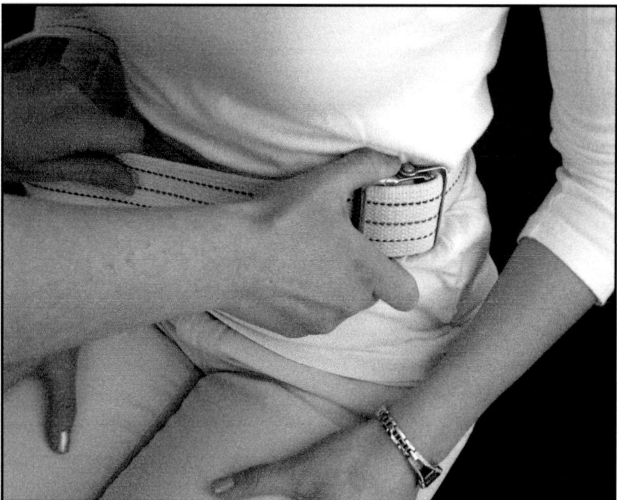

**Figure 33-6.** Secure transfer (gait) belt for safety.

## Transfers

The next step in the occupation-based mobility pyramid is teaching your client with mobility limitations to move from one surface to another. This is called *transferring*. Some facilities and occupational therapy departments require use of a transfer belt for safety when transferring clients. Occupational therapy practitioners need to be aware of the protocol of their facility or department regarding use of a transfer belt or any protocol (Figures 33-5 through 33-8).

### General Safety Considerations

- Be aware of the client factors and context
- Set up the physical environment
- Recognize the dynamic nature of your own physical abilities and limitations
- Use optimal body mechanics
- The client should be wearing shoes with a nonslip sole
- Transfers are most efficient when the surfaces are the same height
- A client with hemiparesis or other one-sided impairment will most easily transfer toward his or her stronger side

### Wheelchair Safety Considerations

- The wheelchair brakes should be locked during all transfers
- The wheelchair footrests are not for the client to stand on and should be moved or removed before a transfer

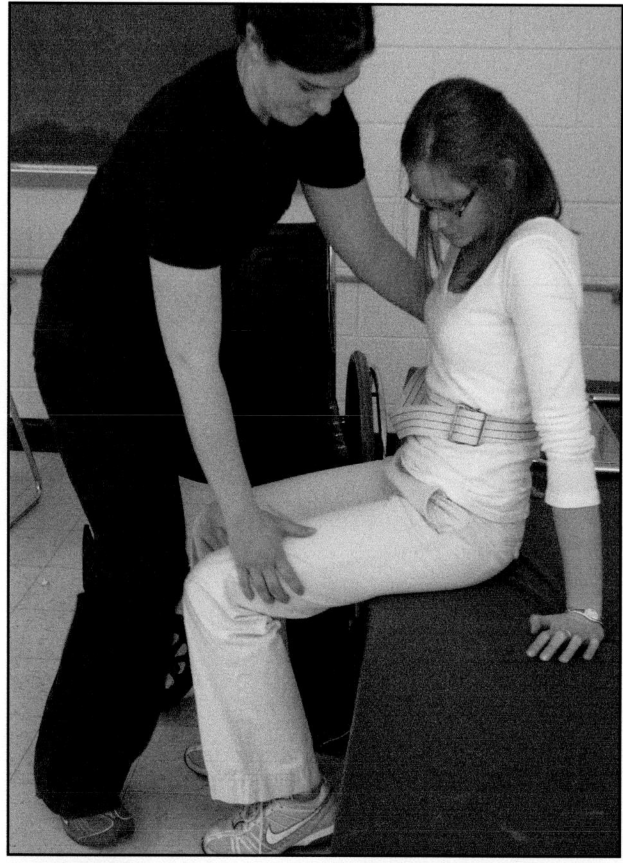

**Figure 33-7.** Facilitate the client to safely scoot forward.

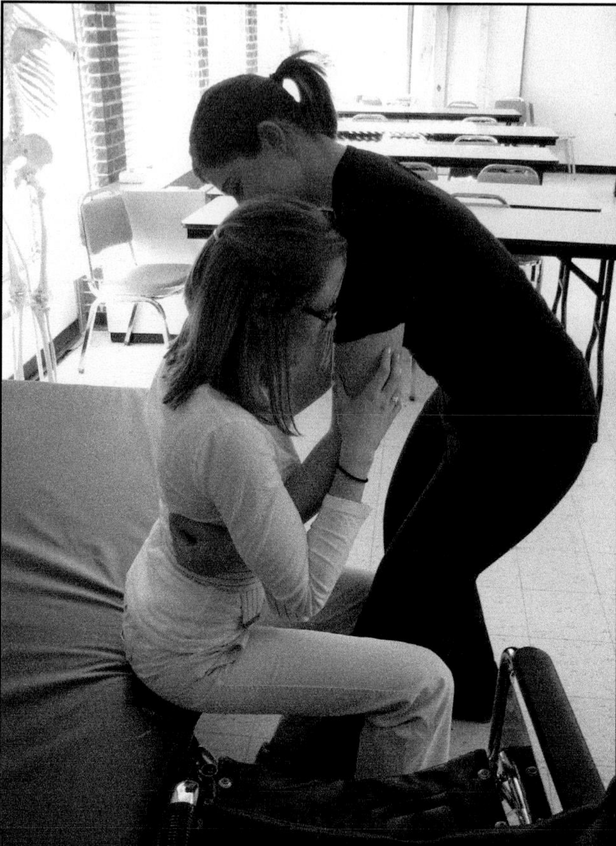

**Figure 33-8.** Facilitate the client into the "nose over toes" position; block the knee or knees if there is weakness.

- All persons involved in the transfer need to have non-skid soles for stability during the transfer (Bolding et al., 2013)

## Therapeutic Principles Incorporated in the Transfer

Therapeutic approaches and client factor remediation can be incorporated into the occupation of transferring. The following can be related to the occupational therapy intervention plan, model, or frame of reference:

- Pelvic tilt and position
- Trunk alignment
- Weight bearing and weight shifting
- Use of manual cues (Neurodevelopmental Treatment; Runyan, 2006)
- Lower extremity positioning
- Upper extremity positioning and functional use
- Cognitive, perceptual, and visual awareness
- Facilitating independence by encouraging the client to do as much of the process him- or herself as possible; the occupational therapy practitioner should provide the minimal amount of physical assistance for safe transfer
- In the case of a client who is interdependent with a caregiver, teach the client how to teach others including his or her family, caregivers, and paid attendants

## Preparation for the Transfer

- Communicate with the client about the procedure and provide rapport and meaning to this mobility occupation
- Position the wheelchair at a 0- to 30-degree angle to the surface to which you are transferring
- Be certain that the surface is stable and the wheelchair brakes are locked; facilitate the client's awareness and participation in the safety process
- The client should wear a transfer belt as facility policy indicates
- Remove the armrest closest to the transfer site (if necessary)
- The client should scoot forward
- The client should lean forward (nose over toes)

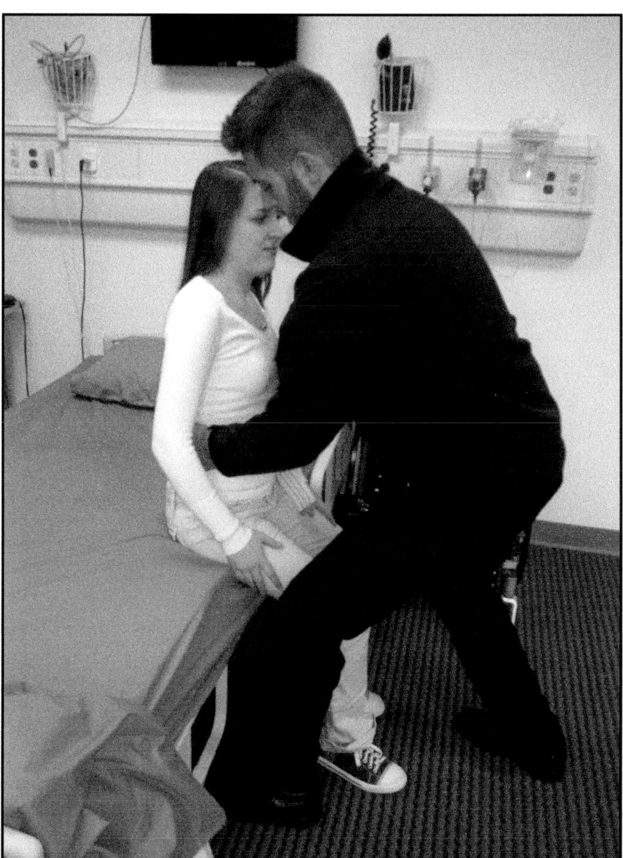

**Figure 33-9.** The client is seated at the edge of the bed ready to stand. Note the body mechanics of the occupational therapy practitioner, including bent knees, straight back, and a wide base of support (stance).

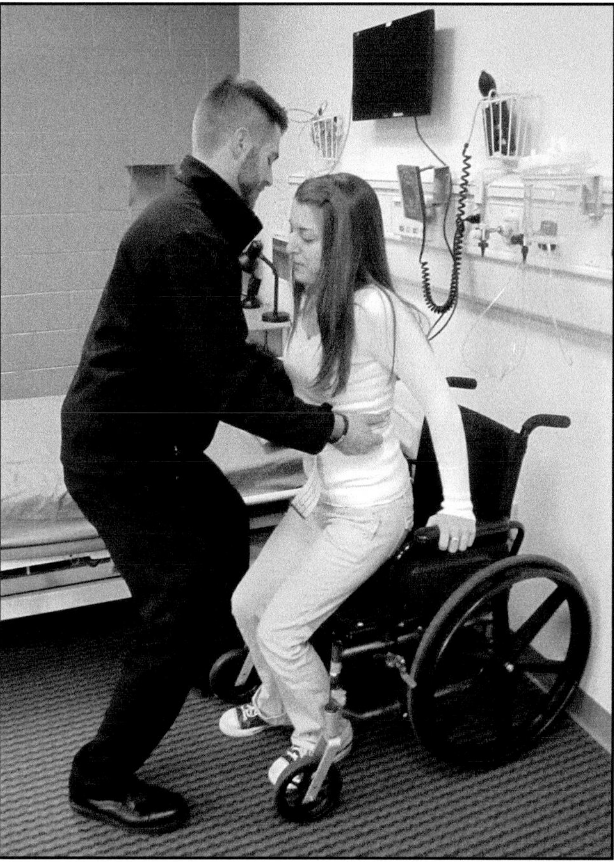

**Figure 33-10.** After the client is standing, the occupational therapy practitioner facilitates the client to pivot to align with the wheelchair. The client is encouraged to reach for and use the wheelchair arms to assist in the transfer.

- Stabilize the lower extremities or the hemiplegic leg (if necessary)
- Support any upper extremity limbs with abnormal tone

## Levels of Assistance in Transfer

If an assistive device or adaptive equipment is necessary, this should be identified in any related documentation. The following are the common levels of assistance required for transfers (Smith, 2013):

- Dependent: 75% to 100% assistance
- Maximum assist: 50% to 74% assistance
- Moderate assist: 25% to 49% assistance
- Minimum assist: up to 24% assistance
- Contact guard: Practitioner has her or his hand on the client at all times
- Supervised: Requires supervision for safe completion; no hands-on assistance, although a verbal cue may be required
- Modified independence: Client requires additional time, adaptive equipment, or assistive devices for completion of task
- Independent: The client is independent in the task (no assistance or cueing is needed)

## Transfer Techniques

The first three types of transfers can be performed as an intervention progression and are often used for clients with hemiparesis or other central nervous system impairments (Figures 33-9 through 33-11):

- Squat or bent pivot
- Stand pivot
- Stand step

The following are equipment used for transfers:

- Sliding board: Commonly used for people who have a spinal cord injury, overall weakness, or an above-knee or double amputation
- Dependent transfers: Use of mechanical device such as a Hoyer lift (Figure 33-12)

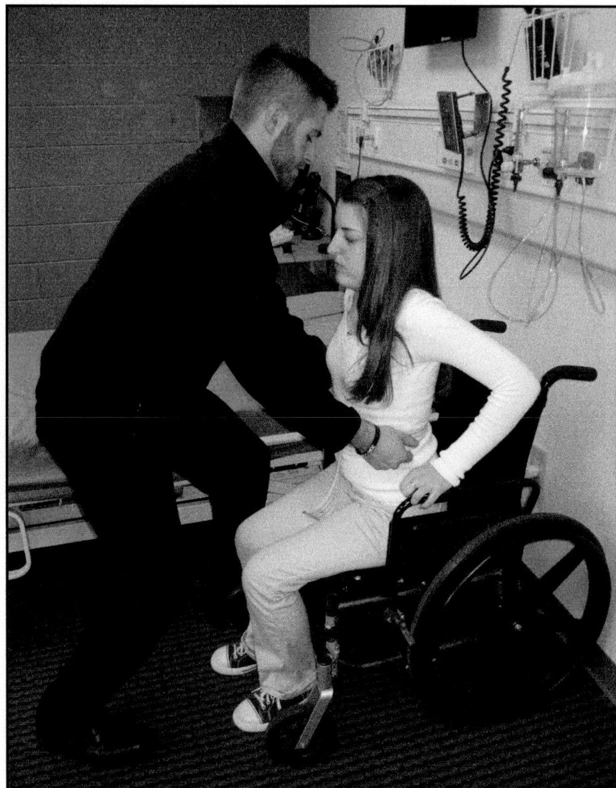

**Figure 33-11.** The client is safely transferred into the wheelchair while the occupational therapy practitioner maintains sound body mechanics.

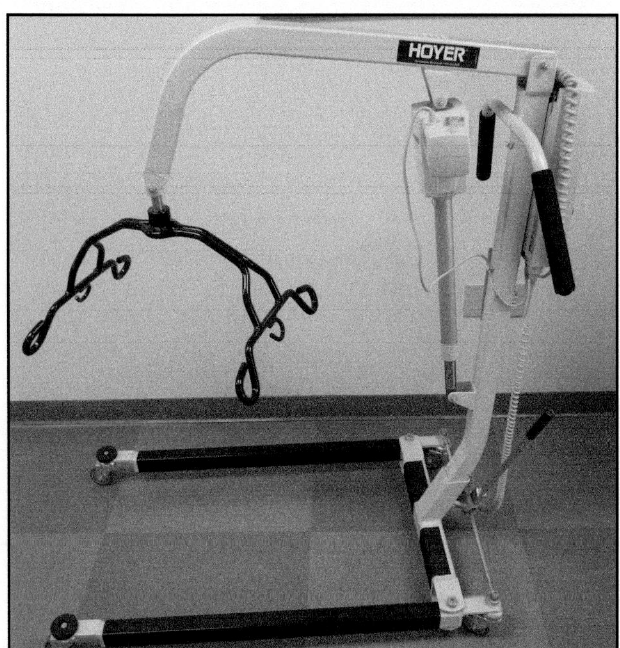


**Figure 33-12.** Dependent lift system.

- Cueing systems: Clients with cognitive impairments may be physically able but may need verbal, tactile, or visual cues to break down the steps of the task for safety

### Bent (Squat) Pivot

- Remove armrest
- Scoot forward and lean forward (nose over toes)
- Position affected arm
- Support affected leg
- Transfer, keeping the client in a bent forward position

### Stand Pivot

- Same as bent (squat) pivot, although you do not need to remove armrests
- Bring client to a standing position, gain equilibrium, do not rush
- Client pivots on unaffected leg, or both
- Reach back for the chair
- Lean the client forward as you descend as well

### Stand Step

- Same as stand pivot, with weight shift of the lower extremities
- Should need less physical assistance

### Sliding Board Transfer (Figures 33-13 through 33-15)

- Set up wheelchair as described previously
- Shift weight to the opposite side of the transfer and maneuver the sliding board under the leg and buttock closest to the wheelchair (when there are sensation losses, male clients need to be careful of the positioning of their genitalia)
- Block the client's knees with your own knees (the practitioner may be seated during the transfer)
- The client should make sure the board is in a good position to travel into the chair
- Instruct the client to lean forward and put his or her hands on the board (clients with a spinal cord injury who are preserving the tenodesis grasp should keep their hands fisted to not overstretch the wrist and hand extensors)
- The client slowly and carefully scoots or moves toward the wheelchair with the practitioner directly in front of him or her (the transfer should become more independent as the client's skill progresses)

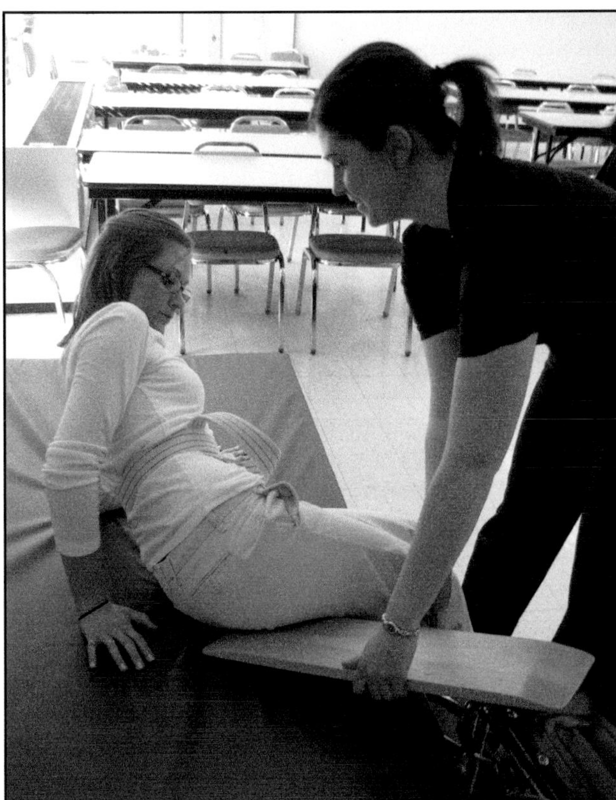

**Figure 33-13.** Sliding board transfer. The client supports herself in a tripod arm position while unweighting the hip closest to the wheelchair.

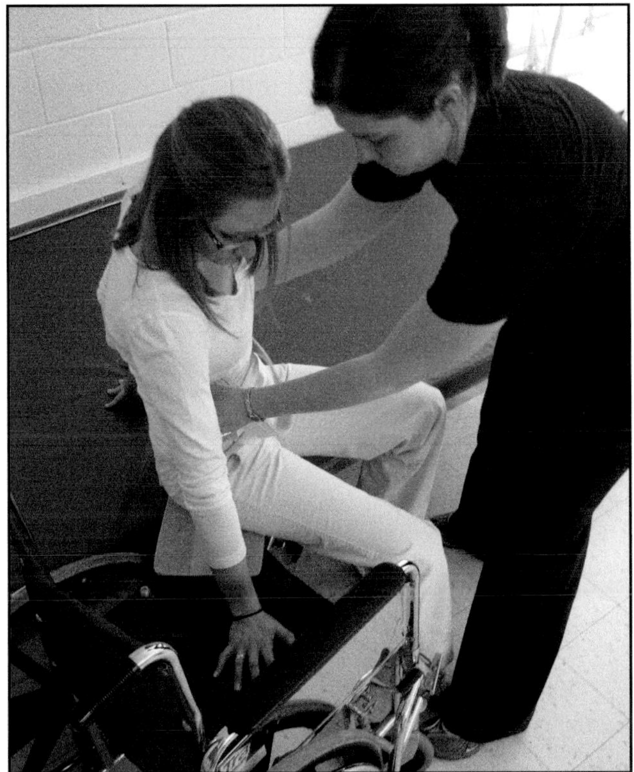

**Figure 33-14.** The occupational therapy practitioner facilitates the client to slide across the board from the mat to the wheelchair. Comparing this sliding process to entering a booth seat at a restaurant may be helpful to the client.

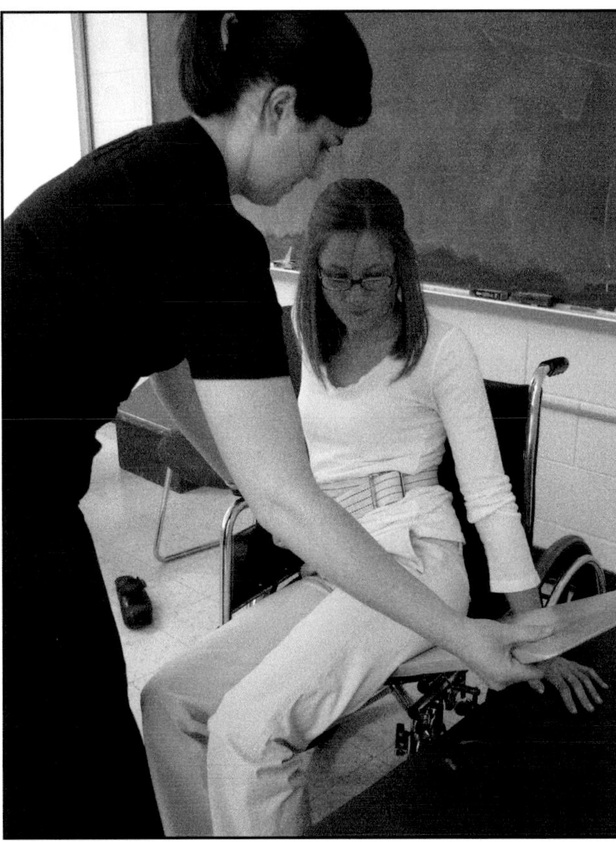

**Figure 33-15.** After the client has transferred to the chair, she continues to lean in the direction of the transfer to unweight the slideboard for removal. It is important to ensure that the client is properly positioned in the wheelchair at the conclusion of the transfer, which includes a neutral pelvic position and being seated deeply enough in the chair.

## Dependent Transfers

Many clients with significant client factors will be dependent in their transfers. It is important for occupational therapy practitioners to know their own limitations and protect their own bodies when attempting dependent transfers for clients. Dependent transfers can be accomplished by use of a team approach. However, if a client needs to transfer dependently long term, the best solution is a client lift system. If a client is very heavy, there are bariatric lift systems available to lift up to 1000 pounds. The role of the occupational therapy practitioner then becomes selection and training of the family or caregiver to use the device. The occupational therapy practitioner can work with more involved clients to ensure that they have the skills to do their own transfer training over the lifespan as caregivers may come and go. An example of this is a client with quadriplegic cerebral palsy making a digital recording of a caregiver performing a model transfer to train others.

# Occupation-Based Mobility Considerations

## Bathroom Mobility

To maintain independence at home, clients must be able to safely move and complete various transfers in the bathroom. Although the transfer process may be similar, environmental factors that affect safety such as throw rugs, steam, temperature changes, and water on surfaces can increase the risk of falls. Changes in client factors can magnify this risk and result in the necessity of using a mobility device to access the bathroom or various pieces of adaptive equipment to assist with bathing and toileting tasks. Home modifications may facilitate safety and occupational performance in the bathroom (AOTA, 2011). Elevated toilet seats, shower chairs or benches, and grab bars are common client-centered adaptations or may be part of universal design to enhance independence with bathroom mobility. If architectural barriers or movement precautions prevent access to the bathroom, a bedside commode may be necessary for toileting purposes. It is essential that the occupational therapy practitioner review bathroom mobility and address the necessary contextual elements to maximize occupational performance in these areas (Bolding et al., 2013).

## Home Mobility

Various instrumental activities of daily living (IADLs), including home management tasks, require dynamic balance and occupation-based mobility skills. In addition to the general safety considerations mentioned previously in the chapter, the home layout, furnishings, clutter, varied floor surfaces, poor lighting, and the presence of pets should be considered. During the intervention process, the occupational therapy practitioner may explore adaptations such as the use of a rolling cart during meal preparation, a long-handled duster to safely clean bookshelves, an automated pet feeder, or a walker basket to transport objects around the house (Bolding et al., 2013; Santucci, 2008).

## Car Transfers

One of the more complex transfers to consider during occupational therapy intervention is car transfers (Bolding et al., 2013). Contextual considerations for car transfers include the skill level of the client or caregiver, the vehicle being used, the use of a mobility device, and if the client will be a passenger or driver. A variety of transfer techniques may be used for this process, and typically, the client will enter the car using a backward approach, swinging his or her legs into the car after being seated (Meriano & Latella, 2008). Some clients find that riding in the back seat, if available, is an easier option than negotiating the front seat. When the client will be driving, it is important to consider the steering wheel during the transfer process as well as management of any mobility devices. There are various adaptations available to promote independent driving that will be discussed later in this chapter.

# Occupation-Based Mobility for Persons of Size

Occupational therapy practitioners are often called on to meet the needs of a large, heavy, or obese client. In the areas of beds, mats, transfer aids, adaptive equipment, and lift systems, specialized equipment is often needed to meet the needs of large, difficult-to-mobilize clients. It is important to use equipment that can handle the individual's weight for maximal safety and comfort of our larger clients. Occupational therapy practitioners should work with their interprofessional team, including durable equipment vendors and manufacturing representatives, to keep current with the evolving adaptive equipment and assistive technology available to meet client needs.

# Wheelchair Management

The occupational therapy practitioner respects the physical and psychosocial difficulties a client may have with use of the wheelchair. The wheelchair is a wonderful tool to facilitate occupational mobility. However, it also carries with it stigma regarding disability and loss of ambulation, whether it is temporary or permanent. The occupational therapy practitioner who is skilled in both physical and psychosocial aspects of human life should be attuned to the client as he or she begins to be mobilized by a wheelchair. Language is essential to acceptance of mobility using a wheelchair. The occupational therapy practitioner should refer to the client as "using" or being "mobilized" by a wheelchair. Care should be taken that clients are not referred to as "confined" to a wheelchair because this statement is limiting and stigmatizing. The occupational therapy practitioner should speak to clients at wheelchair height when possible and not stand over the client to talk (Loukas, 2008).

## Wheelchair Selection

The occupational therapy practitioner works with the interprofessional team to collaboratively select the appropriate wheelchair with the client. The most common types of wheelchairs are manual and electric or power chairs. Considerations in the wheelchair selection process include specific condition and disability needs,

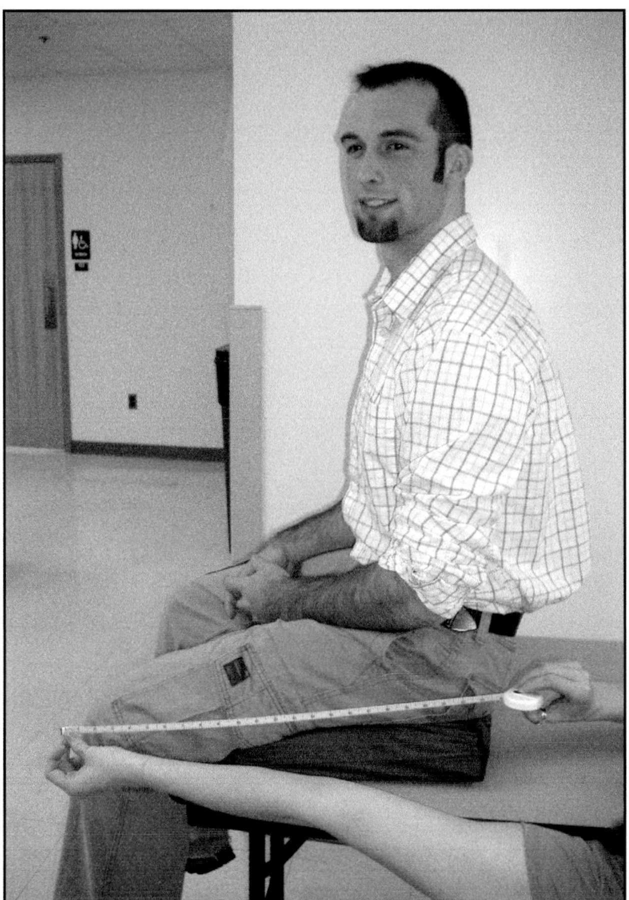

**Figure 33-16.** Measurements for a wheelchair should be made while the client is in the optimal sitting position.

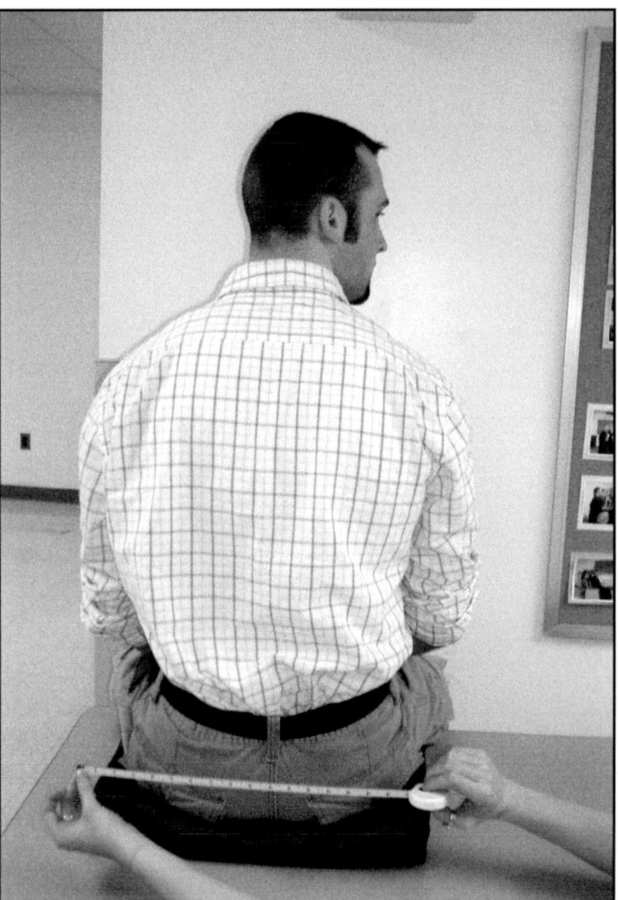

**Figure 33-17.** Hip measurements for wheelchair width.

client lifestyle, context of use, necessary accessories and modifications, payment, size and growth needs, and client factors (especially strength and functional use of the upper extremities). The occupational therapy practitioner often works with the client, physical therapist, and assistive technology professional or durable medical equipment supplier in this process (Bolding et al., 2013). The occupational therapy practitioner uses critical thinking to ensure that the mobility device facilitates the client's occupational performance, enabling the client to participate as fully as possible in occupations in the home, worksite, and community (Figures 33-16 through 33-19).

Manual wheelchairs are commonly used in medical facilities, especially for short-term use. These chairs come in a variety of frame styles that range from a standard wheelchair (Figure 33-20) to more customized chairs with reclining backs or lightweight frames to enhance agility. Power wheelchairs provide a wide range of customization that can enhance independence for individuals who are unable to self-propel a manual wheelchair. The client must have adequate strength and control to mobilize the wheelchair. For clients who will propel their wheelchairs manually, techniques include giving clients protective gloves or lacing the wheelchair with rubber tubing to improve grip. Other techniques, such as using wheeled mobility or electric devices, can conserve energy and improve occupational functioning and community participation for many clients. For clients with high-level paralysis, a breath-controlled or head-controlled electronic system can be used to operate the wheelchair, thus providing important independence and mobility. For children with mobility impairments, there are a myriad of pediatric mobility devices. These include push chairs, positioning chairs, and adaptable level chairs for school-based occupations.

## *Wheelchair Seating and Accessories*

After a manual or power wheelchair has been selected, additional considerations include seating and accessories. The appropriate selection of a seating system that promotes a safe and functional body position is essential. Goals for proper wheelchair seating and positioning include the following:

- To facilitate postural control and head stability
- To provide symmetry and prevent deformity

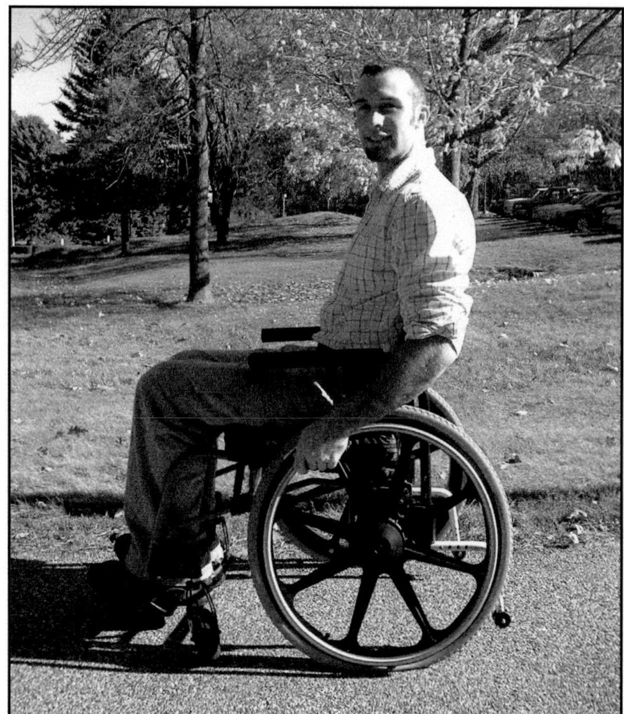

Figure 33-18. The proper type and fit of a wheelchair is necessary for optimal occupation-based community mobility and participation.

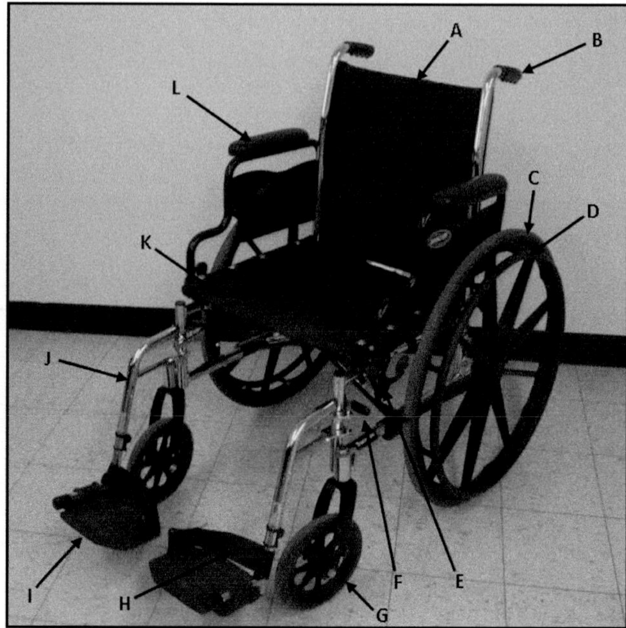


Figure 33-20. Standard wheelchair components. (A) Backrest. (B) Push handle. (C) Drive wheel. (D) Handrim. (E) Brake. (F) Front rigging release. (G) Caster wheel. (H) Heel loop. (I) Flip-up foot rest. (J) Front rigging. (K) Seat. (L) Armrest.

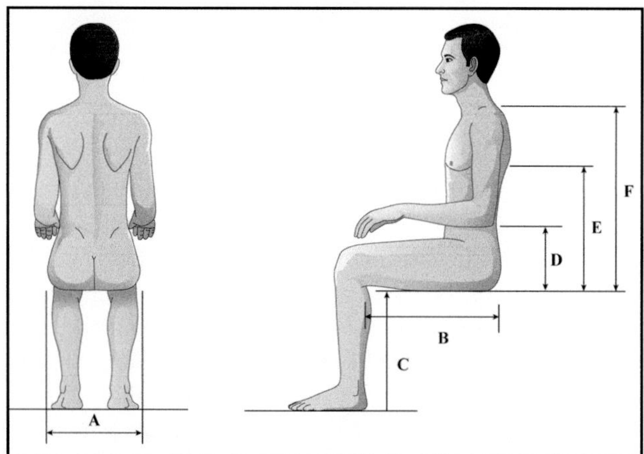


Figure 33-19. Wheelchair measurements.

- To normalize muscle tone and facilitate postural control
- To maintain skin integrity and pressure management
- To promote occupational performance and function to maximize sitting endurance and stamina for activity
- To optimize respiratory function (Bolding et al., 2013)

A variety of specialized cushions are available to clients who use a manual or power wheelchair for mobility. Sling seats in a wheelchair are for very short-term, occasional use. Common cushion types include foam, gel, or air-based systems, which are recommended based on various client factors and physical assessment that may include pressure mapping. If a client requires additional postural support, various positioning devices may be added to the wheelchair frame to maintain body alignment and promote body functions and occupational performance.

Wheelchairs can be customized to meet the specific needs of each individual client. A wide variety of leg rests, armrests, and wheel styles and configurations are available. Various components of the wheelchair, especially on power chairs, can be mechanized to promote skin integrity, respiratory status, blood pressure, and circulatory issues. An interprofessional team can include the client, his or her family or caregiver, a physician, a physical therapist, an assistive technology professional or durable medical equipment supplier, respiratory therapist, and an occupational therapy practitioner. Other specialists such as a speech-language pathologist may be involved when the client uses an electronic communication device. In this circumstance, the positioning and attachment of the device becomes essential to functional use of the communication system (Bolding et al., 2013; Pierson & Fairchild, 2008; Wilson et al., 2006).

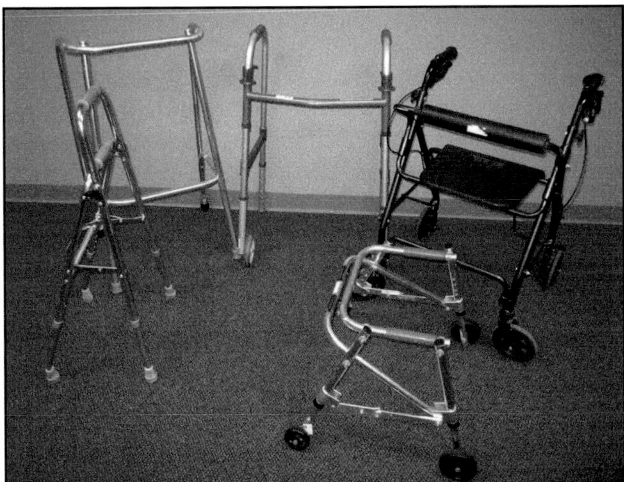

**Figure 33-21.** An assortment of walkers.

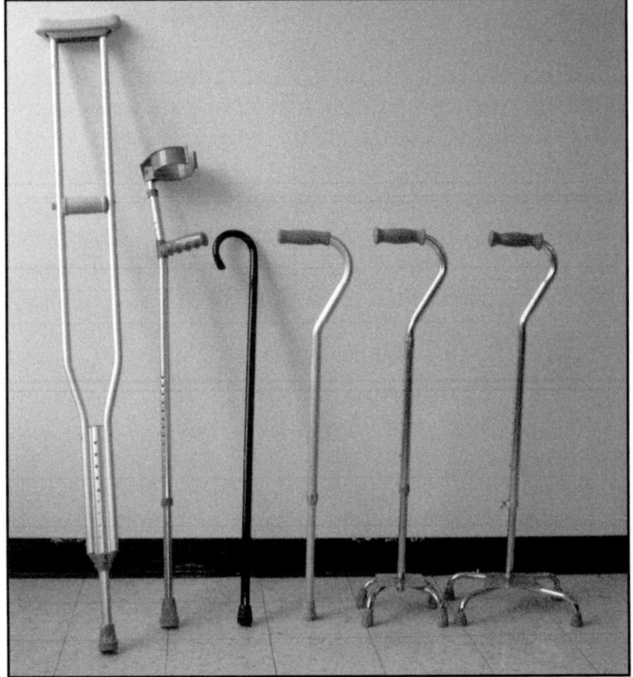

**Figure 33-22.** An assortment of canes and crutches.

## Mobility Devices

During occupation-based mobility, clients may use a variety of mobility devices. The type of device is typically recommended by the physical therapy practitioner based on the diagnosis, prognosis, and ambulation assessment. Occupational therapy practitioners work closely with physical therapists during the intervention process and must be familiar with not only the device but also its proper fit and use. The recommended mobility device will vary in the amount of support provided to the client. Walkers provide more support than canes and include standard and various wheeled varieties (Figure 33-21). A variety of crutches and canes are available, with a quad cane providing greater support than a single-point cane (Bolding et al., 2013; Pierson & Fairchild, 2008; Figure 33-22).

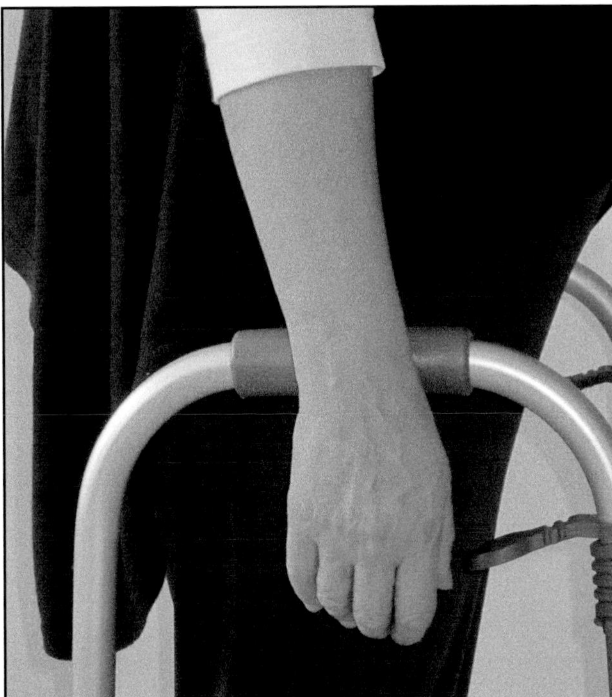

**Figure 33-23.** A properly fit walker or cane should place the handle of the device at the client's wrist crease.

Mobility devices can enhance occupational performance if the device is fitted and used properly. It is not uncommon for clients to attempt using mobility devices recommended for friends and family members, but these often do not fit the client properly. One simple way to ensure that a walker or cane is properly fit to the client is the wrist test. When the client is standing with the walker or cane at the side, the handle should be level with the patient's wrist crease (Pierson & Fairchild, 2008; Figure 33-23). Physical therapy practitioners address ambulation patterns with the client during his or her treatment session, so it is important to collaborate with the team to ensure consistency. Generally speaking, the client will hold a cane in the hand opposite the affected lower extremity. The cane and the affected leg should hit the ground simultaneously. When negotiating a step or stairs, the client should typically step up with the unaffected leg and "down" with the affected leg. Mobility devices for children include posterior walkers, dynamic prone standers, and other specialized equipment (Figure 33-24).

## Driving and Community Mobility

Community mobility continues to be included in multiple official documents for the profession of occupational therapy including the *Framework* and the *Scope of Practice* documents (AOTA, 2014a, 2014b). The title of

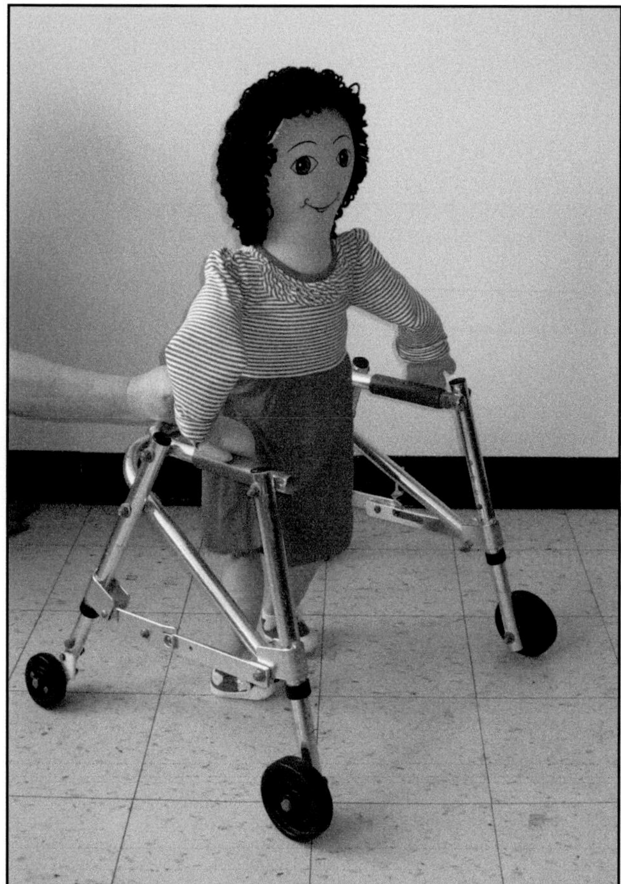

**Figure 33-24.** A pediatric posterior walker.

this IADL has been changed to driving and community mobility in the Third Edition of the *Framework* (AOTA, 2014a) and is defined as "planning and moving around in the community and using public or private transportation, such as driving, walking, bicycling, or accessing and riding buses, taxi cabs, or other transportation systems" (p. S19). The inclusion of driving in the title of this IADL occupation further illustrates the importance that the AOTA has placed on driving, which has become recognized as both an occupation and occupation enabler (Stav, 2014a; Stav & Lieberman, 2008).

Client-centered community participation is a very important aspect to a full life and occupational functioning for individuals across the lifespan (AOTA, 2010). The Americans with Disabilities Act of 1990 has provided important accessibility rights for people with mobility challenges, and this continues to improve (U.S. Department of Justice, n.d.). For children and youth, the Individuals with Disabilities Education Act of 1990 and 1997 and the Individuals with Disabilities Improvement Act of 2004 support both physical and attitudinal accessibility changes in our communities and create more opportunities for people with disabilities (AOTA, 2006). Occupational therapy practitioners are at the forefront of these advocacy efforts. Facilitation of clients to return or emerge into the community is an important aspect of a full life and full participation (Baum, 2006).

For persons with functional mobility impairment, the first important step is for clients to have insight regarding their own abilities, opportunities, and obstacles. A client who can realistically judge his or her own strength and mobility challenges will have more success in planning for community mobility. For clients with cognitive challenges or lack of insight into their own abilities, the occupational therapy practitioner must help them understand and judge their own needs and abilities. The next step is planning. The occupational therapy practitioner can assist his or her client to plan an outing into the community, such as grocery shopping, visiting a friend, going out to eat, or attending church. Planning includes thinking about transportation, devices, safety and equipment needs, medication management, and many other client-specific factors. Finally, going out into the community in graded steps is achieved. The client should be encouraged to reflect on the experiences and to plan and adjust as he or she progresses in community participation. The occupational therapy practitioner may accompany the client on several community outings to foster mobility independence and community participation.

For infants, children, and youth, community participation includes day care centers, preschools, schools, work sites, and social events. Mobility and positioning devices can enhance the opportunities for inclusive participation of children in the community. Adaptive play equipment can facilitate community mobility on the playground or in the gym.

### *Transportation*

Many wheelchair-accessible vans, entry systems, and driving controls are available to clients with mobility challenges. There is also increasingly more public transportation that provides accessibility to people who use wheelchairs and other mobility devices such as independent transportation networks. Children traveling in school buses should have accessible and safe systems in place for transport. Parents with young children who have mobility impairment often transfer their children into a car seat and have portable wheelchairs or push chairs (strollers) for community mobility. It is important for the occupational therapy practitioner to assist the family to explore their adaptive equipment options as the child grows and needs a more accessible system that allows him or her to continue using a wheelchair.

## Driver Rehabilitation

Driving is an integral part of independent living and is essential to a person's success in employment, education, socialization, community participation, and aging in place (American Medical Association [AMA], 2010; Bolding et al., 2013). Occupational therapy practitioners are influencing the practice of driver rehabilitation for persons with physical disabilities in greater numbers. An entry-level occupational therapy education program addresses content related to driving and community mobility (Stav, 2014a). The degree to which this content is covered is up to each individual program but may include lecture and lab content, field trips, experiential learning, and Level I fieldwork rotations (Yuen & Burik, 2011). Occupational therapy assistant programs are also responsible for including training related to driving and community mobility once an established treatment plan has been established by an occupational therapist (AOTA, 2014b, 2015).

Entry-level occupational therapists have the ability to complete IADL evaluation in the areas of driving. The goal is primarily to determine the client's occupational performance and safety while driving (AOTA, 2010). Vehicle features are also an important part of driving for older drivers and those with specific disabilities. Recommendations regarding entering and exiting the vehicle, opening and closing doors, and seat belt use are areas that occupational therapy practitioners can address specific to client needs.

Many independent living centers and rehabilitation centers offer driving assessment and training services. They assist the client in choosing options such as car or vehicle considerations and the adaptive equipment needed to safely operate a motor vehicle. From there, occupational therapists develop a full plan of care to help the client return to driving, begin to drive, or recommend that driving is not a safe option (AMA, 2010; Bolding et al., 2013). Programs that address person-to-vehicle fit, such as the AARP/AAA CarFit program (Thate, Gulden, Lefebvre, & Springer, 2011), can address the needs of aging drivers in vision, location of devices and controls, and emerging technology (Shaw, Polgar, Vrkljan, & Jacobson, 2010; Figure 33-25).

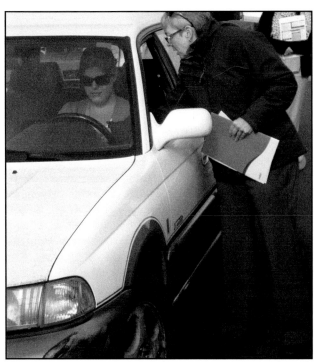

**Figure 33-25.** An occupational therapy practitioner works with older adults to ensure safe and efficient driving using the CarFit program.

Issues that are red flags for medically impaired driving include the following:

- Acute events: A stroke or brain injury, seizure, surgery, or delirium of any type
- Patient or family member concern
- Medical history that includes chronic conditions, particularly those that affect vision, cardiovascular disease, neurologic disease, psychiatric disease, metabolic disease, musculoskeletal disabilities, chronic renal failure, and respiratory disease
- Medical conditions with unpredictable, episodic events
- Medications that can impair performance (AMA, 2010)
- A pattern of motor vehicle accidents

Advanced training and certification is available and encouraged for occupational therapy practitioners who wish to specialize in this area of practice. Advanced practitioners with specialized training in driving-based occupations conduct a thorough evaluation that includes vision, perception, mobility, hand and foot function, and cognition. One option is the driver rehabilitation specialist and optional certification process, which is awarded by the Association for Driver Rehabilitation Specialists (ADED). The driver rehabilitation specialist or certified driver rehabilitation specialist "plans, develops, coordinates, and implements driving services for individuals with disabilities" (ADED, 2016, para. 1). The AOTA has a specialty certification in driving and community mobility available for both for occupational therapists and occupational therapy assistants (Stav, 2014a). Practitioners may also wish to become a certified driving instructor, which is awarded by state or federal agencies based in local laws and regulations. This credential is required in many states to ensure safety of the public on the roadways (Stav, 2014a). Together, these specialists help determine fitness to drive and provide necessary rehabilitation services (AOTA, 2016a).

# Issues Related to Driver Rehabilitation and Recommendations

## The Aging Driver

Motor vehicle injuries are the leading cause of injury-related deaths for the 65- to 74-year-old age bracket and the second leading cause (after falls) for the 75- to 84-year-old age bracket (AMA, 2010). Many older drivers begin to change their own habits by limiting driving to familiar places, driving only during the daylight hours, and avoiding busy or congested areas of traffic. Client factors, particularly regarding vision, are important to assess and address as adults age into their elder years. The loss of the ability to drive has been correlated with risk of entering a long-term care facility in the elder population (Freeman, Gange, Munoz, & West, 2006).

Occupational therapy practitioners have the training and understanding to assist older adults engage in driving and community mobility safely. It is very important that existing programs and services not only assist older drivers to continue driving, but facilitate successful driving retirement when necessary (Golisz, 2014; Stav, Weidley, & Love, 2011). To assist with this process, the AOTA has resources available to consumers and practitioners including the practitioner's toolkit (AOTA, 2016b). Greater involvement of occupational therapy practitioners in policy development and revision of driver licensure laws will provide additional opportunities for the profession and the clients we serve (Stav, 2014b).

## Adolescents and Young Adults With Disabilities

Learning to drive is a rite of passage and important means to community participation as children and youth with disabilities transition to young adult roles and responsibilities. Students with autism spectrum disorders, physical disabilities, or other impairments are often capable of driving. It is important that occupational therapy practitioners encourage safety in all areas of transportation for the students with whom they work. Independence in transportation improves opportunities for employment, housing, social events, and educational and recreational involvement (AOTA, 2012).

## Adaptations to Facilitate Driving

Occupational therapy practitioners with advanced certification can recommend adaptive devices and vehicle modification to maximize occupational performance. Clients with paralysis or right-sided impairment may switch to hand controls. These are manufactured and can be used to help a client with paralysis return to the safe occupation of driving. Behind-the-wheel driving instruction is essential for those individuals who are reestablishing their safe driving skills using adaptive devices.

A number of devices are now being used to assist drivers who are visually impaired. Most states require a visual acuity of 20/40 to 20/70 or better and visual fields of about 140 degrees, although different states vary in their requirements (AMA, 2010). Bioptic telescopes are legal in many states, and may correct acuity to 20/70 or better, but practitioners and consumers should refer to local regulations (AMA, 2010).

## Adapted Vehicles and Lifts

Many companies have a line for adapted vehicles and lifts. These can be very expensive for clients, so it is important to make good decisions for the best overall occupational outcomes. There has been an expansion in vehicle adaptations to such a degree that it is imperative occupational therapy practitioners collaborate with durable medical equipment vendors regarding up-to-date equipment options. Behind-the-wheel assessments are vital to assess the actual adaptive equipment needs so that money is not needlessly spent. Nationwide, there are alternative financing programs available for low-interest loans so that individuals can borrow the money needed to buy adapted vehicles.

### Case Study

An occupational therapist and an occupational therapy assistant have worked together at Madeline-Sadie Rehabilitation hospital for the past 3 years. You are working with Carl, a client who is now 4 weeks status-post a traumatic motor vehicle accident. Carl is a 58-year-old man who sustained multiple rib fractures leading to internal injuries, a mid-shaft fracture in his dominant (right) humerus, and a closed head injury. Carl lives alone in a single level apartment and works full time as customer service specialist at a large electronics retailer. He is excited that his brother managed to get him a new vehicle because it is his main means of transportation. He is currently able to complete all of his basic ADL tasks independently and he is independently using a single-point cane while completing functional mobility. The interdisciplinary team thinks that Carl will be ready for discharge home within the next 3 to 5 days. The occupational therapy department has been asked to determine if Carl is capable of driving safely. Determine the priorities, considerations, and the role for each level of practitioner within the next 3 to 5 days and beyond.

## Evidence-Based Research Chart

| Issue | Description | Evidence |
|---|---|---|
| **Functional Mobility** | | |
| Elders | Elders who fell within 6 months after a hip fracture demonstrate poorer balance, slower gait, and decline in ADLs<br>Leisure engagement student of older adults | Restoring elders to full health after a hip fracture is indicated, including addressing mobility and balance deficits (Shumway-Cook, Ciol, Grubon, & Robinson, 2005).<br>Fear of falling and using mobility devices have a significant effect on leisure engagement of older adults (Nilsson, Nyqvist, Gustafson, & Nygard, 2015). |
| Mobility device use | Qualitative, longitudinal study to assess how frequently older women use their mobility devices<br>Pilot study to explore falls and the fear of falling among elders using rolling walkers<br>Qualitative study about safe patient handling equipment in rehabilitation settings | Assumptions of mobility device use in the home, if recommended, are not always followed. Practitioners should consider the contextual considerations of device use in home during treatment (Porter, Matsuda, & Benson, 2011).<br>Fear of falling is greater among those who have fallen in the past. Inappropriate walker fit and use was identified and may be associated with falls (Liu, Grando, Zabel, & Nolen, 2009).<br>Safe patient handling equipment used with 10% to 25% of caseload during therapy sessions to increase options during therapy sessions. Participants identified significant potential for expanded use for low-level, dependent, and bariatric clients (Darragh et al., 2013). |
| Individuals with spinal cord injury (SCI) | Functional mobility was found to be one of the top three problems identified by clients with SCI | Client-centered approaches have the best results (Donnelly et al., 2004). |
| Seating and mobility | Model for persons with SCI that considers the person, wheelchair, and environments of home, work, and community<br>Researchers examined segmented foam and skin protection wheelchair cushion efficacy to prevent pressure ulcers among nursing home residents | Seating and multiple considerations should be used for persons mobilized with a wheelchair (Minkel, 2000).<br>The combination of a properly fit wheelchair and skin protection wheelchair cushion reduce the risk of pressure ulcers (Brienza et al., 2010). |
| Self-perceived physical independence | Activity limitations correlate with perceptions of independence | Community mobility and coping efficacy improve self-perception of independence (Wang, Badley, & Gignac, 2004). |
| Wheelchair design | Wheelchair performance was tested on a community obstacle course | Differences in wheelchair design affect performance, and wheelchair choice is important to community mobility (Rogers, Berman, Fails, & Jaser, 2003). |
| Wheelchair users at home | Researchers found that of 525 respondents, 37.9% of wheelchair users fell in the past 12 months; 17.7% suffered a fall-related injury | Structural modifications and functional mobility–based therapy services for safety are needed (Berg, Hines, & Allen, 2002). |
| Wheelchair mobility | Users' opinions on mobility devices and satisfaction with the devices<br>People with SCI were studied regarding types of wheeled mobility | Positive effect on activity, transportation, security, and participation in social activities (Wresstle & Samuelsson, 2004).<br>Independent use of manual wheelchairs and the ability to travel efficiently have been correlated with community participation (Cooper, Ferretti, Oyster, Kelleher, & Cooper, 2011). |

*(continued)*

## EVIDENCE-BASED RESEARCH CHART (CONTINUED)

| Issue | Description | Evidence |
|---|---|---|
| Powered mobility | Systematic review of the effect of powered mobility on engagement in independent occupations<br>Quantitative study on perceived quality of life after use of a powered wheelchair | Powered mobility devices are associated with increased quality of life and opportunity for engagement in both previous and new valued occupations (Fomiatti, Richmond, Moir, & Millsteed, 2013).<br>Improvements in mobility and reduction in pain and discomfort were reported (Davies, Souza, & Frank, 2003). |
| Children | Children with cerebral palsy were compared across environmental settings in their gross motor performance | Results show differences across settings, indicating that use of the natural context is important in therapy (Tieman, Palisano, Gracely, & Rosenbaum, 2004). |
| Spirituality and occupation-based mobility | Attendance at church by people with functional disabilities correlated with improved functioning<br>Using prayer as a modality for healing is more common among people with mobility limitations | Church-related community mobility is important (Idler & Kasl, 1997).<br>Practitioners should facilitate a client's own spiritual expression and connection to a higher power, or "religious pluralism" (Hendershot, 2003). |
| **Community Mobility** | | |
| Mobility devices | Pilot study indicates skills course improves mobility | Device use in the community should be addressed individually in practice (Walker et al., 2010). |
| Car transfers | Study of wheelchair athletes | Evidence that car transfers are most essential (Fliess-Douer, Vanlandewijck, & van der Woude, 2012). |
| Driving with a disability | Focus groups find arthritis may affect safe driving | Toolkit created to address safety concerns of this population (Vrkljan et al., 2010). |
| Older adult driving and community mobility | Systematic review of 16 studies on driver licensing policy, driving cessation, and community mobility programs<br>Safety risks occur as a result of incongruence between vehicle and driver | It is important to address both driving and driving cessation including alternate modes of community mobility (Stav, 2014b).<br>Intervention is needed to promote vehicle to driver fit (Shaw, Polgar, Vrkljan, & Jacobson, 2010). |
| Older non-drivers (never drivers and former drivers) | Correlated as an independent risk factor for entering long-term care facilities | Discontinuation of driving and/or limited access to community mobility options can impact ability to live independently (Freeman, Gange, Munoz, & West, 2006). |
| Nonstandard controls for disabled drivers | Large study of people with acquired disability; 79% had returned to driving; a significantly higher proportion had accidents | Problems associated with nonfamiliar controls (Prasad, Hunter, & Hanley, 2006). |
| Safety and mobility of people with disabilities in adapted cars | Safety and perceptions of safety, as well as confidence in an adapted car, were reported | One of 10 had accidents, a small number attributed to special equipment in the car (Henriksson & Peters, 2004). |
| Effects of fatigue on driving for people with multiple sclerosis | People with multiple sclerosis report fatigue, leg problems, numbness, and eye problems | Multiple sclerosis population reports driving short distances and shorter driving times because of fatigue (Chipchase, Lincoln, & Radford, 2003). |
| Drivers with dementia | Exploratory study examining drivers with dementia in the media | Significant safety issues are found in drivers with dementia who become lost (Hunt, Brown, & Gilman, 2010). |
| People with Parkinson disease | Effects of cognitive abilities | Cognitive abilities were found not to be associated with fitness to drive (Radford, Lincoln, & Lennox, 2004). |
| Combat veterans with traumatic brain injury and post-traumatic stress disorder | Veterans found to have more critical driving errors | Intervention to address safe driving needed for veterans (Classen et al., 2011). |

## Summary

Occupational therapy practitioners address occupation-based functional mobility in the contexts in which clients engage in social participation. The occupational therapy practitioner and the physical therapist collaborate in the areas of functional mobility to maximize client potential. As indicated in the occupation-based mobility pyramid, skills progress developmentally from bed mobility to transfers to transportation to community mobility. Many client factors are involved in occupation-based mobility across the lifespan and should be evaluated and addressed in occupational therapy interventions. Safety is a priority in the mobility-based intervention progression. Intervention planning should include a holistic model and frames of reference. Client-centered, occupation-based mobility can be addressed within those therapeutic and often interprofessional approaches as occupational therapy practitioners facilitate participation in life.

## Acknowledgments

The authors acknowledge student involvement of Ethan Drouin, Lindsey Holmes, Sarah Hume, Erin O'Brien, and Justin West. Gratitude is extended to Barb Allen, PT, for her consultative advice.

## Student Self-Assessment

1. Body mechanics. The students should put a necklace on with string and a bolt around the string. The necklace should be long enough to hang at the navel of the student. Instruct students to bend and lift items such as books. They should bend with their legs, and the necklace should not go further than 1 or 2 inches forward as they bend. You can also practice keeping the body stable and not allowing any rotation and pulling versus pushing for bed mobility.
2. Wheelchair experience. Each student should spend 1 day using a wheelchair. Students should go to class, go out in the community, and perform other typical activities. They should then write a journal entry regarding the challenges and changes they experienced and their psychosocial responses to the wheelchair experience. It is very important for students to take this experience seriously and to not get out of the wheelchair in public; this could be disrespectful to people who are mobilized by a wheelchair.
3. Bed mobility practice. Students should practice bed mobility for various clients. Practice the basic skills and then apply these bed mobility skills for clients with the following diagnoses: hemiplegia, spinal cord injury paraplegia, and hip fracture or replacement. They should practice different teaching models in this process.
4. Transfer practice. Students practice all of the transfer methods reviewed in this chapter. They progress from bed or mat to wheelchair, from wheelchair to toilet or tub chair, and finally from wheelchair to car.

## References

Alnaser, M. Z. (2007). Occupational musculoskeletal injuries in the health care environment and its impact on occupational therapy practitioners: A systematic review. *WORK, 29*(20), 89-100.

American Medical Association. (2010). *Physicians guide to: Assessing and counseling older drivers* (2nd ed.).Chicago, IL: Author.

American Occupational Therapy Association. (2006). *The New IDEA: Summary of the Individuals with Disabilities Education Improvement Act of 2004 (P.L. 108-446)*. Retrieved from http://www.aota.org.

American Occupational Therapy Association. (2010). Driving and community mobility. *American Journal of Occupational Therapy, 64*(6), S112-S124.

American Occupational Therapy Association. (2011). *Fact sheet: Home modifications and occupational therapy.* Bethesda, MD: AOTA Press.

American Occupational Therapy Association. (2012). *Fact sheet: The occupational therapy role in driving and community mobility across the lifespan.* Bethesda, MD: AOTA Press.

American Occupational Therapy Association. (2014a). Occupational therapy practice framework: Domain and process (3rd ed.). *American Journal of Occupational Therapy, 68*(Suppl. 1), S1-S48. doi:10.5014/ajot.2014.682006

American Occupational Therapy Association. (2014b). Scope of practice. *American Journal of Occupational Therapy, 68*(Suppl. 3), S34-S40.

American Occupational Therapy Association. (2015). *2011 Accreditation Council for Occupational Therapy Education standards and interpretive guide.* Retrieved from http://www.aota.org/-/media/Corporate/Files/EducationCareers/Accredit/Standards/2011-Standards-and-Interpretive-Guide.pdf

American Occupational Therapy Association. (2016a). *Spectrum of driver services.* Retrieved from https://www.aota.org/-/media/Corporate/Files/Practice/Aging/Driving/Spectrum-of-Driving-Services-2014.pdf

American Occupational Therapy Association. (2016b). *Driving and community mobility.* Retrieved from http://www.aota.org/Practice/Productive-Aging/Driving.aspx

Association for Driver Rehabilitation Specialists. (2016). *CRDS certification.* Retrieved from http://www.aded.net/?page=215

Baum, M. C. (2006). Centennial challenges, millennium opportunities: Presidential address, 2006. *American Journal of Occupational Therapy, 60*, 609-616.

Berg, K., Hines, M., & Allen, S. (2002). Wheelchair users at home: Few home modifications and many injurious falls. *American Journal of Public Health, 92*(1), 48.

Bolding, D., Adler, C., Tipton-Burton, M., & Verran, A. (2013). Mobility. In H. M. Pendleton & W. Schultz-Krohn (Eds.), *Pedretti's occupational therapy* (7th ed., pp. 233-294). St. Louis, MO: Elsevier Mosby.

Brienza, D., Kelsey, S., Karg, P., Allegretti, A., Olson, M., Schmeler, M., & Holm, M. (2010). A randomized clinical trial on preventing pressure ulcers with wheelchair seat cushions. *Journal of the American Geriatric Society, 58*, 2308-2304.

Brookside Associates Multi-Media Edition. (2007). Nursing Fundamentals I. Retrieved from http://www.brooksidepress.org/Products/Nursing_Fundamentals_1/Index.htm

Chipchase, S. Y., Lincoln, N. B., & Radford, K. A. (2003). Measuring fatigue in people with multiple sclerosis. *Disability and Rehabilitation, 25*(14), 778-784.

Classen, S., Levy, C., Meyer, D. L., Bewernitz, M., Lanford, D. N., & Mann, W. C. (2011). Simulated driving performance of combat veterans with mild traumatic brain injury and posttraumatic stress disorder: A pilot study. *American Journal of Occupational Therapy, 65*, 419-427.

Cooper, R. A., Ferretti, E., Oyster, M., Kelleher, A., & Cooper, R. (2011). The relationship between wheelchair mobility patterns and community participation among individuals with spinal cord injury. *Assistive Technology, 23*, 177-183.

Darragh, A. R., Campo, M. A., Frost, L., Miller, M., Pentico, M., & Margulis, H. (2013). Safe patient handling equipment in therapy practice: Implications for rehabilitation. *American Journal of Occupational Therapy, 67*, 45-53. doi:10.5014/ajot.2013.005389

Davies, A., Souza, L. H., & Frank, A. O. (2003). Changes in the quality of life in severely disabled people following provision of powered indoor/outdoor chairs. *Disability and Rehabilitation, 25*(6), 286.

Donnelly, C., Eng, J. J., Hall, J., Alford, L., Gianchino, R., Norton, K., et al. (2004). Client centered assessment and the identification of meaningful treatment goals for individuals with a spinal cord injury. *Spinal Cord, 42*, 302-307.

Fliess-Douer, O., Vanlandewijck, Y. C., & van der Woude, L. H. (2012). Most essential wheeled mobility skills for daily life: an international survey among Paralympic wheelchair athletes with spinal cord injury. *Archives of Physical Medicine and Rehabilitation, 93*, 629-635.

Fomiatti, R., Richmond, J., Moir, L., & Millsteed, J. (2013). A systematic review of the impact of powered mobility devices on older adults' activity engagement. *Physical and Occupational Therapy in Geriatrics, 31*(4), 297-309. doi:10.3109/02703181.2013.846451

Freeman, E. E., Gange, S. J., Munoz, B., & West, S. K. (2006). Driving status and risk of entry into long-term care in older adults. *American Journal of Public Health, 96*(7), 1254-1259.

Golisz, K. (2014). From the desk of the guest editor: Occupational therapy and driving and community mobility for older adults. *American Journal of Occupational Therapy, 68*, 654-656. doi:10.5014/ajot.2014.013144

Hendershot, G. E. (2003). Mobility limitations and complementary and alternative medicine: Are people with disabilities more likely to pray? *American Journal of Public Health, 93*(7), 1079-1080.

Henriksson, P., & Peters, B. (2004). Safety and mobility of people with disabilities driving adapted cars. *Scandinavian Journal of Occupational Therapy, 11*, 54-61.

Hunt, L., Brown, A. E., & Gilman, I. P. (2010). Drivers with dementia and outcomes of becoming lost while driving. *American Journal of Occupational Therapy, 64*, 225-232.

Idler, E. L., & Kasl, S. V. (1997). Religion among disabled and nondisabled persons, II: Attendance at religion services as a predictor of the course of disability. *Journal of Gerontology, 52B*, S306-S316.

Liu, H., Grando, V., Zabel, R., & Nolen, J. (2009). Pilot study evaluating fear of falling and falls among older rolling walker users. *International Journal of Therapy and Rehabilitation, 16*(12), 670-675.

Loukas, K. M. (2008). The evolution of language and perception of disability in occupational therapy. *The Education Special Interest Section Newsletter, 18*(2), 1-4.

Meriano, C., & Latella, D. (2008). Activities of daily living. In C. Meriano & D. Latella (Eds.), *Occupational therapy interventions: Function and occupations* (pp. 129-236). Thorofare, NJ: SLACK Incorporated.

Minkel, J. L. (2000). Seating and mobility considerations for people with spinal cord injury. *Physical Therapy, 80*(7), 701-709.

Nilsson, I., Nyqvist, F., Gustafson, Y., & Nygard, M. (2015). Leisure engagement: Medical conditions, mobility difficulties, and activity limitations—A later life perspective. *Journal of Aging Research, 2015*(610154). doi:10.1155/2015/610154

Pierce, S. (2002). Restoring competence in mobility. In C. A. Trombly & M. V. Radomski (Eds.), *Occupational therapy for physical dysfunction* (5th ed., pp. 665-693). Philadelphia, PA: Lippincott Williams and Wilkins.

Pierson, F. M., & Fairchild, S. L. (2008). *Principles and techniques of patient care* (4th ed.). St. Louis, MO: Saunders Elsevier.

Porter, E. J., Matsuda, S., & Benson, J. J. (2011). Intentions of older homebound women about maintaining proximity to a cane or walker and using it at home. *Journal of Applied Gerontology, 30*(4), 485-504.

Prasad, R. S., Hunter, J., & Hanley, J. (2006). Driving experiences of disabled drivers. *Clinical Rehabilitation, 20*(5), 445-450.

Radford, K. A., Lincoln, N. B., & Lennox, G. (2004). The effects of cognitive abilities on driving in people with Parkinson's disease. *Disability and Rehabilitation, 26*(2), 65-70.

Rogers, H., Berman, S., Fails, D., & Jaser, J. (2003). A comparison of functional mobility in standard versus ultralight wheelchairs as measured by performance on a community obstacle course. *Disability and Rehabilitation, 25*(19), 1083-1088.

Royeen, C. B. (2002). Occupation reconsidered. *Occupational Therapy International, 9*(2), 111-120.

Runyan, C. (2006). Neuro-developmental treatment of adult hemiplegia. In H. M. Pendleton & W. Schultz-Krohn (Eds.), *Pedretti's occupational therapy practice skills for physical dysfunction* (6th ed., pp. 769-790). St. Louis, MO: Mosby Elsevier.

Santucci, M. E. (2008). Instrumental activities of daily living. In C. Meriano & D. Latella (Eds.), *Occupational therapy interventions: Function and occupations* (pp. 238-283). Thorofare, NJ: SLACK Incorporated.

Shaw, L., Polgar, J. M., Vrkljan, B., & Jacobson, J. (2010). Seniors' perceptions of vehicle safety risks and needs. *American Journal of Occupational Therapy, 64*, 215-224.

Shumway-Cook, A., Ciol, M. A., Grubon, W., & Robinson, C. (2005). Incidence of risk factors for falls following hip fracture in community dwelling older adults. *Physical Therapy, 85*, 648-655.

Smith, J. (2013). Documentation of occupational therapy services. In H. M. Pendleton & W. Schultz-Krohn (Eds.), *Pedretti's occupational therapy* (7th ed., pp. 117-139). St. Louis, MO: Elsevier Mosby.

Stav, W. B. (2014a). Consensus statements on occupational therapy education and professional development related to driving and community mobility. *Occupational Therapy in Health Care, 28*(2), 169-175. doi:10.3109/07380577.2014.904539

Stav, W. B. (2014b). Updated systematic review on older adult community mobility and driving licensing policies. *American Journal of Occupational Therapy, 68*, 681-689. doi: 10.5014/ajot.2014.011510

Stav, W. B., & Lieberman, D. (2008). From the desk of the editor. *American Journal of Occupational Therapy, 62*(2), 127-129.

Stav, W., Weidley, L. S., & Love, A. (2011). Barriers to developing and sustaining driving and community mobility programs. *American Journal of Occupational Therapy, 65*, e38-e45. doi:10.5014/ajot.2011.002097

Thate, M., Gulden, B., Lefebvre, J., & Springer, E. (2011). CarFit: Finding the right fit for the older driver. *Gerontology Special Interest Section Quarterly, 34*(4), 1-4.

Tieman, B. L., Palisano, R. J., Gracely, E. J., & Rosenbaum, P. L. (2004). Gross motor capability and performance of mobility in children with cerebral palsy: A comparison across home, school and outdoors/community settings. *Physical Therapy, 84*(5), 419-427.

U.S. Department of Justice. (n.d.). *Americans with Disabilities Act*. Retrieved from http://www.ada.gov

Vrkljan, B., Cranney, A., Worswick, J., O'Donnal, S., Li, L. C., Gelinas, I., ... Marshall, S. (2010). Supporting safe driving with arthritis: Developing a driving toolkit for clinical practice and consumer use. *American Journal of Occupational Therapy, 64*, 259-267.

Walker, K. A., Morgan, K. A., Morris, C. L., DeGroot, K. K., Hollingsworth, H. H., & Gray, D. B. (2010). Development of a community mobility skills course for people who use mobility devices. *American Journal of Occupational Therapy, 65*, 547-554.

Wang, P. P., Badley, E. M., & Gignac, M. (2004). Activity limitation, coping efficacy and self-perceived physical independence in people with disability. *Disability and Rehabilitation, 26*(13), 785-793.

Wheelchair Net. (2006). *Wheelchair and seating evaluations*. Retrieved from http://www.wheelchairnet.org/wcn_ProdServ/Consumers/evaluations.html

Wresstle, E., & Samuelsson, K. (2004). User satisfaction with mobility assistive devices. *Scandinavian Journal of Occupational Therapy, 11*(3), 143-150.

Yuen, H. K., & Burik, J. K. (2011). Brief report–Survey of driving evaluation and rehabilitation curricula in occupational therapy education programs. *American Journal of Occupational Therapy, 65*(2), 217-220. doi:10.5014/ajot.2011.000810

Wilson, P. E., Lange, M. L., & Mandac, B. R. (2006). *Seating evaluation and wheelchair prescription*. Retrieved from http://emedicine.medscape.com/article/318092-overview

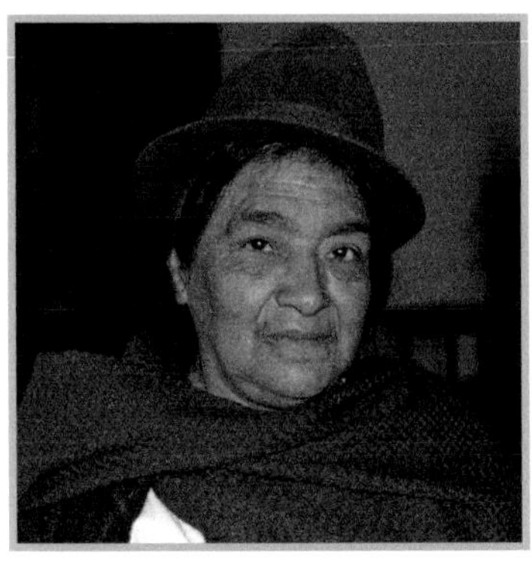

# 34

# Physical Agent Modalities

Alfred G. Bracciano, MSA, EdD, OTR/L, FAOTA

**ACOTE STANDARDS EXPLORED IN THIS CHAPTER**

B.5.13, B.5.14

**KEY VOCABULARY**

- **Deep thermal agents:** Those modalities that penetrate to a depth of 5 cm and cause a change in tissue temperature and biophysiology. Deep thermal agents include, but are not limited to, ultrasound, phonophoresis, diathermy, and other commercially available technologies.
- **Electrotherapeutic agents:** Use electricity and the electromagnetic spectrum to facilitate tissue healing, improve muscle strength and endurance, decrease edema, modulate pain, decrease the inflammatory process, and modify the healing process. Electrotherapeutic agents include, but are not limited to, neuromuscular electrical stimulation, functional electrical stimulation, transcutaneous electrical nerve stimulation, high-voltage galvanic stimulation for tissue and wound repair, high-voltage pulsed current, direct current, iontophoresis, and other commercially available technologies (American Occupational Therapy Association [AOTA], 2012; Bracciano, 2008).

*(continued)*



Jacobs, K., & MacRae, N. (Eds.).
*Occupational Therapy Essentials for Clinical Competence, Third Edition* (pp. 501-519).

KEY VOCABULARY (CONTINUED)

- **Physical agent modalities:** Those procedures and interventions that are systematically applied to modify specific client factors when neurological, musculoskeletal, or skin conditions are present that may be limiting occupational performance. Physical agent modalities use various forms of energy to modulate pain, modify tissue healing, increase tissue extensibility, modify skin and scar tissue, and decrease edema or inflammation. Physical agent modalities are used in preparation for or concurrently with purposeful and occupation-based activities (AOTA, 2012; Bracciano, 2008).
- **Superficial thermal agents:** Those modalities that penetrate to a depth of 1 to 2 cm and cause a change in tissue temperature and biophysiology. Superficial thermal agents include, but are not limited to, hydrotherapy/whirlpool, cryotherapy (cold packs, ice), Fluidotherapy, hot packs, paraffin, water, infrared, and other commercially available superficial heating and cooling technologies (AOTA, 2012).

The profession of occupational therapy has long debated the role and use of physical agent modalities. Misperceptions and misinformation often articulated include that physical agent modalities are passive in nature and beyond the scope of our practice. There has often been heated dialogue over whether physical agent modalities were "occupational" in nature or were the purview of other disciplines and had no role in intervention. There has been controversy regarding training, preparation, and competency, with wide variability in academic and clinical preparation and training (Cornish-Painter, Peterson, & Lindstrom-Hazel, 1997; Glauner, Ekes, James, & Holm, 1997). To some extent, the debate continues between academics, theoreticians, and clinicians. The American Occupational Therapy Association (AOTA) clarified and strengthened the definition of physical agent modalities and their role and use as preparatory agents in the AOTA 2012 position statement. Partially driven by the need to strengthen regulatory oversight of physical agent modalities, the AOTA revised its position statement to assist regulatory bodies and practitioners outline and define physical agent modality use. The 2011 Accreditation Council for Occupational Therapy Education (ACOTE) Standards (B.5.15 and B.5.16) reinforced the need and responsibility of academic institutions and occupational therapy practitioners to provide basic education and theory behind physical agent modality use, though there is great variability in the academic preparation of this content area.

Unfortunately, a broad interpretation of the standards has left many occupational therapy programs providing minimal education and preparation in this area. The Standards (2011) specify that occupational therapy students will: "Demonstrate safe and effective application of superficial thermal and mechanical modalities as a preparatory measure to manage pain and improve occupational performance..." However, the interpretive guidelines for academic programs reduces the intent of the standard by stating: "The word 'demonstrate' does not require that a student actually perform the task to verify knowledge and understanding...." Not only does ACOTE apply a limited interpretation of the Standard (and the definition of demonstrate), but it also minimizes the intent and impact of the standard further by stating that academic programs in States with specific licensing requirements for physical agents need only provide enough preparation to expose the students to modalities used in practice.

In addition, academic programs need only prepare students with enough superficial knowledge and experience to prepare them for, "...the NBCOT Examination and for practice outside of the state in which the educational institution resides" (ACOTE, 2011). From a literal interpretation, an academic program in a state with specific regulatory guidelines for physical agent modalities used by occupational therapists does not have to prepare graduates to meet unique state regulatory requirements specified to practice in their respective state. Failure to prepare graduates to meet the scope of practice and licensing requirements within the academic institution's location/state is incongruous with the AOTA *Occupational Therapy Code of Ethics* (2015), Principle 1E—provide occupational therapy services that are within each practitioner's level of competence and scope of practice (e.g., qualifications, experience, and the law). State licensing regulations are promulgated to protect the consumer/clients from unscrupulous or ill-prepared clinicians. The disconnect between academics and academic programs failing to prepare students to practice in states with specific licensing and regulatory language and clinicians inadequately prepared who are using modalities within the full scope of practice is incongruous, limiting to the profession and contrary to the AOTA's *Code of Ethics*.

Physical agent modalities are a tool for clinicians to use and are one component of the intervention process. Physical agents should always be used preparatory to or concurrently with engagement in occupational activities and tasks The AOTA's position paper (2012) defines physical agent modalities as those procedures and interventions that are systematically applied to modify specific client factors when neurological, musculoskeletal, or skin conditions are present that may be limiting occupational performance. Physical agent modalities use various forms of energy to modulate pain, modify tissue healing, increase tissue extensibility, modify skin and scar tissue, and decrease edema or inflammation. Physical agent modalities are used in preparation for or concurrently with purposeful and occupation-based activities (Bracciano, 2008). An understanding of the classification system for physical agents and their mechanism of action will facilitate selection of appropriate intervention based on the clinical condition and needs of the client.

Physical agent modalities are used as part of clinical intervention to enhance engagement in occupation and to facilitate healing and performance. Many clinicians view the application of physical agents as an external, ancillary intervention with a generalized reaction that may decrease pain or improve client comfort. There is little recognition that by using physical agents we manipulate healing tissue at a cellular level, or at the level of the client factor (AOTA, 2014). Client factors reside within the individual and influence the performance of occupations. Client factors are affected by the presence or absence of disease, disability, or illness and include body functions and structures. Client factors include structures related to the various systems that make up the human body, including the integumentary, cardiovascular, pulmonary, musculoskeletal, and neurological systems—the biophysiological components that provide a foundational level for performance. Physical agent modalities affect client factors at a systems level; the biophysiological, cellular level, affecting the healing process and structures affected by disease, illness, or disability. Clinical consideration of the appropriate timing and application may facilitate the healing process and ultimately improve occupational performance. Physical agents can be a powerful adjunct to intervention and will facilitate outcomes and speed recovery when used appropriately and judiciously. Physical agents should never be used singularly or in and of themselves. To do so is not considered occupational therapy.

Physical agents are often used in the intervention of musculoskeletal injuries, or by therapists whose primary practice is hands. This concept is both limiting to the profession and to the client. The fundamental physiological principles related to healing and the influence of physical agents on that process are consistent whether the tissue is located in the hand, shoulder, knee, or back. An appreciation of the impact physical agents have on physiological and systemic processes (client factors) will facilitate clinical reasoning and generalization of the interventions to other conditions and injuries. Occupational therapy practitioners bring the unique perspective of occupation and performance to the use of these agents as part of the intervention process, and research has demonstrated the effectiveness of pairing movement, valued tasks, and activities with physical agents such as electrotherapy and improved outcomes. There have been dramatic advances in technology, equipment, and research related to physical agents, and to neglect their use as a part of occupational therapy intervention or to overlook their impact to facilitate healing and performance is both limiting to the profession and to the client.

This chapter will provide a broad overview of the different categories of physical agent modalities and their clinical use. Students and practitioners are encouraged to explore additional material and educational opportunities, which can provide the physiological basis and depth of knowledge necessary to safely integrate physical agents into clinical practice and to meet specific state regulatory and licensing requirements. The reader is encouraged to review specific regulatory requirements for the state in which he or she will be practicing as well as any institutional requirements. The terms *physical agent modality, physical agent,* and *physical modality* can be used interchangeably.

## Regulatory Issues and the Role of the Occupational Therapy Assistant

As physical agent modalities have taken on greater significance as an adjunct to occupational therapy intervention, so too have regulatory restrictions. Many states such as Georgia, Florida, Kentucky, Tennessee, Nebraska, Montana, South Dakota, Maryland, New Hampshire, New York, Illinois, and California have specific requirements, language, or separate licensing regulations that must be met before physical agents can be used by occupational therapy practitioners. Most of these states require a specific number of continuing education hours, training, or experience that must be met before physical agents can be used. It is the responsibility of clinicians to know what their respective state requires before using physical agents in clinical practice. Occupational therapy assistants must also meet these regulatory requirements. To date, Nebraska is the only state that restricts occupational therapy assistants to only superficial thermal agents. In all other states with licensing regulations, occupational therapy assistants can apply physical agents under the direction and supervision of the occupational therapist. Some hospitals or clinical settings may also have restrictions or require additional institutional credentialing before using physical agents. It is the ethical and legal responsibility of the occupational therapy practitioner to be aware of all regulatory issues prior to incorporating physical agents as a component of clinical practice and to have documented evidence of competency in the application and safe use of physical agent modalities.

The AOTA's position paper on physical agent modalities (AOTA, 2012) outlines the role and responsibilities of the occupational therapist and occupational therapy assistant. The occupational therapist is responsible for determining physical agent modality use for the specific clinical condition being treated. The occupational therapy assistant can administer physical agent modalities as a part of the intervention plan under the direction and supervision of the occupational therapist. Both the occupational therapist and assistant must meet and comply with all institutional and state regulatory requirements for supervision, licensure, and competency to use physical agents as an adjunct to occupational therapy intervention (AOTA, 2012).

## Physical Agent Modality Classifications

There are four primary classifications of physical agents commonly used by occupational therapy practitioners: superficial thermal agents, deep thermal agents, electrotherapeutic agents, and mechanical devices. The classifications describe the depth of penetration or mechanism of action and provide a convenient method for selection of an agent for the practitioner. Superficial thermal agents are the therapeutic application of any modality that elevates or lowers the temperature of the skin and superficial subcutaneous tissue to a depth of 1 to 2 cm. Common superficial thermal agents include hydrotherapy/whirlpool, cryotherapy, hot packs, paraffin, and Fluidotherapy. Many of these modalities are historically the most commonly used agents by occupational therapy practitioners and are often considered as relatively "safe" in application and effect. However, superficial agents such as hot packs or paraffin can cause serious burns or damage to tissues; care should be used with these applications, and they require close monitoring of the client.

Deep thermal agents include therapeutic ultrasound, phonophoresis, and diathermy and are categorized according to their depth of penetration. Deep thermal agents will affect tissue to a depth of 5 cm and may exert a thermal or mechanical effect. Ultrasound and diathermy are unique in that both modalities can have either a superficial or deep effect depending on the parameters used by the practitioner.

Electrotherapeutic agents are those electrical agents that possess electromagnetic properties and include biofeedback, electrical muscle stimulation, neuromuscular electrical stimulation (NMES), functional electrical stimulation (FES), transcutaneous electrical nerve stimulation (TENS), electrical stimulation for tissue repair (ESTR), high-voltage galvanic stimulation (HVGS), and iontophoresis and low-level light therapy or lasers. Electrotherapeutic agents use electricity and the electromagnetic spectrum to facilitate tissue healing, improve muscle strength and endurance, decrease edema, modulate pain, decrease the inflammatory process, and modify the healing process (AOTA, 2012; Bracciano, 2008). Mechanical devices may include vasopneumatic devices and continuous passive motion (CPM) devices that exert a mechanical force on the underlying tissue (AOTA, 2012).

This chapter will review the mechanism of action and clinical applications of the most commonly used physical agent modalities. The reader is encouraged to continue learning about physical agents through academic preparation, continuing education, reading, and research. Practitioners who will be using physical agents should be able to demonstrate competency and ensure that they have a thorough grounding in the assessment, application, precautions, indications, and contraindications of the physical agents administered. Failure to integrate the theory and application of physical agents as part of the clinical reasoning process will make practitioners mere technicians in using physical agent modalities.

## Biophysiology of Wound Healing—An Occupational Perspective

Occupational therapy practitioners are adept at assessing the client holistically and providing interventions and adaptations to facilitate independence and performance. The interventions and activities we use are very often "visual" to practitioners in that we can physically "see" or visualize what we or the client are doing. We can see how the client is responding in a very concrete way. In effect, we have immediate feedback on our selection of therapeutic intervention or adaptation in an almost linear fashion. As occupational therapy practitioners, we assess and address the performance skills, patterns, contexts, and demands of the client that have been affected by the disease or disorder.

Because of our holistic view of the client's function, we often overlook the ability to influence the unique client factors, body functions, or physiological processes that underlie all performance and function (World Health Organization, 2001, p. 10). Because of our educational training and our theoretical and philosophical approach to illness, injury, or disability, we often fail to take into consideration the primary component of performance—cellular and physiological function at a systems level. We often fail to recognize how selection of appropriate physical agents, preparatory to occupation, can facilitate and influence the healing process in the client. We have become adept at providing holistic adaptations to performance deficits but have failed to appreciate or consider that we may actually be able to "heal" and manipulate at a cellular and physiological level those tissues and structures that have been affected. This may be due, in part, to our profession's historical evolution and movement away from the medical model, which was viewed as limiting and reductionist to the profession and in applying a "top-down" approach to intervention.

Wound healing is an overlapping process of repair that involves a series of events that encompass chemotaxis, cell division, neovascularization, synthesis of new extracellular matrix components, angiogenesis, epithelialization, and the formation and remodeling of scar tissue (Enoch & Harding, 2003; Simon, Romo, Al Moutran, & Pearson, 2016). Because of the impact that physical agents have at a cellular and physiological level, it is crucial for occupational therapy practitioners to have a foundational understanding of the healing process. Any injury to vascularized tissue causes a series of systemic responses that are distinct but overlapping: inflammation, proliferation, remodeling/maturation. This physiological "healing" response occurs to rid the area of any microorganisms, foreign materials, or dead tissues so that the repair process where new tissue will be formed can occur.

Wounds or injuries can be caused by disease; by vascular insufficiency due to compromised venous or arterial flow leading to ischemia or insufficient blood flow; by trauma such as abrasions, lacerations, avulsions, punctures, burns, or even by surgery. These wounds and injuries are often accompanied by pain, limited motion, and decreased motor function and occupational performance. Chronic inflammation, infection, and scarring may also cause complications, preventing a full return to function and performance.

The phases of healing are overlapping and vary in length. A healing wound or injury may demonstrate all three phases at the same time. The three phases of healing include the inflammatory phase (0 to 3 days), proliferative phase (3 to 24 days), and maturation phase (25 to 365 days; Andreadis, 2006; Bolton & van Rijswijk, 1991). Injury to soft tissues below the skin depends on the nature of the causative factor, the location (either superficial or deep), and the material properties of the tissue. Practitioners should understand the phases and timing of healing, because the appropriate physical agent will facilitate or modify the response of the tissue, ultimately affecting outcomes. Improper application of physical agents may negatively influence the healing process and lead to further complications and potential tissue damage (Figure 34-1).

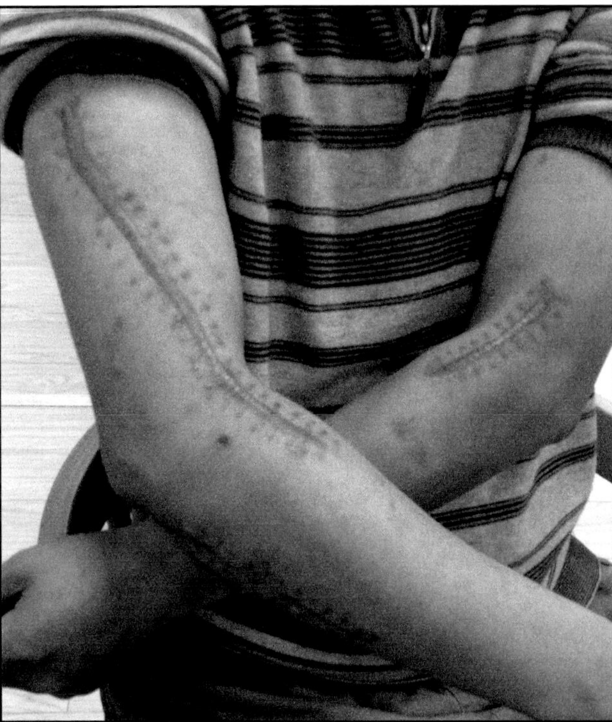

**Figure 34-1.** Example of remodeling phase of healing with imbalance of synthesis lysis process in a 32-year-old man post open reduction and internal fixation (ORIF) secondary to crush injury occurring at work. Note the raised hypertrophic scars within the scar margins.

# Wound Healing

## *Inflammatory Phase*

The inflammatory phase is the initial response of the body to injury and lasts approximately 72 hours. Inflammation is primarily a vascular response to the injury. The initial response to an injury is vasoconstriction, which decreases blood flow to the area, followed by vasodilation and the release of chemicals, nutrients, oxygen, and specialized cells to the site. There are a number of histochemical changes that occur and promote capillary permeability and chemotaxis, which is cell movement along a chemical concentration gradient, positively or negatively. A number of histochemical mediators are released into the tissue at this time, which facilitate formation of the fibrin clot and include histamine,

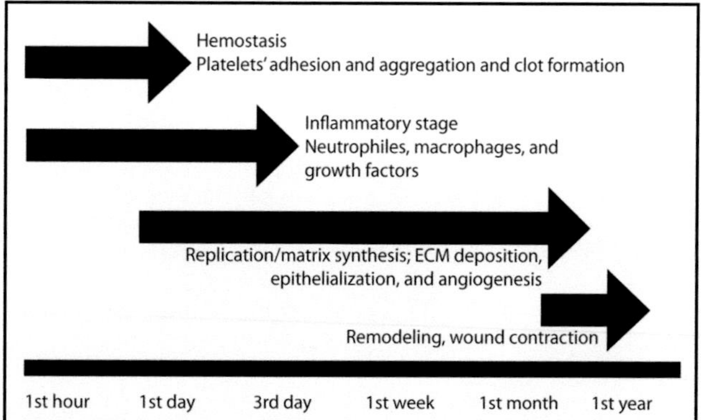


**Figure 34-2.** Representation of the primary phases of the tissue repair process, which occurs traumatically or surgically. Note that there is overlap to the phases, with each phase facilitating the next phase.

prostaglandins, growth factors, and others that stimulate the inflammatory process and facilitate migration of fibroblasts, macrophages, and other specialized cells that form the granulation tissue. A combination of blood exudate and serous transudate creates a reddened, hot, swollen, painful environment in the vicinity of the damaged tissue and wound. The inflammatory edema fills all spaces within the wound, surrounding all damaged or repaired structures, thereby binding them together as a one-wound structure. Some swelling in a wound is necessary to trigger the inflammatory process. However, if too little inflammation occurs, the healing response is slow; if too much inflammation occurs, an excessive scar is produced (Hardy, 1989; Figure 34-2).

## Proliferative Phase

During the proliferative phase of healing, granulation tissue matures to form scar tissue. This phase of healing lasts approximately 3 weeks. Two primary processes occur during this phase: fibroplasia and angiogenesis. Angiogenesis is the process of cell growth or cell budding to form new capillary blood vessels within injured tissue. In the body, angiogenesis is controlled through a balance of growth and inhibitory factors. Cancer is an example of the normal balance of inhibition and growth out of control. Fibroblasts migrate to the area to repair the connective tissue of the skin and are mediated by chemicals released from the macrophages. At the same time, new capillary growth in the damaged tissue is occurring in an effort to establish blood flow and remove the metabolic and repair wastes. Fibroblasts lay down collagen fibers that modify and change as the repair matures. Myofibroblasts are responsible for wound contraction and strength of the repair by drawing the outer edges of the wound together. Collagen fibers are oriented in response to local stress (force) that is applied to them and provide tensile strength in the appropriate or required direction. This force can occur internally or externally and is one of the reasons why occupational therapy practitioners use dynamic or static splinting, physical agent modalities, and grade activities and occupational tasks. The intent of our intervention is to manipulate healing structures through application of forces and energy that facilitate and enhance the healing process and strength and speed of the repair (Kloth & McCulloch, 1995; Figure 34-3).

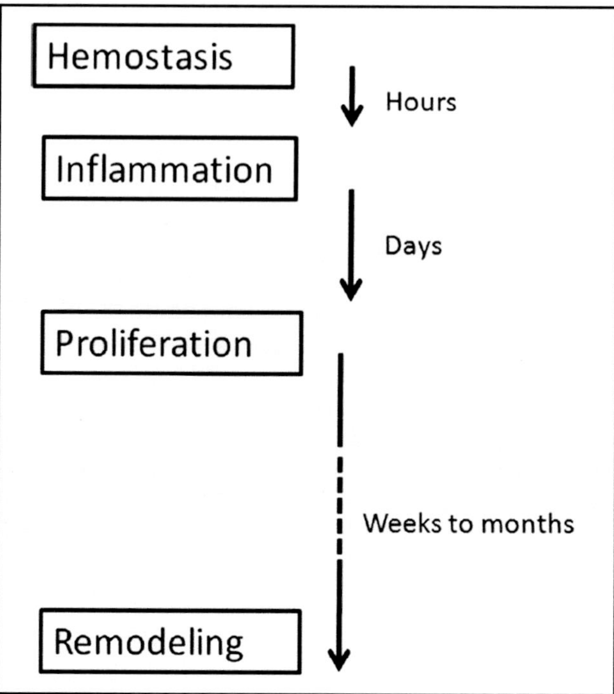


**Figure 34-3.** The phases of healing. Therapeutic interventions manipulate the healing process and structures through application of forces and energy to facilitate or enhance the healing process and tissue.

## Remodeling Phase

The remodeling or maturation phase of the healing process can continue for 1 to 2 years. Epithelialization is an important component of the remodeling phase of healing so that the wound has sufficient skin coverage. During this phase, there is continued fibroblastic activity and laying down of collagen fibers. In addition, there is a balance between the synthesis of the collagen fibers and the subsequent lysis, or breakdown of the collagen. The collagen fibers, healing scar, and tissue continue to realign themselves and differentiate in function based on the tension and forces applied to the healing area. Remodeling overlaps the proliferative phase of healing and can continue for up to 1 year or more. The process of scar remodeling is responsible for the final orientation and arrangement of collagen fibers. Remodeling is influenced by both synthesis–lysis balance and fiber orientation (Rabello, Souza, & Junior, 2014). When the balance

## Case Study

Suzanne was an active and dynamic 85-year-old woman. Her medical history was unremarkable, although she complained of having trouble hearing at times. Suzanne lived independently in a one-floor senior citizens' condominium complex. She no longer drove; however, she did use public transportation extensively to shop, visit her friends for lunch, and attend church services. She was very active in her church and enjoyed socializing with her friends. One wintry day while shoveling snow off the walkway to her door, she slipped and fell. In an attempt to "catch" herself, she put out her arm, extending it fully. When she landed on the ground, she fractured her distal radius, a classic "FOOSH" (fall on outstretched hand). She was taken to the emergency room, where she was placed in a soft splint to accommodate the swelling; 2 days later, she underwent closed reduction of the fracture and was placed in a cast. X-rays indicated good apposition (alignment of the two fragments) of the fractured ends. She healed quickly, and the cast was removed at 7 weeks.

Following removal of the cast, her skin was flaky, dry, and macerated. Although her physician reassured her that the break was "solid" and she should move her wrist and use her hand as much as possible, Suzanne was apprehensive and protective of the extremity. She kept the fingers of her hand closed, and when she moved, she had a tendency to hold her hand in slight flexion at the wrist in a protective, guarded pattern. She was referred for occupational therapy "evaluation and intervention." On the initial visit, the occupational therapy practitioner reviewed the x-rays and report to ensure the fracture was solidly healed and in good alignment and confirmed that there were no biomechanical causes for her hesitancy and guarding of the wrist and hand. When asked to move her hand and wrist, Suzanne politely, but firmly, replied she "couldn't" and was "afraid it was going to hurt." Suzanne's hesitancy to use the hand was limiting her ability to complete her daily routines and self-care activities. She was struggling to dress herself and manipulate fastenings, and she was having difficulty cooking and cleaning because she would use the extremity as a "wedge" to hold objects against her body and forearm rather than grasping objects using her wrist and fingers actively. Passive range of motion appeared to be within functional limits, but Suzanne would not actively use her hand to grasp or manipulate objects. The occupational therapy practitioner was aware that immobilization of the forearm due to the cast could cause disuse atrophy and generalized weakness in the arm and hand and was anxious to get Suzanne moving to prevent fibrosis or adhesions in her shoulder due to lack of movement caused by the guarded position of the arm and hand (Marimuthu, Murton, & Greeenhaff, 2011). The practitioner also realized that the prolonged immobilization may have contributed to distorted sensory perception in kinesthesia and proprioception, which could make Suzanne feel that her arm and hand were not "moving the same" as before the fall.

It was determined by the occupational therapy practitioner to prepare the tissue and area before engaging Suzanne in a variety of activities that would ensure her use of the hand and extremity. Suzanne's skin was dry and flaky, and the skin that was under the cast was "smelly" and macerated. She was motivated to "clean up [her] arm and get rid of the dead skin." The occupational therapy practitioner decided to use a warm hand whirlpool, with the water at a temperature between 102°F and 104°F with a gentle agitation. Suzanne was given a washcloth with which to "scrub" the dry skin off and was assisted by the occupational therapy practitioner in this task. Suzanne diligently "cleaned" the dead slough off her forearm and allowed the occupational therapist to assist. During this time, Suzanne was extending and flexing her fingers and actively moving her wrist in flexion and extension, as well as in supination and pronation of the forearm. After 20 minutes, the practitioner removed Suzanne's extremity from the water, dried the skin, and applied lotion to the forearm and digits, gently mobilizing and manipulating the wrist and fingers in the process. Suzanne mentioned how the warm water "relaxed" her arm and hand, and she was instructed to "soak" her hand in the sink filled with warm water at home, rubbing the extremity with a washcloth to further clean off the dried skin and to provide sensory input into the extremity. Suzanne quickly began to use her healed arm and hand more functionally following a few short interventions, which incorporated the use of superficial warmth in preparing the tissue to engage in a variety of activities, movements, and exercises to strengthen her arm and hand and to improve fine motor control and object manipulation, including donning and doffing a variety of clothing, fastenings, and food preparation. Because of the superficial heating of the tissue, Suzanne was soon functionally independent again, visiting her friends for lunch, and engaging in her active preinjury activities and tasks.

between synthesis and lysis is out of sync, the probability of keloid or hypertrophic scarring increases and may be problematic (Cuzzell, 2002; Gogia, 1995; see Figure 34-1).

During maturation, remodeling of the collagen results in the early, randomly deposited scar tissue arranged in both a linear and lateral orientation approximating the tissues that surround it. During the remodeling phase, the original wound, which resulted in a single scar, now has to differentiate itself to provide a function, such as tendon, muscle, or skin. As occupational therapy practitioners, we attempt to modify this process through our interventions including physical agents, splinting, and engagement in occupational tasks and activities. Induction theory states that the tissue will attempt to mimic the characteristics of the tissue that is surrounding it, whereas tension theory states that a low-load, long-duration stress (force) on the healing tissue—through the application of pressure, dynamic splinting, mobilization, soft tissue loading and unloading, and other techniques—accounts for the differentiation in the healing tissue. The correct and timely selection and application of the physical agent and "force" to the tissue is crucial in effecting positive clinical outcomes (Ankrom et al., 2005).

## Superficial Thermal Agents

Superficial thermal agents are those interventions that cause a temperature change in the underlying tissue. Tissue temperature can be modified through the application of heat to increase tissue temperature, or it can be cooled through the application of cold agents. The use of heat or cold to decrease pain and improve function has a long history. It is important to understand the physiological response to these modalities to determine how they can be used as part of the intervention process. Heat or cold is transmitted to the underlying tissue through the following five primary principles:

1. Conduction refers to heat transfer through direct contact with the underlying tissue. The heat loss or gain occurs when there is contact between materials that possess different temperatures. For example, heat will be absorbed by the body when a hot pack is applied, whereas a cold pack will conduct heat away from the underlying tissue. Both methods of heat transfer through the process of conduction.
2. Convection refers to the transfer of heat or cold to the body through the movement of air, matter, liquids, or particles over and around the extremity or body part. An example of a form of convection is Fluidotherapy, where the air temperature can be adjusted and the cellulose particles are circulated by the force of the air around the treated extremity.
3. Radiation occurs when the radiant energy transfers heat through the air from a warm source, such as an infrared lamp, to a cooler source. The infrared lamps that are often seen in restaurants are an example of this process. Infrared lamps are rarely used in rehabilitation anymore.
4. Conversion occurs when there is a temperature change resulting from the transformation of energy from one form to another. Clinically, this can be seen when thermal ultrasound is used to heat tissue—the sound energy is transformed to thermal or heat energy as the cells respond to the sound waves by vibrating, changing the sound energy into kinetic energy.
5. Evaporation is the transformation of a liquid into a gaseous state. During this change, there is an exchange of energy with the by-product of heat being released when the liquid is transformed into a gas. The most common clinical form of evaporation occurs with the use of vapocoolant sprays, which cause a decrease in skin temperature due to the evaporative effects of the spray.

## Heat Agents

There are a variety of therapeutic heat agents used by occupational therapy practitioners, and these are categorized according to their depth of penetration. These thermal agents are considered either deep or superficial. Superficial heating agents include hot packs, over-the-counter "thermal wraps," Fluidotherapy, paraffin, and warm whirlpool. All of these agents increase the superficial temperatures of the skin and subcutaneous tissues to a depth of approximately 1 to 2 cm. Ultrasound, in its superficial settings (3-MHz frequency), has a depth of penetration of approximately 1 to 2 cm. Short wave diathermy is another physical agent that can increase tissue temperature at deeper levels, but it is rarely used by occupational therapy practitioners.

The extent of temperature change on the underlying tissue depends on four primary factors: the temperature difference between the physical agent being applied and the underlying tissue, the duration of the exposure of the tissue to the agent, the intensity of the heat agent, and the volume or area of the tissue being treated. The thermal conductivity of the tissue is also a factor that must be taken into consideration because adipose or fat tissue will act as an insulator, whereas blood and muscle, due to their blood flow and water content, absorb and conduct heat more efficiently.

### *Tissue Temperature Effect*

The degree of tissue temperature elevation depends on the following:

- Volume or area being treated
- Duration of the application
- Temperature variation between the tissue and the physical agent
- Thermal conductivity of the tissue

### *Physiological Response to Heat*

The primary purpose for applying a thermal agent is to increase the temperature of soft tissue to a specific therapeutic range so a physiological response will occur. When the temperature of soft tissue is increased between the range of 104°F and 113°F, it can have a positive therapeutic effect on the client. If the soft tissue is heated to a temperature of less than 104°F, cell metabolism will not be stimulated adequately enough to elicit a therapeutic response. Conversely, if the same tissue is heated to greater than 113°F, catabolism and cell death may occur. The physiological response to heat will vary according to the duration of the application, the volume of tissue being treated, and how long the modality is applied. Heating doses are considered either mild or vigorous, with the higher temperatures producing more noticeable redness or hyperemia to the underlying tissue. The application of heat causes a number of physiological responses, including increased blood flow to the area due to vasodilation of the blood vessels and increased rate of cell metabolism, oxygen consumption, capillary permeability, inflammation, and muscle contraction velocity. Conversely, the application of heat will decrease fluid viscosity of the tissue, pain, and muscle spasm (Loten et al., 2006). It is important to take into account not only the factors related previously but also the age of the client. Older clients may have an impaired ability to dissipate the heat effectively, and care must be taken to prevent burns or systemic overheating (Petrofsky et al., 2006).

## Clinical Application and Goals

The application of heat as an adjunct to intervention has many therapeutic goals. The application of heat to an extremity can aid in pain relief and decrease the muscle spasms that a client may be experiencing. Because blood flow increases as a result of heat, the outcome will be the removal of the local muscle metabolites and the reduction in sensitivity of the muscle spindles, which tend to stretch and cause pain (Michlovitz, Hun, Erasala, Hengehold, & Weingand, 2004). Heat application can also decrease muscle guarding and muscle spasm, which often lead to the pain-spasm-pain cycle and decrease the client's functional abilities and occupational performance. Heat applications placed on soft tissue also assist in increasing the tissue extensibility (Nadler, Steiner et al., 2003).

Superficial heating agents used in most clinics are typically capable of providing moderate and vigorous thermal dosages. A moderate dose involves elevating the tissue temperature between 102°F and 106°F and will result in only a slight increase of blood flow. This dosage level is effective when heat is indicated, but edema may occur. A vigorous dose results in a marked increase in blood flow. The temperature will increase rapidly, duration will be relatively long, and temperature elevation at the site of pathology will be high (between 107°F and 113°F). This dosage level is beneficial for ischemic conditions and for when heat is indicated and edema is not a concern. Heat will also increase viscosity and elasticity of the soft tissue–muscle tendon and joint capsule when combined with positional or dynamic stretch over a period of time (Robertson, Ward, & Jung, 2005). The average length of time for heat application is between 10 and 20 minutes for physiological effects to occur in the intervention tissue. The length of time depends on the factors identified earlier, the area of tissue being covered, the intensity of the heat, and the duration of application. Although there are different methods used to apply heat, the biophysiological response will always be the same. In addition, it is important to remember that there is a 10-minute window of opportunity following the application of heat within which the load or stretch must be applied, although positional stretch during the heat application can be utilized and is also effective (Kottke, Pauley, & Ptak, 1966; Laban, 1962).

Indications for using superficial thermal agents include the following:

- Stiff joints
- Subcutaneous adhesions
- Soft tissue contractures
- Chronic arthritis
- Subacute and chronic inflammation
- Cumulative trauma
- Wounds
- Neuromas
- Sympathetic nervous system disorders

## Precautions and Contraindications

The choice of heat selection depends on the area of tissue being treated and the goals established for the client. If the area is large and requires the medium to conform to the area (e.g., a shoulder), a hot pack would be an appropriate choice. Hands and wrists can be easily accommodated in either a Fluidotherapy unit or through the application of paraffin. The client's skin should be closely monitored during any heat application because the potential for thermal burns can be high if improperly applied. Heat applications should never be used over open lesions, cuts, lacerations, or sutures of the skin. The area being treated should be inspected prior to application of the thermal agent and the sensation of the area confirmed. The client's cognition, level of awareness, and ability to inform the therapist of any discomfort or pain should also be assessed and reviewed. The skin and treated area should be checked after the first 5 minutes of application to ensure that there are no adverse reactions. Close monitoring of the client is crucial because heat applications are the most common method of burning a client.

Precautions and contraindications for superficial thermal agents include the following:

- Peripheral vascular disease
- Acute inflammation
- Cancer or malignancies
- Acute hemorrhage
- Infection
- Primary repair of tendon or ligaments
- Advanced cardiac disease
- Obesity or fragile clients
- Compromised or limited cognitive status

- External pins/plates/hardware
- Sensory deficits
- Pregnancy

## Cryotherapy

Cryotherapy is the application of a cold agent to selected tissue. The physiological response to cold application is essentially the reverse of heat application. As with heat application, the physiological response to cold application depends on the duration of application, area or volume of the tissue being treated, and the rate at which the agent is being applied. With application of cold, the initial response in the underlying tissue is one of vasoconstriction. Superficial cooling agents are recommended for the inflammatory phase of healing and most acute conditions, producing a decrease in tissue temperature resulting in an analgesic effect (Costello, McInerney, Bleakley, Selfe, & Donnelly, 2012). Cryotherapy can be used clinically to decrease edema, spasticity, muscle spasm, and pain. As the duration of application is increased, the physiological response is one of decreased nerve conduction velocity, decreased delivery of leukocytes and phagocytes, decreased lymphatic and venous drainage, and decreased muscle excitability and muscle spindle depolarization (Barber, 2000; Gracies, 2001; Sanya & Bello, 1999; Welch et al., 2000). With short-duration applications, most clinical applications of cryotherapy will penetrate to a depth of approximately 1 cm, although longer durations may penetrate to a depth of 4 cm (Olson & Stravino, 1972). Commonly used cryoagents include commercially available ice packs, ice cups and ice packs made up of crushed ice, and cryopressure units that are effective following surgery to decrease pain and edema (Singh, Osbahr, Holovacs, Cawley, & Speer, 2001). It is important to recognize that physiological changes will occur when the temperature of the tissue drops below 80.6°F. Care must be taken when cryomodalities are applied for extended periods of time to prevent frostbite and tissue damage.

### *Precautions and Contraindications*

Cryotherapy can be an effective and safe modality when used within the appropriate clinical parameters. However, clients with difficulty in thermoregulation, sensory deficits, or hypersensitivity to cold would be contraindicated or require close monitoring of the application. Cryotherapy is contraindicated in those clients with cryoglobulinemia, Raynaud's disease, or cold urticaria. Systemic responses in clients with cold sensitivity include syncope, increased heart rate, flushing, and a drop in blood pressure. Close monitoring of the client's blood pressure and systemic response should be routinely performed with any thermal application, either heat or cold, with particular attention paid to elderly and obese individuals (Nadler, Prybicien, Malanga, & Sicher, 2003).

Precautions and contraindications include the following:

- Impaired circulation
- Obesity
- Fragile clients
- Peripheral vascular disease
- Hypersensitivity to cold
- Skin anesthesia
- Open wounds or skin conditions
- Infections

## Deep Thermal Agents: Therapeutic Ultrasound

Ultrasound has been used in medicine for diagnosis, in imaging structures for tissue destruction and surgery, and in rehabilitation for its thermal and nonthermal effects. Therapeutic ultrasound uses acoustic or sound energy to produce the physiological effects. There are two primary uses for ultrasound in rehabilitation: to heat deeper structures and tissue and to facilitate healing of soft tissues. The historical use of ultrasound was to raise the temperature of deep structures, such as tendon, ligament, and joint capsules. Ultrasound parameters can be configured to provide either a "superficial" effect, 3-MHz frequency, penetrating to a depth of 1 to 2 cm, or a "deep" effect, penetrating to up to 5 cm using a 1-MHz frequency.

Ultrasound units consist of an ultrasound generator that uses alternating electrical current and creates an acoustic wave at a specific frequency. The ultrasound unit consists of a power supply, oscillator circuit, transformer, coaxial cable, and transducer/sound head (the part that is actually placed on the client to administer the sound energy). The biophysical principle, which is the basis for ultrasound, is known as the *piezoelectric effect*. Essentially, when an alternating electrical current is passed through the crystal located in the sound head of the ultrasound transducer, the crystal responds by oscillating, expanding, and contracting. As the crystal expands and contracts in response to the electric current, it "vibrates," creating sound waves that are then transmitted through the use of a coupling agent (electrode gel) to the underlying tissue.

As the crystal expands and contracts in response to the electrical current, it produces sound waves that, when the transducer is placed on a body part, compress the underlying molecules lying in the path of the sound energy. This movement of the molecules in the underlying tissue, oscillating back and forth against each other, is known as a *longitudinal* or *compressional wave*. This sound wave and molecular movement will continue to expand until the energy is absorbed. When the sound wave reaches bone, it is generated along the periosteum and reflected back toward the surface, creating a shear wave. The sound wave traveling through the body will become attenuated as the energy is either absorbed or dispersed through reflection or refraction (Ter Haar, 1978).

Body tissue is not homogeneous, and each layer will transmit or absorb ultrasound energy according to its own unique properties. Fluid elements of the body have the lowest impedance, or resistance, to the sound energy and lowest acoustic absorption values. Bone has the highest impedance value and highest acoustic absorption coefficient. This means that bone will stop the flow of energy and absorb the energy from the ultrasound wave, causing physiologic changes. With higher energy levels produced by the ultrasound machine, there will be a concurrent effect of heating the tissue. In thermal applications, as the ultrasound is transmitted to the lower tissues coming in contact with the bone, most of the energy will be reflected back, where it will meet the energy that is being transmitted down into the tissue producing a "standing wave" or "hot spot," which can be painful and damage the tissue. To prevent the development of standing waves or hot spots, the sound head should be moved in small circular motions (Dyson, 1987).

To control the amount of energy and the biophysiological effect on the tissue, there are a number of factors that are considered and adjusted when using ultrasound including the frequency, duty cycle, time, and intensity. The frequency of ultrasound determines the number of complete wave cycles that are generated each second and determines the depth of penetration. In the United States, there are two frequencies that can be selected on most ultrasound machines: 1 or 3 MHz. As the number of cycles per second increases, the duration of each cycle and wavelength decreases, which accounts for the difference in the depth of penetration. The frequency of the ultrasound will influence the amount of energy that is absorbed with higher frequencies (3 MHz), delivering more energy but being superficial in depth. Ultrasound using a frequency of 3 MHz leads to a superficial effect (1 to 2 cm deep) compared to an intervention using a frequency of 1 MHz (2 to 5 cm deep; Fyfe & Bullock, 1985). Areas of the body such as the dorsal aspect of the hand, lateral and medial epicondyles, fingers, and other superficial structures would be more effectively treated using a frequency of 3 MHz. Deeper soft tissue structures such as the shoulder joint should be treated with a frequency of 1 MHz (Bracciano, 2008).

The biophysical effects of ultrasound depend on a number of factors, with the primary one being the intensity of the ultrasound and secondary consideration to the duty cycle or pulsing the energy. If the intensity is high enough, it will cause heating of the tissues, a thermal effect; whereas low-intensity and pulsed-mode delivery will result in nonthermal changes due to the "mechanical" effect of the ultrasound energy. Tissues are heated through the transfer of the sound energy into kinetic energy due to the oscillation of the molecules in the tissue responding to the sound waves. To increase the total amount of heat delivered to the targeted tissue, the duration of the ultrasound application and/or the intensity must be increased. Thermal effects of tissue heating will do the following (Enwemeka, 1989; Hong, Liu, & Yu, 1988; Rimington, Draper, Durrant, & Fellingham, 1994):

- Decrease pain perception
- Decrease nerve conduction velocity
- Increase the metabolic rate
- Increase blood flow
- Stimulate the immune system
- Decrease the fluid viscosity in the tissue
- Increase tissue extensibility

Factors influencing the physiological effects of ultrasound include the following:

- Frequency: 1 or 3 MHz (influences the depth of penetration), 1 MHz penetrates to a depth of 5 cm, 3 MHz penetrates 1 to 2 cm
- Duty cycle: On/off time; 10%, 20%, 50%, or 100%
- Time/duration (number of minutes ultrasound is administered)
- Intensity (force or strength of the sound wave; measured in W/cm$^2$)

The thermal effects of ultrasound can be decreased through either lowering the intensity of the ultrasound or by "pulsing" the ultrasound. Pulsing the ultrasound refers to the duty cycle, or that period of time when the sound energy is being delivered to the tissue divided by the pulse period, which is the on time and off time. Most of the ultrasound equipment will have a 50%, 20%, or 10% duty cycle setting.

The nonthermal or "mechanical" effects of ultrasound result in second-order physiological effects, which are effective for wound healing. These mechanical effects occur through the process of acoustic streaming and micromassage at the cell membrane. Benefits have been shown for inflammation, proliferation, and maturation processes, with the primary site of ultrasound interaction and activity occurring at the cell membrane (Nagata, Nakamura, Fujihara, & Tanaka, 2013). From a clinical standpoint, nonthermal ultrasound (pulsed, low intensity) will facilitate tissue repair (Chan et al., 2006; Ebenbichler & Resch, 1994; Fyfe & Bullock, 1985; Giannini, Giombini, Moneta, Massazza, & Pigozzi, 2004; Turner, Powell, & Ng, 1989).

Phonophoresis is the therapeutic application of ultrasound using a topical medication. The intent of phonophoresis is to direct the drug delivery directly to the site where the desired effect is sought. Phonophoresis is noninvasive and essentially painless. There is a discrepancy over whether the mechanism of action is thermal or due to the mechanical effects of the ultrasound. In addition, there are some inconsistencies regarding the effectiveness of ultrasound due to the wide variability of intervention parameters (Casarotto, Adamowski, Fallopa, & Bacanelli, 2004; Klucinec, 1996; Klucinec, Scheidler, Denegar, Domholdt, & Burgess, 2000; Oziomek, Perrin, Herold, & Denegar, 1991; Reshetov, Tverdokhleb, & Bezmenov, 2000). Though used a great deal clinically (Goraj-Szczypiorowska, Zajac, & Skalska-Izdebska, 2007), due to the variability in research parameters and findings, application of topical medications should be a secondary consideration with the thermal or nonthermal effects being primary (Gurney, Wascher, Schenck, Tennison, & Jaramillo, 2011).

## Precautions and Contraindications

Prior to the application of ultrasound, it is important that the practitioner determine which frequency he or she is using as well as whether the intent of the intervention is to "heat" tissue or to "heal" tissue. Many of the contraindications and precautions of therapeutic ultrasound are with thermal, high-intensity applications. As with any physical agent, care must be used when the client has areas of decreased sensation, mentation, or cognitive abilities. Caution should also be used in clients with pacemakers. Ultrasound is contraindicated in clients with malignant tumors, during pregnancy, over epiphyseal plates of children, with joint cement, primary repair of tendons, and thrombophlebitis. Ultrasound should never be applied over the eyes, reproductive organs, or central nervous system tissue.

Precautions and contraindications for ultrasound include the following:

- Malignant tumors
- Joint cement
- Pacemakers
- Primary tendon repair
- Thrombophlebitis
- Reproductive organs
- Eyes
- Central nervous system tissue
- Pregnancy

# Electrotherapy Principles and Applications

There are a variety of therapeutic applications of electrotherapy available to the occupational therapy practitioner. Because of the wide variability in applications and language used in the research and by the manufacturers, there is also a great deal of confusion that exists. The American Physical Therapy Association attempted to standardize the terminology related to electrotherapeutic agents by classifying the agents according to their therapeutic goals. The following applications are the ones most frequently used by occupational therapists in clinical practice:

- Electrical muscle stimulation: Used for denervated muscles, direct current
- NMES: Used with innervated muscles, alternating current
- FES: Use of electrical stimulation as an orthotic substitute, alternating current
- ESTR: Used for tissue healing, decubitus, direct current; also referred to as HVGS
- TENS: Used for decreasing pain, alternating current.
- Iontophoresis: Used for transdermal drug delivery, direct current

The most commonly used applications by occupational therapy practitioners include NMES, FES, TENS, HVGS (used for tissue repair and healing), and iontophoresis (used to administer medications to targeted tissue).

Electricity is a form of energy that exhibits magnetic, chemical, mechanical, and thermal effects. Electrical current involves the flow or movement of ions or electrons from one area to another and from a high concentration to a low concentration. The human body is electrically conductive, and tissue can be either excitable and responsive to the electrical current or nonexcitable and modified by the electrical fields but nonresponsive to the electrical current flow. When electricity is applied to excitable tissue, there is physiological and physiochemical changes that occur due in part to the water in the tissues. If the electrical current is of sufficient intensity, duration, and frequency, a muscle contraction will occur. A primary difference between electrically stimulated movement and voluntary contractions is the sequence of movements. In a voluntary contraction, small motor nerves are recruited first, then larger motor nerves, and finally larger muscles in an asynchronous sequence as gradually greater strength is required. In electrically stimulated movement, however, the reverse occurs with the larger fibers and muscles being recruited first in a synchronous, linear fashion. This accounts for the often "robot-like" movements of electrically stimulated muscles.

## Neuromuscular Electrical Stimulation

The choice of an appropriate electrical device depends on the goals set by the occupational therapist during the evaluation and intervention. NMES uses a pulsed alternating current to stimulate intact peripheral motor nerves to produce a motor response or muscle contraction. This form of stimulation is used to decrease muscle spasms, increase muscle strength, and decrease edema through the pumping action of alternating muscle contractions. NMES is indicated to improve muscle strength without increasing cardiovascular output; it can increase range of motion, decrease or inhibit spasticity, and improve strength and endurance; it is also used for muscle reeducation or facilitation (Baker, Parker, & Sanderson, 1983; Billian & Gorman, 1992; Carmick, 1995, 1997; Chae & Hart, 1998; Scheker & Ozer, 2003). Electrodes are placed on the bulk of the muscle belly over the motor nerve with a second electrode placed distal to the first, usually near the muscle attachment. Correct electrode placement is crucial for effective response, and it is recommended to practice electrode placement on yourself or a colleague to ensure appropriate location. The amplitude or strength of the electrical current is increased until the nerve becomes depolarized and the muscle reaches tetany, causing a muscle contraction.

NMES can also be used for orthopedic injuries, particularly those conditions that have been immobilized such as a Colles' fracture, causing muscle weakness or hesitancy in moving the affected extremity through the available range of motion. Combining NMES with occupational activities and movements facilitates outcomes, strengthens the response, and increases strength more than just by conventional exercise alone (Hesse, Werner, Bardeleben, & Brandl-Hesse, 2002; Weingarden, Kizony, Nathan, Ohry, & Levy, 1997). NMES has also been used to decrease or modulate spasticity in neurologically impaired or orthopedic patients. Success with neurologically involved clients may vary due to the underlying cause. There are two primary methods for improving range of motion and decreasing spasticity: stimulating the spastic muscle to fatigue or stimulating the antagonist muscle to attempt to strengthen it and overpower the spastic muscle. Combining these NMES techniques with static and dynamic splinting, positional stretch, and other "conventional" methods of intervention may facilitate better outcomes (Daly et al., 1996; Detrembleur, Lejeune, Renders, & Van Den Bergh, 2002; Hesse et al., 2002; Scheker, Chesher, & Ramirez, 1999; Scheker & Ozer, 2003).

FES is the use of NMES to activate muscles during functional tasks (Bethoux et al., 2015). FES is a form of NMES, but the targeted stimulation and application is used as a substitute for an orthotic device or to produce a specific motor movement and activity. NMES and FES are frequently used with clients who have suffered from a stroke and hemiplegia. FES has been used as a substitute for the conventional "slings" that clients with shoulder subluxation frequently have following a stroke. Other applications of FES may be for reaching activities of the upper extremity or to strengthen or enhance grasp-and-release activities to allow the client to pick up and manipulate objects. There is a great deal of research and interest in the use of NMES with clients who have suffered a cerebrovascular accident and in the ability to facilitate return and decrease shoulder subluxation and pain in clients at the early stage of recovery (Aoyagi & Tsubahara, 2004; Chae et al., 2005; Liu, You, & Sun, 2005; Yu, 2004). Incorporating FES combining proximal muscle stimulation during reaching activities and distal stimulation during grasp-and-pinch tasks has also been shown to improve hand function and minimize upper extremity impairment in severe stroke patients (Thrasher, Zivanovic, McIlroy, & Popovic, 2008).

As the technology and research continues to expand and progress, occupational therapy practitioners should stay current with these therapeutic applications to facilitate occupational performance and improve outcomes and quality of life in clients with hemiplegia. Electrode placements for shoulder subluxation include over the supraspinatus and the upper trapezius, with a second electrode over the posterior deltoid. FES can also be configured to target two or more muscles to facilitate active movements such as mass extensor patterns or grasp-and-release activities. A creative approach to the intended movement and activity is required to determine the appropriate placement of electrodes. Research assessing the use of electrical stimulation suggests that FES combined with motor learning is beneficial in improving aspects of everyday activity performance after stroke and should be integrated into an intensive treatment protocol (Howlett, Lannin, Ada, & McKinstry, 2015).

## Electrical Stimulation for Wound Healing

It is beyond the scope of this chapter to outline the various parameters of ESTR. It is recommended that the reader interested in this electrotherapeutic application review other materials and information available. There are some factors salient to many of the clinical conditions discussed earlier. Following an injury or surgery, there is a disruption of the body's normally occurring electrical field, with a change in polarity of the adjacent area. The application of electrical stimulation through the use of direct current and high-voltage pulsed current facilitates the transfer of the energy from the electrical current to the wound due to the change in polarity caused by the injury. The electrical current and stimulation affects not only the circulation but also the histochemical effects and functions, as well as the orientation of the cell structures and facilitation of the healing process. ESTR is indicated for pressure ulcers (stages I through IV), diabetic ulcers, venous ulcers, traumatic and surgical wounds, ischemic ulcers, wound flaps, and burn wounds. Precautions and contraindications are essentially the same as those discussed for electrotherapy in general (Baker, Chambers, DeMuth, & Villar, 1997; Bayat et al., 2006; Bogie, Reger, Levine, & Sahgal, 2000; Gardner, Frantz, & Schmidt, 1999; Houghton et al., 2003; Langevin et al., 2006).

## Transcutaneous Electrical Nerve Stimulation

Pain is a complex, multifaceted experience that can have unique social and cultural components. Electrical stimulation in the form of TENS can be an effective adjunct to conventional intervention. Pain is modulated through the use of TENS by affecting the perception and sensation of pain rather than correcting any underlying clinical condition. There are two primary theories related to the efficacy of TENS to modulate pain: the gate control theory and the endorphin or opiate-mediated control theory. The reader is encouraged to explore these theories further to familiarize him- or herself with the intricacies of each. TENS is most often used in the intervention of musculoskeletal disorders, back pain, arthritis, inflammatory disorders of soft tissue, and for postoperative pain. There are a variety of intervention parameters available, and many TENS units are preprogrammed with the regimens that are the most effective.

TENS uses pulsed or alternating current, and the manufacturers have programmed different combinations of stimulation patterns directly into the equipment. There are four common forms of TENS used clinically: subsensory-level, sensory-level, motor-level, and noxious-level stimulation; a combination of all four levels may be used as well.

Subsensory-level stimulation is also known as *microcurrent electrical neuromuscular stimulation, microcurrent electrical stimulation, subliminal stimulation,* or *low-intensity stimulation.* The characteristic of subsensory-level stimulation is that the intensity of the equipment is so low (less than 1 milliamp) that it does not stimulate a muscle contraction and is considered "subthreshold." Much of the research generated by this form of TENS has been in fractures and skin wounds and is based on the movement of the ions in the tissues at such low magnitude that there is no cutaneous sensation (Currier & Mann, 1983; Denegar, 1993). Microcurrent electrical stimulation has gained a great deal of attention for stimulating soft tissues repair as wounds, bones, tendons and ligaments and promising results have been reported, though additional research is needed for clinical applications (Ahmed, Elgayed, & Ibrahim, 2012; Poltawski & Watson, 2010).

Sensory-level stimulation is also known as *conventional* or *high-rate TENS* and is primarily used during the acute phase of injury. This form of stimulation is based on the gate control mechanism or opiate-mediated pain control and uses amplitudes and durations between 50 and 100 pulses per second (Melzack, 1993). Sensory-level TENS activates the cutaneous tactile sensory fibers and causes cutaneous paresthesia or a tingling sensation. The intensity of this form of stimulation does not elicit a motor response, although the client can "feel" the sensation. This form of TENS has a relatively quick response in decreasing pain, but the long-term effects are not usually longer than 1 hour. Extended periods of pain relief may be due to the stimulation interrupting the pain-spasm-pain cycle and through the effect on the opioid and gate pathways (Macedo, Josué, Maia, Câmara, & Brasileiro, 2015).

Motor-level stimulation is also known as *strong low-rate* or *acupuncture-like TENS* and uses a high-amplitude and low-frequency pulse duration. This form of stimulation is also based on the gate control or opiate-mediated theories of pain control. Motor-level stimulation uses an amplitude high enough to produce a motor response in the underlying tissue. As the amplitude is increased, greater numbers of muscle fibers and motor axons are recruited and can reach a titanic contraction. Electrode placement for motor-level stimulation is directly over the motor point, which correlates with the location of the client's pain or on the segmental nerve roots. Motor-level stimulation is often used to treat chronic pain or pain that is caused by damage to deeper tissues, muscle spasms, and myofascial pain (Al-Smadi et al., 2003; Bjordal, Johnson, & Ljunggreen, 2003; Breit & Van der Wall, 2004; Chang, Lin, & Hsieh, 2002).

Noxious-level stimulation is also known as *electro-acupuncture, hyperstimulation,* or *noxious-level TENS.* This form of TENS is of motor-level intensity and uses longer pulse durations and frequencies. As the name suggests, noxious-level stimulation is reached when the stimulation amplitude is increased and perceived by the client to be "painful." This intense stimulation activates the ascending neural mechanisms and is based in part on the endogenous opiate theory. Noxious-level stimulation produces relatively high levels of analgesia. However, the effects are short lived and transitory. Most often, this form of stimulation is used prior to surgical procedures or debridement of tissue (Chandran & Sluka, 2003; Chang et al., 2002; Likar et al., 2001).

Most TENS units have two channels with four electrodes. When used with clients reporting pain, electrodes are positioned over or around the painful site. Other sites that may be used include motor points, which correspond with the area of pain, trigger points, or acupuncture points. These locations are considered electrically active and will facilitate the electrical current flow into the selected tissue. Other potential stimulation sites include areas along the peripheral nerves, the tissue overlying the painful areas, specific dermatomes, or over the spinal segmental myotomes, which correspond to the client's reported pain. Clinically, the practitioner needs to determine whether the desired outcome will involve a motor response, sensory analgesia, or a noxious level of stimulation for analgesia. If the client does not report any improvement in the pain level or is unable to tolerate the stimulation, the practitioner should change the electrode placement or adjust the stimulation parameters. Intervention is continued if the client is able to tolerate the sensation, reports a decrease in pain, and indicates an improvement in occupational performance or movement (Bracciano, 2008). TENS should be a consideration for post-surgical pain during rehabilitation exercises and activities (i.e., as a supplement to routine pharmacologic analgesia) and may have its greatest effect for clients who are not anxious or catastrophizing their pain (Rakel, Zimmerman, Geasland, Embree, & Clarke, 2014).

### *Precautions and Contraindications*

As with any physical agent modality, a thorough examination and assessment of the client is necessary to identify the source of the client's pain and symptoms. Reviewing the past medical history of the client and subjective history of the current condition assists in clarifying and identifying contraindications or precautions that might be required. Precautions and contraindications are essentially the same as those for any form of electrical stimulation. Precautions include those clients with known cardiac disease or cardiac arrhythmias. These clients should be monitored for any sign of distress or adverse effects. Care should be used if TENS is being placed over the lumbar paraspinals or abdominal region during pregnancy, except when used during labor and delivery in uncomplicated pregnancies. If a client has been diagnosed with cancer or malignancies, TENS may be used to assist with pain control. Informed consent of the client and attending physician should be obtained when using electrical stimulation or TENS with both the client with cancer and during pregnancy.

TENS and electrical stimulation are contraindicated in clients with demand-type cardiac pacemakers. Electrical stimulation should never be used over the carotid sinus because stimulation over this region of the neck may cause a hypotensive incident and cardiac irregularities. TENS and electrical stimulation should never be applied over the eye or over areas of decreased or abnormal sensation or used in clients with undiagnosed pain, epilepsy, metastasis, or peripheral vascular disease.

Electrotherapy contraindications include the following:

- Peripheral vascular disease
- Infection
- Impaired cognition or mentation
- Demand-type pacemakers
- Over the carotid sinus
- Over the eye
- Clients with epilepsy
- Cancer malignancies
- Decreased or absent sensation
- Active deep vein thrombosis or thrombophlebitis (Houghton, Nussbaum, & Hoens, 2010)

## Summary

The rehabilitation field has seen a dramatic increase in the use of technology and physical agent modalities. Physical agents can be used as part of the therapeutic intervention for a variety of clinical conditions that affect occupational function and independence. Because of reimbursement, efficacy, and demand for evidence-based practice, research related to physical agent modalities continues to grow, with research and intervention parameters becoming more standardized and objective. Large, randomized controlled trials remain limited, however. The occupational therapy practitioner who is considering the use of physical agents as an adjunct to engagement in occupation needs to consider the context and unique client factors relevant to the disease or impairment to facilitate determination of therapeutic parameters. Rather than using a "technician-like" approach to physical agents, the skilled practitioner needs to determine which client factors and which physiological functions are affected by the impairment or disorder and determine how best to facilitate the desired healing response that will improve occupational performance and function. The ability to discern the underlying physiological components and cause of the impairment or condition, and the clinical experience and knowledge to determine how best to affect that component, requires additional training and experiential learning to ensure that we use physical agents in a timely, systematic, and effective fashion. Failure to consider physical agents and their potential for benefiting our clients through improved occupational functioning not only limits our effectiveness as occupational therapy practitioners and the profession, but also limits our ability to fully help clients achieve their highest level of independence.

## Evidence-Based Research Chart

| Intervention | Keywords | Evidence |
|---|---|---|
| Superficial thermal agents—cryotherapy, heat agents | Cryotherapy/instrumentation, pain, analgesics, superficial heat agent, heat agent, thermal agent, superficial thermal agent, paraffin bath, Fluidotherapy, hot pack, contrast bath, whirlpool, thermotherapy, physical agent modality, hydrotherapy, bath, paraffin embedding, hyperthermia | Conroy & Hayes, 1998; Eversden, Maggs, Nightingale, & Jobanputra, 2007; Hirvonen et al., 2007; Kraeutler, Reynolds, Long, & McCarty, 2015; Martimbianco et al., 2014 |
| Superficial thermal agents—heat | Pain, pain measurement, heat/therapeutic use, intervention outcome | Cruz et al., 2016; Michlovitz et al., 2004; Nagata, Nakamura, Fujihara, & Tanaka, 2013 |
| Therapeutic ultrasound | Ultrasonic therapy, ultrasonic therapy/methods, LIPUS, ultrasound | Citak-Karakaya, Akbayrak, Demirturk, Ekici, & Bakar, 2006; Gurney, Wascher, Schenck, Tennison, & Jaramillo, 2011; Sarrafzadeh, Ahmadi, & Yassin, 2012; Uhlemann, 1993 |
| Electrotherapy—NMES, TENS | NMES, electrical stimulation, FES, task practice, functional activity, practice, repetition, tasks, exercise | Alon, Levitt, & McCarthy, 2008; Hara, Ogawa, Tsujiuchi, & Muraoka, 2008; Howlett, Lannin, Ada, & McKinstry, 2015; Kesar & Binder-Macleod, 2006; Knutson, Hisel, Harley, & Chae, 2009; Lourençao, Battistella, de Brito, Tsukimoto, & Miyazaki, 2008; Macedo, Josué, Maia, Câmara, & Brasileiro, 2015; Mangold, Schuster, Keller, Zimmermann-Schlatter, & Ettlin, 2009; Rakel, Zimmerman, Geasland, Embree, & Clarke, 2014; Thrasher, Zivanovic, McIlroy, & Popovic, 2008 |

## Student Self-Assessment

### *Therapeutic Application of Cold: Determining Clinical Response*

#### Objective

The student will determine the effectiveness of different cold applications in decreasing skin temperature, achieving an analgesic response, and in determining its effect on grip/pinch strength. Students will monitor the form of application, duration, and the client's subjective comments during the application of cold. The student will take a pre- and post-grip and/or pinch test in the same upper extremity to which the cold modality will be applied.

#### Equipment

Select from the various methods of administering cryotherapy, including the following:

- Crushed ice bag
- Ice immersion bucket
- Ice massage cup
- Reusable cold pack
- Stopwatch or watch with second/minute hand
- Dynamometer and/or pinch gauge

#### Procedure

1. Select a method of applying cryotherapy. Identify which upper extremity will be targeted for the application. The modality should be applied to the forearm of the selected upper extremity. Before applying the cold modality, take a baseline grip strength using the dynamometer. Apply the cold modality to the body part for a maximum total of 10 minutes, or less if using the ice massage method (approximately 4 minutes).
2. Using the Numerical Rating Scale (0 = no pain; 10 = unimaginable pain), have the client "rate" his or her pain level at each temperature measurement (each minute).
3. Note the client's response (verbal and behavioral) as well as the skin appearance during each measurement period.
4. Immediately after discontinuing the application, use the dynamometer/pinch gauge and remeasure grip and/or pinch strength in the upper extremity.

5. Using a different area or body part in the upper extremity, apply a different application technique and repeat Steps 1 through 4.
6. Following completion of the lab and measurements, note any differences in grip/pinch strength. What did you find? Was one type of application more effective than another? What were the client's subjective comments? Did you notice any patterns?

## Electronic Resources

Chattanooga University: http://www.djoglobal.com/our-brands/chattanooga/chattanooga-university

Cochrane Library: http://www.cochranelibrary.com/

Electrophysical Agents and Diagnostic Ultrasound Special Interest Group: http://epadu.csp.org.uk/

International Society for Electrophysical Agents in Physical Therapy: http://www.wcpt.org/iseapt

PEDro Evidence Database: http://www.pedro.org.au/

## References


2011 Accreditation Council for Occupational Therapy Education (ACOTE) Standards. (2012). *American Journal of Occupational Therapy, 66*(6 Suppl.). doi:10.5014/ajot.2012.66s6

Ahmed, A., Elgayed, S., & Ibrahim, I., (2012). Polarity effect of microcurrent electrical stimulation on tendon healing: Biomechanical and histopathological studies. *Journal of Advanced Research, 3*, 109-117.

Alon, G., Levitt, A. F., & McCarthy, P. A. (2008). Functional electrical stimulation (FES) may modify the poor prognosis of stroke survivors with severe motor loss of the upper extremity: A preliminary study. *American Journal of Physical Medicine and Rehabilitation, 87*(8), 627-636.

Al-Smadi, J., Warke, K., Wilson, I., Cramp, A. F., Noble, G., Walsh, D. M., et al. (2003). A pilot investigation of the hypoalgesic effects of transcutaneous electrical nerve stimulation upon low back pain in people with multiple sclerosis. *Clinical Rehabilitation, 17*, 742-749.

American Occupational Therapy Association. (2012). Physical agent modalities: A position paper. *American Journal of Occupational Therapy, 66*, S78-S89. doi:10.5014/ajot.2012.66S78

American Occupational Therapy Association. (2014). Occupational therapy practice framework: Domain and process (3rd ed.). *American Journal of Occupational Therapy, 68*(Suppl. 1), S1-S48. doi:10.5014/ajot.2014.682006

American Occupational Therapy Association. (2015). Occupational therapy code of ethics (2015). *American Journal of Occupational Therapy, 69*(Suppl. 3), 6913410030p1-6913410030p8. doi:10.5014/ajot.2015.696S03

Andreadis, S. T. (2006). Experimental models and high-throughput diagnostics for tissue regeneration. *Expert Opinion on Biological Therapy, 6*, 1071-1086.

Ankrom, M. A., Bennett, R. G., Sprigle, S., Langemo, D., Black, J. M., Berlowitz, D. R., et al. (2005). Pressure-related deep tissue injury under intact skin and the current pressure ulcer staging systems. *Advances in Skin and Wound Care, 18*, 35-42.

Aoyagi, Y., & Tsubahara, A. (2004). Therapeutic orthosis and electrical stimulation for upper extremity hemiplegia after stroke: A review of effectiveness based on evidence. *Topics in Stroke Rehabilitation, 11*, 9-15.

Baker, L. L., Chambers, R., DeMuth, S. K., & Villar, F. (1997). Effects of electrical stimulation on wound healing in patients with diabetic ulcers. *Diabetes Care, 20*, 405-412.

Baker, L. L., Parker, K., & Sanderson, D. (1983). Neuromuscular electrical stimulation for the head-injured patient. *Physical Therapy, 63*, 1967-1974.

Barber, F. A. (2000). A comparison of crushed ice and continuous flow cold therapy. *American Journal of Knee Surgery, 13*, 97-101; discussion 102.

Bayat, M., Asgari-Moghadam, Z., Maroufi, M., Rezaie, F. S., Bayat, M., & Rakhshan, M. (2006). Experimental wound healing using microamperage electrical stimulation in rabbits. *Journal of Rehabilitation Research and Development, 43*, 219-226.

Bethoux, F., Rogers, H., Nolan, K., Abrams, G., Annaswamy, T., Brandstater, M., ... Kufta, C. (2015). Long-term follow-up to a randomized controlled trial comparing peroneal nerve functional electrical stimulation to an ankle foot orthosis for patients with chronic stroke. *Neurorehabilitation and Neural Repair, 29*(10). doi:10.1177/1545968315570325

Billian, C., & Gorman, P. H. (1992). Upper extremity applications of functional neuromuscular stimulation. *Assistive Technology, 4*, 31-39.

Bjordal, J. M., Johnson, M. I., & Ljunggreen, A. E. (2003). Transcutaneous electrical nerve stimulation (TENS) can reduce postoperative analgesic consumption. A meta-analysis with assessment of optimal treatment parameters for postoperative pain. *European Journal of Pain, 7*, 181-188.

Bogie, K. M., Reger, S. I., Levine, S. P., & Sahgal, V. (2000). Electrical stimulation for pressure sore prevention and wound healing. *Assistive Technology, 12*, 50-66.

Bolton, L., & van Rijswijk, L. (1991). Wound dressings: Meeting clinical and biological needs. *Dermatology Nursing/Dermatology Nurses' Association, 3*, 146-161.

Bracciano, A. G. (2008). *Physical agent modalities: Theory and application for the occupational therapist* (2nd ed.). Thorofare, NJ: SLACK Incorporated.

Breit, R., & Van der Wall, H. (2004). Transcutaneous electrical nerve stimulation for postoperative pain relief after total knee arthroplasty. *Journal of Arthroplasty, 19*, 45-48.

Carmick, J. (1995). Managing equinus in children with cerebral palsy: Electrical stimulation to strengthen the triceps surae muscle. *Developmental Medicine and Child Neurology, 37*, 965-975.

Carmick, J. (1997). Use of neuromuscular electrical stimulation and [corrected] dorsal wrist splint to improve the hand function of a child with spastic hemiparesis. *Physical Therapy, 77*, 661-671.

Casarotto, R. A., Adamowski, J. C., Fallopa, F., & Bacanelli, F. (2004). Coupling agents in therapeutic ultrasound: Acoustic and thermal behavior. *Archives of Physical Medicine and Rehabilitation, 85*, 162-165.

Chae, J., & Hart, R. (1998). Comparison of discomfort associated with surface and percutaneous intramuscular electrical stimulation for persons with chronic hemiplegia. *American Journal of Physical Medicine and Rehabilitation, 77*, 516-522.

Chae, J., Yu, D. T., Walker, M. E., Kirsteins, A., Elovic, E. P., Flanagan, S. R., et al. (2005). Intramuscular electrical stimulation for hemiplegic shoulder pain: A 12-month follow-up of a multiple-center, randomized clinical trial. *American Journal of Physical Medicine and Rehabilitation, 84*, 832-842.

Chan, C. W., Qin, L., Lee, K. M., Zhang, M., Cheng, J. C., & Leung, K. S. (2006). Low intensity pulsed ultrasound accelerated bone remodeling during consolidation stage of distraction osteogenesis. *Journal of Orthopaedic Research, 24*, 263-270.

Chandran, P., & Sluka, K. A. (2003). Development of opioid tolerance with repeated transcutaneous electrical nerve stimulation administration. *Pain, 102*, 195-201.

Chang, Q. Y., Lin, J. G., & Hsieh, C. L. (2002). Effect of electroacupuncture and transcutaneous electrical nerve stimulation at hegu (LI.4) acupuncture point on the cutaneous reflex. *Acupuncture and Electro-Therapeutics Research, 27*, 191-202.

Citak-Karakaya, I., Akbayrak, T., Demirturk, F., Ekici, G., & Bakar, Y. (2006). Short and long-term results of connective tissue manipulation and combined ultrasound therapy in patients with fibromyalgia. *Journal of Manipulative and Physiological Therapeutics, 29*, 524-528.

Conroy, D. E., & Hayes, K. W. (1998). The effect of joint mobilization as a component of comprehensive treatment for primary shoulder impingement syndrome. *Journal of Orthopaedic and Sports Physical Therapy, 28*(1), 3-14.

Cornish-Painter, C., Peterson, C. Q., & Lindstrom-Hazel, D. K. (1997). Skill acquisition and competency testing for physical agent modality use. *American Journal of Occupational Therapy, 51*, 681-685.

Costello, J., McInerney, C., Bleakley, C., Selfe, J., & Donnelly, A. (2012). The use of thermal imaging in assessing skin temperature following cryotherapy: A review. *Journal of Thermal Biology, 37*(2). doi:10.1016/j.jtherbio.2011.11.008

Cruz, J., Hauck, M., Cardoso, P., Moraes, M., Martins, C., da Silva P., ... Signori, L. (2016). Effects of different therapeutic ultrasound waveforms on endothelial function in healthy volunteers: A randomized clinical trial. *Ultrasound in Medicine and Biology, 42*(2), 471-480.

Currier, D. P., & Mann, R. (1983). Muscular strength development by electrical stimulation in healthy individuals. *Physical Therapy, 63*, 915-921.

Cuzzell, J. (2002). Wound healing: Translating theory into clinical practice. *Dermatology Nursing, 14*, 257-261.

Daly, J. J., Marsolais, E. B., Mendell, L. M., Rymer, W. Z., Stefanovska, A., Wolpaw, J. R., et al. (1996). Therapeutic neural effects of electrical stimulation. *IEEE Transactions on Rehabilitation Engineering, 4*, 218-230.

Denegar, C. (1993). The effects of low-volt microamperage stimulation on delayed onset muscle soreness. *Journal of Sports Rehabilitation, 1*, 95-102.

Detrembleur, C., Lejeune, T. M., Renders, A., & Van Den Bergh, P. Y. (2002). Botulinum toxin and short-term electrical stimulation in the treatment of equinus in cerebral palsy. *Movement Disorders, 17*, 162-169.

Dyson, M. (1987). Mechanisms involved in therapeutic ultrasound. *Physiotherapy, 73*, 116-120.

Ebenbichler, G., & Resch, K. L. (1994). Critical evaluation of ultrasound therapy. *Wiener Medizinische Wochenschrift (1946), 144*, 51-53.

Enoch, S., & Harding, K. (2003). Wound bed preparation: The science behind the removal of barriers to healing. *Wounds, 15*, 213-229.

Enwemeka, C. S. (1989). The effects of therapeutic ultrasound on tendon healing: A biomechanical study. *American Journal of Physical Medicine and Rehabilitation, 68*, 283-287.

Eversden, L., Maggs, F., Nightingale, P., & Jobanputra, P. (2007). A pragmatic randomised controlled trial of hydrotherapy and land exercises on overall well being and quality of life in rheumatoid arthritis. *BMC Musculoskeletal Disorders, 8*, 23.

Fyfe, M. C., & Bullock, M. (1985). Therapeutic ultrasound: Some historical background and development in knowledge of its effects on healing. *Australian Journal of Physiotherapy, 31*, 220-224.

Gardner, S. E., Frantz, R. A., & Schmidt, F. L. (1999). Effect of electrical stimulation on chronic wound healing: A meta-analysis. *Wound Repair and Regeneration, 7*, 495-503.

Giannini, S., Giombini, A., Moneta, M. R., Massazza, G., & Pigozzi, F. (2004). Low-intensity pulsed ultrasound in the treatment of traumatic hand fracture in an elite athlete. *American Journal of Physical Medicine and Rehabilitation, 83*, 921-925.

Glauner, J. H., Ekes, A. M., James, A. E., & Holm, M. B. (1997). A pilot study of the theoretical and technical competence and appropriate education for the use of nine physical agent modalities in occupational therapy practice. *American Journal of Occupational Therapy, 51*, 767-774.

Gogia, P. (1995). *Clinical wound management.* Thorofare, NJ: SLACK Incorporated.

Goraj-Szczypiorowska, B., Zajac, L., & Skalska-Izdebska, R. (2007). Evaluation of factors influencing the quality and efficacy of ultrasound and phonophoresis treatment. *Ortopedia Traumatologia Rehabilitacja, 9*(5), 449-458.

Gracies, J. M. (2001). Physical modalities other than stretch in spastic hypertonia. *Physical Medicine and Rehabilitation Clinics of North America, 12*, 769-92, vi.

Gurney, B., Wascher, D., Schenck, R., Tennison, A., & Jaramillo, B. (2011). Absorption of hydrocortisone acetate in human connective tissue using phonophoresis. *Sports Health: A Multidisciplinary Approach, 3*(4). doi:10.1177/194173811140597

Hara, Y., Ogawa, S., Tsujiuchi, K., Muraoka, Y. (2008). A home-based rehabilitation program for the hemiplegic upper extremity by power-assisted functional electrical stimulation. *Disability and Rehabilitation, 30*(4), 296-304.

Hardy, M. A. (1989). The biology of scar formation. *Physical Therapy, 69*, 1014-1032.

Hesse, S., Werner, C., Bardeleben, A., & Brandl-Hesse, B. (2002). Management of upper and lower limb spasticity in neuro-rehabilitation. *Acta Neurochirurgica, 79*(Suppl.), 117-122.

Hirovnen, J., Kajander, J., Hagelberg, N., Mansikka, H., Någren, K., Hietala, J., & Pertovaara, A. (2007). Correlation of human cold pressor pain responses with 5-HT(1A) receptor binding in the brain. *Brain Research, 1172*(10), 21-31.

Hong, C. Z., Liu, H. H., & Yu, J. (1988). Ultrasound thermotherapy effect on the recovery of nerve conduction in experimental compression neuropathy. *Archives of Physical Medicine and Rehabilitation, 69*, 410-414.

Houghton, P. E., Kincaid, C. B., Lovell, M., Campbell, K. E., Keast, D. H., Woodbury, M. G., et al. (2003). Effect of electrical stimulation on chronic leg ulcer size and appearance. *Physical Therapy, 83*, 17-28.

Houghton, P. E., Nussbaum, E. L., & Hoens, A. M. (2010). Electrophysical agents: Contraindications and precautions. *Physiotherapy Canada, 62*(5).

Howlett, O., Lannin, N., Ada, L., & McKinstry, C. (2015). Functional electrical stimulation improves activity after stroke: A systematic review with meta-analysis. *Archives of Physical Medicine, 96*(5), 934-943.

Kesar, T., & Binder-Macleod, S. A. (2006). Effect of frequency and pulse duration on human muscle fatigue during repetitive electrical stimulation. *Experimental Physiology, 91*(6), 967-976.

Kloth, L. C., & McCulloch, J. M. (1995). The inflammatory response to wounding. In J. M. MuCulloch, L. C. Kloth, & J. A. Feedar (Eds.), *Wound healing: Alternatives in management* (2nd ed., p. 3). Philadelphia, PA: F. A. Davis Company.

Klucinec, B. (1996). The effectiveness of the aquaflex gel pad in the transmission of acoustic energy. *Journal of Athletic Training, 31*, 313-317.

Klucinec, B., Scheidler, M., Denegar, C., Domholdt, E., & Burgess, S. (2000). Transmissivity of coupling agents used to deliver ultrasound through indirect methods. *Journal of Orthopaedic and Sports Physical Therapy, 30*, 263-269.

Knutson, J. S., Hisel, T. Z., Harley, M. Y., & Chae, J. (2009). A novel functional electrical stimulation treatment for recovery of hand function in hemiplegia: 12 week pilot study. *Neurorehabilitation and Neural Repair, 23*(1), 17-25.

Kottke, F. J., Pauley, D. L., & Ptak, R. A. (1966). The rationale for prolonged stretching for correction of shortening of connective tissue. *Archives of Physical Medicine and Rehabilitation, 47*, 345-352.

Kraeutler, M., Reynolds, K., Long, C., & McCarty, E., (2015). Compressive cryotherapy versus ice—A prospective, randomized study on postoperative pain in patients undergoing arthroscopic rotator cuff repair or subacromial decompression. *Journal of Shoulder and Elbow Surgery, 24*(6), 854-859.

Laban, M. M. (1962). Collagen tissue: Implications of its response to stress in vitro. *Archives of Physical Medicine and Rehabilitation, 43*, 461-466.

Langevin, H. M., Storch, K. N., Cipolla, M. J., White, S. L., Buttolph, T. R., & Taatjes, D. J. (2006). Fibroblast spreading induced by connective tissue stretch involves intracellular redistribution of alpha- and beta-actin. *Histochemistry and Cell Biology, 125*, 487-495.

Likar, R., Molnar, M., Pipam, W., Koppert, W., Quantschnigg, B., Disselhoff, B., et al. (2001). Postoperative transcutaneous electrical nerve stimulation (TENS) in shoulder surgery (randomized, double blind, placebo controlled pilot trial). *Schmerz, 15*, 158-163.

Liu, J., You, W. X., & Sun, D. (2005). Effects of functional electric stimulation on shoulder subluxation and upper limb motor function recovery of patients with hemiplegia resulting from stroke. *Di Yi Jun Yi Da Xue Xue Bao, 25*, 1054-1055.

Loten, C., Stokes, B., Worsley, D., Seymour, J. E., Jiang, S., & Isbistergk, G. K. (2006). A randomized controlled trial of hot water (45 degrees C) immersion versus ice packs for pain relief in bluebottle stings. *Medical Journal of Australia, 184*, 329-333.

Lourençao M. I. P., Battistella, L. R., de Brito, C. M., Tsukimoto G. R., & Miyazaki, M. H. (2008). Effect of biofeedback accompanying occupational therapy and functional electrical stimulation in hemiplegic patients. *International Journal of Rehabilitation Research, 31*(1), 33-41.

Macedo, L., Josué, A., Maia, P., Câmara,A., & Brasileiro, J. (2015), Effect of burst TENS and conventional TENS combined with cryotherapy on pressure pain threshold: Randomised, controlled, clinical trial. *Physiotherapy, 101*, 155-160.

Mangold, S., Schuster, C., Keller, T., Zimmermann-Schlatter, A., & Ettlin, T. (2009). Motor training of upper extremity with functional electrical stimulation in early stroke rehabilitation. *Neurorehabilitation and Neural Repair, 23*(2), 184-190.

Marimuthu, K., Murton, A., & Greenhaff, P. (2011). Mechanisms regulating muscle mass during disuse atrophy and rehabilitation in humans. *Journal of Applied Physiology, 110*(2). doi:10.1152/japplphysiol.00962.2010

Martimbianco, C., Gomes da Silva,N., de Carvalho, V., Silva, V., Torloni, M., & Peccin, M., (2014). Effectiveness and safety of cryotherapy after arthroscopic anterior cruciate ligament reconstruction. A systematic review of the literature. *Physical Therapy in Sport, 15*(4), 261-268.

Melzack, R. (1993). Pain: Past, present and future. *Canadian Journal of Experimental Psychology, 47*, 615-629.

Michlovitz, S., Hun, L., Erasala, G. N., Hengehold, D. A., & Weingand, K. W. (2004). Continuous low-level heat wrap therapy is effective for treating wrist pain. *Archives of Physical Medicine and Rehabilitation, 85*, 1409-1416.

Nadler, S. F., Prybicien, M., Malanga, G. A., & Sicher, D. (2003). Complications from therapeutic modalities: Results of a national survey of athletic trainers. *Archives of Physical Medicine and Rehabilitation, 84*, 849-853.

Nadler, S. F., Steiner, D. J., Erasala, G. N., Hengehold, D. A., Abeln, S. B., & Weingand, K. W. (2003). Continuous low-level heatwrap therapy for treating acute nonspecific low back pain. *Archives of Physical Medicine and Rehabilitation, 84*, 329-334.

Nagata, K., Nakamura, T., Fujihara, S., & Tanaka, E. (2013). Ultrasound modulates the inflammatory response and promotes muscle regeneration in injured muscles. *Annals of Biomedical Engineering, 41*, 1095-1105.

Olson, J. E., & Stravino, V. D. (1972). A review of cryotherapy. *Physical Therapy, 52*, 840-853.

Oziomek, R. S., Perrin, D. H., Herold, D. A., & Denegar, C. R. (1991). Effect of phonophoresis on serum salicylate levels. *Medicine and Science in Sports and Exercise, 23*, 397-401.

Petrofsky, J. S., Lohman III, E., Suh, H. J., Garcia, J., Anders, A., Sutterfield, C., et al. (2006). The effect of aging on conductive heat exchange in the skin at two environmental temperatures. *Medical Science Monitor, 12*, CR400-CR408.

Poltawski, L., & Watson, T. (2010). Bioelectricity and microcurrent therapy for tissue healing: A narrative review. *Rehab Med, 14*(3), 42-52.

Rabello, F., Souza, C., & Junior, J. (2014). Update on hypertrophic scar treatment. Clinics, 69(8). doi:10.6061/clinics/2014(08)11

Rakel, B., Zimmerman, B., Geasland, K., Embree, J., & Clarke, C. (2014). Transcutaneous electrical nerve stimulation for the control of pain during rehabilitation after total knee arthroplasty: A randomized, blinded, placebo-controlled trial. *Pain, 155*, 2599-2601.

Reshetov, P. P., Tverdokhleb, I., & Bezmenov, V. A. (2000). The use of hydrocortisone combined with ultrasound with gonarthrosis patients. *Voprosy Kurortologii, Fizioterapii, i Lechebnoi Fizicheskoi Kultury, 4*, 47-48.

Rimington, S. J., Draper, D. O., Durrant, E., & Fellingham, G. (1994). Temperature changes during therapeutic ultrasound in the precooled human gastrocnemius muscle. *Journal of Athletic Training, 29*, 325-327.

Robertson, V., Ward, A., & Jung, P. (2005). The effect of heat on tissue extensibility: A comparison of deep and superficial heating. *Archives of Physical Medicine and Rehabilitation, 86*(4). doi:10.1016/j.apmr.2004.07.353

Sanya, A. O., & Bello, A. O. (1999). Effects of cold application on isometric strength and endurance of quadriceps femoris muscle. *African Journal of Medicine and Medical Sciences, 28*(3-4), 195-198.

Sarrafzadeh J., Ahmadi A., & Yassin M. (2012) The effects of pressure release, phonophoresis of hydrocortisone, and ultrasound on upper trapezius latent myofascial trigger point. *Archives of Physical Medicine and Rehabilitation, 93*(1), 72-77.

Scheker, L. R., Chesher, S. P., & Ramirez, S. (1999). Neuromuscular electrical stimulation and dynamic bracing as a treatment for upper-extremity spasticity in children with cerebral palsy. *Journal of Hand Surgery (Edinburgh, Lothian), 24*, 226-232.

Scheker, L. R., & Ozer, K. (2003). Electrical stimulation in the management of spastic deformity. *Hand Clinics, 19*(4), 601-606, vi.

Simon, P. E., Romo, T., Al Moutran, H., & Pearson, J. M. (2016). *Skin wound healing*. Retrieved from http://emedicine.medscape.com/article/884594-overview

Singh, H., Osbahr, D. C., Holovacs, T. F., Cawley, P. W., & Speer, K. P. (2001). The efficacy of continuous cryotherapy on the postoperative shoulder: A prospective, randomized investigation. *Journal of Shoulder and Elbow Surgery, 10*, 522-525.

Ter Haar, G. (1978). Basic physics of therapeutic ultrasound. *Physiotherapy, 64*, 100-103.

Thrasher, T. A., Zivanovic, V., McIlroy, W., & Popovic, M. R. (2008). Rehabilitation of reaching and grasping function in severe hemiplegic patients using functional electrical stimulation therapy. *Neurorehabilitation and Neural Repair, 22*(6), 706-714.

Turner, S. M., Powell, E. S., & Ng, C. S. (1989). The effect of ultrasound on the healing of repaired cockerel tendon: Is collagen cross-linkage a factor? *Journal of Hand Surgery, 14*, 428-433.

Uhlemann, C. (1993). Pain modification in rheumatic diseases using different frequency applications of ultrasound. *Zeitschrift Fur Rheumatologie, 52*, 236-240.

Weingarden, H. P., Kizony, R., Nathan, R., Ohry, A., & Levy, H. (1997). Upper limb functional electrical stimulation for walker ambulation in hemiplegia: A case report. *American Journal of Physical Medicine and Rehabilitation, 76*, 63-67.

Welch, V., Brosseau, L., Shea, B., McGowan, J., Wells, G., & Tugwell, P. (2000). Thermotherapy for treating rheumatoid arthritis. *Cochrane Database of Systematic Reviews, 4*, CD002826.

World Health Organization. (2001). *International classification of functioning, disability and health* (ICF). Geneva, Switzerland: Author.

Yu, D. (2004). Shoulder pain in hemiplegia. *Physical Medicine and Rehabilitation Clinics of North America, 15*, vi-vii, 683-697.

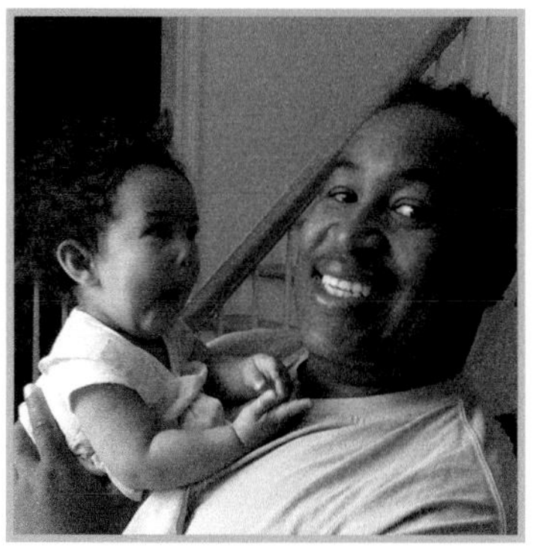

# 35

# Interventions to Enhance Feeding, Eating, and Swallowing

*Kristin Winston, PhD, OTR/L*

**ACOTE STANDARDS EXPLORED IN THIS CHAPTER**

B.5.14

**KEY VOCABULARY**

- **Aspiration:** "Entrance of food or secretions into the larynx below the level of the vocal cords" (Avery, 2014, p. 1349).
- **Bolus:** "Food or liquid in the mouth" (Avery, 2014, p. 1349).
- **Deglutition:** "The act of swallowing" (Avery, 2014, p. 1349).
- **Dysphagia:** "Difficulty with any stage of swallowing (oral, pharyngeal, esophageal)" (American Occupational Therapy Association, 2007, p. 696).
- **Eating:** The ability to keep and manipulate food/fluid in the mouth and swallow it (O'Sullivan, 1995, p. 191).
- **Enteral tube feedings:** Tubes that deliver nutrition directly to the gastrointestinal system (Morris & Klein, 2000).
- **Feeding:** The process of bringing food from plate or cup to the mouth (O'Sullivan, 1995, p. 191).
- **Gastroesophageal reflux disease:** Described as the chronic return of gastric contents into the esophagus.
- **Gastroesophageal scintigraphy:** This medical test looks at stomach emptying as well as the extent and severity of reflux (Morris & Klein, 2000).
- **Gastrostomy tube:** Bypasses the mouth and is inserted directly into the stomach surgically.
- **Jejunostomy tube:** Is placed directly into the jejunum, bypassing the stomach.

*(continued)*



Jacobs, K., & MacRae, N. (Eds.).
*Occupational Therapy Essentials for Clinical Competence, Third Edition* (pp. 521-535).

## KEY VOCABULARY (CONTINUED)

- **Nasogastric tube:** A feeding tube inserted through the oral pharyngeal area, supplying liquid nutrition by passing the mouth.
- **NPO (nil per os):** "Latin for 'nothing by mouth,' no food, liquid, or medication is to be given orally" (Avery, 2014, p. 1349).
- **Parenteral tube feedings:** Tubes that deliver nutrition via bypassing the gastrointestinal system to deliver nutrition into the bloodstream (Morris & Klein, 2000).
- **pH probe:** Medical test used to help identify amount and severity of gastroesophageal reflux.
- **Positioning:** The most important first step in the eating and feeding process.
- **Suck, swallow, breathe synchrony:** The smooth coordination of sucking, swallowing, and breathing to allow for efficient and effective eating.
- **Video fluoroscopy:** "Moving radiographic images of swallowing structure and physiology, also known as 'modified barium swallow study,' recorded on videotape or DVD" (Avery, 2014, p. 1349).

Feeding, eating, and swallowing are important occupations that occur across the lifespan in many different forms. These occupations consist of numerous performance skills, performance patterns, body functions, and body structures (American Occupational Therapy Association [AOTA], 2014b) that can be interrupted or disrupted through a number of neurological, psychosocial, developmental, or orthopedic conditions.

Kedesdy and Budd (1998) stated, "No human activity has greater biological and social significance than feeding" (p. 1). As such, the occupations of feeding and eating have great significance for the practice of occupational therapy. Across the lifespan, feeding, eating, and swallowing are necessary to support nutritional intake and hydration that in turn support growth and overall health (Baer, 2005). For infants and young children, success in the occupations of feeding, eating, and swallowing satisfies their sense of hunger, provides pleasure related to taste and textures of foods, and creates opportunities for parent–child bonding (Kedesdy & Budd, 1998). For the parents of young children, success in the occupations of feeding, eating, and swallowing signifies competence in the role of caregiver and in turn facilitates the bonding experience between parent and young child (Kedesdy & Budd, 1998). From early childhood through adulthood, the occupations related to feeding, eating, and swallowing continue to fulfill a nutritional need, but these occupations also begin to take on strong social and cultural significance (Baer, 2005; Jenks, 2002). The sharing of food and the occupations of mealtimes are frequently a part of celebrations large and small; cultural events; and other social activities at home, at school, in the workplace, and within the community (Figure 35-1).

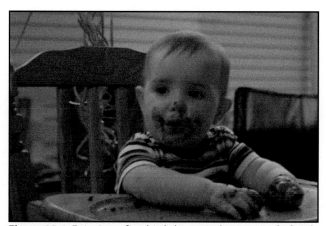

**Figure 35-1.** Enjoying a first birthday cupcake as part of a family celebration.

Secondary to the complex nature of concerns within the occupations of feeding, eating, and swallowing, occupational therapy practice in this area has different levels at which practitioners are able to intervene given varying degrees of competency (AOTA, 2007). Intervention depends on a thorough assessment and evaluation of factors relating to the person, the context and environment, and occupation. The AOTA (2007) states the following: "Occupational therapists and occupational therapy assistants have the knowledge and skills necessary to take a lead role in the evaluation and intervention of feeding, eating, and swallowing problems" (p. 686). As such, occupational therapy practitioners should understand not only the sensory and motor concerns that might be influencing the feeding, eating, and swallowing process but also complex cognitive, perceptual, contextual, and psychosocial factors that influence occupational performance in the areas of feeding, eating, and swallowing. The progression from entry-level practitioner to advanced practitioner in this area of practice is unique for each individual therapist and his or her practice setting. Competence in feeding, eating, and swallowing intervention may involve continuing education, on-the-job training, mentoring, independent study, and practice for the occupational therapy practitioner.

As entry-level practitioners, occupational therapists and occupational therapy assistants are educated to address many concerns related to this area of clinical practice as guided by the theoretical principles that are the foundation for practice. Occupational therapy practitioners provide intervention in this area that relates to occupational performance, performance skills, performance patterns, context, activity demands, and client factors facilitating a holistic approach to intervention (AOTA, 2014b). Entry-level practitioners can refer to AOTA's paper entitled *Specialized Knowledge and Skills in Feeding, Eating, and Swallowing for Occupational Therapy Practice* (2007) for guidelines related to specific roles for each practitioner.

Occupational therapy practitioners are especially skilled to address the performance of feeding, eating, and swallowing from multiple perspectives secondary to the emphasis on client factors, occupational analysis, and contextual factors as outlined by the *Occupational Therapy Practice Framework* (AOTA, 2014b). These factors include but are not limited to motor skills, sensory processing skills, cognitive skills, perceptual skills, contextual factors (such as cultural and social), and performance patterns including habits and routines around meals.

The occupational therapist assumes the primary responsibility for the delivery of assessment and intervention in this practice area. Occupational therapy assistants provide services related to feeding, eating, and swallowing under the supervision of and/or collaboration with the occupational therapist as per the AOTA, as well as individual state rules and regulations regarding the practice of occupational therapy (AOTA, 2014a). "During intervention, both occupational therapists and occupational therapy assistants select, administer, and adapt activities that support the intervention plan developed by the occupational therapist. Practitioners must always adhere to state and agency regulatory laws when providing services across these continua of care" (AOTA, 2007, p. 687). Supervision and/or mentoring that is provided to an occupational therapy practitioner in the area of feeding, eating, and swallowing depends on the individual's training, experience, and competency as well as guidelines within state licensure laws and practice guidelines. "Occupational therapy assistants and entry-level occupational therapists should seek supervision and mentoring from a more experienced occupational therapist or an occupational therapist with advanced knowledge and skills in feeding, eating, and swallowing" (AOTA, 2007, p. 687). As stated previously, the AOTA's specialized knowledge and skills paper on feeding, eating, and swallowing contains detailed information regarding the roles of the occupational therapist and occupational therapy assistant in this practice area (AOTA, 2007).

Occupational therapy practitioners work with individuals who receive their nutritional intake through oral or non-oral means. The following information seeks to clarify issues related to intervention for individuals receiving oral nutrition, non-oral nutrition, or a combination of methods. Non-oral nutrition may be via enteral systems that feed directly into the gastrointestinal tract or via parenteral feeding where nutrition is supplied intravenously.

## Oral Feeding

Oral feeding encompasses the process of gaining nutrition through the intake of fluids and solids by mouth. In the young child, the parent or caregiver facilitates feeding because the young child is dependent in many feeding/eating skills until the motor, sensory, cognitive, and perceptual skills necessary for independence in the area of feeding and eating develop (Case-Smith & Humphry, 2005). Once young children develop the necessary skills, independence in these occupations continues through adulthood, unless illness or disability affects the skills necessary to maintain independence.

Whenever possible, occupational therapy practitioners work with the client to develop the skills needed to feed him- or herself to facilitate occupational performance and promote independence. The occupational therapy practitioner should be aware of the possible stigma of being fed for adults, elders, and older children and move toward self-feeding as soon as possible if this is a meaningful goal.

Examples of adaptive equipment that can facilitate self-feeding include but are not limited to the following (these items can be found in adaptive equipment catalogues; Figure 35-2):

- Dycem to stabilize the plate or bowl
- Plate guards to assist getting food onto a utensil
- Weighted, bendable, strapped, or built-up utensils or self-feeding systems such as the Neater Eater (Sammons Preston) or Stable Slide (Sammons Preston) self-feeding system
- Rocker knives, which can be helpful to cut food when bilateral coordination is compromised
- Universal cuffs, which can be helpful for those with limited hand control
- A cup with a cut-out (nosey cup) to assist those who experience difficulty with head control

Independence and occupational performance may also be promoted in feeding, eating, and swallowing for those who depend on a caregiver for nutritional intake. This is accomplished by assisting the client with

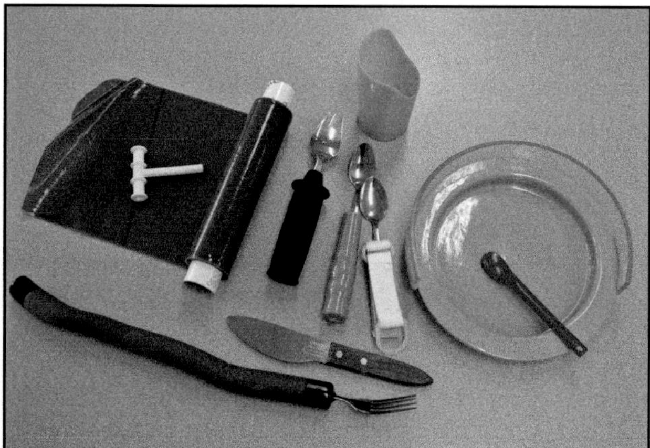

**Figure 35-2.** Assorted adapted equipment commonly used for eating and feeding. Clockwise from left to right: Dycem, chewy stick, built-up utensil, weighted utensil, spoon with universal cuff, nosey cup, weighted plate with plate guard, bolus spoon, rocker knife, and wrap-around utensil.

difficulty in these areas to become an active participant in the relationship that forms between the client and the caregiver.

Expanding the client's options for making choices about types of foods/liquids eaten, times of meals, and other contextual or environmental factors related to feeding and eating fosters independence, engagement, and participation in these occupations. This, in turn, facilitates independence as clients are encouraged to make decisions regarding their own lives (Crittenden, 1990).

# Phases of Oral Eating

## Anticipatory and Pre-Oral Phase

The anticipatory phase of eating is typically described as a precursor to the actual eating of food (Smith & Jenks, 2013). This phase involves addressing a variety of psychosocial factors that may influence a client's participation in mealtime. This may include whether or not the client experiences a sense of hunger, who is preparing the food, where the client is going to eat, with whom the client is eating, and how the food is presented. Intervention in this phase could be directed at performance patterns, performance skills, context and environment, and/or client factors (AOTA, 2014b).

Intervention may focus on the following:

- How the client's routine either supports or hinders participation in mealtime. If the client experiences a decrease in energy or stamina, intervention may focus on developing a routine for meal preparation that utilizes energy conservation techniques to facilitate occupational performance.
- How the social expectations of eating meals out with friends may change if a client is no longer able to feed him- or herself, the occupational therapy practitioner may work with the client and a caregiver to develop skills to negotiate eating out in favored restaurants
- How to present foods for an altered diet consistency so that the food is appealing to the client

The pre-oral phase is described as a "process in which the food or drink is brought to the mouth either by the person engaged in the eating or by the feeder" (AOTA, 2007, p. 698). In this phase the focus may be on how the meal is presented and set up for the client, the ability to grasp a utensil or cup, the ability to bring the utensil or cup to the mouth, or the ability to manipulate finger foods to bring to the mouth. This phase of eating and swallowing is a voluntary process requiring the client to be alert and involved in the process of getting the food to the mouth.

Intervention in this phase may focus on the following:

- Gaining range of motion at the shoulder to facilitate the ability to bring a spoon or cup from the table to the client's mouth.
- Improving strength and coordination to grasp a variety of utensils, cups, and foods for increased independence in mealtimes.

## Oral Preparatory Phase

The phase incorporates a combination of motor and sensory skills that include how the food looks and smells. This phase builds on the client's ability to reach for the food and bring it to his or her mouth with a focus on managing the food once it is in the mouth (AOTA, 2007; Avery, 2014; Smith & Jenks, 2013). This phase also includes the sensory processing skills necessary to assist in determining the taste, texture, and temperature of foods and the initial motor skills needed to prepare and position the food for swallowing. This phase is also voluntary and requires the client to be alert and an active part of the process. Intervention in this phase may be directed at assisting with sensory, motor, cognitive, or perceptual skills that inhibit a client's occupational performance in the areas of feeding and eating.

Examples of intervention techniques in this phase include the following:

- Cheek and jaw support and facilitation of movement can improve feeding effectiveness in preterm infants (Hwang, Lin, Coster, Bigsby, & Vergara, 2010), as well as other clients of all ages who may have weak facial musculature.
- To address weakness of lips or cheeks and concerns regarding range of motion, the use of tapping, vibration, quick stretch or slow stretch, resistive sucking,

and blowing exercises (Avery, 2014; Korth & Rendell, 2015; Smith & Jenks, 2013) may help with strength and range of motion.

- For the presence of atypical oral reflexes, training caregivers to avoid stimulation of the reflex through positioning and adaptive techniques, as well as positioning with stability, may help reduce the impact of atypical reflexes (Avery, 2014).
- To support postural control for muscle efficiency, position with stability in the trunk and pelvis (Korth & Rendell, 2015, Smith & Jenks, 2013). For example, positioning may need to address proximal control at the trunk and pelvis to facilitate distal functioning (utensil use or finger feeding) at mealtimes.
- For concerns related to oral hypersensitivity, try deep pressure or proprioceptive input in and around the mouth, work with food textures that are comfortable for the client (some clients with sensory processing concerns prefer smooth textures, whereas others prefer crunchy), and develop sensory diet activities that calm and organize the oral area before and during a meal or snack (Korth & Rendell, 2015; Logemann, 1998).
- For concerns related to oral hyposensitivity, therapists may try using warmer/colder and more flavorful tastes to stimulate sensation, as well as developing sensory diet techniques that are alerting to increase input to the oral area before and during a meal or snack (Arvedson, Brodsky, & Reigstad, 2002; Logemann, 1998).
- For children experiencing difficulties with the sensory properties of food, food chaining is a technique that is emerging to help children who are restrictive or "picky" eaters (Fraker, Fishbein, Cox, & Walbert, 2007). This technique includes expanding the repertoire of foods by matching color, texture, or context to increase types of food intake in a systematic fashion. Behavioral techniques can enhance this method, which is often used with children who are on the autism spectrum. The Sequential Oral Sensory Approach to feeding may also benefit children who have difficulty with sensory experiences around food and mealtimes (Toomey & Sundeth-Ross, 2011).

## Oral Phase

This phase is described as the phase in which the bolus of food or liquid is propelled by the tongue; masticated by the teeth and gums; and manipulated by the lips, cheeks, and tongue (AOTA, 2007; Avery, 2014; Smith & Jenks, 2013). In this phase, the action is to move the food to the back of the mouth in preparation for initiating the swallow. This phase of the swallow is also voluntary and typically takes about 1 second to complete (Smith & Jenks, 2013). Intervention in this phase for clients who are considered safe for oral feeding is typically directed at assisting with sensory and motor skills that inhibit a client's occupational performance in the areas of feeding and eating.

Examples of intervention techniques in this phase include the following:

- For concerns with slow oral transit time, interventions might include the use of cold or sour boluses, or infusing a sour into foods (such as lemon).
- The occupational therapy practitioner may try thermal stimulation as cold temperatures may facilitate the initiation of the swallow (Avery, 2014; Logemann, Kahrilas, Kobara, & Vakil, 1989).
- For concerns related to positioning of the head and neck for a safe swallow, encourage a chin tuck, which moves the base of the tongue back and protects the airway when the larynx is low and the swallow is weak (Case-Smith & Humphry, 2005; Ohmae, Logemann, Kaiser, Hanson, & Kahrilas, 1996). Korth and Rendell (2015) state that a chin tuck may be contraindicated in some situations, and as such, occupational therapists need to make recommendations based upon comprehensive and individualized assessment (p. 405).
- The occupational therapy practitioner may also try encouraging the individual to use an effortful swallow that helps to facilitate tongue retraction and increase oral and pharyngeal pressure, followed by encouraging the client to squeeze hard with throat muscles while swallowing (Avery, 2014; Pouderoux & Kahrilas, 1995; Smith & Jenks, 2013).
- Following assessment, clients with hemiparesis may use neck rotation to turn the head toward the weaker side, which can help to close the weaker side of the pharynx, utilizing the stronger side (Avery, 2014; Logemann et al., 1989; Smith & Jenks, 2013).
- Therapists may also try intervention strategies aimed at improving oral motor control and coordination as suggested previously in the oral preparatory phase.

Additional references for assessment and intervention in the oral phase include Arvedson and Brodsky (2002), Case-Smith and Humphry (2005), Korth and Rendell (2015), and Wolf and Glass (1992).

## Pharyngeal Phase

This phase is described as the phase in which the swallowing response is initiated and breathing is briefly interrupted (AOTA, 2007; Avery, 2014; Smith & Jenks, 2013). This is an involuntary process, and intervention in the pharyngeal phase is often directed toward working with the individual's team to determine the ability to safely swallow.

This intervention is typically accomplished through facilitated head and neck positioning, including a chin tuck as appropriate for safe swallowing. Diagnostic testing is frequently recommended to examine the individual's ability to safely swallow a variety of food and liquid consistencies without risk of aspiration (i.e., videofluoroscopy). Intervention may involve working with the team to train an individual and his or her caregivers as to what types of foods/liquids are recommended and safe. For example, it may be recommended that the individual have no thin liquids. Strategies would then be discussed to avoid thin liquids and meltables (e.g., ice cream, popsicles, ice), or to thicken liquids to an appropriate consistency as determined by the individual's intervention team (Smith & Jenks, 2013).

Clients with concerns in the pharyngeal phase of swallowing frequently are diagnosed with dysphagia. If the client has swallowing problems or an inability to swallow, the occupational therapist should be aware that continuing education and specialized training is necessary for competent interventions in this area. Specialized medical intervention in addition to individualized precautions are often indicated when a client is experiencing dysphagia. Speech pathologists and occupational therapy practitioners frequently work collaboratively with the client with dysphagia after diagnostic testing is performed. Additional team members may include the physician, a radiologist, a nurse, and nutrition or dietary services (AOTA, 2007).

### *Esophageal Phase*

This phase is described as the phase in which the bolus enters the esophagus and travels through the esophagus and into the stomach (AOTA, 2007; Avery, 2014; Smith & Jenks, 2013). Occupational therapy practitioners do not typically provide direct intervention for concerns identified in this area. However, as a team member working on concerns related to feeding, eating, and swallowing, occupational therapy practitioners need to be aware of concerns that could arise in this phase of eating.

Occupational therapy practitioners may assist in developing interventions focusing on positioning or other factors to improve safety and comfort. In addition, occupational therapy practitioners may assist in team decisions regarding further diagnostic assessment to determine concerns in this phase of eating (AOTA, 2007).

## Non-Oral Feeding

Non-oral feedings are utilized to support nutritional intake when risk of aspiration is a concern and it does not appear to be safe for the individual to eat by mouth.

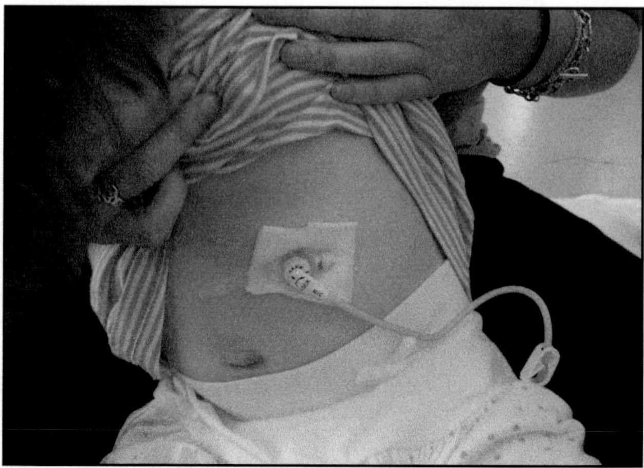

**Figure 35-3.** Placement of a gastrostomy tube for non-oral feeding.

Non-oral feeding may also be utilized to support nutritional intake when the individual is not able to effectively and efficiently take in enough calories by mouth to support growth and overall health (Korth & Rendell, 2015; Morris & Klein, 2000; Smith & Jenks, 2013). Feeding tubes or enteral nutrition may be a temporary or a permanent solution to nutritional intake concerns. Occupational therapy practitioners work with individuals and teams to facilitate the transition from non-oral to oral feedings as appropriate. In addition, occupational therapy practitioners work closely with clients and their families/caregivers to integrate tube feedings into the habits and routines that exist around mealtimes (Korth & Rendell, 2015; Morris & Klein, 2000).

Non-oral feedings are delivered through various tube placements. A few types (defined in the Glossary) include nasogastric tubes, gastrostomy tubes, and jejunostomy tubes. A nasogastric tube is inserted through the nasal cavity into the stomach, a gastrostomy tube bypasses the mouth and is inserted surgically directly into the stomach (Figure 35-3), and a jejunostomy tube is surgically inserted into the jejunum (a branch of the small intestine). For some clients, non-oral feedings will continue secondary to structural issues or neurological issues that prevent safe oral feedings. For others, the goal is to transition from non-oral feedings to oral feedings; however, the process of weaning from non-oral to oral feedings is often complex. Schauster and Dwyer (1996) suggest that promoting a positive relationship between the client and caregiver is an important first step in facilitating the transition to oral feedings. In addition, the transition is facilitated by intervention aimed at normalizing feeding and eating through safe and structured exploration of oral experiences (Figure 35-4).

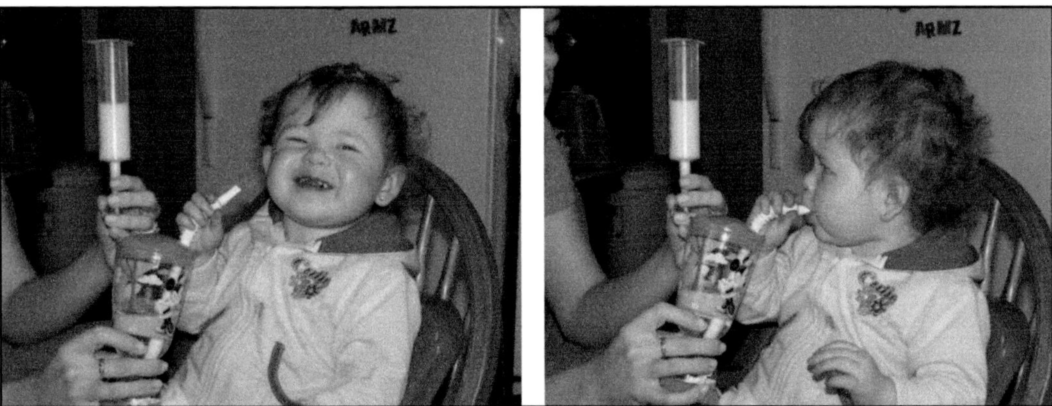

**Figure 35-4.** Providing oral opportunities during non-oral feedings.

# General Factors to Consider

## Developmental Progression

The infant is born with a small oral cavity. The fatty cheek pads and tongue are in close proximity to each other and nearly fill the oral cavity such that a typically developing infant can easily achieve suction and compress a nipple because of the tight fit when placed in the mouth (Korth & Rendell, 2015; Morris & Klein, 2000; Wolf & Glass, 1992). The structures of the throat in the infant are also in close proximity to one another. This arrangement of structures allows for the flow of liquid to pass safely from the base of the tongue to the esophagus. Protection of the trachea from liquid occurs as the larynx elevates the epiglottis and falls over the trachea. The structure of the oral cavity allows for a safe swallow when held in a reclined position for early breast- and bottle-feeding. Aspiration is unlikely in the first 4 months due to these structural arrangements, allowing the safe feeding of infants in a reclined position (Korth & Rendell, 2015; Morris & Klein, 2000). This factor becomes important when working with young children with feeding concerns as structural changes begin to occur between 4 and 6 months and continue through the first year of development (Morris & Klein, 2000). This is important in terms of intervention as therapists need to assist parents in developing options for upright feeding and eating when developmentally appropriate to support safe swallowing without aspiration.

## Positioning

The position of the trunk, head, and neck directly affects the ability to swallow safely in children and adults; therefore, the first and most important aspect of feeding and eating intervention is ensuring that the client is in the proper position for eating (Smith & Jenks, 2013). When positioning a client, the occupational therapy practitioner should typically begin at the pelvis. As feasible, the client should be positioned symmetrically from the head through the neck, trunk, and to the hips. A firm surface is best with the knees and ankles at 90 degrees. The pelvis can be in a slight anterior pelvic tilt with the hips at about 100 degrees (Smith & Jenks, 2013). The trunk should be flexed slightly forward with the back straight. The head should be slightly forward with the chin slightly tucked. Arms can be positioned on the table if necessary for support. It should be noted that in some cases, due to structural or neurological impairments, it might be difficult to achieve symmetry. However, this should be the overall goal to encourage safe swallowing, facilitate postural alignment, and prevent structural deformity (Figure 35-5).

## Suck, Swallow, Breathe Synchrony

An infant as well as a client recovering from neurological diagnosis ideally begins with a suck, swallow, breathe synchrony. The smooth coordination between sucking, swallowing, and breathing is what allows the client to eat effectively and efficiently (Wolf & Glass, 1992). This is evident, as seen with infants suckling from the breast or bottle. It should be noted that clients with respiratory difficulties might experience feeding and eating difficulties because of the necessary breathing component in the rhythm of this synchrony of eating.

## Diet Selection

Diet selection is an important component of the feeding and eating program. Precautions for clients with suspected swallowing difficulties may include avoiding foods with multiple textures; fibrous or stringy vegetables, meats, or fruits; crumbly or flaky foods; foods that liquefy; and foods with skins or seeds (Smith & Jenks, 2013). Diet selection is a team decision that includes the client and caregivers. It is a decision that must be determined following comprehensive evaluation of the client's feeding and eating skills (Smith & Jenks, 2013).

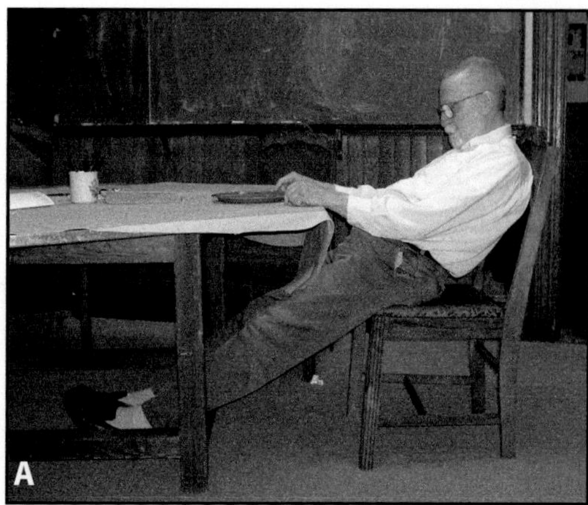


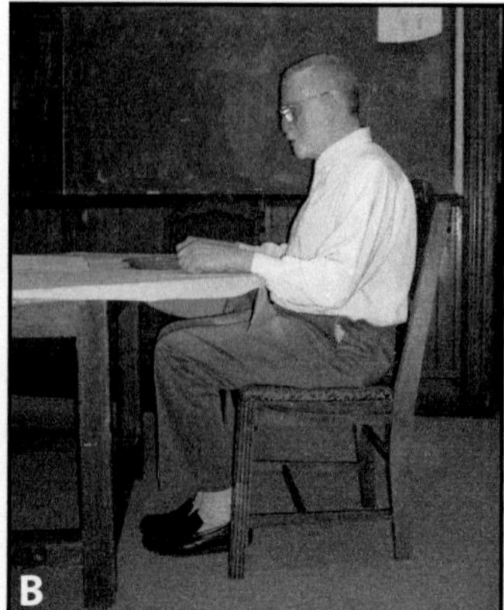


**Figure 35-5.** (A) Improper eating position vs. (B) proper eating position.

## Diet Progression

After making a diet selection, developmental and rehabilitative approaches suggest that, as feasible, the diet should move in the following order from the easiest to manage to the most difficult:

### Solids

Based on recommendations of the National Dysphagia Diet Task Force (2002), as referenced in Smith and Jenks (2013):

- Level 1—Dysphagia puréed (the lowest level of consistency for solids)
- Level 2—Dysphagia mechanically altered (mechanical soft)
- Level 3—Dysphagia advanced
- Regular diet

### Liquids

In general, thickened liquids may be easier to manage based on thorough assessment of swallowing. Liquid consistency may progress to thinner liquids as tolerated by the client. Most dysphagia diet progressions include four liquid consistencies: thin, nectar-like, honey-like, and finally spoon thick. Following consultation with team members, liquids may be thickened with commercial thickeners or with purées such as yogurt or fruit purée. Some commercial thickeners may be contraindicated for young children and for some diagnostic conditions (Korth & Rendell, 2015). Occupational therapy practitioners who are working with clients on dysphagia diets should familiarize themselves with current Food and Drug Administration warnings and information regarding indications and contraindications for use of thickeners.

Ongoing assessment is indicated when considering changing or progressing a client's diet. The decision to move a client to a modified consistency should be a team decision based on diagnostic assessment and clinical reasoning. It should be noted that thin liquids are typically the most difficult consistency to swallow and the easiest to aspirate. Thin liquids should only be given if you are certain the client has an intact swallow. A safe swallow can be determined through videofluoroscopy or a modified barium swallow. Signs and symptoms of possible aspiration include but are not limited to the following (Avery, 2014):

- Prolonged or inefficient cough
- A wet, gurgly quality to the client's voice before, during, or after eating
- Any color change in the client during or after eating
- Breathiness or loss of voice when eating

If the occupational therapy practitioner has any concerns regarding the client's ability to swallow safely, he or she should discuss concerns with the client and his or her team to determine the need for further assessment prior to intervention.

# Additional Issues for Feeding and Eating

## Nil Per Os

*Nil per os,* the Latin term for "nothing by mouth," is a very important and strict precaution. All occupational therapy practitioners should check a client's chart and strictly adhere to this precaution.

## *No Thin Liquids*

Difficulty with thin liquids is common with people after a neurological diagnosis such as a cerebrovascular accident (CVA) or brain injury. The client with aspiration precautions should be watched carefully. Liquids may be thickened with products such as applesauce, Thick-It (Precision Foods, Inc.), or other products. Thickening of liquids should only occur following thorough assessment including appropriate medical testing and team discussion. The client should be closely monitored while eating.

## *Special Diets*

Clients with diabetes, food allergies, or special precautions will be on special diets. The occupational therapy practitioner should be vigilant about knowing precautions and making sure that the client and caregivers fully understand the precautions as well.

## *Sensory Impairment/ Sensory Processing*

An assessment of the client's sensory processing is an important component of feeding, eating, and swallowing evaluation and intervention. Clients with hyposensitivity or decreased sensation will often be unaware of foods in the cheeks or under the tongue. It is important to work with these clients on sensory reeducation or sensory processing strategies to increase awareness and tolerance when eating and drinking. Clients with hypersensitivity or increased sensitivity are often defensive or hyperaware of temperature, taste, and other sensory properties of foods, such as smell, and the visual aspects of foods. A sensory-based intervention program can be helpful to overcome these difficulties (Chatoor, 2009; Korth & Rendell, 2015).

## *General Intervention Techniques*

A variety of techniques might be recommended for the client or for caregiver carryover of feeding, eating, and swallowing strategies. Caregiver programs are individualized and need to be developed based on the client's current areas of need. As occupational therapy practitioners, we must be responsive to creating education materials that are "understandable, accessible and usable by the full spectrum of consumers" (AOTA, 2011, p. 1).

### Positioning

- Ensure proper positioning while feeding, eating, and swallowing by providing the client, caregiver, and/or interprofessional team with a picture or diagram of best positioning for eating. Provide necessary external supports to help facilitate or maintain proper positioning with hips and knees flexed at 90 degrees, feet supported, and trunk symmetrical and erect.
- Positioning to facilitate optimal feeding, eating, and swallowing might include lateral supports, pillows, cushions, or other supports as determined by the intervention team.
- Encourage the client to tuck the chin to better align the head and neck for a safe swallow.

### Presentation of Foods and Liquids

- Assist client and caregivers to follow specifics related to dietary consistency and food choices for each client's nutrition, independence, and safety.
- Consider the pace of the presentation of foods/liquids—some clients will need more time between bites of foods or sips of liquid to process, whereas others will need less time.
- Be aware of the amount of food or liquid being presented—too much or too little food or liquid may affect the client's ability to safely participate in the mealtime and may affect independence as well.

### Sensory Information

- The occupational therapy practitioner may recommend providing sensory input prior to and during feeding to improve sensory awareness in and around the mouth as long as the input is not aversive to the client.
- Provide tactile cues to encourage the use of the correct movement patterns to facilitate the processes of feeding, eating, and swallowing.

### Adaptive Equipment and Adaptive Techniques

- Use adapted equipment as needed to facilitate safety, efficiency, and independence in the occupations of feeding, eating, and swallowing (Figure 35-6).
- Teach the client to clear the throat of food and liquid by coughing, and/or teach the client's caregivers/team to cue the client to clear the throat.

### Contextual Considerations

- Be aware of how cultural considerations may affect your intervention choices. Are there certain foods that are important to the client and/or family? Are there certain routines around mealtimes that need to be addressed?
- You may need to work with the client and caregivers to create an environment that facilitates participation, such as a quieter mealtime, more social interaction, or fewer distractions.

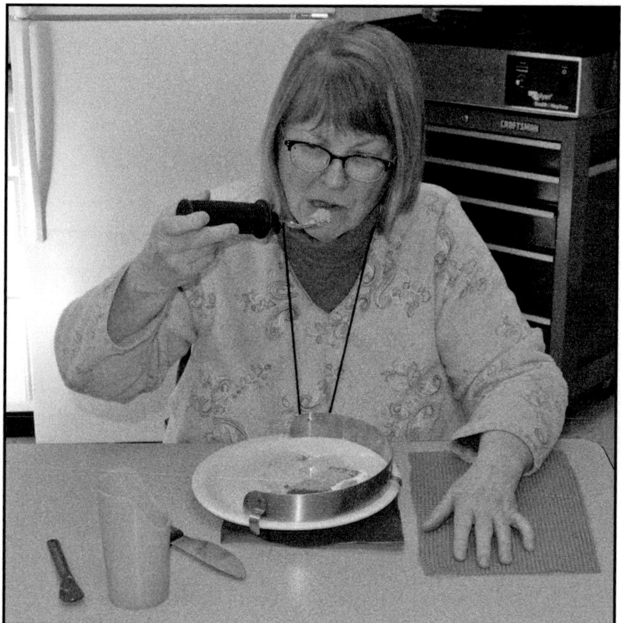

**Figure 35-6.** An adult uses adaptive equipment for independent feeding.

# Professional Reasoning

What are the questions the occupational therapist should ask that begin to guide his or her choice of intervention strategies?

"A profession's domain of concern consists of those areas of human experience in which practitioners of the profession offer assistance to others" (Mosey, 1981, p. 51). The *Framework* (AOTA, 2014b) outlines the domain of practice of occupational therapy "which outlines the profession's purview and the areas in which its members have an established body of knowledge and expertise" (p. S3).

Professional reasoning and evidence-based practice guide the occupational therapist in planning and implementing intervention in the area of feeding and eating using the domain and process established in the *Framework* (AOTA, 2014b). This process is not intended to be prescriptive; each occupational therapy practitioner and client will bring unique areas of strength and areas of concern to be considered. It is also not exhaustive in nature and, as stated previously, is intended to provide a guide for assisting occupational therapy practitioners and the clients with whom they work in planning intervention.

# Occupational Performance

## *Performance Skills*

What motor performance skills and body functions are influencing the client's ability to feed him- or herself or participate in the process of being fed?

Example: There is difficulty with stability and postural control of the trunk, neck, head, and upper or lower extremities while eating.

- Intervention strategies
  - ◊ Remediation/restoration
    - * Therapeutic positioning
    - * Neurodevelopmental Treatment techniques or other facilitation/inhibition techniques to address muscle tone
    - * Graded participation in functional activities to increase occupational performance
  - ◊ Compensation/adaptation
    - * Addition of lateral supports, head/neck supports, or other positioning aids
    - * Mobile arm supports or foot supports

Example: There is decreased strength, coordination, and/or range of motion necessary to bring a cup or a spoon to the mouth.

- Intervention strategies
  - ◊ Remediation/restoration
    - * Therapeutic activities to promote active range of motion as indicated
    - * Therapeutic activities to facilitate muscle strength
    - * Neuromuscular facilitation or inhibition techniques to facilitate active use of the upper extremities in feeding and eating
  - ◊ Compensation/adaptation
    - * Adaptive equipment such as a universal cuff, built-up spoon, or adaptive cup
    - * Self-feeding devices

Example: The client is demonstrating concerns regarding the ability to swallow safely.

This area requires advanced skills and knowledge to intervene. The entry-level practitioner should refer this client to a more experienced team member or seek consult with a feeding and eating specialist.

What process skills, including level of arousal, attention to task, perceptual awareness, impulse control, and cognitive functioning, are influencing the client's ability to feed him- or herself or to be fed?

Example: The client does not have the necessary energy, endurance, and/or breath support to facilitate occupational performance in the areas of eating and feeding.

- Intervention strategies
  - ◊ Remediation/restoration
    - * Postural control activities
    - * Activities designed to improve breath support
    - * Activities designed to build endurance

- ◊ Compensation/adaptation
  - * Positioning
  - * Adaptation of the context to facilitate reduced activity, promote relaxation when eating
  - * Teach the use of energy conservation techniques and pacing techniques

Example: The client lacks the necessary skills to motor plan and sequence the actions needed for occupational performance in the areas of feeding, eating, and swallowing.

- Intervention strategies
  - ◊ Remediation/restoration
    - * Provide consistent instruction during feeding, eating, and swallowing
    - * Establish routines for the client and his or her caregivers around feeding and eating
  - ◊ Compensation/adaptation
    - * Provide checklists for visual cues
    - * Design verbal, written, and/or visual cues to facilitate feeding, eating, and swallowing

Example: For a client who depends on a caregiver for physical assistance or cueing during feeding, eating, and swallowing, there is a concern related to the relationship between the client and the caregiver that does not support occupational performance.

- Intervention strategies
  - ◊ Remediation/restoration
    - * Role model the appropriate level of assistance for the caregiver using a coaching model
    - * Assist the client to be assertive in the feeding, eating, and swallowing process
  - ◊ Compensation/adaptation
    - * Give the caregiver a checklist of appropriate steps
    - * Put verbal cues on a tape recorder
    - * Provide adaptive equipment such as a self-feeder to eliminate the need for assistance

Please note that client factors should be individually evaluated and addressed in the occupational therapy process. Many client factors vary and require advanced practice skills for intervention.

## Performance Patterns

The occupational therapy practitioner may use or develop the client's habits to assist in facilitating his or her occupational performance in the areas of feeding, eating, and swallowing. Establish or facilitate routines that positively influence occupational performance in the areas of feeding, eating, and swallowing. Establish or facilitate roles to positively affect the client's occupations related to feeding and eating. Integrate cultural or religious rituals or functions that are important to this client's occupational performance in the area of feeding and eating into intervention.

## Context

The practitioner should assess the environment for optimal function for each client concerning noise and distractions, visual stimuli, room temperature, and olfactory input. Some clients benefit from the company of others, whereas others eat more efficiently alone, especially if eating is challenging for them. A typical, natural setting is usually best for clients of all ages.

Context includes the following considerations for intervention:

- **Cultural context:** What are the beliefs, values, or attitudes related to feeding and eating? Examples include consideration of religious holidays and family roles for the occupations of feeding and eating.
- **Physical context:** What are the qualities of the environment or objects within the environment as they relate to feeding and eating? Examples include the use of utensils and the ability to eat in noisy or distracting environments.
- **Social context:** What are the relationships that are important in terms of feeding and eating? Examples include individuals who are present at the family table at meals and how relationships change when eating at home versus eating out.
- **Personal context:** Who is the client receiving intervention for concerns related to feeding and eating? Examples include how intervention differs for a parent versus a child.
- **Spiritual factors:** What might inspire or motivate the client receiving intervention? Examples include the natural environment of the client and special meals/foods.
- **Temporal context:** What factors related to time might influence performance in the areas of feeding and eating? Examples include considering when the client is used to eating meals—is a large meal preferred at noon or at 5 p.m.?

## Activity Demands

Consideration of activity demands is an important part of intervention planning for feeding and eating. The occupational therapy practitioner should carefully consider the demands of each activity chosen to ensure that a "just-right challenge" is achieved during the therapeutic process.

## Client Factors

Client factors include body functions and body structures (AOTA, 2014b). Body functions include but are not limited to motor, sensory, cognitive, and perceptual functions; body structures include but are not limited to the structures of the nervous system; structures related to sensory receptors; structures related to movement; and structures related to digestive, cardiovascular, and respiratory systems.

These factors should be considered individually to determine how the factors might affect occupational performance in feeding, eating, and swallowing. Intervention would then be directed at restoration or remediation of areas of concern or at developing compensatory or adaptive strategies to improve performance.

For example, restoration or remediation would be actually improving the ability to bring hand to mouth, whereas compensation would be implementing the use of an assistive device to bring hand to mouth.

## Summary

Feeding and eating are necessary and pleasurable occupations of daily life. Because of the potential loss of independence, loss or change in occupational performance, or risk of safety concerns related to feeding, eating, and swallowing, the occupational therapy practitioner should carefully evaluate and plan intervention for each client in relationship to the model of intervention chosen. The occupational therapy practitioner can carry out that plan with interprofessional input for effective eating and feeding interventions. Independence or effective interdependence in safe feeding and eating are important components of occupational therapy intervention planning.

## Student Self-Assessment

1. Break up into small groups and discuss how context is important to you, your friends, and your family in terms of eating and feeding. Now consider how you would include contextual factors in your intervention planning for clients across the lifespan who are experiencing concerns in the area of eating and feeding. Refer to the *Framework* (AOTA, 2014b).
2. Working in pairs or small groups as an experiential learning exercise, complete an activity analysis of the sensory/motor patterns that are necessary for eating different textures. Fill out the chart in Table 35-1 with your findings. (This chart can be expanded for classroom purposes.)
3. Using Thick-It or another commercially available thickener, thicken water and juice to each of the following thicknesses: honey, nectar, and spoon thick. Try the same activity but use applesauce or another fruit purée. What are the differences between the commercially available thickener and fruit purée? Are there other foods you might be able to use to thicken thin liquids or purées for a modified diet? Discuss the team members and assessment procedures that will determine what modifications need to be made to a client's diet. What are precautions or contraindications to the use of thickeners?
4. For each of the two case studies that follow, students will first fill out Table 35-2 to identify possible options for intervention, and second, role-play to perform the tasks to help your client eat. The instructor will need tables and chairs with armrests, applesauce, graham crackers, lollipops, vibration devices, adaptive equipment of all types, spoons, and paper or nosey cups. Students need to wash their hands and use protective gloves. Hand washing and gloving should be emphasized as a part of infection control. Be sure to ask if any students have latex or food allergies. Students will work in pairs, each taking a turn at being a "client" and a "therapist." Students actually do hands-on set up, positioning, feeding, and facilitation of eating as noted in their completed intervention chart.
   - Client A: Your client, Bob Brown, is a 65-year-old man who had a left CVA about 1 week ago. He has recently been transferred from an acute care hospital to your rehabilitation facility. Bob is a friendly, kind man who served as a police officer until his recent retirement. Bob has right-sided hemiparesis with overall low tone and a low level of alertness. Bob is right dominant. Bob has minimal active movement in his right dominant upper extremity but he is developing some active shoulder elevation and flexion, elbow flexion, and beginning movement of the fingers toward a gross grasp. Bob enjoys spending time with family but is overwhelmed with too much stimulation. Bob sometimes seems embarrassed when he experiences a loss of liquid or food in front of his wife, children, and grandchildren. He has impaired sensation on the right side of his face. He has hypotonia and poor postural control of the trunk, and his head control is weak. Bob has been responding well to facilitation techniques for postural control and head control. You are beginning an eating and feeding program based on the following evaluation results. Prior to the

Table 35-1.

## Activity Analysis of the Sensory/Motor Patterns Form

| Food Type | Motor Patterns Needed (discuss and document motor patterns for the lips, tongue, jaw, cheeks) | Sensory Considerations of Each Food (taste, texture, visual, olfactory, proprioceptive) |
|---|---|---|
| Cracker | | |
| Applesauce | | |
| Carrot stick | | |
| Milkshake | | |
| Rice | | |
| Gummy bear | | |

Table 35-2.

## Feeding, Eating, and Swallowing Interventions

| Intervention Idea | Client A—Bob | Client B—Susan |
|---|---|---|
| Environment or context | | |
| Positioning | | |
| Fine motor skills | | |
| Oral motor skills | | |
| Adaptive equipment or devices | | |
| Additional information needed | | |

CVA, Bob enjoyed many occupations including eating out multiple times per week with friends and family, backyard grilling, and hosting Sunday afternoon football parties where he was involved in the food preparation. Bob hopes to return home in 2 weeks.

Oral motor function: Bob is demonstrating difficulty with lip closure on the right side, and the ability to keep food in his mouth. He has difficulty with lip rounding to drink from a straw or assist with removing food from a spoon. Bob has weakness in the muscles of the lips, cheeks, and tongue. He is demonstrating difficulty with lateral movement of the tongue to clear and position food, more pronounced on the right. He also demonstrates difficulty secondary to jaw weakness.

Swallowing: Bob has had a swallow study completed that revealed some aspiration on thin liquids most likely due to muscle weakness and

## Evidence-Based Research Chart

| Topic | Evidence |
|---|---|
| Behavioral approaches to feeding and eating intervention | Babbitt et al., 1994; Linscheid, 2006; Roche et al., 2011; Twachtman-Reilly, Amaral, & Zebrowski, 2008 |
| Refusal to eat | Bazyk, 2000; Fraker & Walbert, 2011 |
| General feeding intervention | Bober, Humphry, Carswell, & Core, 2001; Case-Smith & Humphry, 2005; Edwards & Martin, 2011; Howe & Wang, 2013; Logemann et al., 2009 |
| Management of drooling | Brei, 2003; Domaracki & Sisson, 1990; Fairhurst & Cockerill, 2011; Iammatteo, Trombly, & Luecke, 1990; Squires, Wills, & Rowson, 2012 |
| Sensory motor concerns related to feeding and eating | Case-Smith, 1989; Overland, 2011; Palmer & Heyman, 1993; Toomey & Sundeth-Ross, 2011 |
| Feeding tube dependency | Schauster & Dwyer, 1996; Tarbell & Allaire, 2002 |

tone changes post CVA. Difficulty was noted in the oral and pharyngeal phases of swallowing. In addition, because of current motor difficulties, he is demonstrating difficulties in the pre-oral and oral phases of swallowing as well. Bob is demonstrating difficulty breaking foods down and forming a bolus to initiate swallowing.

◊ Client B: Susan Smith is a 28-year-old woman who sustained a brain injury 3 months ago because of a car accident. Prior to the accident Susan was living independently and working as a blackjack dealer in Las Vegas. Susan has overall high muscle tone, ataxia, and is hyperalert. She is currently at Rancho Scale Level V. Susan is confused, but is not agitated; however, she is easily distracted. She has difficulty with initiation of activities, remembering activities, and paying attention. She is easily overstimulated, becoming irritated with noise or too many verbal instructions. Susan is able to use both of her upper extremities but has difficulty with coordinated hand function, which affects her independence at mealtimes. She tends to be impulsive at times and will eat quickly, often overstuffing her mouth, which leads to frequent coughing or spitting out food. She is restless and moves around as she eats, sometimes even getting up out of the chair, forgetting what she was doing. As part of her rehab team you are working on a possible discharge plan because Susan cannot live independently at this time.

5. Have students watch a DVD of a videofluoroscopy. These are often available through medical centers with swallowing programs. Watch a typical swallow and have students discuss what they are seeing in the progression. Watch an atypical swallow and see if students can see the areas of difficulty. Discuss the case and why swallowing deficits are dangerous and need to have special attention and a team approach. Occupational therapy practitioners should note the signs and symptoms of an abnormal swallow and make appropriate referrals. Occupational therapy practitioners require further education to perform dysphagia intervention.

## Acknowledgments

Thank you to Kathryn M. Loukas, OTD, MS, OTR/L, FAOTA, for her contribution to this chapter in the Second Edition of this textbook.

## References

American Occupational Therapy Association. (2007). Specialized knowledge and skills in eating and feeding for occupational therapy practice. *American Journal of Occupational Therapy, 61*, 686-700.

American Occupational Therapy Association. (2011). AOTA's societal statement on health literacy. *American Journal of Occupational Therapy, 65*(Suppl.), S78-S79. doi:10.5014/ajot.2011.65S78

American Occupational Therapy Association. (2014a). Guidelines for supervision, roles, and responsibilities during the delivery of occupational therapy services. *American Journal of Occupational Therapy, 68*(Suppl. 3), S16-S22.

American Occupational Therapy Association. (2014b). Occupational therapy practice framework: Domain and process (3rd ed.) *American Journal of Occupational Therapy, 68*(Suppl. 1), S1-S48. doi:10.5014/ajot.2014.682006

Arvedson, J. C., & Brodsky, L. (2002). *Pediatric swallowing and feeding assessment and management.* Albany, NY: Singular Publishing Group.

Arvedson, J. C., Brodsky, L., & Reigstad, D. (2002). Clinical feeding and swallowing assessment. In J. C. Arvedson & L. Brodsky (Eds.), *Pediatric swallowing and feeding assessment and management* (2nd ed., pp. 283-340). Albany, NY: Singular Publishing Group.

Avery, W. (2014). Dysphagia. In M. V. Radomski & C. A. Trombly (Eds.), *Occupational therapy for physical dysfunction* (7th ed., pp. 1327-1351). Philadelphia, PA: Lippincott Williams and Wilkins.

Babbitt, R. L., Hoch, T. A., Coe, D. A., Cataldo, M. F., Kelly, K. J., Stackhouse, C., et al. (1994). Behavioral assessment and treatment of pediatric feeding disorders. *Developmental and Behavioral Pediatrics, 15*(4), 278-291.

Baer, C. T. (2005). Addressing feeding with adults with developmental disabilities: A team approach, part 1. *Developmental Disabilities Special Interest Section Quarterly, 28*, 1-3.

Bazyk, S. (2000). Addressing the complex needs of young children who refuse to eat. *Occupational Therapy Practice, 17*, 10-15.

Bober, S. J., Humphry, R., Carswell, H. W., & Core, A. J. (2001). Toddler's persistence in the emerging occupations of functional play and self-feeding. *American Journal of Occupational Therapy, 55*(4), 369-376.

Brei, T. (2003). Management of drooling. *Seminars in Pediatric Neurology, 10*(4), 265-270.

Case-Smith, J. (1989). *Intervention strategies for promoting feeding skills in infants with sensory deficits. Developmental disabilities: A handbook for occupational therapists*. Philadelphia, PA: Haworth Press.

Case-Smith, J., & Humphry, R. (2005). Feeding intervention. In J. Case-Smith (Ed.), *Occupational therapy for children* (5th ed., pp. 481-520). St. Louis, MO: Elsevier Mosby.

Chatoor, I. (2009). *Diagnosis and treatment of feeding disorders in infants and young children*. Washington, DC: Zero to Three.

Crittenden, P. M. (1990). Toward a concept of autonomy in adolescents with a disability. *Child Health Care, 19*, 162-168.

Domaracki, L. S., & Sisson, L. A. (1990). Decreasing drooling with oral motor stimulation in children with multiple disabilities. *American Journal of Occupational Therapy, 44*(8), 680-684.

Edwards, D. K., & Martin, S. M. (2011). Protecting children as feeding skills develop. *Perspectives on Swallowing and Swallowing Disorders, 29*(3), 88-93. doi:10.1044/sasd20.3.88

Fairhurst, C. B. R., & Cockerill, H. (2011). Management of drooling in children. *Archives of Disease in Childhood: Education and Practice Edition, 96*, 26-30. doi:10.1136/adc.2007.129478

Fraker, C., Fishbein, M., Cox, S., & Walbert, L. (2007). *Food chaining*. Philadelphia, PA: DaCapo Press.

Fraker, C., & Walbert, L. (2011). Treatment of selective eating and dysphagia using pre-chaining and food chaining therapy programs. *Perspectives on Swallowing and Swallowing Disorders, 29*(3), 75-81. doi:10.1044/sasd20.3.75

Howe, T. H., & Wang, T. N. (2013). Systematic review of interventions used in or relevant to occupational therapy for children with feeding difficulties ages birth–5 years. *American Journal of Occupational Therapy, 67*, 405-412. doi:10.5014/ajot.2013.004564

Hwang, Y.-S., Lin, C.-H., Coster, W. J., Bigsby, R., & Vergara, E. (2010). Effectiveness of cheek and jaw support to improve feeding performance of pre-term infants. *American Journal of Occupational Therapy, 64*, 886-894. doi:10.5014/ajot.2010.09031

Iammatteo, P. A., Trombly, C., & Luecke, L. (1990). The effect of mouth closure on drooling and speech. *American Journal of Occupational Therapy, 44*(8), 686-691.

Jenks, K. (2002). Dysphagia. In L. W. Pedretti & M. B. Early (Eds.), *Occupational therapy skills for physical dysfunction* (5th ed., pp. 730-766). St. Louis, MO: Mosby.

Kedesdy, J. H., & Budd, K. S. (1998). *Childhood feeding disorders biobehavioral assessment and intervention*. Baltimore, MD: Paul H. Brookes Publishing Co.

Korth, K., & Rendell, L. (2015). Feeding intervention. In J. Case-Smith & J. C. O'Brien (Eds.), *Occupational therapy for children and adolescents* (7th ed., pp. 389-415). St. Louis, MO: Elsevier Mosby.

Linscheid, T. (2006). Behavioral treatments for pediatric feeding disorders. *Behavior Modification, 30*(1), 6-23.

Logemann, J. A. (1998). *Evaluation and treatment of swallowing disorders*. Austin, TX: Pro-Ed.

Logemann, J. A., Kahrilas, P. J., Kobara, M., & Vakil, N. B. (1989). The benefit of head rotation on pharyngoesophogeal dysphagia. *Archives of Physical Medicine and Rehabilitation, 70*, 767-771.

Logemann, J. A., Rademaker, A., Pauloski, B. R., Kelly, A., Stangl-McBreen, C., Antinoja, J., ... Shaker, R. (2009). A randomized study comparing the shaker exercise with traditional therapy: A preliminary study. *Dysphagia, 24*, 403-411.

Morris, S. E., & Klein, M. D. (2000). *Pre-feeding skills: A comprehensive resource for mealtime development* (2nd ed.). Austin, TX: Therapy Skills Builders.

Mosey, A. C. (1981). *Occupational therapy: Configuration of a profession*. New York, NY: Raven.

Ohmae, Y., Logemann, J. A., Kaiser, P., Hanson, D. G., & Kahrilas, P. J. (1996). Effects of two breath-holding maneuvers on oropharyngeal swallow. *Annals of Otology, Rhinology, and Laryngology, 105*, 123-131.

O'Sullivan, N. (1995). *Dysphagia care: Team approach with acute and long-term patients* (2nd ed.). New York, NY: Cottage Square Press.

Overland, L. (2011). A sensory motor approach to feeding. *Perspectives on Swallowing and Swallowing Disorders, 29*(3), 60-64. doi:10.1044/sasd20.3.60

Palmer, M. M., & Heyman, M. B. (1993). Assessment and treatment of sensory- versus motor-based feeding problems in very young children. *Infants and Young Children, 6*(2), 67-73.

Pouderoux, P., & Kahrilas, P. J. (1995). Deglutitive tongue force modulation by volition, volume, and viscosity in humans. *Gastroenterology, 108*, 1418-1426.

Roche, W. J., Eicher, P. S., Martorana, P., Berkowitz, M., Petronchak, J., Dzioba, J., & Vitello, L. (2011). An oral motor, medical, and behavioral approach to pediatric feeding and swallowing disorders: An interdisciplinary model. *Perspectives on Swallowing and Swallowing Disorders, 29*(3), 65-74. doi:10.1044/sasd20.3.65

Schauster, H., & Dwyer, J. (1996). Transition from tube feedings to feedings by mouth in children: Preventing eating dysfunction. *Journal of the American Dietetic Association, 96*, 277-281.

Smith, J., & Jenks, K. J. (2013). Eating and swallowing. In H. M. Pendelton & W. Schulz-Krohn (Eds.), *Pedretti's occupational therapy practice skills for physical dysfunction* (7th ed., pp. 678-717). St. Louis, MO: Elsevier Mosby.

Squires, N., Wills, A., & Rowson, J. (2012). The management of drooling in adults with neurological conditions. *Current Opinion in Otolaryngology and Head and Neck Surgery, 20*(3), 171-176.

Tarbell, M. C., & Allaire, J. H. (2002). Children with feeding tube dependency: Treating the whole child. *Infants and Young Children, 15*(1), 29-41.

Toomey, K., & Sundeth-Ross, E. (2011). SOS approach to feeding. *Perspectives on Swallowing and Swallowing Disorders, 29*(3), 82-87. doi:10.1044/sasd20.3.82

Twachtman-Reilly, J., Amaral, S. C., & Zebrowski, P. P. (2008). Addressing feeding disorders in children on the autism spectrum in school based settings: Physiological and behavioral issues. *Language, Speech and Hearing Services in Schools, 39*, 261-272.

Wolf, L. S., & Glass, R. G. (1992). *Feeding and swallowing disorders in infancy: Assessment and management*. San Antonio, TX: Therapy Skill Builders.

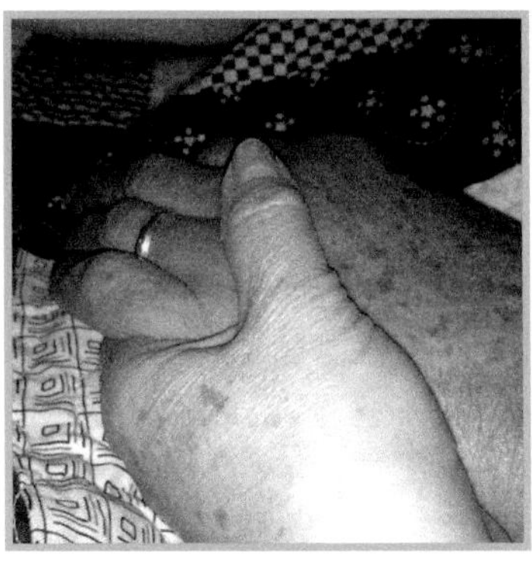

# 36

# Case Management and Coordination

*Diane P. Bergey, MOT, OTR/L and Erica A. Flagg, OT/L*

**ACOTE STANDARDS EXPLORED IN THIS CHAPTER**

**B.5.26–B.5.29**

**KEY VOCABULARY**

- **Care coordination:** A process that facilitates the linkage of individuals and their families with appropriate services and resources in a coordinated effort to achieve good health.
- **Case management:** A collaborative process that assesses, plans, implements, coordinates, monitors, and evaluates the options and services required to meet the client's health and human services needs.
- **Clinical pathway:** A method used in health care settings as a way of organizing, evaluating, and limiting variations in expected client care secondary to diagnosis and other client-specific factors.
- **Interoperability:** A term meaning the ability of diverse systems and organizations to work together in a technical system engineering sense. Alternatively, taking into account social, political, and organizational factors that affect system to system performance, interoperability is synonymous with case management.
- **Managed care:** A variety of methods of financing and organizing the delivery of health care in which costs are contained by controlling the provision of services.
- **Transition services:** A results-oriented process that facilitates movement between settings and providers based on changing client needs. This term is most often used in the school setting but is an essential part of care coordination across the continuum.

Jacobs, K., & MacRae, N. (Eds.).
*Occupational Therapy Essentials for Clinical Competence, Third Edition* (pp. 537-545).

The role of the occupational therapy practitioner in care coordination, case management, and transition services is not only an area of emerging practice, but is already a role that occupational therapy practitioners are filling in traditional practice environments. For instance, it is not uncommon in rural Australia for occupational therapists to work in a dual role as both a case manager and an occupational therapist (Thomasz & Young, 2015). With our education, we are prepared to fill case management roles, utilizing our skills well and meeting the demands of society and our clients effectively. When striving to be marketable in an environment highly influenced by managed care, it is important to realize case management as a career option.

## What Is Case Management?

The Case Management Society of America (CMSA) defines case management as:

> A collaborative process of assessment, planning, facilitation, care coordination, evaluation, and advocacy for options and services to meet an individual and family's comprehensive health needs through communication and available resources to promote quality cost-effective outcomes. (Stricker, 2011)

Case management is both a practice area and a profession; therefore, it allows practitioners from a variety of disciplines and work settings to enter the field. It is a role appropriate for both occupational therapists and occupational therapy assistants. For decades, health care organizations have used case managers to manage resources and reduce costs. This trend in managed care has only increased in recent years, becoming even more relevant. Van Deusen (1995) stated that managed care is here to stay; as such, the issue is how occupational therapy practitioners can function effectively within this system. Case managers are utilized in numerous settings including clinical health care settings, as well as educational programming and community health services. Lohman (1999) proposed that occupational therapy be "proactive" in the current health care environment and take on nontraditional roles, such as case manager.

The term *case manager* is a title; care coordination is the function. Care coordination entails looking at the big picture, assessing needs and goals, identifying resources, and efficiently coordinating services to best meet the client's needs. The case manager's support and coordination facilitates and sustains movement through the health care system toward optimal health. An individual's health care needs often change based on a variety of factors, including nature of condition, age, availability of services, environmental factors, and individual choices. As the single point of entry, the case manager will coordinate care and facilitate transitions. Transition services are an integral part of case management and an area in which occupational therapy practitioners are already providing a vital contribution. For instance, per the Individuals with Disabilities Education Act (2004), a student with an identified disability will receive services through the school system until graduation. This individual will then require transition services that are vocational, residential, and life-skill based. Additionally, a person with a hip replacement will first require acute services in a hospital for stabilization, possible transfer to a skilled facility, and home health services. Each example benefits from the skills of a case manager to ensure a smooth transition. As noted, the occupational therapist, as a member of the team, is currently a vital part of the process.

## How Is Managed Care Affecting Case Management?

"The purpose of managed care is to provide affordable, quality health care with functional outcomes in a reasonable time frame. Access, quality, cost, and satisfaction are the usual goals that exist in health care" (Pope, 1995, p. 110). Case management and managed care are not synonymous. Trends in health care reflect the need for continued and creative resource management, which is driven by managed care. Case managers provide a vehicle to reach these goals. The demand for case management services is likely to increase, given limited financial and human resources. We are living in a society that is aging, clients are returning home after shorter acute inpatient stays, people are living longer with chronic conditions (Markle, 2004), and more children are being identified with persistent medical conditions. With these demands on our system, limited resources are available, necessitating cost efficiency and streamlining of services. Even though insurers use case management to obtain timely and cost-effective outcomes, we need to stress the importance of doing this in a positive way to meet the client's needs (Fricke, 2006). Most importantly, we are there to improve quality of life for the client and family by continued assessment and evaluation. To summarize, managed care is creating a need for case managers, but there is a shortage of nurses and social workers who have traditionally filled this role. This shortage should encourage more allied health professionals such as occupational therapy practitioners to enter the practice area of case management (Baldwin, 2005). Managed care demands more efficient use of resources, ultimately resulting in financial savings; case managers are the means to meet this goal.

The Affordable Care Act (ACA) is driving the need for effective case management. The ACA refers to two pieces of legislation: the Patient Protection and Affordable Care

Act and the Healthcare and Education Reconciliation Act of 2010. These health care insurance reforms address expanded coverage, increased accountability of insurance companies, decreased health care costs, increased choices (for consumers), and enhanced quality of health care for Americans (Medicaid.gov, n.d.). The ACA has affected case management by encouraging a cultural change toward greater patient advocacy and an increased focus on decreasing readmissions and generally keeping patients out of the hospital (AHC Media, 2015). The ACA has placed the functions of case management such as planning, assessing care transitions, and specialty care coordination center stage. There are new models of care that need to be adopted and will ultimately create value. The U.S. Department of Health and Human Services is testing new models of payment to determine if providers can better coordinate care while improving health outcomes and reducing health care costs. Effective case management will be pivotal to payment (Commission for Case Manager Certification [CCMC], 2011).

"The proposed rule includes sixty-five quality measures across five domains—patient safety, prevention, patient experience, caregiver experience, at risk populations—and, significantly, care coordination" (CCMC, 2011).

## Why Is Case Mangement an Appropriate Role for Occupational Therapy Practitioners?

Occupational therapy is the only discipline with the sole focus of understanding function. We evaluate occupational performance, routines, and volition as these factors interact with the client's environment. Our training provides us with strong human interaction skills, knowledge of occupational performance, and the ability to see the "big picture." The *Occupational Therapy Practice Framework* (American Occupational Therapy Association [AOTA], 2014) describes the domain of occupational therapy as focusing on "achieving health, well-being, and participation in life through engagement in occupation." As such, occupational therapy practitioners are a "tremendous untapped talent in terms of case management" (Hettinger, 1996).

There are clear parallels between the criteria for case management and the *Standards of Practice for Occupational Therapy* (AOTA, 2010). Thurkettle and Noji (2003) described case management as a process consisting of assessing, planning, implementing, coordinating, monitoring, and evaluating. These six functions depend on effective communication skills. The case manager must communicate with a number of people including the client, family members, service providers, vendors, insurance companies, and employers. Table 36-1 illustrates the educational standards that prepare entry-level occupational therapy practitioners to take on case management roles. Later, some of the standards of practice for each profession are delineated. Standards such as confidentiality, cultural competency, advocacy, and ethics, although not discussed, are standard components of an occupational therapy practitioner's education as well.

The specific qualities that have supported excellence in occupational therapy will also foster competency as a case manager. The occupational therapy perspective considers meaning in context of the client's condition and environment. The client's medical, spiritual, and psychosocial needs are holistically considered. Consideration of all contexts and participants is essential, both in occupational therapy and case management. All factors, including family interaction, environment, and response to illness and intervention measures, are critical when determining a person's ability to engage in meaningful occupations. Case management's role in transitioning an individual to wellness depends on a clear picture of all the above factors.

Occupational therapy practitioners often consider factors missed by other disciplines. "In the case management role, occupational therapists can help to facilitate a continuum of care from the acute setting to the community by developing clinical pathways that include the whole episode of care that emphasize functional status" (Lohman, 1999, p. 112). Additionally, other professionals may focus more on symptomatic relief and less on functional outcomes. For example, a particular individual with a lower limb amputation may be more functional when utilizing a wheelchair rather than a prosthetic. In the school system, the push to focus on proper grip and handwriting is not appropriate for all. Some students are better served by technology, meeting needs with the use of a keyboard, saving energy, and achieving success in the academic environment.

Clinical pathways are an essential function of care coordination. Occupational therapy practitioners acting as case managers can incorporate their knowledge about work, play, daily activities, disability, and environment into realistic clinical pathways. Accurate assessment is critical in the application of reasonable clinical pathways. Our assessment tools are geared toward understanding occupational effect and can lead to better intervention planning.

Any case manager coordinating the care of a client is concerned with the functional level of the person's ability to complete activities of daily living. The skills that case managers need are an understanding of the injury or illness, ability to act as a lifespan coordinator (i.e., being able to project future care and responsibilities of the person who is ill or injured), knowledge of costs for specific health care procedures and intervention,

Table 36-1.

## Comparison of Case Manager Functions and Standards of Practice

| Case Manager Functions (CMSA, 2010) | Standards of Practice for Occupational Therapy (AOTA, 2010) |
|---|---|
| Standard B—Client Assessment: Client assessment includes but is not limited to physical/functional, mental health, cognitive, spiritual, environmental, and residential, caregiver(s) capability and availability, and self-care capability | Standard II—Screening, Evaluation, Reevaluation: The occupational therapist assesses a client's ability to participate in daily occupations in his or her context through collaboration with the client and support providers |
| Standards C and D—Problem/Opportunity Identification and Planning: Identifies short- and long-term needs, as well as development of appropriate strategies to address needs | Standard III—Intervention: Develops intervention based on evaluation goals, evidence, and clinical reasoning |
| Standard E—Monitoring: Employs ongoing assessment and documentation to determine client's response to the plan of care | Standard IV—Outcomes: Measures, documents, interprets, and monitors expected or achieved outcomes in client-centered plan through achievement of occupational performance |
| Standard F—Outcomes: Utilizes evidence-based guidelines to demonstrate efficacy of interventions in achieving goals | Standard IV—Outcomes: Determines and documents changes in performance and capacities; discontinues services when client has achieved goals and reached maximum benefit or client lacks desire to continue services |
| Standard G—Termination of Case Management Services: Appropriately terminates case management services based on achievement of targeted outcomes | Standard IV—Outcomes: Prepares and implements a transition or discontinuation plan based on client needs and achievement of goals |
| Standard H—Facilitation, Coordination, and Collaboration: Develops and maintains proactive, client-centered relationships with the client and other associated professionals | Standard III—Intervention: Networks with appropriate others to establish progress toward goals including safety, benefits, and risks |

and understanding of clinical pathways (Fisher, 1996). Consequently, better quality of care emerges; these requirements are, again, easily provided by trained occupational therapy practitioners. We are uniquely prepared to provide clear activity analysis as well as understanding of the injury and contextual requirements as they influence clinical pathways.

The basic tenets of occupational therapy have long focused on client-centered planning and care. It is the occupational therapy practitioner's intention to ensure that each individual is able to meet personally chosen goals. "The client/patient is an active partner in care, sharing risk for the effect of choices on quality of life, functional ability, and subsequent income generation" (Thurkettle & Noji, 2003, p. 90). At times, programming goals are created by case managers, based on assumptions of need. However, occupational therapy embraces education as a vital step in including the client in the decision-making process. Clients are provided with information that allows decisions reflective of possible consequences and risks. To remain person-centered, it is important to empower clients, educating them about their disease process and giving them a larger voice in their care delivery and more personalized attention to their needs (Mullahy, 1998).

Occupational therapy's holistic nature allows us to get a broader picture and supports client-centered planning. Our view of the environment does not focus solely on the physical environment. It also considers the sensory environment, recognizing the fact that we all must function within larger systems. There are a number of factors that must be considered in care coordination. Awareness of cultural differences; medical, spiritual, and psychosocial needs; unique gender and role beliefs; and generational norms are essential to client-centered planning. Our holistic view recognizes that we effect change by addressing individual factors as well as the broader system. For instance, when working within the school system, it may be necessary to educate direct care staff, educational technicians, special staff, teachers, and administrators to achieve good outcomes. To support the student, all team members must be working toward a common goal. The holistic focus of occupational therapy allows for case management to occur in the most supportive environment. Although specific clinical pathways are prescribed, it is always necessary to take into consideration the unique characteristics of the individual case that may vary from the norm and influence the success of the plan. Fricke (2006) asserted that the client still remains the priority in an environment of resource management.

Within the current system, which demands cost-effectiveness, the client's needs must be considered foremost. Research shows that cost-effective programming does not exclude good care.

Conscious patient-centered coordination of care not only improves the patient experience, it also leads to better long-term health outcomes, as demonstrated by fewer unnecessary trips to the hospital, fewer repeated tests, fewer conflicting prescriptions, and clearer advice about the best course of treatment. (U.S. Department of Health and Human Services, 2013).

Occupational therapy practitioners are client centered and focus on total care, improving the experience for each individual receiving services.

## Barriers to Case Management

The realm of case management is an exciting area of potential growth for occupational therapy practitioners. However, breaking into a new niche can have its challenges. To be best prepared to meet challenges, it is important for occupational therapy practitioners to be aware of the potential barriers that may be encountered.

Occupational therapy programs are currently providing a good base of education to prepare new therapists for the specialty practice area of case management. However, therapists are likely to find that there will be skills that need to be developed for therapists to be proficient as case managers. As an occupational therapy practitioner enters the realm of case management, weaker skills will become more apparent. Once need areas are determined, further education, networking, mentoring, or exploration can occur. The need areas will highly depend on the setting, client base, community resources, and so forth. Lohman (1999) noted that in her experience as a "participant observer of case management" in an acute care setting, she found that she did not have all of the medical background necessary to be an effective case manager in that particular context. However, through networking with other professionals and reading current journals and textbooks, she was able to gain a better understanding of pertinent issues. She noted that it was important to understand the medical chart by using a functional perspective. This observation is likely to be consistent across many settings. She also noted that advanced training or continuing education addressing the specifics of case management, such as the development of multidisciplinary clinical pathways and economic aspects of interventions, would be beneficial (Lohman, 1999).

Also significant is the current shortage of resources for case managers. For example, there are more nonprofessionals involved in the carry-through of care for our consumers (i.e., personal care assistants, nursing technicians, and other paraprofessionals; Boling & Hoffman, 2001). Paraprofessionals and family members are commonly used at this time to control costs. However, with this trend, more oversight is necessary to ensure good care for our clients. "[C]ase managers must become an even stronger link along the care continuum to oversee the efficient implementation of intervention plans and, at the same time, become instrumental in developing innovative solutions to fill those care gaps already emerging" (Boling & Hoffman, 2001, p. 54).

Case management positions have traditionally been held by social workers and nurses. The current nursing shortage will inevitably affect the provision of case management services. Given the gap in supply and demand, occupational therapy practitioners who choose to fill these roles effectively are likely to have to prove themselves. As outsiders, the challenge is to demonstrate the ability to fill these roles well. Tensions regarding boundaries can be overcome with good interdisciplinary communication. Communication can be enhanced with an understanding of each profession's educational background, values, roles, norms, and thinking differences (Lohman, 1999). An effective interdisciplinary team requires solid communication skills, the ability to resolve conflict, and respect for each team member's role. Occupational therapy practitioners as case managers must be willing to collaborate with those best equipped to address their client's particular needs. Seeking the assistance of other professionals will lead to better care, as well as increased respect from one's peers. Through effective case management, turf barriers should eventually dissolve. "Effective case managers understand the organization's informal political system. They have good communication skills, show a willingness to do a fair workload, respect differences, and have good conflict resolution and negotiating skills" (Lohman, 1999, p. 112).

Barriers to effective care coordination include the following (American Academy of Pediatrics, 2005; Boling & Hoffman, 2001):

- Lack of knowledge with regard to chronic conditions, resources, or the coordination process
- Lack of effective communication
- Poor team building
- Lack of clearly defined roles
- Insufficient acknowledgment for amount of time/work spent
- Inadequate reimbursement
- Lack of an organized system
- Language/cultural barriers
- Decreased client education
- Increased percentage of clinical complications
- Increased nursing/medical error rates

- Decreased client satisfaction
- Decreased clinical outcomes
- Documentation too heavy
- High-volume caseload/burnout
- Interoperability (Stricker, 2011)

## How to Become a Certified Case Manager

Since its inception, case management has evolved as a multidisciplinary specialty practice, with the case manager position filled by those trained in a variety of health care disciplines including nursing, social work, and rehabilitation counseling. Several years ago, case management was not a profession but rather a practice area. Presently, there are accredited degree programs specifically for case management. Traditionally, case managers receive on-the-job training through employee training, supervision, and team meetings. "The Case Management Society of America, through the development of its core curriculum for case managers, established the first national, standardized, basic knowledge and skill set for case managers" (Boling & Hoffman, 2001, p. 54). The CMSA now has standards of practice as noted in Table 36-1. Both methods still allow qualified health care professionals from a variety of disciplines to enter the field. A rehabilitation background will assist a practitioner in becoming a board-certified case manager as the CCMC has identified rehabilitation as one of the knowledge domains in which case managers must demonstrate competency (Jensen, 2012).

In addition to completing a degree program in case management, an occupational therapy practitioner (i.e., an occupational therapist or an occupational therapy assistant) can also become a certified case manager (CCM). The CCM designation is offered through the CCMC (1996). Certification is a voluntary process, as it is possible to fulfill the role of case manager without this credential. If one chooses to become certified, the credentialing process is described next.

- At a minimum, the professional license for certification shall be based on an educational requirement of a post-secondary program in a field that promotes the physical, psychosocial, or vocational well-being of the persons being served. Applicants must hold a current, active, unrestricted license or certification in another health or human services discipline.
- The license must allow the individual to practice independently without the supervision of another licensed professional.
- The individual must show documented employment experience as a case manager or as a supervisor of case management services. The following are three categories of acceptable employment based on time frames for employment and the amount of supervision provided by either a CCM or non-CCM:
    - ◊ Category 1: Twelve months of full-time employment under the supervision of a CCM
    - ◊ Category 2: Twenty-four months of employment as a case manager, with no requirements for supervision
    - ◊ Category 3: A minimum of 12 months directing case management services
- The individual use the eight essential case management activities of assessment, planning, implementation, coordination, monitoring, evaluation, outcomes, and "general" to perform six core practice components, as documented in one's job description.
- The individual must pass a certification examination that covers the six core practice components of psychosocial aspects, health care reimbursement, rehabilitation, health care management and delivery, principles of practice, and case management concepts.
- The individual must display good moral character and reputation.

As it would be in any practice area, it is important to remain educationally current no matter how the credentials of case manager are acquired. The CMSA hosts professional conferences that provide case managers with the opportunity to maintain professional licensure and credentials through continuing education. Training that pertains to a case manager's specific client population is also available to remain current.

## Applications

Case manager skills parallel those used by occupational therapy practitioners in all settings. Occupational therapy practitioners use the skills of case management for best practice in daily decision making, therapeutic intervention, collaboration, and transition planning. Currently, occupational therapy practitioners fill essential roles as team members, providing direct service as needed. They provide information on baseline functioning, work collaboratively with the team, and support the care plan with the ultimate goal of discharge from service. Insurance companies, including workers' compensation and return-to-work programs, depend on occupational therapy to provide the information for planning and coverage.

> Occupational therapy practitioners understand productive living. They understand job analysis, job accommodations, and many of the issues facing injured workers. Because of this knowledge and their background in the psychosocial sciences, occupational therapy practitioners are a natural possibility as case managers for the worker's compensation population . . . understanding a variety of occupations and skills necessary to do certain jobs is an advantage to case management in this area as is understanding specific task modifications and job accommodations. (Fisher, 1996, p. 453)

Occupational therapy practitioners have a unique perspective on functioning, viewing the whole system and the person within their context. They are a valuable asset to case management because of their understanding of function. Occupational therapy practitioners are unique because their education includes the intensive study of all vital components of human functioning, recognizing how the interrelationships of the components affect well-being and quality of life (Hafez & Brockman, 1998). Occupational therapy programming may be helpful in developing services for health promotion. This may include self-care management, cognitive assessments, activities-based programming, and home safety screening for modifications (Chapleau & Meyers, 2011).

An occupational therapy practitioner's education addresses physical and lifestyle factors and their application in the complex task of helping a client continue to live a meaningful and purposeful life. Occupational therapy practitioners are likely to be the only professionals who analyze all factors influencing a client to determine how to build supports that are truly compatible. For instance, a vocational rehabilitation counselor might select a job coach based on availability and not compatibility. If the client required motor-based modeling and demonstration to learn tasks but was paired with a coach who primarily used verbal cueing, success would be diminished. It is the ability of an occupational therapy practitioner to analyze each component of support that increases the potential for success. The cornerstone of a healthy team process must be consumer driven, and all parts must be well matched. Good case management is achieved through a team process. This is well supported by occupational therapy philosophy, making occupational therapy practitioners a natural match for the role.

Presently, occupational therapy practitioners provide care coordination through consultation services. Although not labeled case management, the services provided directly affect the intervention plan, thus driving care coordination. Functional occupational therapy assessment provides recommendations for the client based on the client's occupational capabilities and areas of needs. Clear identification of strengths and weaknesses in the areas of sensory processing, visual perceptual abilities, cognition/learning style, psychosocial engagement, and contextual factors allows the team to use the dynamic process in a truly client-centered approach. Recommendations target areas of need identified by the functional assessment and consider contextual factors and the need for skill building. The format of a typical occupational therapy evaluation reflects an all-inclusive view of a person's functioning. The above sidebar illustrates how this process might unfold.

Case management can also take the form of clinical consultation. For example, on a regular basis, an occupational therapy practitioner can review intervention plans for individuals with mental illness and/or cognitive disability who attend a community-based day program. A care plan, created from information supplied by direct support providers, can be used to guide intervention between scheduled consultation, at which time adjustments are made to the plan to address new or different needs. The plan would provide specific guidelines that drive the direct support for provider interventions as well as a means for documentation and a crisis intervention plan. Team collaboration may reveal the need to bring in additional professionals to address goals and support function.

### Occupational Therapy Evaluation Example

An occupational therapy practitioner would be called in when an individual is not functioning effectively in his or her environment. For instance, a resident with unhealthy eating habits, aggression, and poor hygiene is at risk of losing housing placement. The first step in working with this individual would be to complete a functional assessment. Next, feedback involving the individual and the team would be provided. Through this feedback and the process of collaboration, an intervention plan is developed. This intervention plan needs to address how the system will assist this person, what skill building needs to occur, and how the environment can be set up to facilitate individual growth and functioning. After the completion of a thorough functional evaluation, a number of strategies to address the resident's clinical needs can be determined. For instance, the individual may require more joint compression to calm the nervous system and minimize aggression. It would be important to work with the direct care providers to find appropriate activities to increase deep pressure, weight bearing, and heavy muscle work. The case manager may want to make a referral to vocational rehabilitation services to match this person with an appropriate job with physical components. This would be in addition to helping the individual develop and use strategies to reduce arousal level and minimize aggressive outbursts. In this example, the occupational therapy practitioner is not officially assuming the role of case manager but is acting as a consultant to help direct the provision of services.

## Evidence-Based Research Chart

| Issue | Evidence |
|---|---|
| Effect of managed care on case management | AHC Media, 2015; Baldwin, 2005; CCMC, 2011; Fricke, 2006; Lamb, 2013; Markle, 2004; Medicaid.gov, n.d.; Pope, 1995 |
| Occupational therapy attributes that are a match for case management | Fisher, 1996; Hettinger, 1996; Lohman, 1999; Mullahy, 1998; Thurkettle & Noji, 2003; U.S. Department of Health and Human Services, 2013 |
| Understanding barriers to case management | Boling & Hoffman, 2001; Chapleau & Meyers, 2011; Lohman, 1999; Stricker, 2011 |
| Case management outcomes | Allison, 2004; Blass & Reed, 2003; Jensen, 2012; Lohman, 1999; Van Deusen, 1995 |

Another example of an occupational therapy practitioner's effectiveness in case management can be seen in coordinating transition services for a young person "aging out" of high school or foster care. This is an appropriate role for an occupational therapy practitioner whose expertise in human development facilitates the client's transition from childhood/adolescence occupational roles to those of a young adult.

The goal of case management is to manage limited resources. A means of reaching this goal is to provide comprehensive training to care providers to meet a client's functional needs. If we provide functionally based training with the intent of teaching direct care providers how to better support their clients, we will be supporting more efficient use of resources. For example, a referral for a behaviorally dysregulated client would require functional assessment. Assessment may determine that, to support the least restrictive living environment, additional one-on-one staffing is needed. By providing a structured routine full of motor-based activities, the client would be able to remain calm and organized. For this routine and the interventions to truly be supportive, proper training would need to be offered to direct service providers. This training would identify the needs of persons with sensory defensiveness, detail his or her learning style, and describe sensory interventions and how to structure the environment. As noted above, after an occupational therapy practitioner has provided the necessary training resulting in the provision of effective services, the individual's needs would be met safely and efficiently, enabling significant changes in day-to-day function.

Occupational therapy practitioners are able to look at the big picture by using a systems approach to drive services in an effective manner. The examples presented previously detail how case management can be applied in both traditional settings and in emerging practice areas. Although these are only a few examples, many opportunities exist in our discipline. To recap, occupational therapy practitioners can excel as case managers because of the following skills: our understanding of functional abilities that are needed to match the person to the task; our occupational analysis skills, which allow us to adapt and be creative with support systems and solutions; and our ability to guide support providers to facilitate effective interventions.

## Summary

Understanding the clear connections between the skills of a case manager and the skills of an occupational therapy practitioner highlights the many opportunities that exist. Occupational therapy practitioners can use these skills in roles specifically designated as "case manager." There are also alternative applications that may not carry the title but have the same end result. Occupational therapy practitioners are part of care coordination, transition services, management of resources, and good outcomes in any role that they fill. Good case management demands excellent communication with the client and the interdisciplinary team. It requires comprehensive knowledge of available human, financial, and community-based resources and an ability to use these in the most cost-effective manner. Flexibility as well as ability to adjust the plan based on the client's functional level and changing goals are vital. Occupational therapy practitioners clearly add to these general principles, bringing a truly holistic view of the client and their context.

## Electronic Resources

Case Management Society of America: www.cmsa.org

Commission for Case Manager Certification: www.ccmcertification.org

## References

AHC Media. (2015). Case management, advocacy and the Affordable Care Act. Retrieved from www.ahcmedia.com/articles/134452-case-management-and-advocacy-in-the-era-of-the-affordable-care-act

Allison, L. (2004). Evidence-based practice as tool for case management. *Case Manager, 15*(5), 62-65.

American Academy of Pediatrics. (2005). Policy statement: Care coordination in the medical home: Integrating health and related systems of care for children with special health care needs. *Pediatrics, 116*(5), 1238-1244.

American Occupational Therapy Association. (2010). Standards of practice for occupational therapy. *American Journal of Occupational Therapy, 64*, S106-S111.

American Occupational Therapy Association. (2014). Occupational therapy practice framework: Domain and process (3rd ed.). *American Journal of Occupational Therapy, 68*(Suppl. 1), S1-S48. doi:10.5014/ajot.2014.682006

Baldwin, T. M. (2005). Case management: Entry-level practice for occupational therapists? *Case Manager, 16*(4), 47-51.

Blass, T. C., & Reed, T. L. (2003). Consider case management. *Nursing Management, 34*(10), 81-83.

Boling, J., & Hoffman, L. (2001). The nursing shortage and its implications for case management. *Case Manager, 12*(6), 53-57.

Chapleau, A., & Meyers, S. (2011). Occupational therapy consultation for case managers in community mental health: Exploring strategies to improve job satisfaction and self efficacy. *Professional Case Management, 16*(2), 71-79.

Commission for Case Manager Certification. (1996). *CMM certification guide*. Rolling Meadows, IL: Author.

Commission for Case Manager Certification. (2011). *Center stage in the revolution: A healthcare reform action guide for the professional case manager*. Retrieved from https://ccmcertification.org/sites/default/files/downloads/2011/4.%20Center%20stage%20in%20the%20revolution%20-%20volume%202,%20issue%202.pdf

Fisher, T. (1996). Roles and functions of a case manager. *American Journal of Occupational Therapy, 50*(6), 452-454.

Fricke, K. (2006). Client centered case management in today's health care. *Lippincott's Case Management, 11*(12), 112-114.

Hafez, A., & Brockman, S. (1998). Occupational therapists: Essential team members as service providers and case managers. *Journal of Care Management, 4*(2), 10-20.

Hettinger, J. (1996). Case management: Do OTs have what it takes? Yes! *OT Week, 10*, 12-14.

Individuals with Disabilities Education Act. (2004). 20 U.S.C. 1400.

Jensen, S. (2012). The role of case management and care coordination in improving employee health and productivity. *Professional Case Management, 17*(6), 294-296.

Lamb, G. (2013). Care coordination, quality, and nursing. In G. Lamb (Ed.), *Care coordination: The game changer how nursing is revolutionizing quality care* (pp. 1-3, 8). Silver Springs, MD: Nursebooks.org.

Lohman, H. (1999). What will it take for more occupational therapists to become case managers? Implications for education, practice and policy. *American Journal of Occupational Therapy, 53*(1), 111-113.

Markle, A. (2004). The economic impact of case management. *Case Manager, 15*(4), 54-58.

Medicaid.gov. (n.d.). *Affordable Care Act*. Retrieved from https://www.medicaid.gov/affordablecareact/affordable-care-act.html

Mullahy, C. (1998). *The case manager's handbook* (2nd ed.). Gaithersburg, MD: Aspen.

Pope, T. (1995). Case managers help define managed care. *Case Manager, 6*(4), 109-114.

Stricker, P. (2011). *The quest for case management interoperability*. Retrieved from http://www.cmsa.org/Individual/NewsEvents/HealthTechnologyArticles/tabid/646/Default.aspx

Thomasz, T., & Young, D. (2015). Speech pathology and occupational therapy students participating in placements where their supervisor works in a dual role. *Australian Journal of Rural Health*, 1-5.

Thurkettle, M., & Noji, A. (2003). Case management: A source of support and stability for the client and the health care system. *Lippincott's Case Management, 8*(2), 88-94.

U.S. Department of Health and Human Services. (2013). *2013 annual progress report to Congress: National strategy for quality improvement in health care*. Retrieved from www.ahrq.gov/workingforquality/nqs/nqs2013annlrpt.htm

Van Deusen, J. (1995). What is the role of the occupational therapist in managed care? *American Journal of Occupational Therapy, 49*(8), 833-834.

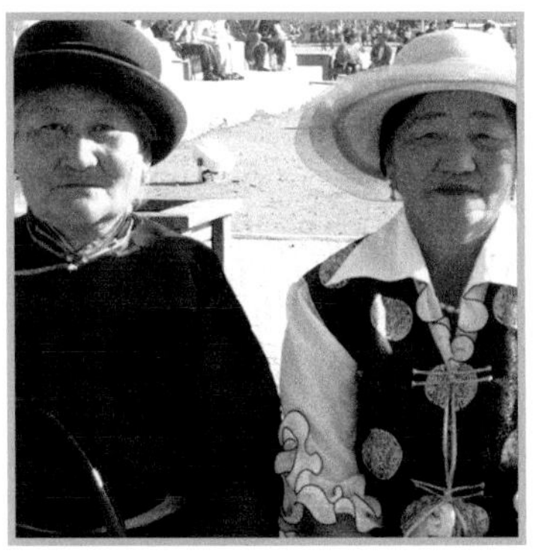

# 37

# Consultation, Referral, Monitoring, and Discharge Planning

*Julie Ann Nastasi, ScD, OTD, OTR/L, SCLV, FAOTA*

**ACOTE STANDARDS EXPLORED IN THIS CHAPTER**

B.5.21, B.5.22, B.5.25, B.5.26, B.5.28, B.5.31

**KEY VOCABULARY**

- **Consultation:** Discussing or meeting with other appropriate resources (medical or non-medical) that provide services that best meet the needs of the client (American Occupational Therapy Association, 2015).
- **Discharge planning:** Determining and preparing for the needs of the client as the client transitions from one setting to another.
- **Monitoring:** Evaluating and assessing the progress of the client during the rehabilitation process.
- **Referral:** Recommending a client to be evaluated by other appropriate resources (medical or nonmedical).



Jacobs, K., & MacRae, N. (Eds.).
*Occupational Therapy Essentials for Clinical Competence, Third Edition* (pp. 547-554).

The Third Edition of the *Occupational Therapy Practice Framework* (American Occupational Therapy Association [AOTA], 2014) addresses the domain and process of occupational therapy. Consultation, referral, monitoring, and discharge planning fall under the process of occupational therapy. While the occupational therapy process is described in a linear manner in the *Framework*, the AOTA acknowledges that the process is dynamic (AOTA, 2014). Please refer to Chapter 6 for more information about the *Framework*. Therefore, it is important to understand how consultation, referral(s), monitoring, and discharge planning facilitate positive outcomes for clients. In this chapter, you will learn more about consultation and referral, monitoring, and discharge planning.

## Consultation and Referral

Occupational therapy practitioners work in numerous settings. Depending on the setting, occupational therapy practitioners may have little to no interaction with other medical and nonmedical professionals or numerous interactions on a daily basis. If an occupational therapist is working in a community setting, the occupational therapist may not work with other medical professionals. If an occupational therapist works in an inpatient hospital setting, the occupational therapist will likely interact with physical therapists, speech therapists, doctors, nurses, respiratory therapists, and other medical professions on a regular basis. Regardless of setting, occupational therapy practitioners should effectively communicate through consultation and referral(s) with medical and nonmedical professionals who provide services to persons, groups, and populations. The following sections will address consultation and referral within the profession of occupational therapy, consultation and referral outside of the profession of occupational therapy, and consultation for persons, groups, and populations.

### Occupational Therapists and Occupational Therapy Assistants

Occupational therapy practitioners are trained to be generalists; however, many go on to specialize in a particular area of practice. The AOTA offers board certification in gerontology, mental health, pediatrics, and physical rehabilitation for occupational therapists. The AOTA also offers specialty certification in driving and community mobility, environmental modification, low vision, school systems, and feeding, eating, and swallowing for occupational therapists and occupational therapy assistants (AOTA, 2016).

In addition to board and specialty certification through the AOTA, occupational therapists also have the ability to earn certifications through professions and organizations outside of occupational therapy. The Hand Therapy Certification Commission (2016) offers certification in hand therapy for occupational therapists, and the Board of Certification in Professional Ergonomics (2016) offers certification in ergonomics. See Table 37-1 for a list of potential board and specialty certification organizations and certifications for occupational therapists.

During the occupational therapy evaluation, the occupational therapist will determine if there is a need to consult or refer a client to an occupational therapist or occupational therapy assistant who has specialized in a particular area of practice. Depending on setting, the occupational therapist might not have specialists onsite. For example, an occupational therapist who works in an acute care setting receives an order to evaluate and treat a client who has sustained a cerebrovascular accident (CVA). During the evaluation, the occupational therapist identifies that the client has double vision because of the CVA. The occupational therapist does not specialize in low vision and does not have a low vision specialist onsite, so the occupational therapist consults with an occupational therapist with specialty certification in low vision to address immediate vision needs while treating the client in the acute care setting. The occupational therapist will refer the client to the specialist upon discharge from the acute care setting. The occupational therapist plans interventions to address double vision based on the recommendations of the consultation and discusses and plans the intervention plan with the occupational therapy assistant at the acute care site. This includes providing proper supervision to the occupational therapy assistant and identifying which techniques the occupational therapy assistant will use during the client's interventions. The occupational therapist and occupational therapy assistant will work together to facilitate the client's intervention plan (Accreditation Council for Occupational Therapy Education [ACOTE], 2011). Effective communication and work between the occupational therapist and occupational therapy assistant will maximize the client's potential during intervention. Information learned from the consultation will allow the occupational therapist and the occupational therapy assistant to provide the best available care to the client while in the acute care setting.

### Consultation With and Referral External to Occupational Therapy

Occupational therapy practitioners need to effectively communicate and work interprofessionally with medical and nonmedical professionals who provide services to their clients. This includes knowing and understanding the roles and responsibilities of the medical and

Table 37-1.

## Advanced Board and Specialty Certification Organizations and Certifications

| Organization | Advanced Board or Specialty Certification |
|---|---|
| Academy for Certification of Vision Rehabilitation and Education Professionals | Certified low vision therapist, certified orientation and mobility specialist, certified vision rehabilitation therapist |
| American Occupational Therapy Association | Board certification: Gerontology, mental health, pediatrics, and physical rehabilitation<br>Specialty certification: Driving and community mobility, environmental modification, low vision, school systems, and feeding, eating, and swallowing |
| Board of Certification in Professional Ergonomics | Ergonomics |
| Hand Therapy Certification Commission | Hand therapy |
| Lymphology Association of North America | Lymphedema therapist |
| National Certification Board for Diabetes Educators | Certified diabetes educator |
| National Stroke Association | Certified stroke rehabilitation specialist |
| Psychiatric Rehabilitation Association | Certified psychiatric rehabilitation practitioner |

nonmedical professionals during the execution of the client's intervention plan. If needed, occupational therapy practitioners should consult with and refer to professionals outside of the field of occupational therapy. Table 37-2 lists a number of medical and nonmedical professionals that occupational therapy practitioners consult with or refer to, but is not all inclusive.

Returning to the earlier example in this chapter, the occupational therapist determined during the occupational therapy evaluation that double vision developed from the CVA. The occupational therapist consulted with an occupational therapist with specialty certification in low vision. The occupational therapist also determined the need to refer the client to a neuro-ophthalmologist at the hospital. The neuro-ophthalmologist evaluates the client's vision and provides appropriate interventions for the client's double vision. The occupational therapist and the neuro-ophthalmologist discuss and determine an intervention plan that will successfully address the client's double vision. This will allow the occupational therapist to work with the client's best available vision while addressing the client's occupations and goals. Occupational therapy practitioners need to communicate and work effectively with interprofessionals. When occupational therapy practitioners consult with and refer to medical and nonmedical professionals, proper interventions are developed and the client's potential is maximized.

### *Providing Consultation to Persons, Groups, and Populations*

Occupational therapists may serve as consultants to persons, groups, and populations. In the *Framework* (AOTA, 2014), consultation has been changed from a type of intervention to a method of service delivery. Consultation is an indirect service. Occupational therapists may serve as consultants to other occupational therapists, teachers, multidisciplinary teams, policymakers, or even businesses. See Table 37-3 for potential persons, groups, and populations for which occupational therapists provide consultations.

Occupational therapy has focused on the specific needs of the clients receiving services. Occupational therapy has evolved to meet societal needs. The role of occupational therapy practitioners has expanded beyond the client receiving direct services to persons, groups, and populations who benefit from the unique perspective that occupational therapy brings to living one's life.

## Monitoring

Monitoring is an integral part of the process of occupational therapy. Occupational therapy practitioners need to continually monitor the client's response to interventions and progress toward the goals desired. Monitoring and reassessment of the client should be in collaboration with the client, caregiver, family, and significant others. It is the occupational therapist's responsibility to

Table 37-2.

## Specialists External to Occupational Therapy

| Medical or Nonmedical Professional | Roles and Responsibilities |
|---|---|
| Acupuncturist | Provides alternative medicine through the use of needles at acupuncture points to address a wide variety of conditions |
| Administrator | Oversees the policies, procedures, and finances of a setting |
| Architect | Plans, designs, and oversees construction; familiar with the Americans with Disabilities Act and universal design |
| Art therapist | Uses art as a therapeutic means to explore feelings and emotions in a mental health setting |
| Athletic trainer | Optimizes performance of athletes through prevention, diagnosis, and intervention for medical conditions |
| Audiologist | Specializes in hearing loss and interventions for hearing loss |
| Care coordinator | Oversees discharge planning |
| Chiropractor (DC) | Specializes in diagnosis and interventions of the musculoskeletal system; manipulates the spine, joints, and soft tissues |
| Dentist (DDS, DMD) | Specializes in diagnosis, prevention, and treatment of conditions in the oral cavity |
| Dietician (RD, DTR) | Promotes healthy eating and nutrition |
| Music therapist | Provides therapeutic interventions through the use of music |
| Neurologist | A physician who specializes in diagnosis and interventions of the nervous system |
| Neuro-ophthalmologist | A physician who specializes in neurology and ophthalmology; provides medical and surgical interventions for the visual system |
| Nurse (LPN, RN) | Responsible for care of individuals in hospitals and community settings |
| Nurse practitioner (NP, DNP) | Provides advanced practice to improve patient and health care outcomes |
| Ophthalmologist | A physician who specializes in the visual system; provides medical and surgical interventions for the eye |
| Optometrist (OD) | An eye doctor who specializes in refraction of the eye and treatment of eye conditions |
| Orientation and mobility specialist | Provides training in safety and navigation for individuals with low vision and blindness |
| Orthopedist | A physician who specializes in treatment of the musculoskeletal system |
| Pediatrician | A physician who specializes in treating children |
| Physical therapist (PT, DPT) | Specializes in assessment and intervention of physical disabilities through strength, endurance, coordination, balance, and mobility |
| Physician (MD, DO) | A medical doctor or doctor of osteopathy |
| Physician assistant (PA) | Provides care under the supervision of an MD or DO |
| Psychiatrist | A physician who specializes in evaluation and treatment of mental illness |
| Recreational therapist | Promotes health through recreational activity |
| Respiratory therapist | Specializes in the cardiopulmonary system, and manages airways and cardiopulmonary support |
| Social worker (LCSW, LICSW) | Coordinates client care to meet client's psychosocial needs |
| Speech and language pathologist (SLP) | Specializes in verbal communication, speech, language, and feeding/swallowing disorders |
| Teacher | Responsible for curriculum development and educating students in a school setting |

## Case Study

An occupational therapist at a low vision clinic prepares to see a new client. The prescription states the client is a 75-year-old woman with glaucoma. The prescriptions states to evaluate and treat the client for decreased participation in occupations and activities. The occupational therapist knows that glaucoma starts off with peripheral field deficits and over time may lead to tunnel vision or complete blindness.

During the occupational profile, the occupational therapist listens to the client and documents the client's occupational history and areas of concern for the client. The client reports problems during ambulation and leaving the home. The client also reports putting objects down and then misplacing the items.

During the low vision evaluation, the occupational therapist notes that the client has decreased peripheral fields in both eyes. Central vision is intact, and the client has moderate low vision. Contrast sensitivity is slightly decreased.

Based on the findings, the occupational therapist and the client identify goals for the client. The client wants to travel safely in the home and in community environments. The client also wants to be able to find and use items in the home. The occupational therapist makes a referral to an orientation and mobility specialist to address safety and navigation outside of the home. The occupational therapist plans to provide low vision occupational therapy services in the client's home.

During occupational therapy intervention sessions in the home, the occupational therapist and the client develop a system to organize items in the home. The client determines locations to place frequently used items. This allows the client to find frequently used items. The occupational therapist and client also identify clutter that does not need to be in the home. The client and the client's family member pack up unused items and store them in the basement of the home. Finally, the occupational therapist trains the client in trailing and squaring off in the home to travel from position to position in the home.

The occupational therapist monitors the client's progress during the follow-up sessions. Based on the client's progress, the client and occupational therapist plan a discharge from occupational therapy on the next visit. The occupational therapist predicts the client will be independent in all of the goals by the last visit.

On the last visit, the client achieves all of her desired goals. The occupational therapist educates the client on signs of progression of the disease, and tells the client to contact her ophthalmologist if there are any changes in her vision. If progression of the disease affects her occupations, the client can be referred back to occupational therapy by her physician. The occupational therapist discharges the client from occupational therapy with all her occupational therapy goals met.

Table 37-3.

### Persons, Groups, and Populations for Which Occupational Therapists Provide Consultations

| Medical or Nonmedical Professional | Roles and Responsibilities |
|---|---|
| Persons | Administrator, architect, builder, lobbyist, nurse, orientation and mobility specialist, parent, physical therapist, physician, politician, speech therapist, spouse, surgeon, teacher, etc. |
| Groups | Families, politicians, students, retirement group, workers, etc. |
| Populations | American Automobile Association, American Association of Retired People, American Association of Motor Vehicle Administrators, Association for Driver Rehabilitation Specialists, American Medical Association, American Society on Aging, National Multiple Sclerosis Society, etc. |

monitor the effect of the occupational therapy intervention and the need for continued or modified intervention (ACOTE, 2011). This includes overall responsibility for the development, documentation, and implementation of the intervention plan (AOTA, 2015). Occupational therapy assistants should implement interventions that have been delegated by the occupational therapist in which the occupational therapy assistant has been deemed competent. The occupational therapist will monitor and modify the intervention plan based on the client's needs and performance. The occupational therapy assistant will contribute to the process by collaborating with the occupational therapist and notifying the occupational therapist of the client's response to interventions and modifications.

Occupational therapists should monitor the client's progress toward established goals. If a client is not progressing, the occupational therapist needs to determine what factors are limiting the client. The occupational therapist will look at the occupations, client factors, performance skills, performance patterns, context and environment, and the activity and occupational demands (AOTA, 2014). The client may need more education and training or benefit from group therapy as well as individual therapy. Modification through simplification of the task may allow the client to succeed at the task. Ultimately, the occupational therapist wants the client to achieve the desired goals and occupations that are important to the client.

## Discharge Planning

Discharge planning will vary depending on the practice setting; however, in all settings occupational therapists should begin thinking about the discharge plan while completing the client's evaluation. During the initial evaluation, the occupational therapist will select specific tools and assessments to measure the client's current abilities (AOTA, 2015). Based on the findings, the occupational therapist will create a problem list and goals that address problems from the problem list. Goals should be client-centered and the client should be active in the goal-setting process. The occupational therapist will establish realistic and measurable goals for a defined period. Goals typically are written as short- and long-term goals. Depending on the practice setting, short-term goals may vary from days to a month in time. Long-term goals are typically written to predict where the client will be at the time of discharge or in a school setting for the next academic year. Discharge planning varies by setting. In the next two sections, the process of discharge planning will be discussed for acute care and outpatient settings.

### Acute Care

In an acute care setting, the occupational therapist may have a social worker or care coordinator who facilitates the discharge process. In this case, the social worker or care coordinator will meet with the client to determine if the client plans to go to an acute rehabilitation facility, a subacute setting, or plans to be discharged home with or without home health services. Based on the client's desires and abilities, the social worker or care coordinator will submit reports from occupational therapy, physical therapy, and speech therapy as applicable to the appropriate settings. The social worker or care coordinator then notifies the client where the client has been accepted upon discharge from the hospital. The client then selects one of the accepted placements.

In the acute care setting, the occupational therapist makes recommendations for discharge on the initial evaluation based on the client's performance during the evaluation and the client's desires for discharge. The occupational therapist notes the client's potential for rehabilitation, establishes goals or outcomes, and plans the frequency of occupational therapy while the client remains in the acute care setting. Upon discharge, the occupational therapist summarizes the client's progress while in the acute care setting and where the client was discharged to for additional services.

### Outpatient

In an outpatient setting, the occupational therapist may be the only person responsible for discharge planning. Outpatient settings typically are the last place services are received along the continuum of care. In an outpatient clinic, the duration of occupational therapy typically varies by diagnosis, need to return to work, and insurance coverage. The occupational therapist needs to understand the client's needs as well as the client's time frame to return to work and the parameters of the client's insurance coverage. The occupational therapist needs to schedule therapy based on the client's needs and the time period for discharge. For example, if a client needs to return to work in a short time, the occupational therapist may schedule the client to come into therapy two to three times a week to maximize the client's recovery over a short time.

Insurance also affects the discharge plan in an outpatient setting. Many clients do not want to incur out-of-pocket expenses for therapy once insurance benefits have run out or if copayments are high. The occupational therapist may need to maximize the client's rehabilitation potential within the limitations of an insurance plan. The client may opt to have an extensive home exercise program and minimize the frequency of visits per week to prolong the time that the client is able to work with the occupational therapist. The occupational therapist and

## Evidence-Based Research Chart

| Topic | Evidence |
|---|---|
| Consultation and referral | Carrier, Freeman, Levasseur, & Desrosiers, 2015; Chapleau, Seroczynski, Meyers, Lamb, & Haynes, 2011; Lauckner & Stadnyk, 2014; Phipps & Cooper, 2014; Raymond, Feldman, Prud'homme, & Demers, 2013 |
| Monitoring | Caizhong, Chunlei, Beibei, Zhiqing, Qinneng, & Tong, 2014; Schnell, 2008; Townsend & Watson, 2013; West, Dunford, Mayston, & Forsyth, 2013 |
| Discharge planning | Atwau & Caldwell, 2003; Drummond et al., 2012; Durocher & Gibson, 2010; Wilson, Atwal, Richards, & McIntyre, 2012 |

the client may also explore exercise classes or activities at community centers that will facilitate the client's recovery at a lower cost to the client.

Many factors go into discharge planning. Obtaining a holistic picture of the client's occupational profile, current abilities, goals, and resources allows the occupational therapist to collaborate with the client and maximize the client's rehabilitation potential prior to discharge. Upon termination of occupational services, the occupational therapist hopes to achieve all of the client's goals and stated outcomes of occupational therapy. The occupational therapist will note the goals and outcomes that have been achieved as well as the ones that were not achieved. The occupational therapist will summarize why goals and outcomes were met or not met. The occupational therapist will also make appropriate recommendations and referrals to the client for post-discharge needs (ACOTE, 2011).

## Summary

Consultation, referral(s), monitoring, and discharge planning are dynamic processes. Occupational therapy practitioners need to understand how consultation, referral(s), monitoring, and discharge planning facilitate positive outcomes for their clients. Consulting with appropriate medical and nonmedical professionals enhances the client's rehabilitation process. By making appropriate referrals, the client's needs should be addressed. Occupational therapy practitioners should keep the client's discharge plan in mind while monitoring and reassessing the client's progress. When executed correctly, occupational therapy will maximize the client's potential to live life to the fullest.

## Student Self-Assessment

1. You see a client with a CVA on an in-patient rehabilitation unit. The client has decreased range of motion and strength in the left upper and lower extremities, swallowing problems, and left neglect.
   - What professions would you expect the client to work with and why?
   - Who would you consult with?
   - Who would you refer the client to?
2. You receive an order to evaluate and treat a client who is status-post left total hip replacement. The client currently is in the hospital and plans to go home upon discharge.
   - What professions should be involved with the client in the hospital?
   - What are the roles of the professions involved?
   - How would you monitor the client's progress?
   - What recommendations would you make and why?
   - What does the client need to do to be discharged home?
   - Why?

## Acknowledgments

I would like to thank Julie Savoyski, MS, OTR/L, MPA, for her contributions to this chapter from her "Consultation, Referral, Monitoring, and Discharge Planning" chapter in the Second Edition of this textbook.

# Electronic Resources

American Occupational Therapy Association: www.aota.org

American Occupational Therapy Association Board and Specialty Certification: http://www.aota.org/education-careers/advance-career/board-specialty-certifications.aspx

American Occupational Therapy Association Official Documents: http://www.aota.org/practice/manage/official.aspx

# References


Academy for Certification of Vision Rehabilitation and Education Professionals. (2016). *ACVREP certifications*. Retrieved from https://www.acvrep.org/ascerteon/control/certifications/landing

Accreditation Council for Occupational Therapy Education. (2011). *2011 Accreditation Council for Occupational Therapy Education (ACOTE®) Standards and Interpretive Guide (August 2014 Intrepretive Guide Version)*. Retrieved from https://www.aota.org/-/media/Corporate/Files/EducationCareers/Accredit/StandardsReview/guide/2011-Standards-and-Interpretive-Guide.ashx

American Occupational Therapy Association. (2014). Occupational therapy practice framework: Domain and process (3rd ed.). *American Journal of Occupational Therapy, 68*(Suppl. 1), S1-S48. doi:10.5014/ajot.2014.682006

American Occupational Therapy Association. (2015). Standards of practice for occupational therapy. *American Journal of Occupational Therapy, 69*(Suppl. 3), 6913410057p1-6913410057p6.

American Occupational Therapy Association. (2016, January 15). *Board and specialty certification*. Retrieved from http://www.aota.org/education-careers/advance-career/board-specialty-certifications.aspx

Atwau, A., & Caldwell, K. (2003). Ethics, occupational therapy discharge planning: Four broken principles. *Australian Occupational Therapy Journal, 50*, 244-251.

Board of Certification in Professional Ergonomics. (2016, January 15). *Why certify?* Retrieved from http://www.bcpe.org/why-certify/

Caizhong, X., Chunlei, S., Beibei, L., Zhiqing, D., Qinneng, D., & Tong, W. (2014). The application of somatosensory evoked potentials in spinal cord injury rehabilitation. *NeuroRehabilitation, 35*, 835-840.

Carrier, A., Freeman, A., Levasseur, M., & Desrosiers, J. (2015). Standardized referral form: Restricting client-centered practice? *Scandinavian Journal of Occupational Therapy, 22*(4), 283-292.

Chapleau, A., Seroczynski, A., Meyers, S., Lamb, K., & Haynes, S. (2011). Occupational therapy consultation for case managers in community mental health. *Professional Case Management, 16*(2), 71-79.

Drummond, A., Whitehead, P., Fellows, K., Sprigg, N., Sampson, C., Edwards, C., & Lincoln, N. (2012). Occupational therapy predischarge home visits for patients with a stroke (HOVIS): Results of a feasibility randomized controlled trial. *Clinical Rehabilitation, 27*(5), 387-397.

Durocher, E., & Gibson, B. (2010). Navigating ethical discharge planning: A case study in older adult rehabilitation. *Australian Occupational Therapy Journal, 57*, 2-7.

Hand Therapy Certification Commission. (2016). *Certification*. Retrieved from https://www.htcc.org/certify

Lauckner, H., & Stadnyk, R. (2014). Examining an occupational perspective in a rural Canadian age-friendly consultation process. *Australian Occupational Therapy Journal, 61*, 376-383.

Lymphology Association of North America. (2016). *Mission statement*. Retrieved from http://www.clt-lana.org/mission-statement.html

National Certification Board for Diabetes Educators. (2016). *Certification information*. Retrieved from http://www.ncbde.org/certification_info/

National Stroke Association. (2016). *Certified stroke rehabilitation*. Retrieved from http://www.stroke.org/we-can-help/healthcare-professionals/improve-your-skills/tools-training-and-resources/csrs

Phipps, K., & Cooper, J. (2014). A service evaluation of a specialist community palliative care occupational therapy service. *Progress in Palliative Care, 22*(6), 347-351.

Psychiatric Rehabilitation Association. (2016). *CPRP certification*. Retrieved from http://www.uspra.org/certification/cprp-certification

Raymond, M., Feldman, D., Prud'homme, M., & Demers, L. (2013). Who's next? Referral prioritisation criteria for home care occupational therapy. *International Journal of Therapy and Rehabilitation, 20*(12), 580-589.

Schnell, G. (2008). Monitoring the progress of young people's occupational performance in an inpatient mental health setting. *New Zealand Journal of Occupational Therapy, 55*(2), 4-10.

Townsend, K., & Watson, A. (2013). Competent use of a motorised mobility scooter: Assessment, training and ongoing monitoring: A vital role for occupational therapy practice. *Australian Occupational Therapy Journal, 60*, 454-457.

West, S., Dunford, C., Mayston, M., & Forsyth, R. (2013). The School Function Assessment: Identifying levels of participation and demonstrating progress for pupils with acquired brain injuries in a residential rehabilitation setting. *Child: Care, Health and Development, 40*(5), 689-697.

Wilson, L., Atwal, A., Richards, C., & McIntyre, A. (2012). Do occupational therapy pre-discharge home visits affect the longer term outcomes of the discharge process? *International Journal of Therapy and Rehabilitation, 19*, 335-343.

# VI

# Context of Service Delivery

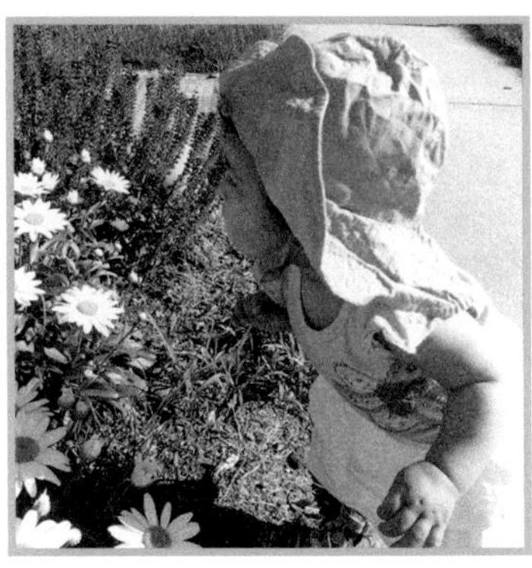

# 38

# EMERGING AREAS OF PRACTICE

Jeffrey L. Crabtree, OTD, MS, FAOTA and Leanna W. Katz, MS, OTD, OTR/L

**ACOTE STANDARDS EXPLORED IN THIS CHAPTER**

B.2.1, B.3.4, B.6.1–B.6.3, B.6.5, B.6.6, B 7.11, B.8.1

**KEY VOCABULARY**

- **Client-centered practice:** [A]n approach to service that embraces a philosophy of respect for, and partnership with, people receiving services (Law, Baptiste, & Mills, 1995, p. 253).
- **Evidence-based occupational therapy:** Client-centered enablement of occupation based on client information and a critical review of relevant research, expert consensus, and past experience (Canadian Association of Occupational Therapists, 2009, p. 1).
- **Population health:** The health outcomes of a group of individuals including the distribution of such outcomes within the group (Kindig & Stoddart, 2003, p. 381).
- **Technology:** A general term that refers to tools and technologies developed to solve human-related problems.



Jacobs, K., & MacRae, N. (Eds.).
*Occupational Therapy Essentials for Clinical Competence, Third Edition* (pp. 557-568).

This chapter will discuss some of the significant changes or trends within the profession and the impact of demographic changes and technology on current practice. It explores the various emerging areas of practice for occupational therapy practitioners, as affected by the changing health care reform of current day. Many would agree that the world, society, and the occupational therapy profession—virtually everything—changes. On the other hand, not all agree whether a particular change is good. The concept of a trend is no more objective. Statistically, we know that it takes several data points to establish a trend. For example, in the case of consumer spending, when one has data about a dozen holiday seasons of consumer spending, one can estimate a trend. However, it is quite another thing to understand why the trend line went in one direction or another, whether the trend will continue, or whether any causal relationship between the trend and background forces can be established. The field of occupational therapy is no different. We see changes and have glimpses of what are likely trends, but it is still quite difficult to understand the forces behind those trends, what the trends predict, or whether the trends will continue. Consequently, the changes and trends discussed here are a combination of the authors' personal perspective and literature supporting that perspective.

## A Professional Perspective

In this section, select changes and trends occurring in occupational therapy within the United States, within other Western English-speaking countries, and—to a lesser extent—within other countries are reviewed. To accomplish this, documents from the American Occupational Therapy Association (AOTA) and English-speaking journals were reviewed. In most cases, the journals are instruments of national occupational therapy or related professional associations. Consequently, these journals contain not only scholarly works, but also information about the professional association and its members. It is important to keep in mind that as the world shrinks because of technology such as the Internet, traditional distinctions between national and international ideas become blurred. So in the strict sense of the word, and from an American perspective, the Canadian, British, and Australian journals of occupational therapy could be considered foreign or international journals, yet a search of English-speaking literature on a particular topic would likely yield pertinent articles in at least one if not all occupational therapy journals from Canada to Australia. These journals publish authors from a variety of countries, and the studies and evolving ideas published in these journals have become an integral part of Americans' notions of occupational therapy.

One example that shows the international quality of our current domestic notions about effective occupational therapy is the concept of client-centered practice (Canadian Association of Occupational Therapists [CAOT], 1997; Law et al., 1995). In addition to many articles published in the *Canadian Journal of Occupational Therapy* (the developers of this concept are Canadian), client-centered practice has been discussed in the *Indian Journal of Occupational Therapy* (Morgan, Kelkar, & Vyas, 2002), the *British Journal of Occupational Therapy* (Unsworth, 2004), the *Scandinavian Journal of Occupational Therapy* (Hammell, 1995), *Occupational Therapy International* (Rigby, Ryan, From, Walczak, & Jutai, 1996), and the *American Journal of Occupational Therapy* (Snodgrass, 2011), just to cite one example from each of these journals.

Emerging areas of practice, which will be discussed later in this chapter about occupational therapy practice in the United States, are also appearing in the international literature. This is evidence that occupational therapy practitioners across the globe are facilitating change related to current ideals and practice within the health field. A prime example is the role of occupational therapy in mental health. The role of occupational therapy in mental health has expanded in areas such as the United States (Arbesman, Bazyk, & Nochajski, 2013), Canada (Hitch, 2016), Israel (Weintraub, Reiss-Poraz, Levy, Saban, & Erez, 2012), Sweden (Pooremamali, Persson, & Eklund, 2011), and Bangladesh (Nahar, Habib, & Nayan, 2011), to name a few. Occupational therapy practitioners are gaining attention in an increasing number of settings, working with populations across the lifespan all over the world.

While it is important to acknowledge the global influence of occupational therapy, for the purposes of this chapter, the remaining sections will focus primarily on occupational therapy practice in the United States.

## Change and Trends Within Occupational Therapy in the United States

To put into perspective the changes and trends that have led to what we understand as occupational therapy today, it is useful to briefly describe the social and medical context of the turn of the 20th century when occupational therapy was a fledgling profession (see Chapter 5).

Medicine and health care during the decades before and after 1900 were changing at a fast rate. On July 9, 1893, Dr. Daniel Hale Williams performed the world's first open heart surgery (Buckler, 1968; Cobb, 1953); the Curies shared the Nobel Prize in physics with Henri Becquerel for their work on radioactivity; vitamins were discovered; Robert Kotch discovered the tubercle bacillus; Wilhelm Conrad Röntgen discovered x-rays (Sutcliffe & Duin, 1992); and only a few "resurrectionists," or grave robbers, were still supplying some medical schools with cadavers. Hospital care changed rapidly during this time. These discoveries, activities, and new approaches to health care only begin to characterize the changes that took place in medicine and health care around the turn of the 20th century.

Around the turn of the 20th century, occupational therapy was being provided by teachers and craftspeople to individuals with mental illness (Licht, 1949). The educational programs were composed of a few weeks post–high school training until the early 1920s when the education grew to 1 year after high school (West, 1979). In March 1917, a group of supporters met in Clifton Springs, New York, to form the National Society for the Promotion of Occupational Therapy (Quiroga, 1995). By 1921, the name was changed to the AOTA, and the association started publishing the *Archives of Occupational Therapy* in that year. Furthermore, the types of clients seen by occupational therapy practitioners were becoming more diversified, and by the early 1900s, practitioners were providing services to clients with physical problems such as arthritis and tuberculosis as well as those with mental illness (Bing, 1981; Quiroga, 1995).

By the 1970s, some of the leaders in the profession were concerned about the quality of professional education and the influence of formal education on practitioners (Gillette, 1979; Johnson, 1979; Wiemer, 1979). Others expressed the need for developing client assessments that were unique to occupational therapy (West, 1979), and for developing research upon which to base our interventions (Yerxa, 1979). Therein, established the foundation of occupational therapy as we know it today—based on principles in education, research, and practice. It is important to note that education, research, and practice compose dynamic parts of a whole. To be a practitioner, one must be educated in the theories and skills of the profession. Sound theories and skills are founded on evidence from research and on the clinical expertise that comes from practice.

At the turn of the 21st century, the same ideals hold true regarding education, research, and practice. Occupational therapy today is grounded in evidence-based, occupation-based, and client-centered practice. However, the field of occupational therapy continues to evolve into the 21st century. One can argue that current trends and changes in occupational therapy in the United States are directly related to the trends in health care. With the passing of the Affordable Care Act in 2010, trends in health care and occupational therapy practice emphasize the importance of prevention and health promotion (Cason, 2015). According to Cason (2015), trends in practice today focus on "improving the health care experience, the health of populations, and the affordability of care" (p. 1). Generally speaking, the overarching goal of occupational therapy is to improve the health of our clients through participation in occupations. Herein, the concept of population health is introduced to occupational therapy. Population health is defined as "the health outcomes of a group of individuals including the distribution of such outcomes within the group" (Kindig & Stoddart, 2003, p. 381). According to Braveman (2016), occupational therapy practitioners may improve the overall health of the population "through the development of occupational therapy interventions at the population level and through advocacy to address occupational participation and the multiple determinants of health" (Braveman, 2016, p. 1). The official documents of the AOTA (found on their website) and the Third Edition of the *Occupational Therapy Practice Framework* support interventions at the population level, especially those that are cost effective and contextually relevant (AOTA, 2014).

Considering the impact occupational therapy may have on the health and well-being of the larger population, the approaches to practice briefly described in the following section may shed a new light on current trends in the United States.

## Client-Centered Practice

The client-centered practice approach in occupational therapy was developed in Canada over the past two decades (CAOT, 1997). As Law et al. (1995) stated, this approach "is a philosophy of practice built on concepts that reflect changes in the attitudes and beliefs of clients and occupational therapists" (p. 253). These attitudes and beliefs include the notion that clients need to express their needs and make choices regarding their occupations, that clients share responsibility for the therapeutic process, that the client-centered approach represents a shift from seeing the person as disabled to seeing the person as enabled, and that clients' "roles, interests, environments, and culture are central to the occupational therapy process" (Law et al., p. 252; Table 38-1). The client may in fact be a singular individual, or it can be groups or "collective of groups of individuals living in a similar locale or sharing the same or like characteristics or concerns" (AOTA, 2014, p. S3).

## Occupation-Based Practice

It is important to note that the concept of occupation as a special form of doing has been part of the occupational therapy ethos since the profession's infancy. Just to cite an example from one of the early proponents of occupational therapy, Dr. Adolf Meyer maintained that "occupation is, with good right, called the most essential side of hygienic treatment of most insane patients" (Meyer & Winters, 1951, p. 46).

Table 38-1.

**Contributions of the Client and Therapist in Evidence-Based Occupational Therapy**

| Client's Contributions | Occupational Therapy Practitioner's Contributions |
|---|---|
| Knowledge, beliefs, hopes, and so forth, necessary for determining meaningful occupational intervention priorities | Knowledge of client's environment and other information relevant to enabling occupational performance |
| Beliefs about what medical, developmental, or social problems prohibit meaningful occupational performance | Using evidence-based occupational therapy principles and professional expertise, assists client to identify and prioritize occupational performance goals |
| Subjective evaluation of present occupational performance | Offers suggestions and encourages client to explore new ways of viewing occupational performance deficits |
| Knowledge and perceptions of personal and environmental resources and limitations | Offers suggestions and encourages client to consider new uses of personal and environmental resources |
| Hopes for outcomes and agreement with possible therapy plans and measures of success | |
| With the therapist, identifies intervention outcomes and commits to the proposed intervention and measures of desired outcomes | |
| Adapted from Canadian Association of Occupational Therapists. (1999). *Joint position statement on evidence-based occupational therapy.* Toronto, Ontario, Canada: CAOT Publications. Retrieved from http://www.caot.ca/default.asp?ChangeID =166 & pageID =156 | |

A number of current models exist that espouse the notion that occupation should form the basis of occupational therapy intervention, and that in addressing occupations, practitioners address not only functional deficits but broader issues of meaning, purpose, and spirituality—issues that must be addressed if we are going to assist in a client's construction or reconstruction of the self (Baum & Christiansen, 1997; Christiansen, 1999; Crabtree, 2003; Howard & Howard, 1997; Mattingly & Fleming, 1994). These include the Canadian Occupational Performance Measure (CAOT, 1997) and the Occupational Performance Model (Australia; Chapparo & Ranka, 1997). In addition, the concept of occupational performance forms the core of the *Framework* (AOTA, 2014). Suffice it to say, these models place occupation, or purposive doing, at the center of occupational therapy intervention and assume that humans are occupational beings who express their meaning and purpose through their occupations. Many of these models are discussed in more depth in other chapters.

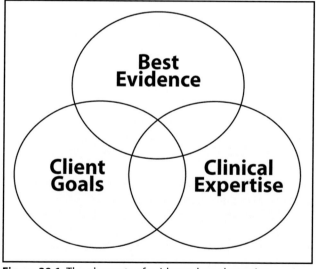


**Figure 38-1.** The elements of evidence-based practice.

## Evidence-Based Occupational Therapy

As discussed earlier, recognition of the need for evidence-based occupational therapy has now reached an international level (Ilott, Taylor, & Bolanos, 2006). Essentially, evidence-based occupational therapy is a collaborative effort between the client and the occupational therapy practitioner in which the client contributes what is uniquely his or hers to offer, and the practitioner contributes his or her expertise (see Table 38-1).

As one might imagine, the application of evidence-based practice across all health care disciplines, many of which have limited research-based knowledge, can be challenging at best and discouraging at worst. Consequently, each profession needs to identify an appropriate blend of the best evidence, clinical expertise, and the client's goals to its practice (Figure 38-1). The concept of best evidence in some ways may pose the greatest challenge to evidence-based occupational therapy. Best evidence is generally based on the idea that certain research designs provide a stronger level of evidence, or greater control of bias, than other research designs. However, there is disagreement among researchers, whether they are part of qualitative or quantitative traditions, as to the precise definitions of evidence, let alone which types of research designs provide the best evidence (Bannigan & Moores, 2009; Cicerone, 2005; Hammell, 2002; Law & MacDermid, 2007; MacDermid, 2004; Sackett, Rosenberg, Muir Gray, Haynes, & Richardson, 1996).

## Emerging Practice Areas

According to the 2015 AOTA member data survey, most occupational therapists (approximately 66%) practiced in traditional settings such as acute hospitals, rehabilitation hospitals, and school systems (AOTA, 2016). The largest trend from the previous year was reflected in the number of occupational therapists and occupational therapy assistants practicing in long-term care facilities or skilled nursing facilities (AOTA, 2016). This upward trend directly reflects the growing population as individuals are living longer and facing more challenges related to aging and disease.

The AOTA has identified a number of what they call emerging niches that fit well within the occupational therapy scope of practice in the United States (AOTA, n.d.). This section identifies only a few of these areas of practice. The reader is encouraged to go to the AOTA members' area on the AOTA website (www.aota.org) for detailed information about these emerging practice areas. With each area, the website includes hot links to more detailed information useful to the practitioner.

Within the emerging practice areas as identified by AOTA, the underlying concept of population health is better understood. Occupational therapy practitioners are trained to analyze client factors, performance skills and patterns, contexts and environments, and the activity demands that affect health and engagement in occupations. This ability to broadly analyze people and their environment allows for the promotion of population health in the various emerging niches at a global scale.

The following briefly explores three of these emerging niches: childhood obesity, prevention, and depression.

### Childhood Obesity

Berwick, Nolan, and Whittington (2008) introduced the concept of the Triple Aim in 2008. The authors proposed that to improve population health, practitioners must simultaneously pursue "three aims: improving the experience of care, improving the health of populations, and reducing per capita costs of health care" (Berwick, Nolan, & Whittington, 2008, p. 759). Occupational therapy practitioners may pursue "The Triple Aim" when working with at-risk populations, such as children with obesity. Occupational therapy practitioners have the ability to promote healthy behaviors through education and participation in physical activities related to meaningful occupations. Persch, Lamb, Metzler, and Fristad (2015) provided an occupational therapy intervention that "analyzed and adapted sleep, physical, and eating routines in ways that enhance[d] health and well-being" (p. 1). The authors successfully targeted an at-risk group at the population level, while ensuring interventions were meaningful and appropriate to the individual. For this particular population, education within a supportive institution is essential to the success of such a program to ensure carryover of consistency of learned behaviors. Furthermore, while the institution plays a large role in the success of the program, as does the child's social network and support. Occupational therapy practitioners have the capacity to integrate all contexts—physical, mental/emotional, and social—to promote participation and buy-in of a healthy habits program.

### Prevention

As mentioned previously, the Affordable Care Act has influenced the trends in occupational therapy programing and funding. One of the emerging areas corresponding to these trends in health care is the prevention of health problems. One can prevent health problems through increased participation in health and wellness promotion programs (Reitz & Scaffa, 2010). Health and wellness promotion is one of the core principles that define occupational therapy practice. According to the *Framework* (2014), "achieving health, well-being, and participation in life through engagement in occupation is the overarching statement that describes the domain and process of occupational therapy in its fullest sense" (p. S4). Health and wellness promotion emphasizes the importance of targeting health-promoting behaviors. In essence, prevention uses a behavioral approach to change the way people think about health at the population level. As the World Health Organization (1986) defines it, health promotion is "the process of enabling people to increase control over, and to improve, their health" (p. 1).

### Depression

According to Pratt and Brody (2014), "almost 43% of persons with severe depressive symptoms reported serious difficulties in work, home, and social activities" (p. 1). The role of occupational therapy can address these difficulties related to occupational performance at the individual level and population level. For example, an occupational therapy practitioner may promote participation in specific social activities for an individual with depressive symptoms by facilitating change in personal and environmental factors. At the population level, occupational therapy practitioners may promote quality of life in individuals with depression. An example at the population level includes older adults living in long-term care facilities. Older adults living in assisted living facilities or nursing homes experience increased depression (Ouyang, Chong, Ng, & Liu, 2015). Risk factors for the elderly population include loneliness, social isolation, and functional decline (Mezuk, Rock, Lohman, & Choi, 2014). The aforementioned risk factors lead to poor health outcomes and a potentially decreased overall quality of life. To promote increased health and well-being in older adults living in long-term care facilities, it is important to address the health factors and occupational participation that influence an individual's well-being. This focus on population health may involve addressing systemic environmental factors within an institution.

# Demographics and Technology

The practice of occupational therapy does not exist in a vacuum. Practitioners and what they practice are situated in political, cultural, social, geographical, religious, and many other contexts. Of the many possible contexts to consider, this chapter focuses on demographics and technology. These appear to likely have significant implications for occupational therapy practitioners in this century.

## Demographics of the United States

There are five trends related to health care that will have a significant impact on the United States population and, by extension, will have important implications for occupational therapy practitioners:

1. Americans are getting older
2. Americans are becoming more ethnically diverse
3. Access and affordability of health care services
4. The rise of more chronic diseases resulting in the increased need for long-term care
5. The U.S. population will likely peak in the mid- to late 21st century

According to the 2014 U.S. Census data and projections, the nation's population will increase to 417 million in 2060 compared to 319 million in 2014 (Colby & Ortman, 2015). In 2060, nearly 20% of Americans will be foreign born. Those 65 years and older will increase from 44.7 million in 2013 to 98 million in 2060, representing more than 20% of the total population (U.S. Department of Health and Human Services, 2013). There is no way of knowing today whether these trends will come to pass exactly as predicted, but regardless of the precision of these trends, demographic changes in the United States are likely to have a significant impact on occupational therapy in varying degrees and ways. The aging and increased ethnic diversity of Americans, in particular, will have an impact on occupational therapy in that the increase in the number of older adults will create an increased demand for occupational services, and the increase in the ethnic diversity of our clients will require increased skill on the part of practitioners to be culturally proficient (Royeen & Crabtree, 2006). When you add the increasing numbers of U.S. citizens with disabling conditions to this equation, the demand for occupational therapy services increases even more.

For example, according to the National Health Interview Survey, January-March 2015, approximately 3.5 million adults over the age of 65 needed help with at least one personal care task from another person because of a physical, mental, or emotional issue (Centers for Disease Control and Prevention, 2015). More than 5 million adults (ages 18 and older) required the help of another person with activities of daily living such as eating, dressing, or bathing, and more than 9 million adults required help with instrumental activities of daily living such as household chores or shopping.

As our nation becomes increasingly ethnically diverse, so will our clinics, hospitals, schools, and other occupational therapy service settings. With this diversity comes differences between practitioners and clients or clients' basic values, attitudes, and beliefs about what it means to be an individual; the importance (or lack of importance) of independence or the ability to make decisions; and many other aspects of culture. Disagreement concerning such values and beliefs need not confound the occupational therapy practitioner's efforts to provide effective services. However, to minimize the chances of such conflicts undermining therapy, occupational therapy practitioners need to be culturally proficient, as discussed in Chapter 2.

## Technology

In this section, there is a focus on technology in general, not on the technology that is available for use in therapy. For specific information on assistive technology, please see Chapter 32; for information on telehealth, please see Chapter 39.

Technology is forever advancing in the health field, from adaptive equipment for individuals with spinal cord injuries to the use of three-dimensional printing in surgical interventions and prosthetics (Kuehn, 2016). Many individuals value the use of technology in everyday tasks. It is no wonder that occupational therapy practitioners strive to use technology with clients to ensure meaningful and goal-oriented care. Occupational therapy practitioners incorporate technology in everyday practice across the lifespan in various practice settings. When using technology in practice, however, it is important to consider the impact technology may have on occupational performance and overall long-term well-being because it has the potential to promote independence or to the contrary, decrease participation in everyday activities.

There is no question that technology has made doing some things easier (Smith, 2000). In most cases, the use of technology is seen as a great addition to short-term and long-term treatments. However, perhaps technology may cause more harm than good. For instance, an adolescent with autism working on social participation may benefit from the use of a virtual environment to interact with other individuals who may have increased difficulty conversing and socializing in person. However, one can easily spend hours in virtual environments and consequently decrease participation in other meaningful and health-promoting activities. The direct and indirect effects of technology as related to overall health and well-being must be considered from the start.

One challenge that occupational therapy practitioners face is meeting a just-right challenge that is not too easy, nor too difficult, for our clients (DeCleene, 2013). While technology may make things a bit easier, the goal of occupational therapy treatment is not to make life easy. Occupational therapy practitioners must not lose sight of the importance of interventions that are meaningful, cost-effective, goal-oriented, and healthful for the individual.

For many, the use of technology can make the difference between isolation and participation and between independence and dependence. However, what might be a liberating technology, a sense of independence, for one person might be a form of subtle enslavement for another.

## Summary

This chapter discusses some of the significant changes, or trends, within the profession and situated occupational therapy in the broad context of the 21st century. The authors address changes in occupational therapy practice as related to the changes in the health care reform and population health. We continue to provide services to those who have been seriously disabled due to illness, accidents, disease, and other factors. These people, as Jennings (1993) suggested, still need "the restoration of wholeness and integrity ... and the preservation of a meaningful life" (p. S25)—the essence of occupational therapy. Regardless of the era, people want to be happy, well, and satisfied with their lives; to participate in the daily course of social and economic events; and to be able to construct worthy goals and meet those goals. As the occupational therapy profession has grown and matured, it has become more able to meet the needs of those people. Now more than ever, the essential value of occupational therapy practice includes more cost-effective, health-promoting interventions that focus on the greater good of the population at large.

### Case Study

Paul is a 78-year-old man residing in a long-term care facility. He moved in 3 months ago, after his wife died. He sees an occupational therapy assistant twice a week to work on increasing participation in activities of daily living and instrumental activities of daily living, which have become increasingly more difficult since a diagnosis of osteoarthritis 3 years ago. During the past 3 weeks, Paul has declined to participate in his occupational therapy sessions. He told his occupational therapy assistant, Sara, that he is "feeling down." Sara has heard others report similar feelings over the past few months, so she decided to talk to her colleagues about addressing a potential population health issue. After consulting her interprofessional team (including social work, psychology, physical therapy, speech therapy, medicine, and nursing), Sara confirms that perhaps residents are demonstrating signs and symptoms of depression. Sara hopes to improve the morale of Paul, her clients, and the other residents, which may subsequently improve overall health. With approval from her superiors, Sara decides to run a weekly group for residents that promotes social participation and quality of life. Sara provides the residents with surveys for possible group topics, to ensure groups are client-centered and meaningful. Sara found that residents who filled out the survey appreciated being included in the process and felt more inclined to participate in the weekly groups than in individual therapy sessions. Sara successfully addressed the community needs, while maintaining client-centered and occupation-based care for those residing in the long-term care facility. Paul found that the groups related to gardening "lifted [his] spirits" and "reminded [him] of [his] wife." For Paul, participating in the groups subsequently decreased his symptoms of depression and increased his quality of life.

## Student Self-Assessment

1. Search the literature on an occupational therapy assessment or intervention and then identify how many professional journals from other countries have published articles on that topic. Were there significant differences in the ways the topic was addressed? If so, how were they different or similar?
2. Compare and contrast two journal articles on a given occupational therapy topic—one from an article published prior to 1970 and one from an article published after 2000.
3. Using U.S. Census data, examine the demographics of your state or county. Explain the implications of your findings related to the need for occupational therapy services in your area. Find examples of people's need for assistive technology in your local newspaper. What were the needs, and who provided the services or applied the technology? Did an occupational therapy practitioner provide the service? If not, speculate why.

## Evidence-Based Research Chart

| Topic | Evidence |
|---|---|
| Population health | Braveman, 2016 |
| Childhood obesity | Persch, Lamb, Metzler, & Fristad, 2015 |
| Prevention | Reitz & Scaffa, 2010 |
| Depression | Kim, Irwin, Kim, Chin, & Kim, 2015 |

## Electronic Resources

Client-centered practice resources: www.caot.ca

Evidence-based occupational therapy resources, American Occupational Therapy Association official documents, and emerging practice areas: www.aota.org

Information about international resources and international occupational therapy programs: www.wfot.org.au

Information about the American Occupational Therapy Foundation and the Wilma West Library: www.aotf.org

## References

American Occupational Therapy Association. (n.d.). *Emerging niches in practice.* Retrieved from https://www.aota.org/practice/manage/niche.aspx

American Occupational Therapy Association. (2014). Occupational therapy practice framework: Domain and process (3rd ed.). *American Journal of Occupational Therapy, 68*(Suppl. 1), S1-S48. doi:10.5014/ajot.2014.682006

American Occupational Therapy Association. (2016). *AOTA salary and workforce survey.* Bethesda, MD: AOTA Press.

Arbesman, M., Bazyk, S., & Nochajski, S. M. (2013). Systematic review of occupational therapy and mental health promotion, prevention, and intervention for children and youth. *American Journal of Occupational Therapy, 67,* e120-e130. doi:10.5014/ajot.2013.008359

Bannigan, K., & Moores, A. (2009). A model of professional thinking: Integrating reflective practice and evidence based practice. *Canadian Journal of Occupational Therapy, 76*(5), 342-350.

Baum, C., & Christiansen, C. (1997). The occupational therapy context: Philosophy-principles-practice. In C. Christiansen & C. Baum (Eds.), *Occupational therapy: Enabling function and well-being* (2nd ed., pp. 27-45). Thorofare, NJ: SLACK Incorporated.

Berwick, D. M., Nolan, T. W., & Whittington, J. (2008). The triple aim: Care, health, and cost. *Health Affairs, 27,* 759-769. doi:10.1377/hlthaff.27.3.759

Bing, R. K. (1981). Occupational therapy revisited: A paraphrastic journey. *American Journal of Occupational Therapy, 35*(8), 499-518.

Braveman, B. (2016). Health policy perspectives—population health and occupational therapy. *American Journal of Occupational Therapy, 70,* 7001090010. doi:10.5014/ajot.2016.701002

Buckler, H. (1968). *Daniel Hale Williams. Negro surgeon.* New York, NY: Pitman Publishing Corporation.

Canadian Association of Occupational Therapists. (1997). *Enabling occupation: An occupational therapy perspective.* Toronto, Ontario, Canada: CAOT Publications.

Canadian Association of Occupational Therapists. (2009). *Joint position statement on evidence-based occupational therapy.* Retrieved from http://www.caot.ca/default.asp?ChangeID=166&pageID=156

Cason, J. (2015). Health policy perspectives—Telehealth and occupational therapy: Integral to the triple aim of health care reform. *American Journal of Occupational Therapy, 69,* 6902090010. doi:10.5014/ajot.2015.692003

Centers for Disease Control and Prevention. (2015). *QuickStats: Percentage of adults with activity limitations, by age group and type of limitation—National Health Interview Survey, United States, 2010.* Retrieved from http://www.cdc.gov/mmwr/preview/mmwrhtml/mm6114a4.htm

Chapparo, C., & Ranka, J. (1997). *Occupational performance model (Australia): Monograph 1.* Sydney, Australia: Total Print Control.

Christiansen, C. H. (1999). Eleanor Clarke Slagle Lectureship—1999. Defining lives: Occupation as identity: An essay on competence, coherence, and the creation of meaning. *American Journal of Occupational Therapy, 53*(6), 547-558.

Cicerone, K. D. (2005). Evidence-based practice and the limits of rational rehabilitation. *Archives of Physical Medicine and Rehabilitation, 86,* 1073-1074.

Cobb, W. M. (1953). Medical history. *Journal of the National Medical Association, 45*(5), 379-385.

Colby, S. L., & Ortman, J. M. (2015). *Projections of the size and composition of the U.S. population: 2014 to 2060. U.S. Census Bureau.* Retrieved from https://www.census.gov/content/dam/Census/library/publications/2015/demo/p25-1143.pdf

Crabtree, J. L. (2003). On occupational performance. *Occupational Therapy in Health Care, 17*(2), 1-18.

DeCleene, K. E., Ridgway, A. J., Bednarski, J., Breeden, L., Mosier, G. G., Sachs, D., & Stephenson, D. (2013). Therapists as educators: The importance of client education in occupational therapy. *The Open Journal of Occupational Therapy, 1*(4). doi:10.15453/2168-6408.1050

Gillette, N. (1979). Practice, education and research. In *Occupational therapy: 2001 AD.* Papers presented at the special session of the Representative Assembly, November 1978 (pp. 18-25). Rockville, MD: AOTA Press.

Hammell, K. W. (1995). Application of learning theory in spinal cord injury rehabilitation: Client-centered occupational therapy. *Scandinavian Journal of Occupational Therapy, 2*(1), 34-39.

Hammell, K. W. (2002). Informing client-centred practice through qualitative inquiry: Evaluating the quality of qualitative research. *British Journal of Occupational Therapy, 65*(4), 175-184.

Hitch, D. P. (2016). Attitudes of mental health occupational therapists toward evidence-based practice. *Canadian Journal of Occupational Therapy, 83,* 27-32. doi:10.1177/0008417415583108

Howard, B. S., & Howard, J. R. (1997). Occupation as spiritual activity. *American Journal of Occupational Therapy, 51*(3), 181-185.

Ilott, I., Taylor, M. C., & Bolanos, C. (2006). Evidence-based occupational therapy: It's time to take a global approach. *British Journal of Occupational Therapy, 69*(1), 38-41.

Jennings, B. (1993). Healing the self: The moral meaning of relationships in rehabilitation. *American Journal of Physical Medicine and Rehabilitation, 72*, 401-404.

Johnson, J. (1979). Reorganization in relation to the issues. In *Occupational therapy: 2001 AD*. Papers presented at the special session of the Representative Assembly, November 1978 (pp. 60-68). Rockville, MD: AOTA Press.

Kim, J., Irwin, L., Kim, M., Chin, S., & Kim, J. (2015). The role of leisure engagement for health benefits among Korean older women. *Health Care for Women International, 36*, 1357-1374. doi:10.1080/07399332.2015.1077843

Kindig, D. & Stoddart, G. (2003). What is population health? *American Journal of Public Health, 93*, 380-383. doi:10.2105/AJPH.93.3.380

Kuehn, B. M. (2016). Clinicians embrace 3D printers to solve unique clinical challenges. *Journal of American Medical Association, 315*, 333-335.

Law, M., Baptiste, S., & Mills, J. (1995). Client-centered practice: What does it mean and does it make a difference? *Canadian Journal of Occupational Therapy, 62*(5), 250-257.

Law, M. C., & MacDermid, J. (2007). *Evidence-based rehabilitation: A guide to practice*. Thorofare, NJ: SLACK Incorporated.

Licht, S. (1949). The changing role of the occupational therapist. *Occupational Therapy and Rehabilitation, 28*(3), 260-264.

MacDermid, J. C. (2004). An introduction to evidence-based practice for hand therapists. *Journal of Hand Therapy, 17*(2), 105-117. doi:10.1197/j.jht.2004.02.001

Mattingly, C., & Fleming, M. H. (1994). *Clinical reasoning: Forms of inquiry in a therapeutic practice*. Philadelphia, PA: F. A. Davis Company.

Meyer, A., & Winters, E. E. (Eds.). (1951). *The collected papers of Adolf Meyer* (Vol. 2). Baltimore, MD: Johns Hopkins Press.

Mezuk, B., Rock, A., Lohman, M. C., & Choi, M. (2014). Suicide risk in long-term care facilities: A systematic review. *International Journal of Geriatric Psychiatry, 29*, 1198-1211. doi:10.1002/gps.4142

Morgan, S. B., Kelkar, R. S., & Vyas, O. A. (2002). Client-centered occupational therapy for acute stroke patients. *Indian Journal of Occupational Therapy, 34*(1), 7-12.

Nahar, N., Habib, M., & Nayan, J. (2011). Occupational therapy mental health service development through supervised fieldwork in Bangladesh. *World Federation of Occupational Therapists Bulletin, 63*, 44-47. doi:10.1179/otb.2011.63.1.008

Ouyang, Z., Chong, A. M. L., Ng, T. K., & Liu, S. (2015). Leisure, functional disability and depression among older Chinese living in residential care homes. *Aging and Mental Health, 19*, 723-730. doi:10.1080/13607863.2014.962009

Persch, A. C., Lamb, A. J., Metzler, C. A., & Fristad, M. A. (2015). Healthy habits for children: Leveraging existing evidence to demonstrate value. *American Journal of Occupational Therapy, 69*, 6904090010. doi:10.5014/ajot.2015.694001

Pooremamali, P., Persson, D., & Eklund, M. (2011). Occupational therapists' experience of working with immigrant clients in mental health care. *Scandinavian Journal of Occupational Therapy, 18*, 109-121. doi:10.3109/11038121003649789

Pratt, L. A. & Brody, D. J. (2014). *Depression in the U.S. household population, 2009-2012. NCHS data brief, 172*. Hyattsville, MD: National Center for Health Statistics.

Quiroga, V. A. M. (1995). *Occupational therapy: The first 30 years: 1900 to 1930*. Bethesda, MD: AOTA Press.

Reitz, S. M., & Scaffa, M. E. (2010). Public health principles, approaches, and initiatives. In M. E. Scaffa, S. M. Reitz, & M. A. Pizzi (Eds.), *Occupational therapy in the promotion of health and wellness* (pp. 70-95). Philadelphia, PA: F. A. Davis Company.

Rigby, R., Ryan, S., From, W., Walczak, E., & Jutai, J. (1996). A client-centered approach to developing assistive technology with children. *Occupational Therapy International, 3*(1), 67-79.

Royeen, M., & Crabtree, J. L. (2006). *Culture in rehabilitation: From competency to proficiency*. Upper Saddle River, NJ: Prentice Hall.

Sackett, D. L., Rosenberg, W. M. C., Muir Gray, J. A., Haynes, R. B., & Richardson, W. S. (1996). Evidence-based medicine: What it is and what it isn't. *British Medical Journal, 312*, 71-72.

Smith, R. O. (2000). The role of occupational therapy in a developmental technology model. *American Journal of Occupational Therapy, 54*(3), 339-340.

Snodgrass, J. (2011). Effective occupational therapy interventions in the rehabilitation of individuals with work-related low back injuries and illnesses: A systematic review. *American Journal of Occupational Therapy, 65*(1), 37-43.

Sutcliffe, J., & Duin, N. (1992). *A history of medicine*. New York, NY: Barnes & Noble Books.

Unsworth, C. A. (2004). Clinical reasoning: How do pragmatic reasoning, worldview and client-centredness fit? *British Journal of Occupational Therapy, 67*(1), 10-19.

U.S. Department of Health and Human Services. (2013). *Administration of aging*. Retrieved from: http://www.aoa.acl.gov/aging_statistics/index.aspx

Weintraub, N., Reiss-Poraz, O., Levy, G., Saban, E., & Erez, A. B. (2012). Occupational therapy in the field of mental health rehabilitation—Processes of learning and growing. *Israeli Journal of Occupational Therapy, 21*, E52-55.

West, W. (1979). Historical perspectives. In *Occupational therapy: 2001 AD*. Papers presented at the special session of the Representative Assembly, November 1978 (pp. 9-17). Rockville, MD: AOTA Press.

Wiemer, R. (1979). Traditional and nontraditional practice arenas. In *Occupational therapy: 2001 AD*. Papers presented at the special session of the Representative Assembly, November 1978 (pp. 42-53). Rockville, MD: AOTA Press.

World Health Organization, Health and Welfare, Canada, Canadian Public Health Association. (1986). *Ottawa charter for health promotion*. Geneva, Switzerland: World Health Organization.

Yerxa, E. (1979). The philosophical base of occupation. In *Occupational therapy: 2001 AD*. Papers presented at the special session of the Representative Assembly, November 1978 (pp. 26-30). Rockville, MD: AOTA Press.

## Suggested Readings

Adams, P. F., Martinez, M. E., Vickerie, J. L., & Kirzinger, W. K. (2011). Summary health statistics for the U.S. population: National Health Interview Survey, 2010. *Vital and Health Statistics, 10*(251), 1-117.

Allen, S., Strong, J., & Polatajko, H. J. (2001). Graduate-entry masters' degrees: Launch pad for occupational therapy in this millennium? *British Journal of Occupational Therapy, 64*(11), 572-576.

American Occupational Therapy Association. (1974). *The 1974-1975 yearbook*. Rockville, MD: AOTA Press.

American Occupational Therapy Association. (1979a). *Occupational therapy: 2001 AD*. Papers presented at the special session of the Representative Assembly, November 1978. Rockville, MD: AOTA Press.

American Occupational Therapy Association. (1979b). Uniform terminology for occupational therapy (1st ed.). *Occupational Therapy News, 35*, 1-8.

American Occupational Therapy Association. (1989). Uniform terminology for occupational therapy (2nd ed.). *American Journal of Occupational Therapy, 43*, 808-815.

American Occupational Therapy Association. (1994). Uniform terminology for occupational therapy (3rd ed.). *American Journal of Occupational Therapy, 48*, 1047-1054.

American Occupational Therapy Association. (1999). ACOTE sets timeline for post-baccalaureate degree programs. *OT Week, 13*(33), i, iii.

American Occupational Therapy Association. (2006). *AOTA 2006 occupational therapy workforce and compensation report*. Bethesda, MD: AOTA Press.

American Occupational Therapy Association. (2008a). Occupational therapy practice framework: Domain and process (2nd ed.). *American Journal of Occupational Therapy, 62*, 625-683.

American Occupational Therapy Association. (2008b). AOTA's societal statement on youth violence. *American Journal of Occupational Therapy, 62*, 709-710.

American Occupational Therapy Association. (2012). *Academic programs annual data report, academic year 2011-2012*. Retrieved from http://www.aota.org/~/media/Corporate/Files/EducationCareers/Accredit/47682/2011-2012-Annual-Data-Report.ashx

American Occupational Therapy Association. (2013). *Chronic disease management*. Retrieved from http://www.aota.org/Practice/Health-Wellness/Emerging-Niche/Chronic-Disease-Management.aspx

Amini, D. (2006). Repetitive stress injuries and the age of communication. *OT Practice, 11*(9), 10-15.

Bakhtin, M. M., Liapunov, V. (Trans. & Ed.), & Holquist, M. (Ed.). (1993). *Toward a philosophy of the act*. Austin, TX: University of Texas Press.

Bear-Lehman, J. (2012). Comparison of the occupational therapy research agenda with the National Institutes of Health roadmap for medical research. *American Journal of Occupational Therapy, 66*(2), 250-253.

Beard, K. W., & Wolf, E. M. (2001). Modification in the proposed diagnostic criteria for internet addiction. *Cyberpsychological Behavior, 4*(3), 377-383.

Bockoven, J. S. (1971). Legacy of moral treatment—1800s to 1910. *American Journal of Occupational Therapy, 25*(5), 223-225.

Bonder, B., & Christiansen, C. (2001). Editorial: Coming of age in challenging times. *Occupational Therapy Journal of Research, 21*(1), 3-11.

Boyer, G., Hachey, R., & Mercier, C. (2000). Perceptions of occupational performance and subjective quality of life in persons with severe mental illness. *Occupational Therapy in Mental Health, 15*(2), 1-15.

Bundy, A. C., Luckett, T., Naughton, G. A., Tranter, P. J., Wyver, S. R., Ragen, J., Singleton, E., & Spies, G. (2008). Playful interaction: Occupational therapy for all children on the school playground. *American Journal of Occupational Therapy, 62*(5), 522-527.

Canadian Association of Occupational Therapists. (2002). *CAOT announces professional master's degree as entry requirement starting 2010*. Retrieved from http://www.caot.ca/pdfs/mastersentry-facts.pdf

Centers for Disease Control and Prevention. (2012). *Chronic disease prevention and health promotion*. Retrieved from http://www.cdc.gov/chronicdisease/overview/index.htm.

Chen, Y-H. (2002). Experiences with the COPM and client-centered practice in adult neurorehabilitation in Taiwan. *Occupational Therapy International, 9*(3), 167-184.

Committee on the Initial Assessment of Readjustment Needs of Military Personnel, Veterans, and Their Families. (2010). *Returning home from Iraq and Afghanistan: Preliminary assessment of readjustment needs of veterans, service members, and their families*. Atlanta, GA: National Academies Press.

Council on Medical Education and Hospitals of the American Medical Association. (1947). Approved schools for occupational therapy technicians. *Occupational Therapy and Rehabilitation, 26*(3), cover 3.

Council of Occupational Therapists for the European Countries. (n.d.). *History of COTEC: Introduction*. Retrieved from http://www.cotec-europe.org

Council of Occupational Therapists for the European Countries. (2012). *Summary of the occupational therapy profession in Europe, 2012*. Retrieved from http://www.cotec-europe.org/

Crabtree, J. L. (2010). No one dresses accidentally: A research synthesis on intentional occupational performance. *OTJR: Occupation, Participation, and Health, 30*(3), 100-110.

Crabtree, J. L. (2011). Neuro-occupation: The confluence of neuroscience and occupational therapy. *Japanese Journal of Occupational Therapy, 45*(7), 879-886.

Curt, A., Schwab, M. E., & Dietz, V. (2004). Providing the clinical basis for new interventional therapies: Refined diagnosis and assessment of recovery after spinal cord injury. *Spinal Cord, 42*, 1-6.

Dance, S. (2012). Amputee eager for arm moved by thought. *Indianapolis Star*, A9.

Darden, L., & Maull, N. (1977). Interfield theory. *Philosophy of Science, 44*(1), 43-64.

Deutsch, J. E., Borbely, M., Filler, J., Huhn, K., & Guarrera-Bowlby, P. (2008). Use of a low-cost, commercially available gaming console (Wii) for rehabilitation of an adolescent with cerebral palsy. *Physical Therapy, 88*(10), 1196-1207.

Dielacher, S., & Höss, V. (2011). Occupational therapy in vocational rehabilitation of adults with mental illness. *Die Rehabilitation, 50*(5), 308-315.

Dunkel, L. M. (1983). Moral and humane: Patients' libraries in early nineteenth-century American mental hospitals. *Bulletin of the Medical Library Association, 73*(3), 274-281.

Ethridge, D. A., & McSweeney, M. (1970). Research in occupational therapy, part 1. *American Journal of Occupational Therapy, 24*(7), 490-494.

European Network of Occupational Therapy in Higher Education. (n.d.). *Organization: Introduction*. Retrieved from http://www.enothe.hva.nl

Farnworth, L. (2003). Sylvia Docker lecture. Time use, tempo and temporality: Occupational therapy's core business or someone else's business? *Australian Occupational Therapy Journal, 50*(3), 116-126.

Fidler, G. (1979). Professional or nonprofessional. In *Occupational therapy: 2001 AD*. Papers presented at the special session of the Representative Assembly, November 1978 (pp. 31-36). Rockville, MD: AOTA Press.

Finlay, L. (2006). "Rigour", "ethical integrity" or "artistry"? Reflexively reviewing criteria for evaluating qualitative research. *British Journal of Occupational Therapy, 69*(7), 319-326.

Fleming, M. H., Johnson, J. A., Marina, M.-H., Spergel, E. L., & Townsend, B. (1987). *Occupational therapy directions for the future. Report of the Entry-Level Study Committee of the American Occupational Therapy Association*. Rockville, MD: AOTA Press.

Gergen, K. J. (1991). *The saturated self: Dilemmas of identity in contemporary life*. New York, NY: Basic Books.

Gillette, N. (1990). Guest editorial: 10th anniversary volume of OTJR: An update of research programs. *Occupational Therapy Journal of Research, 10*(6), 67-73.

Griffiths, Y., & Padilla, R. (2006). National status of the entry-level doctorate in occupational therapy (OTD). *American Journal of Occupational Therapy, 60*(5), 540-550.

Hall, E. T. (1981). *Beyond culture*. New York, NY: Anchor Press.

Haltiwanger, E., Lazzarini, I., & Nazeran, H. (2007). Application of nonlinear dynamics theory to neuro-occupation: A case study of alcoholism. *British Journal of Occupational Therapy, 70*(8), 349-357.

Hamzei, F., Liepert, J., Dettmers, C., Weiller, C., & Rijntjes, M. (2006). Two different reorganization patterns after rehabilitative therapy: An exploratory study with fMRI and TMS. *Neuroimage, 31*(2), 710-720.

Hansen, S. (2002). Excessive Internet usage or "Internet addiction"? The implications of diagnostic categories for student users. *Journal of Computer Assisted Learning, 18*(2), 235-236.

Haynes, R. B. (2001). Of studies, summaries, synopses, and systems: The "4S" evolution of services for finding current best evidence. *Evidence Based Mental Health, 4*(2), 37-38. doi:10.1136/ebmh.4.2.37

Hermann, V. H., Herzog, M., Jordan, R., Hofherr, M., Levine, P., & Page, S. J. (2010). Telerehabilitation and electrical stimulation: An occupation-based, client-centered stroke intervention. *American Journal of Occupational Therapy, 64*(1), 73-81. doi:10.5014/ajot.64.1.73

Hiemstra, G. (2003). *Population myths, trends and transportation planning*. Retrieved from http://www.futurist.com

Hilton, C. L. (2005). The evolving postbaccalaureate entry: Analysis of occupational therapy entry-level master's degree in the United States. *Occupational Therapy in Health Care, 19*(3), 51-71.

Jansa, J., Sicherl, Z., Angleitner, K., & Law, M. (2004). The use of Canadian Occupational Performance Measure (COPM) in clients with an acute stroke. *World Federation of Occupational Therapists Bulletin, 50*, 18-23.

Jantzen, A. (1979). The current profile of occupational therapy and the future—professional or vocational? In *Occupational therapy: 2001 AD*. Papers presented at the special session of the Representative Assembly, November 1978 (pp. 71-75). Rockville, MD: AOTA Press.

Jonas, H. (1982). *The phenomenon of life*. Chicago, IL: University of Chicago Press.

Jonas, H. (1984). *The imperative of responsibility*. (H. Jonas & D. Herr, Trans.) Chicago, IL: University of Chicago Press.

Kawamoto, K., Houlihan, C. A., Balas, E. A., & Lobach, D. F. (2005). Improving clinical practice using clinical decision support systems: A systematic review of trials to identify features critical to success. *BMJ, 330*(7494), 765. doi:10.1136/bmj.38398.500764.8F

Kim, K., Colgate, J. E., Santos-Munne, J. J., Makhlin, A., & Peshkin, M. A. (2010). On the design of miniature haptic devices for upper extremity prosthetics. *IEEE/ASME Transactions on Mechatronics, 15*(1), 27-39. doi:10.1109/TMECH.2009.2013944

Kindig, D. A. (2015). *What is population health?* [Blog post]. Retrieved from http://www. improvingpopulationhealth.org/blog/whatis-population-health.html

Knight, K. L., & Draper, D. O. (2007). *Therapeutic modalities: The art and science with clinical activities manual*. Baltimore, MD: Lippincott Williams and Wilkins.

Kuiken, T., Li, G., Lock, B. A., Lipschutz, R. D., Miller, L. A., Stubblefield, K. A., & Englehart, K. (2009). Targeted muscle reinnervation for real-time myoelectric control of multifunction artificial arms. *Journal of the American Medical Association, 301*(6), 619-628. doi:10.1001/jama.2009.116

Laver, K., Ratcliffe, J., George, S., Burgess, L., & Crotty, M. (2011). Is the Nintendo Wii Fit really acceptable to older people?: A discrete choice experiment. *BMC Geriatrics, 11*(1), 64.

Law, M., Baptiste, S., Carswell, A., McColl, M. A., Polatajko, H., & Pollock, N. (1998). *The Canadian Occupational Performance Measure* (3rd ed.). Toronto, Ontario, Canada: CAOT Publications.

Lazzarini, I. (2004). Neuro-occupation: The nonlinear dynamics of intention, meaning and perception. *British Journal of Occupational Therapy, 67*, 342-352.

Library of Congress. (n.d.a). *The decade of the brain 1999-2000*. Retrieved from http://www.loc.gov/loc/brain

Library of Congress. (n.d.b). *Presidential proclamation 6158*. Retrieved from http://www.loc.gov/loc/brain/proclaim.html

Licht, S. (1947). Modern trends in occupational therapy. *Occupational Therapy and Rehabilitation, 26*(6), 455-460.

Liepert, J. (2006). Motor cortex excitability in stroke before and after constraint-induced movement therapy. *Cognitive and Behavioral Neurology, 19*(1), 41-47.

Lilleleht, E. (2002). Progress and power: Exploring the disciplinary connections between moral treatment and psychiatric rehabilitation. *Philosophy, Psychiatry, and Psychology, 9*(2), 167-182.

Lohman, H., & Royeen, C. (2002). Posttraumatic stress disorder and traumatic hand injuries: a neuro-occupational view. *American Journal of Occupational Therapy , 56*(5), 527.

Luchins, A. S. (1992). The cult of curability and the doctrine of perfectibility: Social context of the nineteenth century American asylum movement. *History of Psychiatry, 3*, 203-220.

Madhill, H., Brintnell, S., & Stewin, L. (1989). Professional literature: One view of a national perspective. *Australian Occupational Therapy Journal, 36*, 110-119.

McAllister, A. K. (2000). Cellular and molecular mechanisms of dendrite growth. *Cerebral Cortex, 10*(10), 963-973.

Mckinnon, A. L. (2000). Client values and satisfaction with occupational therapy. *Scandinavian Journal of Occupational Therapy, 7*(3), 99-106.

Medical Surveillance Monthly Report. (2012). Medical surveillance monthly report. In F. L. O'Donnell (Ed.), *The medical surveillance monthly report* (Vol. 19). Silver Spring, MD: Armed Forces Health Surveillance Center.

Mejias, U. A. (2006). *Technology without ends: A critique of technocracy as a threat to being*. Retrieved from http://blog.ulisesmejias.com/2006/06/03/technology-without-ends-a-critique-of-technocracy-as-a-threat-to-being

Michaels, R. J. (1988). Addiction, compulsion, and the technology of consumption. *Economic Inquiry, 26*(1), 75-88.

National Center for Health Statistics. (2005). *Health, United States, 2005 with chart book on trends in the health of Americans*. Hyattsville, MD: Author.

Northrop, H. (2014). Occupation-focused family intervention and expanding the role of occupational therapy in childhood obesity. *Physical and Occupational Therapy in Pediatrics, 34*, 335-337. doi:10.3109/01942638.2014.932613

Oestergaard, L., G., Maribo, T., Bünger, C. E., & Christensen, F. B. (2012). The Canadian Occupational Performance Measure's semi-structured interview: Its applicability to lumbar spinal fusion patients. A prospective randomized clinical study. *European Spin Journal 21*(1), 115-121.

Padilla, R., & Peyton, C. B. (1997). Neuro-occupation: Historical review and examples. In C. B. Royeen (Ed.), *Neuroscience and occupation: Links to practice*. Bethesda, MD: AOTA Press.

Passel, J. S., & Cohn, D. (2008). *U.S. population projections: 2005-2050*. Washington, DC: Pew Research Center.

Peloquin, S. M. (1989). Moral treatment: Contexts considered. *American Journal of Occupational Therapy, 43*, 537-544.

Peloquin, S. M. (1994). Moral treatment: How a caring practice lost its rationale. *American Journal of Occupational Therapy, 48*, 167-173.

Rescher, N. (1980). *Unpopular essays on technological progress*. Pittsburgh, PA: University of Pittsburgh Press.

Rivers, J. R. (1993). *Contra technologiam: The crisis of value in a technological age*. Lanham, MD: University Press of America.

Rivers, J. R. (2005). An introduction to the metaphysics of technology. *Technology in Society, 27*, 551-574.

Roberts, P. S., Vegher, J. A., Gilewski, M., Bender, A., & Riggs, R. V. (2005). Client-centered occupational therapy using constraint-induced therapy. *Journal of Stroke and Cerebrovascular Diseases, 14*(3), 115-121.

Rogers, J. C. (1983). Eleanor Clarke Slagle Lectureship—1983. Clinical reasoning: The ethics, science, and art. *American Journal of Occupational Therapy, 37*(9), 601-616.

Saposnik, G., Mamdani, M., Bayley, M., Thorpe, K., Hall, J., Cohen, L., & Teasell, R. (2010). Effectiveness of Virtual Reality Exercises in STroke Rehabilitation (EVREST): Rationale, design, and protocol of a pilot randomized clinical trial assessing the Wii gaming system. *International Journal of Stroke, 5*(1), 47-51.

Sayer, N. A., Cifu, D. X., McNamee, S., Chiros, C. E., Sigford, B. J., Scott, S., & Lew, H. L. (2009). Rehabilitation needs of combat-injured service members admitted to the VA Polytrauma Rehabilitation Centers: The role of PM&R in the care of wounded warriors. *PM & R: The Journal of Injury, Function, and Rehabilitation, 1*(1), 23-28.

Schiller, J. S., Lucas, J. W., Ward, B. W., & Peregoy, J. A. (2012). Summary health statistics for U.S. adults: National Health Interview Survey, 2010. *Vital and Health Statistics, 10*(252), 1-207.

Sheffler, L. R., & Chae, J. (2007). Neuromuscular electrical stimulation in neurorehabilitation. *Muscle and Nerve, 35*(5), 562-590. doi:10.1002/mus.20758

Simmons, D. C., Crepeau, E. B., & White, B. P. (2000). The predictive power of narrative data in occupational therapy evaluation. *American Journal of Occupational Therapy, 54*(5), 471-476.

Sluka, K. A., & Walsh, D. (2003). Transcutaneous electrical nerve stimulation: Basic science mechanisms and clinical effectiveness. *Journal of Pain, 4*, 109-121.

Spadaro, A., Lubrano, E., Massimiani, M. P., Gaia, P., Perrotta, F. M., Parsons, W. J., ... Valesini, G. (2010). Validity, responsiveness and feasibility of an Italian version of the Canadian Occupational Performance Measure for patients with ankylosing spondylitis. *Clinical and Experimental Rheumatology, 28*(2), 215-222.

Tandon, P. N. (2000). The decade of the brain: A brief review. *Neurology India, 48*(3), 199-207.

Taub, E. (2004). Harnessing brain plasticity through behavioral techniques to produce new treatments in neurorehabilitation. *American Psychologist, 59*(8), 692-704.

Taub, E., & Uswatte, G. (2006). Constraint-induced movement therapy. *NeuroRehabilitation, 21*(2), 93-176.

Teasell, R. W., Foley, N. C., Bhogal, S. K., & Speechley, M. R. (2002). An evidence-based review of stroke rehabilitation. *Topics in Stroke Rehabilitation, 10*(1), 29-58.

Thaut, M. H., & Abiru, M. (2010). Rhythmic auditory stimulation in rehabilitation of movement disorders: A review of current research. *Music Perception, 27*(4), 263-269.

Thaut, M., Leins, A., Rice, R. R., Argstatter, H., Kenyon, G. P., McIntosh, G. G., Bolay, H. V., & Fetter, M. (2007). Rhythmic auditory stimulation improves gait more than NDT/Bobath training in near-ambulatory patients early poststroke: A single-blind, randomized trial. *Neurorehabilitation and Neural Repair, 21*(5), 455-459.

Tuke, S. (1813). *Description of the retreat, an institution near York, for insane persons.* London, England: Oxford University. [Digitized May 3, 2007].

Tyler, E., Caldwell, C., & Ghia, J. N. (1982) Transcutaneous electrical nerve stimulation: An alternative approach to the management of postoperative pain. *Anesthesia and Analgesia, 61*(5), 449-456.

Warren, A. (2002). An evaluation of the Canadian Model of Occupational Performance and the Canadian Occupational Therapy Measure in mental health practice. *British Journal of Occupational Therapy, 65*(11), 515-522.

Wolf, S. L., Thompson, P. A., Winstein, C. J., Miller, J. P., Blanton, S. R., Nichols-Larsen, D. S., ... Sawaki, L. (2010). The EXCITE stroke trial comparing early and delayed constraint-induced movement therapy. *Stroke, 41*(10), 2309-2315.

World Federation of Occupational Therapists. (n.d.). *History.* Retrieved from http://www.wfot.org.au

Wressle, E., Samuelsson, K., & Henriksson, C. (1999). Responsiveness of the Swedish version of the Canadian Occupational Performance Measure. *Scandinavian Journal of Occupational Therapy, 6*(2), 84-89.

Wuang, Y. P., Chiang, C. S., Su, C. Y., & Wang, C. C. (2011). Effectiveness of virtual reality using Wii gaming technology in children with Down syndrome. *Research in Developmental Disabilities, 32*(1), 312-321.

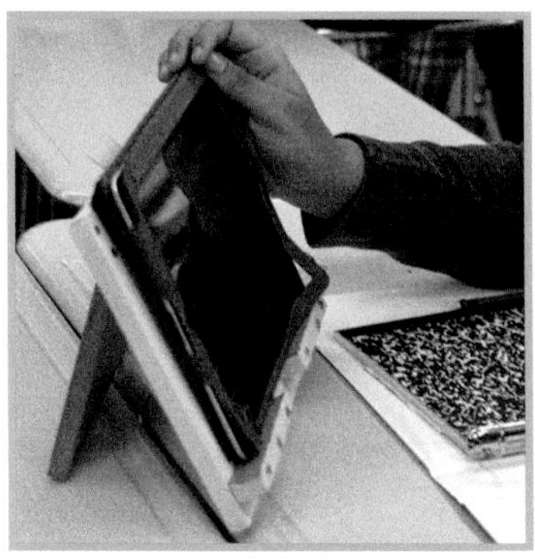

# 39

# Telehealth

*Nancy Doyle, OTD, OTR/L*

**ACOTE STANDARDS EXPLORED IN THIS CHAPTER**

B.1.8, B.2.1, B.3.4, B.6.1–B.6.3, B.6.5, B.6.6, B.8.1

**KEY VOCABULARY**

- **Encrypted communication technologies:** Communication technologies that are encoded to protect client privacy and confidentiality across the lines of communication between service provider and client.
- **In-person:** Where the service provider and client are in the same location and work together face to face.
- **Service delivery model:** A method for providing services to clients.
- **Telehealth:** The delivery of health services using telecommunication technology by providers who are at a distance from clients.
- **Telerehabilitation:** Area of telehealth that is focused on rehabilitation with clients who have had an illness or injury.



Jacobs, K., & MacRae, N. (Eds.).
*Occupational Therapy Essentials for Clinical Competence, Third Edition* (pp. 569-576).

Telehealth is a service delivery model used across various health professions, including occupational therapy. It is a "mode of delivering health care services and public health utilizing information and communication technologies to enable the diagnosis, consultation, treatment, education, care management, and self-management of patients at a distance from health care providers" (Telehealth Advancement Act of 2011, p. 3). Within occupational therapy, telehealth is an emerging niche (American Occupational Therapy Association [AOTA], 2015a) that can be used in any practice area (Cason, 2012b), including children and youth, health and wellness, mental health, productive aging, rehabilitation and disability, and work and industry (AOTA, 2015c). It has been used, for example, to provide early intervention services to children in rural areas (Cason, 2009) or to provide energy conservation educational courses to individuals with multiple sclerosis (Dunleavy, Preissner, & Finlayson, 2013; Holberg & Finlayson, 2007). Typically, it is used to provide occupational therapy services to clients who would otherwise have difficulty accessing services in person. Such difficulties may include remote location, mobility or transportation, and long travel distances to specialists (Schein, Schmeler, Brienza, Saptono, & Parmanto, 2008; Whelan & Wagner, 2011; World Federation of Occupational Therapists, 2014). It has additional benefits of providing cost-effective services in the natural environment of a client (Clawson et al., 2008; LoPresti, Jinks, & Simpson, 2015).

Research has shown telehealth to be at least as therapeutically effective as in-person services in many settings (Jacobs, Blanchard, & Baker, 2012; Sanford et al., 2006) with high client satisfaction ratings (Criss, 2013; Steel, Cox, & Garry, 2011). It has also been shown to be cost effective and efficient for practitioners and clients alike (Cason, 2009; Dreyer, Dreyer, Shaw, & Wittman, 2001; Hermann et al., 2010). When guided by clinical reasoning, evidence, and appropriate technical training (AOTA, 2013), it can be a positive and efficacious model for delivering occupational therapy services. Certainly, it provides an additional method for providing services across the country and around the globe to promote "health, well-being, and participation in life through engagement in occupation" (AOTA, 2014, p. S4).

This chapter will define telehealth; present how it is currently being used in occupational therapy; and discuss practical, legal, ethical, and reimbursement issues related to telehealth. These topics are intended to demonstrate how telehealth can be used to support the "performance, participation, health and well-being" (Accreditation Council for Occupational Therapy Education [ACOTE], 2012, p. S34) of occupational therapy clients. Additionally, this chapter will analyze the telehealth service delivery model and its "potential effect on the practice of occupational therapy" (ACOTE, 2012, p. S52).

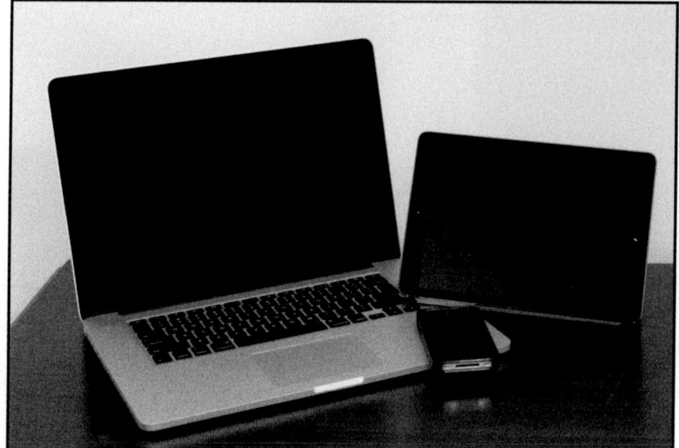

**Figure 39-1.** Examples of telehealth communication devices.

## Terminology

Traditionally, health services have been provided when the provider and client are face to face in the same physical location, termed *in-person services.* In contrast, telehealth allows health services to be provided when the practitioner and client are in different physical locations. *Telehealth* is a broad term that encompasses many different aspects of promoting and providing health and public health services using telecommunication technology. Telecommunication technology is technology that allows communication at a distance. Today, interactive technologies such as synchronous videoconferencing and streaming of video and audio media through the Internet and wireless devices can provide access to face-to-face telehealth for many practitioners and clients (Health Resources and Services Administration, 2012).

*Telemedicine* and *telerehabilition* are related terms that fit under the umbrella of telehealth. Telemedicine focuses specifically on providing medical care and services using telecommunication technology. Telerehabilitation is the provision of rehabilitation services by allied health professionals using telecommunication technology. Cason (2012a) advocates that occupational therapy use the term telehealth to fully represent what we can and do provide to clients via telecommunication technology (Figure 39-1). Our services are more than just rehabilitative for clients with disabilities; they may also include education, habilitation, prevention, health promotion, and wellness services.

## History of Telehealth

Telemedicine was first introduced in the 20th century. Early instances include a published illustration of a physician remotely viewing his patient on a "radio-screen" in a 1924 issue of *Radio News*, a cross-state demonstration of telemedicine at the 1951 New York

World's Fair, and teleradiology in 1957 by Albert Jutras in Montreal, Canada (Dreyer et al., 2001). The National Aeronautics and Space Administration began using telemedicine to monitor the health of astronauts in space as early as the 1960s (Dreyer et al., 2001). Hospitals in the United States began using telemedicine in the late 1960s and in Australia in the early 1980s (Dreyer et al., 2001).

AOTA president Mary Foto began introducing the concept of telerehabilitation to occupational therapists in the United States in the late 1990s (Foto, 1996, 1997). Use of and research about telecommunication technology began in the 21st century (Dreyer et al., 2001) and is growing as an emerging service delivery model in occupational therapy (AOTA, 2015a).

The AOTA has published position papers on telehealth and occupational therapy's role in and contributions to this model of service provision (AOTA, 2005, 2010c, 2013). As telehealth evolves, the position papers will continue to be revised and published every 5 years to keep current with evidence-based provision of occupational therapy through telecommunication technologies. The American Telemedicine Association (ATA) has also worked across disciplines to develop a blueprint, or guidelines, for "providing effective and safe services that are based on client needs, current empirical evidence, and available technologies" (Brennan et al., 2010, p. 263). ATA also has developed many discipline- and technology-specific guidelines. The guidelines from AOTA (2013) and the ATA (see www.americantelemed.org) should be reviewed when implementing a telehealth service provision model; they provide strong guidance for developing the appropriate administrative, clinical, technical, and ethical aspects of telehealth services.

### Case Study

In April, a sophomore college student sustained a hand injury due to colliding with an opening car door while riding her bicycle. She experienced partial lacerations of extensor tendons on her middle and ring fingers and a fracture of the fifth metacarpal of her dominant hand. After tendon repair surgery, she began in-person occupational therapy to rehabilitate the injured tendons and problem solve adaptations and accommodations for performing daily occupations, particularly school-related ones, one-handed with her nondominant hand. Adaptations and accommodations included obtaining a note-taker for her classes and using voice-recognition software for typing her school assignments.

At the beginning of June, the student was scheduled to begin a summer internship across the state, several hours' drive from the location of her occupational therapy services. The occupational therapist investigated state licensure, state laws, institution-specific guidelines, and insurance policies to ensure that telehealth could be used as a service delivery model for this client to continue occupational therapy intervention. Then the occupational therapist and client discussed continuing therapy via telehealth technologies. The client agreed that this option would provide good continuity of treatment, especially because she had a positive working relationship with the occupational therapist and was making progress in achieving her occupational therapy goals. The occupational therapist and client continued occupational therapy intervention via telehealth technologies to rehabilitate strength and flexibility and reduce swelling in the injured hand while problem solving adaptations and accommodations for nondominant, one-handed work. Once the hand injuries had healed and the client had met her goals of regaining strength, flexibility, and function in her dominant hand, occupational therapy services were concluded.

## Telehealth and Occupational Therapy

Telehealth has the potential to be used in all areas of occupational therapy practice (AOTA, 2013; Cason, 2012b). Just as with in-person occupational therapy services, telehealth provided by occupational therapy practitioners focuses on occupational performance. The overall goal of occupational therapy provided through telehealth is to support clients' work toward "achieving health, well-being, and participation in life through engagement in occupation" (AOTA, 2014, p. S4). Telehealth may be used for occupational therapy services at the person, group, and population client levels (AOTA, 2014) that include evaluation, consultation, health promotion, prevention, habilitation, rehabilitation, and long-term monitoring of health (AOTA, 2013).

Research has shown that a variety of assessments are valid and reliable when using telehealth technologies (AOTA, 2013; Cason, 2012a). These include the Kohlman Evaluation of Living Skills, Canadian Occupational Performance Measure, Functional Reach Test, European Stroke Scale, Functional Independence Measure, Jamar Dynamometer, Preston Pinch Gauge, Nine-Hole Peg Test, Unified Parkinson's Disease Rating Scale, and Functioning Everyday With a Wheelchair.

Telehealth has been used across the occupational therapy domain to provide interventions that are preventative, habilitative, and rehabilitative (AOTA, 2013). This service delivery model has been used to provide early intervention, school-based intervention, stroke rehabilitation, and ergonomic services; long-term monitoring of chronic conditions; and virtual reality interventions for individuals with cognitive impairments (AOTA, 2010c; Cason, 2012b). Practitioners have used telehealth to provide services to clients with a variety of concerns including traumatic brain injuries, multiple traumas, prostheses, autism spectrum disorders, cerebral palsy, stroke, and post-stroke fatigue (Boehm, Muehlberg, & Stube, 2015; Cason, 2012a, 2012b; Jacobs et al., 2012; Linder et al., 2015).

Telehealth is included in the Patient Protection and Affordable Care Act of 2010 (ACA; P.L. 111-148) as a means to "expand capacity" (Section 10333) and "better coordinate and manage, and improve access to, care" (Section 10410). This law works to "improve access, quality, efficiency, and transparency of health care services" (Cason, 2012b, p. 131). In a study of telehealth occupational therapy services for children receiving early intervention in rural Kentucky, telehealth provided quality services at a lower cost to families, practitioners, and companies in terms of travel time and cost (Cason, 2009), thereby improving access, quality, efficiency, and transparency. Additionally, the ACA has a Triple Aim to improve individual care experiences, improve population health, and reduce population health costs on a per capita basis. Cason (2015) highlights how occupational therapy delivered via telehealth can and must contribute to all three portions of this Triple Aim to contribute to the changing health care system in the United States.

## Efficacy of Telehealth

Occupational therapy interventions have also been shown to be effective in a variety of practice settings and geographical locations around the world (Heimerl & Rasch, 2009). These include early intervention services for children (Cason, 2009), school-based fine- and visual-motor intervention for handwriting (Criss, 2013), ergonomic computer station redesign (Baker & Jacobs, 2014), metacognitive intervention to address executive dysfunction after traumatic brain injury (Ng, Polatajko, Marziali, Hunt, & Dawson, 2013), and post-stroke rehabilitation (Hermann et al., 2010). Heimerl and Rasch (2009) report on additional telehealth occupational therapy services as diverse as for school children in Hawaii, individuals with mental illness in rural Japan, and clients with neurological issues in rural Minnesota and American Samoa.

Researchers and practitioners must continue to develop and study occupational therapy telehealth services to build our evidence base. In addition to our own profession, we are able to pull from telehealth studies across disciplines that look at mental and physical health. For example, a recent systematic review examines telehealth studies published since 2000 by occupational therapy, psychiatry, counseling, and physical therapy researchers (Steel et al., 2011). Studies comparing the efficacy of in-person and telehealth service provision have found no significant difference in clinical outcomes (Jacobs et al., 2012; Steel et al., 2011). In addition to clinical efficacy, telehealth may reduce costs for some clients and interventions, particularly if in-person services require significant therapist time and travel (Cason, 2009; Clawson et al., 2008; Lopresti et al., 2015). Costs may also be reduced in long-term monitoring of chronic health conditions (Darkins et al., 2008; Jacobs et al., 2012) and by reducing hospital and nursing home stays (Bendixen, Levy, Olive, Kobb, & Mann, 2009).

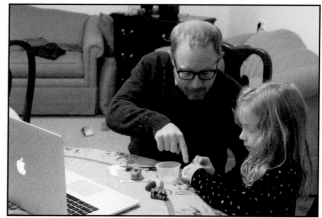

**Figure 39-2.** Client and parent participating in telehealth occupational therapy services.

Overall, clients are satisfied with telehealth services (Darkins et al., 2008; Jacobs et al., 2012; Figure 39-2). It can improve access to services, reduce costs, and improve communication with professionals (Jacobs et al., 2012). Clinicians are also generally satisfied by service delivery by telehealth, although they may be more affected by challenges managing the telecommunication technology than their clients (Jacobs et al., 2012).

## Selecting Telehealth

The decision to use telehealth with occupational therapy clients must be based on sound clinical reasoning and must use the best available evidence for effective service provision. It enables occupational therapy services for clients who otherwise might experience significant access barriers, and who will, in the best judgment of the occupational therapist, positively benefit from services provided through telecommunication technologies.

Cason (2012a) presents three main reasons to select telehealth occupational therapy services for a client. This service delivery model may (1) enable clients to receive services when there are significant barriers to in-person services, (2) allow consultation with "expert practitioners with specialized knowledge and skills" (Cason, 2012a, p. CE2), and (3) provide occupational therapy services in the natural contexts and environments of the client. First, barriers to receiving in-person services may include a shortage of occupational therapy professionals in a given location, distance to services, difficulty with transportation to services, and a client's preference for discreet evaluation or services (Cason, 2012a). Second, telehealth allows clients and generalist occupational therapy professionals to consult with expert practitioners to provide more specialized care (Cason, 2012a). An added benefit to this specialized consultation process is the potential for increasing the knowledge and ability of generalist occupational therapy professionals; this may be particularly helpful when generalists are working in areas where specialized clinicians are not readily available (Schein et al., 2008; Whelan & Wagner, 2011). Third, telehealth also affords the opportunity to work with clients in their natural contexts and environments. This can enhance occupational therapy services by helping a client apply new strategies and adaptations to their daily occupations and natural settings. For example, telehealth may be used for in-home consultation regarding fall prevention and other modifications for older adults who wish to age in place.

It is important to keep in mind that telehealth may present particular barriers to certain clients and practitioners, and therefore is not a panacea for clients who cannot access in-person services. Individuals who have difficulty using telecommunication technology, maintaining such technology, or sustaining participation when utilizing such technology may not be ideal candidates for telehealth services (AOTA, 2010c).

## Technology

The ability to deliver telehealth occupational therapy services is undergirded by the telecommunication technology selected. Technology can range from telephone use, to asynchronous communication through voice or written memos, to face-to-face live interaction using cameras by both therapists and clients. The latter is the most akin to in-person occupational therapy service delivery and therefore may be most satisfactory to many clients and therapists. Today, the cameras used are often web-based and rely on wireless or Internet access, computer and camera hardware, and some type of webcam communication software. Clients may have the ability to use their own home computers and webcams; others may benefit from another service provider's access to these resources; still others may travel short distances to telehealth centers set up by their state's public health department (Cason, 2009).

As with any technology, telecommunication technologies can present opportunities for, but also sometimes challenges to, communication. For example, the speed of an Internet connection can determine whether the video and audio communication between therapist and client are seamless and efficient or halting and time-consuming. Additionally, difficulty with hardware or software can present challenges on either side of the telehealth partnership. It is helpful to have technical support available to both parties before and during the scheduled sessions. It is important to note that this technical support should be involved only to problem solve any technical issues. In order to maintain client confidentiality and privacy, occupational therapy services such as assessment and intervention should be provided when only the therapist and client are present.

Occupational therapy practitioners can benefit from understanding the technology requirements of the telecommunication technologies they will use in providing telehealth services (AOTA, 2013). They may engage in formal or informal training with more experienced telehealth providers or with technical support staff (AOTA, 2005). Finally, occupational therapy professionals who wish to become experts in providing telehealth services can seek out mentorship from other professionals who are advanced in their use of telecommunication technologies and knowledge of best practice and evidence in telehealth (AOTA, 2010b).

## Legal Considerations

It is important to be aware of legal considerations before engaging in telehealth. Such considerations include appropriate state licensure, state laws, institution-specific guidelines, and insurance for providing occupational therapy through telecommunication technologies. Occupational therapy professionals must "comply with the licensure and regulatory requirements" (AOTA, 2013, p. S74) in their physical location as well as the physical location of their client. For example, if a therapist in Virginia is working with a client in West Virginia, the therapist must follow licensure and regulatory requirements in West Virginia as well as Virginia to provide such services legally.

In addition to licensure, occupational therapy professionals should check with the state laws in any states where they are providing telehealth services. It is critical to know any rules and regulations guiding the provision of services, and whether it is legal to provide occupational therapy services through telecommunication technologies.

Finally, occupational therapy professionals should work with their employers and insurers to determine the extent of coverage for professional liability, malpractice, and other applicable forms of insurance. It is important to be clear with insurers about how telehealth services are provided and whether they will be provided to clients in the same or different state as the location of the occupational therapy professional.

## Ethical Considerations

Using telehealth as a service delivery model for occupational therapy necessitates consideration of two main categories of ethics: those pertaining to the profession generally and those related to telehealth specifically. As in all areas of practice, occupational therapy professionals must adhere to the code of ethics related to their professional organization; certification and/or licensure; and national, state, and/or local regulations. For example, in the United States, occupational therapy professionals are guided by the AOTA's *Occupational Therapy Code of Ethics* (2015b). The main elements of this code and set of standards are beneficence, nonmaleficence, autonomy, justice, veracity, and fidelity.

There are aspects of the AOTA's *Code of Ethics* (2015b) that have particular resonance when utilizing a telehealth service delivery model. In terms of caring for others (beneficence), occupational therapy professionals are obligated to practice telehealth only if it is within their range of competence (Principle 1.E), if it utilizes best available evidence (Principle 1.C), and if they have current knowledge of this service delivery model and are able to "weigh potential for client harm when generally recognized standards do not exist in emerging technology or areas of practice" (Principle 1.F; AOTA, 2015b, p. S3). In terms of not causing harm to clients (nonmaleficence), telehealth may be a way to "avoid abandoning the service recipient by facilitating appropriate transitions" such as continuing intervention with telehealth opportunities (Principle 2.B).

In terms of autonomy and veracity, an occupational therapy professional should be sure to "disclose the benefits, risks, and potential outcomes of any intervention" (Principle 3.A; AOTA, 2015b, p. 5) provided to clients through telehealth. Particularly critical when using telecommunication technologies in telehealth is to ensure the privacy and confidentiality of clients (Principles 3.H and 5.J). Encrypted telecommunication across interfaces such as the Internet are important to ensure the security, privacy, and confidentiality of clients (Chiu & Henderson, 2005) and compliance with Health Insurance Portability and Accountability Act (HIPAA) regulations (Cason & Brannon, 2011). It is also essential that only individuals given permission by the client to participate in the session, such as therapist, client, and family members, are able to participate. For example, although there may be technical support staff available to troubleshoot telecommunication technology issues in real time with the therapist and client, they are not included in the actual session's therapeutic interaction and conversation between therapist and client.

The use of telehealth to deliver occupational therapy services and its ability to reach underserved populations resonates particularly strongly with the ethical principle of justice. In particular, occupational therapy personnel will "assist those in need of occupational therapy services to secure access through available means" (Principle 4.B; AOTA, 2015b, p. 6); one such mean may be through telehealth. In delivering such services, it is critical that not only ethical standards but also procedural standards are addressed, including meeting any legal obligations (e.g., institutional policies, state licensure, national certification, state laws) and reimbursement regulations (Principles 4.L and 4.O).

## Reimbursement

Reimbursement for services rendered through telehealth may vary for type of service provider, clients, and clients' health insurers. For example, although some states' Medicaid programs reimburse for occupational therapy delivered through telehealth, Medicare does not provide reimbursement for telehealth occupational therapy services at this time (Cason & Brannon, 2011). The Department of Defense and the Veterans Administration do currently provide funding for some occupational therapy telehealth services to active military and veterans, respectively (Cason, 2012a). Some third-party insurance companies will reimburse for telehealth services; however, it is critical to determine whether occupational therapy practitioners can deliver telehealth services, and if there are only certain services delivered by telehealth that will be reimbursed. Finally, it is important to be sure that when services are delivered through telecommunication technologies, that they are billed accordingly under telehealth codes (AOTA, 2010c; Brennan et al., 2010).

## Summary

Telehealth is a viable, efficacious, cost-effective service delivery model for occupational therapy. It is particularly useful for clients who might not otherwise be able to access occupational therapy services in person. This chapter defined telehealth, described current research and practice areas using telehealth, and discussed legal, ethical, and reimbursement implications for using a telehealth service delivery model in occupational therapy practice. Of particular note is the ability of this emerging niche in occupational therapy practice to provide new ways for clients to access services. This service delivery model may therefore promote social justice (AOTA, 2010a) by adding to in-person services and facilitating the occupational engagement of at-a-distance individuals, groups, and populations.

## Student Self-Assessment

1. Consider a recent fieldwork experience. How could you translate this area of practice to a telehealth service delivery model? What would be the benefits of or barriers to such implementation?

## Evidence-Based Research Chart

| Topic | Evidence |
|---|---|
| AOTA's position on telehealth | AOTA, 2013 |
| AOTA statement on specialized knowledge and skills in technology | AOTA, 2010b |
| Developing telehealth services | Chiu & Henderson, 2005; Dreyer et al., 2001; Heimerl & Rasch, 2009 |
| Efficacy of telehealth | Baker & Jacobs, 2014; Cason, 2009; Criss, 2013; Dreyer et al., 2001; Heimerl & Rasch, 2009; Hermann et al., 2010; Jacobs et al., 2012; Ng et al., 2013; Steel et al., 2011 |

2. List at least two areas of practice that are of interest to you. How could using telehealth increase the range of clients you would be able to serve in each area?
3. Imagine that in your first job, you advocate for the inclusion of telehealth as a service delivery model for your practice. Your manager asks you to create a presentation on this topic. How would you define telehealth? What evidence would you cite to argue for the implementation of telehealth? What state licensure, legal, ethical, and reimbursement considerations for utilizing telehealth technologies would you include in your presentation?

## Electronic Resources

American Occupational Therapy Association: www.aota.org

American Telemedicine Association: www.americantelemed.org

Center for Connected Health Policy: www.cchpca.org

International Journal of Telerehabilitation: http://telerehab.pitt.edu

Office for Advancement of Telehealth: https://www.hrsa.gov/ruralhealth/telehealth/

## References


Accreditation Council for Occupational Therapy Education. (2012). 2011 Accreditation Council for Occupational Therapy Education (ACOTE) standards. *American Journal of Occupational Therapy, 66*, S6-S74. doi:10.5014/ajot.2012.66S6

American Occupational Therapy Association. (2005). Telerehabilitation position paper. *American Journal of Occupational Therapy, 59*, 656-660. doi:10.5014/ajot.59.6.656

American Occupational Therapy Association. (2010a). Occupational therapy code of ethics and ethics standards. *American Journal of Occupational Therapy, 64*, S17-S26. doi:10.5014/ajot.2010.64S17

American Occupational Therapy Association. (2010b). Specialized knowledge and skills in technology and environmental interventions for occupational therapy practice. *American Journal of Occupational Therapy, 64*, S44-S56. doi:10.5014/ajot.2010.64S44

American Occupational Therapy Association. (2010c). Telerehabilitation. *American Journal of Occupational Therapy, 64*, S92-S102. doi:10.5014/ajot.2010.64S92

American Occupational Therapy Association. (2013). Telehealth. *American Journal of Occupational Therapy, 67*(6, Suppl.), S69-S90. doi:10.5014/ajot.2013.67S69

American Occupational Therapy Association. (2014). Occupational therapy practice framework: Domain and process (3rd ed.). *American Journal of Occupational Therapy, 68*(Suppl. 1), S1-S48. doi:10.5014/ajot.2014.682006

American Occupational Therapy Association. (2015a). *Emerging niche: Telehealth*. Retrieved from http://www.aota.org/Practice/Rehabilitation-Disability/Emerging-Niche/Telehealth.aspx

American Occupational Therapy Association. (2015b). Occupational therapy code of ethics (2015). *American Journal of Occupational Therapy, 69*(Suppl. 3), 6913410030p1-6913410030p8. doi:10.5014/ajot.2015.696S03

American Occupational Therapy Association. (2015c). *Practice areas*. Retrieved from http://www.aota.org/Practice.aspx

Baker, N. A., & Jacobs, K. (2014). The feasibility and accuracy of using a remote method to assess computer workstations. *Human Factors, 56*(4), 784-788. doi:10.1177/0018720813503985

Bendixen, R. M., Levy, C. E., Olive, E. S., Kobb, R. F., & Mann, W. C. (2009). Cost effectiveness of a telerehabilitation program to support chronically ill and disabled elders in their homes. *Telemedicine and e-Health, 15*(1), 31-38. doi:10.1089/tmj.2008.0046

Boehm, N., Muehlberg, H., & Stube, J. E. (2015). Brief report—Managing poststroke fatigue using telehealth: A case report. *American Journal of Occupational Therapy, 69*, 6906350020. doi:10.5014/ajot.2015.016170

Brennan, D. M., Tindall, L., Theodoros, D., Brown, J., Campbell, M., Christiana, D., ... Lee, A. (2010). A blueprint for telerehabilitation guidelines—October 2010. *Telemedicine and e-Health, 17*, 662-665. doi:10.1089/tmj.2011.0036

Cason, J. (2009). A pilot telerehabilitation program: Delivering early intervention services to rural families. *International Journal of Telerehabilitation, 1*(1), 29-37. doi:10.5195/ijt.2009.6007

Cason, J. (2012a). An introduction to telehealth as a service delivery model within occupational therapy. *OT Practice, 17*(7), CE1-CE7.

Cason, J. (2012b). Telehealth opportunities in occupational therapy through the Affordable Care Act. *American Journal of Occupational Therapy, 66*, 131-136. doi:10.5014/ajot.2012.662001

Cason, J. (2015). Health policy perspectives—Telehealth and occupational therapy: Integral to the Triple Aim of health care reform. *American Journal of Occupational Therapy, 69*, 6902090010p1-6902090010p8. doi:10.5014/ajot.2015.692003

Cason, J., & Brannon, J. A. (2011). Telehealth regulatory and legal considerations: Frequently asked questions. *International Journal of Telerehabilitation, 3*(2), 15-18. doi:10.5195/ijt.2011.6077

Chiu, T., & Henderson, J. (2005). Developing Internet-based occupational therapy services. *American Journal of Occupational Therapy, 59*, 626-630. doi:10.5014/ajot.59.6.626

Clawson, B., Selden, M., Lacks, M., Deaton, A. V., Hall, B., & Bach, R. (2008). Complex pediatric feeding disorders: Using teleconferencing technology to improve access to a treatment program. *Pediatric Nursing, 34*(3), 213-216.

Criss, M. (2013). School-based telerehabilitation in occupational therapy: Using telerehabilitation technologies to promote improvements in student performance. *International Journal of Telerehabilitation, 5*(1), 39-46. doi:10.5195/ijt.2013.6115

Darkins, A., Ryan, P., Kobb, R., Foster, L., Edmonson, E., Wakefield, B., & Lancaster, A. (2008). Care coordination/home telehealth: The systematic implementation of health informatics, home telehealth, and disease management to support the care of veteran patients with chronic conditions. *Telemedicine and e-Health, 14*(10), 1118-1126. doi:10.1089/tmj.2008.0021

Dreyer, N. C., Dreyer, K. A., Shaw, D. K., & Wittman, P. P. (2001). Efficacy of telemedicine in occupational therapy: A pilot study. *Journal of Allied Health, 30*(1), 39-42.

Dunleavy, L., Preissner, K. L., & Finlayson, M. L. (2013). Facilitating a teleconference-delivered fatigue management program: Perspectives of occupational therapists. *Canadian Journal of Occupational Therapy, 80*(5), 304-313. doi:10.1177/0008417413511787

Foto, M. (1996). Presidential address—Trends, tools, and technology. *American Journal of Occupational Therapy, 50*, 619-625. doi:10.5014/ajot.50.8.619

Foto, M. (1997). Preparing occupational therapists for the year 2000: The impact of managed care on education and training. *American Journal of Occupational Therapy, 51*, 88-90. doi:10.5014/ajot.51.2.88

Health Resources and Services Administration. (2012). *Telehealth.* Retrieved from http://www.hrsa.gov/telehealth/

Heimerl, S., & Rasch, N. C. (2009). Delivery developmental occupational therapy consultation services through telehealth. *Developmental Disabilities Special Interest Section Quarterly, 32*(3), 1-4.

Hermann, V. H., Herzog, M., Jordan, R., Hofherr, M., Levine, P., & Page, S. J. (2010). Telerehabilitation and electrical stimulation: An occupation-based, client-centered stroke intervention. *American Journal of Occupational Therapy, 64*, 73-81. doi:10.5014/ajot.64.1.73

Holberg, C., & Finlayson, M. (2007). Factors influencing the use of energy conservation strategies by persons with multiple sclerosis. *American Journal of Occupational Therapy, 61*, 96-107. doi:10.5014/ajot.61.1.96

Jacobs, K., Blanchard, B., & Baker, N. (2012). Telehealth and ergonomics: A pilot study. *Technology and Health Care, 20*, 445-458. doi:10.3233/THC-2012-0692

Linder, S. M., Rosenfeldt, A. B., Bay, R. C., Sahu, K., Wolf, S. L., & Alberts, J. L. (2015). Improving quality of life and depression after stroke through telerehabilitation. *American Journal of Occupational Therapy, 69*, 6902290020. doi:10.5014/ajot.2015.014498

LoPresti, E. F., Jinks, A., & Simpson, R. C. (2015). Consumer satisfaction with telerehabilitation service provision of alternative computer access and augmentative and alternative communication. *International Journal of Telerehabilitation, 7*(5), 3-13. doi:10.5195/ijt.2015.6180

Ng, E. M. W., Polatajko, H. J., Marziali, E., Hunt, A., & Dawson, D. R. (2013). Telerehabilitation for addressing executive dysfunction after traumatic brain injury. *Brain Injury, 27*(5), 548-564. doi:10.3109/02699052.2013.766927

Sanford, J. A., Griffiths, P. C., Richardson, P., Hargraves, K., Butterfield, T., & Hoenig, H. (2006). The effects of in-home rehabilitation on task self-efficacy in mobility-impaired adults: A randomized clinical trial. *Journal of the American Geriatric Society, 54*(11), 1641-1648. doi:10.1111/j.1532-5415.2006.00913.x

Schein, R. M., Schmeler, M. R., Brienza, D., Saptono, A., & Parmanto, B. (2008). Development of a service delivery protocol used for remote wheelchair consultation via telerehabilitation. *Telemedicine and e-Health, 14*(9), 932-938. doi:10.1089/tmj.2008.0010

Steel, K., Cox, D., & Garry, H. (2011). Therapeutic videoconferencing interventions for the treatment of long-term conditions. *Journal of Telemedicine and Telecare, 17*, 109-117. doi:10.1258/jtt.2010.100318

Teleheath Advancement Act of 2011. (2011). Assembly Bill No. 415. Retrieved from http://www.leginfo.ca.gov/pub/11-12/bill/asm/ab_0401-0450/ab_415_bill_20111007_chaptered.pdf

Whelan, L. R., & Wagner, N. (2011). Technology that touches lives: Teleconsultation to benefit persons with upper limb loss. *International Journal of Telerehabilitation, 3*(2), 19-21. doi:10.5195/ijt.2001.6080

World Federation of Occupational Therapists. (2014). World Federation of Occupational Therapists' position statement on telehealth. *International Journal of Telerehabilitation, 6*(1), 37-40. doi:10.5195/ijt.2014.6153

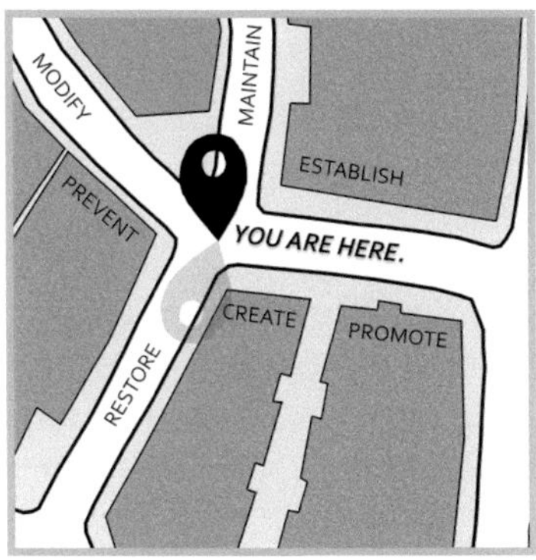


# 40

# Occupational Therapy in Primary Care

*Karen Duddy, OTD, MHA, OTR/L and Nicole Villegas, OTD, OTR/L*

**ACOTE STANDARDS EXPLORED IN THIS CHAPTER**

B.2.4, B.2.5, B.2.9, B.5.17, B.5.21, B.5.27, B.6.5

**KEY VOCABULARY**

- **Generalist:** One who is competent across all age spans and the entire domain of occupational therapy practice as well as knowledgeable about the full scope of practice (Muir, 2012, p. 509).
- **Interprofessional collaborative practice:** When multiple health workers from different professional backgrounds work together with patient, families, carers [sic], and communities to deliver the highest quality of care (World Health Organization [WHO], 2010).
- **Primary care:** "The provision of integrated, accessible health care services by clinicians who are accountable for addressing a large majority of personal health care needs, developing a sustained partnership with patients, and practicing in the context of family and community" (Institute of Medicine, 1994, p. 15).
- **Primary care medical home health:** "The patient-centered medical home (PCMH) is a care delivery model whereby patient treatment is coordinated through their primary care physician to ensure they receive the necessary care when and where they need it, in a manner they can understand" (American College of Physicians, n.d.).
- **Primary health care:** Primary health care is a broader concept. In addition to primary care services, it includes health promotion and disease prevention, and also population-level public health functions. It reflects the approach to service provision for a community proposed in the WHO 1978 Alma-Ata Declaration (Metzler, Hartmann, & Lowenthal, 2012).

Jacobs, K., & MacRae, N. (Eds.).
*Occupational Therapy Essentials for Clinical Competence, Third Edition* (pp. 577-590).

Primary care is an emerging practice area for the profession of occupational therapy. Occupational therapy enhances team-based models of primary care that place the client at the center of care and seek to provide a holistic approach to better meet the needs of individuals and communities. Health care systems are restructuring to organize and coordinate primary care to reduce costs, by focusing on disease prevention and care management for individuals with complex conditions (Calman, Golub, & Shuman, 2012). Treating chronic disease has become a dominant feature of health care in the United States as half of adults have at least one chronic condition (Centers for Disease Control and Prevention [CDC], n.d.). According to the CDC, the health care costs for individuals with chronic conditions account for approximately 86% of health expenditures in the United States, and this number is expected to rise as the population ages. The American Occupational Therapy Association (AOTA) affirms that occupational therapy practitioners are well suited to contribute to interprofessional teams addressing the primary care needs of individuals across the lifespan, particularly those persons living with one or more chronic conditions. Occupational therapy practitioners' distinct expertise regarding the significant impact that habits, routines, and environmental influences have on individuals' health and wellness will make their contribution to primary care unique (Metzler, Hartmann, & Lowenthal, 2012).

This chapter begins with an overview of the emergence and characteristics of new primary care models. Next, the role of occupational therapy in primary care is conceptualized from a historical perspective and in terms of the World Health Organization's (WHO) *International Classification of Functioning, Disability and Health* (ICF) and AOTA's *Occupational Therapy Practice Framework*. The *Framework* is presented in detail in Chapter 6. Then, examples of current occupational therapy clinical practice in primary care settings in the United States are presented. Demonstrating the distinct value of occupational therapy services through achievement of outcomes is essential to support expansion into emerging practice settings as well as to sustain service in current practice areas. The chapter continues with a focus on the importance of outcomes and clinical competence for a value-based health care model. Finally, a review of future directions and strategies for the promotion of occupational therapy in primary care and in other innovative care delivery models is presented in terms of the key tenets of AOTA's Vision 2025.

# What Is Primary Care?

## *Defining Occupational Therapy and Primary Care*

Occupational therapy in primary care is an emerging area of practice within the profession. Primary care is defined as "the provision of integrated, accessible health care services by clinicians who are accountable for addressing a large majority of personal health care needs, developing a sustained partnership with patients, and practicing in the context of family and community" (AOTA, 2014, p. S25). In the declaration of the Alma-Ata, primary care is described as being "the first level of contact of individuals, the family, and community with the national health system bringing health care as close as possible to where people live and work, and constitutes the first elements of a continuing health care process" (WHO, 1978, p. 2). It is important to differentiate between primary care and primary health care. For the purposes of this chapter, primary health care is understood as encompassing public health interventions and population-oriented programs and services that target various determinants of health (WHO, 1978). Primary care focuses on the health of individuals and families.

Occupational therapy's distinct value in primary care was identified in response to changes in the health care system, and the lack of specifically trained professionals on primary care teams to address occupational development, adaptation, prevention, and management. Without occupational therapy practitioners to address these needs, there is a gap between primary care providers and the social determinants of health, potentially creating barriers to wellness for individuals and families. Occupational therapy practitioners' comprehensive education and training from prevention to intervention within the framework of human development can enhance primary care services (Killian, Fisher, & Muir, 2015; Metzler et al., 2012; Roberts, Farmer, Lamb, Muir, & Siebert, 2014). Occupational therapy practitioners are a vital component as part of interprofessional primary care teams.

The conceptualization of occupational therapy in primary care involves consideration of the occupational therapy approach, interprofessional care teams, and types of practice settings. The occupational therapy approach is client centered and addresses a large majority of personal health care needs for clients across the lifespan in areas such as chronic disease management, addressing daily living challenges, and patient care coordination, to name a few (Muir, 2012). Practicing alongside interprofessional primary care providers creates the opportunity for all team members to contribute distinct perspectives, collaborate, and affirm the vision of health care as a coordinated system of care emphasizing holistic service delivery. Interprofessional primary care teams work within

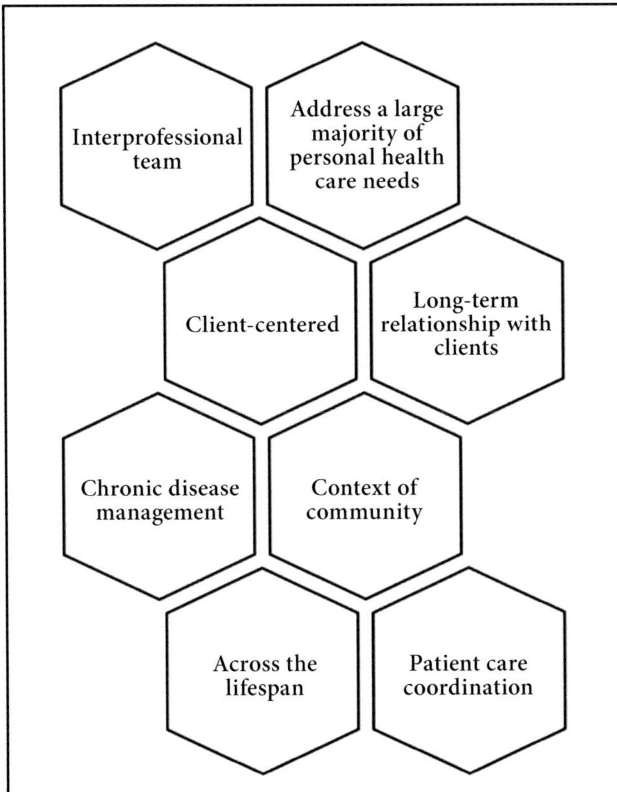


**Figure 40-1.** Defining characteristics of primary care.

a variety of physical practice settings such as in clients' homes, private practices, community-based clinics, and within large hospital systems. As the role of occupational therapy expands to meet the needs of individuals across the care continuum, distinguishing occupational therapy in primary care from other services and settings in which occupational therapy is currently practiced will help to clearly advocate for and communicate occupational therapy's role in the various practice contexts.

Comparison to established practice areas can help define occupational therapy in primary care. An occupational therapy practitioner may perceive that he or she is delivering primary care services when providing prevention-based interventions. This is misleading because practitioners provide health promotion, disease prevention education, and self-management training in many settings, including acute care, inpatient rehabilitation, and in community health clinics. In order to form a common understanding, primary care can be defined in terms of the system of care that focuses on the individual, functions as a patient's first point of entry into the health care system, and serves as a point of care coordination for all needed health care services (Agency for Healthcare Research and Quality, n.d.). While there are specialty primary care practices such as women's health, spinal cord injury, mental health primary care, and geriatric evaluation and management, primary care physicians are typically specialists who are board certified in pediatrics, family medicine, or internal medicine and are practicing as part of a larger accountable care organizations (ACO), university-affiliated practice, or other coordinated care model. Similarly, occupational therapy practitioners in primary care practice as generalists (Devereaux & Walker, 1995; Muir, 2012). Figure 40-1 illustrates the defining characteristics of primary care relevant to occupational therapy.

## Primary Care as a System

To appreciate the impetus and necessity of defining the role of occupational therapy in primary care, it is important to understand the transformation of the primary care system. The Institute of Healthcare Improvement's (IHI) Triple Aim and the subsequent passing of the Patient Protection and Affordable Care Act (ACA) created a window of opportunity for occupational therapy to advocate for a role in the new patient-centered primary care approaches. The new primary care approaches are based on shared principles of whole-person and community-based care. Primary care has traditionally been delivered in a wide variety of settings, from small provider-owned private practices and community health centers to larger integrated organizations with multispecialty practices. However, steadily increasing costs of care and fragmentation of services prompted the need for system-wide improvement initiatives. This broader vision of a health care system, guided by dimensions to improve the individual experience of care, improve the health of populations, and reduce the per capita cost of care, was initially defined by Donald Berwick of the IHI and became known as the Triple Aim (Berwick, Nolan, & Whittington, 2008). The IHI asserts that the dimensions of the Triple Aim must be simultaneously considered when developing or optimizing health system performance.

Despite awareness that the current volume-driven model of primary care was not effective in improving the health of populations, it was not until the ACA defined the value-driven principles of the Triple Aim that change began to occur in the United States (Leland, Crum, Phipps, Roberts, & Gage, 2015). The Triple Aim provided the foundation for the system-wide health care transformation known as the Patient Protection and Affordable Care Act of 2010 (P.L. 111-148). The implementation of Public Law 111-148, marked the beginning of an ongoing transformation in the way that health care services are organized, delivered, reimbursed, and experienced in the United States (Killian et al., 2015).

The ACA created incentives for health care provider organizations to reduce fragmentation of care by reorganizing and coordinating care for Medicare recipients in order to deliver high-quality services, reduce duplication of high-cost services, and reduce medical errors.

ACOs and other innovative models outlined in the ACA place primary care at the center of these reforms. ACOs are groups of providers, such as hospitals, primary and specialty care practices, and outpatient facilities, who voluntarily come together to be responsible for improving the health of a defined population of patients (Fisher & Friesema, 2013). ACOs are measured on quality and cost of care, thus providing the emphasis on health promotion, disease prevention programs, and the integration and coordination of care across providers (Agency for Healthcare Research and Quality, n.d.). The increased accountability for the personal health of a population has encouraged most ACOs to base their model of care on the new primary care medical home model, also referred to as the patient-centered medical home (PCMH). The Institute of Medicine (IOM) has described medical homes as providing continuous healing relationships in which patients' needs and values are central to the physician-patient partnership. The five key functions or attributes of the PCMH are (1) comprehensive care, (2) patient-centered, (3) coordinated care, (4) accessible services, and (5) quality and safety (Agency for Healthcare Research and Quality, n.d.).

These newer interprofessional team-based models of primary care delivery are expected to be the best way to provide care from health promotion to managing the dynamic complex needs of persons with multiple chronic conditions (Piette et al., 2011). The Veterans Health Administration, which is the largest integrated health care system in the nation, began a nationwide implementation of its own version of the PCMH model in 2010 called the Patient Aligned Care Team (Rosland et al., 2013). Primary care teams such as this are comprised of core members including primary care physicians, nurse practitioners, registered nurses, licensed practical nurses, and medical assistants. Other health care professionals such as social workers, occupational therapists, pharmacists, psychologists, and dieticians may provide consultation services to multiple teams (Calman et al., 2012).

Despite health care reform, the care processes in these new models continue to reflect traditional primary care practices that can be characterized as provider-centered, acute, reactive, and episodic. These linear diseased-based models make the principal duties of entering referrals, ordering screenings, completing documentation, and fulfilling performance measures a priority during client visits (Kennedy et al., 2013; Tuepker et al., 2014; Zulman et al., 2014). Fulfilling these priorities leaves the provider little opportunity to effectively consider common concerns presented by the client, such as limitations to daily living occupations resulting from chronic conditions. Addressing limitations and restrictions that impact daily occupations is a distinct focus of occupational therapy. In order to optimize the expansion and contribution of occupational therapy in primary care, it is helpful to explore the history and current international examples of occupational therapy in primary care and frame these experiences within the context of guiding frameworks.

## *History of Occupational Therapy in Primary Care*

The pursuit of occupational therapy in primary care is rooted the WHO's Declaration of the Alma-Ata, presented at the International Conference in Primary Health Care in 1978. The declaration affirms that health is a fundamental human right and describes primary health care:

> Primary health care is essential health care based on practical, scientifically sound and socially acceptable methods and technology made universally accessible to individuals and families in the community through their full participation and at a cost that the community and country can afford to maintain at every stage of their development in the spirit of self-reliance and self-determination. (WHO, 1978, p. 1)

The Alma-Ata was a call-to-action for a national and international collaboration to introduce, develop, and maintain primary care services for all people (WHO, 1978). Occupational therapy literature from around the world has highlighted the significance of the Alma-Ata in recognizing health inequities and recommending the multidimensional approach toward addressing primary health care through promotive, preventive, curative, and rehabilitative services (WHO, 1978). Despite the imperative nature of the Alma-Ata declaration, there are few occupational therapy practitioners in primary care settings. The relative absence of occupational therapy in primary care and differences in practice settings has largely been attributed to funding, countries' established and changing health systems, health attitudes, and priorities. Using a comparative approach and examining the history, best practices, and similarities across countries, an understanding of the role of occupational therapy in primary care can be strengthened and a foundation for optimizing occupational therapy services in primary care worldwide can be established.

The emergence of occupational therapy in primary care was first recognized in the 1980s. Bumphrey (1989) described occupational therapy services in the context of a community care group in Britain, where older adults were referred for functional assessments and health promotion. This is one of the first examples of occupational therapy services provided in the context of primary care. Over the past decade, the Canadian Association of Occupational Therapists (2013) has collected examples of current practices and efficacy research, and provided resources for occupational therapists in Canada to advocate for occupational therapy's role on primary care teams. Additionally, the Council of Occupational Therapists for the European Countries surveyed its 39 member countries and concluded that "the major contribution of occupational therapy seems to be the client-centered and holistic approach, the occupational perspective focused on the enablement of daily living and participation of individuals of all ages, their caregivers and groups in society" (Baaijen, Bolt, Ikking, & Saenger, 2016, p. 11).

The role for occupational therapy in the United States was first identified by thought leaders Elizabeth B. Devereaux and Robert B. Walker in 1995. Devereaux and Walker (1995) summarized the health care climate of the time and identified the need and potential for occupational therapy in primary care. In the following decade, there was little traction in implementing occupational therapy in primary care. In fact, it was not until 2014 that the AOTA released an official position paper asserting that "occupational therapy practitioners are well prepared to contribute to interprofessional care teams addressing the primary care needs of individuals across the lifespan, particularly people living with one or more chronic conditions" (Roberts et al., 2014). Current occupational therapy thought leaders are guiding the development of practice by publishing literature that identifies a need for and provides examples of occupational therapy in primary care (Killian et al., 2015; Metzler et al., 2012; Muir, 2012).

A growing body of research can be cited that supports the efficacy of occupational therapy and expanded practice in primary care in the United States and other countries (Clark et al., 2012; Donnelly, Brenchley, Crawford, & Letts, 2013; Donnelly, Leclair, Wener, Hand, & Letts, 2016; Garvey, Connolly, Boland, & Smith, 2015; O'Toole, Connolly, & Smith, 2013). Research about the relevant client factors, conditions, and specialty populations can also be used to inform evidence-based practice in primary care. For instance, research regarding fall prevention, at-risk populations such as individuals with chronic conditions, and community mental health programs can be utilized to inform occupational therapy practice across a variety of settings, including primary care (Arbesman, Lieberman, & Metzler, 2014; Arbesman & Mosley, 2012; Eklund & Leufstadius, 2007). As occupational therapy programs in primary care from around the globe continue to be implemented and described in literature, a more comprehensive review on the effectiveness of these programs can be undertaken. Exploring the various possibilities for occupational therapy practitioners to participate on interprofessional primary care teams and in the community will enhance the profession and improve client outcomes.

## Guiding Frameworks for Occupational Therapy in Primary Care

As occupational therapy continues to expand its role in primary care, community, and population health, an opportunity is presented to develop professional identity and demonstrate the principles that guide occupational therapy assessment and intervention. The *Framework* "describes the central concepts that ground occupational therapy practice and builds a mutual understanding of the basic tenets and vision of the profession" (AOTA, 2014, p. S3). When integrating with primary care providers, having a shared framework and common language can strengthen collaboration and role clarity. The WHO's ICF framework is a fitting model for conceptualizing interprofessional primary care practice. Both the ICF and the *Framework* emphasize the transactional relationships between the person and contextual factors, but the *Framework* shifts the emphasis to the desired outcome, which is occupational performance. The ICF model is presented next, followed by a description of using the *Framework* to guide occupational therapy practice in primary care.

### International Classification of Functioning, Disability and Health

The ICF uses a classification system to illustrate the effect of health conditions on the individual and explain the interplay of factors that can limit or promote health and function (WHO, 2001). The ICF recognizes the inextricable role of the environment and other contextual factors in the creation of disability and as a support for health promotion. Moreover, the framework portrays functioning as a dynamic interaction between a person's health conditions, environmental factors, and personal factors. The model is organized into three levels illustrating the interrelationship and direction of influence of the factors:

1. The level of the disease or condition
2. The whole person (body structures/functions, activity, and participation)
3. The whole person in context (environment and personal factors)

Figure 40-2 illustrates the levels and interaction of the components in the ICF model in the gray boxes, while also including the corresponding domains from the *Framework* in the white boxes.

In the ICF body functions and structures include systems and functions at the level of the body such as physiologic systems, sensory function, pain, and anatomic structures. Problems affecting body structures and functions are considered impairments and are commonly the focus of rehabilitation efforts. Activities are understood as the performance of tasks such as walking, moving, and self-care. Disease, impairments in body structures and functions, restrictions in participation, and contextual influences alone or collectively can result

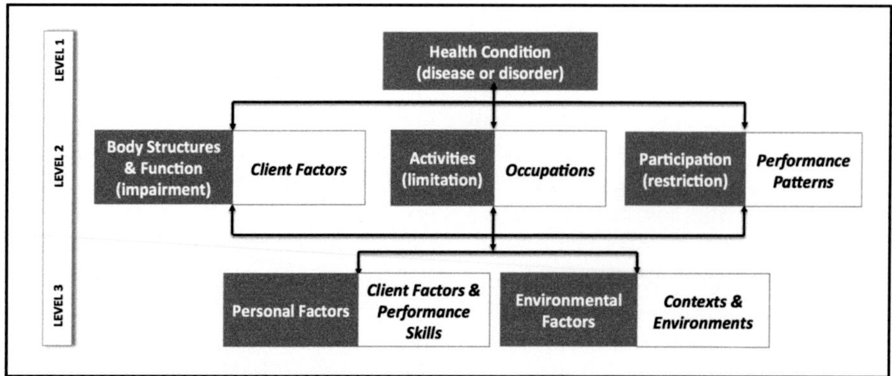


**Figure 40-2.** Interaction between components of ICF and corresponding domains of occupational therapy (AOTA, 2014; WHO, 2001).

in activity limitations. Participation refers to involvement in life situations and as a member of society, and can similarly influence and be influenced by the other components. According to Hemmingsson and Jonsson (2005), "the concept of participation not only plays an important role in the ICF classification but has also become a central construct in health care, rehabilitation and in occupational therapy" (p. 569). Contextual factors, both environmental and personal, include variables such as social, attitudinal, and physical environments, and also include a person's habits, lifestyle, coping styles, social background, and are assumed to impact on all three components (WHO, 2001).

The ICF framework illustrates the interplay of the person and contextual level factors and their effect on participation. More importantly, the ICF explicitly recognizes the relationship between health and participation, which underscores occupational therapy's core assumption that occupation influences health. The WHO describes health in its 1986 Ottawa Charter by stating:

> Health is created and lived by people within the settings of their everyday life; where they learn, work, play and love. Health is created by caring for oneself and others, by being able to make decisions and have control over one's life circumstances, and by ensuring that the society one lives in creates conditions that allow the attainment of health by all its members. Health is, therefore, seen as a resource for everyday life, not the objective of living. Health is a positive concept emphasizing social and personal resources, as well as physical capacities. (p. 2)

In other words, the WHO is affirming that health is created through engaging in occupation and participation in society. Furthermore, if health is a resource for everyday life or occupations, and everyday life influences health, then there is a reciprocal relationship between health and occupation. From this perspective, it becomes clear that if the goal is to restore or promote health, interventions should focus on enabling engagement in meaningful occupations and supporting participation in life roles and society. Improving the health of individuals by focusing on their daily habits, routines, and rituals represents a fundamental shift from a disease-centered to a person-centered approach. The importance of engaging in occupations as a means of promoting, sustaining, and restoring health is the principal tenet and feature of occupational therapy services in primary care.

## Occupational Therapy Practice Framework: Domain and Process Third Edition

The *Framework* complements the ICF asserting that "achieving health, well-being, and participation in life through engagement in occupation is the overarching statement that describes the domain and process of occupational therapy in its fullest sense" (AOTA, 2014, p. S4). The domain of occupational therapy is described in the *Framework* as including occupations, client factors, performance skills, performance patterns, and context and environment. Together, these aspects of the domain impact occupational performance. Aspects of the domain of occupational therapy correlate directly with elements of the ICF. Whether considered together or independent of one another, occupational therapy's language from the *Framework* and components of the ICF highlight the dynamic relationship between factors that impact clients' health and function. The correlation between the ICF and the occupational therapy domains are demonstrated in Figure 40-2. The *Framework* is described in more detail in Chapter 6.

Interprofessional teammates are not expected to have a thorough understanding of occupational therapy domains, so using a shared language and conceptual model can improve interprofessional communication and collaboration on primary care teams. The WHO's ICF provides a common lexicon across professions to understand health, thereby serving as an effective template to illustrate the relationship between the domains of occupational therapy and the ICF factors. For example, when an occupational therapist explains his or her assessment results and recommendations, using the term *participation* instead of *performance patterns*, or using *activities* in lieu of *occupations*, may be more effective toward increasing understanding and reducing confusion. Exploring the overlapping frameworks can facilitate understanding of the dynamic nature of health and disablement and occupational therapy practitioners' distinct skills in promoting health by addressing impairments in body structures, reducing activity limitations, and resolving restrictions to participation. The levels of the ICF introduce consideration of the whole person in the context of his or her life, furthering the aim to provide more person-centered, rather than disease-centered, primary care.

## Occupational Therapy Process in Primary Care

The practice of occupational therapy in primary care follows the established occupational therapy process outlined in the *Framework*. The distinct value of occupational therapy is derived from the occupational therapy process and the profession's focus on occupation while addressing the primary needs of clients across the lifespan (AOTA, 2014).

### Evaluation

Similar to other occupational therapy areas of practice, in primary care the occupational therapy practitioners can gain an understanding of the factors impacting occupational performance through the evaluation process. Depending on the primary care setting, the practitioner may be required to do a focused evaluation for a particular condition whereas in another setting a comprehensive evaluation of activities of daily living (ADLs) and instrumental activities of daily living (IADLs) is required. For example, when the client complains about arthritis pain limiting his or her abilities in a specific activity, the primary care provider may request occupational therapy to specifically address the physical impairments and pain. Similarly, a provider may request a fall risk assessment to determine the need for further intervention. Perhaps only a screening is appropriate in such cases; however, the occupational therapist's actions support the goals of primary care to serve as a point of coordination for health care services. In both examples, an abbreviated and focused evaluation of specific body structures and performance skills is all that is requested.

The occupational therapist may recommend a more comprehensive evaluation to determine additional needs, or may advise that the client be referred for outpatient or specialty services if needed. For example, a client may be referred to occupational therapy for training in self-management of chronic conditions. In this situation the occupational therapist will complete an occupational profile and a more comprehensive evaluation of occupational performance in order to understand the client and environmental factors that impact performance. Occupational therapists use their clinical reasoning to identify and select specific assessments, taking into consideration the physical practice setting, funding structure, resources, and client population. Evaluation may be completed with informal and formal interviews, nonstandardized and standardized assessments, and/or observation of occupational performance. A special consideration in primary care is how to communicate evaluation information with the interprofessional team. Knowing the type of information that is important to the primary care provider or health care professionals on the team may guide the occupational therapy practitioner in choosing the most appropriate assessments and methods. This is also an area where occupational therapists can demonstrate distinct value as part of the interprofessional team and clients' primary care.

### Occupations Addressed

Occupational therapy in primary care addresses a variety of occupations. Evaluations and thorough clinical reasoning are necessary to determine if the occupational performance needs can be appropriately met in the primary care practice area. It may be helpful for occupational therapy practitioners to actively reflect on goals of their practice setting and definition of primary care during this process. The definition of primary care includes addressing a large majority of personal health care needs and providing chronic care coordination, in the context of family and community (Roberts et al., 2014). Defining characteristics of primary care are illustrated in Figure 40-1. Inherently, many occupations are within in this scope, including ADLs, IADLs such as health management and maintenance, sleep and rest, all of which are routinely addressed by occupational therapy in primary care. Occupational therapists have the skills to evaluate, report, and provide interventions appropriate to daily life activities and a variety of occupations, often times discovering client factors or environments otherwise undetected without evaluation of occupational performance. Overall, occupational therapy practitioners in primary care may address all occupations directly, indirectly, or by requesting referrals to appropriate specialty service providers. The scope of primary care, goal of the practice setting, and practitioners' clinical reasoning guide the occupational therapy process.

# Intervention

## Approaches to Interventions

Primary care seeks to promote health, prevent or delay the onset of disease, and provide treatment when disease is detected. According to the *Framework*, approaches to interventions "inform the selection of practice models, frames of references, or treatment theories" (AOTA, 2014, p. S33). Approaches to intervention include create/promote (health promotion); establish/restore (remediation, restoration); maintain/modify (compensation, adaptation); and prevent (disability prevention; AOTA, 2014). Approaches to intervention may vary within occupational therapy interventions in primary care. The approach depends on the client-centered goals and aspects of the domain that are being addressed.

Primary care approaches can be organized along continuum of prevention where interventions are determined based on the presence or absence of disease (Association of Faculties of Medicine of Canada, n.d.). There are three primary care prevention targets: primary, secondary, and tertiary prevention.

1. Primary prevention is intended to prevent disease or injury before it ever occurs. Primary care team interventions at this level focus on hazard reduction, education about healthy and safe habits, immunizations, lifestyle counseling, and fostering safe environments, for example.
2. Secondary prevention focuses on early detection and treatment of disease or injury as soon as possible to halt or slow its progress. Secondary prevention efforts aim to reduce the impact of a disease or injury that has already occurred. Examples of interventions at this level include encouraging personal strategies to prevent reinjury or recurrence and interventions or programs to return people to their original health and function to prevent long-term problems.
3. Tertiary prevention seeks to reduce impairments and lessen the impact of an ongoing illness or injury that has lasting effects. This is done by helping individuals manage long-term, often complex health problems and injuries (e.g., chronic diseases, permanent impairments) in order to optimize their quality of life, improve ability to function, and extend life expectancy.

Occupational therapy services in acute care, rehabilitation, and skilled nursing settings are focused on rehabilitative services following an injury or illness. In these settings, interventions commonly target problems affecting body structures and function and focus on restorative activities to lessen the degree of impairment. Occupational therapy services are often terminated when the individual has recovered from his or her acute condition to allow discharge from the hospital or upon completion of an outpatient course of therapy for a particular condition. Then, occupational therapy delivered as part of a primary care approach would continue to work with individuals and family members providing secondary and tertiary prevention interventions. These interventions may include self-management of lifelong conditions, environmental adaptations, coping strategies, work modification, and creating healthy habits and routines to optimize an individual's ability to participate in life roles and society. In this sense, occupational therapy primary care prevention approaches can be delivered before the need for acute care or rehabilitation services to help prevent or reduce worsening of disease or debility, and again at the point where rehabilitation ends to enhance a person's ability to thrive in his or her home and community.

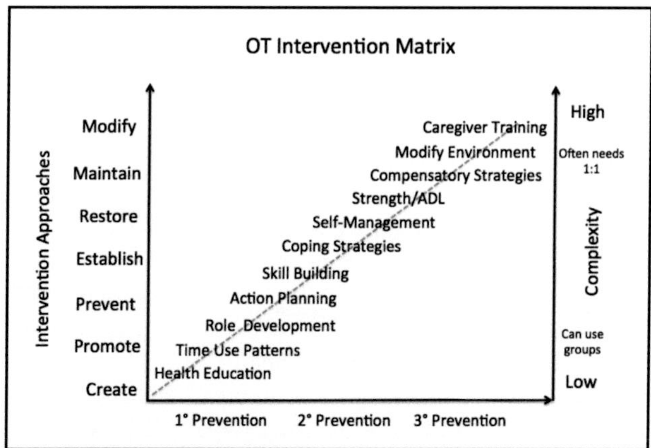


**Figure 40-3.** Occupational therapy intervention matrix.

Ideally, occupational therapy practitioners intervene at the primary and secondary prevention level to address occupational performance challenges prior to the onset of disease, in order to improve the health of individuals and families, and at a tertiary level to minimize debilitating effects of disease and facilitate optimal functioning. Figure 40-3 illustrates common occupational therapy intervention approaches organized along a continuum ranging from simple to more complex treatments and reflecting the level of prevention. The vertical axis on the left side of Figure 40-3 lists the general intervention approaches described in the *Framework*. The right axis suggests that the complexity of the interventions increases at the level of tertiary prevention after disease is identified and impairments are present. In other words, the greater the extent of impairment to body functions, structures, performance skills, and performance patterns resulting from disease and debility, the more complex the intervention plan must be to optimize participation in daily life.

As an example, when performance of ADLs is compromised due to peripheral neuropathy and low vision, a variety of longer term intervention approaches are required, which may include modification of tasks and environment, treatment to reduce pain, and creation and promotion of new routines designed to minimize

## Case Study: Establishment of Health Routines and Medication Management

Sam is a 26-year-old transgender woman living with an anxiety disorder who was starting hormone replacement therapy. She was receiving services from an interprofessional primary care team providing home visits. She was referred to occupational therapy to address management of her new medical treatments. During an informal interview, Sam described how she was fearful of making sure that she took her new medications as directed. Her prescriptions required that she take the medications on a consistent schedule throughout the week, and administer them orally and through intramuscular injections. This was the first time that Sam had multiple medications to manage and the first time she had medication to self-inject. Through a semiformal interview and the completion of a weekly activity time log, the occupational therapist evaluated Sam's strengths, potential challenges, and current routines. The occupational therapist provided education on the benefits of creating a relaxing space when Sam could complete the injection, to cope with her symptoms of anxiety and create the best opportunity for her muscles to be relaxed and prepared for the medication. Sam identified that she feels most comfortable at home in the evenings. With cues from the occupational therapy practitioner to guide problem solving, Sam identified that Tuesday evenings were a time that she would not have engagements with friends or community activities; this was an ideal time to schedule for administering her medication. With occupational therapy instruction and guidance, Sam created a weekly schedule for her medication routine. The occupational therapy practitioner then provided education around self-care, equipment preparation (e.g., gathering alcohol swabs, needles), and clean-up. Sam identified that injecting after the shower may be both relaxing and ensure that the injection site was clean; she would then be able to rest after the injection. A new medication routine was created through occupational therapy, and the occupational therapy practitioner followed up with Sam over the phone using a telehealth approach and in home to support implementation. The occupational therapist consulted with the primary care team nurse to share the plan for medication management and approaches to education that were effective when working with Sam.

effects of peripheral neuropathy. In contrast, a student struggling to balance work and school demands may require short-term intervention to clarify priorities and values, create more effective organization and study strategies, and promote use of stress management techniques. Ultimately, the intervention plan is developed in collaboration with the client and based on preventing or reducing health risks and barriers to occupational performance.

### Service Delivery

Reimbursement structures directly influence many aspects of service provision, including which services can be provided, where these services are delivered, and the amount of service that is allowed. Reimbursement is seen as a principal limiting factor for occupational therapy in primary care (Muir, 2012). Chapter 41 explains the various payers and reimbursement models and should be consulted for a more detailed explanation. In the simplest terms, from a provider perspective, reimbursement structures can be considered as being direct or indirect. Direct reimbursement can be seen as a fee-for-service arrangement where a bill is rendered to an individual or organizational entity outlining the cost of services provided. In contrast, indirect reimbursement occurs when services are rendered as part of an overall set of services. That is, individual services or elements are not billed or reimbursed separately.

The new primary care team–based practice models are funded in a variety of ways. Occupational therapy services can be billed and reimbursed directly or indirectly. In school settings, occupational therapy practitioners are often paid indirectly as employees of the school system or perhaps directly as an independent contractor on a fee-for-service basis. Reimbursement to providers for services delivered in an outpatient clinic setting can be reimbursed either directly or indirectly depending on whether the provider is a salaried employee or independent contractor. Additionally, individual clients can pay directly for occupational therapy services. Common across these examples is the assumption that occupational therapy services are essential and valuable toward achieving the overall outcomes expected. That is, if occupational therapy services were not seen as valuable or not distinctly contributing to the overarching goals of the school, the hospital, the clinic, or the client, then occupational therapy services would not be included in these settings. Demonstrating the distinct value of occupational therapy services is essential to support expansion into emerging practice settings such a primary care, as well as to sustain service in current practice areas (Arbesman et al., 2014).

Occupational therapy in primary care may be delivered in a variety of physical practice settings. Occupational therapy practitioners are beginning to participate in primary care practices that are university-affiliated or are part of a large ACO, such as the Veterans Health Administration, where health care is already being delivered in a comprehensive manner (Leland et al., 2015; Muir, 2012). Conversely, smaller primary care practices, community-based clinics, and those that provide services to specialty populations have begun to recognize the value of occupational therapy services for specific conditions and interventions to promote health and minimize debility (Donnelly et al., 2013). These interventions are common to occupational therapy and may include strategies to address low vision, fall prevention, homelessness, reintegration to work and community living, self-management of chronic conditions, healthy habits and routines, and home adaptation for independent living (Frenchman, 2015). Occupational therapy practitioners who provide services in smaller primary care practices or community settings are often providing services specific to the identified needs of the practice and clients served (Metzler et al., 2012). An example may be a nonprofit program that provides in-home interprofessional primary care services to clients living with HIV or a community clinic that provides primary care occupational therapy groups to address parental strategies for caring with children with physical developmental disabilities.

### Types of Interventions

As in all areas of practice, occupational therapy practitioners in primary care use clinical reasoning to determine the most effective interventions based on client needs and preferences and characteristics and resources of the practice setting. According to the *Framework*, occupational therapy "include[s] the use of occupations and activities, preparatory methods and tasks, education and training, advocacy, and group interventions to facilitate engagement in occupations to promote health and participation" (AOTA, 2014 p. S29). Interventions such as these allow the occupational therapy practitioner to focus on primary health promotion, as well as secondary and tertiary prevention strategies, by addressing the barriers to occupational engagement and promoting self-management. Occupation-based interventions also demonstrate the distinct value of occupational therapy to interprofessional team members.

Helping clients self-advocate or advocating on behalf of clients and providing group workshops are effective community-minded interventions for occupational therapy in primary care. Addressing contexts and environments that limit occupational engagement is also an essential part of advocacy. For instance, an occupational therapy practitioner may advocate for a pediatric client's needs by educating and facilitating change within the family dynamic that is impacting the child's occupational engagement. An occupational therapy practitioner may also represent the needs and concerns of primary care clients by addressing barriers to community mobility and facilitating access to public spaces. Group interventions allow occupational therapy practitioners in primary care to provide cost-effective services to multiple clients, and often address primary and secondary prevention needs. As demonstrated in Figure 40-3, groups may be most appropriate for interventions designed to create, promote, establish, and restore health and occupational performance. For example, an urban PCMH specializing in serving low-income adults experiencing housing instability provides multiple groups that correlate with various prevention levels. These include groups such as understanding addiction, depression and anxiety problem solving, spirituality and healing, gentle yoga, and Qigong.

### Case Example: Lifestyle and Management of Chronic Conditions

Darrell is a 54-year-old man living with diabetes who was referred to occupational therapy by his primary care physician to address issues related to nutrition. Darrell's health status was worsening and he was eating a lot of fast food. Darrell brought his 14-year-old daughter to the initial occupational therapy evaluation. He explained that his doctor told him his blood glucose levels were extremely high, poor circulation in his legs was worsening, and that he had to start eating better and exercising. Through evaluation, the occupational therapist learned that 6 months ago Darrell's wife passed away from cancer leaving Darrell to care for his daughter on his own. His wife had done all the cooking and taking care of the household. Darrell confided that the main reason he wanted to learn how to prepare healthy food at home was so that his daughter wouldn't end up with diabetes like him. He wanted to protect his daughter's health, but didn't know how to do so. Further discussion revealed that Darrell and his daughter were struggling with redefining their roles as father and daughter and what it meant to be a family of two instead of three. Neither Darrell nor his daughter knew how to manage the household tasks and realized that they needed to learn together and work as a team. They both agreed that a shared occupation-based goal of being able to prepare food together and eat dinner at the table would help them feel more like a family again, and also would benefit their health goals. His daughter suggested that they could start by preparing a healthy meal that her mother often cooked. The occupational therapy practitioner helped them to plan this meal by reviewing the necessary steps and identifying and resolving problems, such as when and where to go shopping, making grocery lists, and adjusting work and school schedules so they could be home together and prepared to cook. The following week they wanted to know about other food options so they could continue building the new family dinner routine. The occupational therapy practitioner introduced Darrell's daughter to several meal planning apps and coordinated care with the dietician and health educator to facilitate diabetes education. To address exercise needs, Darrell and his daughter identified that they liked to take the dog out for a walk. They decided on specific times when they could do that together and picked a walking route that Darrell could manage. Subsequent sessions focused on how to successfully incorporate new activities or behaviors into their current routines so they could more readily take care of themselves and each other.

## Outcomes

Measuring outcomes is an essential component of occupational therapy practice. The outcome of occupational therapy is client-centered, family-focused care that improves quality of life, function, and participation. These outcomes align very well with the principles of the Triple Aim and team-based models of care. The *Framework* describes outcomes as being "the end result of the occupational therapy process; they describe what clients can achieve through occupational therapy intervention" and that "outcomes are directly related to the interventions provided and to the occupations, client factors, performance skills, performance patterns, and contexts and environments targeted" (AOTA, 2014 p. S16). Measuring outcomes is important in facilitating mutual goal setting, directing the focus of therapy on the client, and monitoring client progress, as well as demonstrating that therapy is valuable and cost effective.

Outcome measures are determined early in the intervention process and must be congruent with client goals and consistent with targeted outcomes. Sources of outcomes can include client self-report, results from standardized tests, and occupational therapist observations. Service data such as number, length, and cost of interventions can also be considered when evaluating outcomes. It is essential for occupational therapists to realize that it is primarily through the achievement of targeted outcomes that the distinct value of occupational therapy is demonstrated.

## Occupational Therapy Practitioners' Skills

Primary care calls for occupational therapy practitioners to work as generalists, rather than exclusively with specialty populations (Devereaux & Walker, 1995; Muir, 2012). Occupational therapy in primary care expands the scope of assessments and interventions beyond those focused on medical impairments to also encompass behavioral and social determinants of health for the purposes of engaging in meaningful occupations and participation. This focus on occupational performance as being the outcome of intervention is fundamental to occupational therapy, and fulfills the profession's overarching domain, stated as "achieving health, well-being, and participation in life through engagement in occupation" AOTA, 2014, p. S2). The shift to understanding occupational therapy practitioners as generalists challenges the schema of practice for many practitioners who have been working with specialty populations. Muir (2012) asserts that practicing in primary care is not an endeavor suitable for all occupational therapists. More specifically, Muir (2012) states, "To be successful in primary care, an occupational therapist must be a true generalist who is competent across all age spans and the entire domain of occupational therapy practice as well as knowledgeable about the full scope of practice."

### Case Example: Fall Prevention

Dominic is a 79-year-old man who had presented to his primary care doctor complaining of difficulty getting out of bed. After a physical exam, the physician determined there was acute injury and then called the occupational therapist into the exam room to screen for balance issues while she attended to her next patient. The occupational therapist performed the Timed Up and Go test with Dominic and found that the results were normal. Additional assessment of daily living routines revealed that Dominic had fallen several times when trying to go to the bathroom at night. Dominic confided that balance wasn't as much of an issue as was the urgency to go to the bathroom. Recently, he'd experienced several "accidents" in bed and felt ashamed that his wife had to change the sheets in the middle of the night. Both he and his wife thought this was a normal part of aging. Dominic reported having difficulty seeing in the dark and that he would trip over the chair leg or throw rug on his way to the bathroom, which was causing his falls. The occupational therapist provided education on safety issues regarding furniture placement, throw rugs, and lighting. Dominic did not want to use a urinal or a bedside commode, but agreed to discuss this issue with the doctor. The occupational therapist conveyed the recent urinary frequency and incontinence to the physician who gathered more pertinent history and referred Dominic to urology. The occupational therapist recommended a home visit to assess for further safety issues, and Dominic agreed to a video telehealth visit with assistance from his grandson, as he lived a far distance from the clinic. Dominic and his grandson had already made the changes recommended by the occupational therapist at the time of the delivery of service through telehealth technology. Dominic reported he had no additional falls, but wanted to talk about the shower. Through telehealth technology, the occupational therapist was able to recommend use of a grab bar and provided education to Dominic about the placement and requirements regarding safe installation. Dominic was also grateful that he had an open invitation to call the occupational therapist with any additional questions regarding household safety. In this example, positive outcomes were achieved in fall prevention, self-care performance, coordination of care and client satisfaction.

Since primary care is the first point of contact with the health care system for most clients, it follows that occupational therapists should be prepared to serve multiple roles and address a wide variety of occupational performance issues. To illustrate, Eichler and Royeen (2016) provide occupational therapy in a university student health clinic and in a primary care physician's office. In those settings they reported, "We find ourselves drawing on every aspect of our education and experience while working with the breadth of patient needs that present themselves in each of our clinics. We use formal and informal assessments, therapeutic techniques, high-tech and low-tech assistive technology, and knowledge of orthopedics as we partner with the primary care team to achieve optimal patient outcomes" (p. 289). However, the main populations served and characteristics of the primary care clinics are not always the same and will vary depending on whether the clinic is a small community-based clinic in a farming community, a large university-affiliated clinic in a metropolitan area, or an inner-city clinic for underserved populations, for instance. Therefore, it is important to examine the mission and characteristics of the organization to determine the skills and experience necessary to be competent in addressing the occupational needs of the clients served in a particular primary care setting, as one would when appraising self-competency relative to any practice setting. Ultimately, it is the occupational therapy practitioner's ethical responsibility to ensure that service delivery is congruent with his or her credentials, qualifications, experience, competency and scope of practice (AOTA, 2015).

Occupational therapy practitioners in primary care function as part of an interprofessional team, provide consultation to providers, and deliver individual and group interventions for a variety of conditions. For this reason, occupational therapy practitioners must be able to self-advocate, communicate and collaborate with other providers, accurately assess their own self-competency, and understand and articulate the focus and role of occupational therapy in primary care. Most importantly, occupational therapy must be able to demonstrate the positive outcomes delineated by the Triple Aim, including reducing costs, optimizing health outcomes, and improving quality. This area of practice is a good fit for creative occupational therapy practitioners who can thrive as part of an interprofessional team and guide their practice with theories and evidence encompassing health and wellness and participation in meaningful occupation across the lifespan.

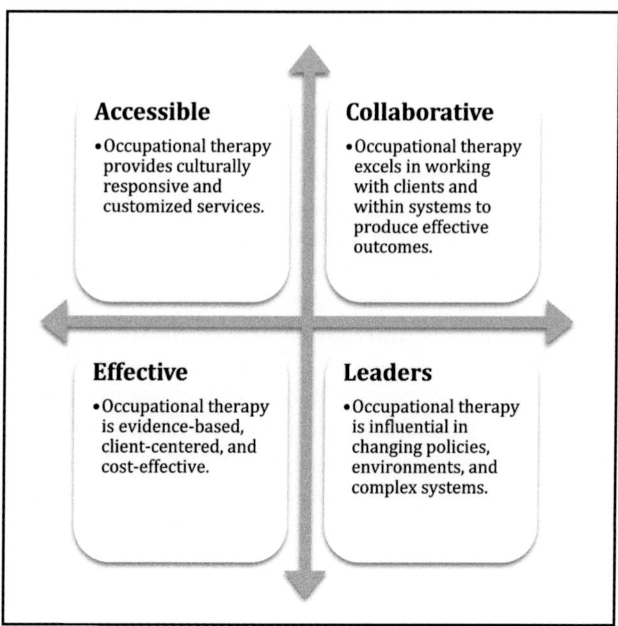


**Figure 40-4.** Vision 2025 (AOTA).

## Future Directions

The AOTA's Vision 2025 is that occupational therapy maximizes health, well-being, and quality of life for all people, populations, and communities through effective solutions that facilitate participation in everyday living (AOTA, 2016). Providing occupational therapy in primary care allows practitioners to deliver interventions throughout the lifespan to prevent the onset of disease or debility and resolve barriers to participation once they occur. The emphasis on the client and engagement in occupations that hold meaning for that client in the context his or her life makes the contribution of occupational therapy distinct.

There are currently a small number of occupational therapy practitioners providing services as part of primary care practices in the United States. However, advocacy is necessary to promote legislation specifying inclusion of occupational therapy as a principal member of primary care interprofessional teams and other innovative models of care. Observing the key tenets of the AOTA's Vision 2025 will help occupational therapy practitioners demonstrate the value of occupational therapy services and support the need for expansion in primary care and other emerging practice areas. Figure 40-4 illustrates the four key tenets of occupational therapy service.

It is not enough for occupational therapists in primary care to advocate for the promotion of the profession. Practitioners in all practice areas must engage in practice promotion in their own area of practice as well as for the profession in general. It is through sharing and communicating a common vision and achieving performance-based outcomes that the value and necessity of occupational therapy services will be known.

## Summary

A system-wide transformation of the organization and delivery of primary care services is underway in the United States. The new systems of care are built on the principles of the Triple Aim and are intended to reduce the cost of care, to avoid duplication of services, and to decrease fragmentation of care across the system. The responsibility for client care coordination is placed with the primary care providers. The overarching goal is to create value-based primary care programs and health centers to meet the primary care needs of individuals by maintaining long-term relationships and providing chronic care management across the lifespan.

## Evidence-Based Research Chart

| Topic | Evidence |
|---|---|
| Recent research studies of occupational therapy interventions in primary care | Arbesman, Lieberman, & Metzler, 2014; Donnelly, Brenchley, Crawford, & Letts, 2013; Garvey, Connolly, Boland, & Smith, 2015 |
| Occupational therapy practitioner experiences in primary care | Donnelly, Leclair, Wener, Hand, & Letts, 2016; Eichler & Royeen, 2016 |
| Describing the role of occupational therapy in primary care | Dahl-Popolizio, Manson, Muir, & Rogers, 2016; Killian, Fisher, & Muir, 2015 |

Recently, occupational therapists in the United States have begun providing direct services in primary care programs or health centers and consulting with PCMH teams in larger health systems to address a variety of occupational performance issues. Preliminary outcomes indicate that, "An occupational therapist, with skills in providing assessment and intervention for physical dysfunction, behavioral and mental health, and the ability to work with individuals across the lifespan, contributes significant value to the health care team" (Dahl-Popolizio, Manson, Muir, & Rogers, 2016, p. 271). Occupational therapy practitioners in primary care function as generalists to address a variety of occupational performance limitations and restrictions. When in fast-paced primary care clinic settings, the therapist must be able to provide rapid, targeted evaluations and focused brief interventions (Muir, 2012, p. 273). Alternately, health promotion programs, ergonomic education, or stress management and relaxation training, for example, can be provided in a community setting using individual training, groups, or through telehealth technology. In addition to providing client-centered interventions and achieving high-value outcomes, it is important for occupational therapy practitioners to understand the practice setting, culture, priorities, and funding sources in order to successfully advocate for occupational therapy services.

In closing, the occupational therapy practitioner's skills to improve function, enable participation, and promote health through occupation offer significant value to the client and contribute to key primary care outcomes. This client-centered approach fundamentally aligns with the defining characteristics of primary care. Use of the *Framework* helps to inform practice and underscores the importance of engaging in occupations as a means of promoting, sustaining, and restoring health. Ultimately, continued implementation of occupational therapy in primary care, dissemination of outcomes and research evidence, and ongoing practice promotion will influence the future of occupational therapy's role in primary care as part of a comprehensive health system providing a full complement of programs geared toward optimizing health and well-being.

## Student Self Assessment

1. Choose a case study in the chapter and identify the following:
   - ◊ Approach(es) to intervention described
   - ◊ Level(s) of prevention addressed
2. Ask friends and family members about their recent visits to primary care. What were their experiences like? Were there personal health care issues or concerns that they did not get addressed or did not bring up? How could occupational therapy address those needs?

## Acknowledgments

Chapter illustration (p. 577) created by Quinn Lindstrom.

## References

Agency for Healthcare Research and Quality. (n.d.). *Defining the PCMH*. Retrieved from https://pcmh.ahrq.gov/page/defining-pcmh

American College of Physicians. (n.d.). *What is the patient-centered medical home?* Retrieved from https://www.acponline.org/practice-resources/business/payment/models/pcmh/understanding/what-pcmh

American Occupational Therapy Association. (2014). Occupational therapy practice framework: Domain and process (3rd ed.). *American Journal of Occupational Therapy, 68*(Suppl. 1), S1-S48. doi:10.5014/ajot.2014.682006

American Occupational Therapy Association. (2015). Occupational therapy code of ethics (2015). *American Journal of Occupational Therapy*, 69(Suppl. 3), 6913410030p1. doi:10.5014/ajot.2015.696S03

American Occupational Therapy Association. (2016). *Vision 2025*. Retrieved from http://www.aota.org/AboutAOTA/vision-2025.aspx

Arbesman, M., Lieberman, D., & Metzler, C. A. (2014). Using evidence to promote the distinct value of occupational therapy. *American Journal of Occupational Therapy, 68*(4), 381. doi:10.5014/ajot.2014.684002

Arbesman, M., & Mosley, L. J. (2012). Systematic review of occupation- and activity-based health management and maintenance interventions for community-dwelling older adults. *American Journal of Occupational Therapy, 66*(3), 277-283. doi:10.5014/ajot.2012.003327

Association of Faculties of Medicine of Canada. (n.d.). *Primer on population health*. Retrieved from http://phprimer.afmc.ca/Part1-TheoryThinkingAboutHealth/

Baaijen, R., Bolt, M., Ikking, T., & Saenger, S. (2016, June). *COTEC Position Paper: Occupational therapy and primary care*. Retrieved from https://www.aoti.ie/attachments/fd742f39-e943-4ddf-9dfc-9e2c2d4e63c7.PDF

Berwick, D. M., Nolan, T. W., & Whittington, J. (2008). The Triple Aim: Care, health, and cost. *Health Affairs, 27*(3), 759-769. doi:10.1377/hlthaff.27.3.759

Bumphrey, E. (1989). Occupational therapy within the primary health care team. *British Journal of Occupational Therapy, 52*(7), 252-255.

Calman, N. S., Golub, M., & Shuman, S. (2012). Primary care and health reform. *Mount Sinai Journal of Medicine, 79*(5), 527-534. doi:10.1002/msj.21335

Canadian Association of Occupational Therapists (2013). *CAOT position statement: Occupational therapy in primary care (2013)*. Retrieved from http://www.caot.ca/pdfs/positionstate/PS_PrimaryCare.pdf

Centers for Disease Control and Prevention. (n.d.). *Chronic disease prevention and health promotion*. Retrieved from http://www.cdc.gov/chronicdisease/

Clark, F., Jackson, J., Carlson, M., Chou, C.-P., Cherry, B. J., Jordan-Marsh, M., ... Azen, S. P. (2012). Effectiveness of a lifestyle intervention in promoting the well-being of independently living older people: Results of the Well Elderly 2 Randomised Controlled Trial. *Journal of Epidemiology and Community Health, 66*(9), 782-790. doi:10.1136/jech.2009.099754

Dahl-Popolizio, S., Manson, L., Muir, S., & Rogers, O. (2016). Enhancing the value of integrated primary care: The role of occupational therapy. *Families, Systems and Health: The Journal of Collaborative Family Healthcare, 34*(3), 270-280.

Devereaux, E. B., & Walker, R. B. (1995). The role of occupational therapy in primary health care. *American Journal of Occupational Therapy, 49*(5), 391-396.

Donnelly, C., Brenchley, C., Crawford, C., & Letts, L. (2013). The integration of occupational therapy into primary care: A multiple case study design. *BMC Family Practice, 14*, 60. doi:10.1186/1471-2296-14-60

Donnelly, C. A., Leclair, L. L., Wener, P. F., Hand, C. L., & Letts, L. J. (2016). Occupational therapy in primary care: Results from a national survey. L'ergothérapie dans les soins primaires: Résultats d'un sondage national. *Canadian Journal of Occupational Therapy, 83*(3), 135-142. doi:10.1177/0008417416637186

Eichler, J., & Royeen, L. (2016). Occupational therapy in the primary health care clinic: Experiences of two clinicians. *Families, Systems, and Health, 34*(3), 289-291. doi:10.1037/fsh0000226

Eklund, M., & Leufstadius, C. (2007). Relationships between occupational factors and health and well-being in individuals with persistent mental illness living in the community. *Canadian Journal of Occupational Therapy, 74*(4), 303-313. doi:10.1177/000841740707400403

Fisher, G., & Friesema, J. (2013). Implications of the affordable care act for occupational therapy practitioners providing services to medicare recipients. *American Journal of Occupational Therapy, 67*(5), 502-506. doi:10.5014/ajot.2013.675002

Frenchman, K. (2015). The health promoting role of occupational therapy in primary health care: A reflection and emergent vision. *New Zealand Journal of Occupational Therapy, 61*(2), 64-69.

Garvey, J., Connolly, D., Boland, F., & Smith, S. M. (2015). OPTIMAL, an occupational therapy led self-management support programme for people with multimorbidity in primary care: A randomized controlled trial. *BMC Family Practice, 16*. doi:10.1186/s12875-015-0267-0

Hemmingsson, H., & Jonsson, H. (2005). An occupational perspective on the concept of participation in the International Classification of Functioning, Disability and Health—Some critical remarks. [Miscellaneous article]. *American Journal of Occupational Therapy, 59*(5), 569-576.

Institute of Medicine. (1994). *Defining primary care: An interim report*. Washington, DC: National Academies Press. Retrieved from http://www.nap.edu/catalog/9153

Kennedy, A., Bower, P., Reeves, D., Blakeman, T., Bowen, R., Chew-Graham, C., ... on behalf of the Salford National Institute for Health Research Gastrointestinal Programme Grant Research Group. (2013). Implementation of self management support for long term conditions in routine primary care settings: Cluster randomised controlled trial. *BMJ, 346*, f2882. doi:10.1136/bmj.f2882

Killian, C., Fisher, G., & Muir, S. (2015). Primary care: A new context for the scholarship of practice model. *Occupational Therapy in Health Care*. doi:10.3109/07380577.2015.1050713

Leland, N. E., Crum, K., Phipps, S., Roberts, P., & Gage, B. (2015). Advancing the value and quality of occupational therapy in health service delivery. *American Journal of Occupational Therapy, 69*(1), 6901090010p1-6901090010p7. doi:10.5014/ajot.2015.691001

Metzler, C., Hartmann, K., & Lowenthal, L. (2012). Defining primary care: Envisioning the roles of occupational therapy. *American Journal of Occupational Therapy, 66*(3), 266-270. doi:10.5014/ajot.2010.663001

Muir, S. (2012). Occupational therapy in primary health care: We should be there. *American Journal of Occupational Therapy, 66*(5), 506-510. doi:10.5014/ajot.2012.665001

O'Toole, L., Connolly, D., & Smith, S. (2013). Impact of an occupation-based self-management programme on chronic disease management. *Australian Occupational Therapy Journal, 60*(1), 30-38. doi:10.1111/1440-1630.12008

Piette, J. D., Holtz, B., Beard, A. J., Blaum, C., Greenstone, C. L., Krein, S. L., ... on behalf of the Ann Arbor PACT Steering Committee. (2011). Improving chronic illness care for veterans within the framework of the patient-centered medical home: Experiences from the Ann Arbor Patient-Aligned Care Team Laboratory. *Translational Behavioral Medicine, 1*(4), 615-623. doi:10.1007/s13142-011-0065-8

Roberts, P., Farmer, M., Lamb, A., Muir, S., & Siebert, C. (2014). The role of occupational therapy in primary care. *American Journal of Occupational Therapy, 68*(Suppl. 3), S25. doi:10.5014/ajot.2014.686S06

Rosland, A.-M., Nelson, K., Sun, H., Dolan, E. D., Maynard, C., Bryson, C., ... Schectman, G. (2013). The patient-centered medical home in the Veterans Health Administration. *American Journal of Managed Care, 19*(7), e263-272.

Tuepker, A., Kansagara, D., Skaperdas, E., Nicolaidis, C., Joos, S., Alperin, M., & Hickam, D. (2014). "We've not gotten even close to what we want to do": A qualitative study of early patient-centered medical home implementation. *Journal of General Internal Medicine, 29*(2), 614-622.

World Health Organization. (1978). *Declaration of Alma-Ata*. Retrieved from http://www.euro.who.int/__data/assets/pdf_file/0009/113877/E93944.pdf?ua=1

World Health Organization. (2001). *International classification of functioning, disability and health*. Geneva, Switzerland: Author.

World Health Organization. (2010). *Framework for action on interprofessional education and collaborative practice*. Retrieved from http://whqlibdoc.who.int/hq/2010/WHO_HRH_HPN_10.3_eng.pdf

Zulman, D. M., Asch, S. M., Martins, S. B., Kerr, E. A., Hoffman, B. B., & Goldstein, M. K. (2014). Quality of care for patients with multiple chronic conditions: The role of comorbidity interrelatedness. *Journal of General Internal Medicine, 29*(3), 529-537. doi:10.1007/s11606-013-2616-9

# VII

# Management of Occupational Therapy Services

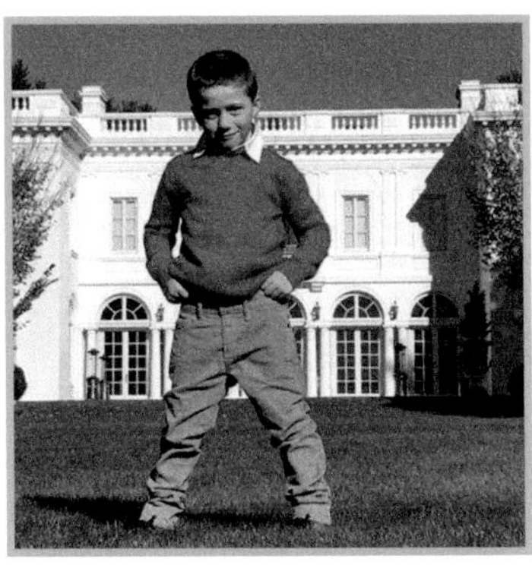

# 41

# Legislation and Reimbursement of Occupational Therapy Services

*Liat Gafni Lachter, OTD, OTR/L*

**ACOTE STANDARDS EXPLORED IN THIS CHAPTER**

B.6.2, B.7.1, B.7.2, B.7.4

**KEY VOCABULARY**

- **Habilitative services:** Services to help one develop, maintain, or improve skills and functioning for daily living. Habilitative services are now mandates as an essential health benefit in most new health care policies. Because these services are often provided by occupational therapy professionals, this legislation presents an opportunity for our profession to better define its role and necessity within the health policy.
- **Managed care:** A system of health care in which patients agree to visit only certain health care providers and locations to control quality and cost.
- **Policy:** A course or principle of action adopted or proposed by a government, party, business, or individual.
- **Reimbursement:** Repayment for money spent.
- **Third-party payers:** Insurance coverage in which a third party, namely the insurance company, pays the actual provider of health care services for services rendered to the consumer/client.



Jacobs, K., & MacRae, N. (Eds.).
*Occupational Therapy Essentials for Clinical Competence, Third Edition* (pp. 593-604).

Occupational therapy practitioners work in a constantly changing environment constructed and framed by policy and legislation. Occupational therapy practitioners have always been involved in working with our clients to enable them to achieve "health, well-being, and participation in life through engagement in occupation" (AOTA, 2014, p. S2). Yet, our work would not have been possible without policy and legislation that acknowledges our important role in health and rehabilitation care, education, and in the community and specifies the funding for our services. These current policies are a direct outcome of more than 100 years of ongoing efforts to advance access to occupational therapy services and adaptations of our profession facilitating our ability to meet society's changing needs.

While public policy often seems to be a remote concept, it in fact directly affects every one of us as a practitioner, student, educator, business owner, entrepreneur, and health care consumer. Federal policy governs how we are credentialed, where we practice, what services we can offer, in what niches we can become involved, and how we are reimbursed. Federal policy will also determine the future of our profession (AOTA, n.d.-a). Some might argue that understanding policy is as essential as "understanding anatomy, physiology, or psychology" (Dimond, 2011, p. IV), because it ensures informed practice in a wider sense and maximizes the services that we can provide to our clients in both the short and long term.

The goal of this chapter is to introduce readers to the current health policies that have shaped occupational therapy, describe various payment systems, and discuss the influence on occupational therapy management and delivery.

## What Is Public Policy?

Birkland (2014) defines public policy as what government, or any part of it (such as public officials, school officials, city council members, county supervisors, etc.), does or does not do about a problem that comes before them for consideration and possible action. More specifically, Birkland names a number of key attributes:

- Policy is made in response to a certain issue that requires attention.
- Policy might take the form of laws or regulations.
- Policy is made on behalf of the "public."
- Policy is oriented toward a goal or desired state, such as the solution of a problem.
- Policy is ultimately made by government, even if the ideas come from outside government or through the interaction of government and the public.
- Policymaking is part of an ongoing process that does not always have a clear beginning or end, since the outcomes of a policy are continually reassessed, revisited, and revised.

## How Is Policy Made?

Policymaking is a complex, long, and continuous process. Understanding the way policy is formed can enable occupational therapy practitioners and students, as professionals and as citizens, to realize their influence on the formation of policy. Switzer (2003) describes the cycle of activities that constitutes the public policymaking process using the policy cycle model that consists of six stages (Figure 41-1):

1. **Agenda setting:** This phase consist of problem recognition. Professional organizations or special interest groups work to bring their area of interest to the awareness and attention of the public and policymakers.
2. **Policy formation:** This stage includes a proposal for a solution. Policy formation is a process that is often trial and error, and might include efforts to modify existing policies. Political forces, particularly key stakeholders, attempt to exert significant influence. For example, the American Occupational Therapy Association (AOTA), as our representative association, has been involved in the advocating and shaping of many policies that relate to occupational therapy practice.
3. **Policy legitimation:** The proposed policy is typically in the form of a bill. Legitimation takes place at the federal or state level legislature, county government, and/or city council. At this stage, interested citizens can lobby their representatives, send letters, or testify at hearings in an attempt to make their views known. The policy is reviewed, voted upon, and then becomes a law or statute.
4. **Policy implementation:** In this stage, the decisions are put into effect. Availability of funding and personnel, court cases and judicial rulings, and continued input from special interest groups often affect implementation.
5. **Policy and program evaluation:** At some point after a policy has been implemented, an assessment is made to determine how well the policy and its resulting programs are working and meeting objectives. Outcomes are analyzed, particularly cost-effectiveness, numbers served, litigation, and satisfaction or dissatisfaction expressed by the media, the public, and those whom the policy affects directly.
6. **Policy change:** Based on the results of the evaluation, the policy might be revised or even terminated. The reasons can be practical or political.

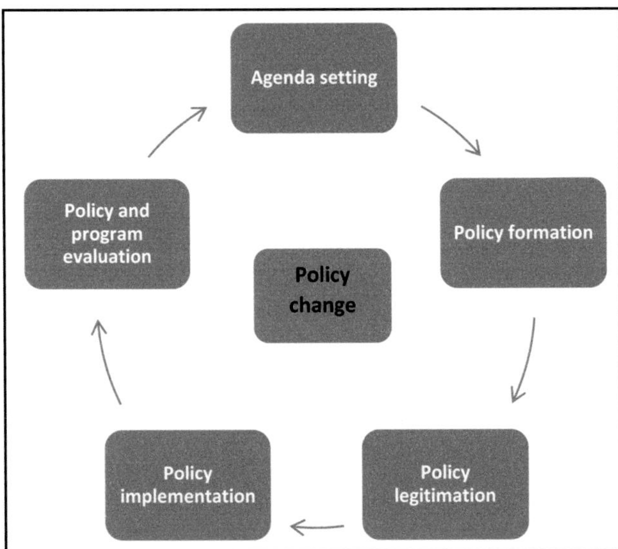


**Figure 41-1.** The policy cycle. (Adapted from Switzer, J. V. [2003]. Disabled policy making/disabled policy. In J. V. Switzer (Ed.), *Disabled rights: American disability policy and the fight for equality.* Washington, DC: Georgetown University Press.)

The evolution of policy can be a long process, but interested citizens and groups may have meaningful influence. It is our responsibility as professionals and citizens to stay up to date about policy that influences our practice and our clients. One opportunity to become involved as a student is participation in Capitol Hill Day in person or virtually. Organized by the AOTA, Hill Day is an opportunity for health care professionals to bring their concerns straight to their state's lawmakers, offer solutions, ask questions, and listen to guest speakers on the topics that affect their work. In 2015, more than 550 occupational therapy practitioners and students from across the United States visited Capitol Hill to make their voices heard (AOTA, 2015b). You can take part in this annual national day or initiate meeting with your local legislators year round to make your own impact about issues that you care about.

## Current Health Policy in the United States: Health Care Reform

The Patient Protection and Affordable Care Act of 2010 (P.L. 111-148)—often referred to as the ACA or Obamacare—has brought health care reform that focuses on provisions to expand coverage, control health care costs, and improve the health care delivery system (Kaiser Family Foundation, 2015a). ACA refers to two separate pieces of legislation: the Patient Protection and Affordable Care Act and the amendments made by the Health Care and Education Reconciliation Act of 2010 (P.L. 111-152). The ACA has expanded access to health insurance coverage for millions of uninsured Americans by expanding eligibility for Medicaid and by developing health insurance marketplaces where uninsured persons may be eligible for subsidies to make private health plans more affordable (Kaiser Family Foundation, 2015a). In addition to expanding access to health insurance, the law includes provisions intended to reform the health care delivery system to produce better patient outcomes at lower cost.

Consisting of 10 separate legislative titles, the ACA has several major aims. The first and central aim is to achieve near-universal health care coverage by establishing a shared responsibility among government, individuals, and employers. A second aim is to improve the fairness, quality, and affordability of health insurance coverage. A third aim is to improve health care value, quality, and efficiency while reducing wasteful spending and making the health care system more accountable to a diverse patient population. A fourth aim is to strengthen primary health care access while bringing about longer term changes in the availability of primary and preventive health care. A fifth and final aim is to make strategic investments in the public's health through both an expansion of clinical preventive care and of community investments (Rosenbaum, 2011).

As a result, the ACA has been greatly altering the health policy landscape in which the occupational therapy practice exists (Lamb & Metzler, 2014). ACA has made more payment options available for new delivery system models, such as primary care, patient-centered medical home, health home, and accountable care organization (Kaiser Family Foundation, 2015a). All of these areas present new and exciting opportunities for emerging models of practice and engagement of occupational therapists in key roles. However, our ability to take part in this reform relies on our ability to understand the policies and our advocating for our profession. The AOTA was been active in the legislative process leading up to the passage and signing of the ACA, working to achieve victories such as inclusion of rehabilitation and habilitation in the essential health benefits package. The AOTA has also been monitoring the regulatory process at the federal and state levels as the ACA has been implemented, and has been advocating for occupational therapy practitioners and consumers. In summary, the dynamic environment created by health care reform creates many opportunities, but also necessitates vigilant monitoring of implementation activities and carefully executed advocacy efforts to ensure that occupational therapy is valued and protected in the future (AOTA, n.d.-b). Among the most influential outcomes of policies are the dollar amounts that are allotted to cover specific expenses; in this case, it is health care services. Because of its importance, the remainder of this chapter will focus on a review of payment systems for occupational therapy services.

Table 41-1.

**PRIVATE INSURANCE COMPANY PLANS***

| | Consumer-Directed Health Care Plan (high-deductible health plan) | Preferred Provider Organization | Health Maintenance Organization |
|---|---|---|---|
| Cost of premiums for client | $ typically low. | $$$ typically the highest cost options. | $$ higher than high-deductible health plan, lower than PPO. |
| Out-of-pocket costs for client | $$$ the consumer must reach a relatively high deductible before insurance benefits begin to take effect. | $$ consumer pays coinsurance and copay. | $ copay, coinsurance, and deductible are typically lower. |
| Flexibility and choice for client | Consumer can see any provider without referral. Out-of-network providers typically cost more. | Consumer can see any provider without referral. Out-of-network providers may cost more. | HMO will only cover services rendered by in-network providers. If the occupational therapy practitioner is out of network, the client will most likely not receive coverage. |
| Reimbursement for services | Providers may initially receive all payments directly from the client, until the deductible is met. Consider a payment program to help your client make payments that are doable. | Client will pay copay or coinsurance according to his or her plan, and the majority of the payment will come later from the insurance company. | Client will pay copay or coinsurance according to his or her plan, and the majority of the payment will come later from the insurance company. |
| Appeal | An appeal is a request for the health insurer or plan to review a decision or a grievance again. The ACA has mandated that all insurance companies provide an explanation for any denied coverage, with a clearly defined appeal process. | | |

*This includes companies offering services in the marketplace; they may offer one or more of these types of plans.

# PAYMENT FOR OCCUPATIONAL THERAPY SERVICES

Health care policy specifies the various services that people are eligible for, including occupational therapy. Most services today are offered via health insurance companies that are managed care systems. Managed care is a health care delivery system organized to manage cost, utilization, and quality. Services are offered according to different plans, including preferred provider organizations (PPOs), health maintenance organizations (HMOs), and point-of-service (PoS) plans, which are a combination of a PPO and HMO. See Table 41-1 for more information about basic managed care/health insurance. Occupational therapy services may be paid for directly by the client, but are typically paid for by a third-party payer. A third-party payer is a managed care company (i.e., a health insurance agency), which could be public or private. To a certain extent, third-party payers define the scope of occupational therapy by identifying what services they will pay for (Howard, 1991). Third-party payers emphasize cost control, effectiveness, and efficiency that lead to critical examination of interventions by the therapists and interventions. There are even some that argue that reimbursement systems shape practice more powerfully than theory (Howard, 1991; Jongbloed & Wendland, 2002). Therefore, understanding the way that third-party payers such as Medicare, Medicaid, health insurance marketplace, workers' compensation, Individuals with Disability Education Act (IDEA), and private health insurance reimburse occupational therapy services is critical for practitioners to optimally provide services and maximize benefits.

## *Documentation and Coding*

All payers require that health care providers justify and communicate the services provided using specific documentation. As noted in the chapter on documentation (Chapter 23), written documentation is the true and legal record of the occupational therapy evaluation, plan of care, interventions, and outcomes. It is a tool to support and manage reimbursement (Holms & Clark, 2014).

Effective documentation is part of our ethical obligations, as stated in the AOTA's (2015a) *Occupational Therapy Code of Ethics.* Principle 4.O. of the *Code of Ethics* states that occupational therapy personnel shall "ensure that documentation for reimbursement purposes is done in accordance with applicable laws, guidelines, and regulations." (p. 6). AOTA's (2010) *Standards of Practice for Occupational Therapy* states that an occupational therapy practitioner documents the occupational therapy services and "abides by the time frames, format, and standards established by the practice settings, government agencies, external accreditation programs, payers, and AOTA documents" (p. S108). These requirements apply to both electronic and written forms of documentation. Documentation should reflect the nature of services provided and the clinical reasoning of the occupational therapy practitioner, and it should provide enough information to ensure that services are delivered in a safe and effective manner (AOTA, 2013).

The majority of third-party payers request the use of specific diagnostic and procedural codes as part of the documentation. Different types of codes are used to communicate diagnoses and interventions with different payers. The *International Classification of Diseases, 10th Revision, Clinical Modification* (ICD-10-CM) is the diagnosis code set used to report diagnoses in all clinical settings, typically assigned by a physician (and not an occupational therapist). The *International Classification of Diseases, 10th Revision, Procedure Coding System* (ICD-10-PCS) is the procedure code set used to report hospital inpatient procedures only. Current Procedural Terminology (CPT) and Healthcare Common Procedure Coding System (HCPCS) are used to report services and procedures in outpatient and office settings (American Medical Association, n.d.). Although the physician must assign the medical diagnosis code, occupational therapists may provide treatment diagnosis codes and should include codes to the greatest level of specificity possible. The codes are used to support medical necessity in documentation, which is essential to reflect the value of skilled services and can affect whether the payer reimburses the claim (AOTA, 2015c). It is recommended that you consult with a local workplace billing specialist to learn about how to use the most appropriate codes to describe the services provided to a client. The AOTA offers many resources on the association's website and in workshops to help practitioners with these decisions.

Health care coverage offered under different programs varies immensely and changes constantly. Consequently, occupational therapy practitioners must take the time to learn about each client's individual coverage and stay up to date with changes. The following sections provide an overview of the major reimbursement options and suggest helpful resources to empower occupational therapists to obtain the knowledge they need to understand and maximize proper utilization of their clients' health medical coverage to provide services that are appropriate and affordable. Note that this is not an exhaustive description of each payment option, and that each practitioner is expected to inquire regarding his or her unique setting. Helpful resources are listed at the end of the chapter.

## Medicare

Medicare, Title XVIII of the Social Security Act enacted in 1965, is the U.S. federal health insurance program for people who are 65 or older, certain younger people with disabilities, and people with end-stage renal disease (Centers for Medicare and Medicaid Services [CMS], 2015a). On its 50th anniversary in 2015, more than 55 million Americans were covered by Medicare (CMS, 2015c), making it the principal financier of health care in the United States, and as such, it has a major influence on the health care system (Sandstrom, Lohman, & Bramble, 2014). The enactment and subsequent amendments of the Medicare act have had significant influences on the development of the occupational therapy profession and our role in hospitals, skilled nursing facilities, hospice, and outpatient practices (Lohman, 2014). Medicare legislation continues to change in a way that directly affects occupational therapy services, including where they can be offered, who is eligible to provide them, what specific services are covered, and the amount that will be reimbursed.

Medicare reimburses skilled occupational therapy services that are reasonable and necessary, according to specific guidelines determined by law or by the payer. Skilled services mean that the intervention requires the unique professional abilities of an occupational therapy practitioner. Occupational therapists prove their skills by obtaining a national and state licensure and in some cases additional specific certifications. All providers that bill under Medicare must obtain a National Provider Identification number from the CMS. Medicare coverage is limited to items and services that are reasonable and necessary for the diagnosis or treatment of an illness or injury, and are within the scope of a Medicare benefit category. National Coverage Determinations are made through an evidence-based process conducted by the CMS, information from the public, and data from the Medicare Evidence Development and Coverage Advisory Committee. In the absence of a national coverage policy, an item or service may be covered at the discretion of the Medicare contractors based on a local coverage determination (CMS, 2015a). Therefore, it is important for us as professionals to be informed of what has been established as evidence based, and continue to demonstrate the value of our services by collecting evidence to demonstrate our distinct value (Lamb & Metzler, 2014).

Medicare is managed regionally via intermediaries, which are insurance companies contracted to review and manage Medicare expenditures. Facility billing may go to the regional intermediary, so there is a possible range of interpretation of reimbursement rules for Medicare based on each intermediary (Holms & Clark, 2014).

Medicare includes four parts that specify different health care coverage and benefits, as follows.

- **Medicare Part A (hospital insurance):** All Medicare enrollees are covered under Part A. This part covers inpatient hospital stays, care in a skilled nursing facility, hospice care, and some home health care. In these settings, services are reimbursed at a predetermined rate system that classifies client conditions into categories. These groups are based on how much medical care a person usually needs given each particular diagnosis. The payment is to cover the usual and customary services for the person according to his or her diagnosis and condition. Occupational therapy services are part of the bundle of services. Table 41-2 presents detail regarding the different classification groups used for each setting.
- **Medicare Part B (medical insurance):** Part B covers certain health services and outpatient care including occupational therapy, medical supplies (including durable medical equipment), and preventive services. Part B will not cover all people who have Medicare Part A. Even with the coverage, the client is responsible for 20% of the costs after the deductible is met. The amount of reimbursement for services rendered under Part B is limited by therapy caps. The therapy cap limit for 2015 was $1,940 for occupational therapy. However, when therapy services are medically reasonable and necessary, the provider can apply for an exceptions process. As part of the exceptions process, there are additional limits (called *thresholds*). If outpatient therapy services are higher than the threshold amounts, a Medicare contractor may review relevant medical records to check for medical necessity. The threshold amount for occupational therapy in 2015 was $3,700 (Medicare.gov, n.d.). If a provider thought there was a need to offer services that were not covered, then he or she was required to provide the client with a written notice, called an Advance Beneficiary Notice of Noncoverage, before providing generally covered therapy services that are not medically reasonable and necessary according to Medicare for the client at the time. This allows the client to choose whether he or she wants the therapy services. Remember that providing uncovered services may result in significant financial stress for the client and/or the practice.
- **Medicare Part C (Medicare Advantage plans):** This is a type of Medicare health plan offered by a private company that contracts with Medicare to provide the client with all Part A and Part B benefits. Medicare Advantage Plans include HMOs, PPOs, private fee-for-service plans, special needs plans, and Medicare medical savings account plans. Enrollment in a Medicare Advantage plan typically means that Medicare services are covered through the plan and are not paid for under original Medicare. Most Medicare Advantage plans offer prescription drug coverage.
- **Medicare Part D (prescription drug coverage):** Part D adds prescription drug coverage to plans offered by insurance companies and other private companies approved by Medicare. Medicare Advantage Plans may also offer prescription drug coverage that follows the same rules as Medicare prescription drug plans.

One of the main challenges of working with Medicare is that funding and guidelines are highly intricate and constantly changing. In the past, the AOTA supported legislative efforts underway at the time of the writing of this chapter to reform Medicare Part B payment policies to provide stability to Medicare beneficiaries and providers and ensure that the program could meet the health and therapy needs of its beneficiaries. Updates are provided via the AOTA Legislative Action Center online and biweekly in the Capital Briefing section in *OT Practice Magazine*.

## Medicaid and Children's Health Insurance Program

Medicaid and Children's Health Insurance Program (CHIP) provide free or low-cost health coverage to millions of Americans, including some low-income people, families and children, pregnant women, the elderly, and people with disabilities. Medicaid is the largest source of funding for medical and health-related services for low-income people in the United States. It is a means-tested program, and eligibility is determined by that test. It is jointly funded by the state and federal governments and managed by the states, with each state currently having broad leeway to determine who is eligible for its implementation of the program. CHIP provides low-cost health coverage to children in families that earn too much money to qualify for Medicaid. In some states, CHIP covers parents and pregnant women. Each state offers CHIP coverage, and works closely with its state Medicaid program. The ACA significantly expanded both eligibility for and federal funding of Medicaid. Under the law, all U.S. citizens and legal residents with income up to 133% of the poverty line, including adults without dependent children, would qualify for coverage in any state that participated in the Medicaid program. States are not required to participate in the program, yet currently all states do.

Individual states establish and administer their own Medicaid programs and determine the type, amount, duration, and scope of services within broad federal

Table 41-2.

**MEDICARE BASIC TERMS**

| Legislation | Service Location | Term | Explanation |
|---|---|---|---|
| Medicare Part A | Acute hospital setting | Diagnosis-Related Groups (DRGs) | Patients can be assigned to a DRG based on their diagnosis, surgical procedures, age, and other information. Hospitals provide this information on their bills, and Medicare uses this information to decide how much the hospitals should be paid. The DRGs reflect the amount of medical care needed by a person with a particular diagnosis. |
| | | Inpatient Prospective Payment System (IPPS) | The base payment rate is divided into a labor-related and non-labor share. The labor-related share is adjusted by the wage index applicable to the area where the hospital is located, and if the hospital is located in Alaska or Hawaii, the non-labor share is adjusted by a cost of living adjustment factor. This base payment rate is multiplied by the DRG relative weight. |
| | Inpatient rehabilitation facility | Case Mix Groups (CMGs) | CMGs classify client discharges into rate system categories to determine reimbursement, based on rehabilitation impairment categories, functional state (both motor and cognitive), age, and other comorbidities. |
| | Skilled nursing facility | Minimum Data Set (MDS) | The MDS is part of the federally mandated process for clinical assessment of all residents in Medicare and Medicaid certified nursing homes. This process provides a comprehensive assessment of each resident's functional capabilities and helps nursing home staff identify health problems and needed resources. |
| | | Resource Utilization Groups (RUG) | A patient classification system that categorizes skilled nursing home patients by functional status and anticipated use of services and resources. The RUG score is used to determine a per diem rate of reimbursement. |
| | | Prospective Payment System (PPS) | With the onset of PPS, payments were made based on a daily rate (per diem). |
| | Inpatient rehabilitation facility, home health | Case Mix Groups | A patient classification system to group patients with similar characteristics and in terms of resources used during care. |
| Medicare Part A or B | Home health | Outcome and Assessment Information Set | Sets the payment rate for each 60 days of service; rates are based on skilled need. |
| Medicare Part B | Outpatient care | Medicare Physician Fee Schedule | Each individual service is coded, reported, and reimbursed accordingly. |
| | | National Provider Identifier (NPI) | Practitioners who have private practices with Medicare reimbursement must apply for an NPI to submit payment requests. Proof of a practitioner's credentials is needed to obtain NPI. |

guidelines. States are required to cover certain mandatory benefits and can choose to provide other optional benefits through the Medicaid program (Medicaid.gov, n.d.). Occupational therapy is an optional benefit, which means that not all states cover occupational therapy services. When applicable, Medicaid funds can be used to cover services through managed care delivery systems, long-term care services in home and community settings, in institutional settings, telehealth services (see Chapter 39), or together with services provided under IDEA as will be discussed later in this chapter. The Kaiser Family Foundation website provides a helpful chart describing each state coverage (http://kff.org/medicaid/state-indicator/occupational-therapy-services/).

## Private Insurance and Health Care Marketplace

Since January 1, 2014, consumers and small businesses have had access to new health insurance marketplaces (or exchanges). Consumers in the 50 states and District of

Columbia are able to buy qualified health plans available through their state's marketplace, and about 18 million Americans may be eligible for tax credits to help pay for their health insurance (CMS, 2015b). States operate their own marketplaces (state-based marketplace) or a state partnership marketplace, in partnership with the federal marketplace. A partnership marketplace allows states to make key decisions and tailor their marketplaces to local needs and market conditions. The federal government is operating a marketplace in those states that did not establish their own (CMS, 2013). The marketplace plans are made for people who do not have health insurance through a job, Medicare, Medicaid, CHIP, or another source that provides qualifying coverage. Some small businesses elect to offer their employees health insurance through the marketplace.

Insurance companies help consumers manage their risk. In exchange for a constant stream of premiums, insurance companies offer to pay consumers a sum of money upon the occurrence of a predetermined event, such as a natural catastrophe, a car crash, or a health care visit. In other words, a large group of people make small routine contributions to a big pot with the guarantee that if they need a larger sum of money to cover a specific event they will be able to pull it out of that pot, under specific circumstances.

Private insurance companies within a range of prices and features offer the different plans. All plans cover essential health benefits including habilitative services, preexisting conditions, pregnancy, and preventive care. A dental plan may be added as well. To encourage enrollment in a health plan, people who do not have coverage in 2017 will pay a penalty.

Occupational therapy is not consistently defined and paid for across plans or within specific companies. Health care insurance plans, whether publicly or privately funded, consist of contracts that specify the rules or conditions under which they will cover an array of services.

Payers often impose limitations or restrictions on covered services and payment. Thomas (2002) suggests the following questions to obtain information necessary for the occupational therapist to provide the optimal covered care and to assist clients in making decisions about continuing care that their insurance may not cover. Practitioners should inquire for each client's health plan:

- What is the plan's definition of occupational therapy?
- Are there limitations in number of visits, sites at which services may be received, or yearly costs incurred for occupational therapy services?
- Is there a network of providers that an occupational therapist must join to bill? Can a patient "opt out" of the network, and if so, what financial disincentives may exist?
- Does the plan offer case management services for some conditions?

### Health Insurance Terms

**Coverage:** A certain service that would be reimbursed under the policy. However, merely having coverage does not mean that all expenses are paid in full. Most often, the client will be responsible for some portion of the health care fees according to their specific health plan.

**Reimbursement:** Paying someone back. It could be paying back a person who made a payment (a client) or someone who rendered services (a practitioner).

**Premium:** The cost one pays each month for insurance.

**Deductible:** A certain amount of money that one needs to pay out of pocket, which may have to occur before he or she begins to receive reimbursement for services. Some people may be unaware of the need to pay the deductible before their coverage begins to take effect.

**Copay:** A flat fee (e.g., $15) paid for every office visit.

**Coinsurance:** A percent of the charges for care (e.g., 20%).

- Does the plan pay a fee for service or is payment for occupational therapy "bundled" into a group of services (e.g., a set amount for all rehabilitation services)?
- Does the payer require specific credentials for occupational therapists?
- Does the payer require that the therapist or health care facility or clinic join a provider network?
- Is the client responsible for copayments, deductibles, or other out-of-pocket expenses? Under what circumstances?

Thomas (2002) reminds us that therapy departments and practices must develop expertise in multiple payer requirements for such issues as network enrollment, coding, billing, and appeals, to be able to provide their clinical expertise. AOTA's Private Practice Packet at www.aota.org provides many helpful resources for work with insurance companies.

Remember that insurance policies change every year. It is important to stay informed and inquire about changes that can affect occupational therapy services.

## Military Health Care

The U.S. Department of Defense and the U.S. Department of Veterans Affairs (VA) operate as two of the largest health care organizations in the nation serving active duty personnel, retirees, survivors, and their dependents. Components of the system include Army, Air Force, and Navy military treatment facilities, and the TRICARE program, which offers both managed care and fee-for-service options for almost 9.5 million beneficiaries worldwide (Development Health Clinical Center, n.d.). On October 1, 2013, the U.S. Department of Defense established the Defense Health Agency to manage the activities of the military health system. The military has developed the most comprehensive medical record in the U.S. health system, including the master client record, which travels with the enlistee (Holms & Clark, 2014). Should a health issue become long term and the enlistee cannot return to active duty, the individual receives a medical discharge and is referred to the VA. The VA is the single largest employer of occupational therapists, with a wide range of clinical care practice settings (U.S. Department of Veterans Affairs, n.d.-a). VA facilities have experienced a 50% growth in the number of their enrollees between 2002 and 2014, as aging veterans have developed medical issues (U.S. Department of Veterans Affairs, n.d.-b).

## School Systems and Early Intervention

The Individuals with Disabilities Education Improvement Act of 2004 (P.L. 108-446), and the Elementary and Secondary Education Act, also known as the No Child Left Behind Act of 2001 (P.L. 107-110), regulate occupational therapy services offered at school systems and in early interventions.

IDEA is a United States federal law that governs how states and public agencies provide early intervention, special education, and related services to children with disabilities ages 0 to 21 to ensure free appropriate public education that is tailored to their individual needs. IDEA is an evolution of the Education of All Handicapped Children Act of 1975 and was improved and amended multiple times since. Part B of the law specifies that students with disabilities must have access to occupational therapy if they need it to benefit from special education (Rep Castle, 2003). This section was the original stimulus for school-based occupational therapy. In 1986, the early intervention program for ages 0 to 3 years was added to the legislation and became Part C with the reauthorization of IDEA in 1997. Part C of the IDEA names occupational therapy as a primary service to collaborate with early childhood and school teams to promote the physical, communication, cognitive, adaptive, and social-emotional domains of infants and toddlers (AOTA Response to Intervention Workgroup, 2012). The 2004 amendments extended the availability of occupational therapy services to all students, not just those with disabilities, to fully participate in school.

The No Child Left Behind Act was passed by the U.S. Congress in 2001. This act requires schools to improve the academic achievement of all students, including those with disabilities, and describes the role of occupational therapy practitioners in supporting children and youth by promoting participation in home, school, and community life (AOTA Response to Intervention Workgroup, 2012).

IDEA specifies that services to eligible children are rendered according to the child's Individualized Education Program (IEP), for children 3 to 21 years old or the Individualized Family Service Plan (IFSP), for children 0 to 3 years old. The IEP is designed to meet the unique educational needs of that one child in the least restrictive environment appropriate to the needs of that child. It is formulated by an interprofessional team that often includes an occupational therapist. The IFSP focuses on the needs of the child and family. Funding for these services is jointly provided by federal, state, and districts, and therefore may change (Lohman, 2014). Medicaid or a specific state medical assistance program may cover some services that are provided at the school or by early intervention services. In these cases, occupational therapy practitioners submit specific documentation to the districts that bill the respective Medicare agencies.

## Uninsured People

Although ACA has made significant improvements, there are still many people who do not have access to coverage through a job, and some people, particularly poor adults in states that did not expand Medicaid, remain ineligible for public coverage (Kaiser Family Foundation, 2015b). Additionally, undocumented immigrants are ineligible for Medicaid or marketplace coverage. Most of the remaining uninsured people are in low-income working families that earn too much to be eligible for the subsidized coverage. In 2014, more than 8 in 10 were in a family with a worker. Non-Whites were at higher risk of being uninsured than non-Hispanic Whites. In 2014, 48% of uninsured adults said the main reason they were uninsured was because the cost was too high (Kaiser Family Foundation, 2015b).

Going without health coverage can have serious health consequences for the uninsured because they receive less preventive care, and delayed care often results in more serious illness requiring more advanced treatment. The uninsured are generally less healthy as compared to those with private coverage. The uninsured are at higher risk for preventable hospitalizations and for missed diagnoses of serious health conditions. The lack of care results in significantly higher mortality rates for the uninsured than those with insurance (Truglio et al., 2012; Wilper et al., 2009). To date, only emergency departments are required by federal law to screen and stabilize all individuals. Health providers can choose to not provide care to the uninsured. However, many providers pursue ways to enable uninsured people to pay and receive services by offering payment plans or seeking grants. Practitioners should learn about their communities and supports that are available. Community religious or fraternal organizations can offer financial support to people with significant health care needs. Contact with local agencies such as the United Way can inform the practitioner of myriad community offerings (Holms & Clark, 2014).

## Meaning for the Practice of Occupational Therapy

Some would say that reimbursement shapes practice more powerfully than theory (Jongbloed & Wendland, 2002). From the historical and public health perspectives, reimbursement issues resulted in many changes in practice over the years. The push to move care from acute hospital settings to other (less expensive) levels of care has significantly shortened the length of stay in acute settings. This shift has also increased the medical acuity of clients moving on to skilled or rehabilitative care, home health care, and even nursing home care. Occupational therapy practitioners have had to learn new skills, reflect on practice, and adapt to new documentation as these changes have infiltrated their workplaces (Holms & Clark, 2014).

Among the ethical dilemmas that result from reimbursement issues is a situation in which individuals who require or could benefit from occupational therapy services cannot and will not receive them since there is no coverage for these services. A demand to keep occupational therapy services financially sustainable leads to concerns from practitioners working in health care settings. Occupational therapy practitioners describe administrative pressures for productivity and revenue that conflict with independent clinical judgment for appropriate patient care (AOTA, American Physical Therapy Association, American Speech-Language-Hearing Association, n.d.). Occupational therapy practitioners need to stay informed and current regarding their code of ethics and state and federal regulations regarding practice and reimbursement to be able to manage these conflicts effectively. State and national occupational therapy associations are aware of these issues, and representatives may offer helpful guidance and support.

However, external demands and restrictions have also resulted in improvements of the efficiency of our occupational therapy practices. Managed care has resulted in a reduced number of therapy sessions, and the need to show results and change. This has motivated therapists to carefully examine what they are doing, to do efficient evaluations, and to work quickly. Patients today are discharged from hospitals as soon as possible, with an emphasis on treatment in the community and homes, focused on function and on outcomes. Family members and occupational therapy assistants assume more responsibility for the interventions (Walker, 2001). As part of our professional survival, occupational therapists must stay current, relevant, and demonstrate results and potential of our work. As part of our pursuit to meet the needs of our communities, we need to take part in the forefront of health care by expanding and strengthening our evidence-based practice to advocate and demonstrate the importance of our role in current and emerging practice niches, such as telehealth and habilitation services (see the Evidence-Based Research Chart).

### Case Study 1

Amy is a 3-year-old girl with significant developmental delays. Although there are many signs that might indicate autism spectrum disorder, Amy's parents are hesitating to accept an autism spectrum disorder diagnosis because they think it will be considered an uncovered preexisting condition. Carrie, a private practice occupational therapist, decided to investigate this issue to determine if there is a risk of denied coverage due to autism spectrum disorder. Researching documents from the National Conference of State Legislatures, she found that 37 states and the District of Columbia have laws related to autism and insurance coverage, at different coverage rates. She also discovered that the ACA has made the coverage of all preexisting conditions mandatory. Carrie advised the parents to discuss their concerns with their employer's benefits manager and also contact their state's department of insurance. For more information, see: http://www.ncsl.org/research/health/autism-and-insurance-coverage-state-laws.aspx.

## Summary

Our greatest professional commitment is to our clients for whom we provide services with a promise of best practices. However, without mindfulness regarding funding for these services, they will not be available. It is therefore the occupational therapy practitioner's responsibility to stay well informed, to provide services thoughtfully and responsibly, and to have the confidence to ask questions about reimbursement. It is also essential that each professional be committed to the standards of practice set by the AOTA and be knowledgeable about optimizing the use of evidence-based interventions (Holms & Clark, 2014). Awareness, adherence, and promotion of policy issues can be best facilitated by engaging with state and national membership associations. These groups advocate for the profession and provide education regarding reimbursement considerations, best practices, and how to make these work together for the benefit of our clients.

## Evidence-Based Research Chart

| Topic | Relevance | Source |
|---|---|---|
| Emerging opportunities within health care policy | The use of evidence to define and promote the position of the profession with consideration of different opportunities that exist with current health care policy | Lamb & Metzler, 2014; Leland, Crum, Phipps, Roberts, & Gage, 2015 |
| Habilitation services | Information about essential Health Benefits Rule including habilitation and the advocacy process to include occupational therapy as a habilitation provider | Brown, 2014 |
| Telehealth | Evidence to support telehealth as an integral component in achieving the goals of current care policy, and the role of occupational therapy | Cason, 2015 |
| Client-centered care | Key issues in client-centered care and research within the health care reform | Mroz, Pitonyak, Fogelberg, & Leland, 2015 |

### Case Study 2

Jacob is an occupational therapist working with Mr. Smith in a skilled nursing facility. Mr. Smith is diagnosed with advanced stages of dementia. Although there is no expectation for functional improvement, Mr. Smith can benefit from skilled occupational therapy to maintain some of his existing skills such as certain self-care and mobility capacities. Jacob was concerned that these maintenance goals will not be deemed reasonable and appropriate by Medicare and therefore will not be covered. Jacob consulted with his supervisor who informed him that as of December 2013, Medicare covers skilled maintenance services. This revision resulted from the Jimmo vs. Sebelius settlement that was approved on January 24, 2013 after a fairness hearing, marking a critical step for thousands of beneficiaries nationwide. The settlement stipulates that skilled services to maintain an individual's condition or prevent or slow his or her decline are covered by Medicare. Following the settlement, the CMS revised its benefit policy manual and numerous other policies, guidelines, and instructions to ensure that Medicare coverage is available for skilled maintenance services in the home health, nursing home, and outpatient settings. Jacob was pleased to learn that he could provide Mr. Smith with needed services and was also excited to learn how policy can be changed according to court rulings. Read more about it at http://www.medicareadvocacy.org/medicare-info/improvement-standard.

## Student Self-Assessment

1. Explore your own or a family member's insurance policy. Can you understand it? Does the policy provide for occupational therapy service reimbursement? Try to answer the questions posed by Thomas (2002).
2. Explore the following websites: http://www.state.gov/policy/ and http://www.aota.org/Advocacy-Policy/Congressional-Affairs/Legislative-Issues-Update.aspx.
   - What are current public policy issues in the United States? Identify three of these policies and describe how they affect you or your practice directly.
   - How can you become involved to promote policies that will support yourself and your clients?

## Electronic Resources

American Occupational Therapy Association: http://www.aota.org/Advocacy-Policy.aspx

Centers for Medicare and Medicaid Services: https://www.cms.gov/

Healthcare.gov Glossary: https://www.healthcare.gov/glossary/

Henry J. Kaiser Family Foundation: http://kff.org/

Medicaid: http://www.medicaid.gov

Medicare: https://www.medicare.gov

U.S. Department of Education: idea.ed.gov

U.S. Department of Health and Human Services: www.HHS.gov

## References

American Medical Association. (n.d.). *ICD-10 frequently asked questions*. Retrieved from http://www.ama-assn.org/ama/pub/physician-resources/solutions-managing-your-practice/coding-billing-insurance/hipaahealth-insurance-portability-accountability-act/transaction-code-set-standards/icd10-code-set/icd10-faq.page

American Occupational Therapy Association. (n.d.-a). *Congressional affairs*. Retrieved from http://www.aota.org/Advocacy-Policy/Congressional-Affairs.aspx

American Occupational Therapy Association. (n.d.-b). *Health care reform implementation*. Retrieved from http://www.aota.org/Advocacy-Policy/Health-Care-Reform.aspx

American Occupational Therapy Association. (2010). Standards of practice for occupational therapy. *American Journal of Occupational Therapy, 64*(Suppl. 6), S106-S111.

American Occupational Therapy Association. (2013). *The reference manual of the official documents of the American Occupational Therapy Association, Inc.* (18th ed.). Bethesda, MD: AOTA Press.

American Occupational Therapy Association. (2014). Occupational therapy practice framework: Domain and process (3rd ed.). *American Journal of Occupational Therapy, 68*(Suppl. 1), S1-S48. doi:10.5014/ajot.2014.682006

American Occupational Therapy Association. (2015a). Occupational therapy code of ethics (2015). *American Journal of Occupational Therapy, 69*(Suppl. 3), S1-S10.

American Occupational Therapy Association. (2015b, September 15). *Occupational therapy practitioners headed to Capitol Hill.* Retrieved from http://www.aota.org/Publications-News/ForTheMedia/PressReleases/2015/091415-HillDayAdvisory.aspx

American Occupational Therapy Association. (2015c). *Federal and regulatory affairs; ICD-10 Codes: Resources for diagnosis coding and transition from ICD-9.* Retrieved from http://www.aota.org/Advocacy-Policy/Federal-Reg-Affairs/ICD-10-Diagnosis-Coding.aspx

American Occupational Therapy Association, American Physical Therapy Association, American Speech-Language-Hearing Association (n.d.). *Consensus statement on clinical judgment in health care settings.* Retrieved from http://www.aota.org/Practice/Ethics/Consensus-Statement-AOTA-APTA-ASHA.aspx

American Occupational Therapy Association Response to Intervention Workgroup. (2012). *AOTA practice advisory on occupational therapy in response to intervention.* Retrieved from https://www.aota.org/-/media/Corporate/Files/Practice/Children/Browse/School/RtI/AOTA%20RtI%20Practice%20Adv%20final%20%20101612.pdf

Birkland, T. A. (2014). *An introduction to the policy process: Theories, concepts and models of public policy making.* New York, NY: Routledge.

Brown, D. (2014). Habilitative services: An essential health benefit and an opportunity for occupational therapy practitioners and consumers. *Journal of Occupational Therapy, 68*(2), 130-138. doi:10.5014/ajot.2014.682001

Cason, J. (2015). Telehealth and occupational therapy: Integral to the triple aim of health care reform. *American Journal of Occupational Therapy, 69*(2), 6902090010p1-8. doi:10.5014/ajot.2015.692003

Centers for Medicare and Medicaid Services. (2013). *Federal marketplace progress fact sheet.* Retrieved from https://www.cms.gov/CCIIO/Resources/Fact-Sheets-and-FAQs/ffe.html

Centers for Medicare and Medicaid Services. (2015a). *Medicare coverage determination process.* Retrieved from https://www.cms.gov/Medicare/Coverage/DeterminationProcess/

Centers for Medicare and Medicaid Services. (2015b). *State health insurance marketplaces.* Retrieved from https://www.cms.gov/CCIIO/Resources/Fact-Sheets-and-FAQs/state-marketplaces.html

Centers for Medicare and Medicaid Services. (2015c). *On its 50th anniversary, more than 55 million Americans covered by Medicare.* Retrieved from https://www.cms.gov/Newsroom/MediaReleaseDatabase/Press-releases/2015-Press-releases-items/2015-07-28.html

Development Health Clinical Center. (n.d.). *DoD/VA Healthcare Services.* Retrieved from http://www.pdhealth.mil/hss/healthcare_services.asp

Dimond, B. C. (2011). *Legal aspects of occupational therapy.* West Sussex, United Kingdom: John Wiley and Sons.

Holms, D. E., & Clark, L. (2014). Laws, credentials, and reimbursement. In K. Jacobs, N. MacRae, & K. Sladyk (Eds.), *Occupational therapy essentials for clinical competence* (2nd ed.). Thorofare, NJ: SLACK Incorporated.

Howard, B. S. (1991). How high do we jump? The effect of reimbursement on occupational therapy. *American Journal of Occupational Therapy, 45*(10), 875-881.

Jongbloed, L., & Wendland, T. (2002). The impact of reimbursement systems on occupational therapy practice in Canada and the United States of America. *Canadian Journal of Occupational Therapy, 69*(3), 143-152.

Kaiser Family Foundation. (2015a). *Medicaid delivery system and payment reform: a guide to key terms and concepts.* Retrieved from http://kff.org/medicaid/fact-sheet/medicaid-delivery-system-and-payment-reform-a-guide-to-key-terms-and-concepts/

Kaiser Family Foundation. (2015b). *Key facts about the uninsured population.* Retrieved from http://kff.org/uninsured/fact-sheet/key-facts-about-the-uninsured-population/

Lamb, A. J., & Metzler, C. A. (2014). Defining the value of occupational therapy: A health policy lens on research and practice. *American Journal of Occupational Therapy, 68*(1), 9-14.

Leland, N. E., Crum, K., Phipps, S., Roberts, P., & Gage, B. (2015). Advancing the value and quality of occupational therapy in health service delivery. *American Journal of Occupational Therapy, 69*(1), 6901090010p1-7. doi:10.5014/ajot.2015.691001

Lohman, H. (2014). Payment for services in the United States. In B. A. Boyt Schell, M. Scaffa, G. Gillen, & E. Cohn (Eds.), *Willard and Spackman's occupational therapy* (12th ed.). Baltimore, MD: Lippincott Williams and Wilkins.

Medicaid.gov. (n.d.). *Benefits.* Retrieved from http://www.medicaid.gov/medicaid-chip-program-information/by-topics/benefits/medicaid-benefits.html

Medicare.gov. (n.d.). *Physical therapy/occupational therapy/speech-language pathology services.* Retrieved from https://www.medicare.gov/coverage/pt-and-ot-and-speech-language-pathology.html

Mroz, T. M., Pitonyak, J. S., Fogelberg, D., & Leland, N. E. (2015). Client centeredness and health reform: Key issues for occupational therapy. *American Journal of Occupational Therapy, 69*(5), 6905090010p1-8. doi:10.5014/ajot.2015.695001

Rep Castle, M. N. (2003). *H.R.1350: Individuals with Disabilities Education Improvement Act of 2004.* Retrieved from http://thomas.loc.gov/cgi-bin/bdquery/z?d108:HR01350:@@@L&summ2=m&

Rosenbaum, S. (2011). The Patient Protection and Affordable Care Act: Implications for public health policy and practice. *Public Health Reports, 126*(1), 130-135.

Sandstrom, R., Lohman, H., & Bramble, J. D. (2014). *Health services: Policy and systems for therapists.* New York, NY: Pearson Higher Education, Inc.

Switzer, J. V. (2003). Disabled policy making/disabled policy. In J. V. Switzer (Ed.), *Disabled rights: American disability policy and the fight for equality.* Washington, DC: Georgetown University Press.

Thomas, J. (2002). Understanding health insurance: Who's paying the bill? *OT Practice Magazine, June 24*, 10.

Truglio, J., Graziano, M., Vedanthan, R., Hahn, S., Rios, C., Hendel-Paterson, B., & Ripp, J. (2012). Global health and primary care: increasing burden of chronic diseases and need for integrated training. *Mount Sinai Journal of Medicine: A Journal of Translational and Personalized Medicine, 79*(4), 464-474.

U.S. Department of Veterans Affairs. (n.d.-a). Become a VA occupational therapist. *Veterans Health Administration.* Retrieved from http://www.vacareers.va.gov/assets/common/print/ot_brochure.pdf

U.S. Department of Veterans Affairs. (n.d.-b). *Selected Veterans Health Administration characteristics: FY2002 to FY2014.* Retrieved from http://www.va.gov/vetdata/

Walker, K. F. (2001). Adjustments to managed health care: Pushing against it, going with it, and making the best of it. *American Journal of Occupational Therapy, 55*(2), 129-137.

Wilper, A. P., Woolhandler, S., Lasser, K. E., McCormick, D., Bor, D. H., & Himmelstein, D. U. (2009). Health insurance and mortality in US adults. *American Journal of Public Health, 99*(12), 2289.

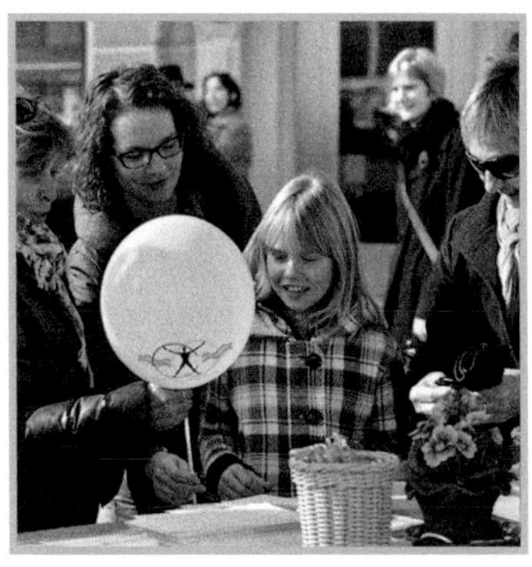

# 42

# Marketing and Management of Occupational Therapy Services

Karen Jacobs, EdD, OTR/L, CPE, FAOTA

**ACOTE STANDARDS EXPLORED IN THIS CHAPTER**

B.6.4, B.6.5, B.7.11, B.9.3

**KEY VOCABULARY**

- **Market:** All actual or potential buyers of a product, service, or idea and can be considered in its entirety.
- **Marketing:** "Marketing is the activity, set of institutions, and processes for creating, communicating, delivering, and exchanging offerings that have value for customers, clients, partners, and society at large" (American Marketing Association, 2013).
- **Promote:** Support or actively encourage; further the progress of something.
- **Promotion strategies:** These can be used to influence the demand for a product or service.
- **Social marketing:** A method used to create activities focused at changing or maintaining people's behavior for the benefit of individuals and society.



Jacobs, K., & MacRae, N. (Eds.).
*Occupational Therapy Essentials for Clinical Competence, Third Edition* (pp. 605-614).

> We are on the verge of an era when the needs for our services are so great as to push us to the brink of glory, if we can only deliver; or we may stumble, because we shall, I fear, cling tenaciously to what we have done without looking at what we might do if we were to take bold new directions. (Cromwell, 1984)

If the concept of marketing had been applied to the profession of occupational therapy over 40 years ago, just imagine how much more of a significant role we may have been playing in the health care marketplace today!

The need for occupational therapy practitioners and students to fully understand and apply the concepts of marketing has become even more critical today.

> We live in a world of limited resources that is technologically complex, economically competitive, and growing more politically accountable with consumer power on the rise. The good news is that this is a world of limitless opportunities for occupational therapy. However, we must work diligently—individually and collectively—to ensure that occupation is recognized as our central construct and to communicate how it shapes and informs our methods and outcomes through infusion in education, research, and practice. We must be aggressive in our support of, and advocacy for, scientific inquiry and pragmatic investigation that build the profession's evidence-based body of knowledge. We must participate in strategic partnerships and interprofessional teams [see Chapter 4] to construct communities where human occupation is recognized as fundamental to quality of life and social participation, as well as central to social, educational, and health care policies in the United States and the global community. We can and will reach this envisioned future. (Jacobs, 2012, p. 652)

We will reach this by understanding and incorporating marketing into our daily activities. Indeed, it will help us reach the 2017 American Occupational Therapy Association's (AOTA) Centennial Vision for the profession: "We envision that occupational therapy is a powerful, widely recognized, science-driven, and evidence-based profession with a globally connected and diverse workforce meeting society's occupational needs" (AOTA, n.d.), as well at the AOTA Distinct Value Statement: "Occupational therapy's distinct value is to improve health and quality of life through facilitating participation and engagement in occupations, the meaningful, necessary, and familiar activities of everyday life. Occupational therapy is client-centered, achieves positive outcomes, and is cost-effective" (AOTA, 2015).

## What Is Marketing?

*Marketing* has been a misunderstood term, most often used synonymously with public relations, selling, fundraising, or development. However, according to marketer Peter Drucker, "The aim of marketing is to make selling superfluous" (Kotler & Murray, 1975).

Marketing consists of meeting people's needs in the most efficient and, therefore, profitable manner (Cromwell, 1984). Kotler and Clarke (1987) defined marketing in the following manner:

> Marketing is the analysis, planning, implementation, and control of carefully formulated programs designed to bring about voluntary exchanges of values with target markets for the purpose of achieving organizational objectives. It relies heavily on designing the organization's offering in terms of the target markets' needs and desires, and on using effective pricing, communication, and distribution to inform, motivate, and service the markets.

Successful marketing planning begins with an idea that serves as the framework for all marketing efforts. It is an orientation that makes satisfying the customer's needs the integrating organizational principle. Although the first impulse of the marketing novice is to design a program, such as a school-based, work-related occupational therapy program, and then look for customers (e.g., adolescents with developmental disabilities), effective marketing dictates that the process be reversed. One first looks at the market and listens carefully to potential customers, and then designs the program to match the needs and desires of these potential customers.

## Marketing Planning

The main benefits of marketing planning can be summarized as follows (Branch, 1962):

- Encourages systematic thinking ahead
- Leads to better coordination of organizational efforts
- Leads to the development of performance standards for control
- Causes the individual/organization to sharpen its guiding objectives and policies
- Results in better preparedness for sudden developments

Marketing planning can be viewed as a three-step process. Figure 42-1 delineates this process with planning as the first step. It encompasses identifying attractive markets and developing marketing strategies and programs. Execution is the second step. It includes carrying out the action programs. The third and final step involves

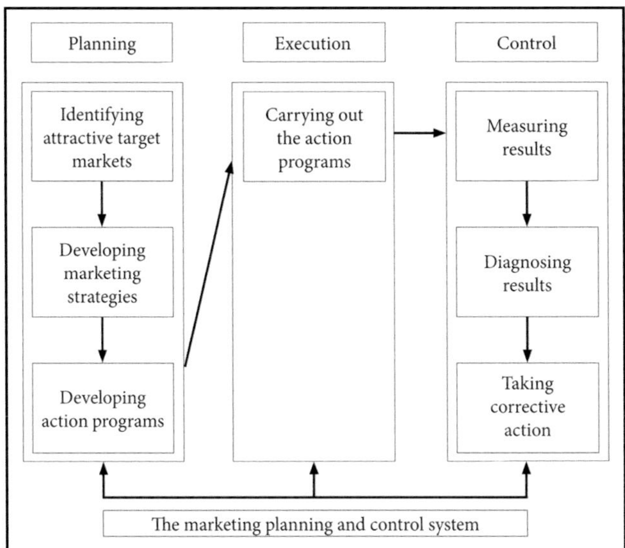


**Figure 42-1.** Example of marketing planning as a three-step process.

marketing control. This final step requires measuring results, analyzing the causes of poor results, and taking corrective action. Adjustments in the plan, its execution, or both would include corrective actions that could be implemented.

# Identifying Attractive Target Markets

Identifying the demands of the market is the first step in marketing. The *market* is defined as all actual or potential buyers of a product, service, or idea and can be considered in its entirety, such as all referral sources to an early intervention program, or divided into relevant segments according to variables, such as types of professionals (e.g., physicians, special education teachers, nurses). Identifying attractive target markets includes the analysis of marketing opportunities. This analysis consists of the following:

- A self-audit
- Consumer analysis
- An analysis of other providers of similar services
- An environmental assessment

## Self-Audit

A self-audit assesses the strengths, weaknesses, opportunities, and threats (SWOT analysis) of your department and/or specific program. Factors to be assessed may include the following:

- The reputation of your facility in the community
- The staff and their qualifications, such as certification as a hand therapist, or board-certified professional ergonomist, or any of the specialty certification available through the AOTA
- Physical size of the program
- Location of the program (e.g., hospital/rehabilitation setting, community-based)
- Convenience of your location to mass transit, highways, and parking
- Type and quality of equipment
- Available budget
- Support from administration. This self-audit assists in understanding how well or poorly prepared you are to meet the marketplace demands. Ascertaining what you do well and maintaining that product (service) at an optimal level is part of marketing.

## Consumer Analysis

It is important to assess the potential consumers of your occupational therapy department's services within your catchment area. An analysis of some of the consumers who might use your products may include the following:

- Physicians
- Rehabilitation managers and consultants
- Other health and rehabilitation professionals
- Nurses
- Vocational counselors
- Special education teachers
- Attorneys
- Business and industry
- Administrators
- Workers with injuries
- Social workers
- Business and industry
- Third-party payers
- Colleagues, such as physical therapists and athletic trainers

## Analysis of Other Providers of Similar Services

How adequately the needs of the marketplace are being met, what areas are not being served, where duplication and overlap are occurring, and where opportunities for collaboration or joint venture exist can be ascertained through an analysis of other providers of similar services. One simple way to obtain information is to place your name on the mailing list of facilities/companies providing a similar product line. Reading through newsletters and brochures from the competition can be insightful. You want to learn as much as possible about the providers of similar services so you can be 10% better or 10% different from them.

## Environmental Assessment

The changes and trends that may have an effect on occupational therapy services and perhaps the future of the profession comprise an environmental assessment. These include the following:

- Demographic variables
- Political and regulatory systems
- Cultural environment
- Economic/financial environment
- Psychographics
- Technological developments

### Demographic Variables

Demographics is the study of human populations according to variables such as age, sex, family size, family life cycle, income, occupation, education, religion, race, and nationality. For example, the increasing number of aging Baby Boomers is a demographic trend that is having an affect on occupational therapy services.

### Political and Regulatory Systems

Both political and regulatory systems may have an affect on occupational therapy services. The Patient Protection and Affordable Care Act of 2010 (P.L. 111-148), Physician Fee Schedule Final Rule for CY 2013, Multiple Procedure Payment Reduction, and the Americans with Disability Act Amendments Act of 2008 (P.L. 110-325) are some examples that affect occupational therapy. Reasonable accommodations are in place so that the individual with a disability can perform the essential functions of the job (U.S. Department of Justice, 2007). You can keep up-to-date on political and regulatory issues as a member of AOTA by going to their website at www.aota.org.

### Cultural Environment

Culture is a force that affects behaviors, values, perceptions, and preferences of individuals within a society. The United States is becoming a more multicultural society, and it is imperative that occupational therapy practitioners and students develop an understanding of and sensitivity to the culture profiles of clients within their catchment area. Having practitioners and students who are bilingual can be most beneficial and may be the variable that assists in making our services even more successful.

### Economic/Financial Environment

An analysis of the economic/financial environment is important because it allows occupational therapy practitioners and students to target occupational therapy services to trends. Some interesting health care trends include the following:

- Compliance with the Affordable Care Act
- Increased number of retail health clinics

The number of U.S. retail health clinics is expected to exceed 2,800 by 2017, increasing 47% since 2014. Walk-in retail clinics, located in pharmacies, retail chains and supermarkets, will add capacity for 25 million patient visits in 2017, up from 16 million in 2014 (Accenture, 2015).

Companies such as Stayhealthy HealthCenter Kiosk are accelerating this trend by providing health kiosks that offer services that would otherwise be provided in a doctor's office. Health kiosks can be used to take basic readings, perform primary care, and even deliver minor urgent care. Schools, worksites, prisons, health clubs, and pharmacies are all potential locations for these kiosks.

### Psychographics

Psychographics is the technique of measuring consumers' social class, lifestyle, and personality characteristics and can provide information on activities, interests, and opinions of these individuals. Understanding the psychographic profile of your clients helps provide information to assist in strategizing products and services to them.

### Technological Developments

The technology arena is greatly advancing and has an almost daily effect on the type of assessment and intervention used by occupational therapy practitioners. Specifically, information technology allows for information to be exchanged in a more efficient manner.

# Selecting Target Markets and Market Segments

Once analysis is completed, there are three steps in target marketing. Market segmentation refers to the act of dividing a market into distinct groups of buyers who might require separate products and marketing mixes. For example, physicians can be segmented into pediatricians or neurologists, and health and rehabilitation professionals can be segmented into speech pathologists, physical therapists, and athletic trainers. Market targeting is the act of evaluating and selecting one or more of the markets to enter. An example of this is targeting orthopedic surgeons as the main referral source for a hand therapy program. Product positioning is the act of formulating a competitive position for the product and a detailed marketing mix.

## Developing Marketing Strategies

Developing marketing strategies includes the development of objectives for each identified target market and its implementation. The 4 P's—product, place, price, and promotion—are the strategies that can be used to influence the demand for a product (Kotler, 1983a; McCarthy, 1999). Here is how each of these P's is used in the marketing mix.

### *Product*

Simply stated, what we do as occupational therapy practitioners is our product. That is, we help people, organizations, and populations through engagement in occupation. Ideally, the goal is to offer a product line—a variety of products associated with one another by an overall theme. For example, an occupational therapy department may have an industrial rehabilitation or occupational health program product line that includes post-offer screening, functional capacity evaluation, and ergonomics consultation. A school-based occupational therapy program may offer a product line identifying assessment accommodations for the Every Student Succeeds Act, which reauthorized the 50-year-old Elementary and Secondary Education Act.

How a product is packaged may influence its success. It is important to make sure all paperwork (e.g., brochures, business cards, stationary, reports) have a professional appearance. The ability to access information quickly and be able to present it in a professional manner to the target markets is an asset.

Many new product ideas are generated by understanding our clients' needs and wants through direct surveys, projective tests, focus group discussions, and letters and complaints received. It is important to note that for every unhappy customer, you lose 50 others, and that 80% of your business is coming from 20% of your customers (Baum & Luebben, 1986).

### *Place*

Occupational therapy services can be provided in a variety of places. Some of these include the following:

- Free-standing facilities located in professional buildings, industrial parks, and shopping centers
- Free-standing facilities affiliated with outpatient service departments, rehabilitation centers, and hospitals
- As part of a comprehensive rehabilitation or acute-care facility/program/hospital
- At worksite programs provided by a company to serve the needs of a specific business or industry
- Schools
- Skilled nursing facilities
- Subacute/transitional care unit

When analyzing the place aspect of marketing planning, other variables that should be considered are the hours the program is offered for business. For example, is your program open during hours convenient to your markets or your staff?

### *Price*

The price or fee schedule for occupational therapy services (products) should be based on cost, competitive factors, geographic area, and what the consumer is willing to pay. It is important for the price to be commensurate with perceived value (Miller & Jacobs, 2007).

### *Promotion*

Promotion is the vehicle of communicating information to your markets about the product's merits, place, and price. Instruments of promotion are advertising, sales promotion, publicity, and personal selling.

#### Advertising

Advertising involves the use of a paid message presented in a recognized medium and by an identified sponsor, with the purpose of informing, persuading, and reminding. Some advertising vehicles include the following:

- Print ads found in newspapers, journals, and magazines
- Brochures
- Direct mail
- Broadcasts
- Transits
- Billboards
- Quarterly newsletters
- Business cards
- Bumper stickers (Figure 42-2)

#### Sales Promotion

Sales promotion is the use of a wide variety of short-term incentives to encourage the purchase of the product. This approach is most effective when used in conjunction

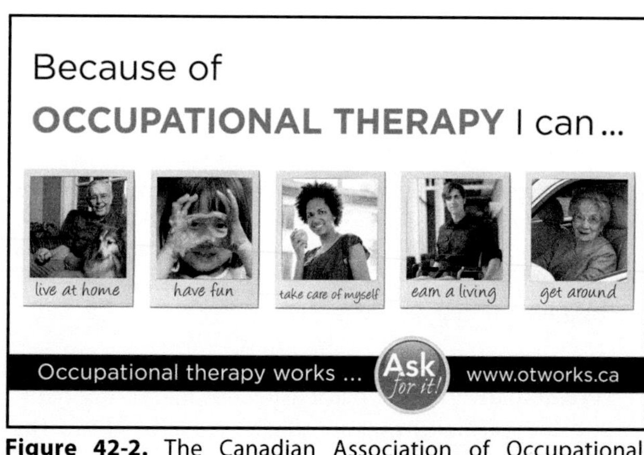


**Figure 42-2.** The Canadian Association of Occupational Therapists (CAOT) promotional campaign. (Reprinted with permission from the Canadian Association of Occupational Therapists.)

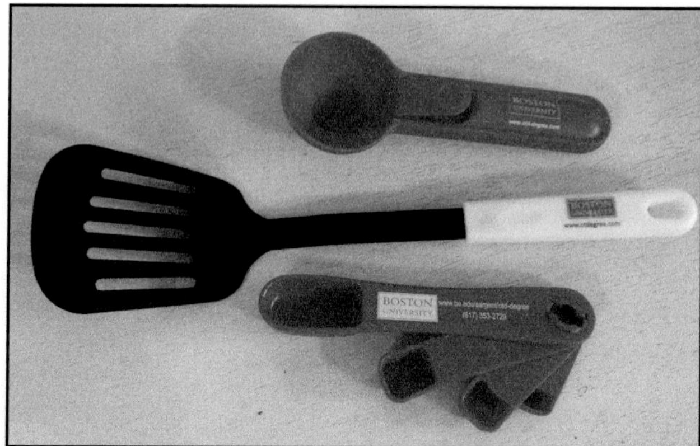


**Figure 42-3.** Examples of sales promotion items that might be given away at a conference.

### Case Study

Since 2000, the AOTA has sponsored National School Backpack Awareness Day on the third Wednesday of September. It is actually one of the most successful and sustainable national promotion initiatives for occupational therapy. Larry is an occupational therapy assistant student enrolled in a course on the analysis and adaptation of occupation. The instructor for the course included an assignment where each student is responsible for planning a National School Backpack Awareness Day event in his or her local community. Larry knows that, as an AOTA member, he can sign up for the AOTA's Backpack Forum on OT Connections at www.otconnections.org. He thinks this will be a good place to network, exchange ideas, and share experiences with other AOTA members participating in National School Backpack Awareness Day. He is considering contacting a local occupational therapy academic program to see if he might collaborate with occupational therapy students to create a weigh-in at a local elementary school.

with advertising. Some examples of sales promotions are pens, pencils, magnets, tote bags, Post-it notes, and mousepads that you might pick up when going into the exhibit halls at your state conference or the annual AOTA conference. Some examples of sales promotions can be seen in Figure 42-3.

For example, at an open house for an occupational therapist in a solo ergonomics practice, a successful sales promotion was giving out mousepads with tips for setting up a computer workstation. Of course, the occupational therapist's contact information was printed on the mousepad, too. In the case study about AOTA's National School Backpack Awareness Day, Larry decided to give out hangtags for backpacks. He will give each child who participates in the backpack weigh-in at a local elementary school a hangtag. The hangtag will promote occupational therapy by having a definition of the profession on the hangtag along with the AOTA's logo and backpack tag line: Pack it Right! Wear it Light! While students are waiting in line to have their backpacks weighed, he will give them a coloring page of the AOTA backpack mascot, OT Rex (see Figure 52-3).

### Publicity

Publicity is often a relatively underused aspect of promotion in relation to the real contribution it can make (Kotler, 1983b). The most positive aspect of publicity is that it is free. However, one has little control over the placement of it and thus it becomes difficult to focus publicity on specific target markets. An example of publicity might be for Larry, the occupational therapy assistant student in the case study, to contact the local newspaper and television and radio stations through submitting a press release about his planned AOTA's National School Backpack Awareness Day event at a local elementary school. He was delighted to find an example of a press release networking on the Backpack Forum on the AOTA OT Connections (Figure 42-4).

If the media finds the event newsworthy and are not understaffed, they will often send a reporter to cover the event. When interacting with a reporter, always share the definition of occupational therapy: Occupational therapy is a health and wellness profession that assists people in developing the skills they need to participate in everyday life where they live, work, and play. Another strategy is to offer to be a resource to them about occupational therapy. Send the reporter(s) your résumé and biosketch for their files (Figure 42-5). Always follow up your interaction with a reporter by sending a thank you via an email, telephone call, or handwritten card or letter. With cards or letters, you should always include two business cards—one for the reporter to keep and the other for him or her to pass along to another person who might be interested in learning more about occupational therapy. It's a "pay it forward" approach.

**News Release**

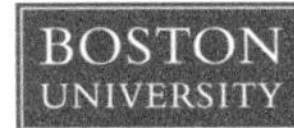


**Boston University** College of Health & Rehabilitation Sciences: Sargent College

**FOR IMMEDIATE RELEASE**:
**CONTACT:** Stephanie Rotondo, (617) 353-7476, rotondos@bu.edu

**BU SARGENT COLLEGE ERGONOMIC EXPERT ASKS STUDENTS 'WHAT'S IN YOUR BACKPACK?'**

***BU Professor Raises Awareness about Health Risks of Overloaded Backpacks***

(Boston) — In honor of National School Backpack Awareness Day™ on Wednesday, September 17, 2014, Dr. Karen Jacobs, a Boston University Sargent College occupational therapy professor and former president of the American Occupational Therapy Association (AOTA), will be conducting "weigh-ins" at a Boston area school to ensure that the weight of kids' backpacks exceeds no more than 10% of their body weight. This annual event helps educate children, parents, school administrators, teachers, and the community about the serious health problems associated with wearing a backpack incorrectly.

Jacobs and 62 graduate OT students from Boston University College of Health and Rehabilitation Sciences: Sargent College will be at the Jackson Mann School in Brighton, MA from 10 a.m. to 11:30 p.m. on September 17th. Jacobs and her graduate students will weigh the backpacks of elementary school students and offer guidance on the best way to wear a backpack. Carrying too much weight in a pack or wearing it the wrong way can lead to aching back and shoulders, weakened muscles, and stooped posture.

"More than 72 million American school children will be wearing a backpack to and from school every day this academic year. And as OT's, we're concerned about the increasingly serious problem posed by improper school backpack use," says Jacobs. "We risk doing long-term damage to our kids' growing bodies by remaining silent on this public health issue."

Jacobs advises minimizing long-term health problems by loading the heaviest items closest to the child's back and arranging books and materials so they won't slide around in the backpack.

Jacobs supports the effectiveness of backpack education. In a study, almost 8 out of 10 middle school children who had been educated on backpack safety subsequently changed how they loaded their backpacks and ultimately, reported less pain and strain in their backs, necks, and shoulders.

Dr. Karen Jacobs is a sought after ergonomics expert who champions backpack and computer safety for children and teens. She conducts research, writes, and speaks about these topics regularly. She is a clinical professor of occupational therapy at Boston University College of Health and Rehabilitation Sciences: Sargent College, the former president of the American Occupational Therapy Association (AOTA), and a recent winner of the Eleanor Clarke Slagle Award, the highest academic honor given by the AOTA. Jacobs is the recent author of the children's book *How Full is Sophia's Backpack* which integrates tips on proper backpack usage into its imaginative story.

Boston University **College of Health and Rehabilitation Sciences: Sargent College** is an institution of higher education, which fosters critical and innovative thinking to best serve the health care needs of society through academics, research, and clinical practice. As reported by *U.S. News and World Report*, its graduate programs in Speech-Language Pathology and Physical Therapy are ranked in the top 8% of all programs while Occupational Therapy is #2 in the nation. For more information and to learn about degree programs in occupational therapy, physical therapy, speech, language and hearing sciences, health science, athletic training, human physiology, behavior and health, and nutrition, visit bu.edu/sargent.

Founded in 1839, Boston University is an internationally recognized private research university with more than 30,000 students participating in undergraduate, graduate, and professional programs. BU consists of 16 colleges and schools along with a number of multi-disciplinary centers and institutes which are central to the school's research and teaching mission.

###

**Figure 42-4.** Example of a press release.

**Biographical Sketch of Karen Jacobs**

Karen Jacobs, EdD, OTR/L, CPE, FAOTA* is a past president and vice president of the American Occupational Therapy Association (AOTA). She is a 2005 recipient of a Fulbright Scholarship to the University of Akureyri in Akuryeri, Iceland; the 2009 recipient of the Award of Merit from the Canadian Association of Occupational Therapists (CAOT); received the Award of Merit from the American Occupational Therapy Association in 2003; and the 2011 Eleanor Clarke Slagle Lectureship Award. The title of her Slagle Lecture was: *PromOTing Occupational Therapy: Words, Images and Action*.

Dr. Jacobs is a clinical professor of occupational therapy and the program director of the distance education post-professional occupational therapy programs at Boston University. She has worked at Boston University for 30 years and has expertise in the development and instruction of online graduate courses.

Dr. Jacobs earned a doctoral degree at the University of Massachusetts, a Master of Science at Boston University, and a Bachelor of Arts at Washington University in St. Louis, Missouri.

Dr. Jacobs' research examines the interface between the environment and human capabilities. In particular, she examines the individual factors and environmental demands associated with increased risk of functional limitations among populations of university and middle school aged students, particularly in notebook computing, use of tablets such as iPads, backpack use, and the use of games such as WiiFit.

In addition to being an occupational therapist, Dr. Jacobs is also a certified professional ergonomist (CPE) and the founding editor-in-chief of the international, interprofessional journal *WORK: A Journal of Prevention, Assessment and Rehabilitation* (IOS Press, The Netherlands) and is a consultant in ergonomics, marketing, and entrepreneurship.

*EdD: Doctorate in Education; OTR/L: registered and licensed occupational therapist; CPE: Certified Professional Ergonomist; FAOTA: Fellow of the American Occupational Therapy Association

**Figure 42-5.** Example of a biosketch.

## Personal Selling

Face-to-face communication between you and your audience is the most effective form of promotion, the most expensive, and also the method most used by occupational therapy practitioners (Jacobs, 1987). Word-of-mouth recommendation by staff and consumers of occupational therapy products and services is a powerful sales pitch. Other successful personal selling methods include the following:

- Exhibiting at various conferences
- Developing a free speakers' bureau
- Presenting in-service training to physicians and health and rehabilitation professionals
- Presenting continuing education workshops
- Lecturing
- Attending professional meetings for various organizations
- Holding an open house
- Holding continuing education seminars for referral sources

## Social Marketing

> Social marketing takes the techniques of marketing and deploys them to create a positive social change...The AOTA National School Backpack Awareness Day campaign is a good example of social marketing. Rebuilding Together (a nonprofit providing rebuilding services to low-income homeowners) and CarFit (an educational program for older drivers) are other examples. (Jacobs, 2012, pp. 663-664)

### Social Media

Social media, which includes social networking sites such as Facebook and LinkedIn, microblogs such as Twitter, and content communities such as YouTube, may be used for effective marketing. Social media are considered a hybrid of promotion and a highly magnified form of word of mouth. Consumers are turning more frequently to social medical outlets to conduct information searches that aid in health care or purchasing decisions (Lempert, 2006; Vollmer & Precourt, 2008). That is not to say that all sources have equal effect. Sillence, Briggs, Harris, and Fishwick (2007) found that individuals preferred sites that were run by reputable organizations or had a medical or expert "feel." They especially trusted the information when the credentials of the site and its authors were made explicit. They also appreciated inclusion of "familiar" (plain) rather than "technical" language and personalized content (i.e., stories from clients like themselves)" (Jacobs, 2012, p. 664).

Check out a YouTube video that was created by an occupational therapist in the AOTA emerging leaders program. Through this type of social media, many people are learning about the distinct value of occupational therapy: https://www.youtube.com/watch?v=17xFZ8UOhE&feature=youtu.be.

In the case study, Larry is using Facebook to promote the AOTA National School Backpack Awareness Day event at the local elementary school. Larry is very careful to avoid using professional jargon in his postings on Facebook and when discussing occupational therapy with the elementary students and their teachers.

## Focus Groups

Focus groups have been found to be an effective marketing technique. These techniques can be used with primary referral sources, such as physicians and employers, or with reimbursement agencies or the direct recipient of our services to provide feedback on current programming efforts and recommendations for future program modifications. The use of focus groups allows you to quickly incorporate this feedback into the delivery of your product and services or the product itself. This in turn should generate an increased commitment on the part of the referral sources to the program.

Focus group interviewing is one of the major marketing research tools for gaining insight into consumer thoughts and feelings (Kotler, 1983a). Focus group interviewing consists of inviting 6 to 10 participants to spend a few hours with a skilled interviewer to discuss any designated subject matter, such as the feasibility of developing a school-based occupational therapy work program. Focus group practitioners are usually paid a small sum for attending the meeting. These are typically held in pleasant surroundings, with refreshments served. The interview begins with broad questions such as, "What do you think about occupational therapy services for elementary school-aged students?" leading to focusing in on more specific questions on the subject matter such as, "What do you think about the feasibility of an occupational therapy ergonomics program addressing the use of information and communication technology being established at Butler Elementary School?" The interviewer encourages free and easy discussion among participants, hoping that the group dynamics will bring out deep feelings and thoughts (Kotler & Clarke, 1984). Although the results cannot generalize the market as a whole due to its small sample size, the information gathered can provide insight into participants' perceptions, attitudes, and satisfaction. Information obtained can help define what issues need to be researched more formally or may provide the foundation for being able to develop a product that will meet the consumer's needs (Kotler & Clarke, 1984).

## Execution of the Marketing Plan

Once you have selected your target market, develop a specific marketing mix (product, price, place, and promotion) for your market that stresses the benefits of your product(s). When executing action programs, a timeline should be delineated, such as a 12-month period, to measure whether objectives and goals are being met. The action plan should be dynamic and able to be changed throughout the year as new opportunities and problems arise. Ideally, actions should be assigned to specific individuals who are given exact completion dates. For example, an action that might be assigned to an occupational therapy practitioner can include developing a single paragraph description of the violence prevention programs provided by the occupational therapy department. The practitioner is given a 1-week timeline to complete this action. Once the description is completed, the supervisor has 2 weeks to incorporate this information into a brochure being developed to promote the expanded product line of occupational therapy to potential referral sources. In this case, as in all aspects of promotion, it is important to communicate in a language that is familiar to your market. Avoid professional jargon.

## Marketing Control

Marketing is an area where rapid obsolescence of objectives, policies, strategies, and programs is a constant possibility (Kotler & Clarke, 1984). Marketing control attempts to circumvent this dilemma and assists in maximizing the probability that a product will achieve

## Evidence-Based Research Chart

| Topic | Evidence |
|---|---|
| Marketing | Fortune et al., 2016 |
| Social media | Feick & Price, 1987; Kietzmann, Hermkens, McCarthy, & Silvestre, 2011; Sillence, Briggs, Harris, & Fishwick, 2007; Vollmer & Precourt, 2008 |
| Social marketing | Chou, Hunt, Beckjord, Moser, & Hesse, 2009; Kotler & Zaltman, 1971 |

its short- and long-term objectives. It is important to measure program results, diagnose these results, and take corrective action, if necessary. There are three types of marketing control (Kotler & Clarke, 1984):

1. Annual plan control consists of the steps used during the year to monitor and correct deviations from the marketing plan to ensure that annual sales and profit goals are being achieved.
2. Profitability control refers to the efforts used to determine the actual profit or loss of different marketing entities such as the products (services) or market segments.
3. Strategic control is a systematic evaluation of the organization's market performance in relation to the current and forecasted marketing environment.

## Summary

A bright future can be a certainty for occupational therapy practitioners and students who are prepared to accept the reality of today's and tomorrow's health care environment. It will be increasingly competitive with various professions vying for control of limited resources that are increasingly complex and increasingly controlled by third-party payers and the government.

Occupational therapy practitioners' and students' abilities to market their skills and knowledge to those who control the dollars will be an ever-present requirement for success. It will likely make the difference between encroachment by other professions, a resulting second-class specialty, and a proud and effective profession placed squarely in a leadership position within the health care industry (Pickelle & Ramos, 1991).

Having access to an expert in marketing to assist in the development of a marketing plan would be the ideal situation, but this is not always the case. On the other hand, the worst possible scenario would be one where even an informal market analysis does not precede product or service development. If this is the case for you, a word of caution: Remember that designing a program and then looking for customers typically leads to facing an uphill battle to success. At the very least, before investing a great deal of useless time, effort, and money, attempt to perform a market analysis on your own following the guidelines presented in this chapter and in other available literature.

## Student Self-Assessment

1. Describe, design, and discuss content for a webpage promoting occupational therapy to high school students.
2. Write a biosketch about yourself using Figure 42-5 as an example.
3. Create a brochure about occupational therapy's contribution to any of the six broad areas of practice: mental health; productive aging; children and youth; health and wellness; work and industry; or rehabilitation, disability, and participation. Be sure to describe occupational therapy's distinct value.

## Electronic Resources

American Marketing Association: https://www.ama.org/Pages/default.aspx

Entrepreneur: http://www.entrepreneur.com/marketing

Introduction to Marketing (free course from the University of Pennsylvania—Wharton): https://www.coursera.org/course/marketing

## References

Accenture. (2015). *Number of U.S. retail health clinics will surpass 2,800 by 2017, Accenture forecasts.* Retrieved from https://newsroom.accenture.com/news/number-of-us-retail-health-clinics-will-surpass-2800-by-2017-accenture-forecasts.htm

American Marketing Association. (2013). *About AMA.* Retrieved from https://www.ama.org/AboutAMA/Pages/Definition-of-Marketing.aspx

American Occupational Therapy Association. (n.d.). *The road to the Centennial Vision*. Retrieved from http://www.aota.org/News/Centennial.aspx

American Occupational Therapy Association. (2015). *Articulating the distinct value of occupational therapy*. Retrieved from http://www.aota.org/Publications-News/AOTANews/2015/distinct-value-of-occupational-therapy.aspx#sthash.waETbONn.dpuf}

Baum, C. M., & Luebben, A. J. (1986). *Prospective payment systems: A handbook for health care clinicians*. Thorofare, NJ: SLACK Incorporated.

Branch, M. (1962). *The corporate planning process*. New York, NY: American Management Association.

Chou, W., Hunt, Y., Beckjord, E., Moser, R., & Hesse, B. (2009). Social media use in the United States: Implications for health communication. *Journal of Medical Internet Research, 11*(4), e48.

Cromwell, F. (1984). The changing roles of occupational therapists in the 1980s. *Occupational Therapy in Health Care, 1*(1), 8.

Feick, L., & Price, L. (1987). The market maven: A diffuser of marketplace information. *Journal of Marketing, 51*, 83-97.

Fortune, T., Ennals, P., Bhopti, A., Neilson, C., Darzins, S., & Bruce, C. (2016). Bridging identity "chasms": Occupational therapy academics' reflections on the journey towards scholarship. *Teaching in Higher Education, 21*(3), 313-325.

Jacobs, K. (1987). Marketing occupational therapy. *American Journal of Occupational Therapy, 41*(5), 315-320.

Jacobs, K. (2012). PromOTing occupational therapy: Words, images, and actions (Eleanor Clarke Slagle lecture). *American Journal of Occupational Therapy, 66*, 652-671.

Kietzmann, J., Hermkens, K., McCarthy, I., & Silvestre, B. (2011). Social media? Get serious! Understanding the functional building blocks of social media. *Business Horizons, 54*, 241-251. Retrieved from http://dx.doi.org/10.1016/j.bushor.2011.01.005

Kotler, P. (1983a). *Principles of marketing* (2nd ed.). Englewood Cliffs, NJ: Prentice Hall.

Kotler, P. (1983b). *Principles of marketing—Instructor's manual with cases*. Englewood Cliffs, NJ: Prentice Hall.

Kotler, P., & Clarke, R. (1984). *Marketing management* (5th ed.). Englewood Cliffs, NJ: Prentice Hall.

Kotler, P., & Clarke, R. (1987). *Marketing for health care organizations*. Englewood Cliffs, NJ: Prentice Hall.

Kotler, P., & Murray, M. (1975). Third sector management: The role of marketing. *Public Administration Review, 35*(5), 469.

Kotler, P., & Zaltman, G. (1971). Social marketing: An approach to planned social change. *Journal of Marketing, 35*, 3-12. Retrieved from http://dx.doi.org/10.2307/1249783

Lempert, P. (2006, September 1). Caught in the web. *Progressive Grocer, 85*, 18.

McCarthy, E. J. (1999). *Basic marketing: A managerial approach* (13th ed.). Homewood, IL: Irwin.

Miller, D., & Jacobs, K. (2007). Economics and marketing of ergonomic services. In K. Jacobs (Ed.), *Ergonomics for therapists*. St. Louis, MO: Elsevier.

Pickelle, C., & Ramos, T. (1991). Publishers' message. *Rehab Management, 9*.

Sillence, E., Briggs, P., Harris, P. R. & Fishwick, L. (2007). How do patients evaluate and make use of online health information? *Social Science and Medicine, 64*, 1853-1862. Retrieved from http://dx.doi.org/10.1016/j.socscimed.2007.01.012

U.S. Department of Justice. (2007). *U.S. Department of Justice website*. Retrieved from http://www.usdoj.gov

Vollmer, C., & Precourt, G. (2008). *Always on: Advertising, marketing and media in an era of consumer control*. New York, NY: McGraw-Hill.

## Suggested Readings

Borger, C., Smith, S., Truffer, C., Keehan, S., Sisko, A., Poisal, J., et al. (2006). Health spending projections through 2015: Changes on the horizon. *Health Affairs, 25*(2), w61-w73.

Catlin, A., Cowan, C., Heffler, S., Washington, B., & National Health Expenditure Accounts Team. (2006). National health spending in 2005: The slowdown continues. *Health Affairs, 26*(1), 142-153.

National Center for Education Statistics. (n.d.). *National Center for Education Statistics website*. Retrieved from http://nces.ed.gov

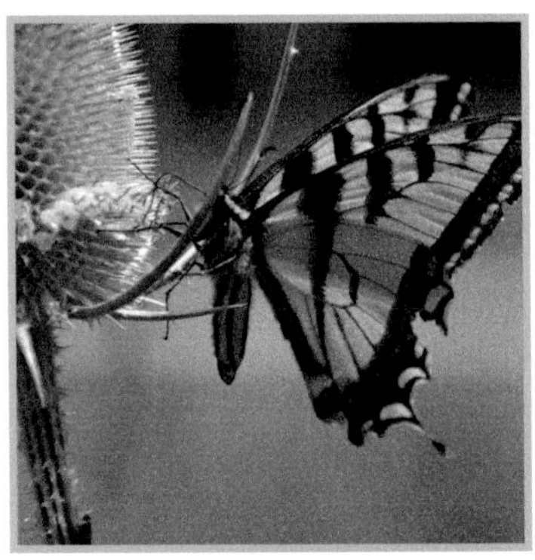

# 43

# Quality Improvement

Elizabeth W. Crampsey, MS, OTR/L, BCPR

**ACOTE STANDARDS EXPLORED IN THIS CHAPTER**

B.7.6

**KEY VOCABULARY**

- **Benchmark:** Quantifiable measures of the outcomes of a process used as comparison to current performances or targets for an improved outcome (Braveman, 2006, p. 289).
- **Quality:** "The degree to which health care services for individuals and populations increase the probability of desired health outcomes and is consistent with current professional knowledge of best practice" (Institute of Medicine, 2001, p. 232).
- **Quality assessment:** Measure of quality against a standard.
- **Quality improvement:** Management philosophy and method for structuring problem solving.



Jacobs, K., & MacRae, N. (Eds.).
*Occupational Therapy Essentials for Clinical Competence, Third Edition* (pp. 615-625).

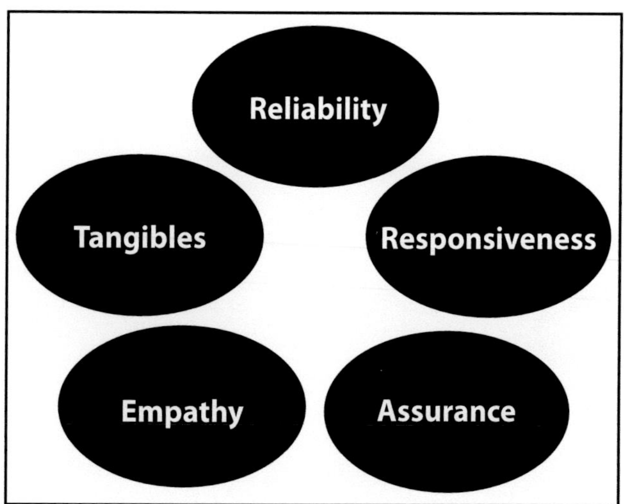


**Figure 43-1.** Five dimensions of quality.

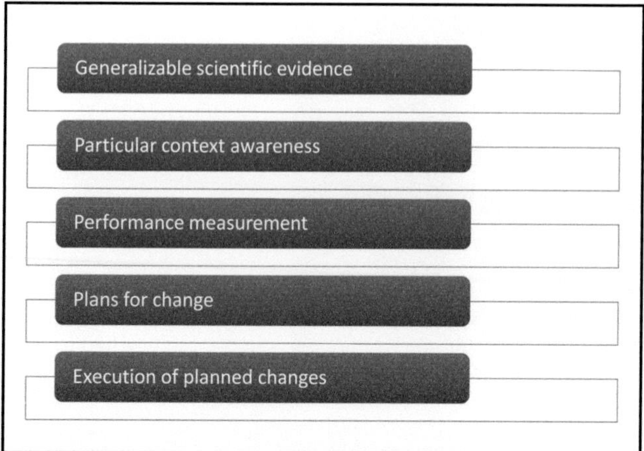


**Figure 43-2.** Five elements of quality improvement.

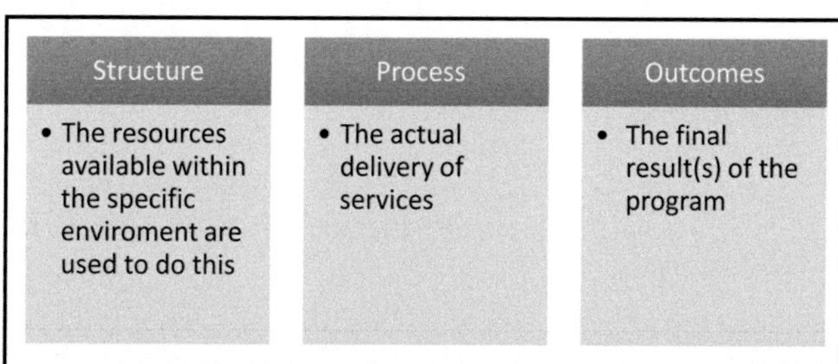


**Figure 43-3.** Examination and evaluation of quality health care. (Adapted from Donabedian, A. [1980]. *Explorations in quality assessment and monitoring: The definition of quality and approaches to its assessment* [Vol. 1]. Ann Arbor, MI: Health Administration Press.)

Quality is a complex concept with innumerable definitions. Quality depends on the individual and the context, for both definition as well as methods of measurement. When discussing quality, it is impossible to underestimate the value component, which is typically the relationship between cost and quality. A critical movement in occupational therapy as a profession is articulating the distinct value of occupational therapy. To that end, a distinct value statement was approved by the American Occupational Therapy Association's (AOTA) Board of Directors:

> Occupational therapy's distinct value is to improve health and quality of life through facilitating participation and engagement in occupations, the meaningful, necessary, and familiar activities of everyday life. Occupational therapy is client-centered, achieves positive outcomes, and is cost-effective. (AOTA, 2015a)

Adding to the complexity of the construct of quality is the fact that health care players (clients, providers, and payers) define quality differently, usually from their unique perspectives. Some of the possible defining concepts of quality include safety, timeliness, courtesy, availability, technical support, accessibility, reliability, economic impact, accuracy, waste, durability, flexibility, and follow-up. The Institute of Medicine defined quality as "the degree to which health care services for individuals and populations increase the probability of desired health outcomes and is consistent with current professional knowledge of best practice" (2001, p. 232). Service is also a likely consideration. Figure 43-1 provides five dimensions often cited as important (Parasuraman, Berry, & Zeithaml, 1991): they are related to the reliability of service, tangible product or service, responsiveness of service to client/customer, assurance of quality to consumer, and empathy exercised toward consumer.

Embedded within quality, there are levels of quality for a product provided or received or a service rendered. There is the expected quality, the perceived quality, and the actual quality. Expected quality is influenced by opinion, whereas perceived quality is subjective; both are difficult to measure. Actual quality can consider multiple factors and be based on statistical data, so it tends to be more easily and reliably measured (Snoby, 2004, p. 69).

Quality improvement is also a management philosophy and method for structuring problem solving. The goal is to meet/exceed customer/client requirements for quality services through a process of improvement. The process is a continuous, nonlinear process and always involves change. However, all change is not improvement, so the process needs to be carefully and intentionally implemented. Batalden and Davidoff (2013) propose five elements by which improvement can be produced (Figure 43-2).

The data that are gathered are used to make decisions, just as for evidence-based practice. A frequently used model developed by Donabedian (1980) is shown in Figure 43-3, which lists three portions of a quality improvement program.

All aspects of both of these models are complementary. In addition, quality for practitioners can be

Table 43-1.

## Client-Driven Actions

| Becoming a Client-Driven Entity Means Moving | |
|---|---|
| **From** | **To** |
| Motivation through fear and loyalty | Motivation through shared vision |
| An attitude of "It's their problem" | Ownership of every problem that affects the client |
| "That's the way we've always done it" | Continued improvement |
| Making decisions based on assumptions | Making decisions based on client data |
| Everything begins and ends with management | Everything begins and ends with the client |
| Organizational foxholes | Cross-functional cooperation |
| Being good at crisis management and recovery | Doing it right the first time |

Adapted from Whiteley, R. C. (1993). *The customer-driven company: Moving from talk to action.* New York, NY: Basic Books.

understood from both a micro, as well as a macro, view. The micro view deals with clinical aspects of care and the technical quality with which they are delivered. Interpersonal aspects of care have significance for clients—the provider's interest in and concern for the client makes an indelible impression. Quality-of-life definitions usually involve the client's sense of overall well-being and ability to participate in those activities/occupations found to be most meaningful (Shi & Singh, 2012).

The macro view of quality includes a broader view of the system-wide efficiencies and outcomes, such as cost, access, and population health status (Shi & Singh, 2012, pp. 515-517). National initiatives, as well as state and community actions, and concerns are addressed using the macro view.

For a quality improvement process to be successful, the following components need to be in place:

- Administrative support of this philosophy
- Training of all staff on the concepts, strategies, tools, and techniques of quality improvement
- Adoption of the norm of customer preferences being the primary determinant of quality (Table 43-1)
- Support for a team approach that encourages all to work together to improve quality; motivation must be apparent for this approach to process analysis and change to be effective

Successful quality improvement efforts work because consumers discern a greater value from the service/product than from that of the competition and a number of the following components. Five "C" components of valid customer requirements are as follows (Braveman, 2006):

### Case Study 1

A health care organization in northern New England demonstrated innovation when looking at quality improvement in a specialized group of patients. These patients are considered to be lower in frequency and higher in risk because in this setting there were few patients needing a tracheostomy, and typically patients with a tracheostomy have higher risk. With careful selection, an interprofessional team of stakeholders was selected and the topic dissected. During this root cause analysis, it is important to understand that the stratification of stakeholders includes all levels within the health care hierarchy. Along with the lower frequency and higher risk, a confounding factor was there was no clear continuum of care for patients to transition from inpatient hospital settings to inpatient rehabilitation settings. The group met consistently, first identifying the concerns from all perspectives, prioritizing them, and finally devising an action plan to address each problem. This required a partnership of all levels of care from the top down and bottom up inclusive of all of the stakeholders. Although at times arduous, this group was able to accomplish considerable client-centered positive change, as well as fiscal responsibility to ensure that this subset of clients had well-trained staff, as well as smoother transitions throughout the health care system. This included appropriate health care team communication, hand-offs, and inclusion of the client and support system to solidify the processes, protocols, and procedures. Tracking the process and progress of both the small tests of change and larger initiatives within this project demonstrated considerable and statistically significant positive change for this group of clients and their families.

1. Product is current
2. Outcome is calculable
3. Plan can be completed
4. Plan is consumer based
5. Plan is consistent with organizational goals

Quality improvement plans are often dictated by improving client safety and outcomes in health care. In organizations quality improvement initiatives are associated with less waste, improved services, lower costs, higher profit margins, recalibration of asset utilization, and competitive positioning. All of this improves the "bottom line," thereby satisfying shareholders and key supporters, without losing sight of the consumers.

## Stages and Principles

Just as outcomes are an integral part of the occupational therapy process, the outcome assessment process in quality improvement is a critical part of evaluating and improving quality. The process consists of the following:

- Identifying goals for organization, program, client, or self
- Developing a plan to achieve goals
- Implementing the plan
- Measuring and reporting outcomes

A widely used method is a quality chain reaction, consisting of a four-part cycle (Deming, 2000). The PDCA cycle, or sometimes referred to as the PDSA cycle, is as follows:

1. **Plan:** Determine what will be measured
2. **Do:** Collect data on chosen indicators
3. **Check/study:** Analyze data and identify areas for improvement
4. **Act:** Implement improvements, first in pilot program; provide rewards and recognition for the team (Figure 43-4)

Critical is that this is a continual process, with these domains integrated and used in conjunction (Deming, 2000). In addition, users of this system need to have an appreciation for a systems approach, the likelihood of variation of performance, the theory of the scientific method of knowledge generation, and an understanding of both intrinsic and extrinsic factors affecting motivation and participation in change within an organization (Braveman, 2006).

In addition to following Deming's organized cycle, the rationale for such a plan needs to address queries such as the following:

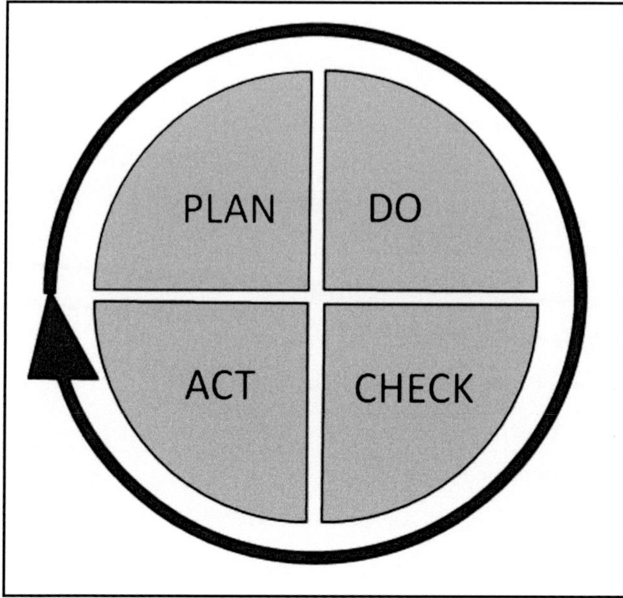


**Figure 43-4.** Plan-Do-Check/Study-Act cycle.

- Who are the stakeholders?
- How do you improve responsiveness of the program?
- How do you ensure high quality standards?

Another effective, widely used system in health care quality improvement is the microsystems approach. The premise of a clinical microsystem is that patient care is complex and includes clients, clinicians, facilities, culture, processes, equipment, and the like (Disch, 2006). Using the microsystems approach, care is interconnected as the basis and foundation for client care delivery. Nelson et al. (2008) asserted that a clinical microsystem is defined as

> A small group of people who work together on a regular basis to provide care to discrete subpopulations of patients. It has clinical and business aims, linked processes, and a shared information environment, and it produces performance outcomes. Microsystems evolve over time and are often embedded in larger organizations. They are complex adaptive systems, and as such they must do the primary work associated with core aims, meet the needs of internal staff, and maintain themselves over time as clinical units. (p. 474)

Further, Disch (2006) acknowledged there is a growing body of research based on the clinical microsystem and that buy in related to the incorporation of "systems theory, complexity science, holistic thinking and chaos theory" (p. 13). This is a departure from focusing on just the individual, and allows for an understanding of the context of care, with the ultimate goal being on the improvement of the client and family, or the client population (Disch, 2006). Nelson et al. (2008) identified the characteristics of high performing and efficient clinical microsystems in Table 43-2.

Table 43-2.

### Characteristics of High Performance and Efficient Microsystems

- The leadership of the microsystem
- The culture of the microsystem
- The support from the macrosystem
- Focus on clients
- Focus on staff
- Interdependence of the care team members
- Information and information technology
- Process improvement
- A performance pattern to track outcomes

Knowing that quality, safety, and costs are on the forefront of quality in health care, a microsystems approach provides a framework for the client and family; it needs to be interconnected with the health care teams (Nelson et al., 2008).

> Clinical microsystems is shorthand for a comprehensive approach to providing value for individuals and families by analyzing, managing, improving, and innovating in health care systems—and can offer senior leaders a strategy and execution framework for competing in an increasingly competitive, data transparent, and value-seeking medical marketplace. (Nelson et al., 2008, p. 367)

More information on clinical microsystems can be found at clinicalmicrosystem.org/.

Along with the PDCA cycle and clinical microsystems, one can also see the value in measuring that work against the 5 Ps. The 5 Ps—purpose, patients, professionals, processes, and patterns (Godfrey, Nelson, Wasson, Mohr, & Batalden, 2003)—focus on patient, people, processes, and patterns as knowing your patients, knowing your people, being familiar with your processes, and the patterns of care are insightful pillars of a functional and effective microsystem. Studies regarding microsystems in health care demonstrate that the most authentic and meaningful microsystems "intentionally designed patient-centered services to support patients and families and the staff providing care" (Godfrey et al., 2003, p. 166).

## Application to Clinical Settings

In an environment of constant change, health care reform, cost containment, mergers, and managed health care, professionals must strive to provide quality care. Examining efficiency, effectiveness, and adherence to standards of quality management in health care is a systematic process for evaluating health care services (The Joint Commission, 2013). Efficiency refers to services that are both cost effective and timely in their delivery. Clinical services must be effective in achieving set objectives or outcomes for care.

Quality improvement or management programs are designed to measure and assess performance to ensure adherence to preestablished standards. These standards are established by state, federal, and accreditation organizations, such as the The Joint Commission and the Commission on Accreditation of Rehabilitation Facilities. Hospitals and other health care facilities refer to this process with many terms: *continuous quality improvement, total quality management, quality assurance,* and *performance improvement.* The processes of quality assurance, quality improvement/assessment, and performance are all methods of assessment. Motivations (external vs. internal), focus (problem-based vs. quality processes), delegation (departmentally vs. interdepartmentally), and outcomes (hiding problems vs. improvement) may vary (Jacobs & Logigian, 1999).

Table 43-3 provides the differences among quality assurance, similar to quality improvement but a step beyond quality assessment; quality assessment, a measure of quality against standards; and performance improvement, a combination of both.

There are many methods for evaluating quality, such as the following:

- Clinical audits refer to a group of peers working collectively to review case records for adherence to standards preestablished by the peer group.
- Peer review is a type of record review based on criteria established by the individual department, for what is determined to be quality care (JCAHO, 1995; Longest & Darr, 2014). Maslin (1991, p. 177) stated: "Common to both peer review and clinical audit procedures is the term process criteria, referring to the activities or procedures undertaken as part of good patient care."
- Accreditation is sought by many hospitals and health care organizations as proof of providing services that meet established minimum standards for Medicare reimbursement (Jacobs & Logigian, 1999; JCAHO, 1995). When performance fails to meet these standards, the organization must assess the performance and attempt to improve the areas of deficit. Changes can occur organizationally, departmentally, or individually. When discussing quality improvement, we must not only look to the organization, but to each individual occupational therapy practitioner who is providing the services.

Table 43-3.

**Differences Among Quality Improvement and Quality Assurance**

| Quality Improvement | Quality Assurance |
|---|---|
| "Why" focus | "Who" focus |
| Prospective | Retrospective |
| Internally directed | Externally directed |
| Focused on patients and the many involved in care | Focused on the organizational structure, delegated to the few |
| Bottom up | Top down |
| More proactive | More reactive |
| Process approach | Events based |
| Quality is integral, focus on all processes to ensure quality | Focus is on meeting clinical criteria, solving problems |

Adapted from Longest, B. B., & Darr, K. (2014). *Managing health services organizations* (6th ed.). Baltimore, MD: Health Professions Press.

Table 43-4.

**Indicators and Thresholds**

| Indicator | Threshold | Data Collection Method | Possible Causes for Thresholds Not Being Met |
|---|---|---|---|
| Falls prevention education was completed and thoroughly documented | 95% | Quarterly chart review of 30 records by the occupational therapist<br>Reports to occupational therapy director and QM committee | Short length of stay<br>Illness<br>Family<br>Client refusal |
| Clients received | 95% | Falls assessment | |
| Documentation | 95% | Documentation of education and client/family understanding | |
| Treatment | 98% | Testing/procedures 3 hours of therapy daily to include occupational therapy and physical therapy and at times, speech-language pathology as documented in client's chart | |

## Data Collection Methods

Data collection methods include qualitative or quantitative methodology, or a combination of both, as well as the use of benchmarks. Benchmarks are the quantifiable measures of the outcomes of a process used as comparisons to current performances or targets for an improved outcome (Braveman, 2006, p. 289). Many methods can be used to collect data. They include observation, interviews, surveys/questionnaires, and focus groups.

Data analysis drives change and closes the loop of quality improvement. A determination about whether the data support the focus on the goals of an organization or its view of success must be determined with an adjustment plan conceived based on the data. Data can also be used to indicate the effectiveness of a practitioner's performance (Table 43-4).

The ultimate goal of quality improvement programs is to have a continuous focus on quality to become the norm of doing business. Success occurs when there is a constant focus on clients and their satisfaction, a constant readiness for change and process improvement, the daily use of quality improvement tools, an abiding belief that use of data to make decisions is the right way to proceed, and a commitment to balance these tasks with those of the needs of people as standard operating procedures (Braveman, 2006).

### *FOCUS-PDCA Model*

A method used by many organizations to implement a quality improvement process is the one developed by the Hospital Corporation of America in 1980. It is known as FOCUS-PDCA. It is a "stepwise approach to teach how to design, implement, and evaluate a quality

Table 43-5.

## The Monitoring and Evaluation Process for Assessment and Improvement

| | |
|---|---|
| Assign responsibility | The organization leaders oversee the design and foster an approach to continuously improve quality including the use of intra- and extradepartmental activities |
| Delineate the scope | The organization, as a whole or as a department, delineates its scope of care and service |
| Identify importance | The organization, as a whole or as a department, identifies high-priority key functions, processes, activities, etc., to be monitored |
| Identify indicators | Teams of experts, inter- or intradepartmental, identify indicators for the important aspects of care and service; indicators pertaining to structures of care are no longer emphasized |
| Establish evaluation | Teams of experts establish the level, pattern, or trend triggers in data for each indicator that will trigger intensive evaluation; statistical methods are emphasized, as is the fact that thresholds are not the only way evaluation is triggered |
| Collect and organize | The data collection methodology often includes a data means by which feedback from sources other than ongoing monitoring is used to indicate areas for evaluation and improvement |
| Initiate evaluation | When thresholds are reached and when other feedback (e.g., client reports) identifies other opportunities for improvement, leaders set priorities for evaluation and establish teams, which evaluate the client care or service function in question |
| Take action | Greater emphasis is placed on focusing actions on processes, especially the "hands off" between departments and services |
| Assess effectiveness | A greater emphasis is placed on ensuring that improvement is sustained over time |
| Communicate results | Findings of those performing monitoring and evaluation of the findings are forwarded to the leaders and affected individuals and groups |
| Other feedback | Receive surveys, comments, suggestions, and complaints |

Adapted from Logigian, M. K. (1999). In K. Jacobs & M. K. Logigian (Eds.), *Functions of a manager in occupational therapy* (3rd ed., p. 124). Thorofare, NJ: SLACK Incorporated.

improvement initiative" (Skledar & McKaveney, 2009, p. 80). The acronym FOCUS is described below:

- Find ways to improve by identifying areas in need of improvement
- Organize a team of individuals who understand both the process and the area to be addressed
- Clarify issues of specified area, addressing who, what, when, and where information
- Understand causes of targeted area, addressing the "why" question
- Select most appropriate method for improvement

The PDCA portion is based on Deming's process, described earlier.

Departmental communication is essential in facilitating a process, such as the preceding, fostering team development, and motivating staff members to maximize efficiency and effectiveness of intervention.

Occupational therapy practitioners who are involved in the quality improvement process will have increased understanding of the indicators and their potential effects on the client, the department, and the organization. Blending this micro and macro view can be empowering to the practitioner. Understanding the factors that affect care from all perspectives should serve to improve the client experience and overall care. Being part of quality improvement projects, when embarked on from an authentic and meaningful perspective, should be a passionate and invigorating process for those involved. Change is not for change's sake, but comes from a deep understanding of the process and problem with the intention to improve and facilitate change.

Table 43-5 provides a more detailed outline of such a process for monitoring and evaluating assessment and improvement programs.

With a strong quality improvement program, departments and organizations will show improved efficiency with decreased cost and waste and improved productivity and effectiveness, with positive outcomes and client satisfaction. Quality care should always be thought of as an ongoing process for the organization as a whole and for each individual working within the organization.

# Impact on the Profession

The Patient Protection and Affordable Care Act of 2010 (ACA; P.L. 111-148) is a volume-based payment system with the emphasis on client-centered care, as well as quality and value of care. Referred to as the Triple Aim, it endeavors to incentivize providers to deliver evidenced-based best practices by linking pay to performance with the ultimate goal to improve population health, enhance consumer satisfaction, and reduce health care costs (Leland, Crum, Phipps, Roberts, & Gage, 2015). Leland et al. (2015) further explored the premise of value-based care within the context of occupational therapy, and delineated how occupational therapy and occupational therapy practitioners can define high-quality care processes to enhance client outcomes while solidifying a sustainable future for the profession. They further contended that defining evidence and client-centered care processes would improve and inform client outcomes, essentially demonstrating the value and contribution of occupational therapy and its practitioners. Occupational therapy practitioners should have a role in quality metrics, such as in inpatient settings, catheter-associated infections, decreasing skin integrity concerns, readmissions rates, minimization of falls, and similar topics. This truly is a team sport because financial incentives are provided to high-quality care, whereas poor performance incurs financial penalties. Occupational therapy can further develop measures that are reliable and valid, as well as add to the body of evidence for both evaluation and intervention. Practitioners need to document accurately and appropriately using client- and occupation-centered language. Documentation should be evidenced base, reflective of the care provided and inclusive of data assessing the quality of care provided (Leland et al., 2015). Demonstrating value across settings and populations within various contexts will aid in demonstrating the efficacy of occupational therapy.

Quality improvement processes are important to the profession of occupational therapy. The principles mirror those of evidence-based practice. Quality improvement and evidence-based practice support the strengthening and growth of our profession and recognize its foundation of occupation. Our profession maintains a unique definition of quality outcomes: occupational therapy outcomes need to be based on engagement in occupation (O'Sullivan, 2004). Measures can include the following (Case-Smith, 2005, pp. 8-9):

- Occupational performance
- Client satisfaction
- Role competence
- Adaptation
- Health and wellness
- Prevention
- Quality of life

Clinical assessment tools need to be critically analyzed with a determination made as to what they assess, how they will be used, and their limitations. Tools also need to be reliable, valid, and sensitive. Some examples of currently used tools are as follows:

- Functional Independence Measure: A national tool used in rehabilitation settings
- Minimum Data Information Set: Used to determine level of intervention needed in nursing homes
- Outcomes Assessment Information Set: Home health standardized assessment
- SF-36: National quality of life assessment
- Canadian Occupational Performance Measure: Can be used with multiple populations

# Outcome Measures

Rather than just at the macro and micro levels, quality outcome measures also need to be applied at the individual practitioner level to ensure quality care for the clients and the continuing competence of practitioners. Looking at quality care, occupational therapy practitioners must look at the overall outcomes of client intervention and their individual professional competence as occupational therapy practitioners. Hinojosa et al. (1998) defined continuing competence as "a dynamic multidimensional process in which the professional develops and maintains the knowledge, performance skills, interpersonal abilities, critical reasoning skills, and ethical reasoning skills necessary to continue in his or her evolving roles throughout a professional career" (p. 4). This process requires the occupational therapy practitioner understand the continuous process of improvement.

The AOTA, the national organization for occupational therapy practitioners, is committed to assisting its members in keeping abreast of advancements in the profession and establishing standards that define quality services. AOTA has a wealth of information to help practitioners to remain confident and competent practitioners. AOTA has established a council, the Committee on Continuing Competence and Professional Development, as a committee of the Representative Assembly to develop and maintain Standards for Continuing Competence (AOTA, 2010) and offer guidelines and tools to support professional development. With financial and time constraints commonly experienced by many occupational therapy practitioners, AOTA has developed continuing education (CE) articles, self-paced clinical courses, workshops on DVD/CD, webinars, and online courses to assist its members in meeting CE requirements and obtaining CE units (CEUs) to stay current in a growing profession. Additionally, the Committee on Continuing Competence and Professional Development has implemented the opportunity for board certification for practitioners in specialty areas.

Occupational therapy practitioners must maintain and demonstrate the appropriate knowledge and skill level for client intervention in varied roles. Many state licensure boards require documentation of CE (refer to your state licensure laws) to maintain current licensure. These CE credits should be related to the occupational therapy practitioner's individual roles within his or her position.

Since 2002, the National Board for Certification in Occupational Therapy (NBCOT) requires practitioners to accrue 36 hours of professional development units (PDUs) over a 3-year period to maintain certification. The requirement is intended to complement state licensure terms. Of the 36 units, two-thirds (24 PDUs) must be directly related to the delivery of occupational therapy services (NBCOT, 2016). CEUs are converted to PDUs according to a formula established by NBCOT. In addition, NBCOT offers a listing of a wide variety of professional activities that may be applied to PDUs. Practitioners must keep records, usually in the form of a portfolio of their professional development activities. At recertification time, NBCOT randomly audits recertification applicants for the required PDUs (NBCOT, 2016).

## Skills Needed by Practitioners

Occupational therapy practitioners must be able to demonstrate appropriate communication (The Joint Commission, 2013), interpersonal abilities, and problem solving to maintain professional relationships with clients, family members, peers, and other health care professionals. Being able to adapt to meet the needs of the client, family, or health care professional will foster greater understanding and may improve overall intervention outcomes. Lastly, occupational therapy practitioners must always adhere to the *Occupational Therapy Code of Ethics* established by the AOTA (2015b). This code guides our practice and allows occupational therapy practitioners to make appropriate decisions and actions. Each occupational therapy practitioner, whether a registered occupational therapist or a certified occupational therapy assistant, is responsible for his or her own ethical practice.

Given the demand for accountability within the health care field and the rapid changes within the profession of occupational therapy and areas of technology, it becomes essential for occupational therapy practitioners to continuously update individual skills and knowledge level. Whether as a new graduate or an advanced practitioner, it is important to have a professional development plan to compete in an ever-changing health care environment. AOTA has a Professional Development Tool (2003) online that enables the occupational therapy practitioner to assess his or her own strengths and weaknesses, develop goals and objectives to improve skills or knowledge, implement the plan, create a space to document credentials and continuing competency, identify possible resources to meet the goals, and engage in cyclical self-reflection. Further, the NBCOT website houses the NBCOT Navigator, a web-based platform for assessment and competency of certificants to maintain their clinical competency and keep abreast of their professional development (NBCOT, 2016).

There are many skills that you will apply to the quality improvement process, including the following:

### Case Study 2

The occupational therapy department in a 32-bed inpatient rehabilitation unit has developed a quality management program to review the following:

- Splinting schedules and adherence to the schedules by the staff
- Falls prevention education and carry-over of the information for the clients
- Intervention minutes

The department, including the occupational therapy director, occupational therapists, and occupational therapy assistants, collected data and completed a chart review. Splinting schedules were to be placed in the chart and documented in the nursing daily sheets for adherence to the schedule. Falls prevention education was to be documented in the occupational therapy daily notes, including client understanding and carry-over. Intervention documentation was to be documented in the daily notes and billing records for a minimum of 45 minutes twice a day.

Annual implementation goals were established as follows:

- Splinting schedules and compliance to the schedule were documented 95% of the time
- Falls prevention education was completed and thoroughly documented with client understanding 95% of the time
- Clients received occupational therapy intervention in 45-minute sessions twice daily 95% of the time; if therapy was missed, thorough documentation was included for missed session 100% of the time.

Thresholds for splinting and falls prevention were met at 95%, whereas thresholds for intervention minutes were not met and achieved 85% compliance. The occupational therapy department held a meeting to discuss the results. The occupational therapy department has two full-time occupational therapists, two full-time occupational therapy assistants, and an occupational therapy aide. Department hours are from 8 a.m. to 5 p.m., Monday through Saturday, and Sunday from 8 a.m. to 12 p.m.

## Evidence-Based Research Chart

| Topic | Evidence |
|---|---|
| Evidence-based quality improvement | Chassin, Loeb, Schmaltz, & Wachter, 2010 |
| Effectiveness of quality improvement strategies and programs | Grimshaw et al., 2003; Leland, Crum, Phipps, Roberts, & Gage, 2015; Mittman, 2004; Shojania & Grimshaw, 2005; Skledar & McKaveney, 2009; Snoby, 2004 |
| Occupational justice as a quality indicator for occupational therapy services | Riegel & Eglseder, 2009 |
| Intervention effectiveness research | Persch & Page, 2013 |
| Clinical microsystem | Dartmouth Institute for Health Policy and Clinical Practice, 2015 |

- Effective communication is necessary in organizing, implementing, and reporting quality improvement activities, whether this is the initial idea of the project or in sharing information with colleagues who are also involved in the study. Effective communication should occur with all levels of the quality improvement team, whether another member of the team, clients, families, or administration.
- The tasks associated with management are frequently part of a quality improvement study. Therefore, knowledge of their procedures and purpose will be of benefit to the practitioner who participates in quality improvement activities.
- Leadership can be displayed in numerous ways. Occupational therapy practitioners may lead the entire study or a portion of it, they may conceptualize the idea needing attention, or they may have more of a peripheral role.

Quality improvement activities are frequently a requirement of accrediting bodies and state regulatory boards. Assessing and improving the quality of care to the clients we serve is an ethical responsibility, as is continually improving and upgrading our own skills. Results of quality improvement activities provide a sound basis for change, improvement, and growth. Practitioners' participation in quality improvement activities will hopefully make the resultant changes easier to implement.

## Summary

A key to success in a quality improvement endeavor is to recognize it as a multidimensional, continuous, and circular process. Such a process requires a culture change to ensure commitment from all affected, interested, and concerned parties. These stakeholders should, at a minimum, include administration, professionals, and consumers. Devising the end results (outcomes) can lead to increased satisfaction for the stakeholders, as well as making the task even more meaningful and worthwhile to all participants.

The end product should always focus on the highest quality care possible. To sustain quality, administration and professionals must communicate and actively participate in the process. The FOCUS-PDCA, 5 Ps, and microsystem approaches demonstrate how the development of a comprehensive quality improvement program can be used to monitor and evaluate quality standards. Assessment of quality does not stop at the clinic or organization; occupational therapy practitioners must strive to provide quality, ethical services while taking responsibility for their own professional development.

Leland et al. (2015) stated:

> Quality improvement presents an opportunity for clinicians, researchers, and educators to collaboratively contribute to defining quality care measures, promote the adoption of these standards of service, and evaluate the delivery of care that occupational therapy provides. By using data to reflect our contribution to improved patient outcomes and recognizing areas for future progress, the profession will be strengthened. (p. 5)

## Student Self-Assessment

1. Identify the FOCUS-PDCA process for monitoring and evaluating quality standards.
2. Consider a clinical experience that you are familiar with. Reflect on the value-added aspects of patient/client care within the system or organization you were working. Which aspects would you define as

value-added for the patient/client? Where are the opportunities for meaningful change?

3. Next, consider your role within the care system for the client. What was most value-added? In other words, when would you have been willing to reach into your own pocket (had you been the client) and endorse the value of provided services? Can you identify further opportunities for change?
4. Discuss possible solutions to remedy the intervention calculation of therapy units problem within the department.

## Acknowledgments

Thanks to Nancy MacRae, MS, OTR/L, FAOTA, and Karen Jacobs, EdD, OTR/L, CPE, FAOTA, for their work on this chapter in the Second Edition.

## References

American Occupational Therapy Association. (2003). *Professional development tool*. Retrieved from http://www1.aota.org/pdt/p2_4.htm#

American Occupational Therapy Association. (2010). Standards for continuing competence. *American Journal of Occupational Therapy, 64*(Suppl. 6).

American Occupational Therapy Association. (2015a). *Articulating the distinct value of occupational therapy*. Retrieved from http://www.aota.org/Publications-News/AOTANews/2015/distinct-value-of-occupational-therapy.aspx

American Occupational Therapy Association. (2015b). Occupational therapy code of ethics. *American Journal of Occupational Therapy, 69*(Suppl. 3).

Batalden, P. B., & Davidoff, F. (2013). *What is "quality improvement" and how can it transform healthcare?* Retrieved from http://qualitysafety.bmj.com/content/16/1/2.full?sid=60556d89-bb15-4c47-8e54-edc85fe71af4

Braveman, B. (2006). *Leading and managing occupational therapy services: An evidence-based approach*. Philadelphia, PA: F. A. Davis Company.

Case-Smith, J. (2005). Using client outcome data to guide your professional development. *OT Practice, 10*(4), 8-9.

Chassin, M. R., Loeb, J. M., Schmaltz, S. P., & Wachter, R. M. (2010). Accountability measures: Using measurement to promote quality improvement. *New England Journal of Medicine, 363*, 638-688.

Dartmouth Institute for Health Policy and Clinical Practice. (2015). *Transforming microsystems in health care*. Retrieved from https://clinicalmicrosystem.org/

Deming, D. E. (2000). *Out of crisis*. Cambridge, MA: The MIT Press.

Disch, J. (2006). Clinical microsystems: The building blocks of patient safety. *Creative Nursing, 12*(3), 13-14.

Donabedian, A. (1980). *Explorations in quality assessment and monitoring: The definition of quality and approaches to its assessment* (Vol. 1.). Ann Arbor, MI: Health Administration Press.

Godfrey, M. M., Nelson, E. C., Wasson, J. H., Mohr, J. J., & Batalden, P. B. (2003). Microsystems in health care: Part 3. Planning patient-centered services. *Joint Commission Journal on Quality and Safety,29*(4), 159-170.

Grimshaw, J., McAuley, L. M., Bero, L. A., Grilli, R., Oxman, A. D., Ramsay, C., et al. (2003). Systematic reviews of the effectiveness of quality improvement strategies and programmes. *Quality and Safety in Health Care, 12*, 298-303.

Hinojosa, J., Bowen, R., Epstein, C., Scwope, C., Davis Rourk, J., Berg Rice, V., et al. (1998). *Continuing competency task force report to the executive board*. Bethesda, MD: AOTA Press.

Institute of Medicine. (2001). *Crossing the quality chasm: A new health system for the twenty-first century*. Washington, DC: National Academy Press.

Jacobs, K., & Logigian, M. K. (Eds.). (1999). *Functions of a manager in occupational therapy* (3rd ed.). Thorofare, NJ: SLACK Incorporated.

The Joint Commission. (2013). *Facts about patient-centered communications*. Retrieved from http://www.jointcommission.org/assets/1/18/Patient_Centered_Communications_7_3_12.pdf

Joint Commission on the Accreditation of Healthcare Organizations. (1995). *Using performance improvement tools in home care and hospice organizations*. Oakbrook Terrace, IL: Author.

Leland, N. E., Crum, K., Phipps, S., Roberts, P., & Gage, B. (2015). Advancing the value and quality of occupational therapy in health service delivery. *American Journal of Occupational Therapy, 69*(1), 1-7. doi:10.5014/ajot.2015.691001

Longest, B. B., & Darr, K. (2014). *Managing health services organizations* (6th ed.). Baltimore, MD: Health Professions Press.

Maslin, Z. B. (1991). *Management in occupational therapy*. San Diego, CA: Singular Publishing Group.

Mittman, B. (2004). Creating the evidence base for quality improvement collaboratives. *Annals of Internal Medicine, 140*(11), 897-901.

National Board for Certification in Occupational Therapy. (2016). *Self-assessment tool*. Retrieved from http://www.nbcot.org/navigator

Nelson, E. C., Batalden, P. B., Huber, T. P., Mohr, J. J., Godfrey, M. M., Headrick, L. A., et al. (2008). Microsystems in health care: Part 1. Learning from high-performing front-line clinical units. *Joint Commission Journal on Quality Improvement, 28*(9), 472-497.

O'Sullivan, G. (2004). Leisure activity programming: Promoting life satisfaction and quality of life for residents in long-term care. *New Zealand Journal of Occupational Therapy, 51*(2), 33-38.

Parasuraman, A., Berry, L. L., & Zeithaml, V. A. (1991). Understanding customer expectations of service. *Sloan Management Review, 32*(3), 39-48.

Persch, A. C., & Page, S. J. (2013). Protocol development, treatment fidelity, adherence to treatment, and quality control. *American Journal of Occupational Therapy, 67*(2), 146-153.

Riegel, S. K., & Eglseder, K. (2009). Occupational justice as a quality indicator for occupational therapy services. *Occupational Therapy In Healthcare, 23*(4), 288-299.

Shi, L., & Singh, D. (2012). *Delivering health care in America: A systems approach* (5th ed.). Burlington, MA: Jones and Bartlett Publishers.

Shojania, K., & Grimshaw, J. (2005). Evidence-based quality improvement: The state of the science. *Health Affairs, 24*(1), 138-150.

Skledar, S. J., & McKaveney, T. P. (2009). A method for teaching continuous quality improvement to student pharmacists through a practical application project. *Currents in Pharmacy, Teaching, and Learning, 1*, 79-86.

Snoby, P. (2004). Performance improvement boot camp. *Radiology Nursing, 23*(3), 68-77.

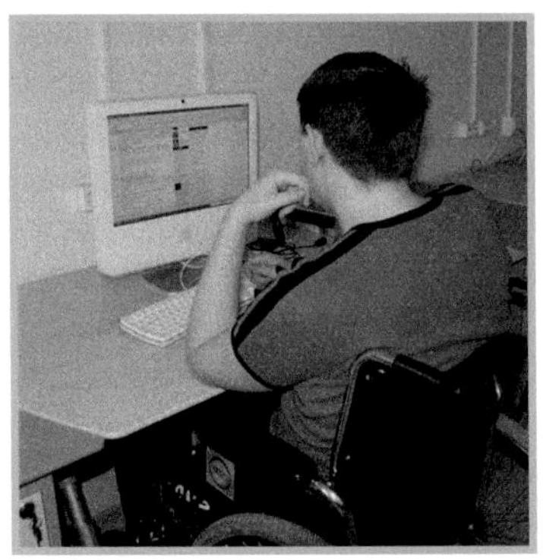

# 44

# Supervision of Occupational Therapy Personnel

*Amy Lamb, OTD, OT/L, FAOTA*

**ACOTE STANDARDS EXPLORED IN THIS CHAPTER**

B.7.7, B.7.12

**KEY VOCABULARY**

- **Intraprofessional:** A team of professionals that are all from the same profession.
- **Occupational therapists:** Based on education and training, with initial certification and appropriate state licensure, are autonomous practitioners who deliver occupational therapy services independently.
- **Occupational therapy assistants:** Based on education and training, with initial certification and appropriate state regulation/licensure, provide occupational therapy services under the supervision of a licensed occupational therapist.
- **Occupational therapy practitioners:** Term used to encompass occupational therapists and occupational therapy assistants.
- **Service competency:** The ability of an occupational therapy assistant to obtain the same information in evaluation tasks or perform treatment procedures in a manner that outcomes and documentation are equivalent to that of the supervising occupational therapist.
- **Site:** Setting in which practice occurs.
- **Supervisee:** One who receives direction and undergoes evaluation by a qualified practitioner.
- **Supervision:** Direct and evaluate performance.



Jacobs, K., & MacRae, N. (Eds.).
*Occupational Therapy Essentials for Clinical Competence, Third Edition* (pp. 627-633).

The advancement of the occupational therapy profession is multifaceted. At the heart of this advancement is the necessary intraprofessional collaborations of occupational therapy professionals of all levels. This chapter identifies the participants in the supervisory relationship; examines the professional guidelines for supervision in occupational therapy; and provides an overview of strategies for effective, competency-based, legal, and ethical supervision of occupational therapy and non-occupational therapy personnel.

## Participants in the Supervisory Relationship

The term *occupational therapy professional* includes occupational therapists, occupational therapy assistants, and students of occupational therapy. In some practice settings, occupational therapy or rehabilitation aides are also a part of the supervisory relationship. The functions of a supervisor are primarily in three areas: educational, administrative, and supportive.

The official documents of American Occupational Therapy Association (AOTA) define supervision as a:

> Cooperative process in which two or more people participate in a joint effort to establish, maintain, and or elevate a level of competence and performance aimed at ensuring the safe and effective delivery of occupational therapy services and fostering professional competence and development. (2014a, p. S16)

## General Supervision Issues

Supervision is a continuing and dynamic process that encourages professional development in both the supervisee and supervisor. Supervision is considered a professional responsibility and, therefore, an important aspect of good clinical practice. Both the occupational therapy assistant and occupational therapist should seek supervision according to the *Occupational Therapy Code of Ethics* and good clinical judgment (Sladyk, 2005). As workforce trends evolve, it is important that appropriate supervision strategies be in place between intraprofessional members of the team to ensure that high-quality occupational therapy services are received by the beneficiaries in need.

Being a supervisor for another practitioner is best designed as a collaborative process that holds the ability to spark development and growth in both the supervisor and the supervisee. Communication is a key factor in the supervisory process. It is often the supervisor who takes the lead in initiating this process. It is best accomplished by scheduling time to sit together and discuss how each of you communicates. For example, if the supervisor is very direct in his or her communication, a supervisee who is more timid may read that as a lack of openness and may refrain from engaging in dialogue or asking questions out of fear. As you prepare to participate in a supervisory relationship, whether as the supervisor or supervisee, it is recommended you spend some time reflecting on how you prefer to give and receive feedback so dialogue can occur between all parties and promote good lines of communication. Opening the lines of communication allows for each party to share how he or she communicates up front before any issues emerge and grow. These open lines also provide a good avenue to offer feedback. Frequent feedback is essential to learning. How does your supervisee prefer feedback? Perhaps he or she prefers it immediately or perhaps all lumped together at the end of the day or week in a summary session. Does the supervisee prefer the nuts and bolts of what needs to be worked on, or does he or she prefer a cushioned approach to feedback, such as stating areas of development in between comments about strengths he or she has in his or her practice? This information can all be discovered by keeping open communication lines.

As a supervisee, putting your best foot forward first is a great way to build a strong relationship with your direct supervisor. Prior to starting the position, examine what it is you need and expect from the supervisor. Reflect on how you prefer to receive feedback and share this information with your supervisor on the first day to help define what you look for from the supervisory relationship. Know what to expect, review the materials the facility has regarding clients and department organization, as well as your job description. Write down questions and ask for clarification; do not assume. Use the documents reviewed for your own reflection as to what kind of supervision you are expecting and in what manner you would prefer to receive supervision. A positive attitude by both parties is fundamental to success. When supervisors and supervisees approach the relationship with a positive attitude, are open to feedback, and participate with open communication, good things happen for the clients, departments, and facilities. Supervision is fundamental to skill development and learning, and being open to the process is the first step toward a successful relationship.

### *Supervision of the Occupational Therapist*

Although no supervision is required, supervision by an occupational therapist with advanced skills is recommended and will enhance clinical practice for entry-level practitioners. Novice practitioners can benefit from supervision from mid-career and advanced practitioners, as they develop their practice and manage the dynamics of the environments in which they work. Mid-career practitioners can often benefit from occasional supervision by advanced practitioners as they continue to grow in their practice and skill set, while identifying emerging opportunities that may benefit from occupational therapy, such as program development and outcome management. The regular interaction of practitioners at all experience levels enhances the practice of all involved and encourages the use of best practices, evidence, and innovative treatment approaches.

### *Supervision of the Occupational Therapy Assistant*

Services of occupational therapy assistants are provided under supervision from an occupational therapist who is ultimately responsible for the occupational therapy services provided. Supervision of the occupational therapy assistant by an occupational therapist is a requirement both professionally and legally. Both the supervising occupational therapist and the occupational therapy assistant should always refer to state practice acts and regulations for detailed information regarding specific supervisory requirements. In addition, "the supervising occupational therapist and occupational therapy assistant are equally responsible for developing a collaborative plan for supervision which is essential for a strong intraprofessional partnership" (AOTA, 2014a, p. S17).

## Professional Guidelines for Supervision

The manner in which this supervision occurs is guided by the general principles outlined by the AOTA in the *Guidelines for Supervision, Roles, and Responsibilities During the Delivery of Occupational Therapy Services.* Key principles in the occupational therapist/occupational therapy assistant supervisory relationship include the following:

- Provision of safe and effective service delivery is essential; therefore, the occupational therapist and occupational therapy assistant should collaborate to determine the manner and frequency of supervision.
- Both the occupational therapist and occupational therapy assistant should recognize when supervision is needed and also build in regular times for supervision to ensure quality occupational therapy services are provided.
- Frequency, methods, and content of supervision is dependent on the practice setting, state laws and regulations, complexity of the clientele, and knowledge and skill level of both the occupational therapist and occupational therapy assistant.
- Supervision that is more stringent than the facility or regulatory body requires may be necessary in settings where clients are complex.
- Methods of supervision should vary and include both direct and indirect contact.
- Occupational therapists and occupational therapy assistants must adhere to facility and state requirements for supervision.
- Occupational therapists must recognize and be responsive to occupational therapy assistants' professional growth and support their advancing practice skill set. (AOTA, 2014a, p. S18)

It is important to recognize that the guidelines provided are to serve as a blueprint as you develop the framework for the occupational therapist/occupational therapy assistant partnership. It is essential that you look at state licensing and reimbursement agency requirements for supervision, as they supersede the preceding guidelines from AOTA.

## Roles and Responsibilities in the Delivery of Occupational Therapy Services

There are several points that are important to emphasize in the roles and responsibilities of occupational therapists and occupational therapy assistants in the delivery of occupational therapy services as it pertains to the supervision process.

- The occupational therapist is responsible for all aspects of occupational therapy service delivery.
- The occupational therapist must be involved in the initial evaluation and regularly throughout the client's intervention.
- The occupational therapy assistant delivers occupational therapy services under supervision of an occupational therapist.
- The occupational therapist determines when to delegate responsibilities to an occupational therapy assistant when service competency has been demonstrated.
- The occupational therapist and occupational therapy assistant demonstrate and document service competency for clinical reasoning and judgment, as well as treatment techniques and interventions. (AOTA, 2014a, p. S18)

Within this area it is important to recognize that service competency means that an occupational therapy assistant gets the same information or performs treatment procedures in a manner that the outcome and documentation are equivalent to what would have been achieved if the supervising occupational therapist had performed the services. Service competency is often established by the occupational therapist and occupational therapy assistant working together to establish such competencies. In the establishment of service competency, open communication is important as is consistent feedback between both the supervisor and supervisee. It is also helpful to document service competencies established in a supervisory file to reflect the partnership between the occupational therapist and the occupational therapy assistant.

### Occupational Therapy or Rehabilitation Aides

Aides are individuals who provide support services to the occupational therapist, occupational therapy assistant, physical therapist, or physical therapist assistant. They are trained by the skilled rehabilitation professional and must demonstrate competency to complete delegated client and nonclient tasks (AOTA, 2014a, p. S21). When aides are being used in any practice setting, the occupational therapist is responsible for developing, documenting, and implementing a supervisory plan for the aide. Either the occupational therapist or the occupational therapy assistant can provide supervision to the aide. Client-related tasks an aide may assist with include routine tasks where processes have been clearly established and will not require judgment, interpretations or adaptations to be made by the aide (AOTA, 2014a, p. S21).

## Skills for Supervisory Success

Supervision is a process by which both the supervisor and supervisee are learning from the other. The supervisory relationship provides partners with a planned opportunity to talk about practice, exchange ideas, and ensure appropriate delivery of services. Supervisors should clarify expectations surrounding their responsibilities as a supervisor within their profession at large and also within their organization to develop a foundation for success.

### Communication

Communication is a must in a successful supervisory relationship. Being successful in your occupational therapy role is not limited to the technical aspects of the job or being willing to work hard. Success is intricately related to being able to transmit information and ideas to others (with clients, occupational therapy team members, and other health care practitioners alike). The ability to communicate in a clear, consistent manner is vital to the supervisory process. Supervisors also need to recognize the importance of listening, establishing rapport, and motivating others. Effective communication leads to productive relationships. Communication should occur regularly to ensure quality occupational therapy services are being provided.

### Appropriate Delegation

It is the responsibility of the supervisor to ensure that when tasks are delegated to a supervisee that they are ready for that responsibility and qualified to adequately complete the task. Delegating does not take responsibility away from the supervisor. When delegating, it is important to consider the practice context, knowledge and skill level of the supervisee, and complexity of the task. It is often helpful to use a method frequently used in documentation for communication in delegating tasks. The SMART method (specific, measurable, achievable, realistic, and time bound) can be used as a framework in which you delegate tasks to a supervisee; this method supports clear communication so both the supervisor and supervisee understand the task and its associated responsibilities.

### Feedback

Clear, consistent, regular feedback is useful in keeping the supervisory/supervisee relationship moving forward. Feedback encourages growth among both parties and is essential to learning and development. Feedback should not just happen once a year at an annual performance review, but is most effective when it occurs regularly and is consistent. Feedback should also be mixed; things the supervisee is doing well should be emphasized along with the areas for growth. It is also recommended that you observe your supervisee in a variety of venues, such as a treatment session, documentation, communication with clients and/or families, and communication with other professionals in the setting, to provide feedback in each of these areas.

Create multifaceted mechanisms for delivering feedback. Each of us processes information differently. Provide avenues to reach the supervisee in multiple ways. Written feedback can be provided in weekly progress forms and shared with the supervisee. Feedback in writing allows the supervisee to reflect back on your comments. Verbal feedback can be provided in conjunction with the written feedback and ideally reviewed in a weekly meeting. Verbal feedback can also occur immediately after an observation session, and depending on the observation setting, you can ask the supervisee to reflect on what happened, what went well, and what he or she would have done differently. This sparks reflective thinking and opens the door for you to offer feedback after he or she has shared his or her reflections with you. Finally, demonstrations can effectively serve as feedback as well. Establish opportunities for staff to learn from one another. It creates a strong sense of team and builds the culture within in a department while promoting strong intraprofessional partnerships.

### *Supporting Professional Growth*

Each occupational therapy practitioner has his or her own desires and interests for professional growth. Working together as a team does not mean that both the supervisor and supervisee need to have similar professional growth interests. One of the benefits of working as a team is supporting one another in professional growth. As a supervisor, when an individual under your supervision expresses an interest in gaining additional skills in a particular area or seeking increased experience in an area he or she finds intriguing, it is your responsibility to assist the supervisee in identifying and supporting appropriate professional growth opportunities.

## Evaluation of Performance

Almost all facilities require a minimum yearly written review of work productivity. Feedback on this form should not come as a surprise to the supervisee, as a good supervisor has talked about the issues well before a formal written evaluation is completed. Feedback should be specific, balanced, and focused on behaviors. The supervisee should initially develop professional goals for the next review period that fit the program's mission statement. Then together the supervisor and supervisee should develop a plan to meet these goals (Sladyk, 2005). A helpful strategy for supervisors to use is to provide the supervisee with a copy of the annual performance documents to utilize as a self-evaluation tool prior to the meeting, as it opens the door to enhanced dialogue in the meeting and allows the supervisee to have done some reflection on his or her performance in a more organized way. From there time should be set aside for the supervisor and supervisee to meet and discuss strengths of performance, areas for improvement, and strategies to support professional development.

## Reflective Learning in Supervision

Reflection is defined as "a thought, idea, or opinion formed or a remark made as a result of meditation" (*Merriam-Webster's Online Dictionary*, 2016). Reflection is a primary vehicle for learning, but it is not a process that comes easily for all. The process of supervision aims to facilitate reflection to deepen understanding (Davys & Beddoe, 2009). When reflection occurs as a part of the supervisory process, the supervisee is driven to learn from the experience and thought rather than pure knowledge of the supervisor. When a supervisor provides opportunity for the supervisee to reflect, he or she encourages the supervisee to take ownership of experiences while enhancing learning and development.

## Generational Differences

Another important factor in the supervisory process is found in understanding the generational differences currently found in practice and in our upcoming generation of occupational therapists and occupational therapy assistants.

When examining generations, we look at the commonalities among individuals from hugely different backgrounds within a defined period of time (Stollings, 2015). How does this information play a role in occupational therapy supervision? Consider who we are often pairing together within the supervisory relationship. Think about how practice has evolved and changed and how rapidly the system in which we practice is changing. Areas of practice have shifted, educational programs have evolved, and the entry-level practitioner today is different from that of 20 years ago. For this discussion, we will focus on three generations, all of which are key players within occupational therapy clinical education: Baby Boomers, Generation X, and Millennials. Table 44-1 explores these generations further.

Generational differences cannot go ignored as we examine the supervisor/supervisee relationship. Let us examine the supervisor/supervisee concept further and then look at a case study that includes the generational mixes found in practice today.

## Ethical Dilemmas in Supervision

It is inevitable that we will encounter ethical challenges in practice. When ethical issues emerge around supervisory relationships, each person is watching the other to see how it will be handled. There are models of decision making related to ethics that can be of use in demonstrating the process of handling ethical dilemmas. Gervais (2005) identified six steps to assist practitioners in this process. These steps include gathering background knowledge of the situation; examining the case based on its facts and context; completing a self-assessment, including the personal capacity for your decision; weighing options for what is most right; acting on the option you feel is ethically correct; and evaluating via reflection to examine what you learned in your review and handling of this situation; and what you would do the same or what you would do differently should the situation arise again.

Table 44-1.

**TRAITS ACROSS THE GENERATIONS**

| Generation (born between) | Outlook | Work Ethic | View of Authority | Leadership Through | Perspective |
|---|---|---|---|---|---|
| Baby Boomers (1940-1960) | Optimistic | Driven | Love/hate | Consensus | Team |
| Generation X (1961-1980) | Skeptical | Balanced | Unimpressed | Competence | Self |
| Millennial (1981-2000) | Hopeful | Ambitious | Relaxed, polite | Achievement | Civic |

Adapted from Raines, C., & Ewing, L. (2006). *The art of connecting: How to overcome differences, build rapport, and communicate effectively with anyone.* New York, NY: American Management Association.

Supervisors should model ethical reasoning to supervisees to assist them in learning how they will approach ethical situations that arise. When an ethical issue arises with a client with whom both you and your supervisee have both been working, it is helpful to engage the supervisee with you as you navigate your decision making.

With the implementation of the Patient Protection and Affordable Care Act, health care is undergoing many transitions in both traditional and emerging areas of practice. This may increase the demands placed on occupational therapists and occupational therapy assistants. It is essential that the focus on delivering high-quality occupational therapy services stay on the forefront at all times (AOTA, 2010, p. 1).

## SUMMARY

Supervision is a process through which both the supervisor and supervisee can develop professionally. The process of supervision is one that when done with open communication, consistent and frequent feedback, and in a manner that promotes professional growth can enhance the intraprofessional relationship and quality of care for clients served. Using reflection in the supervision process enhances the learning for the supervisee and should be utilized regularly to promote professional development. In establishing supervisory partnerships, it is important to consider the generational differences to allow those of different generations to appreciate their colleagues' approach to the supervisory process.

**Case Study**

You are a new occupational therapist working for a rehabilitation company that contracts with skilled nursing facilities, assisted living and independent living facilities, and home health agencies. Your time is often split primarily between two assisted living facilities and home health visits. There is an occupational therapy assistant with more than 15 years of experience and 6 years with the company who also works in these buildings and you will be supervising. It is important to note that the occupational therapy assistant has not had a consistent occupational therapy supervisor for the past 2 years and only on-call staff do occupational therapy evaluations, reevaluations, and discharges as needed. You have been hired to build the occupational therapy caseload and will be handling the occupational therapy services in partnership with the occupational therapy assistant. How will you begin your partnership and supervisory responsibilities with the occupational therapy assistant?

## STUDENT SELF-ASSESSMENT

1. In pairs, practice verbalizing what you envision to be the ideal supervisor/supervisee relationship.
2. On paper, write out how you would best describe your learning style, how you prefer feedback, and your communication style.
3. Practice communicating with a partner and focus on clear, direct communication to get him or her to complete a task.

## Evidence-Based Research Chart

| Issue | Evidence |
|---|---|
| Supervision | AOTA, 2014a, 2014b, 2015a, 2015b, 2015c; Davys & Beddoe, 2010; Gervais, 2005 |
| Reflective learning | Davys & Beddoe, 2009; Thorpe, 2004 |
| Generational differences | Raines & Ewing, 2006; Zemke, Raines, & Filipczak, 2013 |

## References

American Occupational Therapy Association. (2010). OT/OTA *Partnerships: Achieving high ethical standards in a challenging healthcare environment.* Retrieved from https://www.aota.org/-/media/corporate/files/practice/ethics/advisory/ot-ota-partnership.pdf

American Occupational Therapy Association. (2014a). Guidelines for supervision, roles, and responsibilities during the delivery of occupational therapy services. *American Journal of Occupational Therapy, 68*(Suppl. 3), S16-S22. doi:10.5014/ajot.2014.686S03

American Occupational Therapy Association. (2014b). Occupational therapy practice framework: Domain and process (3rd ed.). *American Journal of Occupational Therapy, 68*(Suppl. 1), S1-S48. doi:10.5014/ajot.2014.682006

American Occupational Therapy Association. (2015a). *Occupational therapy code of ethics (2015).* Retrived from http://ajot.aota.org/article.aspx?articleid=2442685

American Occupational Therapy Association. (2015b). *Standards of practice for occupational therapy.* Retrieved from http://ajot.aota.org/article.aspx?articleid=2477354

American Occupational Therapy Association. (2015c). *Value of occupational therapy assistant education to the profession.* Retrieved from http://ajot.aota.org/article.aspx?articleid=2478994

Davys, A., & Beddoe, L. (2009). The reflective learning model: Supervision of social work students. *Social Work Education, 28*(8), 919-933.

Davys, A., & Beddoe, L. (2010). *Best practice in professional supervision: A guide for the helping professions.* Philadelphia, PA: Jessica Kingsley Publishers.

Gervais, K. G. (2005). A model for ethical decision making to inform the ethics education of future health care professionals. In R. B. Purtilo, G. M. Jensen, & C. B. Royeen (Eds.), *Educating for moral action: A sourcebook in health and rehabilitation ethics.* Philadelphia, PA: F. A. Davis Company.

Raines, C., & Ewing, L. (2006). *The art of connecting: How to overcome differences, build rapport, and communicate effectively with anyone.* New York, NY: American Management Association.

Reflection. (2016). *Merriam-Webster's online dictionary.* Retrieved from http://www.merriam-webster.com/dictionary/reflection

Sladyk, K. (Ed.). (2005). *OT study cards in a box.* Thorofare, NJ: SLACK Incorporated.

Stollings, J. (2015). *ReGenerations: Why connecting generations matters and how to do it.* CreateSpace Independent Publishing Platform.

Thorpe, K. (2004). Reflective learning journals: From concept to practice. *Reflective Practice, 5*(3), 327-343.

Zemke, R., Raines, C., & Filipczak, B. (2013). *Generations at work: Managing the clash of Boomers, Gen Xers, and Gen Yers in the workplace.* New York, NY: American Management Association.

## Suggested Reading

Barnfield, H., & Lombardo, M. (2014). *FYI: For your improvement: Competencies development guide* (6th ed.). Los Angeles, CA: Korn-Ferry Publishing.

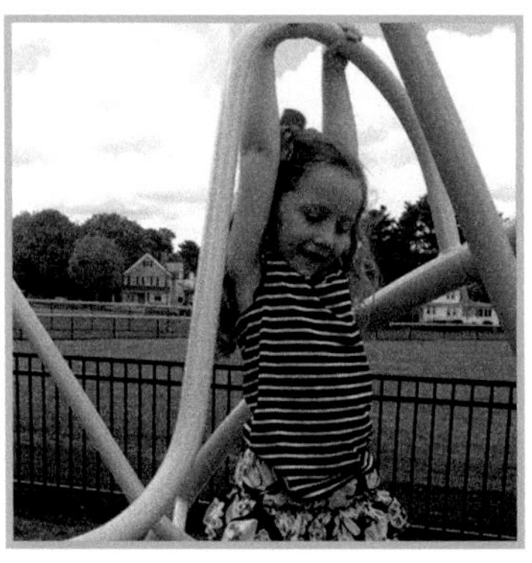

# 45

# Fieldwork Education

*Julie Ann Nastasi, ScD, OTD, OTR/L, SCLV, FAOTA*

**ACOTE STANDARDS EXPLORED IN THIS CHAPTER**

B.7.8

**KEY VOCABULARY**

- **Fieldwork coordinator:** A faculty member who is responsible for overseeing student fieldwork placements.
- **Fieldwork supervisor:** An occupational therapy practitioner who provides supervision to the student during the fieldwork placement.
- **Level I fieldwork:** Introduces the student to the fieldwork experience.
- **Level II fieldwork:** Transitions the student to the role of an entry-level practitioner.



Jacobs, K., & MacRae, N. (Eds.).
*Occupational Therapy Essentials for Clinical Competence, Third Edition* (pp. 635-643).

Fieldwork education is crucial to the field of occupational therapy. Occupational therapy relies on fieldwork supervisors, who work in collaboration with fieldwork coordinators, to train and evaluate students to meet the minimal standards for entry-level practice (Accreditation Council for Occupational Therapy Education [ACOTE], 2011). Successful completion of fieldwork is required to graduate from an accredited program and to sit for the national board examinations (ACOTE, 2011; National Board for Certification in Occupational Therapy [NBCOT], 2015). Occupational therapy practitioners have a professional responsibility to ensure the future of the profession through fieldwork education. Roles, criteria, and components of fieldwork education will be explored in this chapter.

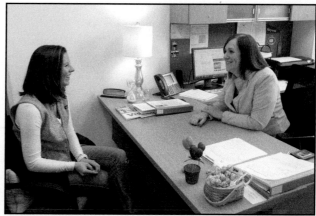

**Figure 45-1.** A fieldwork coordinator advising an occupational therapy student.

## Occupational Therapy Education Programs

Occupational therapy education programs are responsible for training students in the fundamental knowledge and skills necessary to become occupational therapists and occupational therapy assistants. Each occupational therapy education program designs its curriculum to address its mission and vision for the program. The fieldwork coordinator selects fieldwork sites for students that match the program's mission and vision.

### *Fieldwork Coordinator*

Each occupational therapy education program has a fieldwork coordinator who is responsible for the program's compliance with fieldwork education requirements (Figure 45-1). The fieldwork coordinator serves as a liaison between the program and the fieldwork sites to ensure that students are being properly trained and the fieldwork placement aligns with the program's curriculum. The fieldwork coordinator oversees the fieldwork placements and works with the fieldwork supervisor and student in facilitating fieldwork placements.

### *Fieldwork Supervisor*

The fieldwork supervisor is the person responsible for supervising occupational therapy students on Level I or Level II fieldwork placements. The fieldwork supervisor is responsible for the student completing the fieldwork placement. The supervisor guides, facilitates, and evaluates the student throughout the placement. At the end of the placement, the fieldwork supervisor evaluates if the student has accomplished the requirements of the fieldwork placement. If the student achieves the requirements, the student passes the fieldwork placement. If the student does not meet the requirements, the fieldwork supervisor collaborates with the fieldwork coordinator and the student for the purpose of preparing for another placement. They discuss the areas that the student needs to improve prior to securing a new placement.

### *Eligibility Requirements for Fieldwork Supervisors*

ACOTE (2011) requires that Level II fieldwork supervisors have successfully completed initial certification through the NBCOT and have a minimum of 1 year of practice prior to supervising Level II students on fieldwork placements. In addition, the fieldwork supervisor must be adequately prepared to supervise the student. Training in fieldwork supervision may be provided by the academic program or the fieldwork site. The requirements for Level I fieldwork supervisors are less stringent. Occupational therapists and occupational therapy assistants may supervise students on Level I fieldwork as well as other qualified professionals, including psychologists, physician assistants, teachers, social workers, nurses, and physical therapists (ACOTE, 2011).

### *Students*

Students on fieldwork must first complete their academic program's requirements to be eligible for a fieldwork placement. In addition, some fieldwork sites may require students to complete additional requirements. Some of these requirements may include, but are not limited to, a physical examination, cardiopulmonary resuscitation training, a criminal background check, child abuse clearance, fingerprinting, and individual malpractice insurance. The fieldwork coordinator or the fieldwork supervisor typically notifies the students of the requirements for specific fieldwork placements. Some fieldwork sites also require students to complete orientation through their human resources department prior to starting fieldwork. Students need to check to ensure that all requirements are met prior to starting fieldwork to avoid a delay or cancellation in the placement.

While on fieldwork, the students report directly to their assigned fieldwork supervisor. In some settings, students may have more than one supervisor. Students should collaborate and communicate with their assigned fieldwork supervisor(s). If students find they are having problems at their fieldwork site, they should notify their program's fieldwork coordinator. The fieldwork coordinator serves as a liaison between the students and the fieldwork site where the students are placed. It is in the students' best interest to communicate with their fieldwork coordinator about their fieldwork progress.

## Fieldwork

Fieldwork should provide students "with the opportunity to carry out professional responsibilities under supervision of a qualified occupational therapy practitioner serving as a role model" (ACOTE, 2011, p. 33). Students have the opportunity to participate in Level I and Level II fieldwork experiences.

### *Level I Fieldwork*

"The goal of Level I fieldwork is to introduce students to the fieldwork experience, to apply knowledge to practice, and to develop understanding of the needs of clients" (ACOTE, 2011, p. 34). During Level I fieldwork, students complete observations in an assigned setting. Settings are often associated with a particular practice course that the students have taken. For example, some programs have students complete Level I fieldwork in pediatrics during or following their pediatric practice course. The Level I fieldwork experience allows the students to observe and participate in clinical practice settings that relate to their coursework. Students are not required to be supervised by an occupational therapist or occupational therapy assistant during Level I fieldwork. Other qualified professionals for supervision include psychologists, physician assistants, teachers, social workers, nurses, and physical therapists (ACOTE, 2011).

ACOTE now requires students to complete a Level I or Level II fieldwork experience that focuses on "psychological and social factors that influence engagement in occupation" (ACOTE, 2011, p. 34). Students should expect to be placed in a Level I or Level II fieldwork placement that addresses psychological and social factors that impact engagement in occupation.

### *Level II Fieldwork*

The goal of Level II fieldwork is to develop competent, entry-level, generalist occupational therapists and occupational therapy assistants (ACOTE, 2011). "Level II fieldwork must be integral to the program's curriculum design and must include an in-depth experience in delivering occupational therapy services to clients, focusing on the application of purposeful and meaningful occupation and research, administration, and management of occupational therapy services" (ACOTE, 2011, p. 35). Occupational therapy students must complete a minimum of 24 weeks of full-time Level II fieldwork. Typically, the occupational therapy students complete two 12-week fieldwork placements in two different practice settings. Occupational therapy assistant students must complete a minimum of 16 weeks of full-time Level II fieldwork, which typically is in two different practice settings for 8 weeks each.

### *Specialty Level II Fieldwork*

Some programs allow students the option to select a third Level II fieldwork placement in a specialty area, while other programs require students to complete a third Level II fieldwork placement. The third Level II fieldwork placement provides students with the opportunity to complete a fieldwork placement that is in a specialized practice area. Programs are required to prepare students as entry-level generalists (ACOTE, 2011). The third fieldwork placement goes beyond the accreditation requirements, thus providing students with the opportunity for specialization (Nastasi, 2012, 2013). For example, a student may want to complete a third Level II fieldwork placement in low vision rehabilitation or in a neonatal intensive care unit.

### *Doctoral Experiential Component*

Occupational therapy students enrolled in an entry-level occupational therapy doctoral program are required to complete a doctoral experiential component. To complete the doctoral experiential component, students must successfully complete their academic program and Level II fieldwork. In addition, students must pass a competency requirement. The competency requirement varies by academic program and may include a comprehensive examination or oral examination. The doctoral experiential component should provide students with advanced skills beyond the generalist level. The experiential component should align with the program's curriculum design and should further develop skills in clinical practice, research, administration, leadership, program and policy development, advocacy, education, or theory development (ACOTE, 2011).

The doctoral experiential component requires that students complete a minimum of 16 weeks (640 hours), and previous fieldwork experiences may not be counted toward the experience. The experience takes place in a mentored practice setting, and no more than 20% of the experience can take place outside of the mentored practice setting. The mentor must have expertise in the area of focus and does not have to be an occupational therapist. A formal evaluation of the student must take place during and at the completion of the experience (ACOTE, 2011).

# Steps for a Successful Fieldwork Placement

The goal for fieldwork coordinators, fieldwork supervisors, and students is to have students pass their fieldwork placements. Some steps for a successful fieldwork placement include a pre-fieldwork interview, formal orientation, student self-assessment, formative assessment, feedback, shared supervision by two fieldwork supervisors, and technological tools to promote independent learning.

## *Pre-Interview*

Fieldwork supervisors should request that students complete an interview prior to their fieldwork placement. The interview provides the students and the fieldwork supervisors with the opportunity to meet and gain a better understanding of the expectations of the placement, as well as to determine if there will be a good working relationship. Research has found that students benefit from a pre-fieldwork interview (Gutman, McCreedy, & Heisler, 1998; Holloway & Neufeldt, 1995). Grades are not effective indicators for fieldwork success. When students communicated with fieldwork supervisors, they were more successful on their fieldwork placements (Gutman et al., 1998). Students who are interpersonally attractive to their supervisors have been rated as being more effective by their supervisors than by their clients (Holloway & Neufeldt, 1995). The personality fit of the fieldwork supervisors and students played a critical role in the scores that the students received from their fieldwork supervisors. Therefore, scheduling an interview prior to a fieldwork placement allows the fieldwork supervisors and the students to determine if there is a good fit, as well as establish strong communication and a good working relationship (Nastasi, 2013).

## *Formal Orientation*

Students also benefit from formal orientation at their fieldwork sites (Cameron et al., 2013; Hanson & Deluliis, 2015; Nastasi, 2013). Formal orientation provides students with a better understanding of the expectations of the fieldwork supervisors and the fieldwork site. Kirke et al. (2007) used focus groups to determine the key elements of fieldwork education. The groups identified that fieldwork supervisors need to have a planned orientation where the requirements of the placement are covered. Providing role clarity, team members' responsibilities, and a better understanding of the skills required during fieldwork facilitates the fieldwork placement (Robertson & Griffiths, 2009). In addition, structure is needed for continual development of students' skill progression during the fieldwork placement (Cameron et al., 2013; Kleiser & Cox, 2008). Formal orientation provides a way to communicate the expectations of the fieldwork placement and provides students with key training and resources to support their participation in fieldwork education.

## *Student Self-Assessment*

During fieldwork, students need to assess their performance and determine if they are meeting the expectations of their fieldwork supervisors and the site. Different forms of self-assessment have been incorporated into fieldwork education. Duke (2004) reported "that students who had self-awareness of their own strengths and weaknesses, and were not afraid to ask for help, were more competent than the students who were not able to reflect on their practice and to highlight areas of difficulty" (p. 207). One form of self-assessment includes the use of journals or logs (Buchanan, van Niekerk, & Moore, 2001; Hanson & Deluliis, 2015; Maizels et al., 2008). Students complete a daily log during their fieldwork experience. Then at weekly supervision meetings, the students share portions of their journals with their fieldwork supervisors. This provides the students the opportunity to go over their thoughts and concerns during the previous week. Feedback between the students and fieldwork supervisors facilitates growth of the students (Boudreau & Donnell, 2013; de Beer & Martensson, 2015; Grenier, 2015; Hanson & Deluliis, 2015). Upon completion of fieldwork, students should reread their journals and submit their journals to the program's fieldwork coordinator. The journal provides the students the opportunity to communicate with their fieldwork supervisors and to see their growth over the fieldwork placement. Other forms of self-assessment include learning contracts (Hanson & Deluliis, 2015). Whitcombe (2001) studied the use of learning contracts in fieldwork education among 68 participants. The study found that the majority of respondents supported using learning contracts. Students reported that learning contracts allowed them to control their own learning. The fieldwork supervisors reported that the learning contracts helped them to focus on the individual learner's needs.

## *Formative Assessment*

In conjunction with journals and a learning contract, a formal self-assessment should take place at the mid-term and final evaluations (Nastasi, 2013). These formal self-assessments provide a reflective process allowing the students, via collaboration with their fieldwork supervisors, to identify the progressive skill requirements and assess their performance during the placement, including what they need to do to complete the placement successfully.

### Feedback

Fieldwork supervisors and students should provide each other with feedback throughout the fieldwork experience. Grenier (2015) found students repeatedly reported feedback from fieldwork supervisors as a key learning tool that facilitated learning and a better understanding of their strengths and weaknesses. When feedback is provided with suggestions on how to improve, clinical reasoning skills improve (de Beer & Martensson, 2015). If students are at a fieldwork site with multiple students, students may provide feedback to each other. Hanson and Deluliis (2015) suggest that ground rules for feedback between students should be established at the beginning of the fieldwork placement. Rules should facilitate constructive feedback. Students should allow every student to speak, avoid interrupting each other, and provide constructive feedback on skill performance. Feedback provides opportunities for reflection and facilitates clinical reasoning (Hanson & Deluliis, 2015).

### Structure and Validation for Shared Supervision

Fieldwork coordinators and students know that it is not always easy finding fieldwork placements. A shortage of fieldwork placements and changes in occupational therapy practice have led the field of occupational therapy to examine different models of fieldwork supervision. Literature supports students having one or two fieldwork supervisors during their fieldwork placements (Bonello, 2001; Hanson & Deluliis, 2015; Nolinske, 1995; Thomas et al., 2007). Supervision by two fieldwork supervisors provides students with opportunities to complete fieldwork in settings that do not have full-time occupational therapy practitioners. In addition, it provides students with the opportunity to complete fieldwork in emerging practice settings (Bonello, 2001). A study in Australia reported that 96% of participating students were supervised by one or two supervisors during fieldwork (Thomas et al., 2007). By allowing shared supervision between two fieldwork supervisors, both the shortage in fieldwork placements and the opportunity for students to engage in emerging practice areas are met.

### Technological Tools to Promote Independent Learning

Technology provides students with opportunities to learn and collaborate with their fieldwork coordinator and their fieldwork supervisors. Current research supports the use of technology in fieldwork education and for self-directed learning (Cameron et al., 2013; Scanlan & Hancock, 2010). "A growing body of evidence supports the conclusion that technology-enhanced teaching is equivalent in effectiveness compared with traditional methods when student-learning outcomes are the focus of the measurement" (Fullerton & Ingle, 2003, p. 426). Fullerton and Ingle (2003) reviewed 19 studies that focused on allied health professions and evaluated student grades, grade point averages, self-assessment competencies, practice guidelines, test scores, learner satisfaction, and use of technical support. They concluded that there was no difference in scores or grades for students learning on-campus and students learning through asynchronous learning environments. Overall, the evidence suggests that online learning allows for flexibility in studying in a virtual environment and is playing a more important role in supporting learning (Liu & Wang, 2009). Creating online materials for students during their fieldwork experience enhances their fieldwork experience (Scanlan & Hancock, 2010). The use of web-based instruction during fieldwork provides the fieldwork coordinator with the opportunity to communicate with students during fieldwork. Such instruction may include synchronous or asynchronous discussions, or meetings via webcam. In addition, it provides students with the opportunity to network with each other, gain treatment ideas, and remain updated on the profession. In a study by Creel (2001), 89% of students involved in web-based instruction during fieldwork indicated a strong interest in participating in it again for their next Level II fieldwork.

## Training Materials for Fieldwork Education

Training and training materials are essential to fieldwork education. Training materials help fieldwork supervisors to guide students through the fieldwork experience. Training materials include a manual containing a competency checklist, site-specific objectives, and developmental timeline (Nastasi, 2013).

### Manual

Manuals provide fieldwork supervisors and students with a mechanism to store pertinent information about the fieldwork placement. The fieldwork supervisors may decide to review the materials with the students or have the students review the materials on their own time. Manuals should include a competency checklist, site-specific objectives, and a developmental timeline for the students (Nastasi, 2013).

### Competency Checklist

A competency checklist provides fieldwork supervisors and students with information on the areas that the students need to be competent in to pass a fieldwork placement. The checklist allows the fieldwork supervisors and students to develop a plan on how to achieve the specific requirements during the fieldwork placement. The checklist should be reviewed on a weekly basis to ensure that the students are making progress on the required competencies. Fieldwork supervisors should develop and use a competency checklist that corresponds to the entry-level requirements for occupational therapists and occupational therapy assistants at their site because the goal of Level II fieldwork is to achieve entry-level status. This will assist the fieldwork supervisors at the site and the students in understanding the specific requirements of the fieldwork placement (Nastasi, 2013).

### Site-Specific Objectives

Site-specific objectives should align with the Fieldwork Performance Evaluation (American Occupational Therapy Association [AOTA], 2002). Each fieldwork site should identify specific objectives for each of the items on the evaluation. Some sites may opt to use site-specific objectives that are provided by the educational program sending fieldwork students. Whether the site or the educational program creates the site-specific objectives, ACOTE (2011) requires that fieldwork sites have site-specific objectives. Structure and guidance are needed during fieldwork (Cameron et al., 2013; Grenier, 2015; Hanson & Deluliis, 2015; Kleiser & Cox, 2008; Nastasi, 2013; Scanlan & Hancock, 2010; Whitcombe, 2001). Having written guidelines and assessment criteria for fieldwork students assists the students in meeting their educational goals (Buchanan et al., 2001; Meyers, 1995). Both occupational therapy students and fieldwork supervisors have reported that it was important to have defined objectives focusing on the fieldwork experience and the overall learning experience (Whitcombe, 2001). Site-specific objectives help define the students' fieldwork learning experiences.

### Developmental Timeline

Finally, a developmental timeline provides fieldwork supervisors and students with an understanding of how students should progress through their fieldwork experience. Timelines break down the students' responsibilities in terms of caseload and knowledge. By the end of the fieldwork placement, students should be carrying their supervisor's full caseload. A timeline provides students and fieldwork supervisors with a natural progression for the student's competency development. It provides structure and guidance for supervision (Kleiser & Cox, 2008; Nastasi, 2013).

**Case Study**

Mike is an occupational therapy student completing his first Level II fieldwork placement in an acute rehabilitation setting. Prior to the fieldwork placement, Mike interviewed with his fieldwork supervisor and identified pertinent information that he needed to know for the fieldwork placement. Mike reviewed his textbooks, notebooks, and online resources to prepare himself for the fieldwork placement.

During the first week of Mike's fieldwork placement, he completed a formal orientation and read the site's fieldwork manual. After reading the manual, Mike met with his fieldwork supervisor to discuss how they would address the skills on the competency checklist, site-specific objectives, and developmental timeline. Mike knew that his fieldwork supervisor expected him to be responsible for half of the supervisor's caseload by the sixth week of his placement. Mike also knew that he would be responsible for the whole caseload by his last week of fieldwork.

Each night, Mike wrote in his journal about his fieldwork experiences. As Mike approached his sixth week of fieldwork, he reread all of his entries. Mike realized how much he was progressing as he reread the first 6 weeks of his journal entries. During Mike's mid-term evaluation, he sat down with his supervisor and identified areas that he thought he was excelling and areas that he thought were challenging. Mike and his fieldwork supervisor planned times to go over some of the areas that Mike felt were challenging. Mike's fieldwork supervisor told him that he was right on target and was carrying half of the field supervisor's caseload.

Mike continued to journal and work with his fieldwork supervisor on the areas that he thought were challenging at the mid-term evaluation. Mike and his fieldwork supervisor provided feedback to each other and Mike's clinical reasoning skills improved. As Mike entered the last week of his fieldwork, he reread his journal entries. Mike realized that his meetings with his supervisor paid off. Mike no longer felt challenged in the areas he identified. When Mike and his supervisor met for his final evaluation, the fieldwork supervisor concurred. Mike's supervisor reported that Mike met all of the requirements of an entry-level occupational therapist. Mike successfully completed his first Level II fieldwork placement.

## Training Fieldwork Supervisors

Fieldwork supervisors generally receive on-the-job training to become fieldwork supervisors, as well as training from the educational programs that send students to their sites. Formal training is available through The AOTA's Fieldwork Educators Certificate Workshop

## Evidence-Based Research Chart

| Topic | Evidence |
|---|---|
| Pre-fieldwork interview | Gutman, McCreedy, & Heisler, 1998; Holloway & Neufeldt, 1995; Nastasi, 2013 |
| Formal orientation | Cameron et al., 2013; Hanson & Deluliis, 2015; Kirke, Layton, & Sims, 2007; Kleiser & Cox, 2008; Nastasi, 2013; Robertson & Griffiths, 2009 |
| Student self-assessment | Boudreau & Donnell, 2013; Buchanan et al., 2001; de Beer & Martensson, 2015; Duke, 2004; Grenier, 2015; Hanson & Deluliis, 2015; Kramer & Stern, 1995; Liu & Wang, 2009; Maizels et al., 2008; Nastasi, 2013; Whitcombe, 2001 |
| Feedback | de Beer & Martensson, 2015; Grenier, 2015; Hanson & Deluliis, 2015 |
| Structure and validation for shared supervision | Bonello, 2001; Hanson & Deluliis, 2015; Kleiser & Cox, 2008; Nastasi, 2013; Nolinske, 1995; Thomas et al., 2007 |
| Technology tools to promote independent learning | Cameron et al., 2013; Creel, 2001; Fullerton & Ingle, 2003; Liu & Wang, 2009; Maizels et al., 2008; Nastasi, 2013; Scanlan & Hancock, 2010 |
| Fieldwork manual | Holloway & Neufeldt, 1995; Nastasi, 2012, 2013; Whitcombe, 2001 |
| Competency checklist | Allison & Turpin, 2004; Buchanan et al., 2001; Duke, 2004; Kleiser & Cox, 2008; Maizels et al., 2008; Meyers, 1995; Nastasi, 2012, 2013; Robertson & Griffiths, 2009; Whitcombe, 2001 |
| Site-specific objectives | Buchanan et al., 2001; Cameron et al., 2013; Grenier, 2015; Hanson & Deluliis, 2015; Kleiser & Cox, 2008; Maizels et al., 2008; Meyers, 1995; Nastasi, 2012, 2013; Robertson & Griffiths, 2009; Scanlan & Hancock, 2010; Thomas et al., 2007; Whitcombe, 2001 |
| Developmental timeline | Buchanan et al., 2001; Kleiser & Cox, 2008, Maizels et al., 2008; Meyers, 1995; Nastasi, 2012, 2013; Robertson & Griffiths, 2009; Whitcombe, 2001 |
| Training fieldwork supervisors | ACOTE, 2011; AOTA, 2015; Duke, 2004; Gutman et al., 1998; Kleiser & Cox, 2008; Kirke et al., 2007; Kramer & Stern, 1995; Meyers, 1995; Nastasi, 2012; Robertson & Griffiths, 2009 |

(2015). The workshop provides instruction in administration, education, supervision, and evaluation to fieldwork coordinators and fieldwork supervisors. It is important that occupational therapy practitioners are trained to become fieldwork supervisors because their participation is critical to the continued development and growth of the occupational therapy profession.

The ultimate goal for training fieldwork supervisors is to have a positive impact on practice, education, and research. This is established through collaboration with the fieldwork coordinators. Training ensures the fieldwork supervisors' competency as well as comfort with the tools developed for supervising and evaluating students. By providing ongoing support to fieldwork supervisors, occupational therapy education programs enhance their students' experiences on fieldwork.

## Summary

"The purpose of fieldwork education is to propel each generation of occupational therapy practitioners from the role of student to that of practitioner" (AOTA, 2009, p. 821). If practitioners did not supervise students, the fieldwork of occupational therapy would eventually come to an end. Supervision of students brings forth the next generation of practitioners and leaders for the profession. Without future practitioners, societal needs will not be met. Supervising students on fieldwork placements not only benefits the profession, but also benefits the fieldwork sites that take students, the fieldwork supervisors, and the students. For fieldwork sites, supervision of students brings new ideas to the setting, as well as opportunities to recruit new employees. The fieldwork site benefits from training the students to meet the entry-level requirements specific to their site. The fieldwork site often is the first contact the student will have from an employer offering employment; this may allow students an easy transition into their first position as an occupational therapist or occupational therapy assistant. For the fieldwork supervisor, NBCOT recognizes the value of supervising students (AOTA, 2009). Fieldwork supervisors are eligible to receive credit toward their continuing education requirements for renewing their certification as a registered occupational therapist or certified occupational therapy assistant through NBCOT by supervising students on Level I and Level II fieldwork placements. In addition, serving as a fieldwork supervisor is often a practitioner's first chance to serve in the role of mentor or manager. Fieldwork supervision provides practitioners with the opportunity to develop their own skills for career promotion. Finally, for students, fieldwork education provides the students with the opportunity to complete the final steps to becoming a practitioner. Without fieldwork, students would not be allowed to graduate or to sit for the board exams. "In summary, fieldwork education is an essential bridge between the academic education and the authentic occupational therapy practice" (AOTA, 2009, p. 822).

## Student Self-Assessment

1. At mid-term evaluation, you meet with your fieldwork supervisor. The supervisor reports concern because you have not met a number of competencies and the supervisor would like to see you initiate evaluations and intervention sessions.
   - What steps should you take?
   - Where should you begin?
   - How should you monitor your progress?
2. The fieldwork coordinator contacts you after receiving a call from your fieldwork supervisor. The fieldwork supervisor reports that you have been doing well with the intervention sessions, but you are having a hard time completing the evaluations.
   - What is the fieldwork coordinator's role in this situation?
   - What is the fieldwork supervisor's role in this situation?
   - What is your role in this situation?
3. Your Level I fieldwork experience is cancelled unexpectedly. You were scheduled to complete your Level I fieldwork in pediatrics with an occupational therapy practitioner.
   - Who are other possible supervisors for your Level I fieldwork in pediatrics?
   - What types of settings would you find these supervisors in?

## Electronic Resources

American Occupational Therapy Association:

Fieldwork: http://www.aota.org/education-careers/fieldwork.aspx

Fieldwork Education Resources: http://www.aota.org/education-careers/fieldwork/supervisor.aspx

Fieldwork Related Products: http://www.aota.org/education-careers/fieldwork/products.aspx

Site-Specific Objectives: http://www.aota.org/education-careers/fieldwork/siteobj.aspx

Student Supervision: http://www.aota.org/education-careers/fieldwork/stusuprvsn.aspx

## References

Accreditation Council for Occupational Therapy Education. (2011). *2011 Accreditation Council for Occupational Therapy Education (ACOTE®) Standards and Interpretive Guide (April 2016 Interpretative Guide Version)*. Retrieved from http://www.aota.org/~/media/Corporate/Files/EducationCareers/Accredit/Standards/2011-Standards-and-Interpretive-Guide.pdf?la=en

Allison, H., & Turpin, M. (2004). Development of the student placement evaluation form: A tool for assessing student fieldwork performance. *Australian Occupational Therapy Journal, 51*, 125-132.

American Occupational Therapy Association. (2002). *Fieldwork performance evaluation for occupational therapy students*. Bethesda, MD: AOTA.

American Occupational Therapy Association. (2009). Occupational therapy fieldwork education: Value and purpose. *American Journal of Occupational Therapy, 63*, 821-822.

American Occupational Therapy Association. (2015). *Fieldwork educators certificate workshop*. Retrieved from http://www.aota.org/education-careers/fieldwork/workshop.aspx.

Bonello, M. (2001). Fieldwork within the context of higher education: A literature review. *British Journal of Occupational Therapy, 64*, 93-99.

Boudreau, M., & Donnell, C. (2013). The community development progress and evaluation tool: Assessing community development fieldwork. *Canadian Journal of Occupational Therapy, 80*(4), 235-240.

Buchanan, H., van Niekerk, L., & Moore, R. (2001). Assessing fieldwork journals: Developmental portfolios. *British Journal of Occupational Therapy, 64*, 398-402.

Cameron, D., Cockburn, L., Nixon, S., Parnes, P., Garcia, L., Leotaud, J., ... Williams, T. (2013). Global partnerships for international fieldwork in occupational therapy: Reflection and innovation. *Occupational Therapy International, 20*, 85-93.

Creel, T. (2001). Chat rooms and level II fieldwork. *Occupational Therapy in Health Care, 14*, 55-59.

de Beer, M., & Martensson, L. (2015). Feedback on students' clinical reasoning skills during fieldwork education. *Australian Occupational Therapy Journal, 62*, 255-264.

Duke, L. (2004). Piecing together the jigsaw: How do practice educators define occupational therapy student competence? *British Journal of Occupational Therapy, 67*, 201-209.

Fullerton, J. T., & Ingle, H. T. (2003). Evaluation strategies for midwifery education linked to digital media and distance delivery technology. *Journal of Midwifery and Women's Health, 48*, 426-436.

Grenier, M. (2015). Facilitators and barriers to learning in occupational therapy fieldwork education: Student perspectives. *American Journal of Occupational Therapy, 69*(Suppl. 2), 1-9.

Gutman, S. A., McCreedy, P., & Heisler, P. (1998). Student level II fieldwork: Strategies for intervention. *American Journal of Occupational Therapy, 52*, 143-149.

Hanson, D., & DeIuliis, E. (2015). The collaborative model of fieldwork education: A blueprint for group supervision of students. *Occupational Therapy in Health Care, 29*(2), 223-239.

Holloway, E. L., & Neufeldt, S. A. (1995). Supervision: Its contributions to treatment efficacy. *Journal of Consulting and Clinical Psychology, 63*, 207-213.

Kirke, P., Layton, N., & Sims, J. (2007). Informing fieldwork design: Key elements to quality in fieldwork education for undergraduate occupational therapy students. *Australian Occupational Therapy Journal, 54*, S13-S22.

Kleiser, H., & Cox, D. L. (2008). The integration of clinical and managerial supervision: A critical literature review. *British Journal of Occupational Therapy, 71*, 2-9.

Kramer, P., & Stern, K. (1995). Approaches to improving student performance on fieldwork. *American Journal of Occupational Therapy, 49*, 156-159.

Liu, Y., & Wang, H. (2009). A comparative study on e-learning technologies and products: From the east to the west. *Systems Research and Behavioral Science, 26*, 191-209.

Maizels, M., Yerkes, E., Macejko, A., Hagerty, J., Chaviano, A. H., Cheng, E. Y., et al. (2008). A new computer enhanced visual learning method to train urology residents in pediatric orchiopexy: A prototype for accreditation council for graduate medical education. *Journal of Urology, 180*, 1814-1818.

Meyers, S. (1995). Exploring the costs and benefits drivers of clinical education. *American Journal of Occupational Therapy, 49*, 107-111.

Nastasi, J. (2012). Specialty level II fieldwork in low vision rehabilitation. *OT Practice, 17*(11), 13-16.

Nastasi, J. (2013). Specialty level II fieldwork in low vision rehabilitation. *WORK, 43*, 361-378.

National Board for Certification in Occupational Therapy. (2015). *Eligibility requirements*. Retrieved from http://www.nbcot.org/certification-candidates-eligibility

Nolinske, T. (1995). Multiple mentoring relationships facilitate learning during fieldwork. *American Journal of Occupational Therapy, 49*, 39-43.

Robertson, L. J., & Griffiths, S. (2009). Graduate's reflections on their preparation for practice. *British Journal of Occupational Therapy, 72*, 125-132.

Scanlan, J., & Hancock, N. (2010). Online discussions develop students' clinical reasoning during fieldwork. *Australian Occupational Therapy Journal, 57*, 401-408.

Thomas, Y., Dickson, D., Broadbridge, J., Hopper, L., Hawkins, R., Edwards, A., et al. (2007). Benefits and challenges of supervising occupational therapy fieldwork students: Supervisor's perspectives. *Australian Occupational Therapy Journal, 54*, S2-S12.

Whitcombe, S. W. (2001). Using learning contracts in fieldwork education: The views of occupational therapy students and those responsible for their supervision. *British Journal of Occupational Therapy, 64*, 552-558.

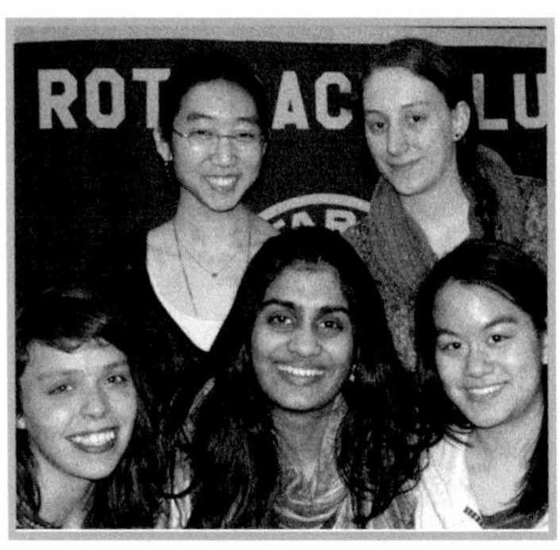


# 46

# LEADERSHIP

*Elizabeth W. Crampsey, MS, OTR/L, BCPR and Caroline Beals, MS, OTR/L*

**ACOTE STANDARDS EXPLORED IN THIS CHAPTER**

B.7.1, B.7.5, B.9.2, B.9.10

**KEY VOCABULARY**

- **Context:** Environment and pragmatic considerations within which leadership takes place.
- **Leader:** A person with authority who influences others toward a set of goals.
- **Leadership:** A process of leading and influencing others, which involves a range of theories of types of leadership.
- **Manager:** A person in a position of power who directs others in their work or tasks.



Jacobs, K., & MacRae, N. (Eds.).
*Occupational Therapy Essentials for Clinical Competence, Third Edition* (pp. 645-660).

> A knowledge of how to support as well as to lead. Some say that leaders are born, others that they are developed, yet whatever you hold to be true you must grant that leaders follow before they lead. (Brunyate, 1957)

What is leadership? In a 1676 letter of Isaac Newton, he states "If I have seen further, it is by standing on the shoulders of giants." When one takes a step back to view the history and evolution of occupational therapy practice, we can identify a multitude of leaders, or "giants," who have shaped the profession into what it is today. These leaders collectively crafted the foundational concepts of occupational therapy for other practitioners to follow in their footsteps. Men and women such as George Edward Barton, Eleanor Clarke Slagle, and Thomas Kidner envisioned a profession that would serve to advance occupation as a therapeutic measure. Robeson (1937) described Slagle's contribution in this way: "Mrs. Slagle has directed and laid the solid foundation stones on which our profession and our national organization rest today." How do we, as occupational therapy practitioners, stand firmly on the shoulders of our founders and ensure the future and success of the profession? It will take bold, innovative, and interprofessional leadership to move forward into the next 100 years of our profession.

What words come to mind when we think of leadership? Do power and authority rise to the top as central characteristics of leadership? Does one need to hold a title to be a leader? Likely each one of us can describe at least one personal or professional experience in which we have engaged with a leader who demonstrates sound leadership skills. Conversely, one could also reflect on an experience working with a leader who provided suboptimal leadership. Our own definitions of leader and leadership may vary somewhat. A commonality would be that true leaders create a vision, move others to believe in it, and aspire to achieve it through the use of shared goals and a tangible, meaningful outcome. Opportunities for leadership present themselves every day. As occupational therapy practitioners, we are in a position to be leaders in our profession, our communities, and our day-to-day interactions with others. A leader is not necessarily in a leadership role, or defined by being a manager.

This chapter explores the importance of leadership in the occupational therapy profession and presents different types of leadership as a necessary background to thinking about effective leading. Personal, social, and cultural contexts are important influences in leadership abilities and styles. Being a leader can be an occupation. The American Occupational Therapy Association's (AOTA) *Occupational Therapy Practice Framework: Domain and Process, Third Edition,* is used to examine the contexts that define leadership (2014). Although leadership occurs in political, community, and global settings, it is also very present in the daily work of occupational therapy practitioners and occupational therapy students. This chapter illustrates several forms of leadership and makes it clear that leadership opportunities—and even obligations—exist for all occupational therapy practitioners in all settings.

## Leadership as Occupation

> It is the privilege and responsibility of a profession to define the kinds of learning which will develop its students' potential for the fulfillment of its educational aims. May we have the courage, the knowledge and the sensitive discernment to measure up to the greatness of this challenge and to prepare professional leaders for tomorrow's practice. (Fidler, 1965)

The *Framework* is an official AOTA published document that is intended to inform internal and external audiences of the unique scope of service of occupational therapy, inclusive of occupational therapy practitioners and students, other health care professionals, educators, researchers, payers, and consumers to summarize the constructs that best describe occupational therapy practice (AOTA, 2014). Please see Chapter 6 for more information on the *Framework*.

AOTA (2014) defines occupational therapy as:

> The therapeutic use of everyday life activities (occupations) with individuals or groups for the purpose of enhancing or enabling participation in roles, habits, and routines in home, school, workplace, community, and other settings. Occupational therapy practitioners use their knowledge of the transactional relationship among the person, his or her engagement in valuable occupations, and the context to design occupation-based intervention plans that facilitate change or growth in client factors (body functions, body structures, values, beliefs, and spirituality) and skills (motor, process, and social interaction) needed for successful participation. Occupational therapy practitioners are concerned with the end result of participation and thus enable engagement through adaptations and modifications to the environment or objects within the environment when needed, using task-oriented, occupation-based activities. Occupational therapy services are provided for habilitation, rehabilitation, and promotion of health and wellness for clients with disability- and non–disability-related needs. These services include acquisition and preservation of occupational identity for those who have or are at risk for developing an illness, injury, disease, disor-

der, condition, impairment, disability, activity limitation, or participation restriction. (AOTA, 2014, p. S1)

The occupation of leadership can be described using the *Framework* as a background.

## Leadership and Context

The *Framework* skillfully outlined the contexts in which occupational therapy occurs within varied environments. Similar to how we assess clients and activity in the clinical world, acting as an effective leader involves performance skills, motor and process abilities, and communication and interpersonal skills. Leadership is a dynamic process that both influences and is influenced by individual roles, habits, and routines. Particular activity demands are involved in leadership, and these demands differ in each situation. Therefore, context significantly influences leadership.

The *Framework* names several types of context: cultural, social, physical, temporal, virtual, and personal. "Understanding the environments and contexts in which occupations can and do occur provides practitioners with insights into their overarching, underlying, and embedded influences on engagement" (AOTA, 2014, p. S8). Below is a brief exploration of each context and its relation to leadership.

- **Cultural context:** The culture in which leadership takes place is important. This context includes beliefs, activity patterns, customs, standards of behavior, and expectations that are all part of an accepted culture of which an individual is a member (AOTA, 2014). These are generally factors that are external to the person. However, much of a cultural context can be internalized by the person as well. Laws that govern employee–employer relations can be part of a leader's cultural context. The internal culture of an organization also influences how leadership is performed.
- **Social context:** Social context includes expectations of other people who are important to the individual, as well as accepted norms of larger social groups (AOTA, 2014). Leaders may have particular ways of dressing or using specific words or language (verbal and nonverbal) as part of their social context. The social context can significantly influence leading.
- **Physical context:** Physical context is the environment, both natural and built, factor typically thought of when discussing context. It includes nonhuman aspects of the environment such as tools, plants, furniture, objects, animals, and natural terrain (AOTA, 2014). The physical context of where an individual engages in leading can greatly influence performance of leadership abilities.
- **Temporal context:** This "time" context refers to the influence time can have on the performance of occupations and is inclusive of stage of life, time of day or year, duration or rhythm of activity, and history (AOTA, 2014). A leader who holds meetings at the end of a long workday may find his or her effectiveness limited by the temporal context. Some leaders may feel influenced in their work by the time of year.
- **Virtual context:** Virtual context has become increasingly important for health care providers and for leaders. This form of leadership occurs in "simulated, real-time, or near-time situations absent of physical contact" (AOTA, 2014, p. S9). The virtual context has greatly influenced how and when communication takes place, as well as how effective it is. Leadership involves a great deal of communication (Hamm, 2006). Leaders must pay attention to the influence of the virtual context on the effectiveness of their leading.
- **Personal context:** According to the *Framework*, personal context is made up of personal factors about the individual—age, gender, and other demographic information such as educational status and socioeconomic status (AOTA, 2014).

## Models and Theories of Leadership

> Occupational therapists will have to learn skills associated with effective consultation, supervision, leadership, and communication. It is not enough to learn the theory and practice of occupational therapy. (Gilfoyle, 1984)

The term *leadership* has taken on many meanings in the history of occupational therapy practice. Much like our evolving profession of occupational therapy, the traditional leadership models and theories are also evolving to meet the needs of the changing health care landscape. As one develops leadership capacity, it is important to consider the foundational concepts of leadership theories, and how these theories evolved over time. While developing leadership abilities, it is useful to understand how leadership theories and models have evolved over time and directly relate to theory and practice. The movement of leadership models to ones of more participatory, or shared, philosophies, as well as transformational constructs, more closely mirrors the way occupational therapy practitioners have been working to interact with people for the past century.

In reviewing the literature, it was found that early models and theories focused on individual traits and characteristics, as well as transactional and managerial leadership. More recent literature focuses on transformational, participatory, and situational leadership. There are countless leadership styles and theories, those listed below present a sample of significant concepts that align well with best practice in the occupational therapy profession.

This is a limited review of theories, and the theories here were chosen to provide a degree of insight into the components of leadership to help us begin to understand the what, why, and how of leadership. The effectiveness of leadership is a complex and ongoing field of study. The most effective leaders are able to use knowledge, experience, and consideration of personal and contextual factors when determining a style of interaction. The issue is not to excel at one particular type of leadership but to determine which approach is best given each particular scenario and context (Pearce, 2004; Shortell & Kaluzney, 2000).

## Trait Theory

Early leadership theorists developed the idea that certain people are born with character traits that predispose them to become great leaders. These earlier trait theories have informed modern leadership, with scholars trying to predict leadership success through the demographic and physical traits, abilities, and personality characteristics of leaders (Bass, 1990; Stogdill, 1948). DeYoung (2005) described how Lewin proposed that most leaders engaged in three leadership styles based on personality traits. These included authoritarian, democratic, and laissez-faire. Trait theory, often referred to as the *great man theory*, proposes that personality traits such as intelligence or cognitive ability, integrity and honesty, ambition, maturity, motivation, and self-confidence influence the emergence and effectiveness of leaders in our society (Walter & Scheibe, 2013). Furthermore, this view implies that these abilities are predetermined, that individuals are born with an innate ability to lead that cannot be learned. Although this theory can be empirically supported through the stories of great leaders in our past, this is the basis for debate as to which traits are most important in effective leadership.

## Behavioral Theory

DeYoung (2005) identified the specific behaviors engaged in by leaders to promote organizational effectiveness when he referred to the Ohio State research, which has been cited by many authors in leadership. According to these studies, leadership behavior can be classified either as consideration behaviors or as initiating structure behaviors. Consideration behavior is defined as behavior indicating that a leader trusts, respects, and values good relationships with his or her followers. Initiating structure behaviors are defined as actions a leader performs to make sure the work gets done. It is important to recognize that these leadership behaviors are not mutually exclusive. Leaders can and do engage in both initiating structure and consideration behaviors. The behavioral models provide insight into leader characteristics but do not address how and why leadership happens (George & Jones, 2002).

## Participatory Leadership

As the evolution of leadership continued over the decades, participatory leadership models gained increasing acceptance (McLagan & Nell, 1995). Given the multitude of societal and cultural change factors in organizations, participatory leadership models have become more popular. “With these changes, coaching and commitment cultures have replaced the command, control, and compartmentalization orientations of the past” (Kets de Vries, 2005, p. 62). Participatory leadership embraces change and readily involves others (Kouzes & Posner, 2007). Leadership in day-to-day work can move from person to person depending on the tasks involved and competencies needed. The leader facilitates and guides transitions (Ackerman & MacKenzie, 2006; McLagan & Nell, 1995). Participatory leaders readily defer to others’ expertise. The parallels with occupational therapy client-centered practice are easily discerned. Engaging in participatory leadership is a powerful way to help people grow their strengths and enable future leaders. In participatory leadership, the focus is on collaboration, commitment, and context.

Participatory leadership incorporates much of the multifaceted tenets of previous leadership theories. Pearce (2004) advocates that the more complex a task is, the more there is a need for shared or participatory leadership. This model is less a body of new work than a coming together of earlier approaches, melding traits, behaviors, and contextual factors. Spreier, Fontaine, and Malloy (2006) recognized that teams working together are more effective than individuals moving toward a goal alone. This is part of participatory leadership. Every time an occupational therapy practitioner works with someone, he or she is leading in a participatory sense. When we embrace this realization, it is a small step to move to leading in a community or global context. Occupational therapy practitioners are especially well positioned to create and influence systems of care and wellness (social and cultural contexts) because of our client-centered beliefs and the leadership abilities that we exemplify every day.

## Servant Leadership

Servant leadership is a relatively new leadership philosophy first coined in 1970 that defines servant leaders as those who put others’ needs before their own (Dillon, 2011). Servant leaders believe in self-knowledge, justice, and caring for the people they lead. Relationships are important. All leaders, in large or small ways, must be in touch with what is meaningful to them (Sadler-Smith & Shefy, 2004). Kouzes and Posner (2007) discussed exemplary leadership as having five important components. One of these is "encouraging the heart." They maintained that leaders need to "hear the heart and see the soul" (Kouzes & Posner, 2007, p. 329). Spirituality is an important factor to consider in terms of how each person participates in leadership behaviors (Stewart, 2007).

## Transformational Leadership

The idea of transformational leadership first appeared in 1978 by Burns, later expanded by Bass in 1985. Transformational leadership is a style of leadership where the leader works with a group to identify the needed change, creates a vision to guide the change, inspires others to participate in the change, and participates in executing the change alongside the group. Transformational leaders also inspire and motivate people in their groups. They tend to be thought of as inspirational and are able to share credit and recognize the people who have contributed to shared work for an organization. This model of leadership serves to motivate, improve overall morale, and ultimately improve the performance capacity of the group. Under the transformational leadership model, the leader tunes into the group's sense of identity, becomes a role model for the group, inspires and raises interest in the change, and challenges the group to take greater ownership for their contributions to the change. The leader strives to understand the strengths and weaknesses of the group, and matches group members with tasks that allow them to function at their optimal capacity. Current evidence and opinion is that a transformational engaging style of leadership is an effective means of leading in today's rapidly changing and evolving health care environment (Firestone, 2010).

## Leadership in Enabling Occupation

Canadian occupational therapy practitioners have long been close colleagues and partners in research related to leadership in occupational therapy practice. A recent leadership effort in 2007 by the Canadian Association of Occupational Therapists was to publish a practice guideline for everyday leadership. From this initiative, *Enabling Occupation II: Advancing an Occupational Therapy Vision of Health, Well-Being and Justice Through Occupation* (Townsend & Polatajko, 2007) was published by the Canadian Association of Occupational Therapists. These generic practice guidelines for leadership consisted of various charts, models, and graphs that portrayed the power for occupational therapy practitioners to engage with others to make decisions and take action. While leadership has been discussed in a variety of publications and models such as this, no model provided a visual tool to represent key elements that will position occupational therapy practitioners for leadership. To remedy this situation, the authors designed the Leadership in Enabling Occupation model with four overlapping ovals that "visually represent the inter-relatedness of four key elements in which all occupational therapists can assert everyday leadership" (Townsend, Polatajko, Craik, & von Zweck, 2011). Through asserting leadership in scholarship, accountability, funding, and workforce planning, occupational therapy practitioners are poised to create optimal conditions for and access to occupational therapy services. For example, the rehabilitation manager of an outpatient clinic who empowers others to provide evidence-based services (scholarship), thoroughly and fairly report their clinical activities (accountability), participates in discussions related to budgeting at the local level (funding), and collaborates with community partners to ensure sustainability (workforce planning) would exemplify all components of the Leadership in Enabling Occupation model.

## Situational Leadership

One of the early theorists credited with considering the context of leadership was Frederick Fiedler (1978). He attempted to explore the interrelationship between leader characteristics and the specific situation in which leadership takes place. The *Framework* (AOTA, 2014) would refer to this as the *influence of context.* Fiedler defined the situation as having three specific dimensions: leader–follower relations, task structure, and the position of the leaders in power. In Fiedler's view, these three relationships, identified as contingency dimensions, significantly affected leadership effectiveness (Fiedler, 1967). Together, the characteristics would determine "situational favorableness" for a particular leadership style (George & Jones, 2002). According to Fiedler, leaders engage in two specific styles of leadership: relationship oriented and task oriented (DeYoung, 2005). Relationship-oriented leaders place primary value on establishing positive working relationships with those they are leading. Leaders who are task oriented primarily emphasize task completion. In this premise of leadership, leaders are most effective in situations that most closely match their leadership styles. It is significant that leadership styles were viewed to be relatively fixed, such that leaders could not easily move from one style to the other.

Developed by Hersey and Blanchard, the situational leadership model examined the relationship among three dimensions: task behavior, relationship behavior, and the maturity of the individuals being led. The task behavior refers to the degree of structure and clarity that the leader provides (clearly defined work roles and responsibilities). The relationship dimension refers to the emotional and psychological relationship between the leader and the individual being led (Hersey & Blanchard, 1982). Related to maturity level of followers, this was characterized by three specific criteria: level of motivation, willingness to assume responsibility, and the individual's experience and education level (Hersey & Blanchard, 1982). Based on these criteria, the leader modifies his or her leadership approach. For example, when working with an entry-level occupational therapy practitioner, a leader will likely provide more structure for a given task to promote success, whereas a practitioner with considerable experience in the same situation may require less direction from the leader. Additionally, this model guides us to take into account the level of motivation of the individual in tailoring his or her leadership behavior and interactions.

## Ethical Considerations

> The new directions in practice allow us to combine our past experience and founders' mandates with the current realities of practice in ways that lead us to realize the future hopes and dreams of our consumers, ourselves as individuals, and the profession as a whole. (Grady, 1995)

The field of occupational therapy is guided by seven core principles: altruism, equality, freedom, justice, dignity, truth, and prudence. In 2015, the *Occupational Therapy Code of Ethics* of the AOTA was revised, acknowledging the changing health care environment, dynamic nature of the profession, and emerging practice areas, as well as the emergence and development of technology that affects research, practice, and education. This official document provides information about the core value of the profession, as well as the principles and standards of conduct that apply to practitioners and volunteers within the profession. The *Code of Ethics* is intended to help members to guide decisions and ethical actions while taking into consideration each multi-faceted aspect of professional behavior, responsibility, practice, and decision making. The *Code of Ethics* should be complementary to licensure board regulations and laws that guide standards of practice. "Recognizing and resolving ethical issues is a systematic process that includes analysis of the complex dynamics of situations, weighing of consequences, making reasoned decisions, taking action, and reflecting on outcomes" (AOTA, 2015, p. 1). Leadership has its place within ethics in occupational therapy. Many of the principles seem to strictly apply to working with clients at first glance. However, the document asks more from practitioners ensuring that we understand that occupational therapy practice involves attention to work with others beyond clients, including the community and greater populations. See Chapter 50 on ethics for more information.

Kronenberg and Pollard (2006) reminded us that, globally, the largest numbers of occupational therapy practitioners reside and work in the United States. This national group "significantly influences thinking, practice, education, and research of occupational therapy practitioners all over the world " (Kronenberg & Pollard, 2006, p. 1). Perhaps in the United States, we are especially obligated to develop new ideas and solutions based upon an original, novel, or unconventional approach given the climate of health care reform. We must critically assess our core professional values and how well they do or do not fit with our social and cultural contexts. Kronenberg and Pollard asserted that our profession's work is "always under construction" and "essentially never finished" (p. 1). They went on to suggest that with our expertise in occupations, perhaps we need to "problematize situations in which 'occupations' contribute to the construction of communities and societies that are exclusive" (Kronenberg & Pollard, 2006, p. 2).

Contextual factors and ethical dilemmas surrounding service delivery, recent health care reformations, and evolution in occupational therapy theory and practice call for a recommitment to leadership that is founded and grounded in competency, relevancy, and currency (Schell & Slater, 1998). Legislation, health care reform, and health care landscape changes for both payers and consumers have provided opportunities for practitioners to commit to a pointed focus on prevention, wellness, and disability management. In addition to creating new venues for leadership, these changes have provided opportunities for the profession to refocus on occupation and occupational performance. Schell and Slater (1998) delineate roles within planning, fiscal management, marketing, personnel management, systems management, and education and research for both the clinical practitioner and the administrative practitioner.

Due to the changes in health care, Schell and Slater (1998) contend that staff are required to manage themselves with less direct supervision as a result of the broader management responsibilities and the flattening of organizational hierarchies. The transition has necessitated a sharper view on the bottom line of fiscally driven service delivery, which has been a paradigm shift for the profession of occupational therapy (Schell & Slater, 1998). With these changes comes trial and error of matrix management models, departmentalization, service extenders, and various other staffing pattern schemes. Accountability, sound management skills, and currency and relevancy of occupation-centered practice and theory are the resounding themes of occupational therapy practice today; both clinical and administrative clinicians will continue to be at the forefront of leadership and innovation (Schell & Slater, 1998). This has implications for the newer practitioner, as well as the seasoned practitioner.

Table 46-1.

**MENTORSHIP PERCEIVED BENEFITS AND CHALLENGES**

| Mentorship Benefits | Mentorship Barriers |
|---|---|
| • Higher employee retention rates<br>• Higher yielding recruitment strategies<br>• Higher productivity<br>• Increased job satisfaction<br>• Increased networking opportunities<br>• Increased salaries<br>• Improved professional confidence<br>• Furthered career and professional goals<br>• Continued competency | • Costs<br>• Time and energy<br>• Challenging (unskilled or toxicity mentor)<br>• Misuse of mentor or mentee role<br>• Reflection on mentor or mentee related to performance |

Adapted from Scheerer, C. R. (2007). Mentoring in occupational therapy: One state's status. *Occupational Therapy in Health Care, 21*(3), 17-33.

## MANAGEMENT VERSUS LEADERSHIP

> We must develop our ability to become leaders; to move with confidence into the community and collaborate in the creation of a healthier environment, contributing our knowledge of activities and human action. We need, therefore, to be able to problem-solve, to understand the factors involved in complex social systems and define the problems where we can make a contribution. (Finn, 1972)

*Leadership* and *management* are often thought of as synonymous terms, implying that leaders manage and managers lead. Although this may be the case in some instances, it is arguably more complex than a title or management role. Effective leaders readily embrace change—they facilitate and guide transitions. Leaders involve others and are aware of their own limitations. Leaders are able to create a shared vision among people. Leaders inspire and coach others to work toward a shared vision of a group or organization.

Managers are often described in terms of the tasks to which they ably attend. They are responsible for resource allocation (staffing and budgets), generating reports, and managing programs (Borkowski, 2005; Grady, 2003).

It is important to note that management and leadership are not mutually exclusive entities, nor is the comparison meant to diminish the functions of a manager. Management functions provide necessary parameters for operations to take place. Leaders may or may not be responsible for managerial components within their situations of leadership.

## *Mentorship: A Critical Role in Leadership*

The role of mentorship in leadership and the sustainability of leadership is widely held through both health-care–related and non–health-care–related professions. Scheerer (2007) conducted a study of Ohio Occupational Therapy State Association members and found that mentoring initiatives strengthen both the individual practitioners and the entire occupational therapy profession. There have been resources provided by health care professions and mentoring from organizations such as the American Speech-Language-Hearing Association, the American Physical Therapy Association, and the AOTA.

It is important to note that there is a literature delineation, as well as a philosophical difference, between the roles of mentoring and supervision. Mentoring is a dynamic, individual, reciprocal relationship rooted in professional development guidance and improvement (Scheerer, 2007), whereas supervision is an authoritative responsibility related to an employee's job responsibilities as it relates to the job description and performance (Kolodner & Hischmann, 1997). It is important to note that the Scheerer (2007) Ohio Occupational Therapy Association study was comprised of a convenience sample of practitioners who were active participants in their state association, indicative that these individuals are more likely committed individuals. This study also indicated that the highest response demographic was practitioners with 1 to 5 years of experience. Although this study outlined the desire for mentor and mentees to have a mentorship relationship, it is to be noted that with the 1 to 5 years of experience, these practitioners may not yet be ready to assume a mentorship role. Mentoring can be a powerful tool to ensure continued practitioner competency as mandated by the *Code of Ethics* and standards of practice that promote life-long learning and best practice (Scheerer, 2007; Table 46-1).

Table 46-2.

| Ways to Practice Leadership | |
|---|---|
| AOTA COOL | Coordinated Online Opportunities for Leadership: https://www.aota.org/aboutaota/get-involved/leadership.aspx<br>Allows AOTA members to voice their areas of interest and be contacted when opportunities arise that meet their personal needs (time commitment, area of interest, etc.). |
| Involvement in state associations | Find out your state association contact here:<br>http://www.aota.org/advocacy-policy/state-policy/state-ot-associations.aspx |
| Monitor state and federal legislative issues | Register for online alerts in http://capwiz.com/aota/home/ to stay informed regarding legislative changes, and write a letter to your representative in support or against certain measures that impact occupational therapy practice. |
| Develop your "elevator speech" | Demonstrate leadership by communicating the value and importance of occupational therapy to your community. Develop a clear, powerful, and brief message about the profession. It is typically about 30 seconds, the time it takes people to ride from the top to the bottom of a building in an elevator. |
| Educational opportunities | Attending and presenting at educational events in your community, both within and externally from the profession of occupational therapy, is an example of practicing leadership. |
| Everyday advocacy | Through evidence-based practice and implementing effective occupational therapy service programs, communicate the distinct value of occupational therapy to members of your team, stakeholders, consumers, and payers. |

# Leadership in Action

## Emerging Practice

As occupational therapy practitioners, our workforce is engaged strategically on the threshold of change within the health care system, emerging practice areas can both be highly rewarding, as well as have embedded challenges to the development and implementation of service delivery (Holmes & Scaffa, 2009). Related to health care change and reform, this has provided both challenges and opportunities for the area of occupational therapy practice. Reimbursement, recruitment, retention, and workforce are all areas that are impacted. Documentation that is reflective of occupational therapy's distinct value, in addition to research of efficacy of provision and service delivery are critical components to understanding and leading the occupational therapy profession into expanding contexts and models of service delivery (Holmes & Scaffa, 2009). Embarking in an area of emerging practice can have both rewards and challenges built into the process of developing and delivering services (Holmes & Scaffa, 2009). The constant transition of health care service delivery and reimbursement leads occupational therapy practitioners to constantly examine the "philosophy of services, current and future roles within the health care system, and methods for service delivery" (Holmes & Scaffa, 2009, p. 190).

Leadership should be, and is, undertaken by occupational therapy practitioners, inclusive of all occupational therapy practitioners, as well as students. Some leadership skills can be similar to skills that practitioners use in their daily practice (McCormack, 2003; Strzelecki, 2007). Practitioners recognize that leadership skills and abilities can be present in everyone. Heard (2014) acknowledged that identified occupational therapy practitioners recognized as leaders had both intrinsic and extrinsic motivations. Further, Heard (2014) identified embedding leadership into curriculum for students; professional cultures that include mentorship, as well as access and awareness of leadership resources, will enable this important paradigm shift for the profession. Many state occupational therapy member associations, such as Maine, Massachusetts, and New York, are free to elect occupational therapists and occupational therapy assistants as president or other executive board positions. Additionally, the AOTA endorses both occupational therapists and occupational therapy assistants as both elected board members, as well as in leadership positions. Table 46-2 provides resources to develop your leadership skills.

## Collaboration Between American Occupational Therapy Association and State Associations

There are countless examples about the symbiotic relationship that AOTA and state associations have forged. Reimbursement relies heavily on our time as practitioners. Being current with varying local and state payment policies, as well as national payment requirements is critical. The AOTA has a Reimbursement and Regulatory Policy department with a primary charge to advocate along with agencies, contractors, and other

Table 46-3.

**Examples of Effective Leadership and Collaboration Between State Occupational Therapy Organizations and AOTA**

| State | Outcomes |
|---|---|
| Washington | The AOTA and Washington Occupational Therapy Association (WOTA) strategized about advocacy efforts, AOTA wrote a comment letter and WOTA worked with lobbyist to get a seat on habilitative services workgroup. |
| Utah | Members of the Utah Occupational Therapy Association testified about the importance of occupational therapy. The AOTA supported Utah's efforts by providing information about essential health benefits and the process taking place in Utah. |
| Kentucky | The Kentucky Occupational Therapy Association with the assist of their lobbyist scheduled a meeting with key decision makers to help advocate for occupational therapy. The AOTA provided support and assisted with drafting a comment letter. |
| California | The Occupational Therapy Association of California, their lobbyist, and AOTA worked in a collaborative process to define habilitative services. Although the definition changed, by being an active part of the process, the outcome was better than having not participated actively. |
| Maryland | The Maryland Occupational Therapy Association in coordination with AOTA attended hearings and provided written and oral testimony to support the habilitative services benefit. |

groups to establish guidelines for payment (Yamkovenko, 2012). The AOTA has a proven track record also of aiding states through research, advocacy, and precedence while tackling local coverage determination. This involvement is helpful to collaborate about payment and documentation requirements. In various states AOTA has worked with volunteer leaders to develop a comprehensive plan to advocate for our clients' needs, as well as those of the occupational therapy practitioner.

Partnership between local, state, and national associations allows for occupational therapy practitioners to remain current on initiatives that are essential to the profession. Changes occur related to practice areas and strategies to ensure that the distinct value of occupational therapy is at the forefront of our leadership opportunities and daily practice. Knowing how to best ensure that our clients are able to access appropriate services allows occupational therapy practitioners to advocate in collaboration, communication, and being a part of the conversation as decisions are routinely made by "state legislatures, local governments, and school districts about how occupational therapy services will be paid for and who will get our services" (Yamkovenko, 2012, p. 5). Health reform advocacy and habilitation services definition has brought about a critical partnership to advocate for occupational therapy (Brown, 2012).

Table 46-3 provides select examples demonstrating effective leadership and collaboration between state occupational therapy organizations and AOTA.

## *Collaboration With National Organization and Official Documents*

There are five categories of official documents published by AOTA: guidelines, position papers, standards, statements, and societal statements. Documents are an invaluable resource to maintain best practice and be current with evidence-based practice for students, as well as new and seasoned practitioners. Table 46-4 differentiates the types of documents within the five categories.

Additional resources are available via the AOTA website including specialized knowledge and skills papers, emerging practice topic areas, and other up-to-date information of importance. Scope of practice, reimbursement and documentation, special interest sections, and licensure details, in addition to multicultural and international affairs, are also available within the website of official documents. The documents that are under review annually are also listed on the site, and feedback is solicited from the membership through surveys on these important, relevant topics. Also of note, through these links are evidence-based practice projects, as well as specific leadership training through the AOTA Emerging Leaders Development Program specifically geared to students and new practitioners, as well as the Leadership Development Program for Managers. Being aware of official documents, conferences and training opportunities, and emerging and best practice initiatives helps each leader remain current and relevant in an ever-changing health care world with a dynamic, innovative field of practice and study.

Table 46-4.

**Five Categories of Official Documents Published by the American Occupational Therapy Association**

| | |
|---|---|
| Guidelines | Provide descriptions, examples, or recommendations of procedures pertaining to the education of occupational therapy practitioners and the practice of occupational therapy. |
| Position papers | Present the official stance of the Association on a substantive issue or subject. They are developed in response to a particular issue, concern, or need of the Association and may be written for internal or external use. |
| Standards | Include a general description of the topic and define the minimum requirements for performance and quality. |
| Statements | Describe and clarify (vs. present an official stance) an aspect or issue related to education or practice and are linked to the fundamental concepts of occupational therapy. They are developed in response to a particular issue, concern, or need of the Association and may be written for internal or external use. |
| Societal statements | Written in the form of public announcements, these statements identify a societal issue of concern; state how the issue affects the participation of individuals, families, groups, or communities in society; and may offer action to be taken by individuals, groups, or communities. |

Adapted from American Occupational Therapy Association. (n.d.). *Official documents.* Retrieved from http://www.aota.org/practice/manage/official.aspx

## *The Centennial Vision and Vision 2025*

> We envision that occupational therapy is a powerful, widely recognized, science-driven, and evidence-based profession with a globally connected and diverse workforce meeting society's occupational needs. (AOTA, 2006)

> We can achieve our Centennial Vision if we emulate the founders as role models of leadership. One quality that stands out in my mind is their personal and professional courage. They were creative risk takers, visionary leaders and tireless advocates for their patients and the profession should serve to remind you that, like our forefathers and foremothers, we all have the potential to be political activists, risk takers, and confident leaders. Indeed, are you so different from the founders? Are you not tireless promoters of occupational therapy? Our founders remind us of what can be done with talent and commitment. And history can strengthen our resolve by helping us to understand that as occupational therapy practitioners of today we have a heritage of strong leaders, from the initial founders through succeeding generations of occupational therapy practitioners whose innovations in clinical practice, theory, measurement, and research reflect the values that the Founding Vision and the Centennial Vision share. Now it is our turn to take up the challenge as we enter a new century of occupational therapy. (Schwartz, 2009)

In 2003, leaders in AOTA began to map the future of the profession to commemorate the Association's 100th anniversary in 2017. The development of this initiative took place from 2003 to 2006, with the implementation phase from 2006 to 2017.

> The purpose of the development of the Centennial Vision was to ensure that individuals, policymakers, populations, and society value and promote occupational therapy's practice of enabling people to improve their physical and mental health, secure wellbeing, and enjoy higher quality of life through preventing and overcoming obstacles to participation in the activities they value. (AOTA, 2006)

In the year 2017, AOTA furthered the intent of the Centennial Vision through the development and implementation of Vision 2025. Occupational therapy maximizes the health, wellbeing, and quality of life for all people, population, and communities through effective solutions that facilitate participation in everyday living (AOTA, 2016). Per AOTA, through the visioning process and creation of Vision 2025, the four core tenets from key stakeholders of occupational therapists, occupational therapy assistants, educators, students, consumers, policymakers, and the general public were identified as accessible, collaborative, effective, and leaders (Table 46-5).

AOTA has long outlined categories for emerging practice, including children and youth, health and

Table 46-5.

| VISION 2025 CORE TENETS | |
|---|---|
| Accessible | Occupational therapy provides culturally responsive and customized services. |
| Collaborative | Occupational therapy excels in working with clients and within systems to produce effective outcomes. |
| Effective | Occupational therapy is evidence based, client centered, and cost effective. |
| Leaders | Occupational therapy is influential in changing policies, environments, and complex systems. |
| Adapted from American Occupational Therapy Association. (2016). *AOTA unveils vision 2025.* Retrieved from http://www.aota.org/AboutAOTA/vision-2025.aspx | |

wellness, productive aging, work and industry, and rehabilitation, disability, and participation. Often, emerging practice areas are an expansion of our historical roots as an occupational therapy profession (Holmes & Scaffa, 2009). Holmes and Scaffa's (2009) survey results of occupational therapy practitioners indicate that the most common description of emerging practice was nontraditional by the respondents and that term was open to various interpretations.

Holmes and Scaffa (2009) found through a survey of current occupational therapy practitioners the following eight elements viewed as relevant to a shared vision of the future:

1. Expanded collaboration for success
2. Power to influence
3. Membership equals professional responsibility
4. Well-prepared, diverse workforce
5. Clear, compelling public image
6. Customers demand occupational therapy
7. Evidence-based decision making
8. Science-fostered innovation in occupational therapy practice

In addition to these eight elements, four strategic directions emerged after a careful analysis of barriers and opportunities:

1. Building the capacity to fulfill the profession's potential and mission, including:
   - ◊ Ensuring an adequate and diverse workforce for multiple roles
   - ◊ Preparing occupational therapists and occupational therapy assistants for the 21st century
   - ◊ Increasing research capacity and productivity
   - ◊ Strengthening our capacity to influence and lead
2. Demonstrating and articulating our value to individuals, organizations, and communities, including:
   - ◊ Meeting societal needs for health and well-being
   - ◊ People understanding who we are and what we do
3. Building an inclusive community of members
4. Linking education, research, and practice

This vision has united practitioners to meet society's occupational needs, with great attention to enhancing the evidence base, increasing global diversity, and diversifying the workforce of occupational therapy practitioners. The ability to create a vision for the future, create energy and momentum through empowering others, and set aspirational goals is truly the definition of leadership. Embedded within the Centennial Vision, AOTA envisions that evidence-based practice is the expectation. The profession's long struggle of bridging the gap between theory and practice remains a challenge to educators, students, and practitioners (Fleming-Castaldy & Gillen, 2013). This becomes a critical discussion point as the National Board for Certification in Occupational Therapy (NBCOT) examination, as well as material in the classroom and in the clinical setting, should be reflective of best and current practice, as the advancement of occupation-based and task-oriented activity are well supported within the literature (Fleming-Castaldy & Gillen, 2013). In addition, academic institutions are required to provide examination pass rate results to the Accreditation Council for Occupational Therapy Education (ACOTE). This is an essential benchmark for institutions to remain accredited and in good standing, as well a significant point of recruitment for prospective students. The *Code of Ethics*, ACOTE Standards, and requirements for certification and licensure all lead occupational therapy practitioners to remain current in their practice patterns.

The therapeutic use of occupation is well established and aligns with the Centennial Vision. Although critical to honor the traditions of occupational therapy and its roots, it is equally critical for leaders to integrate evidence into practice. Not doing so has an undesirable effect on patient outcomes and satisfaction and implications for reimbursement and diminishes the scope of practice of the profession (Fleming-Castaldy & Gillen, 2013). Entry-level practitioners are often on the forefront of creating change through the use of contemporary approaches, comfort level with change, and evidence-based practice.

They can be change agents, instill progress of their peers, and find their leadership role as a stakeholder. Educators must reflect on their courses and their content and take their place in a mentorship role, with mentor and mentee pushing one another to integrate best efficacious practice (Fleming-Castaldy & Gillen, 2013). Extended within that challenge is to authors, editors, publishers, and researchers. Available research and evidence should be used to inform practice; we must appreciate our history, but embrace the future of our profession. With the Vision 2025 unveiled in 2017, these same themes remain central and embedded in this new roadmap for the future of occupational therapy practice. This echoes the profession's strong commitment to preparing and enabling strong leaders to ensure innovation that creates effective solutions for engagement in everyday occupations.

### *Involvement in International Organizations and Other Professional Organizations*

The mission of the World Federation of Occupational Therapists (WFOT) promotes occupational therapy as an art and science internationally. WFOT supports the development, use, and practice of occupational therapy worldwide, demonstrating its relevance and contribution to society. WFOT began in 1951 with discussions with 28 representatives from various countries. The following year, with 10 countries represented, a more formalized organization took shape. In a leadership context, WFOT aims to promote occupational therapy in a global context, unifying various professionals and groups throughout the globe. WFOT provides opportunities for practitioners to exchange information and promotes the education and training of therapists worldwide, for both students and practitioners.

The WFOT provides information including a code of ethics, competencies, and position statements and provides support for awareness opportunities such as World Occupational Therapy Day and Occupational Therapy Global Day of Service annually October 27th. It also provides a wealth of information and advocacy on behalf of the profession worldwide (WFOT, 2011). See Chapter 51 for more information about WFOT.

Depending on practitioners' niche area or areas of interest, there are countless other professional organizations of value to ensure continued competence and knowledge acquisition. These may relate to specific diagnoses or diagnostic categories, populations, or organizations, and may be within state, national, or international venues. Additionally, being aware of the initiatives and best practice of our partners (inclusive of other rehabilitation professionals, educators, and stakeholders) can inform and promote each practitioner to provide their most collaborative and innovative care.

**Clinical Wisdom of a Reflective Practitioner**

A pediatric provider who had worked with leaders in the field of pediatric occupational therapy more than 20 years ago was looking to reenter the field of occupational therapy. However, in her time away to fulfill her occupations as mother, wife, and active community member, she had let her license lapse. In preparation for reentry to the occupational therapy workforce, this individual completed her NBCOT self-assessment, identifying her areas of strengths and opportunities. She then began networking by joining the community of practice for children and youth in Maine. This allowed her to interface with other pediatric practitioners, garner opportunities for continuing education and shadowing to start to fulfill in some of the identified areas of opportunity acknowledged through this process. She also began attending both state and regional continuing education opportunities, allowing her to garner more current continuing education, as well as solidifying more contacts through further networking opportunities. This demonstrated leadership to confront her areas of strength and take ownership for any perceived areas of opportunity, by seeking out resources through AOTA, NBCOT, and her state organization.

## How Leadership Interfaces With Occupational Therapy

### *Professional Development Tools and Self-Assessment Opportunities for Currency in the Profession of Occupational Therapy*

Being a reflective and current practitioner is essential to being an effective occupational therapy practitioner. The AOTA provides a Professional Development Tool that can be accessed at http://www1.aota.org/pdt/index.asp and includes a self-assessment that identifies learning needs through reflection, a professional development plan to develop specific learning objectives for professional growth, and an electronic portfolio to track accomplishments and activities reflective of each individual practitioner. Similarly, the NBCOT has a web-based platform available to certificants that has professional development tools as well. Included are self-assessment tools, resources, performance tracking on assessment tools, and a platform to organize professional development documents to ensure continued competency. More can be found at http://www.nbcot.org/navigator#sthash.yoS2i974.dpuf.

Additional resources at NBCOT.org include access to ProQuest (an online database providing access to evidence-based research) and Refworks (a

## Evidence-Based Research Chart

| Leadership Theory | Foundational Concepts | Evidence |
|---|---|---|
| Participatory leadership | Based upon respect and engagement.<br>Focuses energy in human-to-human encounters.<br>The goal is to harness diversity, build community, and create shared responsibility for action. | Kets de Vries, 2005; McLagan & Nell, 1995; Pearce, 2004; Spreier, Fontaine, & Malloy, 2006; Stewart, 2007 |
| Servant leadership | The servant-leader is servant first, meaning leadership begins with the natural feeling that one wants to serve, to serve first. Then, conscious choice brings one to aspire to lead. Liden et al. (2008) identified these characteristics of a servant leader:<br>• Emotional healing<br>• Creating value for the community<br>• Empowering<br>• Helping subordinates grow<br>• Putting subordinates first<br>• Behaving ethically<br>• Forming relationships with immediate followers<br>• Servanthood | Dillon, 2011; Greenleaf, 1970; Liden, Wayne, Zhao, & Henderson, 2008; Sadler-Smith & Shefy, 2004 |
| Transformational leadership | Leaders and their followers raise one another to higher levels of morality and motivation through:<br>• Integrity and fairness<br>• Clear goals<br>• High expectations<br>• Encouragement of others<br>• Providing support and recognition<br>• Eliciting and encouraging the emotions of people<br>• Encouraging others to look beyond self-interest<br>• Inspiring others to reach beyond the "probable" | Bass, 1985; Burns, 1978; Firestone, 2010 |
| Leadership in Enabling Occupation | Embraces four key elements in which occupational therapy practitioners can assert everyday leadership to create optimal access to and conditions for occupational therapy services:<br>• Scholarship<br>• Accountability<br>• Workforce planning<br>• Funding<br>Optimal leadership occurs when these four elements are integrated into everyday practice. | Townsend et al., 2011 |
| Situational leadership | Influenced by the work of Fiedler (1978), who suggested that leaders are most effective in situations that most closely match their leadership styles.<br>Examines the relationship among three dimensions: task behavior, relationship behavior, and the maturity of the individuals being led (Hersey & Blanchard, 1982). | DeYoung, 2005; Fiedler, 1978; George, 2002; Hersey & Blanchard, 1982 |

citation management tool). Abendstern, Hughes, Tucker, Clarkson, and Challis (2014) investigated self-assessment in occupational therapy services focusing on professional culture and practice specifically related to new tools and approaches. This study used self-assessment through occupational therapy services for both client personalization as well as helping to promote self-help for clientele and assessed the managers responsible for changes and reactions of staff groups following implementation. This study provided an opportunity to identify opportunities and strengths within the service delivery in the United Kingdom, as well as an opportunity to change the implementation of services more individualized to the communities served. Through engaging in professional development, occupational therapy practitioners have the opportunity to provide support to best practice as it relates to service delivery. Having this foundational skill as a cornerstone of leadership has become increasingly important to remain and maintain relevancy as a practitioner.

## Summary

As evidenced by the literature and history of the profession, leadership is not merely an opportunity but an obligation. By carefully increasing awareness and intentional concern for context, all practitioners can engage in leadership. Opportunities for leadership may present themselves in formal ways, such as holding a position as manager or supervisor, but there are other equally important opportunities for leadership (Strzelecki, 2007). Using the information presented about the *Framework* and how leadership can be analyzed as an occupation and having a better understanding of leadership models can engender a discussion about the influence of context on each individual's leadership abilities. Occupational therapy practitioners and students can think about their leadership qualities and desires by reflecting on their process and communication skills in addition to pondering their own individual contextual influences. The ways in which the *Framework* breaks out different contextual influences can be a start in helping individuals assess their leadership abilities and experiences. Most occupational therapy practitioners will find that, upon reflection, many of the tasks they already complete can be viewed as acts of leadership.

This chapter has explored leadership by discussing different leadership theories and analyzing the occupation of leading using the *Framework*. The *Framework* emphasis was on the role of context and the importance of reflection in developing leadership abilities. Participatory leadership and transformational leadership offer particular benefits to occupational therapy practitioners in many situations. Ultimately, leaders need to possess abilities in various types of leadership and use them based on situation and context. Leadership occurs every day in the profession. When we recognize and name these happenings, we are in a position to respond to our obligation to lead in community and global arenas.

## Student Self-Assessment

1. According to your individual context and environment, identify simple and complex leadership actions that can contribute to the future of occupational therapy practice.
2. Choose a leadership scenario from current events in the national or global context. While contemplating this situation, discuss what leadership styles and skills were used. Were they effective? Why or why not? What other leadership abilities could have been used that might have been more effective? Would you have handled the situation in the same or a different manner?
3. Consider one leadership experience you have witnessed or of which you have been a part. Discuss and analyze the different contexts, according to the *Framework*, and how each of them influenced the leadership scenario. What went better than expected? What lessons did you learn for the future? Following your reflection, what opportunities were there?

## Acknowledgments

Thanks to Lisa L. Clark, MS, OTR/L, CLT, and James Marc-Aurele, MBA, OTR/L, for their work on this chapter in the Second Edition.

## References

Abendstern, M., Hughes, J., Tucker, S., Clarkson, P., & Challis, D. (2014). Self-assessment and personalization in occupational therapy services: A managerial perspective on the challenges and opportunities of a service innovation. *British Journal of Occupational Therapy (College of Occupational Therapists Limited), 77*(10), 499-506.

Ackerman, R., & MacKenzie, S. (2006). Uncovering teacher leadership. *Educational Leadership, 63*, 66-70.

American Occupational Therapy Association. (2006). *AOTA's centennial vision*. Retrieved from http://www.aota.org/News/Centennial/Background/36516.aspx?FT=.pdf

American Occupational Therapy Association. (2014). Occupational therapy practice framework: Domain and process (3rd ed.). *American Journal of Occupational Therapy, 68*(Suppl. 1), S1-S48. doi:10.5014/ajot.2014.682006

American Occupational Therapy Association. (2015). Occupational therapy code of ethics. *American Journal of Occupational Therapy, 69*(Suppl. 3).

American Occupational Therapy Association. (2016). *AOTA unveils vision 2025*. Retrieved from http://www.aota.org/AboutAOTA/vision-2025.aspx

Bass, B. M. (1985). *Leadership and performance beyond expectations*. New York, NY: Free Press.

Bass, B. M. (1990). *Bass & Stogdill's handbook of leadership: Theory, research, and managerial applications* (3rd ed.). New York, NY: Free Press.

Borkowski, N. (2005). *Organizational behavior in health care*. Sudbury, MA: Jones and Bartlett Publishers.

Brown, D. (2012). AOTA, state associations collaborate on health reform advocacy. *OT Practice, 17*(17), 6.

Brunyate, R. W. (1957). Powerful levers in common little things. *American Journal of Occupational Therapy, 12*, 193-202.

Burns, J. M. (1978). *Leadership*. New York, NY: Harper and Row.

DeYoung, R. (2005). Behavioral theories of leadership. In N. Borkowski (Ed.), *Organizational behavior in health care* (pp. 173-185). Boston, MA: Jones and Bartlett.

Dillon, T. H. (2011). A legacy of leadership: transforming the occupational therapy profession. In K. Jacobs & G. McCormack (Eds.), *The occupational therapy manager* (5th ed.). Bethesda, MD: AOTA Press.

Fidler, G. S. (1965). Learning as a growth process: A conceptual framework for professional education. *American Journal of Occupational Therapy, 20*, 1-8.

Fiedler, F. E. (1967). *A theory of leadership effectiveness*. New York, NY: McGraw-Hill.

Fiedler, F. E. (1978). The contingency model and the dynamics of the leadership process. In L. Berkowitz (Ed.), *Advances in experimental psychology*. New York, NY: Academic Press.

Finn, G. L. (1972). The occupational therapist in prevention programs. *American Journal of Occupational Therapy, 26*, 59-66.

Firestone, D. T. (2010). A study of leadership behaviors among chairpersons in allied health programs. *Journal of Allied Health, 39*(1), 34-42.

Fleming-Castaldy, R., & Gillen, G. (2013). Ensuring that education, certification, and practice are evidence based. *American Journal of Occupational Therapy, 67*(3), 364-369. doi:10.5014/ajot.2013.006973

George, J., & Jones, G. (2002). *Organizational behavior* (3rd ed.). Upper Saddle River, NJ: Prentice Hall.

Gilfoyle, E. M. (1984). Transformation of a profession. *American Journal of Occupational Therapy, 38*, 575-584.

Grady, A. P. (1995). Building inclusive community: A challenge for occupational therapy. *American Journal of Occupational Therapy, 49*, 300-310.

Grady, A. (2003). From management to leadership. In G. H. McCormack, E. Jaffe, & M. Goodman-Levy (Eds.), *The occupational therapy manager* (4th ed., pp. 331-347). Bethesda, MD: AOTA Press.

Greenleaf, R. K. (1970). *The servant as leader*. Westfield, IN: The Greenleaf Center for Servant Leadership.

Hamm, J. (2006). The five messages leaders must manage. *Harvard Business Review, 84*, 114-123.

Heard, C. P. (2014). Choosing the path of leadership in occupational therapy. *Open Journal of Occupational Therapy, 2*(1), 1-18. doi:10.15453/2168-6408.1055

Hersey, P., & Blanchard, K. (1982). *Management of organizational behavior: Utilizing human resources*. Upper Saddle River, NJ: Prentice Hall.

Holmes, W. M., & Scaffa, M. E. (2009). The nature of emerging practice in occupational therapy: A pilot study. *Occupational Therapy in Health Care, 23*(3), 189-206. doi:10.1080/07380570902976759

Kets de Vries, M. F. R. (2005). Leadership group coaching in action: The Zen of creating high performance teams. *Academy of Management Executive, 19*, 61-76.

Kolodoner, E. L., & Hischmann, C. L. (1997). Mentors and protégés: Partners for professional development. *Administration and Management Special Interest Section Quarterly, 13*(3), 1-4.

Kouzes, J., & Posner, B. (2007). *The leadership challenge* (4th ed.). San Francisco, CA: John Wiley & Sons.

Kronenberg, F., & Pollard, N. (2006). Political dimensions of occupation and the roles of occupational therapy. *American Journal of Occupational Therapy, 60*(6), 617-625.

Liden, R. C., Wayne, S. J., Zhao, H., & Henderson, D. (2008). Servant leadership: Development of a multidimensional measure and multi-level assessment. *The Leadership Quarterly, 19*(2), 161-177. doi:10.1016/j.leaqua.2008.01.006

McCormack, G. (2003). Historical and current perspectives of management. In G. H. McCormack, E. Jaffe, & M. Goodman-Levy (Eds.), *The occupational therapy manager* (4th ed., pp. 331-347). Bethesda, MD: AOTA Press.

McLagan, P. A., & Nell, C. (1995). *The age of participation: New governance for the workplace and world*. San Francisco, CA: Berrett-Koehler Publishers.

Pearce, C. (2004). The future of leadership: Combining vertical and shared leadership to transform knowledge work. *Academy of Management Executive, 18*, 47-57.

Robeson, H. A. (1937). *Eleanor Clarke Slagle: Testimonial to Mrs. Eleanor Clarke Slagle*. 21st annual meeting of the American Occupational Therapy Association. Bethesda, MD: Wilma West Library Archives.

Sadler-Smith, E., & Shefy, E. (2004). The intuitive executive: Understanding and applying "gut feel" in decision making. *Academy of Management Executive, 18*(4), 76-91.

Scheerer, C. R. (2007). Mentoring in occupational therapy: One state's status. *Occupational Therapy in Health Care, 21*(3), 17-33.

Schell, B. A. B., & Slater, D. (1998). Management competencies required of administrative and clinical practitioners in the new millennium. *American Journal of Occupational Therapy, 52*(9), 744-750.

Schwartz, K. B. (2009). Reclaiming our heritage: Connecting the founding vision to the centennial vision. *American Journal of Occupational Therapy, 63*, 681-690.

Shortell, S., & Kaluzney, A. (2000). *Health care management: Organizational design and behavior*. Florence, KY: Delmar Cengage Learning.

Spreier, S., Fontaine, M., & Malloy, R. (2006). Leadership run amok: The destructive power of overachievers. *Harvard Business Review, 84*, 72-82.

Stewart, L. S. P. (2007). Pressure to lead: What can we learn from the theory? *British Journal of Occupational Therapy (College of Occupational Therapists Limited), 70*(6), 228-234.

Stogdill, R. M. (1948). Personal factors associated with leadership: A survey of the literature. *Journal of Psychology: Interdisciplinary and Applied, 25*, 35-71.

Strzelecki, M. (2007). Leaders of the pack. *OT Practice, 12*(7), 16-19.

Townsend, E. A., & Polatajko, H. J. (2007). *Enabling occupation II: Advancing an occupational therapy vision for health, well-being, & justice through occupation*. Ottawa, Ontario, Canada: CAOT Publications ACE.

Townsend, E. A., Polatajko, H. J., Craik, J. M., & von Zweck, C. M. (2011). Introducing the Leadership in Enabling Occupation (LEO) model. *Canadian Journal of Occupational Therapy, 78*(4), 255-9.

Walter, F., & Scheibe, S. (2013). A literature review and emotion-based model of age and leadership: New directions for the trait approach. *The Leadership Quarterly, 24*(6), 882-901. doi:10.1016/j.leaqua.2013.10.003

World Federation of Occupational Therapists. (2011). Retrieved from http://www.wfot.org/

Yamkovenko, S. (2012). AOTA and state associations: Collaborating on local reimbursement issues. *OT Practice, 17*(13), 5-5.

## SUGGESTED READINGS

American Occupational Therapy Association. (2003). *Professional development tool*. Retrieved from http://www1.aota.org/pdt/index.asp

American Occupational Therapy Association. (2015). *Official documents*. Retrieved from http://www.aota.org/practice/manage/official.aspx

American Occupational Therapy Association. (2016). *Cool leadership and volunteer opportunities*. Retrieved from http://www.aota.org/aboutaota/get-involved/leadership.aspx

American Occupational Therapy Association. (2016). *Legislative action center*. Retrieved from http://www.aota.org/advocacy-policy/state-policy/state-ot-associations.aspx

American Occupational Therapy Association. (2016). *State OT associations*. Retrieved from http://www.aota.org/advocacy-policy/state-policy/state-ot-associations.aspx

# VIII

# Scholarship

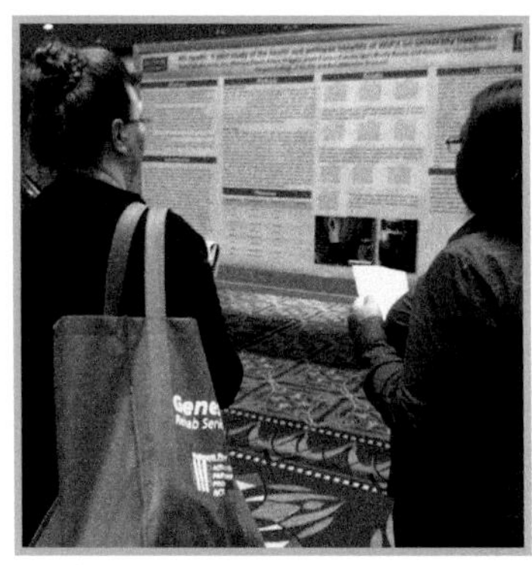

# 47

# THE IMPORTANCE OF SCHOLARSHIP AND SCHOLARLY PRACTICE FOR OCCUPATIONAL THERAPY

*Linda H. Niemeyer, OT, PhD and Karen Duddy, OTD, MHA, OTR/L*

ACOTE STANDARDS EXPLORED IN THIS CHAPTER

B.8.0–B.8.8

KEY VOCABULARY

- **Dependent variable:** One or more clinical findings, behaviors, personal attributes, or internal experiences that are measured in research; the dependent variable might be hypothesized to change as the result of the independent variable or to differ between independent variable groupings.
- **Independent variable:** A factor in research such as an intervention that can be manipulated by the investigator; also, a stable characteristic of individuals by which they can be grouped.
- **Qualitative research:** Exploratory gathering of in-depth, detailed descriptions of problems or conditions from the point of view of the group or individual experiencing them to discover themes and their interrelationships or linkages.
- **Quantitative research:** Use of the scientific method to gather data that can be expressed numerically and analyzed statistically to describe population characteristics or determine the relationship between one or more independent and dependent variables.

*(continued)*



Jacobs, K., & MacRae, N. (Eds.).
*Occupational Therapy Essentials for Clinical Competence, Third Edition* (pp. 663-688).

## KEY VOCABULARY (CONTINUED)

- **Rigor:** Close adherence to experimental research methodology; in broader usage, embedding of sound principles and practices—agreed upon by the scientific community—into each step of the quantitative or qualitative research process to ensure trustworthiness of results.
- **Scholarly practice:** Evidence-based practice; using the knowledge base of the profession in occupational therapy practice and teaching.
- **Scholarship:** Research activities designed to build the knowledge base of occupational therapy to further advance practice and teaching.

At the beginning of the new millennium, Holm (2000), in her Eleanor Clarke Slagle lecture, reflected on the challenges that would face occupational therapy practitioners in the next century. Beginning in the mid-1970s, occupational therapy practitioners had encountered new developments in health care delivery and reimbursement, including managed care, prospective payment, capitation, and changes in staffing ratios, which greatly affected the way services were provided. Moreover, there was an increasing demand for justifying practice patterns via research-based evidence demonstrating that occupational therapy interventions resulted in improved client outcomes. The demand was not only that research evidence should demonstrate positive outcomes but also that it should provide enough information about what was done in the intervention and how it was done so that others could replicate it with comparable clients and achieve similar outcomes.

Indeed, this new emphasis on justifying occupational therapy practice patterns was reflected in an influx of published evidence. On the surface, this was encouraging news, but unfortunately, two problems were created. First, the quantity of the published evidence that practitioners would need to sift through was daunting. Dubouloz, Egan, Vallerand, and von Zweck (1999), based on semistructured in-depth interviews of eight selected participants, identified barriers related to this problem that included a practitioner's perceived lack of skill and feelings of inadequacy with regard to finding, interpreting, and using evidence, as well as lack of time and administrative or organizational support. The authors further noted an attitudinal barrier in the form of practitioner perception that any evidence that was located might threaten routine practice methods perceived to be effective. Second, quantity did not necessarily mean quality. For example, Holm (2000) analyzed the quality of the evidence in articles published by the *Occupational Therapy Journal of Research* between 1995 and 1999 and found that more than 50% provided the weakest evidence in the form of descriptive studies or the opinions of experts, but barely 8% represented what the author would consider the strongest evidence in the form of true experimental studies.

When occupational therapy practice is based on limited or insufficient evidence, this clearly creates an ethical dilemma. Holm (2000) cited sections of the 1994 version of the *Occupational Therapy Code of Ethics* to make her point. This document has been updated, and relevant sections of the 2015 current version of the *Code of Ethics* read as follows (American Occupational Therapy Association [AOTA], 2015, pp. 2-5):

- Beneficence, Principle 1. Occupational therapy personnel shall demonstrate a concern for the well-being and safety of the recipients of their services.
    - Use, to the extent possible, evaluation, planning, intervention techniques, assessments, and therapeutic equipment that are evidence-based, current and within the recognized scope of occupational therapy practice.
    - Take steps (e.g., continuing education, research, supervision, training) to ensure proficiency, use careful judgment, and weigh potential for client harm when generally recognized standards do not exist in emerging technology or areas of practice.
- Nonmaleficence, Principle 2. Occupational therapy personnel shall refrain from actions that cause harm.
    - Avoid inflicting harm or injury to recipients of occupational therapy services, students, research participants, or employees.
- Autonomy, Principle 3. Occupational therapy personnel shall respect the right of the individual to self-determination, privacy, confidentiality, and consent.
    - Establish a collaborative relationship with recipients of service and relevant stakeholders, to promote shared decision-making.

Furthermore, Holm identified what she considered to be key obligations of occupational therapy practitioners to fulfill the ethical responsibilities of the profession, namely to "become competent in, and make a habit of, searching for the evidence, appraising its value, and presenting it to those we serve in an understandable manner" and to "improve our research competencies, to develop the habit of using those competencies in everyday practice, and to advance the evidence base of occupational therapy in the new millennium" (Holm, 2000, p. 584).

As occupational therapy academicians and practitioners tackled this challenge, a new conceptual framework for scholarship emerged that went beyond the traditional association with purely academic study or achievement. In a visionary paper aimed at occupational therapists, Haertlein and Coppard (2003) stated, "An expanded conception of scholarship offers a way for identifying and characterizing an array of methods by which all occupational therapy academicians and practitioners, through collaborative efforts, can succeed at their institutions while contributing to the teaching, research, and service needs of the profession" (p. 641).

## Scholarly Endeavors and Their Contribution to the Occupational Therapy Body of Knowledge

Several types of scholarly endeavors are identified in the occupational therapy literature that can be perceived as being separate yet interrelated. A new conceptual framework for scholarship was outlined in a 2009 AOTA position paper. First, the authors distinguished between scholarly practice and scholarship. Scholarly practice, otherwise known as *evidence-based practice* (EBP), was defined as "using the knowledge base of the profession or discipline in one's practice" and in teaching (AOTA, 2009, p. 790). On the other hand, scholarship was equated with activities designed to build the knowledge base and further advance the practice and teaching of occupational therapy; these activities also came under the heading of research. With regard to the evidence gained through scholarly practice and scholarship, the authors concluded, "All occupational therapists and occupational therapy assistants, regardless of their individual practice roles, have the professional responsibility to not only use that evidence to inform their professional decision making but also to generate new evidence through independent or collaborative research, or both" (AOTA, 2009, p. 793).

The term evidence-based practice had its start as evidence-based medicine in the 1980s at McMaster University Medical School in Ontario, Canada (Law & MacDermid, 2008; Taylor, 2007). Evidence-based medicine was defined by Sackett, Rosenberg, Gray, Haynes, and Richardson (1996) as "the conscientious, explicit, and judicious use of current best evidence in making decisions about the care of individual patients," which entailed "integrating individual clinical expertise with the best available external clinical evidence from systematic research" (p. 71). This concept quickly gained acceptance in the health care field and was soon recognized worldwide. Tickle-Degnen (1999) helped to further the understanding of the role of EBP in occupational therapy by characterizing it as a set of organizing and evaluating tools "designed to integrate research study evidence into the clinical reasoning process" to "help the practitioner select the best assessments and intervention procedures from an array of possibilities" (p. 537) and achieve the best possible outcomes.

According to the classic definition of EBP, the occupational therapy practitioner is asked to integrate his or her own internal clinical expertise with the best available relevant external systematic research to inform practice decisions (Kielhofner, 2006; Law & MacDermid, 2008; Taylor, 2007). The recommended procedure for conducting an EBP inquiry will be discussed later in this chapter. This process calls for a certain amount of flexibility in the practitioner's willingness to modify assessment or intervention in response to the new knowledge gained. The rewards of improved competency in both research skills and clinical practice are much valued by stakeholders, particularly those whose primary focus is consumer protection and judicious use of resources (Christiansen & Lou, 2001; Kielhofner, 2006).

Fortunately, ongoing debate and discussion has led to some evolution regarding implementation of EBP, which has enhanced its applicability to occupational therapy (Christiansen & Lou, 2001; Kielhofner, 2006; Law & MacDermid, 2008). Most notable is the acknowledgment of the importance of the values, needs, and preferences of the client and his or her family. In this adapted format, the occupational therapy practitioner bases clinical decisions on his or her own expertise and the best evidence available while also consulting with the client and family to help determine the most suitable option. The client's perspective is thus taken into account; the evidence and its meaning are translated into user-friendly terms, and choices are made based on client–practitioner collaboration (Dijkers, Murphy, & Krellman, 2012; Tickle-Degnen, 1999). In this way, EBP becomes better suited to the client-centered values and philosophy of occupational therapy.

Let us now turn our attention from scholarly practice, or EBP, to an expanded conception of scholarship. Haertlein and Coppard (2003), as well as the AOTA (2009), described four dimensions of scholarship, which are based on the seminal work of American educator Ernest L. Boyer. These four dimensions are as follows:

1. **The scholarship of discovery.** Conducting original scientific research; this type of scholarship contributes to the growing knowledge base of occupational therapy.
2. **The scholarship of integration.** Seeking new insights from existing original research, both within occupational therapy and across disciplines, by integrating, interpreting and synthesizing in a search for new patterns of connection; this type of scholarship

contributes to the formation of new perspectives and theories in occupational therapy.

3. **The scholarship of application.** Forging a link between theory and practice and between academia and service provision; this type of scholarship contributes to the use of knowledge and insights gained from the scholarship of discovery and integration to address societal problems, occupational therapy assessments or interventions, or classroom teaching of clients or occupational therapy practitioners in a practical way.
4. **The scholarship of teaching and learning.** Systematic study based on the recognition of the complementary nature of teaching and learning; this type of scholarship contributes to the knowledge base needed for high-quality teaching of occupational therapy students and also public sharing of the knowledge of the profession.

The challenge inherent in the scholarship of application dimension opened exciting new opportunities for research but also increased awareness of problems with approaches to occupational therapy research at the millennium (Hammel, Finlayson, Kielhofner, Helfrish, & Peterson, 2002; Kielhofner, 2005a, 2005b; Taylor, Fisher, & Kielhofner, 2005). Of particular concern was the observation that practice tended to lag behind research and that occupational therapy practitioners were disillusioned by theory and research that seemed to be irrelevant to methods used in their everyday work. This observation led to recognition of the need for a more inclusive participatory approach to research that would serve to better connect academicians and practitioners.

One model for enhancing the scholarship of application, termed the *community of scholars*, was designed to incorporate scholarship into the education of occupational therapy students by immersing them in a social context where they could learn "not only from their advisor or instructors but also from a community of scholars that includes student peers, other faculty, staff, clients, practitioners, and community members involved in the scholarship" (Hammel et al., 2002, p. 160). Wilding, Curtin, and Whiteford (2012) used the term *community of practice scholars* to describe an approach wherein a group of occupational therapy academicians worked collaboratively with occupational therapy practitioners. Via monthly teleconference meetings, "members of the community of practice scholars went through a cyclic process of reflection, discovery, planning, implementation, evaluation and re-evaluation" (p. 313). This model made possible an ongoing collaborative interchange that promoted critical reflection on practice and consideration of ways where practice could be improved.

The occupational therapy faculty at the University of Illinois at Chicago developed a model based on what was termed *engaged scholarship* in which institutions

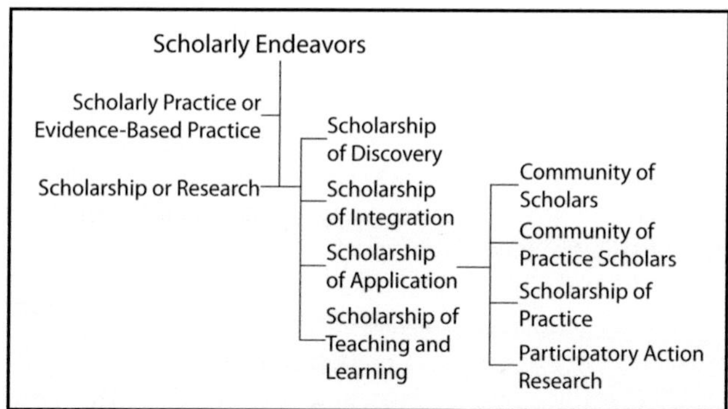


**Figure 47-1.** An expanded conception of scholarship as the means for building the occupational therapy body of knowledge.

of higher education pursued research in collaboration with community settings. In the University of Illinois at Chicago model, called A Scholarship of Practice, long-standing partnerships with multiple community-based organizations were established that became "the foundation for curriculum development, research initiatives, and the development and evaluation of clinical service" (Braveman, Helfrich, & Fisher, 2002, p. 110). A Scholarship of Practice, defined as a "a dialectic in which theoretical and empirical knowledge is brought to bear on the practical problems of therapeutic work and in which the latter raise questions to be addressed through scholarship" (Kielhofner, 2005a, p. 9), represents linking of occupational therapy practitioners and academicians with the community "based on the assumption that those who ultimately will use the knowledge must be partners in its generation" and "begins with the premise that researchers and theorists in the field must work together with practitioners to not only generate the field's theory and research but also to advance practice" (Kielhofner, 2005a, p. 10). This model lays the groundwork for participatory action research. Participatory action research is not so much a research method as an approach that uses the committed involvement of stakeholders to examine how scientific knowledge can be joined with the experiential knowledge inherent in the community, resulting in action that addresses complex social problems (Kielhofner, 2005a; Suarez-Balcazar et al., 2005).

Since the beginning of the new millennium, the breadth and depth of scholarly endeavors has grown, leading to emerging possibilities for expanding the occupational therapy body of knowledge. The types of scholarly endeavors that were discussed in this section are reviewed in Figure 47-1. Ongoing work by occupational therapy academicians and practitioners has led to the understanding that building of the occupational therapy body of knowledge via scholarly practice and scholarship entails an ongoing dialogue that brings together occupational therapy theoretical concepts, empirical research to verify those concepts, and real-world application of those concepts by means of clinical practice and active collaboration with the community. Any occupational therapy practitioner, regardless of his or her role in the profession, thus has the opportunity to help fulfill the ethical responsibility to contribute to the generation of knowledge that leads to steady progression of the profession of occupational therapy.

## Case Study Part 1

Coauthor Karen Duddy, OTD, MHA, OTR/L, while serving as occupational therapy supervisor at the VA Long Beach Healthcare System in California, noticed a gap in service provision for veterans with ongoing chronic health conditions. This population of veterans was not receiving the education, support, or resources through the existing primary care model that were necessary to develop critical health promoting behaviors. There were no interventions available that were specifically aimed at restoring the functional abilities and capacities essential for optimal daily living. Moreover, occupational therapy was not included in the primary care interprofessional team. Because the coauthor knew that occupational therapy is distinctly qualified to address the lifestyle and contextual factors that influence health, she embarked upon the development and implementation of occupation-based occupational therapy services to demonstrate the vital role of occupational therapy in any primary care endeavor aimed at meeting the complex needs of veterans with chronic health conditions. This effort represented the initiation of the scholarship of application.

The scholarship of application begins with a search of the literature. The first step in forging a link between theory and practice and between academia and service provision was to explore the existing body of knowledge. Indeed, veterans have been characterized as "older, sicker, and poorer than the general population" (Lawder, 2014, para. 12). There is a recognized need for programs that support self-management of chronic conditions to mitigate deterioration of health and loss of functional capacity (Darkins, Kendall, Edmonson, Young, & Stressel, 2014). A small body of research was located that demonstrated the effectiveness of occupation-based approaches for people with chronic conditions. Investigators found that positive health behavior strategies are more likely to be adopted and maintained if they are meaningful, relevant to the person's unique daily living challenges and personal motivations, and consistent with the structure and context of his or her life and day-to-day routines (Arbesman & Mosley, 2012; Clark et al., 2012; Kennedy et al., 2013; Linden, Butterworth, & Prochaska, 2010; Skaperdas et al., n.d.; Stav, Hallenen, Lane, & Arbesman, 2012). This and other information confirmed the coauthor's observations and vision for change.

Dr. Duddy next reviewed applicable theories and models of care. Three were selected as best suited to an intervention based on the premise that completion of personal action plans and increasing engagement in activities and occupations supports health. The World Health Organization's (WHO) *International Classification of Functioning, Disability and Health* (ICF; 2001) was chosen as a classification system that illustrates the relationship between health and occupation and the factors affecting functioning and disability. The Ecology of Human Performance framework complemented the ICF and provided structure for designing the intervention by describing the dynamic interaction between person, task, and context and their affect on performance (Kramer, Hinojosa, & Royeen, 2003). The Health Action Process Approach provided a causal model for health behavior change that incorporated important aspects of other established health behavior theories (Schwarzer, Lippke, & Luszczynska, 2011).

Since the aim of the scholarship of application is to address a societal problem, it was imperative to understand the problem, both in terms of the larger context and the inner workings of the VA Long Beach primary care system. The coauthor discovered that the core issue was lack of full implementation of the new primary care team-based model, the Patient Aligned Care Team, which was enacted to promote collaborative care, shared decision-making, and sustained relationships with clients and families in primary care to best address the dynamic and complex needs of Veterans with multiple chronic conditions (Piette et al., 2011). Team-based models were an outgrowth of the Patient Protection and Affordable Care Act of 2010, which encouraged the formation of provider networks to coordinate patient care. As with other health care systems, primary care was overburdened and practitioners encountered barriers to addressing patient behaviors or personal and contextual factors that were central to behavioral management of chronic conditions (Midboe, Cucciare, Trafton, Ketroser, & Chardos, 2011).

The principal outgrowth of the knowledge gained was an innovative, occupation-based approach to intervention entitled the Everyday Matters workshop. This primary care occupational therapy service, which used a group process to achieve secondary and tertiary prevention in primary care, was the first of its kind in the VA. The scholarship of application does not stop here. There are questions to be asked and answered, for example, "Is participation in this program associated with the anticipated positive changes in the population served?" and "What is the impact of an occupation-based self-management program provided by occupational therapists for veterans living in the community with multiple chronic conditions?" The nature and quality of the evidence obtained from research aimed at answering these questions will contribute to the growing body of knowledge about the health-promoting effects of occupation.

# The Nature and Quality of Evidence

The core of any scholarly endeavor, including scholarly practice (or EBP) and scholarship (or research), is the ability to judge the quality of evidence. Basically, quality of evidence might be conceived of as the degree of confidence an occupational therapy practitioner or academician can have in the trustworthiness, accuracy, relevance, and usefulness of information from a published research approach for making practice decisions. An understanding of the quality of evidence is also of critical importance for designing the best possible research approach to substantiate occupational therapy theory or practice methodology. The traditional guideline for judging the quality of evidence was largely established in evidence-based medicine as a single hierarchical system based on study categories and usually termed *levels of evidence* (Law & MacDermid, 2008; Sackett et al., 1996; Taylor, 2007; Tomlin & Borgetto, 2011). This hierarchical system has been widely adopted, sometimes with minor modifications, and is found in AOTA web-based materials (n.d.). It can be visualized as a simple two-dimensional pyramid, as seen in Figure 47-2, with the weakest or lowest quality sources of evidence at the bottom and the strongest or highest quality sources of evidence at the apex.

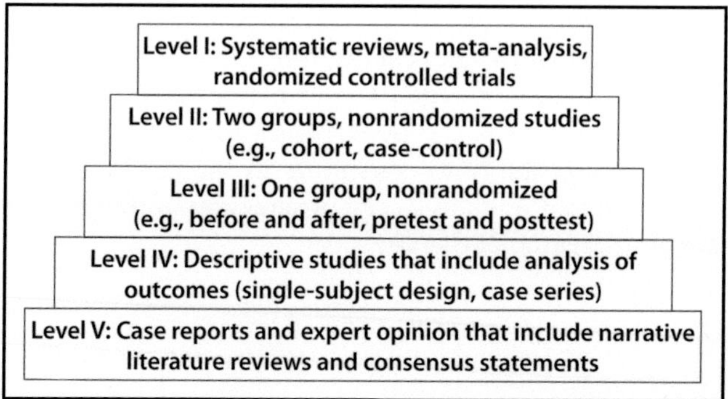


**Figure 47-2.** The single hierarchical system for categorization of levels of evidence (AOTA, n.d.; Tomlin & Borgetto, 2011) shown as a two-dimensional pyramid with the weakest sources of evidence at the base and the strongest sources of evidence at the apex.

However, limitations in the traditional single hierarchical system, as it pertains to occupational therapy scholarly endeavors, have been recognized (Taylor, 2007; Tomlin & Borgetto, 2011). First, this system is mainly directed to research questions about the success of interventions in promoting positive outcomes. It does not take into account the full range of research questions that an occupational therapy practitioner or academician might ask, and different types of research questions might call for different best research approaches. Second, it is rooted in classical experimental methodology in which randomized controlled clinical trials are considered to provide the best evidence. A well-designed, rigorous clinical trial is ideally suited to demonstrate the efficacy of an intervention, meaning the extent to which it can bring about its intended effect under ideal circumstances, such as the controlled conditions of an experiment. This research approach may not always be appropriate for establishing the effectiveness of an intervention, or the extent to which it can achieve its intended effect in a natural clinical, social, or community setting (Newcomer, Hatry & Wholey, 2015; Ottenbacher & Hinderer, 2001).

Occupational therapy practitioners and academicians are often concerned with "outcomes in the real world of physical, social, and spiritual participation" (Tomlin & Borgetto, 2011, p. 189), for which the restrictions of clinical trials may not always be suitable to provide the best evidence. Rather, an occupational therapy research question about the effectiveness of an intervention in a natural setting might call for a single-subject design study. Similarly, a research question about the lived experiences and perceptions of clients might call for a qualitative study, a question about the appropriateness of a screening measure for a comparison group study, or a question about the relationship between home assessment and safety training in elderly community-dwelling adults and incidence of falls over the life course for a longitudinal study (Taylor, 2007).

Tomlin and Borgetto (2011), in response to the recognized need for an alternative model for depicting levels of evidence, proposed the research pyramid. This model was designed to be a more accurate representation of the kinds of evidence needed by occupational therapy practitioners to inform professional decision making. Instead of a single two-dimensional hierarchy, as in the traditional system illustrated in Figure 47-2, the authors' model is three dimensional. It can be seen in Figure 47-3 that the research pyramid portrays three separate hierarchies representing three distinct types of research, each located on one side of the pyramid. Descriptive studies are shown as a flattened pyramid that forms the base or foundation of the main pyramid. As in the single hierarchical model, weaker or lower quality sources of evidence for each type of research occupy lower positions on each side of the pyramid, with the stronger or higher quality sources of evidence approaching the apex.

The authors note that the research pyramid offers theoretical advantages for occupational therapy practitioners over the traditional system in the way that it separates yet values as being equal, experimental, outcome, and qualitative research. They state, "The point of shifting from a single hierarchy model of evidence evaluation to the pyramid model is not to claim that experimental studies are not important for occupational therapists. It is instead to assert that trustworthy evidence of different types can be discovered through disciplined inquiry, and all are important to the profession" (Tomlin & Borgetto,

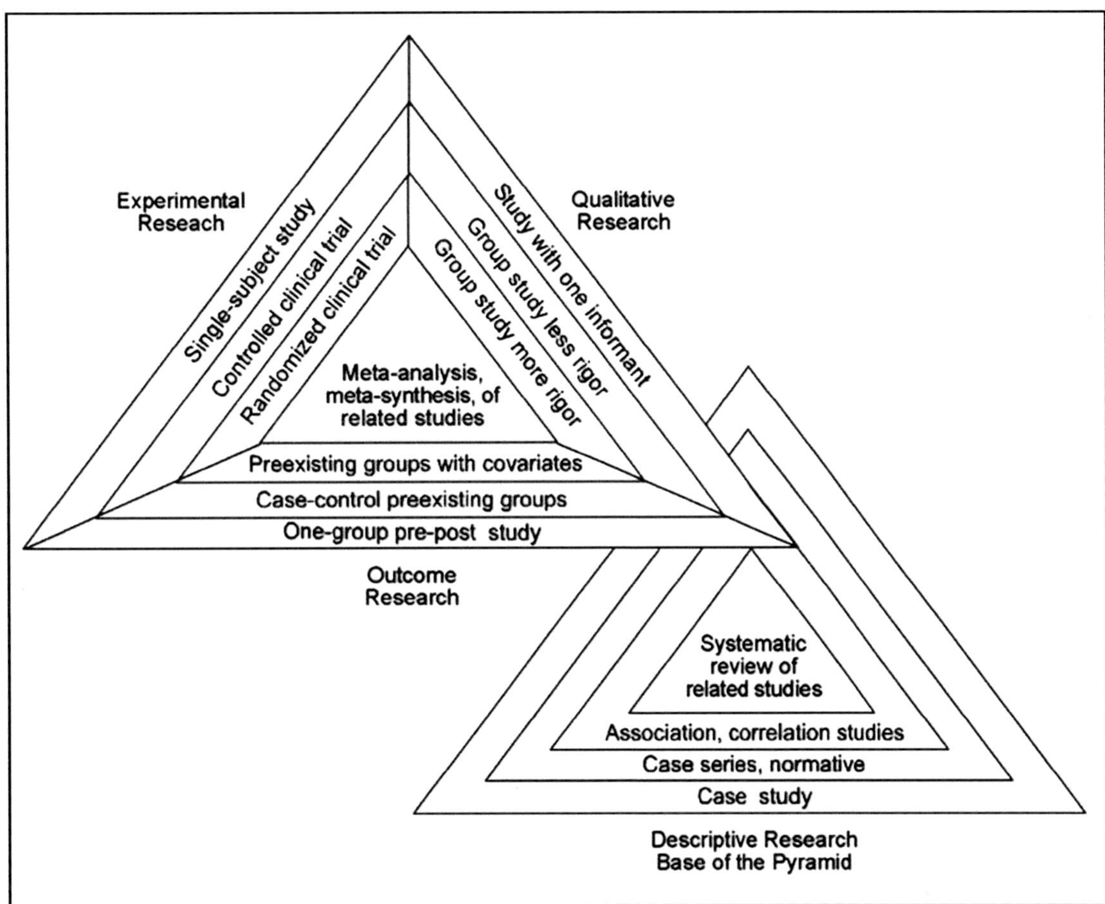


**Figure 47-3.** The research pyramid model for depicting of levels of evidence, drawn as the top view of a three-dimensional pyramid with each of its three sides representing a distinct category of research. The weaker sources of evidence occupy lower positions on each side with the stronger sources of evidence approaching the apex. Descriptive studies are shown as a flattened pyramid forming the base or foundation of the main pyramid. (Adapted from Tomlin, G., & Borgetto, B. [2011]. Research pyramid: A new evidence-based practice model for occupational therapy. *American Journal of Occupational Therapy, 65*[2], 189-196.)

2011, pp. 193-194). Thus, all forms of research have their place, and all contribute to the whole occupational therapy body of knowledge. Although randomized controlled trials may be appraised as the pinnacle of research, in truth what are considered lesser forms of research help provide the foundation that makes the more sophisticated experimental approaches possible. Outcome and qualitative research broaden occupational therapy scholarship to embrace real-world research questions, as well as the lived experiences of clients. Moreover, in larger research projects (e.g., participatory action research), investigators have used mixed methods and gathered both quantitative and qualitative data (Mortenson & Oliffe, 2009; Westhues et al., 2008).

The Tomlin and Borgetto (2011) system is well suited to organize a discussion of the different categories of research approaches. The placement of descriptive research as the base of the research pyramid is fitting because this research approach is very useful for gathering evidence when little is known. Descriptive research "often takes advantage of naturally occurring events or available information in order to generate new insights through inductive processes" (Kielhofner, 2006, p. 58). Its most characteristic function is exploratory, and researchers frequently use preexisting databases. Descriptive studies assemble and organize information on a single individual, population, phenomenon, or problem, typically with no investigator manipulation. The research approaches representing the different levels of evidence for descriptive research, from the highest to the lowest level, are presented in Table 47-1 (Kielhofner, 2006).

The experimental research hierarchy can be seen as residing on one side of the main research pyramid. A detailed explanation of the full variety of experimental designs can easily take up most or all of an entire textbook, yet they characteristically have certain aspects in common. At the core of any experimental design is the intent to establish, by means of statistical tests, the probability that an intervention—called the *independent variable*—caused change in one or more clinical

Table 47-1.

**Descriptive Research**

| | | |
|---|---|---|
| Level I | Systematic review of related descriptive studies | Identification, selection, critical appraisal, and summary of published literature on descriptive studies that address a common research question |
| Level II | Associative, correlational studies | Studies that look at the degree of relationship between two or more naturally occurring phenomena or population characteristics of interest |
| Level III | Multiple-case studies (series) | A collection of individual case studies; a report on a series of clients with a similar characteristic of interest |
| | Normative studies | Research undertaken to establish usual or average values for a characteristic, trait, or performance parameter in a population of interest; related types of studies might document incidence or prevalence data on a health-related condition or patterns of growth or change in a population of interest (e.g., studies of developmental patterns in children) |
| | Descriptive survey | Collection of self-reported information from a population of interest using a structured questionnaire |
| Level IV | Individual case studies | An in-depth report of the experiences or behaviors of a single individual using interviews, observation, testing, or examination of records |

findings—called the *dependent variable(s)*—in a population of interest (Kielhofner, 2006). In classical evidence-based medicine, experimental studies, or clinical trials, the independent variable is a medication, clinical procedure, or treatment, and investigators select the dependent variable(s) based on clinical relevance. True experiments are prospective, meaning that data from measurement of the dependent variable(s) are gathered both before and after the intervention and are used to determine the degree to which the intervention led to change. This is in contrast to retrospective research, wherein data that are collected can refer to both current and past events, phenomena, or clinical findings. Individuals chosen to participate in experimental research ideally can be shown to be representative of a much larger population of individuals based on a close approximation of relevant characteristics such as age, gender, education, diagnosis, or impairment.

Experimental research extends beyond classical applications, particularly in studies conducted by occupational therapy and other allied health professionals. The independent variable can be a treatment, and it also can be a prevention or screening protocol, a form of diagnostic testing, a health care setting, or an educational program. Allied health investigators may select a relevant physical or physiological clinical finding, such as heart rate, breathing patterns, specific laboratory test results, joint range of motion, or muscle strength, as a dependent variable. They may also consider clinical findings that are behaviors or personal attributes, particularly those of importance to clients and their families, caregivers, teachers, or employers, because they are related to functioning in one or more aspects of everyday life. A behavior might be chosen as a dependent variable because it is considered inappropriate, disturbing, or disruptive. A selected personal attribute might be the ability to process sensory information or to perform activities of daily living or might be a skill such as handwriting. Finally, the dependent variable of interest can be an internal experience such as perceived pain or quality of life.

The three key characteristics of true experimental studies, which are also chief considerations for establishing levels of evidence in experimental research, are *control, randomization,* and *blinding.* Control customarily describes the presence of a control group in which participants receive no intervention or engage in neutral activity unrelated to the intervention. Participants can also be assigned to a comparison group in which they receive an alternate intervention. The inclusion of control groups helps support the scientific conclusion that any notable differences in the dependent variable between groups can be attributed to the intervention and not to some other unidentified causal factor. One can conceive of another aspect of control, which is the assurance that all individuals within each experimental group are treated identically. Often the term *fidelity* is used to indicate that the independent variable is administered exactly as planned and is true to the underlying theory of the intervention.

Randomization means that assignment of participants to an intervention or control group is made using a statistical technique such as a random number table, so that each participant has an equal likelihood of being a member of any group. This means that the investigators, the individuals providing the intervention, or the study participants in no way directly influence assignment to group. If randomization is properly carried out, there is

Table 47-2.

## Experimental Research

| Level | Type | Description |
|---|---|---|
| Level I | Meta-analysis or synthesis of related experimental studies | Synthesis: A systematic method of reviewing, critically analyzing, and integrating evidence from published studies that address a common research question. Meta-analysis: Use of statistical procedures to combine the results of multiple related studies to ascertain consistency of findings. Typically, calculation of effect size, or the magnitude of change in a dependent variable as the result of an intervention, is used as a common metric to compare individual studies. |
| Level II | Individual (blinded) randomized controlled clinical trials | A true prospective experimental design in which groups of participants are randomly assigned to intervention and control conditions. Blinding can be single, double, or triple. Tests the efficacy of an intervention. |
| Level III | Controlled clinical trials | A type of prospective experimental study in which an intervention group is compared with a control group. Both the participant and practitioner or researcher may be blinded. The system for assignment to group is not statistically randomized but is based on a quasi-random assignment system (e.g., days of the week or participant Social Security or medical record numbers). |
| Level IV | Single-subject studies | A true experimental design that uses a sample of one participant who serves as his or her own control. The experiment may be replicated with three or four participants. Serial measurements of the behavior or attribute of interest (the dependent variable) are taken before, during, and sometimes after the intervention. Tests the effectiveness of an intervention to change a relevant clinical finding, problem behavior, or attribute. Specific design approaches help to establish causality. |

a high likelihood that the characteristics of participants in each group will be similar. Blinding refers to a process of concealing knowledge of which participant in the experimental population is receiving what intervention or control condition; it can be extended to participants, individuals engaged in providing an intervention or recording dependent variables, or individuals analyzing data from the study. The purpose of blinding is to prevent conscious or unconscious expectations from coloring a participant's response to an intervention, an intervention provider's response to the participant, or the recording or analysis of information by members of the research team. Blinding is not always possible for a number of practical reasons. For example, it might not be feasible to conceal from a practitioner or participant the nature of the intervention that is being administered. The research approaches representing the different levels of evidence for experimental research, from the highest to the lowest level, are presented in Table 47-2 (Cooper, Hedges, & Valentine, 2009; Kazdin, 2010; Kielhofner, 2006; Newcomer et al., 2015).

The outcome research hierarchy occupies a second side of the research pyramid. According to the Agency for Healthcare Research and Quality (2000), outcome research, which is also called *outcomes research*, "seeks to understand the end results of particular health care practices and interventions" (para. 1). As a method of monitoring program performance, outcome research can address, in addition to clinical findings and the internal experiences of recipients of care, a broad array of health care delivery factors such as regulations and reimbursement policies, benefits and risks, cost, timeliness, efficiency, and consumer preferences (Newcomer et al., 2015). "For health care managers and purchasers, outcomes research can identify potentially effective strategies they can implement to improve the quality and value of care" (Agency for Healthcare Research and Quality, 2000, para. 4).

Although the randomized controlled trial has been extolled as the most robust method for providing evidence linking health care to outcomes, conducting this type of experimental research is not always logically feasible for the clinical setting (Ottenbacher & Hinderer, 2001). Clinical trials are demanding of available resources. For example, they call for a large number of participants who have similar characteristics and for highly controlled experimental conditions. Moreover, ethical considerations can arise when participants who are randomly assigned to a control condition receive no intervention. The *quasi-experimental* outcome research designs depicted in Table 47-3 represent viable alternatives that, if conducted with sufficient attention to detail, can provide a quantitative estimate of the affect of an intervention or of certain participant characteristics on outcome (Cooper et al., 2009; Kielhofner, 2006; Newcomer et al., 2015).

Qualitative research, which is represented on the third side of the research pyramid, is an approach that resonates well with the holistic and client-centered worldview and the core concerns, assumptions, and values of occupational therapy (Cook, 2001; Kielhofner, 1982b, 2006; Merrill, 1985). It constitutes a naturalistic method of scientific inquiry that is fundamentally exploratory

Table 47-3.

| OUTCOME RESEARCH | | |
|---|---|---|
| Level I | Meta-analysis or synthesis of related outcome studies | Synthesis: A systematic method of reviewing, critically analyzing, and integrating evidence from published studies that address a common research question. Meta-analysis: Use of statistical procedures to combine the results of multiple related studies to ascertain consistency of findings. Typically, calculation of effect size, or the magnitude of change in a dependent variable as the result of an intervention, is used as a common metric to compare individual studies. |
| Level II | Preexisting groups comparisons with covariate analysis | Also called a nonrandomized comparison group design. Assignment to an intervention or control condition is typically based on naturally occurring preexisting groups (e.g., children in two different classrooms or individuals at the top and bottom of a waiting list for the intervention). A prospective design in which pre- and postintervention measures establish differences between groups in terms of dependent variables or outcomes of interest.<br>A variation is the cohort study, wherein assignment to group is based on differences in key participant characteristics such as certain risk factors. Individuals are followed for a period of time to establish the degree of relationship between these characteristics and subsequent outcome. Lack of random assignment increases the chance of systematic differences between groups that act as confounding variables. A confounding variable is a factor that distorts the actual relationship between the independent and dependent variables or between risk factors and outcomes. Covariate analysis is used to identify and make adjustments for these systematic differences. An alternate strategy is to select individuals that are closely matched between groups in terms of potentially confounding variables. |
| Level III | Case-control studies; preexisting groups comparisons | Also called a case comparison design. A retrospective study with no investigator manipulation. Preexisting groups of individuals (cases) who achieved an outcome of interest are compared with those who achieved a different outcome by means of data gathered from systematic review of relevant records or from participant interview. Often an attempt is made to match the two groups in terms of member characteristics that could be confounding variables. The goal is to determine the degree to which any variables of interest from the past discriminated between the two outcome groups. |
| Level IV | One-group pre–post studies | A prospective study that looks only at the group receiving the intervention. Selected dependent variables are measured before and after the intervention to establish outcome in terms of degree of change. Participants are often selected via convenience sampling, meaning that they were the most available to recruit for the study and therefore may not be representative of the larger population of interest. |

and subjective and whose primary aim is to gather in-depth, detailed descriptions of a phenomenon of interest (e.g., a problem or condition) from the point of view of the group or individual experiencing it. Inquiry does not stop at the level of describing the problem or condition but seeks to interpret each phenomenon in light of physical, social, economic, regulatory, and cultural contexts as well as personal viewpoints, meanings, and perceptions (Kielhofner, 1982a, 2006; Merrill, 1985; Papadimitriou, Magasi, & Frank, 2012). Quantitative experimental and outcome research approaches cannot adequately capture these interwoven and sometimes elusive complexities for a number of reasons (Kielhofner, 1982a; Merrill, 1985). First, when conducting quantitative research, investigators characteristically test hypotheses based on existing theories. Second, quantitative investigators use standardized methods of data collection and numerical analysis to yield findings on preestablished variables. Third, the quantitative discovery process is linear, proceeding from the definition of a research problem through a sequence of steps and concluding with reporting of findings and often generation of new research questions.

In qualitative approaches, however, the discovery process is cyclical and open ended, driven by the perspectives of the participants and not of the researchers (Cook, 2001). Methodology, concepts, and theory develop gradually as the research progresses and are derived as the accumulated data and interpretations lend structure and focus (Kielhofner, 1982a, 2006; Merrill, 1985). Methods of data collection include in-depth unstructured or semi-structured interviews, focus groups, participant or field observation, and review of pertinent records and other documents (Cook, 2001; Mack, Woodsong, MacQueen, Guest, & Namey, 2005). Data are documented via written notes, photos, audio recordings, and video recordings. The goal of analysis and interpretation is to reduce data to recurring patterns of conceptual categories and themes via a painstaking process of review. As meaning and significance emerge, a model is constructed depicting interrelationships or linkages (Newcomer et al., 2015).

Table 47-4.

## Qualitative Research

| | | |
|---|---|---|
| Level I | Meta-synthesis of related qualitative studies | An interpretive process of identifying, extracting, and integrating the findings of related qualitative studies in order to generate new insights, leading to a "fuller understanding of the phenomenon of interest" (Thorne, Jensen, Kearney, Noblit, & Sandelowski, 2004, p. 1346). |
| Level II | Group qualitative studies with more rigor (a, b, c) | Gathering of in-depth and detailed information pertaining to the phenomenon of interest from multiple individuals, using recognized strategies to enhance trustworthiness including (a) prolonged engagement with participants, (b) triangulation of data from multiple sources, and (c) confirmation of data analysis and reinterpretation by means of peer and member checking. |
| Level III | Group qualitative studies with less rigor (a, b, c) | Gathering of in-depth and detailed information pertaining to the phenomenon of interest from multiple individuals but without using recognized strategies to enhance trustworthiness. |
| Level IV | Qualitative studies with single informant | Gathering of in-depth and detailed information from a single key individual judged to be a knowledgeable source of experiences, meanings, and events connected to the phenomenon of interest. |

The qualitative research hierarchy used by Tomlin and Borgetto (2011) and depicted in Table 47-4 takes into account three important strategies that enhance the quality of evidence and that are consistent with a conceptual model proposed by Guba (1981) and discussed by Krefting (1991), which is addressed in the next section. These strategies are as follows:

- **Prolonged engagement with participants:** Spending adequate time observing, speaking with or interviewing, and developing relationships to fully understand the phenomenon of interest and to allow participants to adjust to the presence of investigators.
- **Triangulation of data from multiple sources:** Verifying and cross-checking information by collecting it from several sources, using more than one research, interpretation, or analysis technique, and cross-referencing.
- **Confirmation of data analysis and reinterpretation by means of peer and member checking:** In member checking, the researcher's data, interpretations, and conclusions are repeatedly tested with informants. Peer examination involves the researcher in discussing the research process, emerging assumptions, interpretations, and problems with experienced impartial colleagues.

Another concept addressed by Tomlin and Borgetto is qualitative meta-synthesis, which has been described as an evolving systematic approach to consolidating the findings of a group of qualitative studies to facilitate knowledge development and contribute to an explanatory theory or model (Pearson, Wiechula, & Lockwood, 2005; Thorne, Jensen, Kearney, Noblit, & Sandelowski, 2004; Walsh & Downe, 2005).

Two types of research bear mentioning that do not fit neatly into either the single hierarchical system for assigning levels of measurement or the multidimensional Tomlin and Borgetto (2011) research pyramid. These are cross-sectional and longitudinal designs. Cross-sectional data are gathered during a single defined time period and are used to provide descriptive information on two or more preexisting groups that have certain immediately identifiable characteristics or dependent variables of interest. Typically, there is no investigator manipulation and the primary objective is to statistically identify differences or similarities between the groups (Kielhofner, 2006). Some studies explore factors that may have influenced outcome in a population of interest (Law et al., 1998) or investigate the properties and usability of a newer measure compared with a more established or "gold standard" instrument (DeVellis, 2012). One benefit of using a cross-sectional design is that it allows researchers to address many different characteristics simultaneously.

In longitudinal research, data are collected on selected characteristics or dependent variables in a population of interest at multiple points in time, possibly over months or years. Data might also be collected on interventions or other aspects of health care received by the population, and groups who did or did not receive this care are compared. As in cross-sectional research, there is no investigator manipulation; the primary objective is to detect numerical patterns of stability and change that develop over time and that allow investigators to make statistical inferences regarding how and why change did or did not take place (Kielhofner, 2006). Some sources use the term *cohort designs* for this type of research (Law et al., 1998).

## Case Study Part 2

The Everyday Matters workshop at the VA Long Beach consisted of three sections, each 2 weeks long with one session per week. Lesson content for each section focused on the themes of (1) how occupation influences health and the importance of participating in life and doing what is meaningful, (2) enhancing occupational performance and participation by setting goals to create stable routines, and (3) occupation as empowerment and advocating for one's self and others as well as partnering with providers to optimize care. The occupational therapy practitioners that facililtated the program worked with veterans to explore their occupational interests and capacities, develop skills to address their health concerns and barriers to engagement, and construct daily routines that were satisfying and that optimized well-being. Review of goals, personal reflection, and discussion of "deeper dive" topics took place weekly and participants received a binder that included lesson overviews, worksheets, and resources.

Standardized measurements were administered prior to and following the workshop to quantitatively assess degree of change in important dependent variables as the result of participation in this intervention, which was the independent variable. These were the Stanford Chronic Disease Self-Efficacy Scale measuring perceived ability to manage one's health conditions (Lorig, Sobel, Ritter, Laurent, & Hobbs, 2001), the WHO Disability Assessment Schedule measuring self-identified difficulties due to health conditions (Garin et al., 2010), and the EuroQol, a non–disease-specific instrument measuring self-rated overall health and health-related quality of life (Obradovic, Lal, & Liedgens, 2013). The EuroQol also provides the means to calculate quality-adjusted life years, which can be used for clinical and economic appraisal (EuroQol, n.d.). Nonstandardized measurement was part of data gathering as well. Using weekly goal review sheets, participants listed their goals for that week, their satisfaction with goal accomplishment, obstacles encountered, and outcome. At the end of the final session, facilitators administrated a survey in which participants rated their satisfaction with the program, content, delivery, and relevance on a visual analogue scale. A series of open-ended questions gathered qualitative information from each participant regarding beneficial changes in daily routine as the result of what was learned, aspects or features of the workshop that were most or least useful, and other comments or suggestions.

In the scholarship of application, the coauthor had many factors to consider when planning research to evaluate the Everyday Matters workshop as a completely new intervention. As a rule, evidence is built incrementally via a series of investigations that roughly follow the levels of evidence progression depicted in Figures 47-2 and 47-3. The decision was made to conduct the research in three phases as an ongoing process of discovery. Phase 1 was an exploratory program evaluation study to gather descriptive information for the purpose of fine-tuning the intervention and delivery process. Standardized and nonstandardized quantitative measures were assessed for their usefulness in detecting change. Qualitative feedback from staff and participants provided helpful insights. After appropriate adjustments were made, the program was officially launched in Phase 2. The research design in this phase was a quasi-experimental one-group pre- and post-outcome study that combined quantitative and qualitative methodologies. Phase 3 research is an experimental controlled clinical trial. This phase is expected to take 5 years or more.

## Understanding Validity

Although determining the nature of a research design and its position on a hierarchy are important for judging the quality of evidence, that is just the beginning. Another important hallmark of quality is research validity, which is a core issue for all scientific inquiry, regardless of design (Kielhofner, 1982a). Research validity serves as an indication of the degree to which research methods and findings are sound in that they reflect actual phenomena in the world and are not distorted by inaccuracies in conceptual or theoretical foundations, design, measurement, or analysis. Other terms for research validity are *rigor* and *trustworthiness*. In traditional usage, rigor refers to close adherence to experimental research methodology; in broader usage, it can be described as embedding of sound principles and practices—agreed upon by the scientific community—into each step of a quantitative or qualitative research process to ensure trustworthiness of results (Kielhofner, 2006).

A well-developed conceptual model put forth by Guba (1981) and Krefting (1991) and summarized in Table 47-5 identifies four key criteria for evaluating research validity or trustworthiness that can be applied to both the quantitative and qualitative perspectives. The terminology used reflects the distinct philosophical, conceptual, and methodological differences of these two perspectives. Yet it should be kept in mind that one approach can be used to complement and corroborate the other and thereby extend the scope of inquiry (Mortenson & Oliffe, 2009).

## Making Evidence-Based Decisions

Knowledge of research designs and an understanding of what constitutes rigorous investigation will enhance any occupational therapy scholarly endeavor. In addition to providing a framework for developing an original study, this knowledge underscores the critical appraisal of published research literature, which is essential for making EBP decisions. A number of sources offer specific detailed

Table 47-5.

## Four Criteria for Evaluating the Trustworthiness of Research From Both the Quantitative and Qualitative Perspectives

| Criterion | Qualitative Research Perspective | Quantitative Research Perspective |
|---|---|---|
| Truth value: The level of confidence in the veracity of research findings that the investigators were able to establish, given the study's design, subjects or informants, and context | Credibility: The degree of accuracy in preserving and representing the holistic situation and participants being studied, as well as in describing and interpreting the experiences of participants in way that is immediately recognizable by these individuals | Internal validity: The extent to which a causal connection can be established between an intervention, or independent variable, and one or more outcomes, or dependent variables; identification and ruling out of factors other than the independent variable that could influence or mask the research findings |
| Applicability: The extent to which the findings of a research study can be applied to other contexts, settings, and groups or generalized to larger populations | Transferability: The level of representativeness of the informants or participants for the particular group being studied, such that other program providers can apply the findings to their context | External validity: The extent to which research findings can be generalized or applied beyond the groups or contexts specific to the study |
| Consistency: The degree to which the research findings are reproducible, given that the study is duplicated with the same participants and setting or context | Dependability: The extent to which the uniqueness or repeatability of a study has been established by means of thorough and exact description of the methods of data gathering, analysis, and interpretation, as well as by use of methods to replicate and confirm the accuracy of this information | Reliability: The extent to which an experimental or outcome study would yield the same result if repeated independently; the extent to which a measurement used in a study would produce the same results with different raters or repeat administration over time |
| Neutrality: The level of freedom from bias, meaning that research findings are not influenced by the personal motivations or perspectives of the investigators but are the sole function of the conditions of the study | Confirmability: The degree of understanding how and why decisions were made in a study, such that another researcher would arrive at comparable conclusions given the same data and research context, established using an external or internal auditing process to review data, findings, interpretations, and recommendations | Objectivity: The extent to which judgments made and data recorded during the research process are based solely on observed phenomena without the influence of personal agendas, emotions, prejudices, assumptions, or predispositions |

Adapted from Guba, E. G. (1981). ERIC/ECTJ annual review paper: Criteria for assessing the trustworthiness of naturalistic inquiries. *Educational Communication and Technology Journal, 29*(2), 75-91; Krefting, L. (1991). Rigor in qualitative research: The assessment of trustworthiness. *American Journal of Occupational Therapy, 45*(3), 214-222; and Wholey, J. S., Hatry, H. P., & Newcomer, K. E. (2010). *Handbook of practical program evaluation* (3rd ed.). San Francisco, CA: John Wiley & Sons.

guidelines for scholarly practice, or EBP; these sources include Kielhofner (2006), Melnyk and Fineout-Overholt (2011), and Taylor (2007). This process begins when a clinical situation or problem is encountered in which not all the needed information is at hand. Then inquiry proceeds as a series of steps (Lin, Murphy, & Robinson, 2010).

An occupational therapy practitioner seeking specific knowledge to guide clinical decision making begins by formulating a clear, sufficiently focused, answerable clinical question. PICO, or PICOT (Melnyk & Fineout-Overholt, 2011), is the acronym for a practical structured approach to framing clinical questions pertinent to the care of a specific client or a category of clients seen routinely. P refers to the person, problem, or population of interest; I to the issue or intervention being considered; C to a comparison such as an alternate intervention or no intervention; O to the outcome that would be affected by the intervention; and T to a time frame. Here are two examples:

1. For adolescents with clinical depression receiving antidepressant medication (P), what is the effect of a group occupational therapy program (I) consisting of biweekly 1-hour sessions over 4 weeks (T) on participation in the community (O) compared with antidepressant medication alone (C)?
2. For elders 65 years of age and older with a history of falls who are living at home (P), does in-home fall prevention education by an occupational therapy practitioner (I) result in lower incidence of falls in the home (O) compared with outpatient clinic-based occupational therapy fall prevention education (C) at 6-month follow-up (T)?

The PICO or PICOT system prompts the occupational therapy practitioner to formulate a clinical question that supports an effective systematic search of the published literature for directly related research evidence, which is the second step in the EBP process. Up-to-date published peer-reviewed studies can be located via Internet sources such as Google Scholar or SpringerLink or the electronic database search system of a college or university library. Electronic databases applicable to occupational therapy practice range from specialized (e.g., OTseeker; Bennett et al., 2003) to broad-based compilations of thousands of journals, including EBSCOhost, CINAHL, Medline/PubMed, and PsychINFO. Collected systematic reviews and meta-analyses are published in the Cochrane Library database. The practitioner typically begins the search for relevant literature by using keywords suggested by the clinical question. However, search terms must sometimes be adapted to the standardized medical vocabulary used by some electronic databases. Fortunately, a number of excellent resources teach the often-arduous process of searching the literature and accessing pertinent research articles (Kielhofner, 2006; Melnyk & Fineout-Overholt, 2011; Taylor, 2007).

Step three is critical appraisal of the evidence. The occupational therapy practitioner carefully assesses the quality and trustworthiness of the research evidence in the published literature that has the most direct bearing on the clinical question. Guiding questions for critically appraising a report of quantitative and of qualitative research are presented in Tables 47-6 and 47-7. These tables are based on appraisal questions developed by the McMaster University Occupational Therapy Evidence-Based Practice Research Group.

After the available evidence has been critically appraised, in step four, the occupational therapy practitioner draws an unbiased conclusion, based on integration of information from the multiple studies, as to how the evidence answered the clinical question. This action, sometimes called formulating the "clinical bottom line" (Kielhofner, 2006, p. 680), is followed by step five in which the practitioner integrates the answer to the clinical question with his or her clinical expertise and considers the values, preferences, and unique situation of the client or client group to make a decision regarding the most suitable intervention (Dijkers et al., 2012). Finally, in step six, the practitioner evaluates the outcome of the clinical decision.

## Quantitative and Qualitative Analysis

Knowledge of methods of data analysis for qualitative and quantitative research is essential for both scholarship and scholarly practice. In the former, it supports selection of appropriate analysis procedures or approaches in original research; in the latter, it provides the basis to critically appraise the analyses used by investigators in a published study. This section provides a general overview of important terminology and concepts. Because of the breadth and complexity of the science of data analysis, occupational therapy practitioners embarking on any scholarly endeavor are encouraged to engage in further study.

Quantitative analysis is based on statistics, which "is a branch of applied mathematics that deals with the collection, description and interpretation of quantitative data" (Kielhofner, 2006, p. 213). For a quick reference, readers are invited to explore the Web Center for Social Research Methods at http://www.socialresearchmethods.net. A good first step in selecting the appropriate statistical methodology is to determine whether the core purpose of analysis is descriptive or inferential. *Descriptive statistics* summarize the basic features of study data and are used in the kinds of descriptive research presented in Table 47-1. If a single variable or group is represented in the data, descriptive statistics can be used to depict the frequency or range of individual values, the central tendency, and the spread of values around the central tendency. Descriptive analysis in which there is more than one group or variable consists of computation of the degree of relationship or association between two sets of values. The statistic that is generated is typically called a *contingency* or *correlation coefficient*.

*Inferential statistics* are used to reach conclusions that extend beyond the study data. In experimental and outcome research depicted in Tables 47-2 and 47-3, investigators use this family of analyses to infer the likelihood that what was observed in the study sample is also true for the larger population from which the sample was taken. A key aspect of inferential statistics is the determination of *significance*, which is derived from the probability that the difference between groups or the change seen as a result of an intervention occurred because of random chance. A significant research finding has a high probability of being true.

The additional piece that must be in place before the appropriate statistic can be selected is determination of the type of scale used in the measurement of variables. *Parametric* statistical operations lend themselves to interval or ratio measurement scales, which are based on real numbers. When the measurement scale is nominal, meaning categorical, or ordinal, requiring rank ordering of categories, *nonparametric* statistics must be used. There are additional requirements for use of parametric statistics based on the pattern of distribution of data points around the mean. Each parametric statistic has at least one corresponding nonparametric statistic. Table 47-8 provides a listing of some parametric and corresponding nonparametric statistical operations for basic quantitative research designs, given the core purpose of the analysis, that readers might encounter in a published study or statistics computer program.

Table 47-6.

**Guiding Questions for Appraising Quantitative Research**

| | |
|---|---|
| Study purpose | Was the purpose of the study or research question(s) stated clearly? How does it apply to occupational therapy and the clinical question guiding my efforts to seek evidence for clinical decision making? |
| Literature review | Was relevant background literature reviewed? How well did it justify the need for the study? Was the justification clear and compelling? |
| Design | What was the study design; was it easy or difficult to ascertain? Was it appropriate for the research question(s)? Did the design admit the possibility of the potential influence of biases (e.g., issues of randomization, control, blinding); if so, what might be the direction of their influence on the results? (These questions help to establish internal validity and objectivity.) |
| Study sample population | Was the population sample used in the study described in detail? If a two-group study, was the similarity between groups established? Did the investigators justify the sample size used? Was informed consent obtained? (These questions help to establish external validity and statistical conclusion validity.) |
| Outcomes | What outcome measures did investigators use? What clinical findings (e.g., physical or physiological, behaviors, personal attributes, internal experiences) were measured? Were the measures reliable; were they valid? What was the frequency of measurement (e.g., pretest, post-test, follow-up)? (These questions help to establish internal validity and reliability.) |
| Intervention | Was the intervention described in detail? Could it be replicated in occupational therapy practice? Were steps taken to maintain intervention fidelity? Was contamination bias (members of control group inadvertently exposed to the intervention) or co-intervention bias (other unaccounted for interventions received by participants during the study) avoided? (These questions help to establish internal validity and reliability.) |
| Data analysis | What were the methods of data analysis used? Were the analysis methods appropriate, given the study design? If there were multiple outcomes, was this taken into account in the statistical analysis? (These questions help to establish statistical conclusion validity.) |
| Results | Did any participants drop out from the study; if so, how many dropped out? Were reasons given and dropouts handled appropriately? Were the research findings reported in terms of statistical significance? If results were not statistically significant, was the size of the study population large enough to show an important difference or change if in truth it did exist? Were the differences between groups clinically meaningful (e.g., effect size calculation)? Was the clinical importance or usefulness of the results reported? (These questions help to establish statistical conclusion validity.) |
| Overall rigor | What is the overall degree of rigor of the study, based on the four components of trustworthiness (e.g., internal validity, external validity, reliability, objectivity) plus statistical conclusion validity? How did the investigators ensure each component of trustworthiness? What meaning and relevance does the study have for my clinical question? |
| Conclusion and clinical implications | What did the investigators conclude? Were the conclusions appropriate given the study methods and results? What were the implications of these results for occupational therapy practice? What were the main limitations and biases in the study? |

Statistical conclusion validity refers to the degree to which the investigator's statistical analysis led to a correct decision about the relationship between the intervention and outcome but not to whether a causal relationship exists between these variables (Wholey, Hatry, & Newcomer, 2010).
Adapted from Law, M., Stewart, D., Pollock, N., Letts, L., Bosch, J., & Westmorland, M. (1998). *Guidelines for critical review form: Quantitative studies*. Retrieved from http://www.srs-mcmaster.ca/Portals/20/pdf/ebp/quanguidelines.pdf and Law, M., Stewart, D., Pollock, N., Letts, L., Bosch, J., & Westmorland, M. (1998). *Critical review form: Quantitative studies*. Retrieved from http://www.srs-mcmaster.ca/Portals/20/pdf/ebp/quanreview.pdf

The inferential statistics in Table 47-8 refer to research designs that have one independent and one dependent variable. More complex designs that have two or more independent or dependent variables call for parametric statistics such as two-way analysis of variance, multivariate analysis of variance, analysis of covariance, and multivariate analysis of covariance.

Investigators might also use parametric predictive statistics such as linear regression. In simplest terms, linear regression is a statistical determination of the strength of the relationship between an independent, or predictor, variable and a dependent variable that is being predicted. This means that, given a value of the independent variable, a corresponding value of the dependent variable can be calculated. Regression statistics can determine whether the relationship between the independent and dependent variable is significant and the degree to which one or more predictor variables contribute to change in the dependent variable. An advantage of regression analysis for outcome research is its ease of application with naturally occurring variables, as contrasted with experimentally manipulated variables.

Table 47-7.

## Guidelines for Appraising Qualitative Research

| | |
|---|---|
| Study purpose | Was the purpose of the study or research question(s) stated clearly? How does it apply to occupational therapy and the clinical question guiding my efforts to seek evidence for clinical decision making? |
| Literature | Was relevant background literature reviewed? How well did it justify the need for the study? Was the justification clear and compelling? |
| Study design | What was the basis of the study design (e.g., phenomenology: understanding of a lived experience, ethnography: understanding of a culture, grounded theory: theory construction, participatory action research: knowledge leading to social change); was it easy or difficult to ascertain? Was it appropriate for the research question(s)? Was a theoretical or philosophical perspective related to the phenomenon of interest identified? |
| Methods used | What methods of data collection were used to answer the research question(s) (e.g., in-depth unstructured or semistructured interviews, focus groups, participant or field observation, review of pertinent records and other documents)? Are the methods congruent with the philosophical underpinnings and purpose of the study? |
| Sampling | Was the process of purposive selection of study participants described? Did this sampling maximize the range of information uncovered? Were the sampling methods appropriate to the research purpose and question(s)? Did sampling proceed until redundancy in data was reached? (These questions help to establish credibility and transferability.) Was informed consent obtained? |
| Descriptive clarity | Was there a clear and complete (i.e., "thick" or "dense") description of the study context, site or setting and the participants? Was the description sufficient to impart a sense of personally experiencing the phenomenon being studied? (These questions help to establish transferability.) Was the role of the researcher and his or her relationship with participants explained? Were the assumptions and biases of the researcher identified (e.g., reflexivity via a daily introspective journal)? (These questions help to establish credibility and confirmability.) What information was missing, and how does that influence my understanding of the research? |
| Data collection | Did the researchers provide an adequate "dense" description of data collection procedures (e.g., gaining access to the site, field notes, training of data gatherers)? What flexibility was there in the design and data collection methods? Was there prolonged engagement at the site to allow full understanding of the phenomenon of interest? Were data gathered from multiple sources (e.g., different investigators and methods, documents, video or audio recordings)? (These questions help to establish credibility and dependability.) |
| Data analyses | What were the methods of data analysis used; were the methods appropriate? Did the researchers describe how the findings (e.g., codes, categories, and themes) emerged from the data? Did data analysis include verification and cross checking (i.e., triangulation) of data from multiple sources? Were the researcher's data, interpretations, and conclusions repeatedly tested with informants (i.e., member checking)? Did the investigator(s) discuss the research process, emerging assumptions, interpretations, and problems with experienced impartial colleagues (i.e., peer examination)? (These questions help to establish credibility, dependability, and confirmability.) What were the major findings of the analyses? Were findings logically consistent with and reflective of the data? |
| Auditability | Was the process of analyzing the data sufficiently described, such that an audit could certify that there are data to support every interpretation and that interpretations are consistent with the available data? Did the investigators provide a decision trail (e.g., for any changes in design or data collection methods or for transformation of data into codes, themes, and interrelationships)? What rationale was given for the development of themes? (These questions help to establish dependability and confirmability.) |
| Theoretical connections | Did a meaningful picture of the phenomenon under study emerge? How were concepts under study clarified and refined and relationships made clear? What conceptual frameworks emerged? |
| Overall rigor | What is the overall degree of rigor of the study, based on the four components of trustworthiness (e.g., credibility, transferability, dependability, confirmability)? How did the investigators ensure each component of trustworthiness? What meaning and relevance does the study have for my clinical question? |
| Conclusions and implications | What did the investigators conclude? What were the implications of findings for occupational therapy practice and research? What are the main limitations of the study? Were the conclusions appropriate given the study findings; were they meaningful to me? Did the findings contribute to theory development and future occupational therapy practice and research? |

Adapted from Guba, E. G. (1981). ERIC/ECTJ annual review paper: Criteria for assessing the trustworthiness of naturalistic inquiries. *Educational Communication and Technology Journal, 29*(2), 75-91; Krefting, L. (1991). Rigor in qualitative research: The assessment of trustworthiness. *American Journal of Occupational Therapy, 45*(3), 214-222; Letts, L., Wilkins, S., Law, M., Stewart, D., Bosch, J., & Westmorland, M. (2007). *Guidelines for critical review form: Qualitative studies.* Retrieved from http://www.srs-mcmaster.ca/Portals/20/pdf/ebp/qualguidelines_version2.0.pdf; and Letts, L., Wilkins, S., Law, M., Stewart, D., Bosch, J., & Westmorland, M. (2007). *Critical review form: Qualitative studies.* Retrieved from http://www.srs-mcmaster.ca/Portals/20/pdf/ebp/qualreview_version2.0.pdf

Table 47-8.

## Overview of Some Appropriate Parametric and Nonparametric Statistical Operations Given the Core Purpose of the Analysis

| Core Purpose | Parametric | Nonparametric |
|---|---|---|
| Descriptive: Single group or variable | Mean, percentage, standard deviation | Mode, median, range |
| Descriptive: Association between two groups or variables | Pearson's r correlation coefficient | Pearson's contingency coefficient Phi squared;<br>Cramer's V<br>Goodman and Kruskal's tau<br>Lambda<br>Spearman Rho<br>Kendall coefficient of concordance<br>Kendall's Tau; Stuart's T<br>Gamma coefficient<br>Somers' D |
| Inferential: Experimental and outcomes research<br>Single sample | t or Z test | Binomial test or chi-square |
| Two independent samples | t-test for independent samples<br>One way between groups<br>ANOVA | Chi-square<br>Wald-Wolfwitz runs test<br>Man-Whitney U test<br>Kolmogorov-Smirnov two-sample test |
| Two dependent samples | t-test for dependent samples<br>One-way repeated measures<br>ANOVA | McNemar chi-square<br>Wilcoxon matched-pairs signed-ranks test |
| More than two independent samples | One-way or two-way between groups<br>ANOVA | Chi-square test for k independent samples<br>Kruskal-Wallis one-way analysis of variance |
| More than two dependent samples | One-way or two-way repeated measures<br>ANOVA repeat measures<br>Binomial test or chi-square | Friedman two-way analysis of variance<br>Cochran's Q test |

ANOVA = analysis of variance.
Adapted from Kielhofner, G. (2006). *Research in occupational therapy: Methods of inquiry for enhancing practice.* Philadelphia, PA: F. A. Davis Company and Siegel, S., & Castellan, N. J., Jr. (1988). *Nonparametric statistics for the behavioral sciences.* New York, NY: McGraw-Hill.

In multiple regression there is more than one predictor variable, and in logistic regression, the dependent variable is dichotomous (e.g., example success or failure; Kielhofner, 2006; Newcomer et al., 2015).

An occupational therapy practitioner who is analyzing data from original qualitative research, depicted in Table 47-4, does not use statistical methods but rather might be characterized as playing the role of detective. With the purpose of the research in mind, disciplined examination and creative insight are applied to discover patterns that reveal meaning and significance. Qualitative data analysis and interpretation might be conceived of as separate but interrelated processes. During analysis, the researcher's goals are to bring order to the data and reduce it to manageable components by identifying recurring categories (Bernard & Ryan, 2010; Newcomer et al., 2015). Categories are themes that make sense in the context of the study. A theme that emerges with high frequency in the data is often called a *core category.* Categories that surface are assigned codes, which are essentially labels. By working back and forth between the emerging coded categories and the raw data, the individual conducting the analysis refines the coding system until it appears to contain the existing data. When no new categories are appreciable, it is said that the analysis has reached *saturation.*

In the interpretive process, meaning and significance are attached to the categories, and a model is constructed depicting the interrelationships or linkages between or among them (Bernard & Ryan, 2010). During data collection and data analysis, investigators may write memos consisting of thoughts about an observational theme or category and its relationship to other categories or to the research questions. These thoughts can take the form of preliminary hypotheses, questions, or inferences. Memos are often written in the margins of an interview transcript or a field journal. In published literature, the model might be depicted diagrammatically. Categories can also be described numerically in terms of frequency or proportion of occurrence. It can be seen that analysis of qualitative data requires skill and persistence, yet it allows the occupational therapy practitioner to gain understanding beyond numbers and statistical significance.

# The Process of Scholarly Proposal

Well-known occasions when an occupational therapy practitioner is called upon to write a scholarly proposal are the application for a research grant and completion of the requirements for a graduate degree. However, there is good reason to prepare a detailed proposal for any scholarly project, in particular one aimed at evaluating the effectiveness or efficacy of a program or intervention. The process of writing a scholarly proposal prompts the occupational therapy practitioner to think through the project to explore options and anticipate any difficulties that could arise and thus avoid common pitfalls that would impede successful execution of the research or lessen the trustworthiness of the findings and conclusions (Locke, Spirduso, & Silverman, 2007; Newcomer et al., 2015). "To put it bluntly, one's research is only as good as one's proposal" (Wong, 2005, p. 1).

A scholarly proposal can serve as a mode of communication, a plan of action, and a contract or bond of agreement (Locke et al., 2007). Although the audience may be a panel of experts on a grant review board or faculty members on a thesis or dissertation committee, it can also be composed of stakeholders in the community or practice setting. The primary objective is to convince the audience that the research idea is important, that it is based on a clear grasp of relevant literature and issues, that the methodology is sound, and that the author of the proposal has a well-thought-out plan of action for the project—ideally, within a realistic time frame and incurring reasonable expenses—and sufficient competence to complete it. To achieve this objective, the process of scholarly proposal should effectively convey why the occupational therapy practitioner desires to embark upon the study, what he or she plans to accomplish, and how he or she plans to proceed.

# Case Study Part 3

Because integrating occupational therapy into the primary care team was considered highly innovative at the VA Long Beach, it was imperative to begin developing the scholarly proposal at the outset of the scholarship of application project as a collaborative effort. Representatives of the key stakeholder groups, including primary care providers, administrators, veterans, and occupational therapy practitioners, participated in this effort. Project objectives, as well as long- and short-term goals, were outlined for each group. The agreed overall objectives that supported integration of occupational therapy into primary care were to (1) establish a collaborative relationship with Patient Aligned Care Team providers and define a role for occupational therapy in primary care, (2) highlight best practices in occupational therapy health promotion and prevention and the potential value of occupation-based interventions, and (3) implement occupational therapy services in primary care at the VA Long Beach and nationwide.

Given the objectives identified via collaboration, the first priority was to develop a shared vision with primary care leadership. This entailed recognizing the potential role for occupational therapy practitioner in the primary care teams, establishing a commitment to move forward with the project, and agreeing on a plan of action. This was achieved through use of a formal scholarly proposal or project plan document, which served as both a communication method and an approval mechanism. Once primary care leadership approved the project, the next priority was to identify existing knowledge gaps among primary care providers concerning the scope and practice of occupational therapy and then develop profile- and awareness-raising activities to address those gaps as part of the overall plan. Thus, including primary care providers in the initial development phase of the project was key, as they learned about the vital role of occupational therapy in primary care and about the innovative ways occupational therapy and primary care could partner to optimize function and quality of life for at-risk veteran populations.

Each funding agency or university has its own set of guidelines for submissions, and there are no generally agreed upon rules that dictate the content or order of a scholarly proposal. However, the audience members will universally look for a writing style characterized by precision, simplicity, and clarity as well as the accomplishment of specific communication tasks. "In the mass of detail that goes into the planning of a research study, the writer must not forget that the proposal's most immediate function is to inform readers quickly and accurately" (Locke et al., 2007, p. 6). Fundamental communication tasks that address key elements of the research process and provide any essential information that the writer's audience needs to evaluate the proposed study are presented below (Locke et al., 2007; Wong, 2005).

- **Introduction of the study:** Meticulously prepared opening paragraphs are designed to capture the interest of the readers of the document and lay the foundation for the more detailed discussion that follows. Here the writer familiarizes the readers with the problem or area of concern that prompted the investigation (e.g., the recognition of a gap, deficiency, or need in the field of inquiry), touches upon the theoretical or practical significance of the problem, and sketches the core constructs that will be represented.
- **Statement of purpose:** A declaration, made early in the proposal, of why the writer wishes to embark upon the study and what he or she intends to achieve.
- **Rationale:** Justification of the importance and significance of the proposed study by explaining the potential practical and theoretical effect of findings. In stating his or her case, the writer might bring in applicable facts, use logical reasoning, and provide a diagram of factors and relationships evident in the problem. The aim is to persuade the readers of the proposal that the investigator has sufficiently and correctly defined the problem and that the planned research is unique and worth doing, such that completion of the study will lead to a better understanding of the problem and to opening of new possibilities for a constructive course of action and further investigation.
- **Research questions or hypotheses:** Logical and concise statements that are linked to the purpose of investigation and that identify the specific direction of inquiry; they provide the foundation of the scholarly proposal and identify the independent and dependent variables or the phenomenon of interest. Research questions are most appropriate when the study tends to be exploratory in nature or uses qualitative methodology; they should be foreshadowed by prior studies or theoretical work. In study hypotheses, testable predictions are made about the relationship between two variables (e.g., an intervention and outcome) based on established knowledge and theory. A well-stated research question can lead directly into a study hypothesis. Typically, elements of a scholarly proposal appear in the published study after it is completed. Table 47-9 shows examples of the stated purpose and related research questions or hypotheses in four studies. All were published in the *American Journal of Occupational Therapy* and represent each of the four types of research discussed in this chapter.
- **Delimitations and limitations:** Statements of defined limits in the context of the scholarly proposal. Delimitations refer to factors related to use of constructs or the planned study population that would affect generalizability of findings. Factors in a study that cannot be controlled (e.g., because of feasibility or ethics) may lead to limitations that constrain the conclusions.
- **Definitions:** Clarification of any terms or language specific to the field of research addressed in the scholarly proposal
- **Background of the problem:** Review of relevant research literature and other influential papers such that "the author inserts the proposed study into a line of inquiry and a developing body of knowledge" (Locke et al., 2007, p. 17) and shows how each published source is relevant and contributes to the planned investigation. It is important to demonstrate that the conceptual and theoretical bases and research questions or hypotheses in the proposed study arise from existing knowledge and move inquiry from the answered to the unanswered questions. Discussion might also include critical analysis of methodologies used previously in the area of inquiry as a basis for the selection of procedures for the current study.
- **Explanation of methods:** Precise description, using concrete details, of the research design, study setting and environment, selection and recruiting of participants, and the nature of quantitative tests and measurements, as well as qualitative approaches used to collect data, intervention procedure(s), analytical techniques, and time frame. If financial information is called for, the budget might include such costs as staff and consultants, supplies and equipment, use of recording media, and travel. Information on the planned methodology should be sufficient for the audience to determine its overall degree of rigor.
- **Biographical sketch of the investigator(s):** An overview of the academic, clinical, and research training and experience of the investigators relevant to the area of proposed research

It is important for the occupational therapy practitioner to think of the scholarly proposal as a work in progress. Maintaining openness to new insights and questions that may arise and readiness to modify the project to accommodate this information are often called for. "It is flexibility, not rigidity, that makes strong proposal documents" (Locke et al., 2007, p. 7).

Table 47-9.

## Examples of the Stated Purpose and Related Research Questions or Hypotheses From Four Published Studies Representing Each of the Four Types of Research Discussed in This Chapter

| Source | Type of Research | Purpose of the Study | Related Research Questions or Hypotheses |
|---|---|---|---|
| Duncan-Myers & Huebner, 2000 | Descriptive or associative | "[T]o investigate the relationship between quality of life and personal control as measured by opportunities for choice in self-care and leisure activities among residents of long term care facilities" (p. 505), using two self-report instruments, the Quality of Life Rating and the Duncan Choice Index. | Research questions: "1. What is the relationship between the residents' perceptions of the number of choices available in daily life and how they rate quality of life? 2. What level of quality of life do residents perceive? 3. In which daily tasks do residents have choices in and desire more choice?" (p. 505). |
| Hayner, Gibson, & Gordon, 2010 | Experimental | "[T]o contribute to the understanding of constraint-induced movement therapy (CIMT) by comparing two treatments for chronic UE dysfunction in people in the post-CVA period [namely] (1) a modification of the standard CIMT protocol and (2) bilateral treatment provided with intensity equal to the CIMT condition"(p. 530). | Hypotheses: "1. All participants will demonstrate improved total Wolf Motor Function Test (WMFT) scores after [completion of both interventions]. 2. Participants in the CIMT group will demonstrate greater improvement in total WMFT scores than participants in the bilateral group after treatment of comparable intensity, frequency, duration, and activity selection" (p. 530). |
| Dankert, Davies, & Gavin, 2003 | Outcome | "[T]o evaluate the assumption that occupational therapy provided to preschool children with developmental delays and preschool children without disabilities will significantly improve their visual-motor skills" (p. 544), as measured by the Developmental Test of Visual-Motor Integration. | Research questions: "1. Do preschool children with developmental delays demonstrate significant improvements in visual-motor skills . . . following occupational therapy for 1 school year when compared to their performance . . . prior to therapy? 2. Will preschool children with developmental delays exhibit a rate of gain consistent with typical peers . . . ?" (p. 544). |
| Lyons, Orozovic, Davis, & Newman, 2002 | Qualitative | To study the "occupational nature of a group of persons with life-threatening illnesses, couched within the group's experiences as day hospice program participants, [framed around] a doing-being-becoming conceptualization of occupation [in order to] breathe new life into the profession's occupational gaze" (pp. 293-294). | Research question (phenomenon of interest): "Within an interpretive framework of doing-being-becoming . . . [w]hat are the occupational experiences of the men and women with life-threatening illnesses attending a day hospice program?" (p. 287). |

## Dissemination and Writing a Scholarly Report

After a scholarly project is completed and found to generate new knowledge, the next logical step is dissemination, defined by the National Institutes of Health as "the targeted distribution of information and intervention materials to a specific public health or clinical practice audience. The intent is to spread knowledge and the associated evidence-based interventions" (2007, para. 5). This is in keeping with the stated priorities of the AOTA, which include dissemination of occupational therapy outcomes and evidence. The traditional paths for dissemination are publishing in peer-reviewed journals and presentation at academic or professional conferences. Other dissemination activities can include briefings to stakeholders and educational sessions conducted with clients, colleagues, or policymakers. In addition, there are emerging vehicles for dissemination as promotion, including media coverage, fact sheets, flyers and brochures, web based text and video publications, and social media outlets (Community Alliance for Research and Engagement, 2010; Jacobs, 2012).

However, the gap between new knowledge generated from research findings and its implementation in practice, which was discussed earlier in this chapter, continue to be ongoing concerns in medicine, public health, and rehabilitation, as well as in occupational therapy (Burke & Gitlin, 2012; Cramm, White, & Krupa, 2013; National Center for the Dissemination of Disability Research, 2005). As an outgrowth of this concern, the model of knowledge translation arose as a means to reduce the gap (Backus & Jones, 2013; Bowen & Graham, 2013). Straus, Tetroe, and Graham (as cited by Cramm et al., 2013) define knowledge translation as "a dynamic and iterative process that includes the synthesis, dissemination, exchange and ethically sound application of knowledge to improve health, provide more effective health services and products and strengthen the health care system" (p. 119). This paradigm shift represents movement away from regarding knowledge generated from research as a product to instead seeing it as the result of collaboration between those who conduct the research and those who use the findings.

Dissemination is recognized to be a key element in knowledge translation but is more broadly defined as "a planned process that involves consideration of target audiences and the settings in which research findings are to be received and, where appropriate, communicating and interacting with wider policy and health service audiences in ways that will facilitate research uptake in decision-making processes and practice" (Wilson, Petticrew, Calnan, & Nazareth, 2010, p. 1). It thus behooves the occupational therapy practitioner seeking to disseminate knowledge gained from his or her scholarly project, whether via presentation or publication, to move beyond the assumption that simply informing colleagues about the new knowledge and its benefits will lead to implementation. Rather, inducing colleagues to implement the scholar's evidence-based findings requires communication based on an understanding of what constrains or expedites change in that area of practice. Factors to consider are the health system players in the area of practice (e.g., legislators, regulators, administrators, practitioners, professional organizations, clients, family members), the players' values and beliefs, the culture and climate of practice, and the ways in which new information flows through the system (Burke & Gitlin, 2012).

## Case Study Part 4

The dissemination plan for Everyday Matters at the VA Long Beach was organized according to long- and short-term goals and target audiences. Once the offical launch of the program was well underway and preliminary quantitative and qualitative data were gathered and analyzed, findings were expeditiously disseminated to primary care providers. Personal contact served as the main interaction method, occurring most frequently during informal conversations and planned meetings, as well as through email and the facility instant messaging service. Dissemination activities targeting the VA Long Beach occupational therapy practitioners were provided on an ongoing basis using person-to-person contact as well as electronic and printed materials. The VA Everyday Matters Program and Facilitators Guide was made available via electronic download to occupational therapy practitioners throughout the VA and included key themes from the qualitative data analysis. A VA national Occupational Therapy Monthly Education webinar featuring the VA Long Beach primary care occupational therapy program was attended by 93 occupational therapists and led to an interest in developing a mentorship group to discuss strategies for integration with primary care in other facilities. Poster sessions depicting primary care occupational therapy and the Everyday Matters program to non-VA occupational therapy practitioners were offered at the 2015 and 2016 AOTA conferences.

To increase consumer awareness and create more demand for occupational therapy services, promotional occupational therapy educational activities were offered to benefit veterans with disabilities and chronic health issues. For example, quarterly tabling events were held in primary care, pharmacy waiting areas, and the cafeteria corridor that focused on key topics of interest such as fall prevention and household safety, stress management, low vision, and "occupational therapy life hacks," namely tricks, shortcuts, and new methods that allow a person to more fully participate in meaningful activities. A monthly occupational therapy health promotion quick tip sheet was developed for primary care providers and veterans. Key themes included both work-related and daily living techniques such as alternating between standing and sitting, workstation tips, backpack awareness, mindfulness and stress management strategies, and role balance guidance. Making these tips available organization-wide helped others begin to recognize how occupational therapy can contribute to the health of populations in addition to that of individuals. Community participation helped to shape the identity of occupational therapy as part of primary care as well. Occupational therapy staff took part in annual primary care fairs and other events including the annual Patient Centered-Care Fair and the bi-weekly noontime Health Walk.

This spectrum of creative activities increased organizational and community awareness and disseminated information on the Everyday Matters program to a broad audience both within the VA and beyond. Upon completion of Phase 3 of the scholarship of application research plan, a scholarly report published in a peer-reviewed journal will have the greatest affect on contributing to the occupational therapy body of knowledge.

The most familiar means for an occupational therapy practitioner to disseminate his or her research findings is the full scholarly report, which is a complete description of the study. This format is suitable for presenting the research at an academic conference or submitting a manuscript to a peer-reviewed journal. Practitioners are generally asked to adhere to specific submission guidelines, often based on the current *Publication Manual of the American Psychological Association*. As a rule, a report of this kind begins with a descriptive title and abstract followed by introductory paragraphs and sections presenting methods, results, and discussion (Rudner & Shafer, 1999).

The ideal title of the full scholarly report piques the reader's interest and concisely communicates the essential features of the investigation, for example, by stating the nature and relationship of the targeted intervention and outcome(s). The abstract reproduces the study in about 300 words and usually covers the research question or purpose, design, methods or procedures, participants, measures, findings, and conclusions. A well-crafted scholarly proposal can provide the basis for the introduction and methods sections, with adjustments made to reflect what was actually done in the study. Typically included in the introduction are a description of the nature of problem that led to the investigation; the definition of key terms; a statement of the importance of the study; and review of relevant literature, leading to the research purpose and questions or study hypotheses. The methods section provides a detailed description of the research design, participants, measures, and procedures. Data analysis techniques and results, as well as any problems encountered during analysis, comprise the results section. In the discussion section, the scholar might highlight key results, discuss the limitations of the study, interpret the findings in light of the research questions or hypotheses, draw conclusions regarding implications of the findings, make recommendations, and suggest questions for future research.

Six other formats for reporting the results of a scholarly project, which are listed below, were described by Newcomer et al. (2015). Each has applications for either presentation or publication:

1. **The Mom Test summary:** A statement that effectively conveys the main message of the study. It can be a challenge for a scholar to boil down an entire research project to its essence, but it is that kernel that will attract the attention of the audience members and hold their interest. This short summary works well as a verbal introduction to the study and can also serve as the uniting theme for longer reports.
2. **The compelling paragraph:** A concrete and concise overview of the major research findings and their implications for practice, with highlights of the methodology that was used. A report of this kind can be the basis of a news release, a stand-alone summary that appears on the Internet or in a professional organization's newsletter, an introductory letter or memo sent to a stakeholder with an invitation to read the longer report, or a short oral presentation at a meeting.
3. **The outline:** A set of phrases or sentences that depicts the key topics for the scholarly report and their relative order and importance. The act of composing an outline helps the scholar to set priorities and refine the logical flow of ideas. In a verbal report, the outline can be converted into a slide show and handouts, which provide visual reinforcement for the audience members and help them to focus on the presentation and remember what was said. The outline functions as the backbone of a comprehensive written report and helps to eliminate potential areas of weakness or lack of focus. It can be used on its own to accompany briefings or to create a table of contents.
4. **The two-page executive summary:** A document directed to decision makers or busy higher level stakeholders that highlights the most relevant information while requiring a minimal time commitment to review. Plain language makes it understandable by all readers regardless of their knowledge level or expertise. An executive summary concentrates on findings, implications for practice, and recommendations, with no more than a paragraph devoted to description of the methodology. When used as a means for persuasion, it becomes a call to action that states outcomes and benefits, substantiates benefits using the data, applies the benefits to the reader's particular context, and recommends a solution.
5. **The 10-page report:** A fleshed-out version of the executive summary with added context, supporting facts, and explanation. This format is ideal for Internet publication.
6. **The technical report:** A document aimed at specialists, such as academicians or policy analysts, who need or desire to know the technical details of the methodology, data collection, and data analysis used in the investigation. An important application of the technical report is for research collaboration.

Some additional guiding principles can enhance the affect of a scholarly report directed to consumers, decision makers, or stakeholders (Newcomer et al., 2015). Keep in mind the message, the audience, and the medium. Focus is essential to maintain the interest and attention of the audience; even in a comprehensive report, a good deal of information usually must be omitted. Avoid overly long sentences and paragraphs, technical jargon, and abbreviations and write in the "active voice," wherein the subject appears near the beginning of a sentence and is followed by the verb. Finally, follow the rules of effective document layout and graphic design.

## Evidence-Based Research Chart

| Topic | Evidence |
|---|---|
| AOTA's *Code of Ethics*, which underscore the need for occupational therapy scholarship | AOTA, 2015 |
| AOTA position paper on scholarship | AOTA, 2009 |
| Models for depicting levels of evidence | AOTA, n.d.; Tomlin & Borgetto, 2011 |
| Quantitative research | Kielhofner, 2006; Melnyk & Fineout-Overholt, 2011 |
| Qualitative research | Bernard & Ryan, 2010; Cook, 2001; Mack, Woodsong, MacQueen, Guest, & Namey, 2005 |
| Conducting evidence-based practice | Law & MacDermid, 2008; Taylor, 2007 |
| Writing a scholarly proposal | Locke, Spirduso, & Silverman, 2007 |

Keep the presentation clean and uncluttered; use font styles and sizes that look professional and that are easy to read; use clearly-labeled graphs, tables, and pictures that add relevant information; include judicious use of color where allowed; and be certain that main points are easy to discern. Whether composing a full scholarly report, giving presentations to key audiences, or publishing in peer-reviewed journals, conscientious dissemination of findings from scholarly activities is a critical aspect of translating scholarship to clinical practice.

## Summary

Scholarship and scholarly practice are essential for the professional growth of any occupational therapy practitioner, as well as for developing the knowledge base of the discipline of occupational therapy. Understanding of the types of quantitative and qualitative research designs and their suitable applications, as well as of determinants of level of evidence for each and what constitutes rigorous investigation, is needed to support both research and EBP. Finding the evidence needed for clinical decision making entails following a series of steps from formulating a question to integrating the results of a focused literature search into practice. When an occupational therapy practitioner embarks on a research project, writing a scholarly proposal provides the means to think through the project and make any refinements; after the study is completed, there are a number of vehicles and formats available for dissemination of findings. In any occupational therapy scholarly endeavor, collaboration is a key to narrowing the gap between the new knowledge gained from research and its implementation in everyday practice settings.

## Student Self-Assessment

1. Think of a real-life practice situation that has given rise to a question. For example, it could be a recent clinical event (positive or negative) where you would like to better understand why or how this circumstance occurred. It could also be an assessment or intervention method that you use routinely in your practice for which you would like to have supporting evidence.
2. Develop a clinical question that can be used to gather evidence about the practice situation that you have identified. Compose the question using the PICO or PICOT format. For questions that relate to an assessment or that are exploratory, the "C" or comparison aspect of the question might not be indicated.
3. Consider how you might approach searching for evidence to answer the clinical question that you have decided upon. Options to consider include electronic databases, Internet sources, "brick and mortar" libraries, and contact with colleagues. Decide on the keywords you will use in your search.
4. Locate a research article relevant to your clinical question in a peer-reviewed journal. Determine whether the type of study is quantitative or qualitative. Read the article carefully to discover the following information, as appropriate to the type of study: the purpose of investigation and research questions or hypotheses, the nature of the study participants, the research design, the independent and dependent variables, how the dependent variables were measured, the methods that were used to administer the intervention and gather the data, and the authors' findings.

5. Based on your review of the article, come to a conclusion regarding the trustworthiness of the research findings and their implications for your original clinical question.

## References


Agency for Healthcare Research and Quality. (2000) *Outcomes research. Fact sheet*. Retrieved from http://archive.ahrq.gov/research/findings/factsheets/outcomes/outfact/outcomes-and-research.html

American Occupational Therapy Association. (n.d.). *Guidelines to critically appraised paper (CAP) worksheet evidence exchange*. Retrieved from https://www.aota.org/-/media/Corporate/Files/Practice/EvidenceExchange/CAP%20Guidelines%20for%20Evidence%20Exchange.pdf

American Occupational Therapy Association. (2009). Scholarship in occupational therapy. *American Journal of Occupational Therapy 63*(6), 790-796.

American Occupational Therapy Association. (2015). *Occupational therapy code of ethics (2015)*. Retrieved from https://www.aota.org/-/media/Corporate/Files/Practice/Ethics/Code-of-Ethics.pdf

Arbesman, M., & Mosley, L. J. (2012). Systematic review of occupation- and activity-based health management and maintenance interventions for community-dwelling older adults. *American Journal of Occupational Therapy, 66*(3), 277–283. doi:10.5014/ajot.2012.003327

Backus, D., & Jones, M. L. (2013). Maximizing research evidence to enhance knowledge translation. *Archives of Physical Medicine and Rehabilitation, 94*(1 Suppl.), S1-S2.

Bennett, S., Hoffman, T., McCluskey, A., McKenna, K., Strong, J., & Tooth, L. (2003). Introducing OTseeker (Occupational Therapy Systematic Evaluation of Evidence): A new evidence database for occupational therapists. *American Journal of Occupational Therapy, 57*(6), 635-638.

Bernard, H. R., & Ryan, G. W. (2010). *Analyzing qualitative data: Systematic approaches*. Thousand Oaks, CA: Sage Publications.

Bowen, S. J., & Graham, I. D. (2013). From knowledge translation to engaged scholarship: Promoting research relevance and utilization. *Archives of Physical Medicine and Rehabilitation, 94*(1 Suppl.), S3-S8.

Braveman, B. H., Helfrich, C. A., & Fisher, G. S. (2002). Developing and maintaining community partnerships within "A Scholarship of Practice." *Occupational Therapy in Health Care, 15*(1-2), 109-125.

Burke, J. P., & Gitlin, L. N. (2012). How do we change practice when we have the evidence? *American Journal of Occupational Therapy, 66*(5), e85-e88.

Christiansen, C., & Lou, J. Q. (2001). Ethical considerations related to evidence-based practice. *American Journal of Occupational Therapy, 55*(3), 345-349.

Clark, F., Jackson, J., Carlson, M., Chou, C.-P., Cherry, B. J., Jordan-Marsh, M., ... Azen, S. P. (2012). Effectiveness of a lifestyle intervention in promoting the well-being of independently living older people: Results of the Well Elderly 2 Randomised Controlled Trial. *Journal of Epidemiology and Community Health, 66*(9), 782-790. doi:10.1136/jech.2009.099754

Community Alliance for Research and Engagement. (2010). Beyond scientific publication: Strategies for disseminating research findings. *Yale Center for Clinical Investigation*. Retrieved from https://depts.washington.edu/ccph/pdf_files/CARE_Dissemination_Strategies_FINAL_eversion.pdf

Cook, J. V. (2001). *Qualitative research in occupational therapy: Strategies and experiences*. San Diego, CA: Singular Publishing.

Cooper, H., Hedges, L. V., & Valentine, J. C. (2009). *The handbook of research synthesis and meta-analysis* (2nd ed.). New York, NY: Russell Sage Foundation.

Cramm, H., White, C., & Krupa, T. (2013). From periphery to player: Strategically positioning occupational therapy within the knowledge translation landscape. *American Journal of Occupational Therapy, 67*(1), 119-125.

Dankert, H. L., Davies, P. L., & Gavin, W. J. (2003). Occupational therapy effects on visual-motor skills in preschool children. *American Journal of Occupational Therapy, 57*(5), 542-449.

Darkins, A., Kendall, S., Edmonson, E., Young, M., & Stressel, P. (2014). Reduced cost and mortality using home telehealth to promote self-management of complex chronic conditions: A retrospective matched cohort study of 4,999 veteran patients. *Telemedicine Journal and E-Health*. doi:10.1089/tmj.2014.0067

DeVellis, R. F. (2012). *Scale development: Theory and applications* (3rd ed.). Los Angeles, CA: Sage Publications.

Dijkers, M. P., Murphy, S. L., & Krellman, J. (2012). Evidence-based practice for rehabilitation professionals: Concepts and controversies. *Archives of Physical Medicine and Rehabilitation, 93*(8 Suppl.), S164-S176.

Dubouloz, C., Egan, M., Vallerand, J., & von Zweck, C. (1999). Occupational therapists' perceptions of evidence-based practice. *American Journal of Occupational Therapy, 53*(5), 445-453.

Duncan-Myers, A. M., & Huebner, R. A. (2000). Relationship between choice and quality of life among residents in long-term-care facilities. *American Journal of Occupational Therapy, 54*(5), 504-508.

EuroQol (n.d.). *EQ-5D-5L value sets*. Retrieved from http://www.euroqol.org/about-eq-5d/valuation-of-eq-5d/eq-5d-5l-value-sets.html

Garin, O., Ayuso-Mateos, J. L., Almansa, J., Nieto, M., Chatterji, S., Vilagut, G., ... MHADIE Consortium. (2010). Validation of the "World Health Organization Disability Assessment Schedule, WHODAS-2" in patients with chronic diseases. *Health and Quality of Life Outcomes, 8*, 51. doi:10.1186/1477-7525-8-51

Guba, E. G. (1981). ERIC/ECTJ annual review paper: Criteria for assessing the trustworthiness of naturalistic inquiries. *Educational Communication and Technology Journal, 29*(2), 75-91.

Haertlein, C., & Coppard, B. M. (2003). Scholarship and occupational therapy (2003 concept paper). *American Journal of Occupational Therapy, 57*(6), 641-643.

Hammel, J., Finlayson, M., Kielhofner, G., Helfrish, C., & Peterson, E. (2002). Educating scholars of practice: An approach to preparing tomorrow's researchers. *Occupational Therapy in Health Care, 15*(1-2), 157-176.

Hayner, K., Gibson, G., & Gordon, M. G. (2010). Comparison of constraint-induced movement therapy and bilateral treatment of equal intensity in people with chronic upper-extremity dysfunction after cerebrovascular accident. *American Journal of Occupational Therapy, 64*(4), 528-539.

Holm, M. B. (2000). The 2000 Eleanor Clarke Slagle lecture. Our mandate for the new millennium: Evidence-based practice. *American Journal of Occupational Therapy, 54*(6), 575-585.

Jacobs, K. (2012). PromOTing occupational therapy: Words, images, and actions. *American Journal of Occupational Therapy, 66*(6), 652-671.

Kazdin, A. E. (2010). *Single-case research designs: Methods for clinical and applied settings* (2nd ed.). New York, NY: Oxford University Press.

Kennedy, A., Bower, P., Reeves, D., Blakeman, T., Bowen, R., Chew-Graham, C., ... on behalf of the Salford National Institute for Health Research Gastrointestinal programme Grant Research Group. (2013). Implementation of self management support for long term conditions in routine primary care settings: Cluster randomised controlled trial. *BMJ, 346*, f2882. doi:10.1136/bmj.f2882

Kielhofner, G. (1982a). Qualitative research: Part one. Paradigmatic grounds and issues of reliability. *OTJR: Occupation, Participation, and Health, 2*(2), 67-79.

Kielhofner, G. (1982b). Qualitative research: Part two. Methodological approaches and relevance to occupational therapy. *OTJR: Occupation, Participation, and Health, 2*(3), 150-170.

Kielhofner, G. (2005a). A scholarship of practice: Creating discourse between theory, research and practice. *Occupational Therapy in Health Care, 19*(1-2), 7-16.

Kielhofner, G. (2005b). Scholarship and practice: Bridging the divide. *American Journal of Occupational Therapy, 59*(2), 231-239.

Kielhofner, G. (2006). *Research in occupational therapy: Methods of inquiry for enhancing practice*. Philadelphia, PA: F. A. Davis Company.

Kramer, P., Hinojosa, J., & Royeen, C. B. (2003). *Perspectives in human occupation: Participation in life*. Baltimore, MD: Lippincott Williams and Wilkins.

Krefting, L. (1991). Rigor in qualitative research: The assessment of trustworthiness. *American Journal of Occupational Therapy, 45*(3), 214-222.

Law, M., & MacDermid, J. (2008). *Evidence-based rehabilitation: A guide to practice*. Thorofare, NJ: SLACK Incorporated.

Law, M., Stewart, D., Pollock, N., Letts, L., Bosch, J., & Westmorland, M. (1998). *Guidelines for critical review form: Quantitative studies*. Retrieved from http://srs-mcmaster.ca/wp-content/uploads/2015/05/Guidelines-for-Critical-Review-Form-Quantitative-Studies.pdf

Lawder, D. (2014, July 16). *U.S. veterans agency needs $17.6 billion to clear wait times: Acting head*. Retrieved from http://www.reuters.com/article/us-usa-veterans-idUSKBN0FL26S20140716

Lin, S. H., Murphy, S. L., & Robinson, J. C. (2010). Facilitating evidence-based practice: Process, strategies and resources. *American Journal of Occupational Therapy, 64*(1), 164-171.

Linden, A., Butterworth, S. W., & Prochaska, J. O. (2010). Motivational interviewing-based health coaching as a chronic care intervention. *Journal of Evaluation in Clinical Practice, 16*(1), 166-174. doi:10.1111/j.1365-2753.2009.01300.x

Locke, L. F., Spirduso, W. W., & Silverman, S. J. (2007). *Proposals that work: A guide for planning dissertations and grant proposals* (5th ed.). Thousand Oaks, CA: Sage Publications.

Lorig, K. R., Sobel, D. S., Ritter, P. L., Laurent, D., & Hobbs, M. (2001). Effect of a self-management program on patients with chronic disease. *Effective Clinical Practice, 4*(6), 256-262.

Lyons, M., Orozovic, N., Davis, J., & Newman, J. (2002). Doing-being-becoming: Occupational experiences of persons with life-threatening illnesses. *American Journal of Occupational Therapy, 56*(3), 285-295.

Mack, N., Woodsong, C., MacQueen, K. M., Guest, G., & Namey, E. (2005). *Qualitative research methods: A data collector's field guide*. Research Triangle Park, NC: Family Health International.

Melnyk, B., & Fineout-Overholt, E. (2011). *Evidence-based practice in nursing & healthcare: A guide to best practice* (2nd ed.). Riverwoods, IL: Wolters Kluwer Health/Lippincott Williams and Wilkins.

Merrill, S. C. (1985). Qualitative methods in occupational therapy research: An application. *OTJR: Occupation, Participation, and Health, 5*(4), 209-222.

Midboe, A. M., Cucciare, M. A., Trafton, J. A., Ketroser, N., & Chardos, J. F. (2011). Implementing motivational interviewing in primary care: the role of provider characteristics. *Translational Behavioral Medicine, 1*(4), 588-594. doi:10.1007/s13142-011-0080-9

Mortenson, W. B., & Oliffe, J. L. (2009) Mixed methods research in occupational therapy: A survey and critique. *OTJR: Occupation, Participation, and Health, 29*(1), 14-23.

National Center for the Dissemination of Disability Research. (2005). *Focus technical brief no. 10: What is knowledge translation?* Retrieved from http://www.ncddr.org/kt/products/focus/focus10/

National Institutes of Health. (2007). *NIH conference on: Building the science of dissemination and implementation in the service of public health*. Retrieved from http://www.nimh.nih.gov/research-priorities/scientific-meetings/2007/nih-conference-on-building-the-science-of-dissemination-and-implementation-in-the-service-of-public-health.shtml

Newcomer, K. E., Hatry, H. P., & Wholey, J. S. (2015). *Handbook of practical program evaluation* (4th ed.). Hoboken, NJ: John Wiley and Sons.

Obradovic, M., Lal, A., & Liedgens, H. (2013). Validity and responsiveness of EuroQol-5 dimension (EQ-5D) versus Short Form-6 dimension (SF-6D) questionnaire in chronic pain. *Health and Quality of Life Outcomes, 11*, 110. doi:10.1186/1477-7525-11-110

Ottenbacher, K. J., & Hinderer, S. R. (2001). Evidence-based practice: Methods to evaluate individual patient improvement. *American Journal of Physical Medicine and Rehabilitation, 80*(10), 786-796.

Papadimitriou, C., Magasi, S., & Frank, G. (2012). Current thinking in qualitative research: Evidence-based practice, moral philosophies, and political struggle. *OTJR: Occupation, Participation and Health, 32*(1 Suppl.), S2-S5.

Pearson, A., Wiechula, R., Court, A., & Lockwood, C. (2005). The Joanna Briggs Institute model of evidence-based healthcare. *International Journal of Evidence-Based Healthcare, 3*(8), 207-215.

Piette, J. D., Holtz, B., Beard, A. J., Blaum, C., Greenstone, C. L., Krein, S. L., ... on behalf of the Ann Arbor PACT Steering Committee. (2011). Improving chronic illness care for veterans within the framework of the Patient-Centered Medical Home: Experiences from the Ann Arbor Patient-Aligned Care Team Laboratory. *Translational Behavioral Medicine, 1*(4), 615-623. doi:10.1007/s13142-011-0065-8

Rudner, L. M., & Schafer, W. D. (1999). How to write a scholarly research *report. Practical Assessment, Research and Evaluation, 6*(13). Retrieved from http://pareonline.net/getvn.asp?v=6&n=13

Sackett, D. L., Rosenberg, W. M. C., Gray, J. A. M., Haynes, R. B., & Richardson, W. S. (1996). Evidence based medicine: What it is and what it isn't. *British Medical Journal, 312*(7023), 71-72.

Schwarzer, R., Lippke, S., & Luszczynska, A. (2011). Mechanisms of health behavior change in persons with chronic illness or disability: The Health Action Process Approach (HAPA). *Rehabilitation Psychology, 56*(3), 161-170. doi:10.1037/a0024509

Skaperdas, E., Tuepker, A., Nicolaidis, C., Robb, J. K., Kansagara, D., & Hickam, D. H. (n.d.). Congestive heart failure self-management among US veterans: The role of personal and professional advocates. *Patient Education and Counseling*. doi:10.1016/j.pec.2014.03.002

Stav, W., Hallenen, T., Lane, J., & Arbesman, M. (2012). Systematic review of occupational engagement and health outcomes among community-dwelling older adults. *Journal of Occupational Therapy, 66*(3), 301-310. doi:10.5014/ajot.2012.003707

Suarez-Balcazar, Y., Hammel, J., Helfrich, C., Thomas, J., Wilson, T., & Head-Ball, D. (2005). A model of university-community partnerships for occupational therapy scholarship and practice. *Occupational Therapy in Health Care, 19*(1-2), 47-70.

Taylor, M. C. (2007). *Evidence-based practice for occupational therapists* (2nd ed.). Malden, MA: Blackwell Publishing.

Taylor, R. R., Fisher, G., & Kielhofher, G. (2005). Synthesizing research, education, and practice according to the scholarship of practice model: Two faculty examples. *Occupational Therapy in Health Care, 19*(1-2), 107-122.

Thorne, S., Jensen, L., Kearney, M. H., Noblit, G., & Sandelowski, M. (2004). Qualitative metasynthesis: Reflections on methodological orientation and ideological agenda. *Qualitative Health Research, 14*(10), 1342-1365.

Tickle-Degnen, L. (1999). Organizing, evaluating, and using evidence in occupational therapy practice. *American Journal of Occupational Therapy, 53*(5), 537-539.

Tomlin, G., & Borgetto, B. (2011). Research pyramid: A new evidence-based practice model for occupational therapy. *American Journal of Occupational Therapy, 65*(2), 189-196.

Walsh, D., & Downe, S. (2005). Meta-synthesis method for qualitative research: A literature review. *Journal of Advanced Nursing, 50*(2), 204-211.

Westhues, A., Ochocka, J., Jacobson, N., Simich, L., Maiter, S., Janzen, R., & Fleras, A. (2008). Developing theory from complexity: Reflections on a collaborative mixed method participatory action research study. *Qualitative Health Research, 18*(5), 701-717.

World Health Organization. (2001). *International Classification of Functioning, Disability and Health (ICF)*. Retrieved from http://www.who.int/classifications/icf/en/

Wilding, C., Curtin, M., & Whiteford, G. (2012). Enhancing occupational therapists' confidence and professional development through a community of practice scholars. *Australian Occupational Therapy Journal, 59*(4), 312-318.

Wilson, P., M., Petticrew, M., Calnan, M. W., & Nazareth, I. (2010). Disseminating research findings: What should researchers do? A systematic scoping review of conceptual frameworks. *Implementation Science, 5*(91), 1-16.

Wong, P. T. P. (2005). *How to write a research proposal.* Retrieved from http://ielcass.tripod.com/proposalwriting.pdf

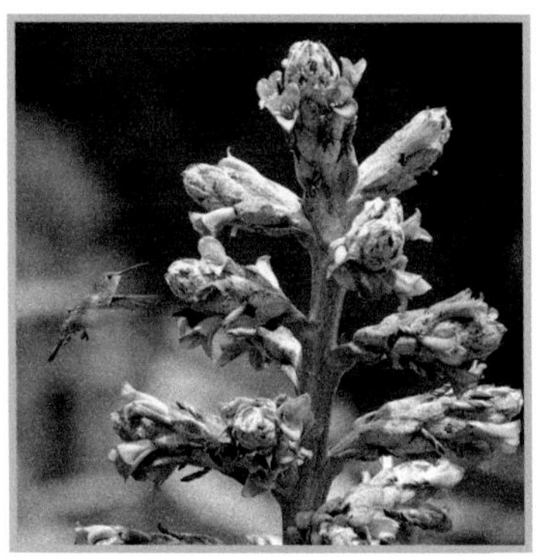

# 48

# GRANTS

Wendy B. Stav, PhD, OTR/L, SCDCM, FAOTA

**ACOTE STANDARDS EXPLORED IN THIS CHAPTER**

B.8.9

**KEY VOCABULARY**

- **Funding agencies:** Federal, state, local, or community organizations, corporations, foundations, and trusts offering monetary support to develop programs or run research projects.
- **Grants:** Monies disbursed by a funding agency to another agency or person for the purpose of a specific program, research study, or products.
- **Proposal:** The collective materials used to apply for a grant including an application and supporting documents.



Jacobs, K., & MacRae, N. (Eds.).
*Occupational Therapy Essentials for Clinical Competence, Third Edition* (pp. 689-698).

The majority of occupational therapy services are reimbursed through third-party payers such as insurance companies or are covered within the larger system in which the clients are treated, as is the case in the school system. However, there are instances in which there is no existing funding mechanism to support the work performed by occupational therapy practitioners or provide the necessary resources. Those instances include research activities, new program development, innovative programs outside of the medical model, and provision of resources to clients necessary for optimal occupational engagement but not deemed medically necessary for third-party payers. While occupational therapy practitioners are generally altruistic and giving of their time and expertise, actual financial support is required to engage in research, develop programs, execute innovative and nontraditional programs, and provide resources to clients. Financial support is available for many of these activities through grant funding from a variety of sources. Grants are funds disbursed by a funding agency to another agency or person for the purpose of a specific program, research study, or products. Grant funds are not loans and do not have to repaid; however, the expectations of the project and reporting of the activity must be completed.

There are several different sources of grant funding including federal agencies, state agencies, corporations, foundations, trusts, and community organizations. Typically, but not exclusively, these funding agencies award grant monies to nonprofit agencies (also referred to as 501[c][3]) and require an application for the funds. The application process is referred to as *grant writing* and requires that applicants adhere to guidelines set forth by the funding agency, including required information to be considered for funding. This chapter will review the types of funding sources, identification of funders, the application process, and deliverables expected by the funders.

## Sources of Grant Funding

A broad range of funding sources can meet a variety of research and programmatic needs. It is important that funding seekers identify the most appropriate funding source for the best chances of successfully receiving a grant. The alignment of the match between the project and funding source is critical and can be the difference between full funding and a rapid rejection letter. Larger agencies such as the federal government and state agencies tend to offer larger grant awards relative to smaller agencies such as a local civic organization (Doll, 2010).

The federal government is the largest grant funder in the United States. A large portion of federal grants come from the National Institutes of Health (NIH), with over $30.1 billion awarded annually for medical research (2015b). The NIH distributes that investment across numerous conditions, including fiscal year 2016 grants of over $2.5 billion on aging, $508 million on rehabilitation, almost $2.3 billion on mental health, $311 million on stroke, $365 million on intellectual and developmental disabilities, $144 million on Parkinson disease, and $789 million on dementia (NIH, 2015a). Choosing the NIH as a funding source is an appropriate selection if one is planning on conducting a research project related to health because they fund only health-related projects and primarily research projects and a smaller number of program and resource grants. The NIH grant funding system includes several types of grants, each of which supports a different type of project. Table 48-1 outlines the types of NIH grants. In addition to selecting the proper type of grant, it is important to submit the grant application to the most appropriate Institute since each has a unique focus and agenda. Table 48-2 lists the different Institutes.

Although the NIH awards a substantial portion of federal funding, there are other federal agencies that support research relevant to and involving occupational therapy, including the Centers for Disease Control and Prevention, the Department of Transportation, and the Department of Education's National Institute on Disability and Rehabilitation Research. A valuable source of available federal grants is grants.gov. Regardless of which agencies are selected, the applicant must be cognizant of the agency's vision, identified gaps, and research agenda to create the best match between the funder's purpose and the project for which funding is sought.

Federal grants typically support projects with budgets in the tens to hundreds of thousands of dollars and even as high as over $1 million dollars. Projects that are smaller in scale, address a statewide issue, or can operate on a smaller budget may benefit from funding from state agencies. Statewide initiatives often parallel federal initiatives or are managed at a state level with federal dollars that have been sent to state agencies for distribution. For example, the campaign to reduce drunk driving–related injuries and fatalities is a national initiative with federal dollars passed to state agencies for distribution via grants from the state departments of transportation. The benefit of applying for state grants is the localized focus on programs and demonstration projects because state agencies are concerned with meeting the needs of the residents of that state through programs and services as opposed to discovering new knowledge through research. The organization and titles of state agencies vary from state to state, so applicants seeking funding should explore their own state agencies to discover the initiatives of each governmental unit to find the best match. In some instances, the identification of a state agency is obvious. For example, therapists wishing to develop a child passenger safety resource center and car seat lending library should apply to the state's department of transportation, whose concern is traffic-related injury prevention. In

Table 48-1.

**TYPES AND PURPOSE OF SELECT NATIONAL INSTITUTES OF HEALTH GRANTS**

| Type | Name | Purpose |
|---|---|---|
| R01 | NIH Research Project Grant Program | Used to support a discrete, specified, circumscribed research project |
| R03 | NIH Small Grant Program | Provides limited funding for a short period of time to support a variety of types of projects, including pilot or feasibility studies, collection of preliminary data, secondary analysis of existing data, small and self-contained research projects, development of new research technology, and so on |
| R13 | NIH Support for Conferences and Scientific Meetings | Support for high-quality conferences and scientific meetings that are relevant to the NIH's scientific mission and to public health |
| R15 | NIH Academic Research Enhancement Award | Supports small research projects in the biomedical and behavioral sciences conducted by students and faculty in health professional schools and other academic components that have not been major recipients of NIH research grant funds |
| R21 | NIH Exploratory/ Developmental Research Grant Award | Encourages new, exploratory, and developmental research projects by providing support for the early stages of project development; sometimes used for pilot and feasibility studies |
| R24 | Resource-Related Research Projects | Used in a wide variety of ways to provide resources for problems for which multiple expertise is needed to focus on a single complex problem in biomedical research or to enhance research infrastructure |
| R41/R42 | Small Business Technology Transfer | Intended to stimulate scientific and technological innovation through cooperative R/R&D carried out between SBCs and research institutions<br>Assists the small business and research communities in commercializing innovative technologies |
| R43/R44 | Small Business Innovative Research | Intended to stimulate technological innovation in the private sector by supporting R/R&D for for-profit institutions for ideas that have potential for commercialization |
| P01 | Research Program Project Grant | Support for integrated, multiproject research projects involving a number of independent investigators who share knowledge and common resources |
| P20 | Exploratory Grants | Often used to support planning activities associated with large multiproject program grants |
| P30 | Center Core Grants | Support shared resources and facilities for categorical research by a number of investigators from different disciplines who provide a multidisciplinary approach to a joint research effort or from the same discipline who focus on a common research problem |

NIH = National Institutes of Health, R/R&D = research/research and development, SBC = small business concern.

Adapted from National Institutes of Health. (2012). *Grants and funding: Types of grant programs.* Retrieved from http://grants.nih.gov/grants/funding/funding_program.htm#PSeries

other instances, the best agency match may not be apparent and could require additional exploration of agency vision and focus. For example, an interprofessional team trying to develop a lifestyle redesign or wellness program for retirees might apply to the state's department of elder affairs or the department of health and human services, depending on the allocation of responsibilities and focus on each agency.

Another source of grant funding is foundations. A foundation is "a nongovernmental entity that is established as a nonprofit corporation or a charitable trust, with a principal purpose of making grants to unrelated organizations, institutions, or individuals for scientific, educational, cultural, religious, or other charitable purposes" (Foundation Center, 2016, para. 1). Each foundation is created with a specific purpose and vision and as such will only fund proposals that are consistent with its agenda. For example, the mission of the Christopher and Dana Reeve Foundation states, "The Reeve Foundation is dedicated to curing spinal cord injury by funding

Table 48-2.

**Institutes in the National Institutes of Health With Relevance to Occupational Therapy**

| Abbreviation | Title of Institute |
|---|---|
| NEI | National Eye Institute |
| NIA | National Institute on Aging |
| NIAAA | National Institute of Alcohol Abuse and Alcoholism |
| NIAMS | National Institute of Arthritis and Musculoskeletal and Skin Diseases |
| NICHD | National Institute of Child Health and Human Development |
| NIDA | National Institute on Drug Abuse |
| NIDCD | National Institute on Deafness and Other Communication Disorders |
| NIMH | National Institute of Mental Health |
| NIMHD | National Institute on Minority Health and Health Disparities |
| NINDS | National Institute of Neurological Disorders and Stroke |

Adapted from National Institutes of Health. (2012). *Institutes, centers, and offices.* Retrieved from http://www.nih.gov/icd/

innovative research, and improving the quality of life for people living with paralysis through grants, information and advocacy" (2016, para. 1) and therefore will only approve grant proposals specific to spinal cord injury research and projects. Other foundations have broader interests, such as the Robert Wood Johnson Foundation, which has program areas including childhood obesity, public and community health, health care quality, uninsured individuals, disease prevention and health promotion, and mental and emotional well-being (Robert Wood Johnson Foundation, 2015). There are hundreds of foundations in existence with each one targeting a different population, need, or problem. Therapists seeking funding can search for individual foundations if a funder with interests in a particular area is known or they can use a foundation search database, such as Foundation Center (www.foundationcenter.org), Foundation Search (www.foundationsearch.com), or Big Online America (www.bigdatabase.com). If a therapist or organization is going to continuously seek foundation funding, investing in a paid membership in these databases is worthwhile. Another option for seeking grant funding from a foundation is through partnerships with occupational therapists in academia because most universities have a grant office with ongoing memberships to these or similar databases.

A final source of funding that can be useful for occupational therapy practitioners is community or civic organizations. Several organizations give back to the community in the form of grant funding and can meet the modest fiscal needs of a community program. CVS, for example, has community grants aimed at inclusive programming for children with disabilities to promote independence and support physical movement and play (CVS Caremark, 2015). Civic organizations, specifically local chapters of Rotary Club, Lions Club, and Kiwanis, often support small one-time grants for the local community, which can be useful in supporting community-based initiatives.

Selection of a potential funding source should involve consideration of several factors, including but not limited to:

- Type of project (research, program/service, resource)
- Size and scope of the project
- Duration of the project
- Population involved
- Amount of money needed to support the project
- Match between project purpose and funding agency vision, mission, and agenda

## Role of Occupational Therapy Practitioners on Grant-Funded Projects

Occupational therapy practitioners can serve in any capacity they would ordinarily fulfill in a clinical practice situation. In some cases, an occupational therapist might perform evaluations on all the study or program participants under the purview of a grant. Under other grants, occupational therapy practitioners might provide intervention or educational services to fulfill the plan of the grant-funded project. The distinction between occupational therapist and occupational therapy assistant roles in a study or grant funded project is consistent with the professional guidelines for practice outlined in the *Guidelines for Supervision, Roles, and Responsibilities During the Delivery of Occupational Therapy Services* (AOTA, 2014). Occupational therapy practitioners are not limited to clinical practice duties under the umbrella of a grant. They can fulfill any role including principal investigator, project director, consultant, data collector, or practitioner as long the individual satisfies the eligibility criteria for the individual position.

## Grant Proposals

Selecting the right potential funding source is an important step in the grant process, but the application process is critical to securing funding. The application document and associated requested material is referred to as a *proposal*. The first determination is whether the funder has sent out a call for grant applications or a request for proposals, commonly referred to as an RFP, or if the funder will accept unsolicited proposals. If the funder's materials state they do not accept unsolicited proposals, they will not award any money for proposals that have not answered a specific RFP. Applicants can increase their chances of getting funding if the proposal is thorough, accurate, includes all the information requested, and strictly adheres to the proposal guidelines.

The guidelines for proposals should be taken very literally and followed exactly. Funders make judgments about an applicant's ability to perform and spend their money wisely by how well the proposal followed the stated guidelines. Therefore, if proposal guidelines identify page length, font size, font style, and margin width, the proposal should follow those guidelines exactly; otherwise the proposal will be immediately rejected prior to reading. Deadlines for submission are another guideline that should not be taken lightly because late submissions will not be accepted. Finally, all sections and information requested on a proposal should be completed because there are no second chances or revisions permitted. All proposals are slightly different depending on the funding source and what information is required to make a decision to award funding, but there are standard elements that exist across most grant proposals. The common parts of a proposal including institutional information, summary of the project with goals and objectives, biographical information of the personnel, budget with budget justification, and a plan for sustainability (Gitlin & Lyons, 2008). Throughout the entire proposal, applicants try to sell themselves and their institutions to the funder by proving the project is worthy of receiving a grant award and the applicant is qualified to see the project completed.

### Institutional Information

Funders ask for information about the institution in which the project will take place to ensure eligibility for funding, as well as to determine whether the institution has the experience, infrastructure, and resources to execute the project. Typically, applicants will be asked to provide general background information about the organization, which is the same content regardless of the grant being sought. This content includes information about the type of institution; size; what type of business is conducted there; and most importantly, the tax status to prove the organization is nonprofit. The sum of this information is referred to as *boilerplate content* and is usually available from the organization's administration.

In addition to the boilerplate information, applicants must demonstrate how the proposed project can be successfully executed based on prior experience in research or program development, expertise with the described population of clients, the size of the organization, proximity to clientele, and available resources. Funders consider grants to be investments in their agenda and toward their vision, so they want to be sure they are making a sound investment.

### Description of the Project

Grant proposals require a detailed description of what will be done with requested funds. For research proposals, this description should detail the population being studied, study design, proposed measurement tools, and planned data analysis. Grant proposals requested for the development of a program or services should demonstrate how the proposed program or service fills an existing gap, identifies the population to be served, and describes the program or services. In addition to a detailed description of the program, applicants identify program or research goals they plan to accomplish. Depending on the nature of the project, the goals may be related to discovering the effect of a certain intervention, identifying the relationships among variables, creating a fully operational program, or serving a specific number of clients. Practitioners who receive grant funding are held accountable for reporting the status toward goal achievement throughout the project. The information in this section of the proposal should illustrate the alignment between the proposed project and the funder initiatives and vision and, if applicable, satisfy the intent of the RFP. Any elements of the proposed project that stray from the funder's mission or initiatives will be grounds for rejection of the request.

**BIOGRAPHICAL SKETCH**

Provide the following information for the Senior/key personnel and other significant contributors in the order listed on Form Page 2.
Follow this format for each person. **DO NOT EXCEED FOUR PAGES.**

| NAME<br>Stav, Wendy Beth | POSITION TITLE<br>Chair and Professor of Occupational Therapy |
|---|---|
| eRA COMMONS USER NAME (credential, e.g., agency login) | |

EDUCATION/TRAINING *(Begin with baccalaureate or other initial professional education, such as nursing, include postdoctoral training and residency training if applicable.)*

| INSTITUTION AND LOCATION | DEGREE *(if applicable)* | MM/YY | FIELD OF STUDY |
|---|---|---|---|
| Quinnipiac University | B.S. | 10/91 | Occupational Therapy |
| Nova Southeastern University | Ph.D. | 1/01 | Occupational Therapy |

**A. Personal Statement**

I have a 17 year history of clinical and scholarly inquiry in the area of driving and community mobility related to program development, medical reporting, licensing guidelines for medically at-risk drivers, predictability of assessments, and clinical practice. My research and professional involvement includes activities at the state and national levels including AOTA's Older Driver Initiative, co-authorship of AOTA official documents and Occupational Therapy Practice Guidelines of Driving and Community Mobility for Older Adult, collaboration with the American Medical Association's Older Driver Project, the American Association of Motor Vehicle Administrator's Older Driver Working Group, and contribution to three separate based literature reviews on older drivers.

**B. Positions and Honors**

Positions

2012 – Chair and Professor, Occupational Therapy Department, Nova Southeastern University
2011 – 2012 Assistant Professor, Department of Occupational Therapy & Occupational Science, Towson University
2006 – 2011 Associate Professor, Department of Occupational Therapy & Occupational Science, Towson University

Honors

2009 American Occupational Therapy Association Roster of Fellow Award
2008 Nova Southeastern University Distinguished Alumni Achievement Award
2008 Maryland Occupational Therapy Association Award of Merit

**C. Selected Peer-reviewed Publications**

Stav, W. (2014). Updated systematic review related to older adult community mobility and driver -licensure policies. *American Journal of Occupational Therapy, 68,* 681-689. http://dx.doi.org/10.5014/ajot.2014.011510

Stav, W., Halleran, T., & Lane, J., & Arbesman, M. (2012). Evidence related to occupational engagement and health outcomes among older adults. *American Journal of Occupational Therapy, 66*(3), 301-310. http://dx.doi.org/10.5014/ajot.111.003699

Stav, W., (2012). Developing and implementing driving rehabilitation programs: A phenomenological approach. *American Journal of Occupational Therapy, 66*(1), e11-e16. http://dx.doi.org/10.5014/ajot.2012.000950

**D. Research Support**

American Occupational Therapy Association Stav (PI) 2/11 – 12/11
Older Driver Evidence-Based Literature Review Update

American Association of Motor Vehicle Administrators Stav (EB Literature Review Contractor) 1/08 – 12/08
Driving Fitness Working Group

National Highway Traffic Safety Administration Stav (PI) 1/07 – 12/09
Barriers to Developing Driving and Community Mobility Programs for Older Americans

**Figure 48-1.** Abbreviated NIH biographical sketch form.

## Biographical Information of the Personnel

Funders request detailed information about the applicant and any members of the project team to determine whether the applicants have the experience and capability to carry out the proposed project. Typically, the RFP identifies exactly what the funder is looking for in terms of education, work experience, prior program development experience, previous scholarship, and often past grant funding received. As in other parts of a grant application, provide all of the information and only the information requested by the funder. This is the applicant's opportunity to sell him- or herself and prove to be a worthy grant recipient. Often a grant funder will provide a format for the applicant's biographical information. If such a form is provided, the applicant should use only that template to provide the requested information. A form commonly completed by grant applicants is the NIH biographical sketch, which includes a template along with open-ended sections to complete including a personal statement, positions and honors, selected peer-reviewed publications, and research support. Figure 48-1 is an example of an abbreviated NIH biographical sketch form.

## Budget With Budget Justification

Development of a budget at the time of the proposal is an important step in the process because the funders will make judgments about the worthiness of the proposed project based on several factors, including the total amount of money being requested, the suggested

Table 48-3.

**EXAMPLE OF A BUDGET**

| Category | Amount | Match | Total |
|---|---|---|---|
| Personnel | $27,560 | $25,825 | $53,385 |
| • Principal investigator @ $67,120 + benefits x 40% | $17,500 | $8,425 | $25,295 |
| • Project associate | $0 | $17,400 | $17,400 |
| • Research assistant | $10,060 | $0 | $10,600 |
| Travel | $2,700 | $0 | $2,700 |
| • Lifesavers conference | $1,500 | $0 | $1,500 |
| • AOTA conference | $1,200 | $0 | $1,200 |
| Contractual services | $4,600 | $0 | $4,600 |
| • Video production @ $500/day for 2 days | $1,000 | $0 | $1,000 |
| • Postproduction @ $40/hour for 90 hours | $3,600 | $0 | $3,600 |
| Equipment | $0 | $5,300 | $5,300 |
| • Computers 3 @ $1,500 | $0 | $4,500 | $4,500 |
| • Printers 3 @ $600 | $0 | $1,800 | $1,800 |
| • Fax machine | $0 | $200 | $200 |
| Other direct costs | $970 | $0 | $970 |
| • Recordable CD-ROMs (100 pack) | $25 | $0 | $25 |
| • Three-ring binders (60) | $180 | $0 | $180 |
| • Packing materials | $240 | $0 | $240 |
| • WebEx account for training | $225 | $0 | $225 |
| • Copying | $300 | $0 | $300 |
| Indirect costs | $1,734 | $1,156 | $2,890 |
| Total | $37,564 | $32,281 | $69,845 |
| Percentage | 53.78% | 46.22% | 100% |

distribution of funds across the categories in the budget, the anticipated tasks to be accomplished with the money, the proposed scope of impact of the project (i.e., local, regional, statewide, or national), adherence to budgetary guidelines in the RFP, and how realistic the request is. Applicants of all grants are required to specify exactly how much money they are suggesting will be spent across several categories within the budget. Some funders identify categories of the budget that are required, whereas other funders allow the applicants to identify the areas of the budget.

Regardless of the structure of the grant application, there are several categories of the budget common to most proposals. Those categories include personnel, materials and supplies, travel, and indirect costs (Gitlin & Lyons, 2008). The more detailed and comprehensive the budget is, the better able the funder will be to make an assessment on whether to fund the proposed project. See Table 48-3 for an example of a budget and Table 48-4 for a sample budget justification. In an effort to provide the detail needed, the above broad categories are often further broken down into individual items. For example, the personnel category, which is often the largest portion of the budget, clearly delineates each individual person involved in the project, each person's salary along with percent of time investment in the project, and the amount of their fringe benefits so all values are understood by the funder. The personnel category includes the principal investigator, who leads the entire project; other team members; subcontractors; graduate assistants; and support staff. Occupational therapy assistants applying for grants should be sure to include an occupational therapist in the project to ensure adherence to state practice guidelines in the jurisdiction of the project. If a project is planned for more than 1 year, the budget needs to reflect all of these values across each individual year of the budget. Another large portion of the budget is the materials and supplies category. This section includes all the items and services necessary to execute the project. The obvious items in this portion of the budget are the clinical instruments for use in the project such as assessment tools, furniture, and intervention equipment. Additional costs covered in this section include phone charges, paper and envelopes, copying, postage, food, marketing materials, consultation fees, computers, and laptops. Travel costs are also covered in a grant budget and incorporate local travel for day-to-day operation of the project as well as distance travel for dissemination of

Table 48-4.

**BUDGET JUSTIFICATION**

| Category and Item | Justification |
|---|---|
| Personnel: Principal investigator | The principal investigator will coordinate the project, oversee development of materials, and supervise the tasks of the other personnel. The principal investigator has more than 20 years of experience as an occupational therapist with associated expertise in the relationship between the person and the environment, as well as more than 15 years of expertise in the area of driver safety. Forty percent of the principal investigator's time will be dedicated to the project. |
| Personnel: Research assistant | The research assistant will assist with the project coordination, information gathering, scheduling of events, and dissemination of materials developed. |
| Travel: Lifesavers conference | Travel to present project experiences and outcomes at a national traffic safety conference. |
| Travel: AOTA conference | Travel to present project experiences and outcomes at a national occupational therapy conference. |
| Contractural services: Video production | The educational curriculum created from the project will be created in a video format, requiring the skilled work of video production. The project will include 2 days of video shooting at $500 per day. |
| Contractural services: Postproduction | After video shooting, all footage will be edited for content and flow with the addition of graphics and text where necessary at a fee of $40 per hour for 90 hours. |
| Direct costs: recordable CD-ROMs | The video format educational program will be copied onto CD-ROMs for distribution statewide. |
| Direct costs: Three-ring binders | Educational materials to supplement the video (handouts, tests, instructions, and so on) will be printed and placed in binders for dissemination to programs statewide. |
| Direct costs: Packing materials | Packing materials will be used to pack CD-ROMs and three-ring binders for shipping via the intrastate mail system. |
| Direct costs: WebEx account | A WebEx account will be used to provide synchronous training program statewide in the use of the program. |
| Copying | Copying services will be used to generate hard copies of the educational materials for dissemination statewide. |

the results. Applicants should plan ahead at the time of the proposal and consider where they would like to present the study results or project outcomes. Preliminary research on the cost of travel to the location of conferences will be necessary for inclusion in the budget. A final area of the budget is indirect costs, which represent the administrative and facility expenses to run a program or project. Some funders state that no indirect costs will be covered, whereas others identify a maximum percentage allowable. Often indirect costs are calculated by a percentage of the direct costs. The monies supporting indirect costs cover expenses such as building costs, utilities, and the administrative fees associated with coordinating a grant within an institution.

Additional considerations when developing the budget for a grant are matching funds and in-kind contributions. Many funding sources require matching funds from the organization to receive an award. Matching funds are dollars or services contributed by the institution equal to a specified percentage of money awarded by the funding agency. In some cases, the institution has money set aside just for the purpose of matching; however, in-kind contributions can add up to a dollar amount required by the funder so long as those contributions are given a value. For example, if an institution offers to contribute a computer and printer worth $1,500 toward a project, that amount is documented. Personnel time can also be considered as an in-kind contribution as in the case of a volunteer working 10 hours per week as an estimate worth of $10 per hour or 25% of an administrative assistant's time not financially supported by the grant.

After each category and year of the budget is subtotaled and the sum of the total money requested is calculated, the applicant must write a budget justification. The justification is a rationale for each individual line in the budget to clarify exactly how the money will be spent. Budget justifications are written in a narrative format, but depending on the funder may also be allowable in a table format infused with budget values. As with any other portion of a grant proposal, it is incumbent upon the applicant to read the instructions and understand the expectation prior to writing the proposal.

## Evidence-Based Research Chart

| Term | Evidence |
|---|---|
| Grants | Cameron & Luvisi, 2012; Cole, 2006; Doll, 2010; Jacob & Lefgren, 2007 |
| Funding | Bear-Lehman, 2011; Lambert, 2001; Lin, 2011 |

### *Plan for Sustainability*

Most proposals for programs will ask the applicants to describe a plan for sustainability of the program. It is not the intention or desire of a funding agency to provide fiscal support for a program into perpetuity. Rather, funding agencies offer grants to programs as a means for start-up and development costs. Applicants must include a plan to generate revenue or another source of sustainability. Without such a plan documented in the proposal, funders may have concerns their investment is not worthwhile over just a short time of the funding. Depending on the nature of the program, applicants should consider several options for sustainability, which may include reimbursement from a third party, out of pocket payments by clients, integration into another existing program, or training and delegation to other practitioners or disciplines.

## Deliverables

After a grant is awarded, the grantee has an obligation to execute what was promised in the proposal. In addition to carrying out the research study or program as proposed, the grantee must provide evidence of his or her activities. This evidence is often referred to as *deliverables*. Any and all products, reports, articles, and materials generated by the project should be sent to the funder for their review. This includes marketing materials created, outcome studies, documents and forms developed, and articles published as a result of the project. In addition, many funders request reports at predetermined intervals, such as annually or quarterly, so they can maintain awareness of how their monies are being spent. Failure to comply with these requests or any other legally mandated or funder-imposed guidelines, such as protection of health information, appropriate allocation of funds, and ethical treatment of study participants, can result in revocation of funds.

### Case Example

The sample budget and associated justification presented in Tables 48-3 and 48-4 represent a portion of the grant proposal written to develop a driver-vehicle fit program for teenage novice drivers. The principal investigator, having significant experience in driver safety and the CarFit program, was approached by the state highway safety office inquiring about driver-vehicle fit for teenage drivers. The RFP was approaching so the principal investigator wrote a proposal for funding to meet the state's needs. The proposed program involved the development of an evidence-based educational curriculum specific to driver-vehicle fit for teenagers. The program included the development of a curriculum with a video, worksheets, informational handouts, tests, and an instructional handbook. The plan and desire of the funder was to disseminate the curriculum to all state-sanctioned driver education schools statewide. The dissemination process would include full copies of the curriculum and associated materials as well as train the trainer sessions delivered by the program staff to the driving schools via a web-based instructional platform. Strengths of the proposal included experienced personnel, collaboration between resource-rich agencies (a state university and the regional office of a national traffic safety organization), and a plan to develop and evidence-based program. This particular grant proposal was very strong in design as well as funder interest; however, it was written and submitted just prior to a significant downward shift in the economy, so all grant funding from the state agency was reduced and the project was ultimately not funded.

## Summary

Receiving a grant comes with a tremendous responsibility to execute the project, sustain professional and ethical standards, manage the funds and personnel properly, and complete the reports in a timely manner. It is not recommended that individuals pursue large grant funding opportunities because it requires a vast skill set and extensive time commitment beyond what an individual can dedicate. Despite the challenges associated with grants, receiving external funding to support research and projects is necessary. Grant funding allows occupational therapy practitioners to grow the profession, discover new and innovative methods to measure and enhance occupational performance, and create new forays into areas of practice that would otherwise not be reimbursed in the traditional health care system.

## References


American Occupational Therapy Association. (2014). Guidelines for supervision, roles, and responsibilities during the delivery of occupational therapy services. *American Journal of Occupational Therapy, 68*(Suppl. 3), S16-S22. doi:10.5014/ajot.2014.686S03

Bear-Lehman, J. (2011). The NIH roadmap: An opportunity for occupational therapy. *OTJR: Occupation, Participation and Health, 31*(3), 106-107. doi:10.3928/15394492-20110428-01

Cameron, K. A. V., & Luvisi, J. (2012, March). Grants: Fulfilling dreams and needs for occupational therapy. *Administration and Management Special Interest Section Quarterly, 28*(1), 1-3.

Christoper and Dana Reeve Foundation. (2016). *About us*. Retrieved from http://www.christopherreeve.org/site/c.ddJFKRNoFiG/b.4409743/k.C825/About_Us.htm

Cole, S. S. (2006). Researcher behavior that leads to success in obtaining grant funding: A model for success. *Research Management Review, 15,* 16-32.

CVS Caremark. (2015). *Our giving*. Retrieved from http://info.cvscaremark.com/community/our-impact/community-grants

Doll, J. (2010). *Program development and grant writing in occupational therapy: Making the connection*. Sudbury, MA: Jones and Bartlett.

Foundation Center. (2016). *Knowledge base*. Retrieved from http://www.grantspace.org/Tools/Knowledge-Base/Funding-Resources/Foundations/What-is-a-foundation

Gitlin, L. N., & Lyons, K. J. (2008). *Successful grant writing: Strategies for health and human service professionals* (3rd ed.). New York, NY: Springer.

Jacob, F., & Lefgren, L. (2007). The impact of research grant funding on scientific productivity. *Journal of Public Economics, 95,* 1168-1177.

Lambert, R. (2001). The money is out there: One route to a major research funding award. *British Journal of Occupational Therapy, 64*(6), 311-313.

Lin, S. H. (2011). Increasing research capacity and advocating for research. *OT Practice, 16*(17), 33.

National Institutes of Health. (2012). *Institutes, centers, and offices*. Retrieved from http://www.nih.gov/icd/

National Institutes of Health. (2013). *Grants and funding: Activity codes*. Retrieved from http://grants.nih.gov/grants/funding/ac_search_results.htm

National Institutes of Health. (2015a). *Estimates of funding for various research, condition, and disease categories (RCDC)*. Retrieved from https://report.nih.gov/categorical_spending.aspx

National Institutes of Health. (2015b). *What we do: Budget*. Retrieved from http://www.nih.gov/about-nih/what-we-do/budget

Robert Wood Johnson Foundation. (2015). *Our topics*. Retrieved from http://www.rwjf.org/en/our-topics.html

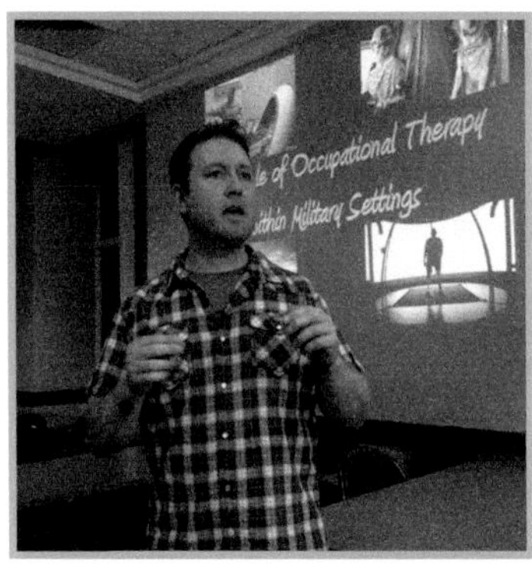


# 49

# PROFESSIONAL PRESENTATIONS

*Christine Sullivan, OTD, OTR/L*

**ACOTE STANDARDS EXPLORED IN THIS CHAPTER**

B.8.8

**KEY VOCABULARY**

- **American Psychological Association format:** The standard format used in health science literature for in-text citation and reference information.
- **Peer review:** A process in which a panel of experts in the field is responsible for judging the merit of a proposal for a scholarly publication or presentation.
- **Plagiarism:** The use of information that was created by another individual as though it were original.
- **Professional presentation:** An oral report of research findings or other evidence-based practice information.
- **Scholarly reports:** Documents that are written by reflective practitioners for the advancement of a profession.



Jacobs, K., & MacRae, N. (Eds.).
*Occupational Therapy Essentials for Clinical Competence, Third Edition* (pp. 699-712).

Occupational therapy practitioners have many roles to fill regarding being a professional. A review of the literature reveals the multitude of activities that are the hallmark of fulfilling a professional role. Braveman (2006) discussed involvement in the professional association as being important, naming professional associations in the United States as being the "primary vehicle" that allows a profession to "promote and develop its services." This sentiment is clearly echoed in the American Occupational Therapy Association's (AOTA) Centennial Vision (2007): "We envision that occupational therapy is a powerful, widely recognized, science-driven, and evidence-based profession with a globally connected and diverse work force meeting society's occupational needs."

This vision was created to be a "roadmap" to commemorate the AOTA's 100th anniversary in 2017. Member and nonmember feedback was sought to ensure that this was a shared vision. Demonstrating the skills to writing a scholarly report for either a presentation or for publication is in direct line with the need for the profession to be visible and science-based throughout the world. The Centennial Vision's goal of linking education, research, and practice will only be reached by ensuring that occupational therapy practitioners are able to communicate effectively both in scholarly writing and in professional presentations. Attendance at conferences is an important part of a professional's life. Information presented at conferences is usually current and many states have continuing education requirements tied in with license renewal in most health professions.

## Scholarship in Occupational Therapy

In the official AOTA document entitled *Scholarship in Occupational Therapy* (AOTA, 2009, p. 790), scholarship is described to be important to the "growth, development, and vitality of the profession" and the necessity for it so that the profession can advance. The document describes "scholarly practice" as the use of "the knowledge base of the profession in one's practice" (p. 790). Scholarly practice is viewed by the AOTA as evidence-based practice that is delivered by "reflective practitioners."

This official document describes scholarship akin to research, in which the emphasis is on an investigation that is made more available to the public, subject to review and evidence that adds or expands the base of knowledge in a professional discipline. Scholarship builds on what has been published before and allows the profession to advance. The belief of the AOTA is that participating in scholarship and scholarly activities is a professional responsibility, similar to the professional responsibility referred to in the introduction regarding the need to belong to professional associations.

The official document describes the work of Boyer's definitions of the various types of scholarship (1990): the scholarship of discovery, the scholarship of integration, the scholarship of application, and the scholarship of teaching and learning. Boyer presented these categories in 1990 in a sentinel work entitled *Scholarship Reconsidered: Priorities for the Professoriate*. Boyer's descriptions of the following classifications were not hierarchical.

### Scholarship of Discovery

This type of scholarship is work in an activity that leads to the development of "knowledge for its own sake" (Boyer, 1990, p. 17). The scholarship of discovery consists of primary, original research, the purpose of which is to expand the base of knowledge of a specific discipline. This is the type of scholarship that is most often completed by faculty members who are engaged in research. The AOTA recognizes the need for this type of scholarship in terms of understanding human occupation and how the participation in meaningful occupations can maintain the physical and mental health of our citizens. This is the "science driven" phrase that is a salient feature of the Centennial Vision.

### Scholarship of Integration

The AOTA official document uses Boyer's (1990) definition of this type of scholarship as "...making creative connections both within and across disciplines to integrate, synthesize, interpret and create new perspectives and theories" (AOTA, 2009, p. 790). The difference between this and the scholarship of discovery is that this type of scholarship poses different research questions. It examines original research findings within a specific discipline and then looks to integrate them in a more interdisciplinary way. Boyer refers to finding information that "...lies in the intersections of disciplinary boundaries," which leads to the formation of new knowledge. In the field of occupational therapy, this type of research would facilitate an improved understanding of how we can meet societal needs. This focus then brings us full circle to the goals of the Centennial Vision.

### Scholarship of Application

In this type of scholarship, practitioners can apply the knowledge gained by the two previously discussed types: scholarship of discovery and scholarship of integration. The scholar then applies how the knowledge gained can be put to practical use at all levels of society. The AOTA official document *Scholarship in Occupational Therapy* gives several examples of this type of scholarship. One example given is "the value of occupations as a health determinant to address health disparities of populations" (AOTA, 2009, p. 791). Some authors (as identified by the

AOTA document) use the term *scholarship of practice* (Braveman, Helfrich, & Fisher, 2001). This type of scholarship focuses on occupational therapy intervention. One final type of scholarship of application has been identified in the AOTA document as the scholarship of engagement (Boyer, 1996). In this type of scholarship, multiple stakeholders (within and without the occupational therapy professional community) produce scholarly works with persons and organizations.

### Scholarship of Teaching and Learning

This type of scholarship has more of a research frame of reference, with the systematic study of teaching and learning. Because of the nature of the subject, it is more prone to public sharing via either publications or presentations (AOTA, 2009). Because it tends to be more open to the public than the other types of scholarship, it is open to outside comment and "critical review."

## Scholarly Writing and Publication

Occupational therapy practitioners must understand not only the importance of scholarly writing, but also the "how to's" of successful writing and all of the component parts: from the inception of the idea to the literature review to the writing and finally to the submission for peer review and, optimally, acceptance for publication. Many skilled clinicians have anxiety about writing. Some of the areas of concern of novice authors are regarding whether they chose a topic that has enough information; that they have done adequate research; and finally, whether or not they are competent in writing at such a professional level.

### What Constitutes Scholarly Writing?

Aitchison and Lee (2006) posited that the purpose of scholarly writing is to "...create knowledge rather than [to write]...merely as knowledge-recording" (p. 270). Their view is echoed by others throughout the literature (Lavelle & Bushrow, 2007) in which writing skills combine with oral skills. Dallimore, Hertenstein, and Platt (2008) coined the phrase *communication competence,* which describes both the written word and the ability to present the ideas after a manuscript or article is written.

### Types of Articles

The American Psychological Association (APA) classifies written works for the behavioral and social sciences according to the study of the subject and content of the manuscript. The *Publication Manual of the American Psychological Association, Sixth Edition* (2010), is the primary source for the health sciences style of source citation and works cited. Readers will see and hear this described as "APA format." The APA manual describes journal articles as "...reports of empirical studies, literature reviews, theoretical articles, methodological articles or case studies" (p. 10). The following is a description of each category as per the manual.

#### Empirical Studies

Empirical studies are always articles that are primary resources, which means that these articles describe original research that is written by researchers. Articles regarding empirical studies follow a typical format in which there is an introduction section followed by a method section, a results section, and finally a discussion section. The methods section must be written so that any scholar or scientist would be able to reproduce the study using the same research design and sequence. The discussion section includes the author's summary of the results, any limitations of the study, and questions for further research study.

#### Literature Reviews

Literature reviews are considered to be a secondary source. This category of scholarly writing analyzes previously published works that have been written by researchers and scholars. Textbooks, such as this, are secondary sources that use literature reviews to draw upon the knowledge base in a discipline. The APA (2010) further defines this category of scholarly writing as being "research synthesis and meta-analyses" (p. 10). In this type of writing, the author searches for previously published writings on a particular topic, organizes the data, and uses quantitative and substantiated data to make comparisons and conclusions about current knowledge.

#### Theoretical Articles

Theoretical articles are those in which the author uses existing literature to propose new hypotheses to advance existing theories. In a theoretical article, the author examines both the "...internal consistency and external validity" (APA, 2010, p. 10) and forms a judgment as to whether the previous theoretical frameworks are sound. Study limitations or research design flaws are considered as the author suggests new or revised theories for study.

### Methodological Articles

Methodological articles introduce new approaches to existing research designs. The focus of methodological articles is on the examination of empirical data and how current methods might be altered for a different research protocol. The intent of methodological articles is to be "user friendly" to readers within the body of the article. More complex information may be included in tables and appendices at the end of the article for more experienced readers to use as a reference.

### Case Studies

Case studies are articles that describe reports of information obtained while the researcher rendered care or services to "...an individual, a group, a community or an organization" (APA, 2010, p. 11). Case studies define a problem, discuss the interventions used to ameliorate the problem, and open the door for further study of similar cases. Confidentiality is an important consideration for authors who choose to write case study articles.

### Other Types of Articles

The *Publication Manual of the American Psychological Association* (2010) lists other less frequently published types of articles, including brief reports, book reviews, letters to the editor, and monographs (p. 11). Anyone considering submission of an article must be aware of the required criteria of a journal before submitting a manuscript.

## Authorship: The Peer Review and Editorial Process

Scholarly articles are always reviewed by a panel of experts in the same field as the submission. This is to ensure authenticity and originality of the work, as well as a determination that the article presents information or research that is significant to broadening the knowledge base in the field. The terms *peer-reviewed, refereed,* and *juried* are generally used interchangeably to describe this process. Scholarly journal articles are expected to be original, primary publications (APA, 2010). Scholarly journal articles have not been published before. In addition, it is also common expectation that an author will not submit an article to more than one journal at a time (Belcher, 2009).

In the peer-review process, an editor is responsible for overseeing the quality and content of a scholarly journal. There may also be associate, consulting, and advisory editors in addition to ad hoc reviewers, who might be brought on to review specialty areas. The associate editor might also assist in the communications with the authors in regard to acceptance, rejection, and edits of the manuscript that might be requested of the author. The editor has the right to reject an article before it is sent for review to others on the peer-review board. Editors may also request a "masked review" (sometimes referred to as a *blind review*) in which all identifying information of the author is removed before the review (APA, 2010; Belcher, 2009).

The amount of time it takes for a review is said by the APA (2010) to be approximately 2 to 3 months. After a manuscript has been reviewed, the author should expect an answer regarding whether the article is accepted or not. There are three answers that an author might expect: acceptance, rejection, or rejection with an invitation to revise the article and resubmit it. If an author has not been informed of any decision after a period of 3 months, it would be acceptable to contact the editor. If the author is ultimately notified that the article is not accepted at all, it is then permissible to submit it to another journal for review (Belcher, 2009).

## Types of Citation Formats

There are several styles, or formats, of citation styles. Style manuals give authors explicit instructions as to how to cite in-text quotations and list references and how to incorporate tables and illustrations in a manuscript, among other requirements. Some styles are designed to identify standards for authors; others are geared more toward providing standards for editors and publishers. Although several science disciplines have developed their own styles (e.g., chemistry and physics), Lipson (2006) and Belcher (2009) list that there are three major citation styles. These are Chicago (sometimes referred to as *Turabian*, after the name of the originator of the system), Modern Language Association (MLA), and APA.

### *Chicago Style*

Chicago style covers a variety of topics from manuscript preparation and publication to grammar, usage, and documentation. This is generally considered the standard for preparation of books (rather than having a focus on journal articles). It covers a wide variety of book publishing issues, ranging from the writing of the book to sections regarding the actual printing and binding of books. For further information, refer to *The Chicago Manual of Style, 16th Edition* (2010).

### *Modern Language Association Style*

MLA style is most commonly used to set the publication standards of manuscripts within the liberal arts and humanities. This style addresses standards for writing books and articles on literature and language. It is geared toward the preparation for authors rather than for editors.

For further information, please refer to the *MLA Style Manual and Guide to Scholarly Publishing, Third Edition* (2008).

## American Psychological Association Style

APA style is most commonly used to cite sources within the social sciences. Because of the nature of the standards, APA format is designed for use by the author more than for that of the editor. This resource centers on the preparation of scholarly journal articles with standards for in-text citations, endnotes and footnotes, and the reference page. For more information, please consult the *Publication Manual of the American Psychological Association, Sixth Edition* (APA, 2010).

Although most writings that are done in the field of occupational therapy require APA format, it is important for scholarly writers to be cognizant of the required citation style for a particular journal, especially at the point of the initial submission. Having a manuscript in the required format may even improve the chances for acceptance of a submission because it allows the publisher the ability to visualize if the work would be appropriate for acceptance.

There are also some reliable and valid online resources that can be helpful for each of the various formats. One valid and frequently updated resource is a webpage designed and maintained by Purdue University. It is called the Online Writing Lab (OWL) and can be found at http://owl.english.purdue.edu/owl.

## Acceptable Time Frame for References

Most editors require references to be used that are no older than 5 to 7 years; however, there can be exceptions. If one of the sentinel works on a particular topic is greater than 7 years old and describes a foundational theory for a particular topic, older references may be appropriate.

# Occupational Therapy and Scholarly Writing

Occupational therapy practitioners have several venues for submission of peer-reviewed publications. The *American Journal of Occupational Therapy* (AJOT) is the "...official peer-reviewed journal of the American Occupational Therapy Association" (AOTA, 2012, p. S104). This journal is published in hard copy and in an online format. The author's responsibilities, types of articles, format, and requirement for APA reference style are listed in the *Guidelines for Contributors to AJOT*, which was published as a supplement to Volume 66 of the journal in 2012 (AOTA, 2012).

This guideline document is especially helpful to novice writers who have not had the experience of submitting manuscripts for review. In addition to providing the specific responsibilities required of all authors, the guideline document lists the various types of articles that will be reviewed by the AOTA peer-review boards.

## Types of Articles Accepted by the American Journal of Occupational Therapy

Several types of articles will be accepted for review, including feature-length articles on original research (25 pages or a maximum of 5,000 words), critical reviews (related to works on occupational therapy), brief reports (15 pages or a maximum of 3,000 words) that address a pilot program or a research need, and case reports (20 pages maximum or 4,000 words) that address a short report of original work on a "case example of a clinical situation."

One interesting possibility for an AJOT submission is called "The Issue Is." These articles address current issues in the field that are being debated in the literature. These submissions have an 18-page or 3,500-word maximum.

Letters to the editor are published only in the online version of the journal. These are the only submissions to AJOT that are not peer reviewed for the journal.

## Manuscript Preparation

There is an entire section devoted to the requirements for manuscript preparation, including a requirement that authors submit a masked (AOTA, 2012) version of the manuscript to ensure that there is no identifying information. This is called a blind review, in which the reviewers do not know the source of the submission. In addition, requirements for the title page and the inclusion of an abstract and key words are described. The author is instructed on how to list practice implications and an acknowledgment page and to use the Sixth Edition of the *Publication Manual of the American Psychological Association* (APA, 2010) for referencing.

Information regarding the inclusion of figures, illustrations, tables, statistics, tests and assessment tools, abbreviations, and permissions is also specifically defined in the author instructions.

The process of how the manuscript is reviewed is described in detail, as well as the fact that after a manuscript is accepted, authors must give AOTA copyright ownership of the publication: "Manuscripts published in the journal are copyrighted by AOTA and may not be published elsewhere without permission" (AOTA, 2012).

Last, there is a reference for the author to complete an online registration at http://ajot.submit2aota.org. This registration includes a checklist so the authors ensure compliance with all of the requirements of a submission.

## *Additional Writing Opportunities for the American Occupational Therapy Association*

The AOTA has a program called the Evidence Exchange for Critically Appraised Papers (Arbesman, Lieberman, & Bondoc, 2012). This program is a storehouse for evidence-based practice articles that are judged for their scientific validity and value to the profession. Articles that are accepted for this program are generally submitted from articles classified as "CATS," which stands for "critically approved topics," through the AOTA. These topics are divided into practice areas that address evidence-based studies and are then posted in the Evidence-Based Practice and Research section of the AOTA's website. Criteria for this submission process are included on the AOTA's website. The criteria include the following:

- The article or study describes an intervention within the scope of occupational therapy practice.
- The article was published in a peer-reviewed journal.
- The article has Level I, II, or III evidence.
- The article was published within the past 10 years of date of critically appraised paper submission.
- Study was published more than 10 years from date of critically appraised paper submission but is considered "classic or seminal" (e.g., influential impact on the field, frequently cited, etc.).
- The critically appraised paper does not duplicate an article currently included in the AOTA Evidence Exchange.
- Finally, the purpose of this program is to support the Centennial Vision by giving practitioners the opportunity to participate in a science and evidence-based practice.

Further information can be found on the AOTA website, if one uses the search function for "Evidence Exchange" or "Author Guidelines."

## Competency in Scholarly Writing

There have been few studies in the literature regarding the perceptions of graduate students and what they have found useful in programs that have taught them how to write scholarly papers (Fallahi, Wood, Austad, & Fallahi, 2006). The little that is documented in the literature discusses the fact that writing skills, in general, are usually taught in undergraduate level composition courses. The level of writing required for scholarly works is certainly beyond what would be acceptable for these lower level courses. Fallahi et al. (2006, p. 171) discussed the "...dearth of evidence-based methods of writing instruction for undergraduate psychology students" as meeting an unmet need in most curricula.

## Reasons to Write a Scholarly Paper

The task before us as professionals is to ascertain how to gain the skills necessary to write in a scholarly manner. Skills for this are not usually taught to occupational therapy practitioners in the same manner as our skills for client assessment and treatment. Rocco and Hatcher (2011) described scholarly writing as "...a difficult undertaking, and a challenge that produces growth and satisfaction—all at the same time." (p. 3). The authors discussed the fact that getting started with a piece of writing is a daunting task—one that can take hours, days, or sometimes months of work just to get started. People choose to write for different reasons, both personal and professional. Academics (especially those in new faculty positions) write to keep their positions, earn promotions in rank, and increase their visibility or prestige within a university or discipline. Some universities and colleges offer merit raises based on a faculty member's productivity in being published. Undertaking scholarly writing with the idea of immediate profit is not supported in the literature (Rocco & Hatcher, 2011). Profit is rather a long-term effect in that a show of advanced knowledge, prominence, and prestige in a field can open the doors to better professional opportunities. In the case of academia, publications in specialty areas can lead to invitations for presentations at conferences that can pay handsomely, as well as provide the opportunity for reimbursement for all expenses and the added benefit of travel to places that one might not otherwise ever visit.

## How to Create Writing Opportunities

Establishing a network of colleagues to serve as mentors is one of the best ways to begin the journey of scholarly writing. Reading the work of good writers and reflecting on what makes it good can help. Attending lectures and seminars given by writers can assist in honing the craft of writing. Networking at conferences is an excellent way to meet new colleagues and share what your skills are and what you would be interested in writing

> **Case Study**
>
> Rocco and Hatcher (2011) discussed a case study in which students became involved in the area of scholarly writing. Two graduate students in a Master in Health Education program decided that they wanted to submit a paper for acceptance at a local conference. Their professor was very experienced in both doing professional presentations and submitting juried scholarly articles. The students worked hard at many rewrites and incorporated the revisions that were suggested by their skilled professor. They were accepted to present their paper at the conference, and then based on feedback from discussions at the conference, they revised their manuscript and submitted it to a peer-reviewed journal. Not only was the paper accepted for publication, but the article won an award for the best student paper.
>
> Having won the award for the best article, the students had many exciting doors open to them. They were both offered positions at an institute that provided continuing education courses on weekends all throughout the United States. So in addition to gaining a lucrative side job (the salary was not quoted, but speaking engagements such as this can pay from $1,000 to $2,000 per day), they traveled the country with all expenses paid. One of them eventually successfully competed for a position as a keynote speaker and was awarded an all-expenses-paid trip to a health conference in South Africa.
>
> Although this is an extreme example, it illustrates what can happen when someone becomes adept and competent in scholarly writing and presentations. The need to determine why a person is doing the scholarly writing can greatly help with the motivation and perseverance it takes to do it. Some scholars write to so they can secure or advance in faculty positions, but most engage in the activity of writing to "...clarify ideas, explore areas, and contribute to [their] profession" (Rocco & Hatcher, 2011, p. 4). This relates back to the section in this chapter that addressed the AOTA's official document on the various types of scholarship.
>
> It is apparent throughout the literature that there are many reasons to write. For most authors, financial reward is the least of all motivators. Most scholars write so they are a part of the professional conversation. The motivation for others may be the sense of power, self-satisfaction, or the pure sense of happiness in seeing their name in print when the work is accepted and published.

about. Some reflection is required in that you need to determine if you would feel more comfortable writing alone or in a group. Certainly, if you are involved in any group research projects, a joint effort is best for publications that are submitted for peer review. You also need to verbalize and let others know that you are interested in this endeavor. It is important to solidify connections and be sure to follow through on any opportunities that might present themselves. In the case of students, it is important to be proactive in setting up and attending meetings. Attend the meeting with an agenda and take notes, being especially careful to pay attention to the process required and the deadlines to be met (Rocco & Hatcher, 2011). Notes taken in an "action item" format with due dates can help keep you on track.

Other opportunities that can arise are the call for papers that are published in professional and trade journals requesting writings for conferences, journals, and books.

The AOTA sends out a call for papers in the late spring for the annual conference each year. Criteria for submission are listed, as well as the need for an abstract to describe the work. Careful detail must be paid to the deadlines. Most conference submissions are now done online via the use of computerized systems. These systems ensure anonymity on the part of the submitter when the application is reviewed.

## The Importance of Correct Citation in Scholarly Writing

Scholarly writing is a challenge to all who attempt it. Not only must the author present information that is based on fact, but the author must also write with the integrity necessary to cite the sources of information and then do so correctly. Sutherland-Smith discussed "... what it means to be an author—and the rights attached to authorship" (2008, p. 3). She further posited that one of the difficulties in original writing and the avoidance of plagiarism is that individuals view it differently (especially in the world of higher education). Proper citations lead to full disclosure of one's sources of information; therefore, the occurrence of plagiarism (whether intended or accidental) can be lessened.

Lipson (2006) outlined three reasons to cite materials used as (1) to give credit to the work of others, (2) to inform the reader as to the source of the material on which you have based your ideas, and (3) to direct the audience on how to find the information so they can either verify a written work or complete further investigations on a topic. Therefore, when an author uses correct citations, this accomplishes several things. It gives the author credit for his or her work and legitimizes the ideas presented by outlining what is current in the literature.

### *Definition of Plagiarism*

Many authors discuss the various intricacies of the meaning of the word plagiarism (Dee & Jacob, 2010; Lipson, 2006; Sutherland-Smith, 2008); all comment on the fact that plagiarism is a complex issue, the base of which is fraud. The following is the definition of plagiarism from *Merriam-Webster Online Dictionary*: "The act of using another person's words or ideas without giving credit to that person: the act of plagiarizing something" (2013).

Dee and Jacob (2010) completed a study of more than 1,200 undergraduate student papers. In the experiment, half of the students completed an antiplagiarism tutorial before submitting their papers. The results of the study showed that the rate of plagiarism decreased substantially, and a follow-up study led the authors to theorize that incidents of plagiarism are a student "behavior" that can be changed by increasing knowledge of the act of plagiarism. The authors posited that the act of plagiarism is indicative not just of poor academic integrity, but in more of the cases, a lack of understanding on the part of the student regarding what constitutes plagiarism. Students were less likely to plagiarize because they had a better understanding of what plagiarism is and how it can be avoided.

## *Plagiarism in Today's World*

In a world in which we have unlimited access to sources because of electronic databases and the Internet, novice writers may not understand the importance of avoiding non-citation of sources that are "out there" on the Internet. According to Baehr and Schaller (2010), having the information at our fingertips may be easier than when authors had to physically go to a library, look in card catalogs, and retrieve their sources. With this convenience comes the onus of "mastering many skills... even within the last decade due to shifts in technology, expectations of the [reader] and content" (p. 3). Online searching and use of key words can bring up many results. Many authors do not read entire articles because of the volume of search results. If one is not extremely conscientious about tracking this flood of information, unintended plagiarism might occur.

The AOTA's *Occupational Therapy Code of Ethics* (2015) aligns one of the identified core values with the need for occupational therapy practitioners to "...provide comprehensive, accurate, and objective information when representing the profession" (p. 7). This is identified by the AOTA as Principal 5, Veracity (p. 7). Under this principal, occupational therapy practitioners shall "give credit and recognition when using the ideas and work of others in written, oral, or electronic media (i.e., do not plagiarize)."

## *Tips for Avoiding Plagiarism*

Antiplagiarism programs, such as Turn It In (http://turnitin.com), can be useful tools that are employed primarily by institutions of higher education to evaluate whether written information is original or if it has been plagiarized. Programs such as these can be used not just by academics who are grading papers but also by students or writers who wish to employ online plagiarism and grammar checks. Turn It In also offers online tutoring. All of these services are fee based, according to which portion of the program is selected.

Free online resources that are valid, regularly updated, and reliable can be helpful to writers. Two of these are Thesaurus.com (http://thesaurus.com), which enables writers to search for synonyms, antonyms, and definitions, and OWL (http://owl.english.purdue.edu), an excellent educational website that offers more than 200 free resources, including information on academic writing and source citations in APA, MLA, and Chicago citation formats.

# Professional Presentation of Scholarly Works

An essential part of the scholarly process is the presentation of the work at professional conferences and other venues so an author can share his or her work with others. Conference proposals may be identified as a call for papers, which is posted in both scholarly and trade journals. There may or may not be a required theme for proposals.

## *Initiating the Process for Presentation*

The first thing to consider when you see a call for papers is to read the requirements, criteria, and deadline for submission. If possible, it is advantageous to submit your work before the deadline. Late submissions may make a poor initial impression on the reviewers because it may suggest to them poor planning or time management skills. Most proposals require an abstract of between 250 to 300 words, and these are submitted online with a character limit for each section. It is imperative that the writing be concise and makes an impression on those who will be reviewing the submission. Key words should have high effect and relate directly to the topic being proposed.

## *Important Considerations for Proposal Writing*

The initial item to be considered is who the future audience will be. This will help determine the level of information and how detailed the proposal and eventually the presentation will be. Questions such as whether the presentation will be for all occupational therapy practitioners or for the general public must be considered.

Smith and Gutman (2011) addressed the issue of health literacy as the ability of people to understand the terms connected with health care. This factor must be taken into account if a presentation is delivered to an audience of various types of stakeholders who are not cognizant of scientific or medical terminology. Presentation proposals for large groups require the author to speak in such a way that everyone in the audience will understand and benefit from the information presented.

Quotations should be used judiciously and only to emphasize an idea. It is important that the text in the proposal conveys the meaning of the author's intent and does not overuse quotations from others. If a writer is comparing studies or the work of others, clarity is required that connotes original ideas for the proposal.

# Types of Papers

There are several types of presentations, including paper presentations, panel presentations, roundtables, and poster presentations.

## *Paper Presentations*

Paper presentations are usually read aloud at a conference; most times, the presenter uses audiovisual equipment to illustrate the points. PowerPoint presentations, graphs, tables, and other pictorial images are used to demonstrate the salient points of the presentation. The depth and breadth of the presentation depend on the sophistication and professional level of the audience. Some audiences are well versed in research and interested in the design of a study. Other audiences may be less educated in the topic and might be attending the presentation for more useful and practical information. The speaker will be aware of the level of the audience because of the process of the proposal and from which professional body the call for papers originated.

## *Panel Presentations*

Panel presentations usually consist of three to four participants. Formats vary regarding how the information is presented. Most panels are designed so that each member gives a 15- to 20-minute presentation, which may or may not use PowerPoint or other audiovisual aids. The leader of the panel will generally decide if questions should immediately follow each presentation or if there will be time incorporated into the presentation for questions and answers at the end. It is always best practice (both for the speaker and the audience) to announce at the beginning of the presentation how questions will be handled. Time management and awareness are the responsibility of the panel members, although there may be a leader or moderator assigned to the panel.

## *Roundtables*

Roundtable presentations average five to six speakers. Each speaker is generally allowed 5 to 10 minutes to discuss his or her topic. This format can be slightly less formal than a panel discussion, and the topic is generally a timely issue that is shared by the participants. Written materials may be distributed before the discussion to have more targeted questions posed by the attendees.

## *Poster Presentations*

Poster presentations are those in which the presenter prepares a visual display about his or her research or topic. It is a medium that lends itself well to graphs, tables, artwork, and photographic images. Generally, the author of the poster is present at a specified time and is able to converse with attendees in this most informal style of presentation. Materials used for the poster can range from inexpensive cardboard displays to professionally produced laminated posters. The laminated posters offer the most professional-looking results; however, they can be costly. Printing services such as FedEx or others will charge according to the size of the poster. Poster sizes may be regulated by the organization that is hosting a conference. This might be related to how much space there is for presentation. For example, printing charges for a 24- x 36-inch poster may cost more than $100 (depending on the printing options chosen and shipping and handling costs, with additional fees charged if it is requested to be a "rush").

# General Information About Proposals

Most professional proposals are submitted online and are completed as blind reviews, in which the reviewers do not know who has submitted the proposal. In the case of the AOTA, an online system such as the the Online Abstract Submission and Invitation System is used in which the proposer submits his or her ideas for the paper, including an abstract and learning objectives. Several months later, the proposer receives an email response that will indicate whether the paper has been accepted or not. At that time, the proposer is made aware of the final score that is assigned by the reviewers (AOTA, 2013).

## *Tips for Successful Presentation Submissions*

Proposals should reflect the author's interest, expertise, and enthusiasm for the subject. They should be thoughtfully written, as well as concise and clear. Learning objectives should be written that complete the phrase: "By the end of this presentation, the participant will be able to..." and should end with an action verb such as "explain" or "describe."

Topics that are too broad most likely will lessen the chance of acceptance. Researchers should be sure to do adequate research on the topic in advance so they are aware of the types of topics that are timely and have not been presented before. Rating and acceptance of submissions are completed by experienced scholars and professionals in the field, so the author should be sure to design a proposal that has originality and a topic that has the potential to advance the profession.

For some proposals, the reviewers might be looking for a "theme." If this is the case, that will be outlined in the call for papers. If a theme is part of the criteria for acceptance for a particular conference, be sure that your topic is clearly aligned with the theme and that your explanation illustrates that linkage.

Above all, be sure that your proposal is well written, clear, and free of any grammatical or spelling errors. Proofread, proofread, and proofread again! It is also helpful to have someone else (a colleague within the field) proofread for you. You may know what you mean by a particular section of your proposal, but it might not be as clear as you think. Be willing to take constructive criticism and put your ego aside if you ask the opinion of others; just make sure you ask persons whose opinion you can trust.

### *Submitting a Conference Proposal*

The method in which you submit a conference proposal will vary according to the method used by the reviewing body. Some are submitted via email, and others are submitted via online systems, such as the aforementioned Online Abstract Submission and Invitation System. In any event, be sure to follow the requirements of the proposal and make sure your credentials (and those of any co-presenters) are properly identified. If the proposal is to be sent via email in an attachment, be sure to send it as a Microsoft Word document because this format can be accessed by the majority of computers. Use of double spacing and a clear font (usually Times New Roman) is the preferred style. The document should be saved as a Portable Document Format (pdf) file because these files cannot be edited with free software and are accessible with most computer operating systems. Be sure to review all of the requirements several times and proofread the document before submitting the proposal.

If an electronic system is used, be aware of the character space limits, especially in the box that is usually included for the abstract. Be sure to make the best use of your limited characters in your writing so your proposal topic is clear to the reviewers. With these types of systems, you may be able to go in and out of the system at various times while you craft your proposal. In any electronic submission system, you will be issued a log-in and password that will be necessary to access and edit your entry, so be sure to keep track of this information. The password and log-in will most likely be autogenerated by the system, so they may not be characters that are easy to remember. Either write them down or send them to yourself in an email so you can access your information for later retrieval.

## Presenting the Conference Paper

Congratulations if your paper is accepted! Now you are on to the next steps, which are even more daunting than the proposal. It is important to decide on the purpose of the presentation (Jacobs & Gafni-Lachter, 2015). Are you reviewing a research project, teaching a treatment technique, or merely demonstrating an activity?

Koegel (2007) discusses the fact of being organized from the first notification of your acceptance. He uses the acronym of OPEN UP as representing "...the six characteristics shared by exceptional presenters."

- **O: Be organized.** Koegel believes that the message should be delivered in a structured flow, one that the audience can easily follow.
- **P: Be passionate.** Exceptional presenters "exude enthusiasm and conviction." Convey a positive energy not just about the topic but also about the fact that you appreciate your audience.
- **E: Be engaging.** Build rapport with the audience quickly and engage them immediately. An introduction or short personal anecdote informs your audience who you are, how you are qualified, and why they should listen to you.
- **N: Be natural.** Exceptional presenters convey a conversational feel as they deliver their presentations. They also appear comfortable with their audience, and this comfort level in turn makes the audience more confident.
- **U: Understand your audience.** Taking a poll of the audience (by a show of hands to various questions) can help you understand your audience. For example, in occupational therapy, it would be helpful to know how many participants in the audience are occupational therapists and how many are occupational therapy assistants.
- **P: Practice.** Practice not only improves your delivery of a presentation, but it can also greatly lessen the "stage fright" that many are faced with just before stepping up to the podium. Some presenters memorize the opening and closing remarks so they maintain eye contact with the audience during these two crucial points of the presentation. In addition, if you

are doing your presentation in a hotel or other type of conference room, it is important to visit the room the night before your presentation (if possible) so you can visualize how you will use the room. The day of the presentation, always arrive 1 hour early. Many professional conferences have "speaker's lounges" or other types of resources available if there are issues with any computer or audiovisual equipment. Arriving 1 hour early gives you the opportunity to make sure you are ready as your audience starts to arrive.

Plan ahead and if possible visit the venue the night before your presentation so that you do not encounter any surprises the day of the presentation. Be sure to begin your presentation on time. It is not fair to force those in the audience who have arrived on time to wait for you to begin because some attendees come in late.

Lastly, if one is not provided for you by the persons who are sponsoring the conference, have an evaluation form ready for participants to complete after your presentation as they leave the room. Feedback can be a valuable tool for you the next time you do a presentation. Evaluations should contain comments on the content, delivery, currency of the topic, and general logistics (e.g., was the room temperature comfortable?).

## Some Comments About Style and the Use of PowerPoint

PowerPoint can be a very useful tool when you are giving a presentation, but it should be considered just that—a tool. PowerPoint is an aid to a presentation; it should never be the presentation. The exterior content (what you say to the audience) should be different than the interior content of your slides. The notes function at the bottom of the slides (which are seen by the presenter and not by the audience) can be helpful in ensuring that you just do not read off the slides. Even the best PowerPoint presentation cannot take the place of your voice and eye contact with your audience.

Hoffman and Mittelman (2004) posit that "A successful [presentation] is one in which the speaker is able to strike a balance between conveying ideas in a serious manner and doing so in an entertaining style to maintain the audience's attention." (p. 358). They suggest (p. 359) that the title should be short—no longer than 10 words. They add that the role of the speaker is "…to enlighten the audience rather than to gratify his own ego" (p. 358). They discussed the importance of the speaker's voice (projection and inflection) and of the importance of correct enunciation and pronunciation of words. They warn to be cautious with the use of humor and to be culturally sensitive to the audience in this regard. The adage "when in doubt, leave it out" is a wise way to think about the use of humor during a presentation. Too much joking or funny slides may detract from the seriousness of the topic and may wear old on the audience. Used appropriately, and always in moderation, humor can be appropriate tool in your presentation.

Collins (2004) discussed the fact that "…the effectiveness of any presentation depends …on the ability of the presenter," and that the visual aids should be just that, an aid to the presentation. As with any audiovisual tool, PowerPoint requires planning to be effective. Items to consider are your audience, the subject, and the type of presentation you are doing. For example, if you are doing a panel presentation, the group might decide to use the same slide design for better consistency and a better final product for the audience. Quality PowerPoint presentations are suitable for your audience, the subject, and the type of presentation. Strong opening slides should be crafted to engage the audience immediately at the beginning of the presentation. The opening slide should have the name of the presentation, the author, the date, and the name of the conference or event. The second slide should consist of an outline that serves as the table of contents, and this same slide may be used at the end of the presentation for review. Learning objectives of the presentation are generally the third and fourth slides. Logos are appropriate to use in footers and help to emphasize the speaker's professional affiliation.

As the presenter designs the content slides, there must be awareness that they are appropriate for the subject and the audience. For example, if you are presenting the findings of a research study that has slides with bar graphs and data tables, animated slides with figures flying in would be distracting. They might even be annoying to some in the audience and certainly would not add anything to your presentation. In this case, clear slides without any animation or long transitions would be most appropriate. If, on the other hand, you are doing a public relations piece that explains what occupational therapy is to a community group, then that would be the appropriate place for some fun graphics and animation.

Robinson (2003) made an excellent statement about the use of a laser pointer for reinforcement, which he expressed is most useful when you are illustrating figures and images but not as effective for text. He discussed several points worth thinking about in terms of the use of a laser pointer: (1) be aware of the length of time you leave the pointer on the slide (not too long; just use it for emphasis), (2) be aware of movement while you have the pointer in your hand so that you do not "fire" at the audience, and (3) be aware of keeping your hand steady when you hold the pointer. For the last point, Robinson suggested to hold the laser pointer at the edge of the lectern as you point with it which will help to steady your hand, and the laser will not move all around.

## Specifics Regarding Slide Design in PowerPoint: Fonts and Backgrounds

Fonts used for presentations should be clear and the size large enough that the audience can read. Use of sans serif fonts are almost always the most appropriate. OWL defines a sans serif (or non-serif) font as one that has no "feet" (although both the OWL and others cannot claim the exact derivation of this term). This information can be found at the OWL's website at http://owl.english.purdue.edu/owl/resource/705/02. In essence, it means that the font style is more of a plain block style that does not have any additional "flair." The best examples of sans serif fonts are Calibri and Arial; this is why they are used most often in published works.

Most title slides are best written in a font size of 44, and subtitles are most suitable in a range from 28 to 34. It is distracting to the audience if different font styles are used. Lettering in bold or in italics is generally the preferred way to emphasize points. Bullets, if used, should be consistent. Do not mix alphabetical bullets with numerical bullets; use one or the other. Generally, numbers can be confusing unless you are trying to demonstrate a hierarchical relationship within a list. For example, if the slide is meant to show the prevalence of different types of diseases within a population, it would be appropriate to label the diagnosis that occurs the most with the value 1 and then list the remaining diagnoses with the appropriate sequential numbers.

In terms of the slide's background design, use of contrast allows for greater visibility. The suggestion is to use a light-colored lettering on a dark background or dark lettering on a light background. Keep in mind that to some in the audience, a white screen may cause glare. Colors often appear lighter when projected, and pastel colors may even appear to be white, depending on the projector. Always look at your slide design with a critical eye and imagine how you would react to it if you were in the audience. For example, use of red lettering on a dark blue background can give the optical illusion of the words "dancing" on the page, and this cannot only be an annoyance to the audience but can also detract from the message on the slide. Finally, consistency in the design of the entire presentation creates a more professional appearance. The bottom line is that you want the audience to focus on your presentation, not on your background effects.

One common mistake made in PowerPoint slides is when presenters put too much text on one slide. An excess of text on a slide makes it difficult to read, especially if the presentation is being given in a large room that only has one screen. The goal of a PowerPoint presentation is to have the slides as a reference; the design should allow the audience to attend to what the presenter is saying, not to struggle to see what is up on the screen. Source citations should be included on the slide with the cited information, so be sure to leave room for the entire appropriate citation.

At the conclusion of your presentation, it is helpful to have a slide that says "Thank You" or "Questions and Answers." This is a professional way of closing your presentation and letting your audience know that you are finished. Have you ever attended a presentation and the speaker stands there at the end and says something like, "Well, that's it!"? Don't you find that to be an awkward way to end a presentation? It almost makes it seem as though the end of the presentation was not planned at all. It does not leave the audience with a good impression. Conducting a question-and-answer period followed by a thank you to the audience is the most professional way to complete a presentation.

Be sure to be aware of what you are proficient at with the use of PowerPoint and keep the tips listed in this chapter in mind as you prepare your slides. Koegel (2007) reminds speakers to minimize eye contact with objects in the room (i.e., the screen) and maximize eye contact with the people to ensure an effective presentation. Always face forward to your audience; never turn your back while you glance at your slides for reference. To secure the audience's attention, leave time between slides and maintain eye contact with your audience. By following these tips and by practicing and knowing what is on your slides, you can deliver an effective PowerPoint presentation that will hold the attention of the audience from your first word to the final question.

## Summary

This chapter has provided an overview of the definitions and importance of scholarly writing to the growth of the field of occupational therapy and to those who are fortunate enough to practice in this profession. The competence needed for the completion of scholarly writing was explored with an emphasis on the types of scholarship available to occupational therapy practitioners. Discussion of the AOTA's Centennial Vision further illustrated why scholarly writing and the ultimate presentation of the work at conferences will advance the profession of occupational therapy for future generations of practitioners. Occupational therapy practitioners are charged with the responsibility of attaining the goals that were delineated by the leaders in the profession on the occasion of the 100th year of the profession. Occupational therapy scholarly writers must strive to be recognized as individuals who base their writings in sound, evidence-based science and who are competent in assisting the advancement of the profession into the next centennial.

## Evidence-Based Research Chart

| Topic | Evidence |
|---|---|
| Occupational therapy scholarship | AOTA, 2009, 2012, 2015 |
| Scholarly writing | AOTA, 2009; Rocco & Hatcher, 2011 |
| APA format for source citation | APA, 2010; Lipson, 2006 |
| Plagiarism | Beins, 2012; Harris, 2005; Sutherland-Smith, 2008 |
| Professional presentation | Koegel, 2007 |

## Student Self-Assessment

1. What does "scholarship" consist of in the field of occupational therapy?
2. Identify the components that must be included to complete an article that will be submitted for a peer-reviewed journal.
3. How did this chapter help you to understand the definition of plagiarism? Can you explain how the appropriate use of citations lessens the chance of unintended plagiarism?
4. You have been given an assignment to do a 15-minute presentation on osteoarthritis. The professor requires that you include evidence-based data and that you create a PowerPoint presentation that will be given in class. What steps would you take to plan this project? How would you design your PowerPoint slides?

## Acknowledgments

I would like to thank Karen Jacobs, EdD, OTR/L, CPE, FAOTA, and Nancy MacRae, MS, OTR/L, FAOTA, for their guidance and support in the writing of this chapter.

## Electronic Resources

American Occupational Therapy Association: http://www.aota.org

American Psychological Association: http://apastyle.org

FedEx: http://www.fedex.com/us

Merriam-Webster Online Dictionary and Thesaurus: http://www.merriam-webster.com

Purdue Online Writing Lab: http://owl.english.purdue.edu

Thesaurus.com: http://thesaurus.com

Turn It In: http://turnitin.com

## References

Aitchison, C., & Lee, A. (2006). Research writing: Problems and pedagogies. *Teaching in Higher Education, 11*, 265-278.

American Occupational Therapy Association. (2007). AOTA's Centennial Vision and executive summary. *American Journal of Occupational Therapy, 61*, 613-614.

American Occupational Therapy Association. (2009). Scholarship in occupational therapy. *American Journal of Occupational Therapy, 63*, 790-796.

American Occupational Therapy Association. (2012). Guidelines for contributors to AJOT. *American Journal of Occupational Therapy, 6*(Suppl.), S104-S107.

American Occupational Therapy Association. (2013). Retrieved from http://www.aota.org.

American Occupational Therapy Association. (2015). Occupational therapy code of ethics (2015). *American Journal of Occupational Therapy, 69*(Suppl. 3).

American Psychological Association. (2010). *Publication manual of the American Psychological Association* (6th ed.). Washington, DC: Author.

Arbesman, M., Lieberman, D., & Bondoc, S. (2012, December 17). Evidence exchange: Writing a critically appraised paper. *OT Practice*, 8.

Baehr, C., & Schaller, B. (2010). *Writing for the internet: A guide to real communication in virtual space*. Santa Barbara, CA: Greenwood Press

Beins, B. C. (2012). *APA style simplified*. Hoboken, NJ: John Wiley & Sons. Retrieved from http://mercycollege.eblib.com/patron/FullRecord/aspx?p=822040

Belcher, W. L. (2009). *Writing your journal article in 12 weeks: A guide to academic publishing success*. Thousand Oaks, CA: Sage Publications.

Boyer, E. L. (1990). *Scholarship reconsidered: Priorities of the professoriate*. San Francisco, CA: Jossey-Bass.

Boyer, E. L. (1996). The scholarship of engagement. *Journal of Public Service and Outreach, 1*, 11-20.

Braveman, B. (2006). *Leading and managing occupational therapy services: An evidence-based approach*. Philadelphia, PA: F. A. Davis Company.

Braveman, B. H., Helfrich, C. A., & Fisher, G. S. (2001). Developing and maintaining community partnerships within "a scholarship of practice." *Occupational Therapy in Health Care, 15*, 109-125.

Collins, J. (2004). Giving a PowerPoint presentation: The art of communicating effectively. *Radiographics, 24*, 4, 1-7.

Dallimore, E. J., Hertenstein, J. H., & Platt, M. B. (2008). Using discussion pedagogy to enhance oral and written communication skills. *College Teaching, 56*, 163-172.

Dee, T. S., & Jacob, B. A. (2010). *Rational ignorance in education: A field experiment in student plagiarism. National Bureau of Economic Research, working paper 15672*. Retrieved from http://www.nber.org/papers/w15672

Fallahi, C. R., Wood, R. M., Austad, C. S., & Fallahi, H. (2006). A program for improving undergraduate psychology students' basic writing skills. *Teaching of Psychology, 33*(3), 171-175.

Harris, R. A. (2005). *Using sources effectively: Strengthening your writing and avoiding plagiarism* (2nd ed.). Glendale, CA: Pyrczak Pub.

Hoffman, M., & Mittelman, M. (2004). Presentations at professional meeting: Notes, suggestions and tips for speakers. *European Journal in Internal Medicine, 15*, 358-363.

Jacobs, K., & Gafni-Lachter, L. (2015, October 26). Best presenters: Public speaking for occupational therapy practitioners. *OT Practice*, 7-12.

Koegel, T. J. (2007). *The exceptional presenter: A proven formula to open up and own the room*. Austin, TX: Greenleaf Book Group Press.

Lavelle, E., & Bushrow, K. (2007). Writing approaches of graduate students. *Educational Psychology, 27*, 807-822.

Lipson, C. (2006). *Cite right: A quick guide to citation styles—MLA, APA, Chicago, the sciences, professions, and more*. Chicago, IL: University of Chicago Press.

Modern Language Association. (2008). *MLA style manual and guide to scholarly publishing* (3rd ed.). New York, NY: Author.

Plagiarism. (2013). In *Merriam-Webster online dictionary*. Retrieved from http://www.merriam-webster.com

Purdue University. (2012). *Purdue online writing lab: OWL*. Retrieved from http://owl.english.purdue.edu

Robinson, J. P. (2003, February 2012). *Presentation 101 for graduate students: A guide to giving a quality presentation*. Message posted to http://www.cyto.purdue.edu/education

Rocco, T. S., & Hatcher, T. (2011). *The handbook of scholarly writing and publishing*. San Francisco, CA: Jossey-Bass.

Smith, D. L., & Gutman, S. A. (2011). Health literacy in occupational therapy practice and research. *American Journal of Occupational Therapy, 65*(4), 367-369.

Sutherland-Smith, W. (2008). *Plagiarism, the internet and student learning*. New York, NY: Routledge.

University of Chicago Press. (2010). *The Chicago manual of style* (16th ed.). Chicago, IL: Author.

## Suggested Reading

Venkatraman, V. (2010, April 16). *Conventions of scientific authorship*. Retrieved from http://www.sciencemag.org/careers/2010/04/conventions-scientific-authorship.

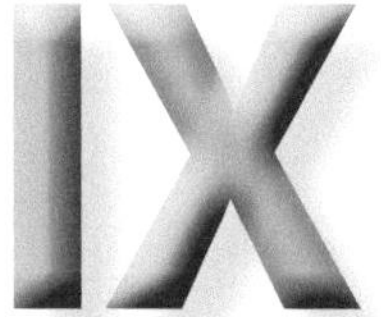

# Professional Ethics, Values, and Responsibilities

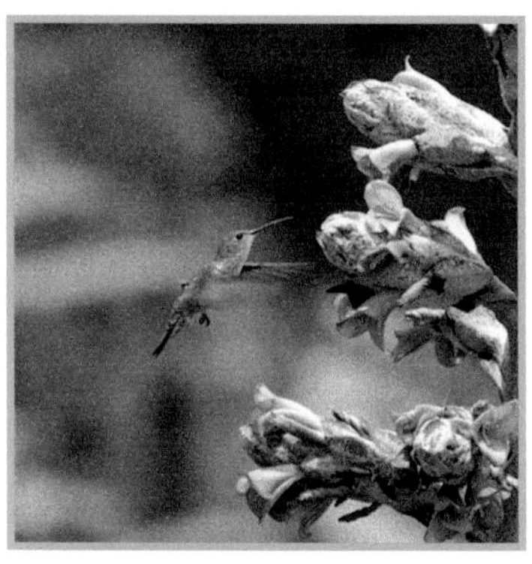

# 50

# Ethics and Its Application to Occupational Therapy Practice

*Gail M. Bloom, OTD, MA, OTR/L*

**ACOTE STANDARDS EXPLORED IN THIS CHAPTER**

B.9.1, B.9.2

**KEY VOCABULARY**

- **Code of Ethics:** A collection of formal explicit statements forming a moral guide for an identified group outlining right and valued behavior, principles, and values.
- **Ethics:** A set of value-based principles to assist the individual in making moral decisions. Ethics examines how an individual should think and behave toward others.
- **Morality:** The accepted standards of right or wrong that direct the conduct of a person or a group.
- **Principles:** Basic rules of conduct.
- **Values:** Ethical principles that set a standard of quality or a worthwhile ideal.



Jacobs, K., & MacRae, N. (Eds.).
*Occupational Therapy Essentials for Clinical Competence, Third Edition* (pp. 715-731).

Occupational therapy is firmly rooted in ethical concepts and principles and has a long tradition of caring about morality-based social values. The earliest practitioners were concerned with concepts such as autonomy and independence and issues such as meaningful and productive. Occupational therapy professional values are fundamentally linked to quality of life (QOL) issues. Central to the practice of occupational therapy is a commitment to these ethical QOL issues. The promotion of maximum independence by enhancing functional ability and adapting the environment is basic to promoting QOL. The profession has always emphasized self-sufficiency through occupation that is meaningful to the individual.

Philosophers place an emphasis on concepts such as fairness, equality, goodness, justice, consequence, and obligation. These moral concepts provide a traditional foundation to create a practical, function-based approach to ethics. This chapter begins by establishing a foundation of understanding through an examination of some basic ethical concepts. The chapter looks at societal groups and organizations for the structural hallmarks or characteristic building blocks necessary for the implementation of ethical principles. This chapter shows how everyday practice provides opportunity for the direct application of ethics.

## Ethics and Its Application to Occupational Therapy Practice

In the rapidly changing health care environment, occupational therapy practitioners are confronted with complex ethical issues. As professionals, occupational therapy practitioners must take responsibility for understanding applicable policies, federal and state laws, and association principles. Occupational therapy practitioners must maintain high standards of professional competence, including an understanding of ethics. The moral aspects of practice require professionalism. Professional competencies include knowing how to obtain informed consent, knowing what to do if a client refuses intervention, and knowing how to communicate confidential material. Development of professional skills assists occupational therapy practitioners to make ethical decisions for moral behavior.

Occupational therapy and the study of ethics share common ground because both are concerned with individual choice. Both the ethical decision-making process and the clinical problem-solving approach of occupational therapy can rely on a process for function-based analysis. Ethical reasoning is a part of clinical decision making.

Critical thinking requires carefully weighing alternatives. Deliberate analysis is a part of solving problems. An implicit or explicit judgment guides decisions about which problems are worthy of attention. Ethical decision making is, of necessity, woven among the threads of clinical decision making. Ethical decision making is a mandatory component of clinical problem solving. Both involve the identification of the principles specific to the particular case situation, contemplation, negotiation, and reaching a resolution. The conceptual understanding of ethics is critical to decoding the complexity of specific situations. Occupational therapy practitioners should take all case-specific factors into consideration before making reasoned decisions. Daily clinical issues provide opportunity for the direct application of ethics in everyday practice. Ethical action is the product of ethical decision making.

An understanding of ethics can assist in sorting out complicated health and social issues. The same ingredients can be useful for ethical problem solving in all areas of practice, including the clinical, corporate, and academic settings. Perhaps the secret recipe is seeking a balance of theoretical knowledge and practical application well seasoned with humanistic empathy and caring. An understanding of ethics helps occupational therapy practitioners know how to cope with QOL issues and quality of care problems.

## A Foundation of Understanding

Essentially, ethics is a set of value-based principles to assist the individual in making moral decisions. Ethics examines how an individual should think and behave toward others. Morality is the accepted standard of right or wrong that directs the conduct of a person or group. Morality is learned early. Personal concepts of right and wrong are gathered from a variety of sources. The social environment is filled with influences that affect moral choice, including family, school, religion, and the media. A choice, or conversely, avoidance of a particular choice, made as a mature adult could be influenced by moral rules learned as a child at home or in kindergarten (Fulghum, 1988): share, work cooperatively, do not cheat, treat others with respect. We learn morality by example from role models and by analogies shared through narratives (Cowley, 2005).

A basic rule of conduct is known as an *ethical principle*. An ethical principle that sets a standard of quality or a worthwhile ideal is a value. Most people consider certain values such as caring, honesty, and respect to be morally worthy. Tradition and custom have assigned worth to certain actions. Social norms set the expectation for certain behaviors and avoidance of other behaviors. Some social norms have been codified into law.

The practical application of knowledge is as fundamental to the study of ethics as it is to the practice of occupational therapy. There is an obligation to examine one's own personal values and belief system with recognition and insight of oneself as a moral agent. The honorable occupational therapy practitioner must have self-awareness. The process of becoming self-aware allows for an organization of one's belief system. The organization of ethical principles into an orderly system of beliefs assists the individual in making ethical decisions for determining rightness, morality, and praiseworthy behavior from wrongness, immorality, and blameworthy behavior. As an occupational therapy practitioner there is a social and legal obligation to consider the consequences of one's actions. A moral individual must focus on the questioning that results in making a decision to act or to not take action. Moral occupational therapy practitioners must focus on the case-specific human factors toward a process of clinical reasoning resulting in ethical decisions. An ethical decision is based on a thoughtful judgment, resulting in the production of action or the inhibition of action. Judgment is the act of deciding after considering alternatives. Ethics involves right and wrong conduct as determined by a reasoned thought process.

## Theories of Fundamental Characteristics

Some philosophical schools of thought promote the idea that belief systems are based on basic rules. The deontological theory of reasoning relies on an acceptance of universal law or accepted truths. Proponents of these belief systems suggest that fundamental objective principles of morality exist. When making a decision, the fundamental principles of morality are examined for guidance to determine the best plan of action. An action is judged either "good" or "bad" because of the intrinsic nature of the action to be good or bad. There is an objective understanding of what is accepted as "good" or "bad." There is an obligation for action or inaction simply because some deeds are praiseworthy or blameworthy. Action is either right or wrong. One is obligated to a course of action that promotes goodness. There is an explicit call to duty. Awareness of moral standards is necessary to choose in accordance with inherent moral guides. The correct course of action can be determined by applying the appropriate obligatory rule to the situation. Rules based on universal law set standards. Universal imperatives include natural order and the Golden Rule. According to these sets of ethical rules, goodness or worth does not change with the circumstances of a specific situation.

For an example of this type of process, consider the concept of "fairness." To be "fair," all decisions must be based on a rule to treat all persons in an equitable, impartial way independent of any particular circumstances those persons might be facing. Therefore, fairness does not change with the circumstances of a specific situation. A standard of "justice" has a duty to be fair and equitable or it is "unjust" by definition.

## Theories of Comparative Characteristics

Some philosophical schools of thought do not promote the idea that belief systems should be based on inherent and unchangeable basic rules. This type of teleological theory of reasoning does not rely on an acceptance of universal law or accepted truths. Proponents of these belief systems do not suggest that fundamental principles of morality exist. The teleological theory of reasoning demands a comparative evaluation of the particular unique circumstances of a specific situation. These thinkers do not believe any rule can be valid for every possible application. Theories of teleological ethics apply a methodical process of reasoning to assess the subjective nature of "good" and "bad." One must define what is meant by "good." One must decide which action will result in the most good. Additionally, "bad" must be defined. Thought must be given to determine which action will result in the most harm. An obligation or duty to weigh the benefits and costs of any potential action must be considered with each event.

Consequentialism is based on the idea that the right or wrong action is determined by the result of that act. Actions have consequences, and consequences are compared to evaluate relative merit. Moral worth is determined with an evaluation of the consequences of an action. Careful weighing of all of the benefits and all the costs of an action is required before choosing an action judged most likely to maximize good relative to harm. An action is worthwhile if the resulting consequences are valued with more good consequences than bad consequences. The consequences of the action determine if its outcome is primarily good or bad. The outcome must be specified with a measurement of good as a defined goal. The outcome goals (or ends) are evaluated by rating the end product. Quite literally, "the ends justify the means." Ethical dilemma occurs with the acknowledgment that undesirable choices may lead to less than ideal alternatives or a need to choose between the lesser of unappealing options. A justification for action or inaction is derived from a review of options. Choosing one option will produce more benefit than selecting other options, and some options are more or less likely to produce more

Table 50-1.

**Ethical Decision Making: A Sample of a Quantitative Process for Analysis**

| Problem | Pro | Con |
|---|---|---|
| To splint or not to splint? | Avoid contractures<br>Maintain skin integrity | Amount of fabrication time<br>Several clients will not get therapy<br>Cost of material<br>On/off assistance needed<br>Cleaning assistance needed |
| **Result** | | |
| Do not make the splint. | Two pros or good idea components | Five cons or bad idea components |

harm or less harm. A prediction must be made to determine relative benefit (or utility).

Utilitarianism is one type of teleological thought system. Utilitarian thinking compares benefits and costs with an emphasis on utility. Utility is something that provides a useful purpose. Decision making using utilitarian reasoning opts for the choice that promotes the greatest good for the greatest number. Utilitarianism emphasizes achieving the greatest benefit for the largest number of individuals. A utilitarian considers the available resources and develops an objective standard for consequences. A utilitarian approach is reflected in a reliance on a standardized measurement. Contemplate the ethical guidance inherent in a QOL index, productivity report, and cost–benefit forecast. A form of utilitarianism examines the process rather than the final goal, or the "means toward the end" is evaluated. This type of thoughtful assessment relies on a comparison of situational variables. Analysis follows a separation of the whole into elemental parts because it is thought to be important to judge the "good" and "bad" of each of the components. This is an almost mathematical approach. Either a quantitative or a qualitative value is assigned to each situational variable. The variables are compared to resolve the ethical dilemma.

Ethical judgment is required when one thinks about factors such as the allocation of scarce resources. Occupational therapy practitioners rely on an implicit or explicit moral rule for guidance when determining who will get services. An ethical dilemma is present when an occupational therapy practitioner decides how to ration time because time constraints exist, and time is often a scarce resource in an occupational therapy clinic. For example, an occupational therapy practitioner is worried about the amount of time required to fabricate a splint for one client because without sufficient time in the workday, several other clients will not be seen that day. Resolution of an ethical dilemma is based on the assumption that moral value can be determined with the categorization of the arguments for and against an action. A moral decision can be made by creating a list and then counting the pros and cons. Alternatively, a moral decision can be made with a numeric value placed on each variable for a total score. Let us first solve the problem using a quantitative utilitarian analysis. Table 50-1 uses a quantitative process for ethical decision making to resolve this issue. The action (splinting) is assessed to have two good components (pros) and five bad components (cons) in our listing of situational characteristics specific to this dilemma. There are more arguments against the action. The larger amount of five situational variables on the con side of the equation necessitates a resolution against the action. The splint will not be made tomorrow.

Now we will solve the problem using a qualitative utilitarian analysis. We will see that using a qualitative analysis rather than a strictly quantitative analysis can lead to a very different result. Table 50-2 uses a qualitative process for ethical decision making to resolve this issue. The same situational characteristics specific to this dilemma are listed with a 10-point maximum quality rating scale for each factor. A quality rating is used to indicate relative benefit. The comparative numeric weight of the end result will indicate whether an action should be pursued. The action (splinting) is assessed to have a total value of 19 favorable (pros) quality value points and a total of 13 against (cons) quality value points in this situation. The larger amount of 19 points on the pro side of the equation necessitates a resolution in favor of the action. There is an obligation to perform the action in consideration because it will produce more value or benefit. The splint will be made tomorrow.

Table 50-2.

**Ethical Decision Making: A Sample of a Qualitative Process for Analysis**

| Problem | Pro | Quality Value | Con | Quality Value |
|---|---|---|---|---|
| To splint or not to splint? | Avoid contractures<br>Maintain skin integrity | 10<br>9 | Amount of fabrication time<br>Several clients will not get therapy<br>Cost of material<br>On/off assistance needed<br>Cleaning assistance needed | 4<br>5<br>2<br>1<br>1 |
| Total points | | 19 | | 13 |
| **Result** | Make the splint. | | | |

## Theories of Relative Standards

Ethical relativism is another philosophical school of thought. An underlying question asks if any rule can be valid for all people all the time. Ethical relativism is formed around the assumption that rules to guide behavior should change relative to time and place. The values of the society in which people live are recognized as important for establishing norms and community traditions. Moral principles are expected to change over the course of time. Morality is viewed as not static but changing according to the accepted standards of a specific society at a specific point in time. Actions regarded as praiseworthy or blameworthy will be (and should be) different within various cultures, religions, and other communities. There is an acceptance that certain practices are valued as praiseworthy in some communities but that the same type of action would be condemned as blameworthy in other communities. Values differ because judgment of praiseworthy and blameworthy actions is a function of the social order.

Certain actions were socially acceptable in their time but judged immoral from our perspective looking back at the circumstances of history. Historical perspective can stimulate dialogue on the appropriateness of actions. Was child labor a rational socioeconomic product of its time? Were the massive legislative and institutional changes leading to closing of hospitals and the deinstitutionalization and community integration efforts of persons with mental illness during the 1970s and 1980s justified? Well-intentioned people can disagree as to what is right or wrong. There are societal and cultural differences when judging the moral acceptability of life-sustaining measures, euthanasia, abortion, and numerous other topics of controversy. This type of reasoning can lead to incendiary debates. Ethical relativism does not provide universal rules for easy determination of good behavior.

## Making a Distinction Between Ethical and Legal

It is important to note that there are distinct differences between the law and ethics; these terms are not interchangeable. The law and ethics are not one and the same. Legal considerations and ethical concerns are not necessarily the same. Of course, there are times when legal and ethical share the same compatible basis. There are instances when illegal and unethical are consistent. Unequal pay based on gender discrimination is both against the law and unethical. There are examples of legal actions that do not seem ethical. There are historical examples of legislation with unintended ramifications resulting in major unexpected ethical problems. Choices can be legally acceptable but not ethically appropriate. As an example, widespread commercial advertising promoting cheaply made toys to children is legal but not necessarily ethical in motivation. Conversely, illegal activity can be morally defensible. The story of Robin Hood robbing the rich to give to the poor is a classic example of an illegal action that can be defended as ethically acceptable.

Federal, state, and municipal governments have the power to pass legislation and implement policy through regulations. The forces of government have jurisdiction within their own borders. Each jurisdiction monitors for compliance and develops methods of enforcement.

Laws tend to differ from state to state. Age of maturity for minors and other laws intended to safeguard the rights of persons needing special protection vary across state borders. State licensure laws protecting the public by regulating the practice of health care providers, including occupational therapy practitioners, are somewhat different from state to state. It is important to know the state licensure laws in the location of your practice. Obligation exists for a professional to know the laws, regulations, and ethical principles in the community and the place of employment. Each type of work environment can have a set of guidelines specific to place, time, and person. Universities are required by federal law to develop and implement procedures for research, and they have faculty policies.

Legal concerns and ethical issues often overlap in the delivery of health care. Courts have decided that society has an obligation to protect life, and courts have ordered life-saving medical intervention for young persons with parents who refuse intervention. On occasion, the rights of the individual conflict with the rights of society. Both medical law and medical ethics (bioethics) are in dynamic change. New legislation and the latest court decisions interpreting existing legislation create a need for up-to-date understanding of law. Federal and state judicial systems consider and then rule on court cases creating revised analysis of constitutional rights and other laws. Courts analyze specific questions and make an official ruling based on the particular situation presented in the case. Precedent is set with interpretation of influential cases and subsequent generalization to similar situations. Past dilemmas offer guidance for handling current dilemmas.

## Quality of Life

The idea of QOL is a multidimensional and complex variable that has different meaning for each individual. Good QOL is determined by the personal values of the individual. Subjective ideas for what makes a good QOL tend to change over time based on life experiences.

The concept of health-related quality of life (HRQOL) regards the factors that determine the presence or absence of health to be observable and measurable. HRQOL measures the affect of health on QOL. HRQOL measurement tools assess perceptions of wellness through ratings of physical health and mental health. HRQOL population studies can be used to provide insights into broad community needs as well as special populations in clinical settings. Diagnosis of disease, the intervention process, and the side effects of the intervention can disrupt coping strategies and occupational balance. When independence is limited or task accomplishment becomes compromised, occupational roles may be altered. HRQOL measurements assess perceptions of health status and activity performance. The presence of disability may result in limitations in functional independence and decreased opportunities for life satisfaction. QOL may be diminished from the perspective of the individual. Alternatively, enhanced perceptions of control over adverse situations may enhance positive adjustment and improve QOL. Changes in health status can encourage a personal self-assessment with exploration of standards measuring QOL and sometimes causing a reprioritizing of values. An understanding of meaningful engagement in occupation can help assess QOL beyond generalizations based on the presence of disability or cultural or gender implications. Relative independence in functional activities of daily living is not an adequate measure of HRQOL factors. QOL is more than an ability to perform self-care activities. Occupational therapy practitioners must assess beyond a fragmentation of component parts to adequately measure HRQOL.

Social policy often cannot keep pace with scientific discoveries. Advances in medical technology influence change in medical ethics. Improvements in medical technology now let us do the unimaginable. Life-sustaining techniques enable medical teams to prolong life in emergency departments, intensive care units, neonatal centers, and long-term care facilities. This creates an ethical dilemma highlighting QOL issues when the anticipated HRQOL and functional status are poor. The individual, family members, and health care professionals must sort through complex issues as they make important bioethical decisions for themselves or their loved ones.

## Health Care Resource Allocation and Distribution

Community is a source of support representing fundamental access to basic resources. Conversely, community can be a source of barriers limiting access to essential material goods. Community suggests a context surrounding the individual with influence on available choices. Community standards create customs, beliefs, attitudes, expected behaviors, and normative social routines. Public policy establishes social infrastructure. Essential commodities such as housing, food, water, and education are considered basic rights in modern society. The quality and methods of distribution of fundamental commodities vary widely. Health care disparities exist because health care access and service allotment are not always defined as a basic right. Society does not grant equal access to health care services or equality to service delivery. Populations in remote rural locations have limited access to health care because of geographic location. Parts of the population have limited access to health care because of income status or financial limitations. Ethical health care issues focus on questions of entitlement (who can get service), access (which types of services are covered), and allotment (how many services). Access to health care, entitlement, and allotment are determined by public policy. Equitable distribution refers to the moral concept of justice. If we say that benefits should be distributed in fair proportions, then we must decide how "fair" is determined. Similar to other economic-based commodities, some say health care should be a basic right, but others disagree and say that health care is not a right. Many wonder if health care can be allocated or rationed effectively or efficiently. Whether health care can be rationed fairly is a question dependent on ethical judgment.

The overburdened health care system struggles with limited resources and rising expenses. In many places, "business as usual" means doing more with less. The perception of danger or crisis has been known to legitimize organizational behavior the larger society would judge as unethical. There have been instances of price controls having resulted in "padding" allowable expenses by ordering authorized but unnecessary procedures. An organization might be tempted to compromise or abandon values when threatening external forces influence decisions to conduct business outside of accepted standards. Temptation can lure some to increase profits while decreasing quality of service. Some facilities unable to recruit skilled professionals because of staffing shortages might hire untrained workers to fill gaps for the providing of therapeutic services.

Conflict between loyalty to recipients of services and loyalty to employer can result in an ethical "dilemma of the double agent" (Bruckner, 1987). Ethical unease can occur because health care providers have dual goals that could be in conflict: to provide quality services and to generate high profits. Serious ethical dilemmas arise when the role of clinical advocate is compromised against the role of income generator. Pressures for cost containment can influence a replacement of a decision for clinical service delivery with a decision based on financial or allocation factors. Dilemmas are created when practitioners feel that clinical excellence or social responsibility is in opposition to economic reality.

Quality care is the primary goal for occupational therapy practitioners and other care providers. Quality care can be defined as the best possible intervention resulting in the best outcome for the individual recipient of care. Who defines quality? The recipient of care, the provider of care, and the party who pays for the care determine quality.

Ethical issues include concern for modifications of service access, program costs, and reimbursement. Additional focus is placed on determination of approved services and eligibility for services. At least in part, medical decisions are based on somebody's value judgment. Course of action is planned after weighing the competing interests in terms of the benefits and costs to all stakeholders, including the client, facility, insurers, advocacy groups, lawyers, legislators, and society as a whole.

Managers of health care are expected to allocate resources, structure cost-effective practices, encourage efficiency, and increase productivity while simultaneously limiting costs. Incremental changes bring models of health care reform offering lessons for what to do and what not to do because lessons will be taught as innovative ideas are tried. Successes will be replicated, and deficiencies will need corrections as society continues to plan for a fair and affordable system of health care delivery. How do decisions about health care cost, program access, and service quality get made, and who should make them? Who is covered? What is covered? Who pays for it? How much is paid? Funding initiatives fluctuate depending on external macroenvironmental conditions and shifting environmental priorities. Innovations in biotechnology (e.g., new medications, experimental testing), civil emergencies because of the threat of terrorism or epidemic (e.g., tuberculosis, polio, influenza, measles), demographic changes, and weather-related disasters (e.g., hurricanes, floods) have had an affect on the amount of dollars available for public health programs as well as the types of health services funded.

Ultimately, decisions are always made. The moral agents expected to provide the structure for health care benefits and services are governments, businesses, and philanthropic organizations. Organizations in the business of health care service delivery are expected to provide quality services in an equitable way. As a society, we expect a health care business to conduct operations in a manner that creates some good, has social responsibility, and does not harm the greater community. We expect that an ethical society will strive to create a fair system because of a social obligation to maximize justice and equitable consequences. There is a belief that there will be an attempt to form a balance of more good over less harm. Generally accepted social principles form the philosophical foundation for medical ethics. The values that guide behavior in society at large are the basic standards used to make decisions in medical ethics. If fairness is an esteemed value in society as a whole, then fairness will also be an important factor for the resolution of medical ethical dilemmas. If compassion is an important social value, then empathy and caring will guide medical ethical decision making.

## Direct Application in Everyday Practice

From corporations to street gangs, an expected obligation of group membership is an adoption of group values. All groups of all types assume member acceptance of group values. Group membership implies compliance with fundamental principles of the group. Behavioral norms are established through either formal or informal systems. The degree of formal structure does not determine the amount of internalization of values or the extent of compliance to rules. Regulations and laws are examples of formal methods of sharing group values with strong incentives for compliance. Custom and tradition are relatively informal methods of sharing group values, yet they have compelling authoritative commands for observance of principles. A sense of belonging to a group will foster adoption of group norms as personal values. Consequences for noncompliance include a wide variety of sanctions and penalties for infractions handed down in the form of restrictions, fines, or prison time. Compliance based merely on rule recognition rather than an internalized system of values has a focus on the threat of detection and punishment. Drivers who do not obey posted speed limits on interstate highways but slow down in the presence of a marked police vehicle demonstrate this observable truth.

Private entities such as professional associations or corporations create standards of conduct. It is not unusual for an organization policy to go beyond the minimum requirements set by legal standards. We can assume that just like individuals, organizations may rely on more than one type of value-based principle. Customs, principles, and regulations blend to define ethical behavior unique to an organization.

Attitudes and traditions are a part of organizational culture. The creation of an ethical work environment sets the tone for an organization. Constructing an ethical climate is most effective when the people who implement the policies and procedures cooperatively participate in their formation because a realistic, yet rigorous, set of ethical standards is more likely to be adhered to if there is a "buy-in" from those who must live under its authority. A proactive management can support ethical behavior by adopting a policy to lead by example. If management clearly supports ethical behavior, employees will be more likely to view an unethical action as unacceptable.

Either an implicit agreement or an explicit contract is established between an employer organization and its employees. Employees can expect a safe workplace environment, fair work conditions, and an equitable salary with benefits. There is a reasonable expectation of job satisfaction. It is incumbent upon employees to use performance skills and execute a fair amount of work in return.

## Codes and Standards for Occupational Therapy

A code of ethics is a collection of formal explicit statements forming a moral guide for an identified group outlining right and valued behavior, principles, and values. Any formal statement can serve as a code of ethics if it provides group members with an outline of what is right and valued and defines underlying beliefs. A code of ethics creates recognition of the behaviors deemed good or bad within a group context. A code of ethics is a collection of value-based rules forming an impartial guide for making decisions by an identified group.

A code of ethics can be a stand-alone document or a component of an organization's policies and procedures manual. In many cases, a code of ethics is integrated into the organization's mission statement. Typically, an organization creates secondary documents such as an enforcement code to assist in interpretation and implementation of the code of ethics. These supplementary documents are generally safeguards built into the system to encourage compliance. Mechanisms for sanctions and penalties to deal with ethical misconduct in violation of principles specified in the code of ethics are provided in ancillary papers. Auxiliary supportive documents are commonly used to address specific issues as a need becomes evident.

The professional associations for occupational therapy practitioners have clearly identified the value-based principles important to the profession. The World Federation of Occupational Therapists (WFOT), National Board for Certification in Occupational Therapy (NBCOT), and American Occupational Therapy Association (AOTA) have a shared sense of which values are important and what constitutes good practice. In service of a mission with responsibility to protect the public interest, our professional organizations specify criteria for the appropriate conduct of all occupational therapy practitioners and define our responsibilities toward the recipients of occupational therapy services. Official documents for the use of members and nonmembers are available on each of our professional association's websites.

The WFOT's *Code of Ethics* (see Appendix I) presents a general guide for "appropriate conduct . . . in any professional circumstance" (2005). Categories highlighted are personal attributes, responsibility toward the recipient of occupational therapy services, collaboration, continued professional development, and promotion of the profession (WFOT, 2005).

The *NBCOT Candidate/Certificant Code of Conduct* (2013a) and the *Procedures for the Enforcement of the NBCOT Candidate/Certificant Code of Conduct* (2013b) "define and clarify" professional responsibilities to protect the public. The NBCOT requires certified occupational therapy practitioners and students compliance toward the seeking of "high standards for personal and professional conduct" (NBCOT, 2013a, 2013b). Violations can result in certification ineligibility for a specified time or sanctions such as monitoring or supervision. The NBCOT has the authority to impose penalties from a formal reprimand kept on record up to indefinite revocation of certification.

The AOTA has developed and adopted a series of documents to provide guidance for the occupational therapy practitioner. These documents of the AOTA represent a comprehensive ethics guide for all occupational therapy personnel (occupational therapists, occupational therapy assistants, and students). A set of principles for professional conduct is given in the *Occupational Therapy Code of Ethics* (2015b). The *Standards of Practice for Occupational Therapy* (AOTA, 2010) provides practice guidelines for the delivery of occupational therapy services, defining minimum practice standards and giving the occupational therapy practitioner guidance for application of values and principles. *Enforcement Procedures for the Occupational Therapy Code of Ethics* (AOTA, 2015a) establishes a complaint process and sanctions as well as outlines the AOTA's ability to penalize AOTA members who violate the ethics standards (AOTA, 2015b). There are numerous examples of auxiliary documents adopted by AOTA in support of advocacy toward increased access to services or to decrease societal problems; the AOTA statement on end-of-life care (2011) is one example, and its *Societal Statement on Livable Communities* (2009) is another example.

The *Occupational Therapy Code of Ethics* (2015b) highlights the long-standing commitment of the profession to seven core values as first emphasized in *Core Values and Attitudes of Occupational Therapy Practice* (AOTA, 1993). Ethical values and morality-based attitudes form the core foundation for the practice of occupational therapy. These seven concepts are altruism, equality, freedom, justice, dignity, truth, and prudence.

1. Altruism is concerned with creating benefit for others.
2. Equality is the basis for impartial fairness.
3. Freedom is reflected in self-determination and the right to choose.
4. Justice is being objective and unbiased.
5. Dignity places emphasis on the unique characteristics of each person as valuable and worthy of respect.
6. Truth is a requirement for honesty and accuracy.
7. Prudence is the basis for cautious good sense.

The *Occupational Therapy Code of Ethics* (2015b) and the related official documents of the AOTA are intended to assist occupational therapy personnel with moral dilemmas and conflicts. A combination of deontological beliefs and teleological application principles are offered as guidance to sort through conflicting priorities in any type of work setting. With the *Code of Ethics* (2015b), there is a recognition that members of the profession will be called upon to make decisions regarding "situation-specific" ethical issues. The *Code of Ethics* (2015b) defines a set of principles: beneficence, nonmaleficence, autonomy, justice, veracity, and fidelity.

- Principle 1 is based on the concept of beneficence. Maximize positive and good benefits. Perform with compassionate goodwill. Occupational therapy personnel are expected to provide services in a fair manner without discrimination.
- Principle 2 is based on the concept of nonmaleficence. Minimize or avoid causing harm. Occupational therapy personnel are called on to use good judgment and to refrain from taking part in actions that result in injury, abandonment, undue influence, compromise to safety, or exploitation.
- Principle 3 is based on the double obligations of a respect for autonomy and confidentiality or the rights of the individual.
    - ◊ The first is autonomy, free will or self-determination with respect for individuality. There is an obligation to collaborate with respect for individuality and to follow the standards of informed consent. The client has a right to refuse treatment.
    - ◊ Confidentiality must be maintained, including the protection of privacy, information, and communication. This requires guarding information shared in confidence. Discussions must be protected, taking care that conversations will not be overheard. Records are not to be disclosed except under conditions of authorized access in compliance with regulations. Computer security measures must be observed.
- Principle 4 requires the promotion of justice. Social justice or distributive justice obligates occupational therapy practitioners to advocate for fair distribution of resources. We must work toward increased access while limiting barriers. Procedural justice demands compliance and the unbiased following of applicable laws, standards, regulations, and rules.
- Principle 5 is veracity. There is an obligation for being truthful. Accurate and honest communication is a requirement.
- Principle 6 identifies a need for fidelity. An obligation exists for fairness, integrity, and loyalty in professional interactions.

## Informed Consent

Principle 3 of the *Occupational Therapy Code of Ethics* (2015b) speaks to a concern with obtaining informed consent from recipients of services and participants in research. Although facility procedures may only focus on signing an informed consent form, the key to true informed consent is the process of educating with appropriate, relevant, and truthful information so a reasonable person can make a decision regarding the risk (harm) and options for success (benefits). Informed consent is a process that acknowledges the service recipient's right to be directly involved in health care decisions. The informed consent process protects against unwanted intervention and allows for choice, including refusal to participate. Respect for the individual is fundamental to the concept of self-determination. The idea of informed consent is based on the principle of autonomy. Closely linked to beneficence, the process of informed consent relies on recognition of self-determination. A minimum of three components is widely recognized as necessary for informed consent:

- **Disclosure:** Sufficient knowledge for making decisions
- **Competency:** Sufficient capability to understand information
- **Voluntary:** Sufficient freedom to choose

## Disclosure: Sufficient Knowledge for Making Decisions

The occupational therapy practitioner must include the recipient of services as a full participant in the informed consent process. The practitioner must try to understand the situation from the perspective of the recipient of services. An active listening approach can allow the clinician to hear the preferences of the participant while avoiding a compromise to the values of the clinician or, more importantly, the client. Autonomy can be preserved with an appreciation of individual needs. A commitment for respect and honesty should be maintained. Collaboration is a requirement. A dynamic plan for communication should be standard procedure. Information must be shared in a manner that will facilitate communication. There is an obligation on the occupational therapy practitioner to ensure understanding and maximum comprehension. Allow for the asking of questions and answer with honesty.

The feelings, hopes, and fears of the individual must be considered within an environment that fosters open communication. Avoid prejudicing the selection process. Do not use coercive influence and avoid creating a sense of intimidation. Be aware of the unequal power between a caregiving professional and the recipient of care. The paternalistic sentiment of the health care professional's "knowing what is best" for the client is no longer meaningful in today's health care environment.

The practitioner has an obligation to clearly describe the preferred clinical alternative and the other options. The purpose of the recommended intervention must be presented. Available intervention alternatives must be offered. The probability of benefits and risks must be explained for all available options. An exhaustive list of every possible risk no matter how slight the probability is not required nor is it encouraged. Enough information must be given to allow a choice. The client has a right to either accept or refuse the recommended intervention. A refusal of intervention should be honored, but refusal does not necessarily mean the end of discussions because an exploration of the reason for refusal and consideration of alternatives is not only acceptable but also required.

## Competency: Sufficient Capability to Understand Information

The ability to give informed consent involves determination of competency by legal or common law standards. Capacity for reason and deliberation is required. There must be an ability to understand the treatment alternatives and appreciate the risks or benefits. It can be useful to look at decisional capacity instead of reliance on legal standards of competence. Strict adherence to legal standards can have the disadvantage of moving the responsibility for informed consent away from the recipient of service because of an impaired ability to communicate, degenerating or wavering mental status, or the person is a minor below the age of consent. Decisional capacity is based on the determination that the individual is capable of making a decision at a given time. How are intervention decisions made if the person does not have decisional capacity or is determined legally not competent? The question that should be asked in this type of case is, "What would the person do if able to decide independently?" Decisions should be made in the context of the individual's past values and preferences. Decisions should be consistent with earlier life choices. Conversations with family, friends, and staff at residential centers can lead to insights about preferences. Some states recognize a health care proxy, a family member or friend designated by the individual to make medical intervention decisions if the recipient of services is unable to make clinical care decisions and if the preferred option remains unknown. The designated health care proxy has the authority of making decisions on behalf of the individual. Decisions can be made according to the best interests determination when client wishes or attitudes are not known. Often the situation circumstances were not discussed with the surrogate decision maker or the person's wishes were not made clear. In some cases, the courts will assign a legal guardian to weigh all of the facts and determine what is in the client's best interest. Substituted judgment is a form of decision making asking, "If the client could tell us, what would the client's choice be in this situation?" The best intervention option is determined by deciding, "What would this person do in this specific situation?" It is putting yourself in the client's shoes and contemplating, "What if?" Again, the details of the specific situation must be considered. The situation-specific details necessitate the weighing of risks and benefits resulting in an examination of QOL issues. Decisions should not be based on age or presence of disability or generalized stereotypes.

## *Voluntary: Sufficient Freedom to Choose*

Adherence to client autonomy respects the rights of the individual even if the individual chooses to abdicate decision-making control to another person. Each person and each family will have a unique experience based on family roles, education, immigration, assimilation, and personal patterns (Candib, 2002; Gold, 2004; Ho, 2006). Emphasis should be placed on expressed client values and expectations (Leino-Kilpi et al., 2003). It is important to avoid stereotypes and generalizations based on ethnicity. A respectful humanitarian position accommodates multicultural needs by meeting "traditional fundamental standards of ethics while respecting cultural and societal norms" (Crigger, Holcomb, & Weiss, 2001, p. 465).

The health care provider and the client might not speak the same language, creating linguistic challenges to obtaining informed consent. Terminology to describe pathology is lacking by western standards in many cultures (Crigger et al., 2001), making interpretation difficult. Translators have been known to create bias because of dialect or cross-cultural miscommunication (Barnes, Davis, Moran, Portillo, & Koenig, 1998; Crigger et al., 2001) with culture-based differences in maintaining hope (Barnes et al., 1998; Kagawa-Singer, 1993). The presence of unfamiliar translators taking part in personal, emotion-laden conversations can cause additional barriers to communication (Barnes et al., 1998). Family involvement in decision making can necessitate an interdependent approach to obtaining informed consent. Allowing the client to express a clear preference for another (or others) to contribute to the process for making decisions should be accepted as being as valid as an individual's own decision (Barnes et al., 1998; Ho, 2006). Authoritarian forcing of individual decision making is another form of paternalism (Candib, 2002; Ho, 2006). Some cultures believe the rights of the bigger community or family override the rights of the individual. In a family, the cultural expectation may motivate a husband to routinely make decisions on behalf of his wife (Crigger et al., 2001). Decisions by a leader are expected as the norm, and the client will assume a passive role in decisions, leaving authority and control to the expertise of the health care practitioner (Barnes et al., 1998). Some cultures avoid an overt discussion of dying or life-threatening illness. This cultural norm would lead to medical decision making by a trusted family member rather than directly by the client. "Partial disclosure" or "ambiguity" is widely practiced as a way to share information in an indirect manner (Candib, 2002). Only recently, medical culture in western traditions adopted the view that disclosure of a life-threatening diagnosis was a beneficent act. In 1961, the majority of U.S. doctors did not disclose the diagnosis of cancer directly to clients; however, by the mid to late 1970s, most doctors disclosed as a routine practice (Candib, 2002; Gold, 2004).

Criticism of the informed consent form became widespread as facilities attempted to adopt more user-friendly documents. Similar to other medical documents, the informed consent form is viewed as too technical, too complicated, and too lengthy for the typical reader. Studies show that the document is often skimmed or not read in detail (Huntington & Robinson, 2007; Varnhagen et al., 2005). It is hypothesized that in addition to low readability, informed consent documents are not read because of a perception of low risk (Huntington & Robinson, 2007; Varnhagen et al., 2005) because the institution or clinician is trusted. True informed consent is not obtained even with a signature on a document when the document is not fully read and understood. Health messages developed according to universal accessibility standards clarify unfamiliar medical terminology and make complex concepts more comprehensible. Improved readability can be created with simpler text, decreased jargon and technological language, choice of font, and format clarity. Technical jargon should be avoided. At a minimum, terminology should be clearly defined, and layman's terms should be used whenever possible. Lack of comprehension can occur because of a language barrier, literacy level, cognitive deficit, or situation-specific anxiety. The demands of the medical environment can increase stress, often causing a barrier to communication. Attempt to decrease anxiety. Creating an informed consent document that meets universal accessibility standards for improving literacy can honor legal requirements and address ethical concerns for process.

Informed consent guidelines can be developed specific to the specialized needs of researchers. Although there are aspects of clinical informed consent similar to research informed consent, there are differences and implications to consider. The dual roles of researcher and clinician can cause confusion, conflict of interest, and the potential for coercion (Crigger et al., 2001).

Informed consent for research goes beyond the requirements of obtaining a signature on a permission form. Participants in a research study must be provided with sufficient information to understand the benefits and risks associated with becoming a research subject. Research participants have a right to stop participation in the activity under study. Commonly accepted practice understands informed consent to be a process throughout the research participant's experience.

Moral fundamentalism accepts informed consent principles as universal and applicable throughout the world in all research situations (Crigger et al., 2001). Therefore, the protocol for obtaining informed consent should not be modified for populations in different geographic areas. Moral multiculturalism is in contrast to moral fundamentalism. A multicultural ethic does not seek absolutes but rather accepts a more situational approach that varies among communities. Therefore, protocol for obtaining informed consent should be modified to meet the cultural needs to place and time of the studied population.

## Choices! Choices! Decisions! Decisions!

An ethical dilemma exists in a situation in which an argument can be made for opposing decisions or conflicting choices. Sometimes there is more than one "right" solution to a problem. There are situations when there is no clear indication of the "right or wrong" course of action. Rules might be vague or not well established. Sometimes partial good can be found in incompatible trade-offs. At times, dubious pathways lead to "good" end results. Other times, none of the available alternatives appears to be an acceptable option likely to result in a good ending. Rarely are there clearly defined problems with definitive solutions.

The role of ethics in occupational therapy is to assist the practitioner in solving complex problems when there is no clear identification of right or wrong or there is a need to identify the best alternative out of choices. Medical ethics can be a hodgepodge of incompatible values and conflicting regulations. Ethical dilemmas in health care reflect the moral conflicts of the larger society. Proponents and opponents can logically and passionately argue contradictory viewpoints on life and death issues.

Clinical ethics committees have been established in a number of health care facilities, and a study showed that facility employees are most likely to look to clinical ethics committees for legalistic guidance on informed consent and record keeping (Kerridge, Pearson, & Rolfe, 1998). Often dilemmas in the "typical" experience of occupational therapy practitioners are complex, involving a need for consensus among several participants and lasting an extended time period with repetition of episodes (Barnitt, 1998).

Ethical decision making in the work setting can "get stuck" while everyone with a stake in the process waits for someone else on the team to make a decision. Fear of malpractice or other litigation can slow the process further. Occupational therapy personnel are faced with ethical dilemmas along with the other professionals on the workplace team. In some cases, occupational therapy practitioners may feel excluded from the decision-making process; however, practitioners are encouraged to accept or develop a position of responsibility. All occupational therapy personnel inclusive of occupational therapists, occupational therapy assistants, and students have a duty to take an active role in the ethical decision-making process.

Ethics obligates one to judge. Ironically, adopting avoidance maneuvers, advocating for a neutral position, or having no judgment about anything will become a judgmental decision. Saying "I don't want to judge" is making a judgment. A course of action or inaction will result. Consequences will occur even without an acknowledgment of moral beliefs.

Moral occupational therapy practitioners identify and analyze ethical problems. An appropriate response to ethical problems is an exploration of choices. No two cases are ever identical, and "one size fits all" solutions do not exist. Emphasis cannot be placed on learning the "right" concept or replicating the "correct" action. Responsible decisions depend on thoughtful consideration of competing rights, obligations, values, and interests. Occupational therapy practitioners should consider and weigh conflicting and competing agendas, priorities, choices, values, and opinions of relevant stakeholders. The same practical thinking used outside the workplace to do the "right thing," such as being loyal to a friend or treating a grandparent with respect, is useful in the work setting.

Act with goodwill, show compassion, and treat others with integrity and respect, or in other words, beneficence. Altruism is another way to express the importance of sharing. Equality and justice are based on fairness and point to distribution of scarce resources. There is an obligation to community. Do not cause harm and do not hurt anyone. Know the rules and follow them. Judgment necessitates a clarification of values and ethical principles.

## The Ethical Decision SOAP

Is there a fair and just way to sort through conflicting principles to decide on a course of action—or inaction? How should an occupational therapy practitioner determine the best option? Identify the principles specific to the particular case situation, contemplate, negotiate, and reach a resolution. The ethical decision SOAP format is adapted for the purpose of resolving ethical dilemmas. A process for making ethical decisions is derived from clinical practice with a time-honored reporting method: the SOAP progress note.

### How to Write an Ethical Decision SOAP

1. Create an initial problem list.
    - List the central problems or the most significant problems. What is the conflict? List all involved persons.

2. Subjective: Identify the subjective case-specific issues.
    - Identify the ethical issues or problems raised by the case-specific situation. It is critical to understand the clinical and social facts of the particular situation. Are the thoughts and wishes of the participants clear? Recognize the presence of feelings (e.g., acceptance, fear, worry, anger, ambivalence, other emotions). Clarify your own opinion and biases.
3. Objective: Gather objective case-relevant data.
    - Search the literature to identify similar situations. Determine the consensus of experts on prior cases. Examine the interpretation of law through court decisions. Find relevant department or organization procedures. Know professional guidelines and standards of practice. Determine relevant code of ethics principles.
4. Assess: Assess the situation.
    - Contemplate the relevant ethical principles as they apply to the specific people of the particular situation. Articulate the solution alternatives and realistic options.
    - Postulate all of the consequences of each choice. Weigh the competing interests, needs, risks, and benefits of all involved participants. Determine if the options are reasonable. Evaluate if resources for implementation of the alternatives are available.
5. Plan: Articulate a plan of action.
    - Plan for a practical and realistic solution. Formulate an overall strategy and schedule.
6. Implement the plan.
7. Evaluate the need to modify the plan.

## Summary

Many occupational therapy personnel borrow from an assortment of ethical theories to arrive at a balanced approach to a moral making of decisions in the workplace. An eclectic approach is often used to make daily work decisions. The development of an ethical style or "personal compass" is an ongoing process.

Perhaps the highest standard for ethical decision making is a reliance on the principle of beneficence. Virtuous practitioners strive to maximize possible benefits in a fair way. "Superior quality" is a value judgment with an expectation for excellence. Value-based concepts such as dignity and respect can provide a foundation for service delivery.

Everyday occupational therapy practice is based on ethical judgments. Integrate an awareness of ethics into everyday practice. Moral reasoning strategies enhance clinical outcomes. Faced with increasing demands and decreasing resources, occupational therapy practitioners must cope with issues of quality, quantity, access, and allocation. Contemplate the pertinent ethical questions and the implications. Initiate conversations about the relevant moral principles. Proficiency with ethical knowledge develops ability when coping with real-world concerns.

## Student Self-Assessment

1. Personal reflection: Where did you get your sense of morality? Write a four- or five-page biographical narrative describing your values and principles, linking the evolution of your standards to your personal history of past experiences and events.
2. Personal credo: Write your own code of ethics. Create a moral credo defining your personal system of philosophical beliefs.
3. Professional credo: Adapt your personal code of ethics to craft a professional doctrine suitable for use in work environments.

### *Small Group Exercises*

1. Working in teams, think of a situation that raises an ethical dilemma. Concisely describe the situation using an objective descriptive style.
2. Brainstorm as many ideas as possible. Generate a list of alternative solutions to resolve the ethical dilemma described in Exercise 1.
3. List the relevant principles and values in the ethical dilemma described in Exercise 1.
4. Present a role play reflecting the attitudes, opinions, and feelings of the participants involved in the ethical dilemma described in Exercise 1.

### *Document Review*

1. Visit a local health care facility or human services agency. Request a mission statement, code of ethics, or patient bill of rights. Obtain a copy of any document that demonstrates moral concepts. Identify the main ethical principles or standards in the document(s).
2. Search the websites of two types of facilities that might provide occupational therapy services. You can choose a local hospital and a major teaching hospital, or you could select any combination of hospital, rehabilitation facility, home health agency, nursing home, school, or other place of service delivery for occupational therapy. Locate a mission statement, code of ethics, or patient bill of rights for

both facilities. Compare the documents. Do they refer to the same values and standards? Describe two ethics-based components that are the same and two components that are different.

## Ethics Case Study Projects

Answer the following ethics case study questions for each case:

1. What is the most significant ethical dilemma? Explain your answer.
2. Which principles in the *Occupational Therapy Code of Ethics* (2015b) apply to the case? Explain your answer.
3. Write an ethical decision SOAP.
4. Discuss the implications of allocation and distribution of resources.

### Case Study 1: Larry

Leaving the cafeteria after a late afternoon snack, you are rushing toward the elevator to get to a utilization review meeting when Larry, a nurse, taps your shoulder and with a big, friendly grin says, "I'm so glad that I ran into you. Let's ride back up to the unit together because I want your opinion about Mr. Stone's getting discharged next week." As the doors close on the crowded elevator, Larry looks at you and continues speaking, "So, I want to know if Mr. Stone can dress independently yet."

### Case Study 2: Edie

You work in the outpatient unit of a busy rehabilitation hospital. Dropped off in the parking lot by her mom, Edie always arrives promptly for her occupational therapy visits. She is being seen for intervention of a fracture to her left elbow after a slip on the stairs at her piano teacher's home. Her intervention time seems to be shorter than the hour duration because throughout the sessions, she chats about the numerous activities and events typical to an active 17-year-old high school student. Shortly before the end of today's session, Edie confides that she has a handgun bought from another student.

### Case Study 3: Maddy

You are a member of a geriatric medical behavioral assessment team in a large suburban hospital. One of your clients is an 80-year-old woman recuperating from a fall. The cause of her fall remains unknown. During her stay, Maddy presents as frightened, depressed, and anxious. She has ripped out her IVs repeatedly. She thwarts attempts made by staff to keep her seated in a chair and refuses to stay in her hospital bed. The staff considers her "a fall risk." She has multiple chronic conditions, including diabetes and arthritis. She is legally blind secondary to diabetic retinopathy. Significant hearing loss in both ears is somewhat compensated for with bilateral hearing aids. Never married, Maddy lives alone in the house that has been the family home for three generations. Maddy dedicated her adult life to caring for her frail, confused, and incontinent mother in her last years until she passed away about 10 years ago. Health insurance will not cover long-term home care services. Her small pension combined with her Social Security check makes her slightly over income for subsidized programs. Family members (a younger brother and a niece who, coincidentally, is a nurse on another unit) share responsibility of occasional visits, grocery shopping, and helping with mail for bill payments. Both relatives describe Maddy as strong, independent, self-reliant, and proud of it. The brother would like to see Maddy return to independent living in her own home as soon as possible. The niece is worried about Maddy returning home and has asked the assessment team to help decide for long-term planning. A transfer to a long-term care facility such as an assisted living facility, nursing home, or custodial care residence is a possibility being considered. Everyone who enters Maddy's room is asked the same question, "When can I go home?" One staff member said, "Sure, she wants to go home, but this would be for her own good; she will learn to like it." The multidisciplinary team looks to you, the occupational therapy practitioner, to determine the level of independent functioning with activities of daily living and to assess safety in the home. Will this client be safe at home? The discharge meeting starts.

### Case Study 4: The Roommate

You have not seen your old roommate since graduation. You are meeting for a casual lunch on the following Sunday. Your roommate's family owns several skilled nursing facilities in a metropolitan center. After graduation, your friend's father asked you to work in the main facility where the corporate office is housed. After a few months of work at Sunny Meadows, it became obvious that the amount of actual therapy visits did not match what was documented in the medical record. Residents were wheeled into the large therapy area and then returned to the unit dayroom. You were instructed by the rehabilitation services director to document "slow progress" in the medical record so the residents appeared to need more intervention than actually required because health care insurers generally require termination of services if measurable progress halts.

### Case Study 5: Michael and Maria

You are nearing the end of the number of home health visits allowed by Michael's health insurance plan. Michael, a 45-year-old carpenter who experienced a traumatic brain injury, is making measurable therapeutic gains during your home visits. Michael's wife, Maria, often accompanies her husband during the occupational

## Evidence-Based Research Chart

| Topic | Evidence |
|---|---|
| Moral conflict and ethical dilemmas | Barnitt, 1998; Foye, Kirschner, Brady Wagner, Stocking, & Siegler, 2002; Kälvemark, Höglund, Hansson, Westerholm, & Arnetz, 2004; Kassberg & Skär, 2008; Kirschner, Stocking, Wagner, Foye, & Siegler, 2001; Luboshitsky & Weil, 1993; Mukherjee, Brashler, Savage, & Kirschner, 2009; Scheirton, Mu, Lohman, & Cochran, 2007 |
| Principles and values | Dige, 2009; Reed, 2006; Reed & Peters, 2006, 2007, 2008, 2010 |
| Autonomy and independence | Cardol, De Jong, & Ward, 2002; Russell, Fitzgerald, Williamson, Manor, & Whybrow, 2002; Tamaru, McColl, & Yamasaki, 2007 |
| Utilitarianism | Levack, 2009 |
| Ethical decision making and reasoning | Dieruf, 2004; Martinez, 2000; Opacich, 1997 |

therapy sessions in their kitchen. Maria is very worried, saying, "I don't want Michael to go downhill and lose his ability to do things. You know he is trying very hard! Can't you keep visiting? You know he has goals. Hope is important!"

### Case Study 6: Fred

Fred is a 92-year-old man on your caseload. You are providing occupational therapy intervention after a hip fracture secondary to metastatic lung cancer. Fred has no remaining family. He has outlived his wife of 61 years. A drunk driver in a motor vehicle accident killed his only daughter on Christmas Eve 7 years ago. He is obviously depressed. He tells you that he doesn't want occupational therapy or more surgery, radiation therapy, or chemotherapy: "I just want to be left alone." The home health team has learned that his condition is considered terminal.

### Case Study 7: Juan

Juan is well liked by the teachers of the residential school for his quick sense of humor and compassionate demeanor. His obvious empathy for younger kids is frequently shown by his friendly attitude on the school playground. He is an artistically talented 16-year-old with strong academic skills. Juan lives at the school because of a shortage of appropriate foster care homes. His short attention span and periodic fits of rage were too much for his teacher in the traditional classroom environment. Juan's teacher noticed cigarette burn marks along the insides of his arms. When questioned, he revealed he sometimes thought about suicide. Recently, the outpatient mental health unit intervention team completed retesting and tentatively made the diagnosis of bipolar disorder. Intervention suggestions include medication, individual counseling, and stress management techniques. After 2 months of intervention, Juan is saying he wants to quit school and is refusing to take medication. He complains that medication side effects always make him feel tired and thirsty. He says the worst part is no longer feeling "the flow of creativity" and that his "artistic energy is gone." The residential staff members are concerned because Juan is beginning to become "a loner," isolating himself in his bedroom.

You work for the occupational therapy team of the school department in a large urban community. Knowing occupational therapy can provide a range of interventions that could improve functional abilities in the school environment, you know you have a lot to offer kids like Juan. Shortly before his transfer to the residential school, the homeroom teacher requested an "occupational therapy consult for handwriting improvement." Initial contact with Juan was made in his old classroom, where sitting in a corner chair slouched into his oversized black hooded sweatshirt, he avoided eye contact. His only comments were, "My handwriting is just fine like it is. I don't want your help."

An invitation to Juan's IEP meeting arrived in today's mail. You look at your calendar to discover you already agreed to participate in another IEP meeting scheduled at the same time for a student who attends a different school. Sighing, you decide to write a memo to be read into the official meeting minutes outlining your thoughts and recommendations.

## Electronic Resources

American Occupational Therapy Association:

- Ethics Commission Overview and Roles: http://www.aota.org/Practice/Ethics/EC.aspx
- Federal Regulatory Affairs Department: http://www.aota.org/Advocacy-Policy/Federal-Reg-Affairs.aspx

Consensus statement on clinical judgment in health care settings: AOTA, APTA, ASHA. Published on AOTA website 10/14/14. https://www.aota.org/-/media/Corporate/Files/Practice/Ethics/APTA-AOTA-ASHA-Concensus-Statement.pdf

Ethical Issues Around Payment for Services, Advisory Opinion for the Ethics Commission: https://www.aota.org/-/media/Corporate/Files/Practice/Ethics/Advisory/ecadv-pymt.pdf.

Frequently Asked Questions About Ethics: https://www.aota.org/Practice/Ethics/FAQ.aspx

Official Documents page includes *Occupational Therapy Code of Ethics* (2015), *Enforcement Procedures for the Occupational Therapy Code of Ethics* (2015), Guidelines, Standards, Position Papers, Statements, and Societal Statements: https://www.aota.org/practice/manage/official.aspx

Bioethics Research Library and Kennedy Institute on Bioethics at Georgetown University: http://bioethics.georgetown.edu

Ethical Decision Making Resources from the Markkula Center for Applied Ethics, Santa Clara University: https://www.scu.edu/ethics/ethics-resources/ethical-decision-making/

The Hastings Center, a nonpartisan research institution dedicated to bioethics and the public interest: http://www.thehastingscenter.org/Default.aspx

How to File a Complaint to the National Board for Certification in Occupational Therapy: http://www.nbcot.org/file-a-complaint

National Board for Certification in Occupational Therapy

Occupational Therapy State Regulatory Board Contact List: http://www.nbcot.org/state-license-info

Professional Conduct page includes Code of Conduct, Practice Standards, Procedures for Enforcement, Disciplinary Action Overview, and the Disciplinary Action Information Exchange Network (DAIEN, disciplinary actions taken by NBCOT and state regulatory agencies): http://www.nbcot.org/professional-conduct

National Institutes of Health, U.S. Department of Health and Human Services

Glossary of Commonly Used Terms in Research Ethics: http://www.niehs.nih.gov/research/resources/bioethics/glossary/index.cfm

Office of Clinical Research and Bioethics Policy: http://bioethics.od.nih.gov

Research Ethics Timeline (1932-Present): http://www.niehs.nih.gov/research/resources/bioethics/timeline/index.cfm

Presidential Commission for the Study of Bioethical Issues: http://bioethics.gov

Tips on Informed Consent from Office for Protection from Research Risks, Office for Human Research Protections, U.S. Department of Health and Human Services: http://www.hhs.gov/ohrp/policy/ictips.html

UNESCO, Learning To Live Together, Ethics, Science, and Society: http://www.unesco.org/new/en/social-and-human-sciences/themes/

World Federation of Occupational Therapists Position Statements: http://www.wfot.org/AboutUs/PositionStatements.aspx

## References


American Occupational Therapy Association. (1993). Core values and attitudes of occupational therapy practice. *American Journal of Occupational Therapy, 47*, 1085-1086.

American Occupational Therapy Association. (2009). American Occupational Therapy Association's societal statement on livable communities. *American Journal of Occupational Therapy, 63*, 847-848.

American Occupational Therapy Association. (2010). Standards of practice for occupational therapy. *American Journal of Occupational Therapy, 64* (Suppl.), S106-S111.

American Occupational Therapy Association. (2011). The role of occupational therapy in end-of-life care. *American Journal of Occupational Therapy, 59*, 675.

American Occupational Therapy Association. (2015a). Enforcement procedures for the occupational therapy code of ethics. *American Journal of Occupational Therapy, 69.*

American Occupational Therapy Association. (2015b). Occupational therapy code of ethics (2015). *American Journal of Occupational Therapy, 69*(Suppl. 3).

Barnes, D. M., Davis, A. J., Moran, T., Portillo, C. J., & Koenig, B. A. (1998). Informed consent in a multicultural cancer patient population: Implications for nursing practice. *Nursing Ethics, 5*(5), 412-423.

Barnitt, R. (1998). Ethical dilemmas in occupational therapy and physical therapy: A survey of practitioners in the UK National Health Service. *Journal of Medical Ethics, 24*(3), 193-199.

Bruckner, J. (1987). Physical therapists as double agents. Ethical dilemmas of divided loyalties. *Physical Therapy, 67*(3), 383-387.

Candib, L. M. (2002). Truth telling and advance planning at the end of life: Problems with autonomy in a multicultural world. *Families, Systems and Health, 20*(3), 213-228.

Cardol, M., De Jong, B. A., & Ward, C. D. (2002). On autonomy and participation in rehabilitation. *Disability and Rehabilitation, 24*(18), 970-974; discussion 975-1004.

Cowley, C. (2005). The dangers of medical ethics. *Journal of Medical Ethics, 31*, 739-742.

Crigger, N. J., Holcomb, L., & Weiss, J. (2001). Fundamentalism, multiculturalism and problems of conducting research with populations in developing nations. *Nursing Ethics, 8*(5), 459-468.

Dieruf, K. (2004). Ethical decision-making by students in physical and occupational therapy. *Journal of Allied Health, 3*(1), 24-30.

Dige, M. (2009). Occupational therapy, professional development, and ethics. *Scandinavian Journal of Occupational Therapy, 16*(2), 88-98.

Foye, S. J., Kirschner, K. L., Brady Wagner, L. C., Stocking, C., & Siegler, M. (2002). Ethical issues in rehabilitation: A qualitative analysis of dilemmas identified by occupational therapists. *Top Stroke Rehabilitation, 9*(3), 89-101.

Fulghum, R. (1988). *All I really need to know I learned in kindergarten: Uncommon thoughts on common things* (pp. 6-7). New York, NY: Villard Books.

Gold, M. (2004). Is honesty always the best policy? Ethical aspects of truth telling. *Internal Medicine Journal, 34*, 578-580.

Ho, A. (2006). Family and informed consent in multicultural setting. *American Journal of Bioethics, 6*(1), 26-28.

Huntington, I., & Robinson, W. (2007). The many ways of saying yes and no: Reflections on the research coordinator's role in recruiting research participants and obtaining informed consent. *IRB: Ethics and Human Research, 29*(3), 6-10.

Kagawa-Singer, M. (1993). Redefining health: Living with cancer. *Social Science and Medicine, 37*(3), 295-304.

Kälvemark, S., Höglund, A. T., Hansson, M. G., Westerholm, P., & Arnetz, B. (2004). Living with conflicts: Ethical dilemmas and moral distress in the health care system. *Social Science and Medicine, 58*(6), 1075-1084.

Kassberg, A. C., & Skär, L. (2008). Experiences of ethical dilemmas in rehabilitation: Swedish occupational therapists' perspectives. *Scandinavian Journal of Occupational Therapy, 15*(4), 204-211.

Kerridge, I. H., Pearson, S., & Rolfe, I. E. (1998). Determining the function of a clinical ethics committee: Making ethics work. *Journal of Quality in Clinical Practice, 18*, 117-124.

Kirschner, K. L., Stocking, C., Wagner, L. B., Foye, S. J., & Siegler, M. (2001). Ethical issues identified by rehabilitation clinicians. *Archives of Physical Medicine and Rehabilitation, 82*(12 Suppl. 2), S2-S8.

Leino-Kilpi, H., Valimaki, M., Dassen, T., Gasull, M., Lemonidou, C., Scott, P. A., et al. (2003). Perceptions of autonomy, privacy, and informed consent in the care of elderly people in five European countries: Comparison and implications for the future. *Nursing Ethics, 10*(1), 58-66.

Levack, W. M. (2009). Ethics in goal planning for rehabilitation: A utilitarian perspective. *Clinical Rehabilitation, 23*(4), 345-351.

Luboshitsky, D., & Weil, F. (1993). Ethical and moral dilemmas in the treatment of an abusive parent: The occupational therapy perspective. *Med Law, 12*(3-5):221-227.

Martinez, R. (2000). A model for boundary dilemmas: Ethical decision-making in the patient-professional relationship. *Ethical Human Sciences and Services, 2*(1), 43-61.

Mukherjee, D., Brashler, R., Savage, T. A., & Kirschner, K. L. (2009). Moral distress in rehabilitation professionals: Results from a hospital ethics survey. *PM & R, 1*(5), 450-458.

National Board for Certification in Occupational Therapy. (2013a). *NBCOT candidate/certificant code of conduct*. http://www.nbcot.org/code-of-conduct

National Board for Certification in Occupational Therapy. (2013b). *Procedures for the enforcement of the NBCOT candidate/certificant code of conduct*. Revision November 14, 2011. http://www.nbcot.org/procedures-for-enforcement

Opacich, K. J. (1997). Moral tensions and obligations of occupational therapy practitioners providing home care. *American Journal of Occupational Therapy, 51*(6), 430-435.

Reed, K. L. (2006, April 17). Occupational therapy values and beliefs: The formative years: 1904-1929. *OT Practice*, 21-25.

Reed, K. L., & Peters, C. (2006, October 9). Occupational therapy values and beliefs, part II: The Great Depression and war years: 1930-1949. *OT Practice*, 17-22.

Reed, K. L., & Peters, C. (2007, December 24). Occupational therapy values and beliefs, part III: A new view of occupation and the profession: 1950-1969. *OT Practice*, 17-21.

Reed, K. L., & Peters, C. O. (2008, October 6). Occupational therapy values and beliefs, part IV: A time of professional identity: 1970-1985—Would the real therapist please stand up? *OT Practice*, 15-18.

Reed, K. L., & Peters, C. O. (2010, April 5). Occupational therapy values and beliefs, part V: 1986-2000—Is this really occupational therapy? *OT Practice*, 15-18.

Russell, C., Fitzgerald, M. H., Williamson, P., Manor, D., & Whybrow, S. (2002). Independence as a practice issue in occupational therapy: The safety clause. *American Journal of Occupational Therapy, 56*(4), 369-379.

Scheirton, L. S., Mu, K., Lohman, H., & Cochran, T. M. (2007). Error and patient safety: Ethical analysis of cases in occupational and physical therapy practice. *Medicine, Health Care and Philosophy, 10*(3), 301-311.

Tamaru, A., McColl, M. A., & Yamasaki, S. (2007). Understanding "independence": Perspectives of occupational therapists. *Disability and Rehabilitation, 29*(13), 1021-1033.

Varnhagen, C. K., Gushta, M., Daniels, J., Peters, T. C., Parmar, N., Law, D., et al. (2005). How informed is online informed consent? *Ethics and Behavior, 15*(1), 37-48.

World Federation of Occupational Therapists. (2005). *Code of ethics*. Western Australia, Australia: Author.

## Suggested Readings

Atkinson, J. C. (2005). Ethical issues as an occupational therapist and epidemiological researcher. *British Journal of Occupational Therapy, 68*(5), 235-237.

Atwal, A., & Caldwell, K. (2003). Ethics, occupational therapy and discharge planning: Four broken principles. *Australian Occupational Therapy Journal*, 244-251.

Bushby, K., Chan, J., Druif, S., Ho, K., & Kinsella, E. A. (2015). Ethical tensions in occupational therapy practice: A scoping review. *British Journal of Occupational Therapy, 78*(4), 212-221.

Kinsella, E. A., Park, A. J., Appiagyei, J., Chang, E., & Chow, D. (2008). Through the eyes of students: Ethical tensions in occupational therapy practice. *Canadian Journal of Occupational Therapy, 75*(3), 176-183.

Sim, J. (1996). Client confidentiality: Ethical issues in occupational therapy. *British Journal of Occupational Therapy, 59*(2), 56-61.

Wright-St Clair, V. A., & Newcombe, D. B. (2014). Values and ethics in practice-based decision making. *Canadian Journal of Occupational Therapy, 81*(3), 154-162.

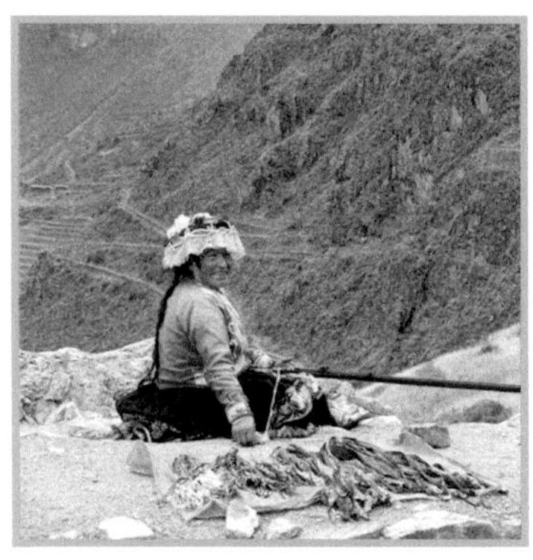

# 51

# Local to Global Resources for the Occupational Therapy Professional

Sarah McKinnon, MS, OTR/L, BCPR, MPA

**ACOTE STANDARDS EXPLORED IN THIS CHAPTER**

B.6.6, B.9.2

**KEY VOCABULARY**

- **Evidence-based practice:** The integration of research, clinical experience, and client preferences in clinical decision making.
- **Global networking:** The communication and connection with resources, groups, or populations from all over the world.
- **Professional development:** The advancement of knowledge, skills, and expertise to succeed in or demonstrate professional growth in a particular profession.
- **Professional engagement:** The act of participating in one's profession to enhance the knowledge, skills, or strength of an individual or group.
- **Trade organization:** Organization founded and funded by members of a profession that operate in a specific industry.



Jacobs, K., & MacRae, N. (Eds.).
*Occupational Therapy Essentials for Clinical Competence, Third Edition* (pp. 733-741).

> Occupational therapy [practitioners] must strive to incorporate resources that are relevant and evidence-based for the benefit of clients. (Metzler & Metz, 2010)

The opportunity for occupational therapy students, clinicians, administrators, and academia professionals to access global resources to influence occupational therapy in one's local setting has evolved extensively over the past two decades, specifically with the advancement of technology and online resources. With increasing internationalization of occupational therapy, clinicians, students, administrators, and members in academia do not only have to rely on national sources of information but also consult international literature that is now much more widely available (Froude & Craik, 2010). Ongoing evolution of the occupational therapy practice has strengthened with increased access to global resources that can promote occupational therapy in one's local setting. In fact, the significance of enhancing global recognition and global connections in occupational therapy practice has led to the incorporation of occupational therapy being "globally connected" as part of the American Occupational Therapy Association's (AOTA) 2017 Centennial Vision (2013). Incorporation of global resources into local practice through the use of research findings and ideas for accessible international resources can bring occupational therapy closer to being a truly evidence-based, science-driven profession (Froude & Craik, 2010). The understanding of the role of local, state, national, and international resources on the occupational therapy profession has also emerged in occupational therapist and occupational therapy assistant education curriculums to align with Accreditation Council for Occupational Therapy Education (ACOTE) Standards.

The purpose of this chapter is to identify the widely known and easily accessible local and global resources that can influence occupational therapy practice and enhance connections between occupational therapy practitioners around the world. Occupational therapy professional organizations, evidence-based resources, and resources to enhance global connections will be discussed.

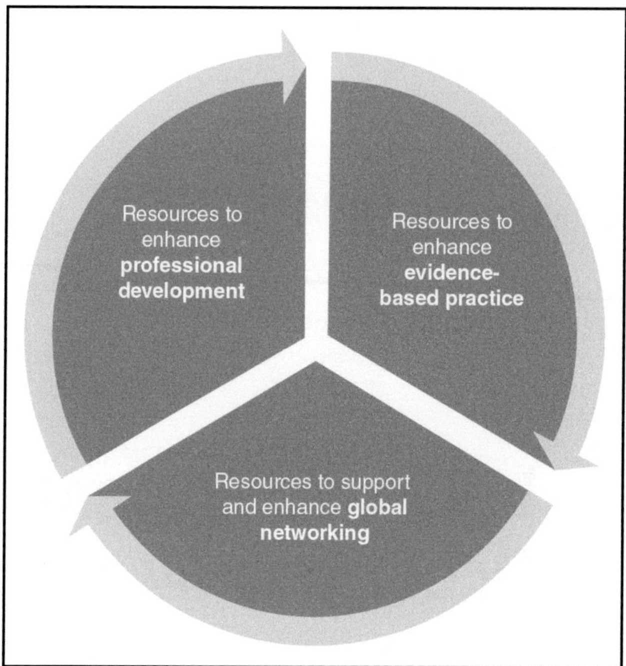


**Figure 51-1.** Categories of local and global resources that can increase professional engagement.

# Linking Occupational Therapy to Local and Global Resources

Professional engagement is the act of participating in one's profession to enhance the knowledge, skills, or strength of an individual or group. Occupational therapy students and practitioners have many strategies for enhancing professional engagement. Engagement, along with exploration and empowerment, are significant practice strategies used by occupational therapy practitioners to understand clients and how to facilitate participation (Stoffel, 2015). In addition to engaging with clients, occupational therapy students and practitioners can engage in seeking resources that can enhance the connection between the clinician and client, but also increase connections between occupational therapy practitioners around the world.

Figure 51-1 shows the various aspects in which an occupational therapy practitioner can demonstrate professional engagement by incorporating local and global resources into practice. Resources that enhance professional development, evidence-based research, and global networking can be categorized into these aspects.

- Professional development can be defined as the advancement of knowledge, skills, and expertise to succeed in or demonstrate professional growth in a particular profession.
- Evidence-based practice is defined as the integration of research, clinical experience, and client preferences in clinical decision making.
- Global networking is the communication and connection with resources, groups, or populations from all over the world.

Targeting professional development, evidence-based research, and global networking are three priorities that have been identified as meeting the AOTA 2017 Centennial Vision (AOTA, 2014). Many of these local and global resources can be accessed through established professional organizations that support occupational therapy and can enhance professional engagement in the field of occupational therapy. The case study at the end of this chapter describes Paula, an occupational therapist with 5 years of experience who used a variety of resources to expand her knowledge and engage with the occupational therapy community globally.

## Professional Organizations

A trade association, also known as an *industry trade group, business association,* or *sector association,* is an organization founded and funded by members of a profession that operate in a specific industry. An industry trade association participates in public relations activities such as advertising, education, political donations, lobbying, and publishing, but its main focus is collaboration between companies or standardization. Associations may offer other services, such as producing conferences, networking, charitable events, or offering classes or educational materials. Many associations are nonprofit organizations governed by bylaws and directed by officers who are also members. Trade associations are often dominated by members of the same discipline and represent a group of common interests. There are many professional organizations that support the occupational therapy profession and that enhance one's access to a variety of resources that can influence relationships between clients, as well as clinicians around the world. For example, occupational therapy practitioners and students may choose to join a variety of trade associations in occupational therapy including the World Federation of Occupational Therapists (WFOT), the AOTA, or the American Occupational Therapy Foundation (AOTF), as all offer resources to support professional development, evidence-based practice, social networking opportunities, and effective, occupation-based interventions. For occupational therapy practitioners and students interested in occupational therapy in European countries, the Council of Occupational Therapists for the European Countries at http://www.coteceurope.eu/ would be a good resource. In the United States, individual states have trade associations that occupational therapy students and practitioners may join. For example, occupational therapy practitioners living in Massachusetts might join the Massachusetts Association for Occupational Therapy. Joining associations on local and global levels helps to keep us informed as global citizens.

### World Federation of Occupational Therapists

The WFOT is the international leader of the occupational therapy profession, composed of 80 national occupational therapy professional organizations globally. Beginning in 1951 with 28 representatives from various countries, WFOT evolved to encompass this current mission, which is "to promote occupational therapy as an art and science internationally...supporting the development, use and practice of occupational therapy worldwide, demonstrating its relevance and contribution to society" (WFOT, 2016a). The World Health Organization formally accepted WFOT into the organization's official relations in 1959.

WFOT offers three types of memberships. To become a member, an individual must have received occupational therapy education from an occupational therapy program from a country that is recognized as one of WFOT's member organizations. The WFOT directly links 84 global member organizations with individual members exceeding 30,000 members and a national organization membership that represents more than 420,000 occupational therapy professionals internationally (WFOT, 2016a).

In addition to membership access to networking opportunities, WFOT creates position papers to identify the official stance from WFOT on important issues. Position papers typically developed in response to an issue or given the growth of a new area of practice. These papers are adopted following a vote by the WFOT Executive Council. The position papers are posted online and are available to nonmembers (WFOT, 2016b). Many of the 30+ position papers are available in more than four languages. They can be accessed online, as summarized in Table 51-1.

There are many opportunities to enhance global networking opportunities through use of social resources from WFOT. World Occupational Therapy Day is held on October 27 each year to heighten the visibility of the profession's development work and to promote the activities of WFOT internationally (WFOT, 2016b). Occupational Therapy Global Day of Service is an annual event in which occupational therapists participate in community service and promote the profession within community (promotingot.org). Occupational Therapy Virtual Exchange (OT24Vx) is an annual virtual conference that is free to anyone with Internet access, which promotes occupational therapy for 24 hours through virtual presentations (http://ot4ot.com/ot24vx.html). Participation in World Occupational Therapy Day, Occupational Therapy Global Day of Service, and OT24Vx is a great way to use global resources to connect with occupational therapy professionals internationally. Use of resources at the official WFOT website, as well as social media, will provide excellent avenues to be globally connected with occupational therapy.

Table 51-1.

**Resources Available From the World Federation of Occupational Therapists to Enhance Professional Engagement**

| Topic | Globally Accessible Resources |
|---|---|
| WFOT position statements | Positions statements provide a platform for WFOT to define its stance on occupational therapy issues. Resource center for official WFOT documents, including 30+ position papers. Most publications are available for immediate viewing in at least four languages. They can be accessed at http://www.wfot.org/AboutUs/PositionStatements.aspx.<br>• Academic Credentials for Occupational Therapy Educators for University Based Education in Occupational Therapy (2008)<br>• Activities of Daily Living (2012)<br>• Client-centeredness in Occupational Therapy (2010)<br>• Community Based Rehabilitation (2004)<br>• Competency and Maintaining Competency (2012)<br>• Consumer Interface with Occupational Therapy (2010)<br>• Diversity and Culture (2010)<br>• Environmental Sustainability Sustainable Practice within Occupational Therapy (2012)<br>• Global Health: Informing Occupational Therapy Practice (2014)<br>• Human Displacement—Revised (2014)<br>• Human Rights (2006)<br>• Inclusive Occupational Therapy Education (2008)<br>• International Collaborative Research in Occupational Therapy—Revised (2012)<br>• International Professionalism (2014)<br>• Occupational Science (2006)<br>• Occupational Therapy in Disaster, Preparedness and Response (2014)<br>• Occupational Therapy Entry-Level Qualifications (2008)<br>• Occupational Therapy—Profession Autonomy (2007)<br>• Professional Registration (2010)<br>• Recruiting Occupational Therapists from International Communities—Revised (2014)<br>• Recognition of Former Educational Status (2014)<br>• Scope and Extension of Practice (2014)<br>• Specialization and Advanced Occupational Therapy Practices (2014)<br>• Telehealth (2014)<br>• Universal Design (2012)<br>• Vocational Rehabilitation (2012) |
| World Occupational Therapy Day | Resources, promotional resources, and details regarding how to be involved in international events that take place on October 27th of each year<br>• Guide to World Occupational Therapy Day<br>• Social media information<br>• Occupational Therapy Global Day of Service examples<br>• OT24Vx information and past presentations |

Reprinted with permission from the World Federation of Occupational Therapists. (2016). *WFOT resource center.* Retrieved from http://www.wfot.org/ResourceCentre.aspx#

## *American Occupational Therapy Association*

The AOTA is located in Bethesda, Maryland. As defined by AOTA, occupational therapy is a rehabilitation profession that aims to enable people across the lifespan to participate in the meaningful activities (occupations) that they need to to maintain optimal quality of lives (AOTA, 2015a). These include addressing challenges such as physical, emotional, or social barriers related to developmental, chronic, or traumatic diagnoses. The AOTA represents "the interests and concerns of occupational therapy practitioners and students of occupational therapy and to improve the quality of occupational therapy services" (AOTA, 2015a). Major programs of this national professional association are focused toward ensuring the quality of occupational therapy services and improving consumer access to occupational therapy services. Additionally, programs are in place to promote the professional development of AOTA members.

AOTA was established in 1917 as the National Society for the Promotion of Occupational Therapy. Currently, AOTA is led by an Executive Director and Board of Directors. Within AOTA are many councils and committees, all of which provide official documents to adhere to the mission of AOTA and the development of AOTA strategies (AOTA, 2015b). The AOTA Official Documents are published each year, available online. These documents offer transparency to the organization and provide information for various priorities including education, practice, and ethics.

The requirements for an acceptable occupational therapy education were first adopted by the American Medical Association in 1935. In the 1990s, AOTA established language for accreditation of occupational therapy assistant programs. By 1994, the accredited occupational therapist and occupational therapy assistant programs transferred into the ACOTE. ACOTE has since established accreditation standards for doctoral, master's, and associate-level programs and is recognized as the accrediting agency for occupational therapy education by both the U.S. Department of Education and the Council for Higher Education Accreditation (AOTA, 2015a).

Within AOTA is the American Occupational Therapy Political Action Committee (AOTPAC), which is a voluntary, nonprofit committee formed by the AOTA to raise and contribute money to the campaigns of candidates to advance the group's interests. AOTPAC is the political action arm of AOTA whose purpose is to further the legislative aims of the Association by influencing or attempting to influence the selection, nomination, election, or appointment of any individual to any federal public office (AOTA, 2015c). AOTPAC contributions help elect candidates who endorse occupational therapy concerns, as occupational therapy is not fully understood in the political arena where health care, education, and funding decisions are being made. By law, AOTA cannot contribute to political campaigns, nor are any portion of candidates' dues used for such lobbying; therefore, all funding toward political campaigns representing AOTA must come from contributions from outside of AOTA membership dues (Figure 51-2).

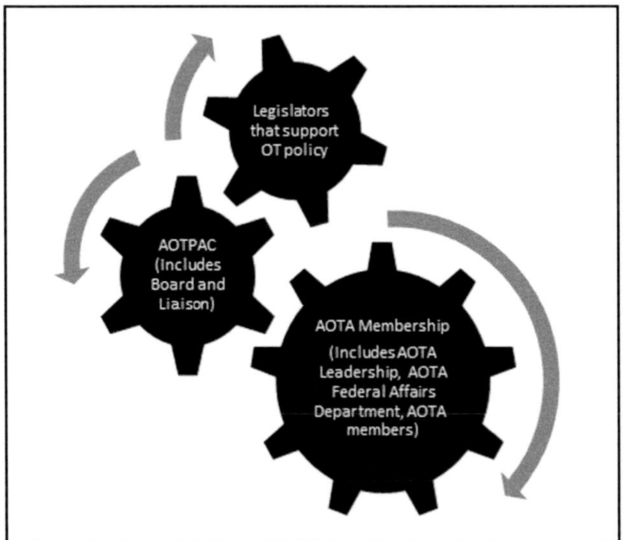


**Figure 51-2.** The continuous relationship between AOTA, AOTPAC, and legislators.

AOTPAC is led by an elected chairperson and five board members who each represent one of five regions of the United States. The AOTPAC chairperson and board members are strongly supported by the AOTA political action administrator, who serves as a liaison between AOTPAC and AOTA, particularly the efforts of the AOTA federal affairs department.

Membership to the AOTA can be one of eight levels including different tiers as an occupational therapist, occupational therapy assistant, student, or individual associate. For occupational therapists and occupational therapy assistants, AOTA provides a reduced rate for both first year and second year new practitioners. An individual associate is a membership for an individual who is an occupational therapist certified exclusively in a foreign country (AOTA, 2015d). Benefits include, but are not limited to, subscriptions to a monthly journal, discounted continuing education, access to professional resources including a job link website, and the access to insurance rates for clinical practice. Additionally, AOTA establishes educational opportunities via online and in-person workshops, including an annual conference during April, which is Occupational Therapy Month. In her presidential address, Dr. Ginny Stoffel (2014) stated, "AOTA is viewed as an organization that provides value to its members and opportunities to enhance their knowledge, skills, and effectiveness while at the same time offering a warm welcome to members engaged in sharing their leadership and talents and developing advocacy and advanced practice skills." Membership to AOTA has been as high as 54,000 members, with growth noted in all membership categories, with an overall growth of almost 6% in 2014 (Stoffel, 2014). There are an estimated 213,000 practitioners and students in the United States (AOTA, 2015d).

Within AOTA, there are multicultural networking groups such as the Asian/Pacific Heritage Occupational Therapy Association that might be an excellent resource to becoming a global citizen. This multicultural networking group in particular strives to create a better understanding of Asian/Pacific cultural issues that affect occupational therapy practitioners. In addition to this networking group, others include National Black Occupational Therapy Caucus; Network for Lesbian, Gay, Bisexual and Transgender Concerns in Occupational Therapy; Network of Occupational Therapy Practitioners with Disability and Their Supporters; Occupational Therapy Network for Native Americans; and Orthodox Jewish Occupational Therapy Chavrusa.

### American Occupational Therapy Foundation

The AOTF is a 501(c)(3) charitable, scientific, and educational organization that supports occupational therapy research, primarily by increasing the understanding of the relationships between health and occupation. Founded in 1965, AOTF accomplishes its mission most notably through grants and scholarships to others who create research and programs to support this mission. These grants and scholarships provided to groups or individuals are supported by contributions, grants, and endowments to AOTF. This organization is governed by an elected board with members of the occupational therapy community and with members from the public (AOTF, 2016a).

Although AOTF is independent of AOTA, the two organizations work closely to support a variety of initiatives to advance research, education, and leadership in occupational therapy. In efforts to network within the profession and better understand research resources, AOTF and AOTA launched a research database for this purpose. OT SEARCH is an AOTF-AOTA project, which is a bibliographic database covering the literature of occupational therapy and related subject areas. Currently, OT SEARCH contains more than 42,000 records of materials, some of which date from 1910. Although the full text of the indexed resources is not in the database, the citation to identify the literature and an abstract exist (AOTF, 2016b). Future initiatives include access to full-text articles. Currently, OT SEARCH is a fee-based subscription service, which is available at a reduced rate for AOTA members. Institutional membership is also available to promote occupational therapy evidence-based practice in clinical and academic settings.

In addition to online databases, AOTF also stores physical copies of all materials cited on OT SEARCH. These physical copies are located in the Wilma L. West library. The aim of this library, which is located in Bethesda, Maryland, is to blend occupational therapy resources from all over the world. In addition to occupational therapy resources, there are also materials from supporting disciplines including health care administration, rehabilitation science, education and psychology. The inclusion of supporting disciplines in the Wilma L. West library, however, remains selective, because AOTF only includes non–occupational therapy journal articles that have been authored by occupational therapy practitioners.

### State Associations

All states in the United States have their own professional occupational therapy association. Membership to the state association in which an occupational therapy practitioner is licensed, in addition to AOTA membership, will assist with support of the profession at the local and state levels. Some states also have an annual conference, website, special interest groups and social media opportunities, so it is important for the occupational therapy practitioner to know, understand, and belong to the appropriate associations related to occupational therapy to become more globally connected. State associations are independent from AOTA, but work together to advance the profession. For example, AOTA provides position statements, practice guidelines, and language for occupational therapy, but the state association must work to get these positions, guidelines, and verbiage into state legislation/licensure (McKinnon, 2015; Phillips, 2014).

## Online Journals

Access to online journals with and without a professional organization membership can enhance professional engagement in occupational therapy. In addition to the OT SEARCH and the Wilma L. West library, journal databases are an excellent way to access professional journals. Access to journal databases is often included with membership to professional organizations, however, many institutions, particularly those in hospital systems or those linked with universities, will have access. In this section, seven journals that promote occupational therapy practice are described: *American Journal of Occupational Therapy* (AJOT), *Canadian Journal of Occupational Therapy* (CJOT), *British Journal of Occupational Therapy* (BJOT), OTJR: *Occupation, Participation, and Health, Occupational Therapy International, Australian Occupational Therapy Journal* (AOTJ), and *Scandinavian Journal of Occupational Therapy*. A summary of these journals is provided in Table 51-2. An additional PDF publication written by Lin and Williams (2013) and published can also be used as an excellent resource, listing more than 100 journals that have published or are relevant for occupational therapy practice.

Increasing global networks of research is evidenced by an agreement between BJOT, AJOT, and CJOT in 2013 allowing 80,000 members of the journals' respective professional bodies to have free online access to each other's journals. Online access is available by members of these professional organizations by visiting each association's website and clicking on the link to the journal (Harries,

Table 51-2.

**Online Journals That Promote the Occupational Therapy Profession**

| Journal | Mission | Access |
|---|---|---|
| *American Journal of Occupational Therapy* | Examines the effectiveness and efficiency of occupational therapy practice, reliability and validity of occupational therapy instruments, and relationship between occupational engagement and participation (publishes six issues/year) | ajot.aota.org |
| *Canadian Journal of Occupational Therapy* | Promotes advancement and growth of research, theory, and practice in occupational therapy (publishes five issues/year) | www.caot.ca |
| *British Journal of Occupational Therapy* | Publishes topics relevant to theory, practice, research, education, and management in occupational therapy internationally (publishes 12 issues/year) | http://www.cot.co.uk/bjot/online |
| *OTJR: Occupation, Participation, and Health* | Reflects commitment to advancing the profession from supporting disciplines including social sciences, neuroscience, nursing, and psychology (publishes quarterly) | http://otj.sagepub.com |

Gutman, & Polatajko, 2013). The agreement between BJOT, AJOT, and CJOT to share the three associations' journals encourages members of all three associations to cite each other's research, as increased citations of occupational therapy research will increase the impact score of all three journals and promote occupational therapy as a valid and respected health care profession (Harries et al., 2013).

## American Journal of Occupational Therapy

AJOT, which started publication in 1947, publishes six issues a year. In addition to six issues a year, AJOT also publishes an annual supplement featuring the AOTA's official documents, which are listed in this chapter. Foci of the journal include research examining the effectiveness and efficiency of occupational therapy practice, reliability and validity of occupational therapy instruments, and relationship between occupational engagement and participation (Harries et al., 2013). In addition, the journal provides an opportunity for scholars to debate professional issues that affect research, clinical, and education issues (Harries et al., 2013). The journal also publishes special issues that focus on particularly topics, which may include, but are not limited to, sensory processing and sensory integration, effectiveness of mental health practice, older driver and community mobility, and productive aging (Harries et al., 2013).

Members of AOTA can access AJOT with written publications sent every 2 months, or online at ajot.aota.org. Currently, online issues are available from 1980. Online access of AJOT can also be found through subscriptions to a variety of research databases.

## Canadian Journal of Occupational Therapy

CJOT, which began publication in 1933, publishes five issues a year. The mission of the journal is to "provide a forum for leading-edge occupational therapy scholarship that advances theory, practice, research, and policy" (Canadian Association of Occupational Therapists, 2015). The journal advances its mission through the publication of articles that promote advancement and growth of research, theory, and practice in occupational therapy (Harries et al., 2013).

CJOT can be accessed online by members of CJOT and reciprocal membership organizations at www.caot.ca. Online issues are available beginning in 1974 and shortly will be available all the way back to 1933. CJOT is excited to be in partnership with BJOT (2008), AOTJ (2011), the *New Zealand Journal of Occupational Therapy* (2009), and AJOT (2013; Harries et al., 2013).

## British Journal of Occupational Therapy

BJOT, which originally commenced as the *Journal of the Occupational Therapists' Association* in 1938, publishes 12 times a year. This journal publishes articles relevant to theory, practice, research, education, and management in occupational therapy internationally (Harries et al., 2013). Special issues have included articles promoting physical activity to enhance quality of life and the Model of Human Occupation, participation in occupations across the life course and occupational performance measures for health and well-being (Harries et al., 2013).

BJOT can be accessed by members of the British Association of Occupational Therapists or by members of reciprocal organizations. Online issues are available from 1998 at http://www.cot.co.uk/bjot/online.

## OTJR: Occupation, Participation, and Health

*OTJR: Occupation, Participation, and Health* is a prominent research journal in occupational therapy published by AOTF. Published quarterly, the journal reflects the AOTF's commitment to advancing the profession through scientific inquiry with contributions from supporting disciplines including social sciences, neuroscience, nursing, and psychology. *OTJR: Occupation, Participation, and Health* was originally entitled the *Occupational Therapy Journal of Research* from 1980 to 2001. *OTJR: Occupation, Participation, and Health* accepts original research articles and systematic review papers "that advance the science of occupational therapy or the understanding of occupation, and will lead to improving the lives of people at risk of being restricted from participating in meaningful activities and roles" (AOTF, 2016c). Access to journal articles published since 2002 can be accessed at http://otj.sagepub.com.

## Occupational Therapy International

*Occupational Therapy International*, which began publication in 1994, publishes four issues a year. Recent publications include how to sustain international partnerships, global partnerships for fieldwork placements, and innovations in global collaborations. This journal focuses on globalization for occupational therapy, expanding knowledge of the influence of culture on occupational performance (Hansen, Munoz, & Suarez-Balcazar, 2013). *Occupational Therapy International* can be accessed by database subscription at http://onlinelibrary.wiley.com/journal/10.1002/(ISSN)1557-0703. Online issues are available since its inception in 1994.

## Australian Occupational Therapy Journal

AOTJ publishes six times per year. The journal aims to promote research and interdisciplinary communication between practitioners, providing a forum for discussion related to occupational therapy practice (Lin & Matthews, 2013). Access to journal articles dating back to the journal's creation in 1952 are available at http://onlinelibrary.wiley.com/journal/10.1111/(ISSN)1440-1630.

**Case Study**

Paula is an occupational therapist who has been practicing for 5 years in physical rehabilitation, primarily working with people with stroke. An opportunity arose for her to travel internationally and work with occupational therapists in South America. Paula planned to visit a nonprofit organization that provided medical and rehabilitation services to individuals with disabilities who do not have the financial resources that cannot otherwise be provided within the government-organized health care system.

Paula decided to prepare her visit by reviewing resources of WFOT and AOTA. In review of WFOT's position statements, she realized that she would print them in Spanish to share with other occupational therapy professionals. She also chose to print information about membership. Additionally, Paula visited AOTA's list of practice guidelines. Knowing that she would be attending AOTA conference in just a few weeks, she decided she would educate herself on what was available, in preparation for sharing with others on her trip.

Lastly, Paula decided to update her knowledge on the most recent evidence for clients with stroke. Specifically, she used OT SEARCH to explore this population, and widened her search to include the impact of culture on practice. Paula then decided to share her favorite article on social media, as she has many occupational therapy connections on her various social media accounts. With preparation of materials from her favorite professional organizations, journals, and social media outlets, Paula felt prepared in a unique way for her trip to South America.

## Scandinavian Journal of Occupational Therapy

The *Scandinavian Journal of Occupational Therapy*, which started in 1994, publishes six times a year. The journal aims to coordinate occupational therapy research efforts in the Nordic countries and in the rest of the world. Like other journals listed in this chapter, this journal provides a forum to disseminate research results in occupational therapy to promote evidence-based practice. Access to this journal is available online at http://www.tandfonline.com/toc/iocc20/current.

# Summary

Local and global resources, particularly those that enhance professional development, evidence-based practice, and global networking, are powerful and necessary components for practice for all occupational therapy practitioners. The importance of identifying and using available resources will allow an occupational therapy practitioner to better provide meaningful relationships with him- of herself, other occupational therapy professionals, and clients. Additionally, the membership to professional organizations including WFOT, AOTA, AOTF, and state associations will increase access to and awareness of global resources.

It is easier than one might think to access occupational therapy resources that can enhance professional development, evidence-based practice, and networking at the local and global levels in occupational therapy advocacy efforts. Identification of resources that meet the needs and interests of the occupational therapy profession, with use of the tables within the chapter, can help initiate opportunities to increase one's own occupational therapy resource database.

## Student Self-Assessment

1. Prior to reading this chapter, how did you demonstrate professional engagement? After reading this chapter, identify a new way to connect with the world of occupational therapy that will connect you to occupational therapy globally. Share your reflection and new resource on social media.
2. Review the professional organizations, evidence-based journal articles, and social connection opportunities. Of the three categories, which do you use most frequently and why? Identify at least one resource in each section that you will explore in the upcoming month. Share this information with your peer.
3. Create a "Favorites" folder on your computer that includes the websites of the identified local and global resources to guide your practice and connection with the world of occupational therapy. How many resources did you include? Discuss your new favorite resource with your colleagues—perhaps they might do the same!
4. Review the case study of a new practitioner using resources from her professional organization. What strategies did she use to expand her network? Although it was not mentioned, how do you think her clients benefited from her use of a variety of resources?

## References

American Occupational Therapy Association. (2013). *2017 and beyond: Mile marker on the road to the Centennial Vision. AOTA Annual Report 2012-2013*. Bethesda, MD: Author.

American Occupational Therapy Association. (2014). *Mile markers on the road to the Centennial Vision*. Retrieved from http://www.aota.org/-/media/corporate/files/aboutaota/2014-annual-report.pdf

American Occupational Therapy Association. (2015a). *About occupational therapy*. Retrieved online from http://www.aota.org/About-Occupational-Therapy.aspx

American Occupational Therapy Association. (2015b). *Administrative standard operating procedures*. Retrieved from http://www.aota.org/-/media/Corporate/Files/AboutAOTA/Governance/Admin%20SOP%20with%20attach%205212.pdf (member log-in required).

American Occupational Therapy Association. (2015c). *AOTPAC*. Retrieved from http://www.aota.org/Advocacy-Policy/AOTPAC.aspx

American Occupational Therapy Association. (2015d). *About AOTA*. Retrieved from http://www.aota.org/AboutAOTA.aspx

American Occupational Therapy Association. (2015e). Official documents available from the American Occupational Therapy Association. *American Journal of Occupational Therapy, 69*(Suppl. 3), 1-3. doi:10.5014/ajot.2015.696Sfm

American Occupational Therapy Foundation. (2016a). *About AOTF*. Retrieved from http://aotf.org/aboutaotf

American Occupational Therapy Foundation. (2016b). *OT SEARCH*. Retrieved from http://aotf.org/resourceswlwlibrary/otsearch

American Occupational Therapy Foundation. (2016c). *OTJR: Occupation, Participation, and Health*. Retrieved from http://www.aotf.org/resourceswlwlibrary/otjroccupationparticipationandhealth.aspx

Canadian Association of Occupational Therapy. (2015). *Canadian Journal of Occupational Therapy (CJOT)*. Retrieved from www.caot.ca

Froude, E., & Craik, C. (2010). Facilitating access to evidence—A benefit to the profession. *British Journal of Occupational Therapy, 73*. doi:10.4276/030802210X12918167234082

Hansen, A., Munoz, J., & Suarez-Balcazar, Y. (2013). The realities of a globally connected profession. *Occupational Therapy International, 20*, 55-57. doi:10.1002/oti.1351

Harries, P., Gutman, S., & Polatajko, H. (2013). Reciprocal access agreements between BJOT, AJOT, and CJOT: New resources for occupational therapists around the world. *American Journal of Occupational Therapy, 67*(2), 138-139. doi:10.5014/ajot.2013.672002

Lin, S., & Matthews, S. (2013). *Occupational therapy and related journals*. Retrieved from https://www.aota.org/~/media/Corporate/Files/Practice/Researcher/ResearchJournalIndexFINAL.ashxa

McKinnon, S. (2015). Leadership and advocacy. In K. Jacobs (Eds.), *Management and administration for the OTA: Leadership and application skills* (pp. 15-32). Thorofare, NJ: SLACK Incorporated.

Metzler, M., & Metz, G. (2010). Translating knowledge to practice: An occupational therapy perspective. *Australian Occupational Therapy Journal, 57*(6), 373-379.

Phillips, S. (2014). Occupational therapy professional organization. In B. Boyt Schell, G. Gillen, & M. Scaffa (Eds.), *Willard and Spackman's occupational therapy* (pp. 1005-1013). Baltimore, MD: Lippincott Williams and Wilkins.

Stoffel, V. (2014). Presidential address—Attitude, authenticity, and action: Building capacity. *American Journal of Occupational Therapy, 68*, 628-635. doi:10.5014/ajot.2014.686002

Stoffel, V. (2015). Engagement, exploration, empowerment. *American Journal of Occupational Therapy, 69*(6), 1-8. doi:10.5014/ajot.2015.696002

World Federation of Occupational Therapists. (2016a). *History*. Retrieved online from http://www.wfot.org/AboutUs/History.aspx

World Federation of Occupational Therapists. (2016b). *WFOT resource center*. Retrieved from http://www.wfot.org/ResourceCentre.aspx#

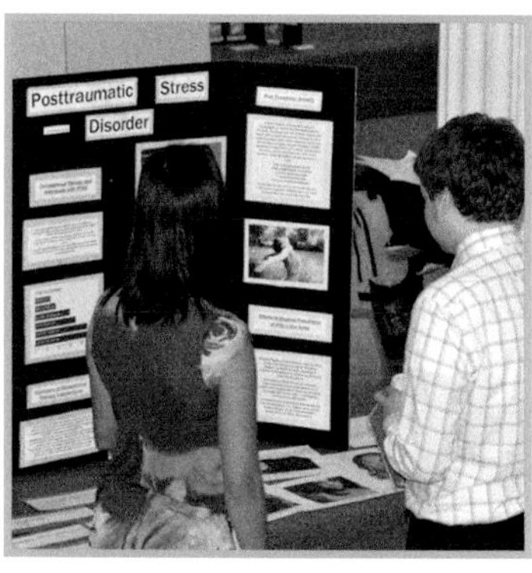


# 52

# Promoting Occupational Therapy to the General Public

Iris Wilbur-Kamien, MS, OTR/L and Jan Rowe, DrOT, MPH, OTR/L, FAOTA

**ACOTE STANDARDS EXPLORED IN THIS CHAPTER**

B.9.3

**KEY VOCABULARY**

- **Advertisement:** Something that is shown or presented to the public to help sell a product or to make an announcement; a person or thing that shows how good or effective something is; the act or process of advertising (Merriam-Webster, 2016).
- **Persuade:** The act of causing people to do or believe something; a particular type of belief or way of thinking (Merriam-Webster, 2016).
- **Promote:** To help (something) happen, develop, or increase (Merriam-Webster, 2016).



Jacobs, K., & MacRae, N. (Eds.).
*Occupational Therapy Essentials for Clinical Competence, Third Edition* (pp. 743-748).

Many years ago, we turned to the radio, magazines, newspaper, or even "snail" mail to gather the latest news and information within our society. In this day and age, we often turn to social media platforms, such as Facebook, Instagram, Twitter, YouTube, Pinterest, and LinkedIn to get the latest updates on what is going on in the world. As technology evolves and becomes more accessible to the general public, so do the means of promoting the profession of occupational therapy. The Internet can serve as a very powerful tool to help us promote our profession in the most effective way possible. In this chapter, we will discuss the importance of promoting our profession and the most effective avenues to do so. Additionally, we will highlight means to promote occupational therapy to survive the changes in health care and to be recognized in community participation.

Occupational therapy practitioners have daily opportunities to define and promote occupation to clients, stakeholders, organizations, and community members. Essential to effectively promoting occupational therapy is accurately defining the profession at its core to the general public in simple, understandable terms, regardless of our niche. It seems as though the term *occupation* is commonly misunderstood, which distracts individuals from the true meaning of our profession. Perhaps occupational therapy would be more clearly understood if the term occupation was explained as any activity that occupies time throughout the day. The *Occupational Therapy Practice Framework* defines occupation as "the daily life activities in which people engage" (American Occupational Therapy Association [AOTA], 2014, p. S6) and occupational therapy as "the therapeutic use of everyday life activities (occupations) with individuals or groups for the purpose of enhancing or enabling participation in roles, habits, and routines in home, school, or workplace, community, and other settings" (p. S1). Occupation is core to our profession. Not using the word occupation in our definition of the profession is a big mistake. Students and practitioners alike have the power to educate the public about occupational therapy and should be doing so on a regular basis.

Many think of occupational therapy very narrowly. Jamnadas, Burns, and Paul (2001) reported that students from physician assistants and nursing professions had perceived knowledge about occupational therapy, but their awareness of the scope of the profession was very narrow. In fact, most of their knowledge regarded activities of daily living. These results imply that more information about our profession is needed with other professional programs, as well as the general public. Additionally, in 1999, Barnhart interviewed different clinicians as part of her attempt to provide strategies for promotion of the profession. She found that practitioners felt that the general public had a lack of awareness about occupational therapy, but certainly the specifics of what we do as occupational therapy practitioners are unknown to most (Barnhart, 1999, p. 26).

This chapter will explore promotion of our profession through the art of persuasion, advertisement, and assessing the profession's image. This chapter will include a review of the literature to provide the reader with information on what has been done to promote our profession both within and external to our field. We will look at literature from occupational therapy as well as other health professions such as nursing and physical therapy. While some literature does exist on promotion of the profession, the majority of what was found was anecdotal or "tips for promotion." Image is also important to the survival of a profession. As occupational therapy practitioners, we have all had the question, "What is occupational therapy?" posed to us. Promotion of a person, product, or service relies on an image. What is our occupational therapy image? If a consistent, representative, and catchy image is lacking, consumers, colleagues, and communities will have difficulty remembering who we are and will therefore have difficulty establishing loyalty to our profession (Scarborough & Zimmerer, 2003).

## Promotion

To effectively promote something, you need to have knowledge or awareness of the item or service, understand what it can do for you, and then believe in it (Barnhart, 1999). Promotion involves savvy persuasion of individuals or groups. Promotion also involves a level of advertisement. Persuasion and advertisement are done in many ways, depending on the personality and skills of the promoter (Scarborough & Zimmerer, 2003).

All occupational therapy practitioners know the value of "selling their goods." Our caseloads, number of community contracts, student recruitments for educational programs, and even number of clients in private practices depend on our skills of "selling." Personal, one-to-one selling does have a significant effect (Jacobs, 1998).

Consider the skills of school children selling candy in their neighborhood to promote and fundraise for a school band. Not all will be promotion savvy, but they believe in the band, and their belief is what drives them. As they make sale after sale, they learn that if you make others believe in your product, they will support it.

## Persuasion

Acts of persuasion are as variable as the persuader. From the skills of a 6-year-old to the skills of an educated, experienced occupational therapy practitioner, persuasion is powerful if effectively employed. Persuasion involves promotion and can include "publicity, personal selling, and advertising" (Scarborough & Zimmerer, 2003, p. 317). Timing is also included in the art of persuasion. As an effective persuader, you have to know when to pitch the idea, when to push or sell hard, and then when to quit. Leave the other party with just enough information (and contact numbers) and the feeling that this has all been under his or her control. Of course, there is also the strategy of the school child: "Believe it and they will buy." Do not stop talking until they buy the candy, agree to see an occupational therapy practitioner, or choose your educational program over others!

Is one-to-one selling of ideas, images, or services effective? Are we able to persuade our clients, customers, or communities that they need occupational therapy services? Consider the "partnership" that takes place during client-centered practice. In this relationship, there is mutual respect for both parties and an agreement to work together to achieve agreed-on goals. In this partnership, there is "buy-in" by the client and practitioner to meet established goals. This is an example of one-to-one selling (Law & Mills, 1998). We also sell one to one when we provide our clients with the evidence that supports our practice. In this one-to-one selling, the client may have an empowered and positive experience with occupational therapy and become a loyal fan. In our education of communities and organizations, occupational therapy is further promoted. Group selling is possibly more powerful and effective than one-to-one selling. Overall, it seems that persuasion is not enough. Advertising our services has become more popular over the past several years. This has been achieved in the national awareness campaign with advertisements about occupational therapy appearing in *People Weekly, Family Circle, Better Homes and Gardens,* and *USA Today* (Jacobs, 1998, p. 620).

## Advertisement

Advertising can have a significant affect for an individual, company, or profession. Advertisements have an agreed-on message by a paid sponsor (Jacobs, 1998, 2011; Scarborough & Zimmerer, 2003). Advertisement includes "calling public attention to something, especially by emphasizing desirable qualities so as to arouse a desire to buy or patronize" (Merriam-Webster, 2016).

The AOTA has launched many advertisement campaigns over the decades. In the early years of our profession, members of AOTA and the founders published in journals like *The Modern Hospital* and *Maryland Psychiatric Quarterly* (Jacobs, 2011). In addition, there have been books written about being an occupational therapist, such as *A Story of Occupational Therapy* by Betty Blake, and public service announcements by famous people (Jacobs, 2011).

You may be aware of the national advertisement campaign launched by AOTA in 1997. In the first phase of the campaign, paid messages appeared in a variety of well-known and common household magazines targeted to women between the ages of 35 and 55. In preparation for the sponsored ads, the marketing agency conducted interviews with occupational therapy practitioners to find out the answer to what their practice involved. The outcome was the byline "skills for the job of living" (Jacobs, 1998; Whiting, 1999). This was in effect a redirection of the question, "What is occupation?" The slogan "Occupational therapy: Skills for the job of living" has provided us mileage as a profession, but do more people actually understand the term occupation?

The answer is a resounding yes. According to Whiting (1999), there was a 44% increase in requests for information about occupational therapy from 1998 to 1999. In addition, "more than 16 million people, most of them members of our target audience, saw the ads" (p. 5). In the second phase of the ad campaign, the target audience included managed care organizations, long-term care facilities, and consumers (again, women between the ages of 35 and 55). The results again were very positive. The advertisements "reached over 2.6 million key decision makers in managed care and long-term care" (Whiting, 1999, p. 12). Hundreds of our practice guidelines were requested by people seeing the advertisements, and almost 1.5 million people saw the Internet ads. The advertising agency working for AOTA remarked that "this campaign has been a huge success!" (Whiting, p. 12).

In 2008, AOTA launched a new promotional campaign, which replaced the previous tag line with "Living Life to Its Fullest." Four years ago, the Nursing Association partnered with Johnson & Johnson (New Brunswick, NJ)—a well-known, family-oriented company. Partnering with a "household name" such as Johnson & Johnson has been a "win-win" situation for both parties. The nursing profession has had significant promotion as a result of the Johnson & Johnson advertisement campaign. Nursing has seen an increase in applicants to the professional educational programs, more than 8 million dollars has been raised for nursing scholarships, and the first-ever "men in nursing scholarship" has been developed. Finally, there has been increased visibility for the profession overall (Johnson & Johnson, 2006). AOTA's partnership with L.L. Bean (Freeport, ME) to promote the first backpack awareness initiative is one such example of partnership in occupational therapy (K. Jacobs, personal communication, February, 2016).

The American Physical Therapy Association (APTA) has a national advertisement campaign as well. They are hoping to recruit physical therapists to promote their own practice or company as part of the "Move Forward" campaign (APTA, n.d.). The organization developed a 15-second television advertisement to "increase consumer awareness of the benefits of physical therapist treatment." Their goal is to direct clients to the www.moveforwardpt.com website to find a physical therapist in their area. This is an excellent way to promote their profession's role while also bringing in business to local physical therapists.

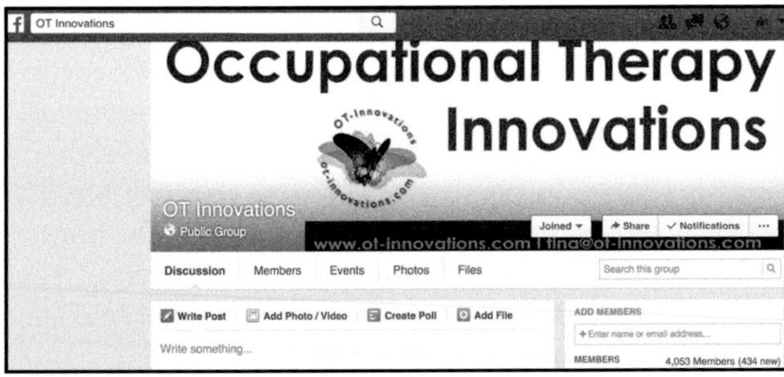


**Figure 52-1.** The Facebook Group "OT Innovations" often posts links to news articles related to occupational therapy and techniques used in practice. There are several contributors who post about various topics, such as sensory rooms, rehabilitation solutions for older adults, and mental health treatment strategies. (Retrieved from https://www.facebook.com/groups/253712334753788/)

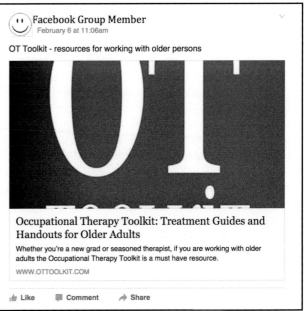


**Figure 52-2.** A group member of the group "OT Connections" on Facebook shares a great resource for occupational therapists to use in practice. (Retrieved from https://www.facebook.com/groups/253712334753788/)

Social media may be an effective way to share information about our profession to the general public. In fact, Giordano and Giordano (2011) found that health care students, including students of occupational therapy, prefer online media as their primary source of information (Figures 52-1 and 52-2). Facebook can be used to share recent articles about occupational therapy with friends and family. Several occupational therapy-based groups exist on social media pages in which members can join and "follow" to gather information and news about a particular area or topic related to occupational therapy practice. These groups often post links and articles on their page sharing information of topics related to various settings within the field, ranging from pediatric interventions to geriatric care. You may decide to create your own group as a platform or share other groups' articles and links to promote knowledge of occupational therapy to your family, friends, and beyond.

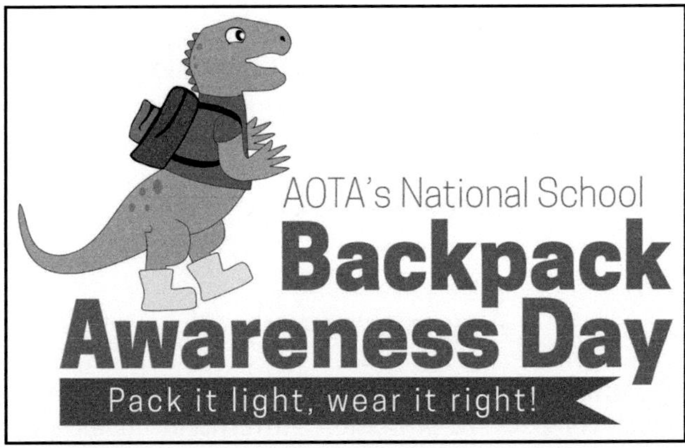


**Figure 52-3.** Using a symbol such as the OT Rex may help catch one's attention, thus drawing more awareness to the profession. (Reprinted with permission from the American Occupational Therapy Association. Retrieved from http://www.aota.org/-/media/Corporate/Images/Conference-Events/Events/Backpack/OT-Rex-Backpack-logo.jpg)

## Our Image

When you think of our profession, what image comes to mind? It is one thing to define our profession in words; it is another to define our profession in images. Maybe the AOTA's logo is our profession's image. Or is our image based on the stories we read and pictures we see during AOTA's occupational therapy month each year? Perhaps our image is that of the former National School Backpack Awareness Day campaign image—Luminie, the lightening bug! Or OT Rex, the 2015 image (Figure 52-3)!

Many occupational therapy practitioners and students often have difficulty stating succinctly what we do in occupational therapy. We must explain to our clients and community what we do, the evidence behind why we do it, and the level of education needed to enter the profession. In the nursing discipline, Lusk (2000) found that nurses from the 1930s to 1950s were seen by the public as subordinate to physicians and hospital administrators. Overall, the nurses of the 1940s were seen as performing more complex activities when compared to the nurses of the 1930s and 1950s. The important message in this article is that nurses of that era were not seen as professional. In the profession of occupational therapy, we want the public to view us as professionals. Image, pride for the profession, and ensuring that people know what occupational therapy is are key.

The old adage "a picture is worth a thousand words" might be useful here. In an *OT Practice* issue, the Oklahoma State Association President, Suzanne

## Evidence-Based Research Chart

| Category of Promotion | Means of Promotion | Evidence |
|---|---|---|
| Recruitment strategy; prospective occupational therapy students | Careers pack | Craik & Ross, 2003 |
| National perspective about occupational therapy | Publication/presentation | Dickinson, 2003; Jacobs, 1998 |
| Promotional ideas | "Mediaspeak," National Awareness Campaign, Occupational Therapy Cruiser, mass media to promote nursing | Collins, 2002; Walls, 1999; Whitehead, 2000; Whiting, 1999 |
| Awareness/knowledge of occupational therapy; nursing | Marketing, survey | Barnhart, 1999; Jamnadas, Burns, & Paul, 2001; Lusk, 2000 |
| Social media | Facebook, YouTube, Twitter, Instagram, LinkedIn | Giordano & Giordano, 2011 |

Bowman, shows off her "OT Cruiser" (Collins, 2002, p. 11). Promoting occupational therapy visually is powerful. Not only does this type of promotion get people talking, but it also can and will convey pride in our profession. Wearing occupational therapy shirts and using pens, note pads, and drink holders with the occupational therapy logo are powerful ways to convey an image of the pride for our profession. Providing clients, consumers, students, and community stakeholders with visual images and "freebies" is a step in the right direction. To equate the profession with an image is memorable and can lead to building a loyal fan base.

## General Promotion

When promoting anything or anyone, the same three principles apply: publicity, personal selling, and advertising (Scarborough & Zimmerer, 2003). We are all capable of doing any or all of these three things. Consider writing an article for *OT Practice* or a letter to the editor for your local newspaper. Sponsor an in-service or seminar for a local agency to promote occupational therapy or go to your child's school and talk to the classmates about occupational therapy. Speaking and "selling" to individuals is another approach. Becoming involved in the Occupational Therapy Global Day of Service is an excellent way to promote the profession while learning what occupational therapists around the world are doing.

Personal selling for occupational therapy enlists the client-centered approach, but in general, personal selling is that one-to-one relationship between salesperson and consumer or customer. Developing the relationship is often what gives one company the "edge" over another. Having good interpersonal skills is a must when engaging in personal selling. Let the other person talk while you listen, be enthusiastic, pay attention to all details, and measure your success by the client's satisfaction. These are good strategies for effective practitioners as well, but in the end, we might have to resort to advertising our wares.

Advertising can encompass various media types, including magazines, newspapers, direct mail, radio, television, and now the Internet. We have previously discussed occupational therapy's past approach to advertising. These attempts will need to continue in assorted ways to ensure that we reach our target populations. These days, understanding the Internet and the use of social media is essential to broaden our means of promoting occupational therapy. The target populations will change over time depending on the message we are sending and, therefore, our media type will have to vary to reach our intended audience. Identify your audience and select the most appropriate media to reach them, then go for it!

## Summary

This chapter provides an overview of promotional strategies that will assist in the promotion of occupational therapy to a broad and complex global community. Please see Chapter 42 for more information on marketing.

## Student Self-Assessment

1. In 15 seconds or less, describe or define occupational therapy. How did you do? Did you get the words occupation, daily living skills, health promotion, and activities of daily living in there? If you were going to do this activity again, what would you change about your definition?

2. As an exercise, browse social media and identify three different accounts or groups used to promote occupational therapy practice. Now search the Internet for a recent news article related to occupational therapy that you could use on your own social media site to spread awareness to your friends and family connected through the platform.
3. Occupational therapy is a diverse and wide-reaching profession. We often define the profession based on what our role is within the discipline. To promote the field of occupational therapy, you need to give your listeners a full range of what the profession is and what it can do for them. As another assignment, jot down the first 10 things that come to mind when you think about what an occupational therapy practitioner can do for a client, student, resident, community, or organization. What commonalities did you find in your lists? How often do you think about occupational therapy serving communities?

## References


American Occupational Therapy Association. (2014). Occupational therapy practice framework: Domain and process (3rd ed.). *American Journal of Occupational Therapy, 68*(Suppl. 1), S1-S48. doi:10.5014/ajot.2014.682006

American Physical Therapy Association. (n.d.). Retrieved from http://www.apta.org/PRMarketing/Consumers/MediaBuying101/

Barnhart, P. D. (1999). Secrets of success: OTs share their strategies. *OT Practice, 4*(3), 26-30.

Collins, L. (2002). Easy ways to promote occupational therapy. *OT Practice, 8*, 11-14.

Craik, C., & Ross, F. (2003). Promotion of occupational therapy as career: A survey of occupational therapy managers. *British Journal of Occupational Therapy, 66*(2), 78-81.

Dickinson, R. (2003). Occupational therapy: A hidden treasure. *Canadian Journal of Occupational Therapy, 70*(3), 133-135.

Giordano, C., & Giordano, C. (2011). Health professions students' use of social media. *Journal of Allied Health, 40*(2), 78-81.

Jacobs, K. (1998). Innovation to action: Marketing occupational therapy. *OT Practice, 52*(8), 618-620.

Jacobs, K. (2011). Eleanor Clarke Slagle lecture. PromOTing occupational therapy: Words, images and actions. *American Journal of Occupational Therapy, 66*(6), 652-671.

Jamnadas, B., Burns, J., & Paul, S. (2001). Understanding occupational therapy: Nursing and physician assistant students' knowledge about occupational therapy. *Occupational Therapy in Health Care, 14*(1), 13-27.

Johnson & Johnson. (2006). *The campaign for nursing's future: A progress report*. Retrieved from http://www.discovernursing.com/progressreport.pdf

Law, M., & Mills, J. (1998). Client-centered occupational therapy. In M. Law (Ed.), *Client-centered occupational therapy*. Thorofare, NJ: SLACK Incorporated.

Lusk, B. (2000). Pretty and powerless: Nurses in advertisements, 1930-1950. *Research in Nursing and Health, 23*(3), 229-236.

Merriam-Webster. (2016). *On-line dictionary* (11th ed.). Retrieved from http://www.merriam-webster.com

Scarborough, N. M., & Zimmerer, T. W. (2003). *Effective small business management: An entrepreneurial approach* (7th ed.). Upper Saddle River, NJ: Prentice Hall.

Walls, B. S. (1999). Sound bite: OT practitioners learn "mediaspeak." *OT Practice, 4*(7), 7, 20.

Whitehead, D. (2000). Using mass media within health-promoting practice: A nursing perspective. *Journal of Advanced Nursing, 32*(4), 807-816.

Whiting, F. (1999). PromOTing OT: Year two of the national awareness campaign. *OT Practice, 4*(6), 5, 12.

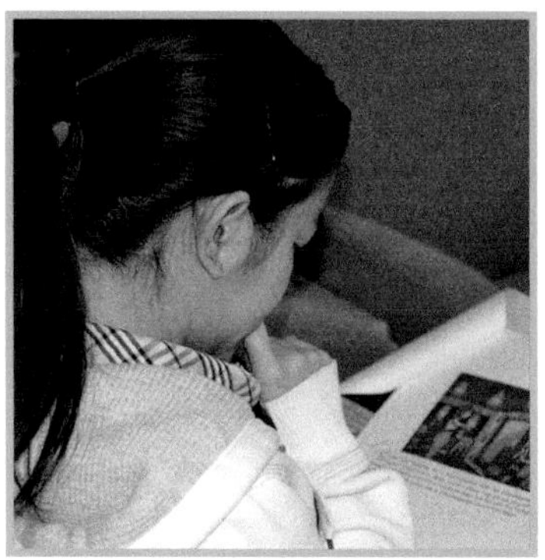

# 53

# Competence and Professional Development
## Learning for Complexity

Penelope Moyers Cleveland, EdD, OT/L, FAOTA

**ACOTE STANDARDS EXPLORED IN THIS CHAPTER**

B.9.3

**KEY VOCABULARY**

- **Competencies:** Explicit statements that define specific areas of expertise and are related to effective or superior performance in a job (Spencer & Spencer, 1993).
- **Continuing competence:** Refers to an individual's ongoing or life-long capacity to perform responsibilities as a part of one's professional role performance.
- **Continuing competency:** Focuses on an individual's actual performance in a particular situation according to standard as a part of one's current professional role performance.
- **Professional development:** A process in which one plans and achieves excellence or establishes expertise when seeking a change in responsibilities, or when assuming more complex professional roles.
- **Self-assessment:** Provides the means to assess performance, abilities, and skills; to analyze demands and resources of the work environment; to interpret information about clients' outcomes; to reassess current learning goals; and to develop goals and plans for professional growth and continuing competence and competency.



Jacobs, K., & MacRae, N. (Eds.).
*Occupational Therapy Essentials for Clinical Competence, Third Edition* (pp. 749-762).

> In today's complex world, we must educate not merely for competence, but for capability (the ability to adapt to change, generate new knowledge, and continuously improve performance). (Fraser & Greenhalgh, 2001)

Rapid incorporation of innovation is driven by the need to improve the client's experience within health care, social, and educational systems; improve the health of individuals and their families and populations; and reduce the per capita cost of health care and social services. These factors are often referred to as the Triple Aim guiding the redesign of health care and social services. It is quite clear that improvement in health care includes a seamless integration of social services and community living. Professionals must demonstrate team-based practice competencies as an essential component of seamless integration. Additionally, in terms of the education of new health care professionals and current professionals, there is growing awareness of the importance of translating evidence into practice. Value-based health care and social services balance efficiency and effectiveness in terms of their cost and quality, which involves professionals working collaboratively with each other and their clients within interdependent health and health care systems (Burwell, 2015). Consequently, the stakes for being competent as occupational therapists and occupational therapy assistants continue to rise not only with the focus on evidence-based practice (Moyers & Hinojosa, 2003), but also on interprofessional collaborative practice (Josiah Macy Jr. Foundation, 2013) and knowledge translation methods (Petzold, Korner-Bitensky, & Menon, 2010). According to the World Health Organization (2010), interprofessional collaborative practice occurs "when multiple health workers from different professional backgrounds work together with patients, families, carers [sic], and communities to deliver the highest quality of care" (p. 7). Implementation science, a type of knowledge translation, is the process of putting to use or integrating evidence-based interventions within a specific setting (Fixsen, Naoom, Blase, Friedman, & Wallace, 2005). As a component of implementation, the organization purposefully designs effective learning approaches for clinicians and staff throughout the organization to achieve full adoption of the practice change.

While quality of care requires occupational therapy practitioners to prevent harm by ensuring that clients are not seriously injured during implementation of services due to practitioner neglect or malpractice or due to poor risk management, harm has a broader meaning. In addition, harm results when our clients receive an ineffective intervention or an intervention that is not as effective as an alternative method in improving health, well-being, and participation in life. Even when using an evidence-based intervention, harm occurs when the intervention is implemented inadequately or in a way that does not reflect adherence to tested protocols or policies. Occupational therapy practitioners who are ineffective in collaborative practice with key team members also create harm when they contribute to unnecessary team conflict, avoid addressing team conflict, do not examine effectiveness of their team performance, and are not reliable and dependable in carrying out team-assigned responsibilities. Harm also results from occupational therapy population- or organization-based services that are poorly designed, implemented, and evaluated. Services that are not interdependent with a range of systems and that do not incorporate input to constantly improve the quality of the client experience contribute to harm as well. The harm that occurs relates to the cost benefit of services in terms of the expenditures made for poor outcomes. Additionally, the client, organization, or population may have to assume other costs associated with intervention continuing over a longer duration than expected, with the additional burden for caregiving resulting from reduced participation in activities of daily living, with the loss of the worker role to support daily living, and with the possible reduction in the economic viability of the community if a large population or organization is negatively affected by ineffective programming. Policy for reimbursement of medically based services is incorporating the concept of paying for performance or the outcome achieved after intervention is delivered within a collaborative-based practice model (Burwell, 2015).

Because of the increasing pressure for accountability related to health care and social service outcomes, employers, third-party payers, community agencies, business, and industry all expect practitioners to remain competent and knowledgeable of the new developments in the field of occupational therapy, collaborative practice, and in related contextual areas involving local, state, national, and global communities. It is not acceptable to believe that an occupational therapist or occupational therapy assistant enters practice thoroughly trained, possessing all the knowledge needed throughout one's career. The career path taken should be punctuated with learning to enhance professional development and continuing competence and competency in occupational therapy, in collaborative practice, and in knowledge translation and management.

In this chapter, the *Occupational Therapy Practice Framework: Domain and Process, Third Edition*, will be used to understand the occupation of education (American Occupational Therapy Association [AOTA], 2014), particularly as learning is important for continuing competence and competency and professional development in occupational therapy and collaborative practice. These terms then are differentiated to highlight the three distinct purposes of the different areas of learning; however, knowledge translation undergirds all learning areas in which the professional engages. A model that proposes how change occurs and how assessment links collaborative practice performance, career growth, and learning is described. Based on a gap between actual and desired collaborative practice performance or gap between desired career development and actual career trajectory, a learning plan is developed that includes feasible strategies thought best to narrow these gaps and most likely to produce a measurable change in client daily life participation outcomes and in achievement of the practitioner's career goals. For collaborative practice, a team learning and development plan is necessary. The roles of administrators, team members and leaders, organizations, professional organizations, universities, continuing education providers, credentialing bodies, and government in fostering this model are described.

## Education as an Occupation

> Lifelong learning means that education converges with (and is influenced by) work, family, and personal development. (Fraser & Greenhalgh, 2001)

Education in the *Framework* (AOTA, 2014) addresses the "activities involved in learning and participating in the educational environment" (p. S42). One can be a learner beyond the formal education years when exploring learning needs and interests and participating in "informal classes, programs, and activities that provide instruction or training in identified areas of interest" (AOTA, p. S20). This chapter is concerned with the education related to the occupation of work after one has completed entry-level formal education as an occupational therapist or occupational therapy assistant. This life-long education throughout one's career requires the practitioner to possess the necessary underlying body functions (movement-related, mental, and sensory) as well as performance skills (motor, process, and social interaction). The occupational therapy practitioner has to have the ability to adapt new knowledge and skills, including advanced interprofessional competencies, to one's professional roles to be a successful learner, knowledge translator, and practice collaborator.

Learning as a part of the educational process is influenced by cultural, personal, and temporal contexts and physical and social environments. For instance, the social expectations from the public and the profession are for the practitioner to be competent and up to date in the knowledge, attitudes, and skills associated with providing a high-quality service, including collaboration with colleagues, clients, and team members. The organization in which one works may have a culture in which learning is left up to the individual practitioner rather than one that values learning as an aspect of organizational performance and collaborative practice. Depending on the learning preferences of the learner, the physical environment could be inadvertently designed where learning is inhibited instead of being facilitated. Often, virtual synchronous or asynchronous contexts, whether in the form of online learning platforms, list serves and discussion groups, online courses, blogs, web-based conferencing technology, and websites, are where learning occurs to accommodate geographical distance and a variety of schedule differences among learners. Thus, virtual contexts allow learners to individually address the temporal contextual needs of their daily lives and biorhythms so that learning can occur at the most opportune time. The personal contextual factors of age, educational level, and socioeconomic status can influence learning in terms of the design of the education (e.g., education with expectations for large amounts of memorization may be difficult for older learners, or learners with young children may have less time to engage in educational offerings occurring over a long duration or requiring travel and overnight stays away from the family). Costs associated with the educational offering may deter participation as well (e.g., participating in some offerings may be cost prohibitive for practitioners with little employer support, lower salaries, and family financial pressures). Team-based learning is influenced by not only the confluence of personal contextual factors of the team members, but also by their access to technologically supported learning that bridges the time pressures when bringing team members together around a learning event. In addition, there is the added complication of what the team considers to be the focus of learning as individuals on the team will have competing interests, needs, and vision about how to improve client-centered care.

## Competence, Competency, and Professional Development

The word *continuing* is typically combined with both competence and competency to denote a life-long learning process. Often, the terms *competence* and *competency* are used interchangeably, when in fact there is an important difference between these two concepts. Competence "refers to an individual's capacity to perform" professional responsibilities, whereas competency "focuses on an individual's actual performance in a particular situation" (McConnell, 2001, p. 14). Professional development is a process in which one plans and achieves excellence, establishes expertise, seeks a change in responsibilities, or assumes more complex professional roles (Moyers & Hinojosa, 2003). Continuing competence and competency are requirements for one's current professional responsibilities in a given role in contrast to professional development, which involves what one aspires to achieve regardless of one's present position or role. Professional development may not focus on what one needs to learn to perform better, but rather may address what one is interested in learning to advance one's career.

Continuing competence is designed to build capacity to perform one's responsibilities in the future for a given role. Occupational therapy practice and health care in general advances rapidly so that a practitioner who does not engage in continuing competence activities will become markedly out of date in a short amount of time. For example, if a new documentation system is going to be implemented, training would be needed to properly prepare for the change. Because neither the systems in which we work nor the external environment will ever be constant (Fraser & Greenhalgh, 2001), educating for capacity is very important.

Continuing competency, in contrast, ensures that the practitioner performs according to standard given that a distinctive set of variables dynamically interact, resulting in each client situation being unique. It is well known that practitioner performance is highly context dependent, such that the practitioner may have better outcomes in one situation compared to another similar situation (Handfield-Jones et al., 2002). With continuing competency, there is also an assumption that all practitioner skills and abilities fade with lack of practice, feedback, or team and administrative/system support.

Another factor important in understanding both continuing competence and competency is that there is not a linear relationship between learning and improved practice performance and changed capacity. Instead, there may be periods of time when there is either no improvement or even a slight decrease in performance. These periods of little change then may be followed by sudden jumps in practice performance (Handfield-Jones et al., 2002). Because most of practice is based on cognitively complex tasks, learning typically requires cognitive reorganization that may involve abandonment of previously held ideas and principles. Therefore, the impact of learning on practice appears to occur in sudden leaps rather than through continuous and gradual change. Consequently, while practice performance improves in some areas, it may simultaneously deteriorate in others. When practicing in teams, learning among team members takes longer to integrate into a smooth practice change that significantly affects client care. Team learning typically involves complex system change to support the changed work of the team.

## Self-Assessment Model

The learning of currently practicing occupational therapists and occupational therapy assistants is different from learning obtained as students within their professional programs: the focus in the latter was on learning generalist practice and a core set of competencies, allowing few opportunities to learn any particular interest area in depth. Level II fieldwork and the first year or two on the job has been the time for specialized learning. More recently, the entry-level doctorate allows time for delving into these interest areas through the doctoral experiential component (Accreditation Council for Occupational Therapy Education, 2011). The first several years in a position in which intensive job training occurs, however, is complicated by the need to not only develop specialization but to focus learning efforts to enhance expected performance. The requirement is to simultaneously keep up with advances in these specialty areas as well as advances in quality improvement and team-based care. As a result, practitioners are expected to engage in and employers must facilitate a systematic approach to learning that considers learning styles, client populations, career stage, and influence of previous learning. For learning to result in a sustainable practice change, the learner and organization must understand the barriers and supports for implementation of evidence to practice, particularly within a climate of collaborative practice, quality improvement, and value-based outcomes (Schreiber, Perry, Downey, & Williamson, 2013). Learning plans maximize the practitioner's educational efforts to enhance therapy and collaborative practice outcomes and to advance one's career (Wilkinson et al., 2002). Learning is thus a process to be managed, one that necessitates a dynamic approach to target the learning needs that arise from daily practice and from one's goals for career development, as well as arise from the organizational goals of translating evidence successfully to value-based service delivery.

In order to link practice performance with learning, the occupational therapist and occupational therapy assistant have to engage in a self-assessment process that increasingly involves their collaborative practice colleagues (Figure 53-1). "Self-assessment provides the means by which therapists and assistants develop goals and plans for professional growth, reassess current goals, assess performance, analyze demands and resources of the work environment, and interpret information about the consumers' outcomes" (Moyers & Hinojosa, 2003, p. 484). In addition, self-assessment focuses on one's capacity to translate evidence to practice for sustainable change (Straus et al., 2011). Self-assessment for the development of a learning plan should primarily be formative in nature as summative assessments are mainly used for employee evaluation, certification programs, or licensure. Self-assessment answers the question, "What can I do to improve competence and competency in my job or role on a collaborative practice team?" Self assessment can also answer the question of what is needed to advance one's career (Smith & Tillema, 2001). Self-assessment not only locates discrepancies in current practice compared to an ideal, but also validates what is going well. In terms of professional development, self-assessment ascertains strengths and how to further develop those strengths in preparation for career advancement.

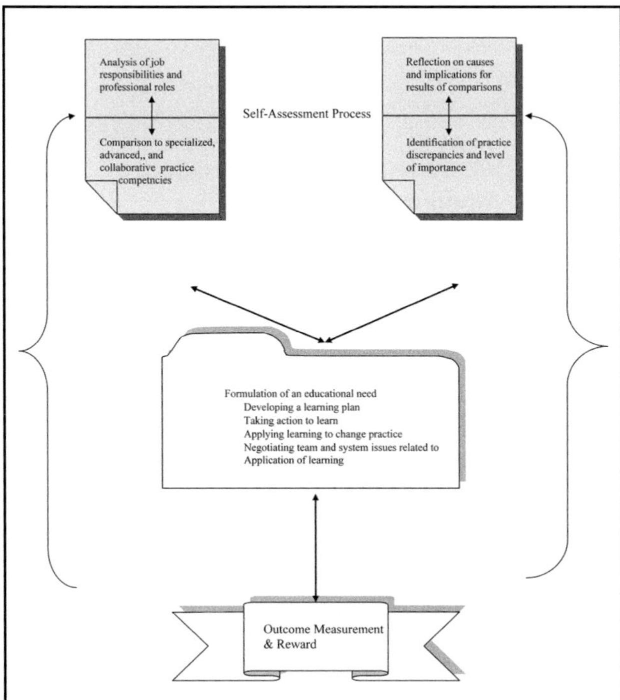


**Figure 53-1.** Linking practice performance and learning.

## Job Responsibilities and Client Outcomes

Self-assessment begins with an analysis of one's job responsibilities and roles, typically answering such questions as the following:

- What are my main responsibilities and roles?
- Within those roles, what are my most significant job tasks?
- What kinds of expertise are required to produce successful client outcomes?
- What are the criteria for successful performance?

Then, the self-assessment incorporates information from one's own work performance and would include answering such questions as the following:

- How does the current evidence, occupational therapy and team outcomes data inform my learning needs and that of my collaborative practice colleagues?
- Is improvement in my performance and the team's performance indicated?
- Are there systems problems and team collaboration issues that I can help modify?
- What can I do to improve efficiency and effectiveness of occupational therapy services and their interdependent integration within collaborative practice environments?

Self-assessment for professional development is slightly different and includes such questions as:

- What are my goals for my career?
- What roles will I need to develop?
- What kinds of tasks might be included in these roles?
- What skills and types of reasoning are involved in these tasks?
- What is my current skill level and reasoning ability in comparison to what might be required for these new tasks?
- What are the criteria for successful performance?

Generally, the practitioner learns to compare his or her current practice performance with some ideal or desired result. To be helpful, self-assessment for the practitioner requires the gathering of valid and reliable information about one's appropriateness and adequacy in working with clients in terms of helping them achieve health, well-being, and participation in life goals within a collaborative practice environment. Self-assessments may include fidelity measures of protocol adherence, knowledge tests, skills checkouts, performance observations, case studies, self-reflection, and peer ratings from team members, record audits, outcomes data, or consumer feedback (Ward, Gruppen, & Regehr, 2002). Self-assessment for professional development typically requires feedback from a mentor or from someone who is in a similar role in comparison to the one in which one hopes to assume.

The question is, how does one determine what is the desirable practice performance or desired level of professional skill development? This requires research into the latest evidence, practice guidelines or standards, recommended competencies, protocols, professional benchmarks, expert recommendations, efficacy and effectiveness studies, and meta-analyses or systematic evidence reviews, as well as expectations of employers, team members, clients, third-party payers, and the public.

## Competencies

Competencies are another type of standard guiding self-assessment. Competencies are explicit statements that define specific areas of expertise or competency (Decker, 1999), of which there are four types (Decker & Strader, 1997):

1. Generic across all jobs in an organization
2. Related to management, supervision, or leadership roles
3. Threshold or minimum requirements of a job
4. Specific to a job

Table 53-1.

## Core Competencies for Interprofessional Collaborative Practice

| Interprofessional Competency Domain | Competency Statement |
|---|---|
| Values of ethics of interprofessional practice | "Work with individuals of other professions to maintain a climate of mutual respect and shared values" (p. 19). |
| Roles and responsibilities | "Use the knowledge of one's own role and those of other professions to appropriately assess and address the health care needs of the patients and populations served" (p. 21). |
| Interprofessional communication | "Communicate with patients, families, communities, and other health professionals in a responsive and responsible manner that supports a team approach to the maintenance of health and the treatment of disease" (p. 23). |
| Teams and teamwork | "Apply relationship-building values and the principles of team dynamics to perform effectively in different team roles to plan and deliver patient-/population-centered care that is safe, timely, efficient, effective, and equitable" (p. 25). |

A sample statement to illustrate how competencies are written is as follows: "Ability to select and use the most appropriate assessment instrument given the client's age, health and disability status, values, goals, and preferences for specific occupations." This is a threshold statement that could be written to be more specific to a specialized area of occupational therapy practice by referring to an age range or other demographics, diagnoses, type of occupations, performance skills and patterns, contexts or environments, or method of intervention.

The Interprofessional Education Collaborative Expert Panel (2011) has developed core competencies for interprofessional collaborative practice that all team practices should use to guide their competency and continuing competence. Within the report of the expert panel, the concept of interprofessionality was defined as "the process by which professionals reflect on and develop ways of practicing that provides an integrated and cohesive answer to the needs of the client/family/population" (p. 8). Because interprofessional practice has unique values, codes of conduct, and ways of working, competencies are categorized in a slightly different framework than that described by Decker. According to Barr (1998), professionals on a team have "common" or overlapping competencies, which are those expected of all health professionals. Each team member may overlap the competencies of other professionals on the team in varying ways depending on the professions involved and their scopes of practice, and on the expertise these professionals have developed within their various scopes. Overlapping competencies can be the source of interprofessional tensions, such as in the debate about overlapping competencies between occupational and physical therapists and speech and language pathologists. Overlap should not be seen automatically as negative; it is, in fact, an important strategy to extend the reach of a health profession whose practitioners are inaccessible for various reasons, or when reinforcement of interventions must occur throughout multiple client sessions.

In addition, team members have "complementary" competencies that enhance the qualities of other professions in providing care. For instance, rehabilitation professionals work well together to achieve the outcomes for clients after a stroke, where gait, cognition, swallowing, and communication are addressed in ways that assist the occupational therapy practitioner's focus on occupations. Important for all team members are "collaborative" competencies, where each profession needs to work (a) within a profession and among professions, (b) with patients and clients and their families, (c) with nonprofessionals and volunteers, and (d) within and between organizations and communities. These interprofessional competencies have been organized within domains with associated competency statements (Interprofessional Education Collaborative Expert Panel, 2011). Table 53-1 lists these competencies and their accompanying statements.

Another set of competencies that are becoming more important include those associated with knowledge translation to execute practice change in a way that leads to the expected client outcomes. Knowledge to Action Process (Graham et al., 2006) is a framework that guides implementation of a practice change where the practitioner first identifies a problem and finds the evidence to guide solution. Then this evidence has to be adapted to the local practice context. Prior to adaptation or implementation, barriers to knowledge use are identified and modified, or removed, when possible. The intervention may require tailoring to fit the context, which is difficult given that the goal is to implement the intervention with the strength needed to produce the expected outcome. The goal is to create or obtain knowledge that delineates the essential components of the intervention. Implementation efforts are monitored to ensure fidelity, and the client outcomes are evaluated. If the client outcomes are expected, then the practitioner works to achieve sustainability of the practice change through embedding the practice within the everyday practices of the organization (e.g., incorporating needed documentation components of the intervention into the electronic health record). Embedding the practice change leads to development of policies, purchasing and storage of supplies and equipment, staff education processes, and strategies to monitor new evidence that may update the new intervention.

## Discrepancies

Practice discrepancies uncovered through self-assessment do not always necessitate a change in practice, but careful analysis is needed to determine whether modification is needed. The practitioner reflects on why the difference exists as perhaps there are team, system, population, or other key circumstances that explain why one's results are dissimilar to the benchmarks. The size of the gap between what exists and what should occur in practice or in professional development contributes to motivation for change in that a small discrepancy may be overlooked as unimportant and a large discrepancy may appear impossible to resolve (Handfield-Jones et al., 2002). Ultimately an educational need is identified that prompts development and implementation of a learning plan. The desired change has to be divisible into small, manageable learning steps.

Learning then has to be applied to practice to bring about a change with thought given to how to measure the impact of the learning application on client satisfaction and outcomes. Application to practice requires removal of team and system barriers and creation of system supports in which administration plays a key role. For instance, if the occupational therapist has learned how to administer a reliable and valid occupational performance assessment tool that has evidence for its effectiveness in developing occupation-based intervention, but there are no funds available to purchase the instrument, space to administer the evaluation, or time allowed to complete the evaluation, nor an intervention philosophy among team members that supports occupation-based practice, then the practitioner will be unable to apply this new learning. Similarly, learning will be difficult to apply to professional development if the new opportunities or roles are not available in one's employment or within one's professional roles.

## Motivation for Learning

Motivation for learning is complicated and is dependent on one's understanding of the ethical nature inherent in the learning process. The competence of the occupational therapist and the occupational therapy assistant provides the moral justification for implementing occupational therapy processes and services (Moyers, 2005). Principle 1 of the AOTA's *Occupational Therapy Code of Ethics* (2015a) indicates the practitioner's responsibility for maintaining high standards of competence. In many states, mandatory continuing education is an aspect of licensure renewal. Similarly, the National Board for Certification in Occupational Therapy (NBCOT) has requirements for achievement of Professional Development Units in the renewal process for the practitioner to use the initials OTR or COTA, whichever is appropriate. The Joint Commission, which accredits hospitals and other health care organizations, has standards that require all employees to update and demonstrate competence to carry out the job tasks assigned.

Motivation to engage in self-assessment and ongoing learning activities, in addition to external requirements of employers, credentialing and accrediting bodies, has an intrinsic component in that it is partially related to the virtues of being a "good" occupational therapist or occupational therapy assistant. The practitioner must display the integrity to self-assess as honestly as possible as a part of one's altruistic responsibility for providing optimal client services (Moyers, 2005). Prudence as a virtue facilitates the disciplined pursuit of competence in which there is a sincere effort to learn what will most likely contribute to excellent client outcomes and high levels of service satisfaction (Moyers, 2005). The practitioner must also have certain underlying abilities to support learning, such as the "requisite intellectual skill and cognitive complexity to understand and synthesize" information, the emotional ability to take risks in applying learning, and the relational abilities to inform clients and team members and to work within systems to implement learning application (p. 28). Obviously, learning application that leads to successful practice change in enhancing service outcomes has the potential for creating an iterative self-assessment process as the result of motivation derived from the quality improvement and collaborative practice process itself.

## Development and Implementation of the Learning Plan

Given the complexity of the roles occupational therapists and occupational therapy assistants assume, the questions guiding the development and implementation of the learning plan, whether for continuing competency and competence or professional development, are listed in Table 53-2.

The job competencies thought most likely to lead to high-quality client outcomes are addressed in the learning plan. These selected competencies are analyzed through the help of AOTA's *Standards for Continuing Competence* (2015b), which includes how knowledge, critical reasoning, interpersonal and performance skills, and ethical practice contribute to successful enactment of each competency. For instance, refer to the sample competency described earlier—to select and use the best assessment given the client's age, health and disability status, and preference for occupations. This competency requires knowledge of assessments available to measure the specific performance in the desired occupation. Critical reasoning involves the ability to select according to best evidence the assessment most likely to accurately and reliably assess the performance in the occupation of interest given the client's characteristics, values, and needs. The performance skill underlying this competency is the ability to administer the assessment according to standardization. Collaboratively selecting the assessment and explaining the evaluation process to promote client and team decision making is the requisite interpersonal ability. Weighing pragmatic issues of the evaluation process against client needs includes ethical practice ability.

Also, to develop an effective learning plan, one needs to be aware of the best methods for learning performance and interpersonal skills, gaining knowledge, and developing critical reasoning and ethical practice. For instance, reading may be appropriate for gaining knowledge, but does not compare to role-playing and simulation strategies that may be more effective in enhancing interpersonal abilities, particularly when improving team interactions and communication. Learning plans typically include learning goals, target dates for completion of the learning activities, specific learning activities, resources needed to implement the plan, how one plans to apply the learning to practice, and how one will determine the effectiveness of learning. Learning goals are derived from the learning needs identified in the self-assessment, related to the job competencies and AOTA's *Standards for Continuing Competence* (2015b), and lead to learning applied to practice. There is enough evidence to indicate lecturing, demonstration, practice, and feedback in a traditional learning context do not lead to application in practice. Instead these learning strategies lead primarily to knowledge retention and ability to return the demonstration (Joyce & Showers, 2002). Coaching outside of the learning context that occurs within practice is most likely to lead to a practice change.

In general, learning for competent performance against standards, for developing capacity, and for professional development must address the intricacy of today's practice environment, regardless of one's roles within that environment. Because occupational therapists and occupational therapy assistants assume roles in which problem solving occurs in complex environments, the cognitive processes are similar to creative thinking (Fraser & Greenhalgh, 2001). Therefore, learning approaches should be designed to facilitate the creative thinking involved in the ability to "appraise the situation as a whole, prioritize issues, and then integrate and make sense of many different sources of data to arrive at a solution" (p. 801). These creative learning approaches are nonlinear in nature or are designed to help learners capture a situation in its "holistic complexity" (p. 801). Nonlinear learning methods typically involve storytelling, case histories, reflection, and problem-based learning strategies. There is an emphasis on self-directed learning, in which the learner is supported in developing his or her own learning goals, receiving feedback, reflecting, and consolidating one's ideas. These self-directed learning goals avoid rigid and prescriptive content in that the subject matter may vary depending on the needs of the learner.

There also should be efforts to capture the benefits of informal and unplanned learning. Some examples of these informal learning methods include experiential learning (e.g., job shadowing, apprenticeships); networking opportunities; reflection exercises; list serves and discussion groups for professional interest groups; "teach-back" opportunities, in which newly skilled practitioners teach others their shared understanding; and feedback on the application of the learning (Fraser & Greenhalgh, 2001, p. 802).

Self-directed learning, however, in collaborative practice requires modification to include team self-directed learning, in which the learning of the team as a whole takes precedence over individual learning needs. In addition, team-based learning is more likely to use work-based learning methods, in which adult learning approaches, small group work, and critical and active learning are central to the learning process (Cameron, Rutherford, & Mountain, 2012). The strategies for team learning that occur within the work context include similar self-directed learning and informal methods described previously, but always include clinical supervision, action learning through project work, and individual and team coaching/mentorship.

Table 53-2.

## Learning Questions and Learning Purposes

| Questions | Continuing Competence | Continuing Competency | Professional Development |
|---|---|---|---|
| Trigger for learning | Does trend information or forecasts indicate that a change in my typical and collaborative practice will be required in the future for my current role? | Is there a gap between my practice and collaborative practice outcomes and what is standard or what is ideal? | In order to assume another position, to be promoted, or to undertake professional leadership, what do I need to learn given my current skills and abilities? |
| Timing | When should learning occur given the likelihood that the prediction about future practice is feasible in my practice context? | When should learning occur given the importance of the standard to outcomes and to safety? | When should learning occur given my career goals and opportunities? |
| Content | What specific content for learning that might be applied in my collaborative practice context is suggested by the trend data or forecasts? | What specific evidence-based learning and collaborative practice content would most likely improve safety or outcomes in my practice? | What specific learning content would best prepare me for my future roles? |
| Learning methods and strategies | How should the learning be organized and delivered given the application feasibility issues and the collaborative practice context? | How should the learning be organized and delivered to ensure application to practice according to standard such that there most likely will be improvements in collaborative practice outcomes or safety? | How should the learning be organized and delivered to assist me in developing potentially applicable skills and abilities needed for assumption of other roles and responsibilities? |
| Location of learning | How important is learning in context of my practice and in collaboration with my team given that feasibility of application may or may not yet be determined? | How can I implement learning in the context of my practice so that I am able to apply the new learning to collaborative practice more effectively and efficiently? | How can I locate opportunities to apply learning so that skills and abilities will not erode before I reach my career goals? |
| Educational providers and role of employer | Who is producing the most up-to-date information on this trend and is conducting the latest research applicable to my collaborative practice? | How can I work with my employer and team to create learning opportunities within the context of my collaborative practice? | Is my employer supportive of my career goals and should I consider locating a mentor outside of work to help me get started? |
| Application | What aspect of the learning could be applied to collaborative practice in the near future? And, do I need more education and training before application? | What aspect of the learning must be applied to collaborative practice in order to better meet standards for safety and for outcomes? | What aspect of the learning could be implemented if I take advantage of upcoming career opportunities? |
| Context, environment, or system | What aspects of the collaborative practice context support or inhibit the feasibility of learning application in the near future? | What barriers in the collaborative practice context require removal and what supports should be put in place in order to assist me in meeting standards and achieving outcomes? | What barriers and supports in my professional context exist that would impact application of learning if I seek specific career opportunities? |
| Modifying context | What are the best strategies to enhance feasibility of learning being applied to collaborative practice in the near future? | What strategies would be effective in modifying the collaborative practice context to support immediate application of learning so that standards are met and outcomes are improved? | What do I need to do to make sure that I can take advantage of opportunities to apply new skills and abilities in order to meet my career goals? |
| Evaluation of the impact of learning | How will I know if my learning has made a difference in collaborative practice given questions of feasibility of application? Should I target evaluation primarily to change in knowledge? | How and when should the impact of learning on client outcomes be measured, or how will I know my learning has been effective in meeting collaborative practice standards? | What formative and summative skill and ability evaluations should I implement to give me feedback about my progress toward my career goals? |

## Portfolios

Portfolios archive the self-assessment process described in the model, including the reflection on the self-assessment to determine learning needs related to job-related competencies or to professional development aspirations (Tillema, 2001). The learning plan devised to address the learning needs is also housed in the portfolio, along with evidence of engagement in the various learning activities, such as specialty certifications or professional recognition and documentation of continuing education, coursework, publications, or presentations. Each of the learning activities is carefully appraised to ensure that the activity contributes to achievement of the learning competencies. The self-appraisal process answers the question, "What evidence would best indicate my potential for possessing the competencies needed for practice?"

The most complete portfolios are reflective in nature, as there is an examination of why one chose a particular learning activity and how participation in that activity affected one's practice relative to the specific competency. Reflection connects learning application to practice with client outcomes. For instance, if the competency is about administering specialized assessments, then why was writing a case study chosen; how did constructing the case study contribute to knowing how and when to administer particular assessments; and how did the client evaluation experience change as the result of applying the learning to practice? Portfolios used to document one's continuing competence or competency or professional development processes are thus quite different in complexity and should not be considered the same as a scrapbook of personal and professional achievements, an archive of all one has ever done in one's life or career, or a collection of random continuing education certificates and program handouts. Portfolios can demonstrate the potential for continuing competence and competency, especially if requiring evidence of the following (Miller, 1990):

- Knowing
- Knowing how (knows the procedures or steps)
- Showing how (can do the procedures or steps)
- Actual doing (actually does the procedures in practice)

Even though portfolios have usefulness in determining potential for continuing competence and competency, safeguards to ensure the quality of the portfolio must be in place because the self-assessment (determining the learning need) and self-appraisal (selecting the best evidence of achieving the competency) skills of a health care professional may be limited under certain conditions. Health care professionals benefit from training in these self-evaluation processes, require experience over time, and need feedback from others who view their performance to become more skilled in self-assessment and in self-appraisal (Kruger & Dunning, 1999). Feedback is needed because high achievers tend to underestimate their abilities and low achievers tend to overestimate their abilities. However, persons who are incompetent may not only reach erroneous conclusions about their level of ability (overestimate), but they may also lack the metacognitive ability to realize their incompetence. Inherent within self-assessment and self-appraisal is the ability to accurately reflect on one's own practice to determine where further learning would be beneficial.

## Mentoring

A key ingredient for effective portfolio review and self-assessment techniques is including professional feedback from a trusted source. This relationship is called *mentorship*, which may occur between an individual mentor and mentee, a mentee and multiple mentors, or a mentor with several mentees. The relationship can be a formal, structured exchange or informal. Regardless of the complexity of mentoring relationships, there is consensus about teaching/learning as a critical component of the mentoring process (Andrews & Chilton, 2000; Eby, Allen, Evans, Ng, & DuBois, 2008; Melnyk, 2007). Milner and Bossers (2005) identified expert knowledge, clinical experience, and guidance skills as desirable characteristics in a mentor. Andrews and Chilton (2000) identified mentor roles as including eye opener, door opener, challenger, giver of feedback, idea bouncer, envisioner, investor, supporter, teacher, standard prodder, problem solver, energizer, and modeler. Abdullah et al. (2014) completed a systematic review to examine the effectiveness of mentoring in knowledge translation where they found only 10 studies from 1988 to 2012. These studies showed there was improvement in knowledge, changes in beliefs about evidence, and successful change throughout the organization as a result of formal mentoring.

## Roles of Stakeholders

A variety of stakeholders are interested in continuing competence and competency and professional development. The stakeholders in the professional community include occupational therapists and occupational therapy assistants, AOTA, state occupational therapy associations, state licensing boards, and NBCOT. Stakeholders in the community at large include clients, the public, state and federal governments, third-party payers, accrediting bodies, other professional organizations, employers, team members, and educators. Some of these stakeholders, such as occupational therapists and occupational therapy assistants, are interested in continuing competence and

## Case Study

Janet is an occupational therapist who works closely with Mark, an occupational therapy assistant. Janet and Mark both work together on an interprofessional team that provides services for older adults in a senior care organization that offers independent and assistive living, as well as long-term care and memory care. Janet and Mark and the team have been discussing with the infection control nurse the increase in ventilator-acquired pneumonia (VAP) that has occurred in the long-term care facility that houses a 15-bed ventilator unit [data input for the team self-assessment of competence and competency]. The team has charged the therapy staff, the respiratory therapist, and the director of nursing to be on a sub-team to design the interventions for the nursing assistant staff in an evidence-based effort to decrease the incidence of pneumonia.

The sub-team met to determine who had the most experience and current competencies in working with ventilator patients in terms of preventing pneumonia [team self-assessment of competence and competency]. The respiratory therapist, the physical therapist assistant, and the director of nursing had the most experience with this issue compared to the knowledge and experience of the occupational therapy staff; however, the occupational and physical therapist had recently finished an educational program in evidence-based practice and implementation science. The occupational therapy assistant recently completed a workshop on positioning several months earlier.

The sub-team members decided to have the respiratory therapist present to them a brief overview about the role of the respiratory therapist in preventing VAP [team learning plan]. Given their new learning in evidence-based practice, the occupational and physical therapists agreed to conduct a literature search about VAP in long-term care [application of learning to practice] and to bring that information to the next sub-team meeting. The occupational therapy assistant and the physical therapist assistant would locate evidence for positioning and prevention of VAP, thereby having the opportunity to work with the therapists in learning more about evidence-based practice [learning methods]. The director of nursing and respiratory therapist planned to review the current nursing policies about care of ventilator patients [system support for competence and competency].

During the second sub-team meeting, the group discovered through appraisal and synthesis of the evidence that specific mouth care interventions could greatly decrease VAP in comparison to positioning interventions. The director of nursing realized that the nursing policies were not specific enough in terms of the type of toothbrush and the type of mouthwash and toothpaste to use. In addition, the policies were not clear about total length and frequency of tooth brushing and whether mouthwash was to be used before or after tooth brushing. The sub-team decided they needed to work with the administrator and purchasing manager to determine cost implications of the needed supplies. The sub-team then decided they needed to develop education programs for the nursing staff that included the new policy for mouth care, documentation methods to note mouth care protocol adherence, other data monitoring methods of adherence to the mouth care protocol, and coaching at the elbow with the nursing assistants to implement the mouth care protocol [organizational learning implementation and practice change sustainability plan].

competency as equally as they are concerned with professional development. Others are primarily interested in continuing competence and competency, with a secondary focus on professional development. Because of their missions to protect the public, state licensing boards and voluntary credentialing programs such as NBCOT have a primary focus on continuing competence and competency. Professional development is encouraged as it intersects with ensuring that the public receives services from competent occupational therapists and occupational therapy assistants.

Providers of continuing education, such as state and national organizations and universities, need to help learners understand the competencies to be addressed in the offering, as well as incorporate learning activities that are more likely to lead to gains in knowledge, skills, or reasoning abilities. The providers should also help the learner devise a transfer of training plan, or how the practitioner hopes to apply the learning to collaborative practice contexts. Suggestions on how to measure the impact of the learning application should be made as well. The learning program should also incorporate time for periodic reflection about what one is learning and how that learning might improve practice.

Employers have a large role in the learning of their employees in terms of facilitating the self-assessment process, the use of portfolios, and the self-appraisal of learning activities. Careful consideration of the resources needed for learning should occur and should be reflected in the budgeting process in terms of ensuring that the employee has time for learning and the money needed to implement the learning plan. Employers are also in the best position to remove barriers to and to create supportive environments for the application of learning. This typically involves changes in the system and in the collaborative practice context so that new approaches and interventions can be tried and measured. Employers can also help employees obtain and interpret client outcomes data both in terms of identifying learning needs and assessing the success of learning application. Reward and incentive systems are also an important way that employers can facilitate the continuing competence and

## Evidence-Based Research Chart

| Topic | Evidence |
|---|---|
| Self-assessment | Finlay & McLaren, 2009; McManus, Rakovshik, Kennerley, Fennell, & Westbrook, 2012; Meretoja & Leino-Kilpi, 2003; Wilkinson, 2013; Wilkinson et al., 2002 |
| Portfolios | Miller & Tuekam, 2011; Mills, 2009; Sowter, Cortis, & Clarke, 2011 |
| Learning methods | Bricker et al., 2010; Happell & Martin, 2004; Khomeiran, Yekta, Kiger, & Ahmadi, 2006; Landers, McWhorter, Krum, & Glovinsky, 2005; McQueen, Miller, Nivison, & Husband, 2006; Vachon & LeBlanc, 2011; Welch & Dawson, 2006; Williams, 2010 |
| System barrier and facilitators | Cochrane et al., 2007; Price, Miller, Rahm, Brace, & Larson, 2010; Rappolt, Pearce, McEwen, & Polatajko, 2005; Sparrow, Ashford, & Heel, 2005 |

competency and professional development of their staff. Finally, employers are crucial in determining the competency of their employees as they can use observational methods to compare actual performance to standards.

## Summary

Portfolios are an important aspect of continuing competence and competency and professional development. Portfolios document the self-assessment process when it becomes clear that a learning need is evident following a systematic investigative process. The learning need then leads to careful selection of learning activities thought more likely to produce an improvement in one or more competencies necessary for not only excellent but collaborative practice. Achieving these competencies through a focus on obtaining knowledge, skills, and reasoning abilities should result in a significant impact on client outcomes. Portfolios designed in this manner are powerful tools in facilitating formative assessment and effective learning; however, the challenge is ensuring that sufficient rigor is maintained throughout the portfolio self-assessment and self-appraisal processes. Portfolios are, more importantly, a way for ensuring that all occupational therapists and occupational therapy assistants undertake an active role in identifying and meeting their own learning needs as an aspect of continuous quality improvement within collaborative practice contexts typical of interdependent health care and social systems. Widespread, rigorous use of portfolios stands to greatly affect the profession in its ability to provide society with quality occupational therapy services.

## Student Self-Assessment

1. Spend time reflecting on your career goals 5 years after you graduate. Identify generally what you would need to learn to achieve this career goal, the resources you would need, and how you would obtain these resources.
2. Suggest some ways that you could incorporate nonlinear learning, self-directed learning, and team-based learning to augment what you are learning in a particular class.
3. Reflect on an unplanned learning event in which you experienced a change in your ability to analyze a client situation. Share this reflection in small groups.
4. If you worked with a practitioner who claimed never having time to read anything about occupational therapy, explain how this would be an ethical dilemma and how you would address this situation as a colleague.

## References

Abdullah, G., Rossy, D., Ploeg, J., Davies, B., Higuchi, K., Sikora, L., & Stacey, D. (2014). Measuring the effectiveness of mentoring as a knowledge translation intervention for implementing empirical evidence: A systematic review. *Worldviews on Evidence Based Nursing, 11*, 284-300. doi:/10.1111/wvn.12060

Accreditation Council for Occupational Therapy Education. (2011). *2011 Accreditation Council for Occupational Therapy Education (ACOTE®) Standards and Interpretive Guide (effective July 31, 2013) August 2015 Interpretive Guide Version*. Bethesda, MD: Author.

American Occupational Therapy Association. (2014). Occupational therapy practice framework: Domain and process (3rd ed.). *American Journal of Occupational Therapy, 68*(Suppl. 1), S1-S48. doi:10.5014/ajot.2014.682006

American Occupational Therapy Association. (2015a). Occupational therapy code of ethics (2015). *American Journal of Occupational Therapy, 69*(Suppl. 3), 6913410030. doi:10.5014/ajot.2015.696S03

American Occupational Therapy Association. (2015b). Standards for continuing competence. *American Journal of Occupational Therapy, 69*(Suppl. 3), 6913410055. doi:10.5014/ajot.2015.696S16

Andrews, M., & Chilton, F. (2000). Student and mentor perceptions of mentoring effectiveness. *Nurse Education Today, 20*, 555-562. doi:/10.1054/nedt.2000.0464

Barr, H. (1998). Competent to collaborate: Towards a competency-based model for interprofessional education. *Journal of Interprofessional Care, 12*(2), 181-187.

Bricker, P., Baron, J., Scheirer, J. J., DeWalt, D., Derrickson, J., Yunghans, S., & Babbay, R. A. (2010). Collaboration in Pennsylvania: Rapidly spreading improved chronic care for patients to practice. *Journal of Continuing Education in the Health Professions, 30*(2), 2010. doi:10.1002/chp

Burwell, S. M. (2015). Setting value-based payment goals—HHS efforts to improve US healthcare. *New England Journal of Medicine, 372*, 897.

Cameron, S., Rutherford, I., & Mountain, K. (2012). Debating the use of work-based learning and interprofessional education in promoting collaborative practice in primary care: A discussion paper. *Quality in Primary Care, 20*, 211-217.

Cochrane, L. J., Olson, C. A., Murray, S., Dupus, M., Tooman, T., & Hayes, S. (2007). Gaps between knowing and doing: Understanding and assessing the barriers to optimal health care. *Journal of Continuing Education in the Health Professions, 27*(2), 94-102.

Decker, P. J. (1999). The hidden competencies of health care: Why self-esteem, accountability, and professionalism may affect hospital customer satisfaction scores. *Hospital Topics, 77*(1), 14.

Decker, P. J., & Strader, M. K. (1997). Beyond JCAHO: Using competency models to improve health care organizations, part 1. *Hospital Topics, 75*(1), 23.

Eby, L. T., Allen, T. D., Evans, S. C., Ng, T., & DuBois, D. L. (2008). Does mentoring matter? A multidisciplinary meta-analysis comparing mentored and non-mentored individuals. *Journal of Vocational Behavior, 72*, 254-267. doi:/10.1016/j.jvb.2007.04.005

Finlay, K., & McLaren, S. (2009). Does appraisal enhance learning, improve practice and encourage continuing professional development? A survey of general practitioners' experiences of appraisal. *Quality in Primary Care, 17*, 387-395.

Fixsen, D., Naoom, S., Blase, K., Friedman, R., & Wallace, F. (2005). *Implementation research: A synthesis of the literature*. Tampa, FL: University of South Florida, Louis de la Parte Florida Mental Health Institute, The National Implementation Research Network (FMHI Publication #231).

Fraser, S. W., & Greenhalgh, T. (2001). Complexity science. Coping with complexity: Education for capability. *British Medical Journal, 323*(6), 799-803.

Graham, I., Logan, J., Harrison, M., Strauss, S., Tetroe, J., Caswell, W., & Robinson, N. (2006). Lost of knowledge translation: Time for a map? *Journal of Continuing Education in Health Professions, 26*, 13-24.

Handfield-Jones, R. S., Mann, K. V., Challis, M. E., Hobma, S. O., Klass, D. F., McManus, I. C., ... Wikinson, T. F. (2002). Linking assessment to learning: A new route to quality assurance in medical practice. *Medical Education, 36*, 949-958.

Happell, B., & Martin, T. (2004). Exploring the impact of the implementation of a nursing clinical development unit program: What outcomes are evident? *International Journal of Mental Health Nursing, 13*, 177-184.

Interprofessional Education Collaborative Expert Panel. (2011). *Core competencies for interprofessional collaborative practice: Report of an expert panel*. Washington, DC: Interprofessional Education Collaborative.

Josiah Macy Jr. Foundation. (2013). *Transforming patient care: Aligning interprofessional education with clinical practice redesign*. Retrieved from http://macyfoundation.org/publications/publication/aligning-interprofessional-education

Joyce, B., & Showers, B. (2002). *Student achievement through staff development* (3rd ed.). Alexandria, VA; Association for Supervision and Curriculum Development.

Khomeiran, R. T., Yekta, Z. P., Kiger, A. M., & Ahmadi, F. (2006). Professional competence: Factors described by nurses as influencing their development. *International Nursing Review, 53*, 66-72.

Kruger, J., & Dunning, D. (1999). Unskilled and unaware of it: How difficulties in recognizing one's own incompetence lead to inflated self-assessments. *Journal of Personality and Social Psychology, 77*(6), 1121-1134.

Landers, M. R., McWhorter, J. W., Krum, L. L., & Glovinsky, D. (2005). Mandatory continuing education in physical therapy: Survey of physical therapists in states with and states without a mandate. *Physical Therapy, 85*, 861-871.

McConnell, E. A. (2001). Competence vs. competency. *Nursing Management, 32*(5), 14.

McManus, F., Rakovshik, S., Kennerley, H., Fennell, M., & Westbrook, D. (2012). An investigation of the accuracy of therapists' self-assessment of cognitive-behaviour therapy skills. *British Journal of Clinical Psychology, 51*, 292-306.

McQueen, J., Miller, C., Nivison, C., & Husband, V. (2006). An investigation into the use of a journal club or evidence-based practice. *International Journal of Therapy and Rehabilitation, 13*, 311-317.

Melnyk, B. M. (2007). The latest evidence on the outcomes of mentoring. *Worldviews on Evidence-Based Nursing, 4*, 170-173. doi:/10.1111/j.1741-6787.2007.00099.x

Meretoja, R., & Leino-Kilpi, H. (2003). Comparison of competence assessments made by nurse managers and practicing nurses. *Journal of Nursing Management, 11*, 404-409.

Miller, G. E. (1990). The assessment of clinical skills/competence/performance. *Academic Medicine, 65*(Suppl.), S63-S67.

Miller, P., & Tuekam, R. (2011). The feasibility and acceptability of using a portfolio to assess professional competence. *Physiotherapy Canada, 63*(1), 78-85.

Mills, J. (2009). Professional portfolios and Australian registered nurses' requirements for licensure: Developing an essential tool. *Nursing & Health Sciences, 11*(2), 206-210.

Milner, T., & Bossers, A. (2005). Evaluation of an occupational therapy mentorship program. *Canadian Journal of Occupational Therapy, 72*(4), 205-211.

Moyers, P. A. (2005). The ethics of competence. In R. B. Purtilo, G. M. Jensen, & C. B. Royeen (Eds.), *Educating for moral action: A sourcebook in health and rehabilitation ethics* (pp. 21-30). Philadelphia, PA: F. A. Davis Company.

Moyers, P. A., & Hinojosa, J. (2003). Continuing competency. In G. McCormack, E. Jaffe, & M. Goodman-Lavey (Eds.), *The occupational therapy manager* (4th ed., pp. 489). Bethesda, MD: AOTA Press.

Petzold, A., Korner-Bitensky, N., & Menon, A. (2010). Using the Knowledge to Action Process Model to incite clinical change. *Journal of Continuing Education in the Health Professions, 33*, 167-171.

Price, D. W., Miller, E. K., Rahm, A. K., Brace, N. E., & Larson, R. S. (2010). Assessment of barriers to changing practice as CME outcomes. *Journal of Continuing Education in the Health Professions, 30*(4), 237-245. doi:10.1002/chp.20088

Rappolt, S., Pearce, K., McEwen, S., & Polatajko, H. J. (2005). Exploring organizational characteristics associated with practice changes following a mentored online educational module. *Journal of Continuing Education in the Health Professions, 25*, 116-124.

Schreiber, J., Perry, S., Downey, P., & Williamson, A. (2013). Implementation of an innovative continuing education program focused on translation of knowledge into clinical practice. *Journal of Physical Therapy Education, 27*, 63-71.

Smith, K., & Tillema, H. H. (2001). Long-term influences of portfolios on professional development. *Scandinavian Journal of Educational Research, 45*(2), 183-203.

Sowter, J., Cortis, J., & Clarke, D. (2011). The development of evidence based guidelines for clinical practice portfolios. *Nurse Education Today, 31*(8), 872-876.

Sparrow, J., Ashford, R., & Heel, D. (2005). A methodology to identify workplace features that can facilitate or impede reflective practice: A National Health Service UK study. *Reflective Practice, 6,* 189-197.

Spencer, L. M., & Spencer, S. M. (1993). *Competence at work*. New York, NY: John Wiley and Sons.

Straus, S. E., Brouwers, M., Johnson, D., Lavis, J. N., Legare, F., Majumdar, S. R., ... for KT Canada Strategic Training Initiative in Health Research (STIHR). (2011). Core competencies in the science and practice of knowledge translation: Description of a Canadian strategic training initiative. *Implementation Science, 6*, 1-7.

Tillema, H. H. (2001). Portfolios as developmental assessment tools. *International Journal of Training and Development, 5*(2), 1360-1376.

Vachon, B., & LeBlanc, J. (2011). Effectiveness of past and current critical incident analysis on reflective learning and practice change. *Medical Education, 45*, 894-904. doi:10.1111/j.1365-2923.2011.04042.x

Ward, M., Gruppen, L., & Regehr, G. (2002). Measuring self-assessment: Current state of the art. *Advances in Health Sciences Education: Theory and Practice, 7*, 63-80.

Welch, A., & Dawson, P. (2006). Closing the gap: Collaborative learning as a strategy to embed evidence within occupational therapy practice. *Journal of Evaluation in Clinical Practice, 12*, 227-238.

Wilkinson, C. (2013). Competency assessment tools for registered nurses: An integrative review. *Journal of Continuing Education in Nursing, 44*, 31-37. doi:10.3928/00220124-20121101-53

Wilkinson, T. J., Challins, M., Hobma, S. O., Newble, D. I., Parboosingh, J. T., Sibbald, R. G., & Wakeford, R. (2002). The use of portfolios for assessment of the competence and performance of doctors in practice. *Medical Education, 36*(10), 918-924.

Williams, C. (2010). Understanding the essential elements of work-based learning and its relevance to everyday clinical practice. *Journal of Nursing Management, 18*, 624-632. doi:10.1111/j.1365-2834.2010.01141.x

World Health Organization. (2010). *Framework for action on interprofessional education and collaborative practice*. Retrieved from http://whqlibdoc.who.int/hq/2010/WHO_HRH_HPN_10.3_eng.pdf

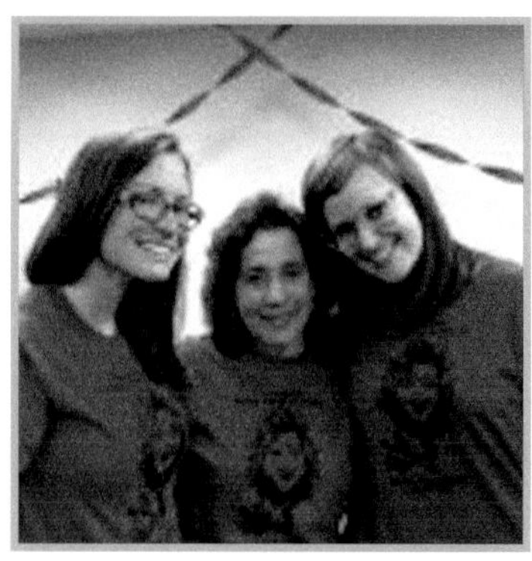

# 54

# Roles of Occupational Therapy Practitioners

*Caroline Beals, MS, OTR/L and Thomas Fisher, PhD, OTR, CCM, FAOTA*

**ACOTE STANDARDS EXPLORED IN THIS CHAPTER**

B.9.7–B.9.9

**KEY VOCABULARY**

- **Consultant:** Provider of services to an organization, individual, or group; not responsible for the outcome of the intervention.
- **Contractor:** Individual not employed by an agency but given a contract for specific services.
- **Educator:** Faculty member in an academic setting.
- **Entrepreneur:** One who is partially or completely self-employed.
- **Practitioner:** One who is engaged in providing direct, indirect, and/or consultative services.
- **Researcher:** Scientist contributing to a body of knowledge.
- **Roles:** Set of behaviors expected by a group.



Jacobs, K., & MacRae, N. (Eds.).
*Occupational Therapy Essentials for Clinical Competence, Third Edition* (pp. 763-775).

Throughout the history of occupational therapy practice, the roles that practitioners fill within the interprofessional team have evolved to meet the occupational need of society. Consistent with the Centennial Vision set forth by the American Occupational Therapy Association (AOTA), the occupational needs of society have been met by occupational therapy practitioners in roles such as a consultant, an educator, a researcher, or an advocate. These role(s) have evolved over the century, and extend beyond reducing the effects of illness, injury, and disease on an individual to the promotion of health and wellness, enabling individuals and groups to increase control over and improve their health and well-being (Wilcock, 2003, 2006).

According to the Accreditation Council for Occupational Therapy Education (ACOTE; 2011), to be a competent contemporary occupational therapist in the 21st century, the following standards must be met:

- Discuss and justify the varied roles of the occupational therapist as a practitioner, educator, researcher, consultant, and entrepreneur (Standard B.9.7).
- Explain and justify the importance of supervisory roles, responsibilities, and collaborative professional relationships between the occupational therapist and the occupational therapy assistant (Standard B.9.8).
- Describe and discuss professional responsibilities and issues when providing service on a contractual basis (Standard B.9.9).

Additionally, ACOTE charges those who enter the field of occupational therapy with a doctoral degree to have a further understanding of the varied roles of the occupational therapist as not only a practitioner, educator, researcher, consultant, and entrepreneur, but also as a policy developer, program developer, advocate, and administrator. While this chapter will focus on the roles of the master's degree level standard (Standard B.9.7), the existence, emergence, and contribution of the occupational therapy practitioner serving as a policy developer, program developer, advocate, and administrator will also be explored and discussed.

Christiansen and Baum (1997) define roles as "a set of behaviors that have some socially agreed upon function and for which there is an accepted code of norms" (p. 603). As we enter the second century of the profession, it is important to look back and view the changes within the professional roles of the occupational therapist.

The profession's official publication, *Occupational Therapy Practice Framework: Domain and Process, Third Edition* (AOTA, 2014b), defines roles as "sets of behaviors expected by society and shaped by culture and context that may be further conceptualized and defined by the client" (p. S45). It is important to note that throughout every iteration that the history has defined as the role of the occupational therapist, a primary role has been to work collaboratively with the person/group we service to identify ways in which to promote functional independence in daily life. Much like the varied roles of the occupational therapy practitioner, each client or group we serve has a vast array of roles he or she fills within the context of his or her daily life. For example, one can fill the role of mother, sister, employee, friend, artist, spouse, and caregiver simultaneously. Consequentially, when that same individual experiences an illness, injury, or disease, an occupational therapy practitioner would assesses that individual's performance within each given role, and design intervention plans that address the skills needed for those specific roles in order for the individual to resume those roles that existed before the injury, illness, or disease. Through these interventions, an individual acquires or redevelops the skills necessary for role performance. With time, these skills translate into habits of behavior, allowing the individual to continue filling these meaningful roles within his or her daily life.

Much research has focused on the importance of roles in everyday life. From an occupational science perspective, roles provide us with an awareness of social identity and related obligations, as well as a framework for appreciating relevant situations and constructing appropriate behaviors. Roles support us in identifying our unique value and contribution to society (Kramer, Hinojosa, & Royeen, 2003). As occupational therapy practitioners, we address roles and role performance with the clients we serve. It is an essential component of the occupational therapy process.

Similarly, an occupational therapy practitioner may assume several different professional roles during a career. These roles may occur simultaneously, or have specific timeframes within the span of one's professional career. Each role is unique and has specific performance expectations. Appreciating and meeting the performance expectations of these roles as an entry-level practitioner will ensure the profession moves strongly into the next century as a valued role on any interprofessional team, regardless of setting.

Roles are important to consider because the environment where we work, and the services we provide, greatly affect client outcomes. Research continues to emerge that shows the distinct value of occupational therapy services in a variety of settings. Shannon (1985) addressed the broadening roles of occupational therapy practitioners in the continuity of care in a special edition of *Occupational Therapy in Health Care*. He expanded on an earlier discussion about occupational therapy beyond hospital-based occupational therapy practice. He reminded practitioners to understand the political, economic, and cultural environment in which they practice, regardless of their role. He suggested that they appreciate their holistic perspective and broad knowledge base, and he emphasized the unique opportunities that community practice brings. In an article for Health Care Policy Perspectives in the *American Journal of Occupational Therapy* in 2012, Muir continues the support of this discussion, and argues "who better to lead a team of health care professionals to improve the lives of members of our communities than the one profession that has always known the critical importance of occupation and the absolute need of humans to be engaged and productive? Who better than occupational therapists?" (p. 509). She further describes the critical importance for research to continue to validate the therapeutic use of role-specific valued occupations in the rehabilitation process.

Alternatively, the emerging roles of occupational therapy practitioners in realms such as preventative health and health promotion remain relatively unknown to the greater public. In 2013, a group of occupational therapy practitioners and researchers out of Norway sought to understand the views of occupational therapy practitioners concerning competence in health promotion strategies, and their perceptions of how they apply these competences in their daily work. They also asked practitioners to consider their ability to fill a role within health promotion and preventative health. The main findings showed that participants rarely engaged in health promotion on a systemic or societal level. They believed that their clients and collaborating partners, as well as public officials, remained unaware of their competences in health promotion. Findings such as this should highlight the importance of discussion among occupational therapy practitioners regarding a more significant contribution to health promotion (Holmberg & Ringsberg, 2014).

Braveman and Page (2012) concluded that roles help one to achieve identity and are associated with "who we are" (p. 40). They suggested that roles are critical for human development. Roles are how individuals see themselves, whether it is worker, student, son, granddaughter, and so on. When discussing or describing them, one will often share the responsibilities and obligations that are associated with the particular role. There are no other disciplines in the health and human services industry that explicitly address this component of humans. It is here we see the distinct role and value of the occupational therapy practitioner.

## Roles

There are a multitude of roles within the profession of occupational therapy. Frequently, an occupational therapist's position with an employer may include more than one role. For example, as an occupational therapy educator, the individual may also function as a researcher, service provider, and consultant. Another example would be an occupational therapist on an inpatient rehabilitation unit who could be functioning as a supervisor to the other occupational therapists, occupational therapy assistants, and students and/or as the team coordinator for the unit (e.g., stroke, spinal cord, brain injury) in addition to providing direct occupational therapy services. Regardless of the employment arrangement, practitioners employed by the organization, independent contractor to the organization, or consultant to the organization, the professional responsibility of the occupational therapy practitioner to perform a specific role and provide services in a accordance with the ethical and professional expectations set forth in the *Occupational Therapy Code of Ethics* cannot be overemphasized (AOTA, 2015a).

Because of the dynamic nature of the occupational therapy practitioner, and the ability of the practitioner to fill multiple roles within an interprofessional team, the professional organization, AOTA, has addressed this officially. There are official documents (ACOTE, 2011) that support occupational therapy practitioners in understanding and appreciating the various roles and describe the supervision of occupational therapists and occupational therapy assistants. The following roles will be examined—practitioner, fieldwork educator, educator, researcher, consultant, and entrepreneur. Table 54-1 outlines and defines these varied roles.

## Practitioner

While there are supervisory relationships between the occupational therapist and the occupational therapy assistant that will be discussed in the content of this chapter, it is important to include both occupational therapists and occupational therapy assistants under the umbrella term of *practitioner*. While the responsibilities of the occupational therapist and occupational therapy assistant differ, both practitioners progress along a continuum in clinical practice. They move from entry-level to intermediate and then into advanced level based on experience, education, and practice skills. In 2014, the AOTA set forth updated *Guidelines for Supervision, Roles, and Responsibilities During the Delivery of Occupational Therapy Services* (2014a). This document is a set of guidelines describing the supervision, roles, and responsibilities of occupational therapy practitioners. According to AOTA, it is intended for both internal and external audiences, and provides an outline of the roles and responsibilities of occupational therapists, occupational therapy assistants, and occupational therapy aides during the delivery of occupational therapy services.

Table 54-1.

**VARIOUS ROLES OF THE OCCUPATIONAL THERAPIST**

| Topic | Definition | Reference |
|---|---|---|
| Practitioner | An individual initially certified to practice as an occupational therapist or occupational therapy assistant, or licensed or regulated by a state, district, commonwealth, or territory of the United States to practice as an occupational therapist or occupational therapy assistant, and who has not had that certification, license, or registration revoked due to disciplinary action. | ACOTE, 2011 |
| Fieldwork educator | The person who supervises and educates entry-level students during Level I or Level II fieldwork. | Jacobs & McCormack, 2011 |
| Educator | The role of educator is a practice area that some occupational therapists assume in their careers that can either be a core, full-time, or part-time position. | AOTA, 2007 |
| Researcher | One who finds discovering the science behind occupational therapy assessments, interventions, and outcomes important and wishes to contribute to the profession by building the science. | Kielhofner, 2006 |
| Consultant | A practitioner, educator, or researcher who is asked to provide a specific service/intervention. The individual is not employed by the organization. As a consultant, one is not responsible for the outcome of the recommendation(s) made. | Braveman, 2006 |
| Entrepreneur | Either partially or fully self-employed individuals, including those in private practice, independent contractors, and consultants. | Braveman, 2006 |

The focus of occupational therapy is to assist the client in "achieving health, well-being, and participation in life through engagement in occupation" (AOTA, 2014b, p. S2). The occupational therapy practitioner delivers services that address the needs and goals of the client related to engaging in areas of occupation. Additionally, consideration of the performance skills, performance patterns, context and environment, and client factors that may influence performance in various areas of occupation is crucial to providing services that are congruent with best practice. In 2015, new *Standards of Practice for Occupational Therapy* were published by the AOTA (2015c). The document outlines the minimum standards for a practitioner to uphold in four areas in which occupational therapy practitioners must demonstrate competence. This document also begins to describe the relationship between the occupational therapist and the occupational therapy assistant. Table 54-2 outlines just a few highlights from the four areas, with examples of behaviors that exemplify this standard. The entire document can be found within the official documents of AOTA (https://www.aota.org/practice/manage/official.aspx).

In some settings, occupational therapy practitioners provide services in groups. In fact, in mental health settings, acute rehabilitation settings, and many community settings (e.g., adult day programs, outpatient facilities, developmental disabilities centers), this is how occupational therapy services are delivered (Scaffa, 2001). There is evidence to support the role of occupational therapy in a supported group setting, such as a group which was formed by occupational therapy practitioners to support caregivers of children with cerebral palsy (Jahagirdar, 2012). It was found that the perceived effectiveness of this parent/peer group was high, supporting the use of a group setting for this educational workshop as a means for inducing learning in caregivers of children with cerebral palsy (Jahagirdar, 2012). Again, the importance of ethical decision making in the group setting, especially in regard to autonomy, beneficence, fidelity, and justice, cannot be emphasized enough (AOTA, 2014a).

The role of occupational therapy practitioner can be seen in a variety of emerging fields, as outlined in the Evidence-Based Research Chart. Although this list is by no means exhaustive, it highlights how the emergence of new roles is yet another way in which occupational therapy practitioners are meeting society's occupational needs (AOTA, 2006).

Table 54-2.

**AMERICAN OCCUPATIONAL THERAPY ASSOCIATION STANDARDS OF PRACTICE FOR OCCUPATIONAL THERAPY**

| Standard | Example of Behaviors |
|---|---|
| Professional Standing and Responsibility | • Delivers occupational therapy services that reflect the philosophical base of occupational therapy and are consistent with the established principles and concepts of theory and practice<br>• Abides by the *Code of Ethics* (AOTA, 2015)<br>• Abides to standards of continuing competence, by establishing, maintaining, and updating performance, knowledge, and skills<br>• Maintaining current licensure, registration, and certification<br>• Maintains current knowledge of legislative, political, social, cultural, societal, and reimbursement issues that affect clients and the practice of occupational therapy<br>• Respects the client's sociocultural background and provides client-centered and family-centered occupational therapy services |
| Screening, Evaluation, and Reevaluation | • Uses current assessments and assessment procedures and follows defined protocols of standardized assessments and needs assessment methods during the screening, evaluation, and reevaluation process<br>• Communicates screening, evaluation, and reevaluation results within the boundaries of client confidentiality and privacy regulations to the appropriate person, group, or population<br>• Educates current and potential referral sources about the scope of occupational therapy services and the process of initiating occupational therapy services |
| Intervention Process | • Collaborates with the client to develop and implement the intervention plan, on the basis of the client's needs and priorities, safety issues, and relative benefits and risks of the interventions and service delivery<br>• Uses professional and clinical reasoning, available evidence-based practice, and therapeutic use of self to select and implement the most appropriate types of interventions; preparatory methods and tasks, education and training, advocacy, and group interventions are used, with meaningful occupations as the primary treatment modality, both as an ends and a means |
| Transition, Discharge, and Outcome Measurement | • Facilitates the transition or discharge process in collaboration with the client, family members, significant others, other professionals (e.g., medical, educational, social services), and community resources, when appropriate<br>• Responsibly reports outcomes to payers and referring entities, as well as to relevant local, regional, and national databases and registries, when appropriate |

Adapted from American Occupational Therapy Association. (2015). Standards of practice for occupational therapy. *American Journal of Occupational Therapy, 69*(Suppl. 3), 6913410057. http://dx.doi.org/10.5014/ajot.2015.696S06

## COLLABORATION WITH OCCUPATIONAL THERAPY ASSISTANTS

In the 1950s, because of the demand for occupational therapy services and the time required to prepare professional occupational therapists, the profession created occupational therapy assistants in the United States (Crampton, 1958). Early on, the occupational therapy assistant education was designed for those individuals who were high school graduates or equivalent and employed as an occupational therapy aide. Many of the earlier occupational therapy assistant graduates were prepared to work in mental health occupational therapy. The training went from strictly technical to additional didactic instruction. Supervised clinical work (as it was called in earlier times) was mandatory. Throughout the history of occupational therapy assistant education, occupational therapists have been careful to include the assistant in the discussion, with recognition that the professional occupational therapist had the formal educational preparation to understand the essence of occupation and its influence on humans (Hirama, 1986). Because of the appreciation of what the occupational therapy assistant brings to practice, the profession has routinely been a voice within the occupational therapy profession through representation within AOTA. Occupational therapy assistants in the AOTA may run for any office of the association, with the exception of chairperson of the Commission on Education. That individual must be an occupational therapist with a doctoral degree. This is the criteria established by the Nominating Committee of the AOTA and approved by the Representative Assembly.

In *Guidelines for Supervision, Roles, and Responsibilities During the Delivery of Occupational Therapy Services* (AOTA, 2014a), it is stated that

> Based on education and training, occupational therapy assistants, after initial certification and meeting of state regulatory requirements, must receive supervision from an occupational therapist to deliver occupational therapy services. Occupational therapy assistants deliver occupational therapy services under the supervision of and in partnership with occupational therapists. Occupational therapists and occupational therapy assistants are equally responsible for developing a collaborative plan for supervision. The occupational therapist is ultimately responsible for the implementation of appropriate supervision, but the occupational therapy assistant also has a responsibility to seek and obtain appropriate supervision to ensure proper occupational therapy is being provided. (pp. S16-S17)

Regardless of the setting in which occupational therapy services are delivered, occupational therapists and occupational therapy assistants assume the following general responsibilities during evaluation; intervention planning, implementation, and review; and targeting and evaluating outcomes. AOTA provides the following guidelines, as outlined in the 2014 document *Guidelines for Supervision, Roles, and Responsibilities During the Delivery of Occupational Therapy Services.*

## Evaluation

- The occupational therapist directs the evaluation process.
- The occupational therapist is responsible for directing all aspects of the initial contact during the occupational therapy evaluation, including:
  - ◊ Determining the need for service
  - ◊ Defining the problems within the domain of occupational therapy to be addressed
  - ◊ Determining the client's goals and priorities
  - ◊ Establishing intervention priorities
  - ◊ Determining specific further assessment needs
  - ◊ Determining specific assessment tasks that can be delegated to the occupational therapy assistant
- The occupational therapist initiates and directs the evaluation, interprets the data, and develops the intervention plan.
- The occupational therapy assistant contributes to the evaluation process by implementing delegated assessments and by providing verbal and written reports of observations, assessments, and client capacities to the occupational therapist.
- The occupational therapist interprets the information provided by the occupational therapy assistant and integrates that information into the evaluation and decision-making process.

## Intervention Planning

- The occupational therapist has overall responsibility for the development of the occupational therapy intervention plan.
- The occupational therapist and the occupational therapy assistant collaborate with the client to develop the plan.
- The occupational therapy assistant is responsible for being knowledgeable about evaluation results and for providing input into the intervention plan, based on client needs and priorities.

## Intervention Implementation

- The occupational therapist has overall responsibility for intervention implementation.
- When delegating aspects of the occupational therapy intervention to the occupational therapy assistant, the occupational therapist is responsible for providing appropriate supervision.
- The occupational therapy assistant is responsible for being knowledgeable about the client's occupational therapy goals.
- The occupational therapy assistant in collaboration with the occupational therapist selects, implements, and makes modifications to occupational therapy interventions, including, but not limited to, occupations and activities, preparatory methods and tasks, client education and training, and group interventions consistent with demonstrated competency levels, client goals, and the requirements of the practice setting.

### *Intervention Review*

- The occupational therapist is responsible for determining the need for continuing, modifying, or discontinuing occupational therapy services.
- The occupational therapy assistant contributes to this process by exchanging information with and providing documentation to the occupational therapist about the client's responses to and communications during intervention.

### *Targeting and Evaluating Outcomes*

- The occupational therapist is responsible for selecting, measuring, and interpreting outcomes that are related to the client's ability to engage in occupations.
- The occupational therapy assistant is responsible for being knowledgeable about the client's targeted occupational therapy outcomes and for providing information and documentation related to outcome achievement.
- The occupational therapy assistant may implement outcome measurements and provide needed client discharge resources (AOTA, 2014a).

Throughout the decades, occupational therapists and occupational therapy assistants providing services together has been important to the profession and society (Hirama, 1986). Because of this relationship, the need for the occupational therapist to possess basic supervision skills is critical. Alternately, the ability of the occupational therapy assistant to openly engage in a supervisory relationship is also crucial to providing best practice. Regardless of the practice setting or service model, the AOTA purports collaboration between occupational therapists and occupational therapy assistants as fundamental and necessary.

As discussed earlier, understanding the importance of the supervisory role and performing the functions of that role competently allow for a successful delivery of occupational therapy services. Being capable of meeting this understanding is an expectation and standard for accrediting an educational program (ACOTE, 2011). To accomplish this important expectation, it becomes necessary for professional entry-level programs to provide examples of the collaborative relationships during the didactic portion of the academic preparation, to have occupational therapy assistants on the faculty or used as guest lecturers, and to facilitate the exposure of student occupational therapists to occupational therapy assistants while doing both Level I and II fieldwork.

## Fieldwork Educator

The role of fieldwork educator is arguably a role that ensures future success of occupational therapy practice. The fieldwork educator needs not only to understand, value, and evaluate the provision of skilled services, but also to understand the components of graduate professional education. It is the responsibility of the fieldwork educator to help the student assimilate the knowledge learned in the classroom environment with the real-time happenings of a clinical setting. While performing both roles (practitioner and educator) challenges a variety of skills, it is an important role in ensuring the next generation of competent and compassionate practitioners. It is important to note that in occupational therapy, an occupational therapist is not permitted to supervise a Level II fieldwork student until the therapist has practiced full-time for 1 year (ACOTE, 2011, Standard C.1.14). However, the therapist can begin taking Level I students soon after graduation. In addition to these two roles, the occupational therapist might also provide an educational offering in the community to families of persons with disabilities, support groups, other health professionals, and so forth. This assists in explaining the continuum of providing occupational therapy education services to individuals and groups.

While the role of fieldwork educator requires responsibilities in addition to that of practitioner, the value of providing fieldwork education to future practitioners is unmeasurable. Recent studies have shown that despite common assumptions that fieldwork educators struggle to meet the role expectations and productivity demands in the workplace, there is no difference in clinician productivity with or without a student. Practitioner years of experience, practice area, and productivity without a student were significant predictors of practitioner productivity while supervising a student, and should be taken into consideration before assuming the role of fieldwork educator (Ozelie et al., 2015). See Chapter 45 for information on fieldwork education.

## Educator

At some point in one's career as an occupational therapist, an individual might consider a role as faculty member in an academic setting. Occasionally, the individual might be considered adjunct faculty by some universities. The profession, through the policymaking body of the organization (Representative Assembly), established a set of standards that articulate the competencies for individuals assuming the role as faculty member in a professional entry-level occupational therapist academic setting or a technical entry-level occupational therapy assistant program as faculty member. These were reaffirmed in the official document *A Descriptive Review of Occupational Therapy Education* (AOTA, 2007). This is a guide to occupational therapy education that was intended for the occupational therapy community to better understand occupational therapy education (doctorates, post-doctorates, residencies, master's, and associate degrees).

Additionally, there are role documents for the program directors and academic fieldwork coordinators. These official documents articulate those competencies long suggested by scholars in the field of occupational therapy (Clark, 1987; Fidler, 1981; Jantzen, 1974; Mosey, 1998). They too believed that occupational therapists practicing in professional education have critical demands placed on them and that their performance influences practice, education, and research.

In fact, Bondoc (2005) suggested that professional accountability begins in the formative and formal educational years of the occupational therapy practitioner, thus making it critical that, as a profession, we recognize that graduate professional education needs to have those individuals who understand evidence-based education and practice. He articulated that education is a connection that binds the profession, and evidence-based education enhances that link. Because of this, it is no surprise that there was and still is a belief that practitioners functioning in the role of occupational therapy educator should be held to certain standards. These standards are important to recognize and understand. Therefore, they are explicitly discussed in this chapter. The development of these standards and subsequent approval were not controversial. It was an expectation from the field. In the future, it would be useful to have similar competencies identified for other roles assumed by occupational therapists (e.g., consultant, researcher).

Competencies based on the AOTA's *Standards for Continuing Competence* (2015b) describe those skills, responsibilities, obligations, and expertise/content knowledge in an area of occupational therapy service that the educator should possess. The standards are knowledge, critical and ethical reasoning, interpersonal skills, and performance skills. Table 54-3 presents these standards.

In terms of applying the standard for knowledge and serving in the academic role, AOTA (2003) applied these standards to the faculty role by declaring that a faculty member must do the following:

- "Demonstrate the knowledge of how to facilitate student development toward leadership roles
- Develop a plan to continue competency in the breadth and depth of knowledge in the profession to incorporate student learning
- Facilitate effective learning processes that can be used to enhance the learning opportunities for students
- Develop a plan to continue proficiency in teaching through investigation, formal education, continuing education and self-investigation" (AOTA, 2003, p. 649)

The standard of critical reasoning declares the faculty member must do the following:

- "Facilitate professional development in teaching through continuing education, research, or self-investigation
- Demonstrate the ability to effectively judge new materials, literature, and educational materials that enhance the lifelong learning of future occupational therapy practitioners
- Demonstrate the ability to critically integrate practice, theory, literature, and research for evidence-based practice
- Demonstrate the ability to critically evaluate curriculum and participate in curriculum development" (AOTA, 2003, p. 649)

The ethical reasoning standard includes acting as a "role model of an occupational therapy advocate and change agent with professional and ethical behavior" (AOTA, 2003, p. 650).

The interpersonal skills standard requires that the faculty member in an academic setting must do the following:

- "Project a positive image of the program both internally (within the college or university) and externally (within the community)
- Demonstrate a competent and positive attitude that will result in the mentoring of students in the beginning skills of scholarship, research, and/or service
- Effectively mentor and advise students and student groups
- Create a positive presence of occupational therapy in the university/college and community through service, scholarship, and/or educational experiences
- Effectively mentor other faculty members in their development of teaching, scholarship/research, and/or service
- Demonstrate positive interactions with diverse faculty, students, and others" (AOTA, 2003, p. 649)

Finally, the standard for performance skills states that the faculty member must do the following:

- "Demonstrate the expertise to contribute to the growing body of knowledge in occupational therapy
- Demonstrate the ability to contribute to the profession, academic community, and/or society through service

Table 54-3.

## Standards for Continuing Competence

| Standard | Description | Example |
|---|---|---|
| Knowledge | Occupational therapists and occupational therapy assistants shall demonstrate understanding and integration of the information required for the multiple roles and responsibilities they assume | Regardless of setting, occupational therapists address the roles that clients assume during their everyday life. |
| Critical reasoning | Occupational therapists and occupational therapy assistants shall use reasoning processes to make sound judgments and decisions | When presented with a client who is critically ill and has had multiple roles, the occupational therapist establishes a rapport with the client, and the client's support system determines an appropriate and safe intervention plan. |
| Interpersonal skills | Occupational therapists and occupational therapy assistants shall develop and maintain their professional relationships with others within the context of their roles and responsibilities | During team meetings (regardless of settings), the occupational therapist presents client-centered, occupation-based, theory-driven, and evidence-based assessments and interventions. |
| Performance skills | Occupational therapists and occupational therapy assistants shall demonstrate the expertise, proficiencies, and abilities to competently fulfill their roles and responsibilities by employing the art and science of occupational therapy in the delivery of services | When working with a client who presents with hemiparesis after a stroke, the therapist utilizes the most recent evidence to support the intervention planning process. |
| Ethical practice | Occupational therapists and occupational therapy assistants shall identify, analyze, and clarify ethical issues or dilemmas to make responsible decisions within the changing context of their roles and responsibilities | The occupational therapy practitioner engages in dialogue with other members of a health care team regarding the ethical implications of a complex case. |

Adapted from American Occupational Therapy Association. (2015). Standards for continuing competence. *American Journal of Occupational Therapy, 69*(Suppl. 3), 6913410055. doi:10.5014/ajot.2015.696S16

- Demonstrate the ability to competently prepare ethical and competent practitioners for both traditional and emerging practice settings" (AOTA, 2003, p. 649)

For the AOTA to have engaged in this level of discussion and then adoption by the Representative Assembly are evidence supporting the notion that occupational therapy practitioners who want a professional career as a faculty member in an academic setting need to be committed to demonstrating the above competencies. The profession has articulated its beliefs about professional occupational therapy education and the competencies that should be demonstrated by occupational therapy practitioners in the role of faculty or academic fieldwork educator. Some individuals in the academic setting may pursue a career in the role of researcher. This role is one that all entry-level occupational therapy practitioners should understand and value.

## Researcher

Another role that occupational therapy practitioners perform is that of researcher. Kielhofner (2006) suggested that occupational therapists who become researchers do this because they "find the process of discovery exhilarating and because they see how it enhances occupational therapy practice" (p. xiii). This specific role had less emphasis in earlier educational standards but then became recognized and required in the ACOTE 1998 Standards. The current standards (ACOTE, 2011) affirm this educational need for research as the profession is now post-baccalaureate entry education (master's or clinical doctorate) for the professional occupational therapy practitioner. Because of research standards for entry level, the expectation for evidence-based practice, and the advancement of the profession, the role of researcher has gained focus by the profession. This particular role should continue to attract those individuals with the formal preparation, interest, and commitment to inquiry. Successful demonstration of the effectiveness and efficacy of occupational therapy interventions will continue during the 21st century.

Like other health professionals, occupational therapy acknowledged the need for research/evidence-based practice and scholarly activity. Because of this appreciation and understanding of the importance of research, the profession agreed that entry-level therapists needed to enter the profession with a graduate professional degree. Educational standards obligated academic programs to recruit and retain faculty with knowledge and skills who could teach this content and role-model the behavior of researcher. As the profession's number of faculty with doctorates increase, the number of faculty assuming the role of researcher/career scientist will also increase.

The major functions for the role of researcher at entry level are to collect, read, interpret, and apply scholarly information as it relates to occupational therapy. In addition to these functions, entry-level research skills include assuming responsibility for ethical concerns related to research and complying with the various institutional research boards and committees (AOTA, 2015a).

As an individual progresses through the research career continuum, it is feasible for a practitioner to acquire a research degree and assume the role exclusively as a researcher, scholar, or scientist. As a scholar, one possesses advanced knowledge and engages in the conceptualization of a research project, develops the proposal independently, and refines the study as needed. Research scholars in occupational therapy advance the profession of occupational therapy through their discovery, knowledge, and evidence. The Academy of Research, through the American Occupational Therapy Foundation, recognizes and inducts individuals who have made substantial contributions to occupational therapy through research. See Chapter 47 on the importance of scholarship and scholarly practice in occupational therapy.

## Consultant

The role of consultant has been assumed by occupational therapy practitioners for some time. Many times, this is the role that the practitioner or researcher is asked to assume given the nature of the relationship. Organizations or individuals may wish to engage the occupational therapy practitioner as a consultant because the service requested is specific or the need for ongoing direct services is not necessary. Therefore, this role was addressed in the *Framework* (AOTA, 2014b) describing the consultation process for either the person, organization, or population. The *Framework* describes:

> Providing services to clients indirectly on their behalf, practitioners provide consultation to entities such as teachers, multidisciplinary teams, and community planning agencies. Occupational therapy practitioners also provide consultation to community organizations such as park districts and civic organizations that may or may not include people with disabilities. In addition, practitioners consult with businesses regarding the work environment, ergonomic modifications, and compliance with the Americans With Disabilities Act of 1990. (AOTA, 2014b, p. S11)

## Entrepreneur

Another role with which the entry-level occupational therapy practitioner should be familiar is that of entrepreneur. Entrepreneurs are either partially or fully self-employed individuals. They include those in private practice, independent contractors, and consultants. Because of the broad scope of services that these individuals may be providing, the structure of their organization may be sole proprietorship, partnership, corporation, group practice, or joint venture. Independent contractors, consultants, and private practice owners are held to the same standard for demonstrating competencies as employees of an organization. This arrangement for demonstrating competence becomes a responsibility for both the contract employee and the employer contracting for the services. Regardless of what the employer or potential employer informs the occupational therapy practitioner, it is that individual's responsibility to perform in an ethical and professional manner. There are several ways in which an occupational therapy practitioner can become an entrepreneur, either through sole proprietorship, partnerships, or corporations. Each has advantages and disadvantages; however, it is recommended that an entrepreneur fully understand the intricacies of each business type. Braveman (2006) supported the role of entrepreneur when he shared the types of common businesses that occupational therapy practitioners can consider, and also suggested that to assume the role of an entrepreneur, one needs to understand the various common types of businesses.

## Advocate

Although each of these roles carries a certain weight and responsibility to the occupational therapy practitioner, it is important to also consider the role of advocate. All entry-level practitioners should be prepared to step into the role of advocate for a client, for the profession,

## Evidence-Based Research Chart

| Emerging Role | Evidence |
|---|---|
| Case management/care coordination | Baldwin & Fisher, 2005; Fisher, 1996; Skinner & Kizziar, 2012 |
| Primary care | Donnelly, Brenchley, Crawford, & Letts, 2013; Killian, Fisher, & Muir, 2015; Muir, 2012 |
| Disaster relief and preparedness | Lee, 2014; Nair & Tyagi, 2014 |
| Telehealth | Gibbs & Toth-Cohen, 2011; Hoffmann & Cantoni, 2008; Jacobs, Blanchard, & Baker, 2012 |
| Productive aging/aging in place | Horowitz, Nochajski, & Schweitzer, 2013; Sheffield, Smith, & Becker, 2012 |
| Bullying/childhood emotional health | Arbesman, Bazyk, & Nochajski, 2013; Gronski et al., 2013 |
| Childhood obesity | Orban, Erlandsson, Edberg, Önnerfält, & Thorngren-Jerneck, 2014; Pizzi & Vroman, 2013 |

or the benefit of the interprofessional care team. While this role may often be seen as only for those in formal leadership positions, the role of advocate extends to the everyday life of the occupational therapy practitioner. The *Framework* defines advocacy as "efforts directed toward promoting occupational justice and empowering clients to seek and obtain resources to fully participate in daily life occupations. The outcomes of advocacy and self-advocacy support health, well-being, and occupational participation at the individual or systems level" (AOTA, 2014b, p. S30). The absence of advocacy in occupational therapy practice would certainly ensure a bleak future. The role of the advocate involves, but is not limited to, facilitating discussions that directly affect everyday practice, bringing issues to light with sensitivity to the political and social environment, engaging in the creation of systems that support engagement in occupation for a particular clientele, and being mindful of legislative and procedural decisions that affect service delivery. Additionally, the *Framework* states "occupational therapy practitioners can indirectly affect the lives of clients through advocacy. Common examples of advocacy include talking to legislators about improving transportation for older adults or improving services for people with mental or physical disabilities to support their living and working in the community of their choice" (AOTA, 2014b, p. S11). By engaging in advocacy, one is able to ensure all other roles discussed within the content of this chapter continue to remain relevant and valued in the future, and emerging roles are continually researched and supported. See Chapter 56 for more information on advocacy in occupational therapy.

## Summary

Understanding the importance of roles assumed by occupational therapists is as important as valuing them from a client perspective. In this chapter, the varying roles of practitioner, researcher, educator, consultant, and entrepreneur were discussed. In addition, the importance of the collaborative relationship with occupational therapy assistants, appreciating the responsibilities associated with providing services on a contractual basis, and the importance of engaging in advocacy were presented. This chapter provided only an overview of issues related to one's role as an occupational therapist. It is the responsibility of occupational therapists to further explore, reflect, and investigate their roles as they move through their careers. Table 54-1 provides definitions of roles and references to the role.

## Student Self-Assessment

1. As you consider your career trajectory, what roles do you see yourself assuming?
2. During your professional education, including all your fieldwork experiences, what roles did you observe occupational therapy practitioners assuming? What are the knowledge and skills necessary to be successful in those roles?
3. What are ways that you can envision assuming the role of "advocate" in your future practice?
4. Identify some roles you can see occupational therapy practitioners assuming that were not considered in this chapter.

# References


Accreditation Council for Occupational Therapy Education. (2011). *Standards and interpretive guide for an accredited educational program for the occupational therapist.* Retrieved from www.aota.org

American Occupational Therapy Association. (2003). Role competencies for a professional-level occupational therapist faculty member in an academic setting. *American Journal of Occupational Therapy, 58*(6), 649-650.

American Occupational Therapy Association. (2006). AOTA's centennial vision. Retrieved from http://www.aota.org/News/Centennial/Background/36516.aspx?FT=.pdf .

American Occupational Therapy Association. (2007). A descriptive review of occupational therapy education. *American Journal of Occupational Therapy, 61*(6), 672-677.

American Occupational Therapy Association. (2014a). Guidelines for supervision, roles, and responsibilities during the delivery of occupational therapy services. *American Journal of Occupational Therapy, 68*(Suppl. 3), S16-S22. doi:10.5014/ajot.2014.686S03

American Occupational Therapy Association. (2014b). Occupational therapy practice framework: Domain and process (3rd ed.). *American Journal of Occupational Therapy, 68*(Suppl. 1), S1-S48. doi:10.5014/ajot.2014.682006

American Occupational Therapy Association. (2015a). Occupational therapy code of ethics. *American Journal of Occupational Therapy, 69*(Suppl. 3).

American Occupational Therapy Association. (2015b). Standards for continuing competence. *American Journal of Occupational Therapy, 69*(Suppl. 3), 6913410055. doi:10.5014/ajot.2015.696S16

American Occupational Therapy Association. (2015c). Standards of practice for occupational therapy. *American Journal of Occupational Therapy, 69*(Suppl. 3), 6913410057. doi:10.5014/ajot.2015.696S06

Arbesman, M., Bazyk, S., & Nochajski, S. M. (2013). Systematic review of occupational therapy and mental health promotion, prevention, and intervention for children and youth. *American Journal of Occupational Therapy, 67,* e120-e130. doi:10.5014/ajot.2013.008359

Baldwin, T., & Fisher, T. F. (2005). Case management: Entry-level practice for occupational therapy practitioners. *Case Manager, 16*(4), 47-52.

Bondoc, S. (2005). Occupational therapy and evidence-based education. *Education Special Interest Section Quarterly, 15*(4), 1-4.

Braveman, B. (2006). *Leading and managing occupational therapy services: An evidence-based approach.* Philadelphia, PA: F. A. Davis Company.

Braveman, B., & Page, J. (2012). *Work: Promoting participation and productivity through occupational therapy.* Philadelphia, PA: F. A. Davis Company.

Christiansen, C., & Baum, C. M. (1997). Glossary. In C. Christiansen & C. Baum (Eds.), *Occupational therapy: Enabling function and well-being* (2nd ed., pp. 591-606). Thorofare, NJ: SLACK Incorporated.

Clark, B. (1987). *The academic life: Small worlds, different worlds.* Princeton, NJ: Carnegie Foundation for the Advancement of Teaching.

Crampton, M. W. (1958). The recognition of occupational therapy assistants. *American Journal of Occupational Therapy, 12,* 269-275.

Donnelly, C., Brenchley, C., Crawford, C., & Letts, L. (2013). The integration of occupational therapy into primary care: A multiple case study design. *Biomed Central, BMC Family Practice, 14,* 60-71. doi:10.1186/1471-2296-14-60

Fidler, G. S. (1981). From crafts to competence. *American Journal of Occupational Therapy, 35,* 567-573.

Fisher, T. F. (1996). Roles and functions of a case manager. *American Journal of Occupational Therapy, 50,* 452-454.

Gibbs, V., & Toth-Cohen, S. (2011). Family-centered occupational therapy and telerehabilitation for children with autism spectrum disorders. *Occupational Therapy in Health Care, 25*(4), 298-314.

Gronski, M. P., Bogan, K. E., Kloeckner, J., Russell-Thomas, D., Taff, S. D., Walker, K. A., & Berg, C. (2013). The issue is—Childhood toxic stress: A community role in health promotion for occupational therapists. *American Journal of Occupational Therapy, 67,* e148-e153. doi:10.5014/ajot.2013.008755

Hirama, H. (1986). The COTA: A chronological review. In S. E. Ryan (Ed.), *The certified occupational therapist: Roles and responsibilities.* Thorofare, NJ: SLACK Incorporated.

Hoffmann, T., & Cantoni, N. (2008). Occupational therapy services for adult neurological clients in Queensland and therapists' use of telehealth to provide services. *Australian Occupational Therapy Journal, 55,* 239-248.

Holmberg, V., & Ringsberg, K. C. (2014). Occupational therapists as contributors to health promotion. *Scandanavian Journal of Occupational Therapy, 21,* 82-89.

Horowitz, B. P., Nochajski, S. M., & Schweitzer, J. A. (2013) Occupational therapy community practice and home assessments: Use of the home safety self-assessment tool (HSSAT) to support aging in place. *Occupational Therapy in Health Care, 27*(3) 216-227.

Jacobs, K., Blanchard, B., & Baker, N. (2012) Telehealth and ergonomics: A pilot study. *Technology and Healthcare, 20,* 445-458.

Jacobs, K., & McCormack, G. (Eds.). (2011). *The occupational therapy manager* (5th ed.). Bethesda, MD: AOTA Press.

Jahagirdar, S. (2012). Occupational therapy psycho-educational group: Empowering caregivers of children with cerebral palsy. *Indian Journal of Occupational Therapy, 44*(2), 15-23.

Jantzen, A. C. (1974). Academic occupational therapy: A career specialty, 1973 Eleanor Clarke Slagle lecture. *American Journal of Occupational Therapy Association, 28,* 73-81.

Kielhofner, G. (2006). *Research in occupational therapy: Methods of inquiry for enhancing practice.* Philadelphia, PA: F. A. Davis Company.

Killian, K., Fisher, G., & Muir, S. (2015). Primary care: A new context for advancing scholarship of practice. *Occupational Therapy in Health Care, 29,* 383-396. doi:10.3109/07380577.2015.1050713

Kramer, P., Hinojosa, J., & Royeen, C. B. (2003). *Perspectives in human occupation: Participation in life.* Philadelphia, PA: Lippincott Williams and Wilkins.

Lee, H. C. (2014). The role of occupational therapy in the recovery stage of disaster relief: A report from earthquake stricken areas in China. *Australian Occupational Therapy Journal, 61*(1), 28-31.

Mosey, A. C. (1998). The competent scholar. *American Journal of Occupational Therapy, 52,* 760-764.

Muir, S. (2012). Health policy perspectives—Occupational therapy in primary health care: We should be there. *American Journal of Occupational Therapy, 66,* 506-510. doi:10.5014/ajot.2012.665001

Nair, P., & Tyagi, N. (2014). Occupational therapy: Metamorphosis with a vision in public health for disaster preparedness, response, and recovery. *Indian Journal of Occupational Therapy, 46*(3), 71-76.

Orban, K., Erlandsson, L.-K., Edberg, A.-K., Önnerfält, J., & Thorngren-Jerneck, K. (2014). Effect of an occupation-focused family intervention on change in parents' time use and children's body mass index. *American Journal of Occupational Therapy, 68,* e217-e226. doi:10.5014/ajot.2014.010405

Ozelie, R., Janow, J., Kreutz, C., Mulry, M. K., & Penkala, A. (2015). Supervision of occupational therapy level II fieldwork students: Impact on and predictors of clinician productivity. *American Journal of Occupational Therapy, 69,* 6901260010. doi:10.5014/ajot.2015.013532

Pizzi, M. A., & Vroman, K. (2013) Childhood obesity: Effects on children's participation, mental health, and psychosocial development. *Occupational Therapy in Health Care, 27*(2), 99-112.

Scaffa, M. (2001). *Occupational therapy in community-based practice settings.* Philadelphia, PA: F. A. Davis Company.

Shannon, P. D. (1985). From another perspective: An overview of the issue. In F. S. Cromwell (Ed.), *The roles of occupational therapists in continuity of care.* New York, NY: Haworth Press.

Sheffield, C., Smith, C. A., & Becker, M. (2012) Evaluation of an agency-based occupational therapy intervention to facilitate aging in place. *The Gerontologist, 53*(6), 907-918.

Skinner, N., & Kizziar, B. K. (2012). The evolving role of care coordination in an acute care environment: Confirming the appropriate utilization of necessary services—Separating tasks from process. *Case Management Society of America Today, 2*, 18-20.

Wilcock, A. A. (2003). Population interventions focused on health for all. In *Willard and Spackman's occupational therapy* (10th ed.). Hagerstown, MD: Lippincott Williams and Wilkins.

Wilcock, A. A. (2006). *An occupational perspective of health* (2nd ed.). Thorofare, NJ: SLACK Incorporated.

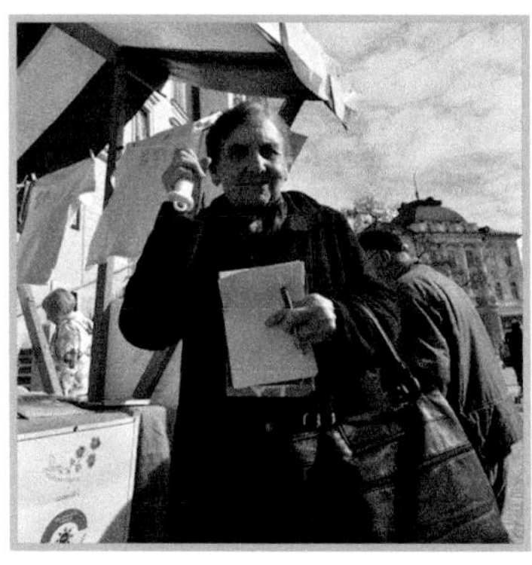

# 55

# RESOLUTION OF ETHICAL CONFLICT

*Susan C. Burwash, PhD, MSc(OT), OTR/L, OT(C) and John W. Vellacott, EdD, MEd, BA*

**ACOTE STANDARDS EXPLORED IN THIS CHAPTER**

B.9.10, B.9.11

**KEY VOCABULARY**

- **Bullying:** Unwanted, repetitive, aggressive behavior that may involve physical, verbal, relational, and/or electronic means of exerting power over another individual.
- **Conflict resolution:** Consciously used communication and problem-solving strategies for addressing conflict.
- **Ethical conflicts:** Disagreements between parties about the ethical resolution to a problem.
- **Ethical dilemmas:** Situations in which there are several alternatives, all of which are ethically somewhat problematic.
- **Moral distress:** Distress occurring when an individual knows what she or he should do but is not able to do it.
- **Moral residue:** Persisting feelings that arise over time from repeated experiences of moral distress.



Jacobs, K., & MacRae, N. (Eds.).
*Occupational Therapy Essentials for Clinical Competence, Third Edition* (pp. 777-790).

Occupational therapists and occupational therapy assistants work with people seeking our services because they or their loved ones are ill, may be suffering, and are unable to do what they need or want to do in their daily lives. Our role as occupational therapy practitioners is to help individuals with whom we work to regain hope for the future; to maintain, restore, or gain the skills they need; to change how they do their occupations; and/or to make environmental modifications—all in the service of moving forward in their lives. Occupational therapy is, at its heart, an inherently moral undertaking. Thus, it should not be surprising that occupational therapy practitioners frequently encounter situations that call on them to recognize and resolve moral and ethical conflicts within practice.

Occupational therapy practitioners are guided by their personal morals as well as professional values and the expression of values that are contained in codes of ethics from national organizations (American Occupational Therapy Association [AOTA], 2015; see discussion in Chapter 50) and state licensing boards. However, no code of ethics is both broad and deep enough to provide specific guidance in every situation in which we encounter ethical conflicts and dilemmas. Furthermore, we work with clients, families, and other health care providers who may hold differing opinions about what is right or wrong and how individuals, groups, and communities should be. Our work occurs within a variety of systems that are governed by laws, policies, and procedures that direct individuals working within them.

It is not surprising, then, that practitioners encounter ethical quandaries on a very regular basis. Respondents to a study done by Kyler (1998), which included occupational therapists, assistants, and students, reported frequent (21% daily, 31% weekly) instances where they had experienced ethical concerns. Slater and Brandt (2009) found high numbers of practitioners who had distress related to ethical issues, including reimbursement constraints, conflict with organizational policies, questionable decisions made by others, and conflicts about discharge decisions, among others. Kinsella, Park, Appiagyei, Chang, and Chow (2008) studied Canadian occupational therapy students' experiences of ethical tensions during fieldwork and found systemic constraints, conflicting values, observing questionable behavior, and failure to speak up as the most common themes reported in students' stories. Penny, Ewing, Hamid, Shutt, and Walter (2014) report moderate levels of moral distress in a survey done with occupational therapy practitioners working in adult physical disability and geriatric settings. Situations contributing most frequently to moral distress included witnessing inadequate care resulting from poor team communication, pressures from administrators to reduce costs, or lack of provider continuity. Almost half (47.4%) of the 224 respondents had either left a job in the past due to moral distress or had considered doing so. A recent review of research on ethical tensions reported by occupational therapy practitioners identified seven themes: resource and systemic issues, upholding ethical principles and values, client safety, working with vulnerable clients, interpersonal conflicts, upholding professional standards, and practice management (Bushby, Chan, Druif, Ho, & Kinsella, 2015).

In this chapter, we will discuss ethical conflicts and ethical dilemmas—what they are, strategies for acting on these concerns (including the pros and cons of action), and general guidelines for reasoning through these challenging situations. We will also briefly explore the special case of bullying, given that this is something that occupational therapy practitioners' clients, or occupational therapy professionals themselves, may have experienced and be responding to. Resources for further learning will also be provided.

The Accreditation Council for Occupational Therapy Education (ACOTE, 2012) Standards ask us to be able to competently identify, reason through, and take action (informal or formal) when we have either personal or organizational ethical issues. Although the primary focus of this chapter is on personal ethical conflicts and how they can be resolved, we acknowledge that ethical conflicts often arise from differences between individual practitioners and the organizations in which they work, and suggest that resolution of ethical issues rests on the shoulders of organizations as well as on practitioners.

## Ethical Conflicts and Dilemmas

As described in Chapter 50, occupational therapy practice is guided by the principles of altruism, equality, freedom, justice, dignity, truth, and prudence. These principles guide us in everyday decisions about confidentiality, informed consent, and, more broadly, about the quality of life concerns that are central to occupational therapy practice. No matter how much we attend to following the code of ethics, we will face personal ethical conflicts and dilemmas that will sometimes cause distress.

### *Ethical Conflicts*

Ethical conflicts arise when what we believe is the best resolution to a problem is either not in accordance with what another person involved in the situation believes and/or when our personal ethical standards collide with values we have committed ourselves to uphold as occupational therapy practitioners. For example, we might not agree with an individual's decision to refuse activities of daily living (ADL) skills training following a stroke because she or he expects that her or his family will provide significant support on a daily basis—an assumption that is part of the individual's cultural norms. Our professional values related to the importance of independence, our own valuing of independence, and the priorities of the health care systems in which we work may make it challenging for us to accept that a client might want to be dependent in ADLs, or, more accurately perhaps, interdependent. Still, it would be possible, having talked with both the client and their caregiver(s), to use the code of ethics to explore this conflict and uphold the principles of freedom of choice. In so doing, the practitioner may decide to support this individual's decision and turn attention away from independence to working with the client and caregiver(s) to support them in completing ADLs interdependently.

A frequently cited conflict from respondents in both Kyler (1998) and Slater and Brandt's (2009) studies was conflict arising from other health care professionals making or recommending discharge plans with which the occupational therapy practitioner disagreed. If the occupational therapy practitioner has strong doubts about the readiness of the client, family, or other caregivers for safe discharge to home, conflict could arise. Again, the code of ethics would provide guidance and direct the practitioner toward taking a stand, using altruism and prudence as guiding principles. Another example of an ethical conflict could occur when a practitioner is asked by his or her employer to use billing codes that do not accurately reflect services provided. In all of these examples, there is a choice that appears to clearly be more closely aligned with occupational therapy values and, in the last case, with legal requirements. Thus, the challenge to the practitioner is mostly in determining how, or if, action can be taken to address the conflict.

### *Ethical Dilemmas*

Ethical dilemmas, in comparison to ethical conflicts, are considerably more complex. They are defined as what happens when occupational therapy practitioners find themselves in situations where a decision must be made between two or more alternatives, all of which have considerable drawbacks (Epstein & Delgado, 2010). For instance, to go back to the example of discharge planning, a dilemma might be having to choose between recommending one of two discharge options, neither of which the client has chosen or is likely to provide the level of ongoing support that you know this client will need to continue to improve. Both options are available now within the client's home community and have a reputation for providing reasonably competent staff. Another example would be the dilemma faced by an occupational therapy practitioner when neither of three adaptive technology options for which funding is available are nearly as good as a more expensive option that is not covered by the client's insurance. A third common example could be balancing the competing demands of seeing more clients during a day but for less time each, or spending more time with certain clients and not seeing other clients that day. Ethical dilemmas can be large or small, but what marks them is the sense that there is no clear answer in the view of the person experiencing the dilemma. The challenge becomes if the practitioner can make a choice and on what grounds to pick one of several nonoptimal options.

## Possible Responses to Ethical Tensions

Just as we have choices in how to address conflicts and dilemmas we encounter in our day-to-day lives outside work, we must also make informed choices within our workplaces about our available options. Most occupational therapy practitioners have had some experience with, or training in, assertive communication to address interpersonal conflicts. Many practitioners even teach social skills, including assertiveness, self-advocacy, and conflict resolution to clients. Our professional standards speak to the importance of occupational therapy practitioners acting as advocates for clients. Even so, the studies cited previously about ethical tensions suggest that occupational therapy practitioners sometimes struggle with taking ethical action. Students, in particular, are faced with tough decisions about whether to (1) ignore ethical issues that arise, (2) avoid discussing them with any of the involved parties and perhaps even their supervising therapist, or (3) take the risk of addressing these issues and potentially jeopardizing successful completion of fieldwork. This ethical predicament has been observed not only in occupational therapy students, but also in medical students (Caldicott & Faber-Langendoen, 2005; Lorris, Carpenter, & Miller, 2009), dietetics students (Tighe & Mainwaring, 2012), and nursing students (Callister, Luthy, Thompson, & Memmott, 2009), among others.

Each of these possible responses has some benefits and costs. Ignoring issues that arise or avoiding discussion of them may feel, particularly to students, like the safest choice. Finding a way to speak out may seem dangerous and requires careful consideration. Suggestions for how to address conflict are presented later in this chapter.

## What Are the Costs of Not Addressing Conflict?

Although it may seem risky to speak up when you encounter ethical dilemmas or conflicts, there are also risks involved in ignoring or avoiding ethical concerns, or as Kinsella et al. (2008) call them, *ethical tensions*.

Possible negative influences may affect not only clients and families but also colleagues, organizations, the community, and the occupational therapy profession. Jameton (1984) talks about *moral distress* as occurring when an individual knows what she should do but is not able to do it. Practitioners or students who see someone discharged who they clearly believe is not able to safely manage in the environment to which he or she is going, or who are unable to provide the number of therapy sessions that they believe will solidify gains made in a neurorehabilitation program, or who see a client being treated disrespectfully and do not intervene might all suffer moral distress. Jameton (1984) and others (Webster & Baylis, 2000) have labeled these long-term feelings as *moral residue*.

Much of the research on moral distress, and the long-term feelings arising from it, has focused on the nursing profession, although there is a recent study of 592 health care providers, including physicians, social workers, pharmacists, physical therapists, and occupational therapists (Whitehead, Herbertson, Hamric, Epstein, & Fisher, 2014). The moral distress research has been briefly summarized by Kirk (2011). Epstein and Hamric (2009) note that nurses experiencing moral distress/moral residue may become morally numbed in the face of new ethical challenges. They often respond by withdrawing and feeling isolated from their colleagues, who they perceive to be better managing these tensions. They may choose more or less productive ways of registering their dissent. They may suffer from *compassion fatigue* or *burnout*. Compassion fatigue and burnout are associated with a variety of physical and behavioral symptoms that compromise practitioner/caregiver health and well-being (Compassion Fatigue Solutions, 2013). Slater and Brandt's (2009) survey of occupational therapy practitioners who reported moral distress found that some had left jobs, were exploring other positions, or had even considered leaving the profession. More than half reported persistent feelings of guilt, anxiety, and depression because of these ethical tensions.

It is clear that unresolved ethical tensions will affect the clients with whom these practitioners are working. It can also affect health care organizations as a whole. Organizations and professional associations are recognizing this, although research on moral distress/residue's impact at the institutional level is somewhat sparse—after all, what organization wants to admit that situations leading to moral distress occur within their organization? Still, there have been institutional responses as organizations have recognized the levels of distress that are occurring. These will briefly be discussed later. However, our primary focus is at the individual practitioner level. Practitioners often cannot completely address these concerns on their own. Kinsella et al. (2008) note "a need for greater attention to the ways in which macro-level policies can shape micro-level practices, and thus raise issues for occupational therapists" (pp. 180-181).

# Individual and Organizational Strategies to Address Ethical Conflict

How can individuals and institutions, as well as professional associations and educational programs, help to reduce ethical tensions and address them when they arise? In this section, we review some general principles for conflict resolution and some specific strategies that have been developed for dealing with resolution of ethical conflict. Some of the general guidelines for resolving ethical conflict come from the work of those interested in improving assertiveness skills and/or nonviolent conflict resolution. Many occupational therapy practitioners may have learned some of these skills prior to entering their professional education or during their coursework. Taylor's (2008) *The Intentional Relationship* text also offers some concrete strategies for occupational therapy practitioners when dealing with therapist–client conflicts. These strategies could be usefully reviewed when considering how to address ethical conflicts with other individuals in the practice setting. Although we review some of these approaches here, in our experience, students and clinicians report that knowing these skills alone is not always sufficient.

# Assertive Communication

People communicate with one another through many different means—verbally, nonverbally, in writing, or in images. In therapy settings, the issue of communication arises in interactions between the practitioner and the client/family, other clinicians, administrators, billing authorities, and so forth. When conflict occurs during the communication process, the use of assertive communication skills can be a critical element in effectively managing the situation. Whitehead et al. (2014) identify "witnessing diminished care due to poor communication" as one of the top three root causes of moral distress reported by the health care professionals they surveyed. Slater and Brandt (2009) note the crucial contribution that effective communication has in preventing and resolving conflicts. This aspect of the chapter will describe what assertive communication is and some specific approaches that occupational therapy practitioners can use in both their own practice and in assisting clients/families.

## What Is Assertive Communication?

Hasan (2008) defines *assertiveness* as a mid-way point between passivity and aggression. He defines *assertive communication* as "the direct expression of an individual's ideas while respecting the rights of others in an atmosphere of trust" (p. 2). Similarly, Kubany, Richard, Bauer, and Muraoka (1992) consider assertiveness as the "expression of feelings, preferences or opinions in ways that respect the rights and opinions of others" (p. 337). Pipas (2010) likewise describes assertive communication as "the ability to represent to the world what you really are, to express what you feel, when you feel it necessary. It is the ability to express your feelings and your rights, respecting the feelings and rights of others" (p. 649). She notes that individuals who have mastered assertive communication skills are usually able to manage or reduce interpersonal conflicts in their lives. How does one communicate assertively? There are a number of possible techniques and approaches.

## Preparing to Communicate Assertively

Before trying to communicate assertively, it is important to lay the groundwork for ensuring that the communication effort is successful. Barnette (2009) suggests the following steps:

- **Assess the situation:** Before engaging in assertive communication, attempt to determine the possible consequences. Although assertive communication usually will result in a positive response, some people might react negatively to it. If that occurs, are you prepared to accept and address this response?
- **Set the stage:** Remember that other individuals may be accustomed to interacting in a certain way. Being presented with a more assertive approach to communicating may be disconcerting or upsetting to them. Advising other people upfront and prefacing the conversation or communication with an acknowledgment that you may be communicating differently than you have in the past may be beneficial.

## Assertive Communication Techniques

There are many different skills and techniques that can be applied to communicate assertively and effectively. Tillman (2007) breaks these down into three sets, which she summarizes as follows:

- **Nonverbal:** These include such things as:
  - Eye contact (maintaining direct eye contact about 50% of the time)
  - Voice tone (well modulated)
  - Posture (straight and relaxed)
  - Facial expressions (reflecting your emotional state—smiling if happy, serious if angry, etc.)
  - Use of gestures (nodding or shaking head, avoiding aggressive gestures such as hands on hips, fists, etc.)
  - Nonverbal listening (attending to the person while he or she is speaking, leaning in slightly to show you are listening, etc.).
- **Verbal:** The use of communication approaches such as:
  - Restatement (restating to the other person what you have heard)
  - Reflection (indicating what you saw, believe the other person said, and how you interpret it)
  - Clarification (asking the speaker to explain a point that he or she is trying to make)
- **Interactive:** Assertive communication is a two-way street, with both parties responding and interpreting each other's verbal and nonverbal cues. To assist in this process, the individual can apply strategies such as:
  - Soft assertion (making statements that do not require anything of the listener, such as compliments and visual images)
  - Basic assertions (simple statements of what the speaker wants or does not want to happen)
  - Empathic assertions (attempts to communicate how he or she thinks the other person may be thinking or feeling)
  - Escalating assertions (a statement with a consequence attached to it)
  - Confrontative assertions (a statement made when an agreement has been violated)

Often, individuals engaging in assertive communications encounter resistance from the other party, who may not be responsive to the techniques described earlier. Barnette (2009) suggested some additional strategies for addressing challenges to assertive communication:

- **Broken record:** Keep repeating your point, using a low-level, pleasant voice. Do not get pulled into arguing or trying to explain yourself. This allows you to ignore manipulation, baiting, and irrelevant logic.
- **Fogging:** This is a way to deflect negative, manipulative criticism. You agree with some of the facts but retain the right to choose your behavior.
- **Content to process shift:** This means that you stop talking about the problem and bring up, instead, how the other person is behaving **right now**. Use it when someone is not listening or is trying to use humor or a distraction to avoid the issue.
- **Defusing:** Let someone cool down before discussing an issue.
- **Assertive inquiry/stop action:** This is similar to the content to process shift. "Let's hold it for a minute, something isn't working, what just happened? How did we get into this argument?" This approach helps to identify the real issue when the argument is actually about something bigger than the immediate topic (p. 4).

Assertive communication involves the effective application of both verbal and nonverbal strategies to ensure that the individual is able to express his or her feelings, preferences, or opinions in a manner that is effective but that also respects the rights and opinions of others (Kubany et al., 1992). Assertive communicators are confident, direct, and honest but also willing to acknowledge the viewpoints of others (Kolb & Griffith, 2009). Effective and assertive communication can go a long way toward addressing and resolving conflict, whether it is about day-to-day differences or ethical issues.

## Anticipating and Addressing Conflict Through the Use of the Intentional Relationship Model

Taylor (2008) discusses some of the anticipated conflicts that practitioners may experience and strategies for dealing with these conflicts. Anticipating what she calls the "inevitable interpersonal events of therapy" (p. 117) and having the skills to understand the client, understand oneself, and being able to shift modes (i.e., from educating mode to empathizing mode) can prevent or reduce practitioner–client conflicts. She also briefly addresses other instances of conflict and provides advice on how to resolve these conflicts, as well as provides learning activities designed to further develop these skills. She links the modes to the ethical principles outlined by AOTA and describes how using these modes can help the practitioner meet these ethical standards.

## A Process for Addressing Ethical Tensions and Moral Distress

The American Association of Critical-Care Nurses (AACN, 2008) outlines a helpful process for those experiencing and addressing ethical conflict. This "4As" model asks that we do the following:

- **Ask:** Reflect on whether we are experiencing moral distress as the result of ethical conflicts or dilemmas.
- **Affirm:** Validate our experience with trusted others, decide that we are willing to take care of ourselves, and review our professional obligations.
- **Assess:** Determine the personal and environmental factors contributing to distress, the severity of distress, our willingness to take action, and pros/cons of taking action.
- **Act:** Prepare, act, and maintain the change you have initiated.

These steps are described in more detail in the AACN publication *The 4A's to Rise Above Moral Distress* (available at no charge) on the AACN website (see the Electronic Resources section for the URL).

## Other Suggestions for Dealing With Ethical Conflicts

Epstein and Delgado (2010) summarize some strategies for addressing moral distress in a variety of work settings. Being willing to speak up, being intentional, being accountable, ensuring that you have support from colleagues, focusing on the system and not just on individuals, and participating in or designing interprofessional ethics workshops are all strategies that they suggest may help. The institution with which they are affiliated has instituted a Moral Distress Consult Service specifically to address these concerns. Most large institutions will have a medical ethicist on staff; such individuals can also be very helpful when individual action seems overwhelming or has not been successful. Ethicist Hilde Nelson (1995) suggests the importance of addressing issues as part of what she calls a *chosen community*; she believes that it is in these communities of peers that individuals can further develop moral agency.

Student practitioners who encounter ethical conflicts and dilemmas should, ideally, address these first with their supervising therapist and also with their educational institutions' fieldwork coordinator. It is important to have support as you work through what is happening and what your next step should be. Document what you are experiencing. Reflect on your options and the pluses and minuses of each. Consider whether the 4A process mentioned previously might help you in your decision making. Many educational programs offer some form of fieldwork "debriefing" sessions following fieldwork. Use these as an opportunity to share your experiences and get support and advice from faculty and student colleagues. Brown and Gillespie (1997) used "theatre of the oppressed" techniques to assist occupational therapy students in practicing moral courage in response to ethical tensions. In this approach, the individual who has experienced ethical tensions describes the incident to peers, who help her or him act out the incident. During subsequent repetitions of the scene, observers may take the part of the protagonist to show alternative ways of dealing with the situation differently.

## The Special Case of Bullying and Conflict Resolution

Conflict takes many forms, and resolving conflicts in a professional and ethical manner is a critical skill for all professionals. However, some types of conflict present more challenging issues than others. One such example is the behavior known as *bullying*. Bullying, in all its manifestations, has been the topic of much attention within the media, academia, and society at large in recent years. Bullying is increasingly being recognized as a problematic and destructive phenomenon that is present in many aspects of society, including within the family, educational settings, academia, the online world, the workplace, and within institutional settings. Bullying is one of the most common forms of violence in our society (Blazer, 2005) and is a phenomenon that is experienced across the age spectrum. Monks and Coyne (2011) note that the term bullying can be used to denote a range of behaviors that take place across a wide range of relationships and social contexts. They can occur across the lifespan from preschool to old age, and encompass relationships within various settings, such the family, workplace, dating, online, institutions, prisons, etc. (p. 4). Monks and Coyne (2011) also note that such behaviors can be described and researched under other terms such as *abuse, harassment,* and *domestic violence*, among others. Although this presents challenges to the practitioner or researcher, it also provides opportunities to draw insight and resources from research spanning a range of disciplines.

In this section, we will briefly explore aspects of bullying in certain contexts where occupational therapy practitioners may be called upon to provide services, such as school settings and online, in workplace settings, and institutional care settings for the aged. Occupational therapy practitioners, in their varied roles, can be called upon as key interveners in addressing bullying behaviors and its impacts. For as Sercombe and Donnelly (2013) observe, "Bullying is not only a psychological concept, but it is also an ethical one. Bullying is a demonstrated risk factor within human development and in the health and safety profile of organizations, but it is also wrong" (p. 491).

### Bullying: Definitions

Although the underlying causes or origins of bullying behavior are not fully understood (Strandmark & Hallberg, 2007), there are many different definitions of what constitutes bullying, depending on the population and setting. Walsh, D'Aoust, and Beamer (2011) state that bullying involves three key elements: power differential, repetition, and motivation. Monks and Coyne (2011) differentiate bullying from other forms of aggression by noting the repetition of the behavior and the power imbalance between the perpetrator and the victim, who is in the weaker and more vulnerable position (pp. 2-3). In children and adolescents, the U.S. Centers for Disease Control and Prevention (CDC; 2015) defines bullying as:

> Any unwanted aggressive behavior(s) by another youth or group of youths, who are not siblings or current dating partners, involving an observed or perceived power imbalance and is repeated multiple times or is highly likely to be repeated. Bullying may inflict harm or distress on the targeted youth including physical, psychological, social, or educational harm. A young person can be a perpetrator, a victim, or both (also known as a "bully/victim." (para. 2)

The National Association of School Psychologists (2012) defines bullying as:

> Unwanted, repetitive, and aggressive behavior marked by an imbalance of power. It can take on multiple forms, including physical (e.g., hitting), verbal (e.g., name calling or making threats), relational (e.g., spreading rumors), and electronic (e.g., texting, social networking). (p. 1)

The U.S. Department of Health and Human Services (n.d.) notes that bullying behaviors involving young adults can also be encompassed under other terms such as *hazing, harassment,* or *stalking* (para. 2).

Significant research in adult bullying has focused on the workplace. Bullying in the workplace is usually more covert than overt, and the construct normally excludes direct physical violence (Bulutlar & Oz, 2009). Rayner and Keashly (2004) identify a range of behaviors as signifying bullying, including social isolation, undermining of professional status, tampering with tools or equipment that people need to do their jobs, intimidation, micromanagement of one's work duties, and personal attacks on credibility. Georgakopoulos, Wilkin, and Kent (2011), building on Leymann and Gustafsson's (1996) constructs, identify workplace bullying as a form of psychological violence that is continuously and persistently repeated and is done with malice.

Bullying among and upon the aged is a relatively new area of research (Selwood, Cooper, & Livingstone 2007). Walsh, D'Aoust, and Beamer (2011) perceive the act of bullying the elderly as a subset within a broader definition of elder abuse, and emphasize the repeated nature of the behavior and that, with each incident, the power differentials between the bully and the victim are reinforced. They also note that while elder abuse can include both intentional and unintentional harm, bullying is by definition both intentional and usually occurs in situations where there is an expectation of trust in the relationship (p. 186). While bullying of the elderly can occur in a variety of settings, research of bullying among the elderly to date has focused primarily on older adults within institutional care facilities (Mapes, 2011). Bullying within this context often involves passive-aggressive behaviors such as gossiping and whispering but is occasionally compounded by direct physical contact and violence, something atypical among younger adults (Bonifas, in Mapes, 2011).

Other definitions of bullying focus less on the age of bully or victim, and more on societal or racial characteristics. Fox and Stallworth (2004) include racial and ethnic bullying under the construct, arguing that racism is often expressed overtly through bullying behaviors. Other researchers focus on the differences in power between perpetrator and victim as the key dynamic (Carbo, 2012; Monks & Coyne, 2011; Strandmark & Hallberg, 2007). For example, Jenkins (2011) differentiates between bullying and normal conflict by noting the power imbalance between the perpetrator and victim, as the victim is placed in an increasingly inferior position to the bully. Jenkins (2011) also notes the role of intent, where the perpetrator deliberately intends to inflict harm of some form on the victim. This behavior can be predatory in nature, with the bully deliberately targeting individuals who he or she knows to be vulnerable.

## Bullying: Prevalence

As noted earlier, bullying is prevalent across age groups. The CDC (2012), citing a 2011 nationally representative sample of youth in Grades 9 through 12, found that 20.1% reported being bullied on school property in the 12 months preceding the survey, and 16.2% reported being bullied electronically (email, chat room, website, texting) in the 12 months preceding the survey. The National Association of School Psychologists (2012), while acknowledging that there is a lack of consensus in the research literature on the prevalence of bullying due to challenges faced with differing methodologies, nonetheless estimates that approximately 70% to 80% of school-aged children have been involved in bullying, either as perpetrator, victim, or bystander.

In adults, the U.S. Workplace Bullying Survey (Workplace Bullying Institute, 2014) states that 27% of respondents reported having experienced some form of workplace bullying, with a further 21% having witnessed abusive behaviors in the workplace and 72% being aware that such behaviors occur at work. The costs to organizations and the economy at large are estimated in the billions of dollars per year (Gardner & Johnson, 2001; Sypher, 2004) through increased absenteeism, turnover, decreased staff commitment, job satisfaction, and productivity (Bulutlar & Oz, 2009; Hague, Skogstad, & Einarsen, 2007). But it is the personal costs to individual workers that are the most alarming. Negative and, in some cases, severe effects on an individual's physical and psychological health can occur, including anxiety, depression, burnout, frustration, eating disorders, heart disease, and stomach ailments (Keashly & Neuman, 2004). Workplace bullying is a silent epidemic causing untold harm to millions of people.

The prevalence of bullying of the elderly is often difficult to estimate, as very often it is undertaken covertly, and perpetrated against vulnerable people (often with memory or other cognitive impairments) by caregivers or others on whom they depend (Selwood et al., 2007, p. 1009). Walsh, D'Aoust, and Beamer (2011), citing Gordon and Brill (2001), likewise note that accurate estimates are difficult to generate due to the hidden nature of the behavior, and that reported cases often involve severe cases of elder abuse involving physical aggression or active neglect (p. 187). Bullying between seniors is equally difficult to estimate given the diversity of the population and settings. Researchers estimates that up to 20% of seniors residing in institutional settings have experienced some form of peer-to-peer bullying (Mapes, 2011; Searson, 2012). Perfett (2013) notes that in institutional environments such as retirement homes or other senior settings, bullying tends to occur more readily because resources are being shared. She also argues that elderly bullies are often reflecting lifelong personality traits, although dementia and other age-related cognitive impairments could also result in behaviors that mimic bullying, though they may not be done with intent.

## Ethical Considerations in Bullying

Rhodes, Pullen, Vickers, Clegg, and Pitsis (2010) note that "bullying is not a simple phenomenon, and nor is it necessarily easy to detect, identify, and categorize" (p. 96). Because the term bullying encompasses such a wide range of behaviors and environments, the ethical considerations for occupational therapy practitioners are many and varied. Although each situation is unique, there are a number of common ethical considerations that can be clustered, which are discussed next.

### Individual

Victims of bullying often seek, or are referred to, assistance from professionals who are perceived as having some ability to intervene or otherwise assist the individual. In these cases, the potential intervener is faced with a number of ethical considerations. Some are associated with the professional role of the intervener, such as professional ethical guidelines, professional skill levels, scope of practice, and so forth. Other ethical considerations are more specific to the situation at hand.

- Can the intervention be effective?
- Does the intervener have the authority (official or inferred) to be effective?
- Could the intervention make things worse?

Functioning as an intervener in bullying situations is not without risks, and the phrase from the Hippocratic Oath, "First, do no harm," should be a driving ethical consideration for any potential intervention.

### Organizational

A considerable amount of research undertaken in the area of bullying has focused on the ethical issues of the organizations in which the bullying takes place. This is particularly true when looking at bullying within the workplace or within senior care facilities. Bullying activities are often seen in the context of poor management (Ontario Safety Association for Community and Healthcare, 2010). Rhodes et al. (2010) argue that another common response is to place responsibility solely on the perpetrator, the so-called bad apple syndrome, which minimizes the organization's ethical responsibility. Other researchers contend that the high-performance expectations and high-pressure environments within today's educational and work environments can predispose some individuals to bullying behaviors (Yamada, 2008). Sercombe and Donnelly (2013), referencing Swain (1996), also note that in adult and particularly workplace contexts, the accusation that an individual is engaging in acts of bullying can have serious implications for an individual's reputation and career, including forming grounds for dismissal. As a result, organizations can be cautious in responding to complaints from victims. Ferris (2004) observed that many organizations responded to allegations of workplace bullying by either (1) determining that the behavior was, in fact, acceptable; (2) ascribing the issue as being equally attributable to both parties as a personality conflict; or (3) assessing that the behavior in question was harmful and inappropriate (p. 389).

Regardless of causal factors within the organization, there is concurrence across the literature that organizations have a moral, ethical, and legal responsibility to ensure the prevention of bullying, and to have policies and mechanisms in place to address specific instances should they occur (Bulutlar & Oz, 2009; Carbo, 2012; Chartered Institute of Personnel and Development, 2004; Fox & Stallworth, 2004; Ontario Safety Association for Community and Healthcare, 2010; Rhodes et al., 2010; Yamada, 2008).

## *Ethical Interventions to Address Bullying*

Interventions to address bullying can be divided into two different categories: (1) preventative, which attempts to establish organizational and environmental constraints that reduce the probability that bullying will occur; and (2) responsive, which attempts to address current or ongoing cases of bullying and ameliorate, to the degree possible, the negative effects on the victim.

### Preventative

Much of the research on bullying focuses on the role of the organization in creating a safe environment wherein bullying behaviors are not only discouraged but also one where they are effectively prevented. Naturally, the differing environments in which the occupational therapy practitioner works and the victim resides will determine the type and scope of preventative interventions possible.

Bennett (2009), citing Harris, Petrie, and Willoughby (2002), identifies a number of elements necessary for effective prevention of bullying in schools:

- A warm, positive environment with involved adults
- Policies setting firm limits on unacceptable behavior
- A commitment by administration and staff to consistent application of nonhostile, nonphysical sanctions on offenders
- Active engagement by authoritative (but not authoritarian) adults (p. 14)

Cecil and Molnar-Main (2011), in their review of the literature, identify a number of elements to an effective anti-bullying approach within schools, including the following:

- A whole systems approach that engages school, community, and family environments
- Specific activities and measures tailored for the particular setting
- The adequate monitoring of program implementation, including multiple sources of data
- Effective and ongoing school staff training
- Educating parents and engaging them in bullying prevention efforts
- Clearly delineated disciplinary methods
- Sufficient program duration (p. 2)

The AOTA (n.d.) tip sheet on bullying prevention and friendship promotion in schools describes how occupational therapy contributions to ensure student participation in enjoyable occupations, teach coping skills and facilitate formation of friendships can serve to prevent, or buffer the effects of, bullying and the consequent impact on mental health. The work of Susan Basyk is also cited by AOTA (2011) as an example of ways in which occupational therapy practitioners can prevent bullying. Leigh (2013) summarizes what occupational therapy practitioners can contribute.

For adults, particularly within workplace settings, much of the research on prevention of bullying has focused on the role of the employing organization. Bulutlar and Oz (2009) argue that the most effective way of preventing workplace bullying is through the establishment of an "ethical climate," encompassing a caring organizational climate combined with a principle-led approach to ethical decision making within the organization. Together, these will produce an organizational environment in which bullying is actively discouraged. Yamada (2008) proposes a two-pronged approach for organizations seeking to prevent workplace bullying. One prong emphasizes a values-based approach to leadership by the organization's managers, which emphasizes honesty and mutual respect at all levels, promotes a level of trust that reduces feelings of helplessness by victims, and supports the belief that organizational leaders can be approached for help. The other prong focuses on educational and policy responses, with information being provided to staff to assist in the recognition of workplace bullying among peers and superiors, combined with clearly identified policies, procedures, and sanctions to address cases of workplace bullying.

Fox and Stallworth (2004) identify four ethical considerations that organizations must address to prevent workplace bullying:

1. Recognizing that workplace bullying exists and that there are environmental factors within the organization that can prevent or encourage bullying behaviors
2. Establishing internal policies and procedures that impose serious and prompt sanctions on workplace bullies
3. Developing effective conflict management and dispute resolution mechanisms to deal with complaints of workplace bullying
4. Supporting anti-bullying efforts at the legislative and community levels

Preventative measures for bullying to and among older adults is a relatively new area of study and closely linked to research on elder abuse and neglect. Fallon (2006), in her review of the literature and international best practices, identifies preventative interventions at both the systemic and organizational level:

- Guidelines on the development and implementation of multiagency policies and procedures to protect vulnerable adults from abuse
- Specific adult protection legislation
- Drawing on community resources to provide a coordinated response; advocacy programs premised on a philosophy that the least restrictive and intrusive interventions should be used

Citing Keys (2003), Fallon refers to three major themes emerging from the literature:

1. A multidisciplinary approach
2. A commitment to preventative measures in addition to direct responses to individual cases
3. Local/community-level responses

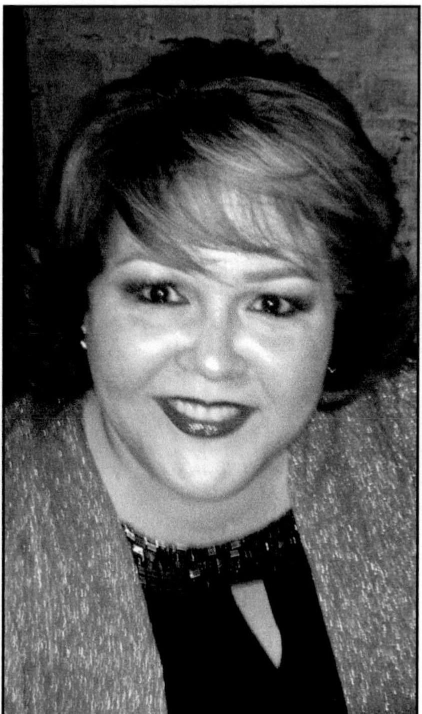

**Figure 55-1.** Terry Olivas-De La O, COTA/L, ROH, founder and CEO, Family Success by Design.

## Responsive

Ethical responses or interventions to addressing specific cases of bullying vary both in terms of approaches and effectiveness. These will hinge in large part on the specifics of the school, workplace, or institution and the individuals involved.

In school situations, a vast range of resources are available both online and in the educational and occupational therapy literature to assist practitioners in developing effective responses to specific cases of bullying by and among children. Of particular note is the pioneering work done by Terry Olivas-De La O, a COTA/L (Figure 55-1) in California who made anti-bullying initiatives one of the primary goals of her practice prior to her death in 2014. Her work included organizing a yearly Young Man's Conference and Young Woman's Summit, which sought to provide young men and women with leadership skills to address bullying within their schools and communities. These summits were supported by a number of southern California businesses and schools. Terry presented on this work at the AOTA conference in San Diego in 2013. A radio interview provides us with a way to learn more about her life and work. http://www.blogtalkradio.com/latino-role-models-success/2013/04/12/terry-olivas-de-la-o-cotal-roh.

Some other relevant discussions of possible ways in which occupational therapy practitioners can address bullying can be found at these sites:

## Evidence-Based Research Chart

| Topic | Evidence |
|---|---|
| Occupational therapy and mental health promotion, prevention, and intervention for children and youth | Arbesman, Bazyk, & Nochajski, 2013 |
| Bullying research | Centers for Disease Control and Prevention, 2015 |
| Moral distress in occupational therapy practitioners | Penny, Ewing, Hamid, Shutt, & Walter, 2014 |
| Ethical tensions in occupational practice | Bushby, Chan, Druif, Ho, & Kinsella, 2015 |

- AOTA on bullying prevention: http://www.aota.org/en/Practice/Children-Youth/Emerging-Niche/Bullying.aspx
- AOTA has a continuing education course based on Bazyk's work on bullying prevention and friendship formation: https://myaota.aota.org/shop_aota/prodview.aspx?TYPE=D&PID=241197935&SKU=WA1080
- AOTA (n.d.) bullying prevention and friendship formation tip sheet describes three levels of possible intervention
- AOTA has held two pediatric virtual chats on occupational therapy and bullying prevention: http://www.talkshoe.com/talkshoe/web/audioPop.jsp?episodeId=380320&cmd=apop and http://recordings.talkshoe.com/TC-73733/TS-934286.mp3

In terms of workplace bullying, Jenkins (2011) notes that mediation (either external or internal) can at times be an effective tool, particularly if supported by legislative or policy authority that helps balance the power discrepancy between parties. Official processes, such as legal proceedings or (in the case of unionized environments) collective agreement grievance procedures are sometimes effective in addressing bullying behaviors or at least intimidating bullies from continuing (Fox & Stallworth, 2004). Training the victim on skills in effective conflict management and bullyproofing are sometimes effective in challenging or managing the bullying behaviors (Ontario Safety Association for Community and Healthcare, 2010), although Strandmark and Hallberg (2007) caution that the power imbalance in many work environments can result in such strategies backfiring by provoking the bully to assert dominance. Lastly, and unfortunately, in situations where neither organizational nor external supports or interveners are available, and personal conflict management and bullyproofing strategies prove ineffective, the victim may need to evaluate the possibility of personally leaving the abusive environment. Workplace bullying is highly complex and involves a host of factors, including personality types, organizational structure, leadership and management styles, cultural values, race, gender, and power. Navigating this minefield and helping the victim (or yourself) is neither easy nor always successful. However, in today's increasingly competitive and globalized work environment, workplace bullying is a phenomenon that will not be going away any time soon.

Effective responses for the cases of bullying among older adults are again determined in large part by the environment in which the behavior is taking place, such

### Case Study

Lindsay is a Level II student occupational therapist completing her fieldwork at a child and adolescent inpatient mental health unit. She has worked hard to establish positive relationships with the young clients she sees, many of whom have been admitted with symptoms of psychosis. In the community in which she is completing her fieldwork, there are limited outpatient mental services for adolescents. She has noticed that during team discussions, her supervising therapist actively contributes to discharge planning for younger clients, but almost always does not contribute ideas unless directly asked when discussing both current status and discharge plans for older adolescent clients. Her practitioner has mentioned how much she loves working with the younger clients. Lindsay wonders if these older adolescent clients are getting the benefit of occupational therapy. She goes home from fieldwork many days feeling frustrated and wondering what she should and could do. She finds herself avoiding her supervising therapist.

**Consider the following questions:**

1. Identify the ethical dilemmas that this student could be experiencing. Refer to the ethical principles in the AOTA's *Occupational Therapy Code of Ethics*.
2. What are the pros and cons of taking action?
3. How could Lindsay prepare herself to address this issue with her supervising therapist? Consider whom she could consult, and what skills she could practice in advance.

as institutional, community, or independent living settings. Perfett (2013) suggests that providing education and training to seniors who are experiencing bullying behaviors on how to manage bullies may be effective. These strategies include the following:

- Determining if the setting has a set of rules or policies in place to address bullying, what they encompass, and how they are enforced
- Discussing the issue with supervisors, staff, or other professionals such as senior advocates or ombudsmen, clergy, social workers, or a family member
- Developing support networks
- Being understanding of the bully, particularly if dementia or other forms of cognitive impairment are evident
- Ignoring or walking away from the bullying

Bullying by staff, family members, or other individuals who are in a position of power over the senior is more complex and may require interventions based on organization policies, legal standards or codes, or even criminal investigations. Occupational therapy practitioners engaged in these types of interventions should reference the ethical guidelines of their professional association and the policies and procedures in place within their own organizational settings.

Bullying is highly complex and involves a host of factors, including personality types, organizational structure, leadership and management styles, cultural values, race, gender, and power. Navigating this minefield and helping the victim (or yourself) is neither easy nor always successful. However, bullying is an issue that will continue to present itself to occupational therapy practitioners in a variety of settings. Being able to ethically address and assist your clients is a key skill in effectively dealing with this destructive behavior.

## Summary

In this chapter, we have examined conflict—particularly ethical conflict. We have discussed how conflict affects individuals and organizations, and possible responses to conflict. The use of a variety of skills, including assertive communication, and strategies for resolving ethical conflict were reviewed. The special case of bullying and how individual clinicians as well as the organizations they work for, or in, can address bullying was also discussed. It is the authors' hope that students and clinicians will explore these ideas and find them useful when they encounter, and need to address, ethical conflicts in their practice.

## Student Self-Assessment

1. Describe the differences between ethical conflicts and ethical dilemmas.
2. Given your context, review local, state, or national regulations regarding bullying.
3. How comfortable are you with resolving conflict? Think of a situation in which you have experienced ethical distress. Describe what happened, what you did, and what you would hope to do differently next time. If possible, share this with a trusted colleague. Ask the colleague to suggest other possible resolutions.
4. How would you describe your approaches to assertively communicating, and how would you deal with someone who is actively resistant to your interpersonal communication styles?

## Electronic Resources

American Association of Critical-Care Nurses' handbook on addressing moral distress: http://www.aacn.org/WD/Practice/Docs/4As_to_Rise_Above_Moral_Distress.pdf

Conflict resolution skills: http://www.helpguide.org/articles/relationships/conflict-resolution-skills.htm

Dealing with workplace bullying: http://occupational-therapy.advanceweb.com/student-and-new-grad-center/student-top-story/dealing-with-workplace-bullies.aspx

Nonviolent communication: http://www.cnvc.org/

## References


Accreditation Council on Occupational Therapy Education. (2012). *ACOTE standards and interpretive guidelines (August 2012).* Retrieved from http://www.aota.org/Education/Careers/Accreditation/StandardsReview.aspx

American Association of Critical-Care Nurses. (2008). *The 4A's to rise above moral distress.* Retrieved from http://www.aacn.org/WD/Practice/Docs/4As_to_Rise_Above_Moral_Distress.pdf

American Occupational Therapy Association. (n.d.). *Bullying prevention and friendship promotion.* Retrieved from https://www.aota.org/practice/children-youth/mental%20health/bullying.aspx

American Occupational Therapy Association. (2011). *Bullying.* Retrieved from https://www.aota.org/practice/children-youth/emerging-niche/bullying.aspx

American Occupational Therapy Association. (2015). Occupational therapy code of ethics (2015). *American Journal of Occupational Therapy, 69*(Suppl. 3).

Arbesman, M., Bazyk, S., & Nochajski, S. M. (2013). Systematic review of occupational therapy and mental health promotion, prevention, and intervention for children and youth. *American Journal of Occupational Therapy, 67*, e120-e130. doi:10.5014/ajot.2013.008359

Barnette, V. (2009). *Assertive communication.* Retrieved from http://www.uiowa.edu/ucs/asertcom.shtml

Bennett, C. (2009). *Literature review of bullying at schools.* Winnipeg, Manitoba, Canada: University of Manitoba.

Blazer, C. (2005). *Literature review on bullying.* Miami, FL: Miami-Dade County Public Schools.

Brown, K. H., & Gillespie, D. (1997). "We become brave by doing brave acts": Teaching moral courage through the theatre of the oppressed. *Literature and Medicine, 16*, 108-120. doi:10.1353/lm.1997.0001

Bulutlar, F., & Oz, E. U. (2009). The effects of ethical climates on bullying behavior in the workplace. *Journal of Business Ethics, 86*, 273-298. doi:10.1007/s10551-008-9847-4

Bushby, K., Chan, J., Druif, S., Ho, K., & Kinsella, E. (2015). Ethical tensions in occupational therapy: A scoping review. *British Journal of Occupational Therapy, 74*, 212-221. doi:10.1177/0308022614564770

Caldicott, C., & Faber-Langendoen, K. (2005). Deception, discrimination and fear of reprisal: Lessons in ethics from third-year medical students. *Academic Medicine, 80*, 866-873. doi:10.1097/00001888-200509000-00018

Callister, L., Luthy, K., Thompson, P., & Memmott, R. (2009). Ethical reasoning in baccalaureate nursing students. *Nursing Ethics, 16*, 499-510. doi:10.1177/0969733009104612

Carbo, J. (2012). *Exploring solutions in workplace bullying*. Retrieved from http://www.aabri.com/OC2012Manuscripts/OC12037.pdf

Cecil, H., & Molnar-Main, S. (2011). Olweus bullying prevention program in high schools: A review of the literature. *Center for Schools and Communities Research Brief No. 5*. Retrieved from http://www.Center-School.org

Centers for Disease Control and Prevention. (2012). *Youth violence: Facts at a glance*. Retrieved from http://www.cdc.gov/violenceprevention/pdf/yv-datasheet-a.pdf

Centers for Disease Control and Prevention. (2015). *Featured topic: Bullying research*. Retrieved from http://www.cdc.gov/violenceprevention/youthviolence/bullyingresearch/

Chartered Institute of Personnel and Development. (2004). *Managing conflict at work: A guide for line managers*. Retrieved from http://www.cardiff.ac.uk/humrs/staffinfo/organisationaldevelopment/leadership/dashboard/Managing%20Conflict%20at%20Work%20-%20a%20guide%20for%20line%20managers.pdf

Compassion Fatigue Solutions. (2013). *Running on empty: Compassion fatigue in professionals*. Retrieved from http://compassionfatigue.ca/article-to-recommend/

Epstein, E., & Delgado, S. (2010). Understanding and addressing moral distress. *Online Journal of Issues in Nursing, 15*(1). doi:10.3912/OJIN.Vol15No03Man01

Epstein, E., & Hamric, A. (2009). Moral distress, moral residue and the crescendo effect. *Journal of Clinical Ethics, 20*, 330-342.

Fallon, P. (2006). *Elder abuse and/or neglect: Literature review*. Wellington, New Zealand: Centre for Social Research and Evaluation, Te Pakapū Rangahau Arotaki Hapori, Ministry of Social Development.

Ferris, P. (2004). A preliminary typology of organizational response to allegations of workplace bullying: See no evil, hear no evil, speak no evil. *British Journal of Guidance and Counselling, 32*(3), 389-395. doi:10.1080/03069880410001723576

Fox, S., & Stallworth, L. E. (2004). Employee perceptions of internal conflict management programs and ADR processes in preventing and resolving incidents of workplace bullying: Ethical challenges for decision makers in organizations. *Employee Rights and Employment Policy Journal of Chicago-Kent College of Law, 8*, 375-405.

Gardner, S., & Johnson, P. R. (2001). The leaner meaner workplace: Strategies for handling bullies at work. *Employee Relations Today, 28*(2), 23-36. doi:10.1002/ert.1012.abs

Georgakopoulos, A., Wilkin, L., & Kent, B. (2011). Workplace bullying: A complex problem in contemporary organizations. *International Journal of Business and Social Science, 2*(3), 1-20.

Gordon, R. M., & Brill, D. (2001). The abuse and neglect of the elderly. *International Journal of Law and Psychiatry, 24*(23), 183-197. doi:10.1016/S0160-2527(00)00076-5

Hague, L. J., Skogstad, A., & Einarsen, S. (2007). Relationships between stressful work environments and bullying: Results of a large representative study. *Work and Stress, 21*(3), 220-242. doi:10.1080/02678370701705810

Harris, S., Petrie, G., & Willoughby, W. (2002). Bullying among 9th graders: An exploratory study. *NASSP Bulletin, 86*(630), 3-14. doi:10.1177/019263650208663002

Hasan, S. (2008). Instructional design and assessment: A tool to teach communication skills to pharmacy students. *American Journal of Pharmaceutical Education, 72*(3), 1-9. doi:10.5688/aj720367

Jameton, A. (1984). *Nursing practice: The ethical issues*. Englewood Cliffs, NJ: Prentice Hall.

Jenkins, M. (2011). Practice note: Is mediation suitable for complaints of workplace bullying? *Conflict Resolution Quarterly, 29*(1), 25-38. doi:10.1002/crq.21035

Keashly, L., & Neuman, J. H. (2004). Bullying in the workplace: Its impact and management. *Employment Policy, 83*(3), 335-373.

Keys, F. (2003). *Responding to elder abuse and neglect: Assessment and referral procedures*. Wellington, New Zealand: Office for Senior Citizens.

Kinsella, E. A., Park, A., Appiagyei, J., Chang, E., & Chow, D. (2008). Through the eyes of students: Ethical tensions in occupational therapy practice. *Canadian Journal of Occupational Therapy, 75*, 176-183. doi:10.1177/000841740807500309

Kirk, S. (2011). Moral distress: A literature review. *Arizona Bioethics Network*. Retrieved from http://abnbp.tapslhi.org/wp-content/uploads/2011/05/Moral-Distress.pdf

Kolb, S. M., & Griffith, A. C. S. (2009). I'll repeat myself again: Empowering students through assertive communication skills. *Teaching Exceptional Children, 41*(3), 32-36.

Kubany, E. S., Richard, D. C., Bauer, G. S., & Muraoka, M. Y. (1992). Impact of assertive and accusatory communication of distress and anger: A verbal component analysis. *Aggressive Behavior, 18*, 337-347. doi:10.1002/1098-2337(1992)18:5<337::AID-AB2480180503>3.0.CO;2-K

Kyler, P. (1998). Putting everyday ethics into practice. *OT Practice, 3*, 36-40. doi:10.1136/inpract.29.4.234

Leigh, I. (2013). Preventing bullying: How occupational therapy practitioners can help make schools a safer place for everyone. *OT Practice*, 18(5),12-16. Retrieved from http://dx.doi.org/10.7138/otp.2013.185f2

Leymann, H., & Gustafsson, A. (1996). Mobbing at work and the development of post-traumatic stress disorders. *European Journal of Work and Organizational Psychology, 5*, 251-276. doi:10.1080/13594329608414858

Lorris, K. D., Carpenter, R. O., & Miller, B. M. (2009). Moral distress in the third year of medical school: A descriptive review of student case reflections. *American Journal of Surgery, 197*, 107-112. doi:10.1016/j.amjsurg.2008.07.048

Mapes, D. (2011). *Mean old girls: Seniors who bully*. Retrieved from http://www.nbcnews.com/id/41353544/ns/health-aging/%20-%20.UQ8_--jZq_4#.UvJboPldXQg

Monks, C. P., & Coyne, I. (2011). *Bullying in different contexts*. Cambridge, United Kingdom: Cambridge University Press.

National Association of School Psychologists. (2012). *A framework for school-wide bullying prevention and safety*. Retrieved from http://www.nasponline.org/resources/bullying/Bullying_Brief_12.pdf

Nelson, H. (1995). Resistance and insubordination. *Hypatia, 10*, 23-40. doi:10.1111/j.1527-2001.1995.tb01367.x

Ontario Safety Association for Community and Healthcare. (2010). *Bullying in the workplace: A handbook for the workplace*. Toronto, Ontario, Canada: HealthForce Ontario.

Penny, N., Ewing, T., Hamid, R., Shutt, K., & Walter, A. (2014). An investigation of moral distress experienced by occupational therapists. *Occupational Therapy in Health Care, 28*, 382-393. doi:10.3109/07380577.2014.933380

Perfett, M. (2013). *Senior bullying: Cliques, harassment, ostracism prevalent among elders*. Retrieved from http://www.thebesttimes.org/aaa/elder_abuse/0811_senior_bullying.shtml

Pipas, M. D. (2010). Assertive communication skills. *Anales Universitatis Apulensis Series Oeconomica, 12*(2), 649-656.

Rayner, C., & Keashly, L. (2004). Bullying at work: A perspective from Britain and North America. In S. Fox & P. E. Spector (Eds.), *Counterproductive work behavior: Investigations of actors and targets* (pp. 271-296). Washington, DC: American Psychological Association.

Rhodes, C., Pullen, A., Vickers, M. H., Clegg, S. R., & Pitsis, A. (2010). Violence and workplace bullying: What are an organization's moral responsibilities? *Administrative Theory and Praxis, 32*(1), 96-115. doi:10.2753/atp1084-1806320105

Searson, L. (2012). *Senior bullying.* Retrieved from http://www.retirement-living.com/senior-bullying/

Selwood, A., Cooper, C., & Livingston, G. (2007). What is elder abuse: Who decides? *International Journal of Geriatric Psychiatry, 22*(10), 1009-1012. doi:10.1002/gps.1781

Sercombe, H., & Donnelly, B. (2013). Bullying and agency: definition, intervention and ethics. *Journal of Youth Studies, 16*(4), 491-502. doi: 10.1080/13676261.2012.725834

Slater, D., & Brandt, L. (2009). Combating moral distress. *OT Practice, 14,* 13-16.

Strandmark, M., & Hallberg, L. R. M. (2007). The origin of workplace bullying: Experiences from the perspective of bully victims in the public service sector. *Journal of Nursing Management, 15,* 332-341. doi:10.1111/j.1365-2834.2007.00662.x

Swain, H. (1996). Bullying claims may lead to dismissal. *Times Higher Education.* Retrieved from http://www.timeshighereducation.co.u /story.asp?storyCode=91266§ioncode=26

Sypher, B. D. (2004). Reclaiming civil discourse in the workplace. *Southern Communications Journal, 69*(3), 257-270. doi:10.1080/10417940409373296

Taylor, R. (2008). *The intentional relationship: Occupational therapy and use of self.* Philadelphia, PA: F. A. Davis Company.

Tighe, B., & Mainwaring, J. (2012). The bioethical experiences of student dietitians on their final clinical placement. *Journal of Human Nutrition and Dietetics, 26*(2), 198-203. doi:10.1111/jhn.12007

Tillman, L. D. (2007). *Effective communication: Speaking up assertively.* Retrieved from http://www.speakupforyourself.com/Powerpoint/BasicAssertiveCommunication.pps

U.S. Department of Health and Human Services. (n.d.). *Young adults: Is it bullying?* Retrieved from http://www.stopbullying.gov/what-is-bullying/related-topics/young-adults/index.html

Walsh, C. A., D'Aoust, G., & Beamer, K. (2011). Elder abuse and bullying: Exploring theoretical and empirical connection. In C. P. Moks & I. Coyne (Eds.), *Bullying in different contexts* (pp. 185-210). Cambridge, United Kingdom: Cambridge University Press.

Webster, G. C., & Baylis, F. (2000). Moral residue. In S. B. Rubin & L. Zoloth (Eds.), *Margin of error: The ethics of mistakes in the practice of medicine* (p. 208). Hagerstown, MD: University Publishing Group.

Whitehead, P., Herbertson, R. K., Hamric, A. B., Epstein, E. G., & Fisher, J. M. (2014). Moral distress among healthcare professionals: Report of an institution-wide survey. *Journal of Nursing Scholarship, 47*(2), 117-125. doi:10.1111/jnu.12115

Workplace Bullying Institute. (2014). *2014 U.S. workplace bullying survey.* Retrieved from workplacebullying.org/multi/pdf/WBI-2014-US-Survey.pdf

Yamada, D. C. (2008). Workplace bullying and ethical leadership. *Journal of Values-Based Leadership, 1*(2), 49. Retrieved from http://papers.ssrn.com/sol3/papers.cfm?abstract_id=1301554

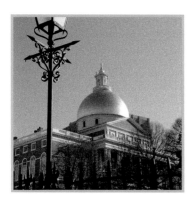

# 56

# Advocacy in Occupational Therapy

Amy Lamb, OTD, OT/L, FAOTA and Elizabeth C. Hart, MS, OTR/L

**ACOTE STANDARDS EXPLORED IN THIS CHAPTER**

B.2.3, B.6.4, B.9.13

**KEY VOCABULARY**

- **Advocacy:** To speak up for or plead the case of another.
- **Coalition:** Individuals or groups joining forces together for a common cause.
- **Grassroots advocacy:** A group effort of like-minded individuals working together to achieve a desired outcome.
- **Policy:** Principle or rule to guide decisions and achieve outcomes.



Jacobs, K., & MacRae, N. (Eds.).
*Occupational Therapy Essentials for Clinical Competence, Third Edition* (pp. 791-800).

Occupational therapy is an integral part of today's dynamic health care system. However, as a profession we are consistently challenged to keep our place in the system. We are consistently advocating for appropriate reimbursement in a health care market that is full of competition and low on resources. We diligently work to demonstrate the value and skill occupational therapy brings to the treatment of clients. In this current era of health care reform, it is vital that we communicate the message that occupational therapy is a worthy investment. We must make the occupational therapy voice heard for our clients, for our profession, and in the larger context of health care reforms. Occupational therapy enables meaningful participation that allows people to "live life to the fullest." As occupational therapy professionals, we must be aware of the changes currently affecting our practice and the system at large, and keep a laser-like focus for our advocacy efforts.

## Advocacy Defined

*Advocacy* means to speak up, or to plead the case of another (Merriam-Webster, 2016). For a practitioner, this may mean speaking up for a client who could benefit from continued services or for an occupational therapy department to be included in a new program within your organization. For a professional association, such as the American Occupational Therapy Association (AOTA), this means championing a cause on behalf of the people it serves, and asking people to help in carrying out the organization's mission. Examples of advocacy include voicing positions about the rights or benefits to which someone is entitled or taking action to ensure that institutions work appropriately.

Why is advocacy important to the occupational therapy profession? Advocacy is about getting listened to, being at the table when decisions are made, and being heard by people who make decisions (Daly, 2011). It is essential for the voices of occupational therapy practitioners to be heard at tables where decisions are being made regarding clients and populations who can benefit from our services. Policymakers, employers, consumers, advocacy groups, health care and education professionals, and the insurance industry will better understand the value of occupational therapy through the advocacy efforts of the profession.

## History of Advocacy in Occupational Therapy

### *Early Efforts*

The pioneers of occupational therapy believed in the profession and were staunch advocates for it. They fought for the survival of occupational therapy because they believed in the benefits of the services. They wanted to create a base for future generations of occupational therapy professionals to build on. Quiroga (1995, p. 15) states that "in the early 1900's the founders defined the profession's boundaries, developed theories of practice, increased the number of practitioners, strategized to convince the American public and the medical world the value of occupational therapy, built many institutions in which to train practitioners and treat patients, and established standards for training and practice." These efforts of our profession's pioneers are examples of their role in advocating for occupational therapy.

Several individuals were extremely active in the advancement and expansion of the occupational therapy profession. Eleanor Clark Slagle, for example, was active in advocacy with medical professionals to help bring to light the importance of occupational therapy intervention in mental health care, as well as tuberculosis prevention and care. These efforts helped occupational therapy move into the medical arena of health care. Quiroga (1995, p. 46) reports that "Slagle made it her business to contact people in other cities who were beginning to see, as she did, that her work had the potential to become its own profession." Contacting people and promoting the benefits of occupational therapy was a demonstration of her involvement in advocacy for the profession and its potential clients.

William Rush Dunton, Jr., a psychiatrist who has come to be known as the "father of occupational therapy," was also instrumental in the advancement of the profession. Quiroga (1995) reported that Dunton participated in nationwide struggles to raise the status of psychiatry in American medicine. He viewed making occupational therapy a profession as an important step in that direction, for he believed that the new profession combined a scientific approach with humanitarian values. Together, Dunton and Slagle were active in the establishment of our first national association, the National Society for the Promotion of Occupational Therapy. This association today is known as the AOTA. Establishing the first national association was a direct result of advocacy efforts and a first step for occupational therapy toward becoming a distinct profession.

Susan Tracy was another advocate of the profession. Tracy is credited for shaping the identity of the new profession by training newcomers to the field, widening the settings in which occupational therapy was practiced, and exposing a variety of clients to the services we provide. In addition, she also helped carve a place for the profession in early 20th-century America (Quiroga, 1995). Susan Tracy was an advocate for the profession through her attempts to train future therapists with a broader domain of practice.

In her 1967 Eleanor Clark Slagle lecture, Wilma West encouraged occupational therapy leaders and professionals to direct advocacy efforts to meet the needs of society. West cited two major purposes of a profession: "to meet external obligations to society" and "to meet the internal loyalties to members on the other" (1968). "Responsibility for awareness and interpretation of those changes which affect any part of our profession, and responsibility for whatever group action is appropriate to facilitate or hasten adjustment to change." She went on to state that "both as individuals and as a professional group we should be assuming a far more frequent and contributing part in the planning of health services. It will be mandatory that we do so if we are to have a part in shaping our own development" (West, 1968). These words continue to provide direction for the profession today.

Occupational therapy was a valuable profession in the past, we are a valuable profession today, and we have every opportunity to continue to be a valuable part of the health care system in the future. To succeed in this ever-changing environment, occupational therapy professionals will need to be advocates within the larger conversation of reform. Some of the changes we see today are different than those faced by our founders, while some are similar. Nonetheless, it is our time to take charge to fight for the same roots of the profession that our founders fought for so many years ago.

## *Instrumental Legislation*

Occupational therapy is included in numerous pieces of legislation that have been instrumental in opening doors and opportunity for occupational therapy; our inclusion is a direct result of advocacy by association leaders and grassroots advocates. These laws have been very influential in the services provided by occupational therapy as well as the rights our clients are entitled to.

The Medicare system was established as an amendment to the Social Security Act of 1965. This landmark legislation provided health insurance to persons who were 65 and older and those under 65 with specific diagnoses. Later, advocacy efforts of the AOTA were successful in including occupational therapy as a reimbursable service under both Medicare Part A and Part B.

The Individuals with Disabilities Education Act (IDEA; 1990) was a landmark piece of legislation that made a place for occupational therapy in the schools and assisted in the reimbursement for such services. Occupational therapy is a related service under Part B of IDEA and provides services to children with special education needs.

The Americans with Disabilities Act (ADA; 1990) was another landmark piece of legislation shifting the way in which society views persons with disabilities. The ADA played a vital role in changing social attitudes about health, disease, and disability since its inception. This legislation has affected the occupational therapy profession and provided standards to increase accessibility for persons with disability.

The Patient Protection and Affordable Care Act (PPACA), more commonly referred to as the Affordable Care Act, was passed in 2010. This law expanded health care coverage to about 31 million uninsured Americans through a combination of cost controls, subsidies, and mandates. The PPACA includes programs aimed at shifting the current health care system from a fee-for-service model to a value-based payment model to improve coordination and patient outcomes, as well as to achieve savings. The PPACA delineates 10 essential health benefits, outlining parameters of what insurance plans are required to cover, including ambulatory patient services, emergency services, hospitalization, maternity and newborn care, mental health and substance use disorder, prescription drugs, rehabilitative and habilitative services and devices, laboratory services, preventive and wellness services and chronic disease management, and pediatric services including oral and vision (PPACA, 2010). While implementation of the PPACA is ongoing, occupational therapy has advocacy opportunities in meeting the needs of newly covered individuals, in ensuring that the insurance plans in state exchanges adequately cover habilitative and rehabilitative services, and in promoting occupational therapy's role in improving health outcomes and reducing costs.

The 10 essential health benefits of the PPACA are also applicable to beneficiaries within the Medicaid program. In the United States, Medicaid has a distinct role in our health care system, including providing health insurance coverage to children, low income families, the elderly, and persons with disabilities. In addition, the PPACA, included language that expanded Medicaid from 133% of the federal poverty level to 138% of the federal poverty level. While Medicaid expansion has not been accepted in all 50 states, the Medicaid program has been strengthened by the passage of the PPACA by providing Medicaid beneficiaries with the 10 essential health benefits and taking a step forward to reduce disparities in care.

The PPACA is moving the U.S. health care system to a value-based system, increasing the need for occupational therapy practitioners to understand the outcomes and benchmarks their organizations are seeking to achieve for the populations and individuals they serve. There are a variety of alternative payment models that are being trialed as the health care system works to enhance the quality of care, enhance the efficiency of the system, and reduce health care spending. With the rapidly changing environment surrounding health care today, advocacy is vital to ensure that occupational therapy services remain accessible to individuals and populations that need them.

These are examples of federal laws that have made improvements in the access to occupational therapy services. Without the advocacy efforts of our professional association and occupational therapy professionals, these

Table 56-1.

**Percentage of Occupational Therapists by Work Setting, 1973-2015**

| | 1973 | 1982 | 1990 | 1998 | 2001 | 2015 |
|---|---|---|---|---|---|---|
| Hospital (non-mental health) | 37 | 36 | 35 | 24 | 28 | 27 |
| Behavioral health | 18 | 10 | 9 | 4 | 3 | 2 |
| School system/early intervention | 11 | 18 | 19 | 22 | 30 | 25 |
| Academic | 7 | 5 | 4 | 6 | 4 | 6 |
| Skilled nursing facility/long-term care | 6 | 10 | 9 | 23 | 14 | 19 |
| Home health | 1 | 4 | 4 | 6 | 6 | 7 |
| Freestanding outpatient | | 3 | 5 | 5 | 5 | 11 |
| Community-based | | 2 | 1 | 2 | 1 | 2 |
| Work/industry/ergonomics | | 1 | 1 | 1 | 1 | |
| Private practice | 1 | 4 | 8 | 6 | 6 | |
| Other | 19 | 8 | 5 | 1 | 2 | 1 |

pieces of legislation may have advanced without the inclusion of occupational therapy. They have also had a significant effect on where occupational therapy is practiced, as illustrated in Table 56-1. Notice the decline in behavioral health practice following the deinstitutionalization of mental health facilities during the 1970s, the growth in school-based practice after the passage of the Education for All Handicapped Children Act of 1975, the expansion of skilled nursing practice in the 1990s after these facilities began providing Medicare Part B services, and the decline in skilled nursing practice when the Medicare Part B therapy cap was implemented in the 2000s. These trends demonstrate the effect of public policy on occupational therapy practice and the importance of professional advocacy to ensure occupational therapy has a voice in a changing health care environment.

## A Changing Society

It is essential for us to examine the societal context in which we live, work, and play to understand what advocacy is needed to promote occupational therapy. The U.S. health care system is undergoing reforms emphasizing systems that support increased efficiency in the health care system, increased quality of services provided, and decreased costs. There is a growing emphasis on creating a culture of personal responsibility for one's health and attempts to shift the system to focus on prevention and wellness. There is a shift toward primary care in an effort to reduce costs and increase system efficiency. We face continuing challenges to our reimbursement structure and system as it currently exists. This context of the U.S. health care system is essential for us to understand in our advocacy efforts. It is imperative that as we grow as a profession we set our path within the external societal issues we face. Occupational therapy practitioners will be required to go beyond performing direct services and step forward to articulate a clear message outlining the value and distinctiveness of occupational therapy.

The AOTA has provided a vision statement for where occupational therapy will be in its centennial year of 2017. It states, "We envision that occupational therapy is a powerful, widely recognized, science-driven, and evidence-based profession with a globally connected and diverse workforce meeting society's occupational needs" (AOTA, 2006). The Centennial Vision was the first of its kind developed by AOTA and provided occupational therapy professionals with a laser-like focus for their advocacy efforts moving forward. Significant progress has been made, all centering around building capacity within the profession to meet society's occupational needs and demonstrate our value. The Centennial Vision served as a platform for all volunteer leaders to work together on our journey to 2017, and we are working to build upon the progress we have made with the Centennial Vision as we embark on Vision 2025.

## Importance of Grassroots Advocacy

Grassroots advocacy is a group effort of like-minded individuals working together to achieve a desired outcome. Grassroots advocacy may occur as part of our daily practice, within our professional organizations, and at the health systems level. As occupational therapy professionals, our grassroots advocacy efforts are enhanced when we share a clear and consistent message with our target audience.

## Therapy Level

Earlier, we defined advocacy as the act of speaking up for or pleading the case of another. This definition clearly fits the grassroots advocacy efforts of occupational therapy practitioners in their daily practice. This may occur in clinical, education, community-based, or research settings depending on where you put your occupational therapy knowledge and skills to work on a daily basis.

In our practice, we often engage in advocacy on behalf of the clients we serve as well as assisting them in developing their own advocacy voice. Opportunities for advocacy are endless in our daily practice, regardless of what setting that may be.

### Practical Examples of Therapy Level Advocacy

- Ensure that clients have access to the services for which they are eligible
- Make the client's requests known to other members of the health care team and promote coordinated care
- Take complex information and provide the necessary client education to increase the client's understanding and ability to apply the information into the habits and routines of his or her everyday life
- Take the time to explain the role of occupational therapy in our setting to our clients, help them see the link to occupation (the meaningful, familiar tasks of their everyday life)
- Provide evidence-based, occupation-centered interventions to our clients and document the distinct value of occupational therapy services to payers

### Case Study 1

David is an occupational therapist who works in home-based primary care for the VA. His client, Mr. A, is an 82-year-old veteran with a diagnosis of type 2 diabetes, diabetic retinopathy, osteoarthritis, and mild intellectual disability. While he no longer drives, he uses his four-wheeled walker to walk to a local shopping center every day, where he likes to visit shop owners and other patrons, visit the movie theater, and grab a slice of pizza at his favorite restaurant. He was referred to the home-based primary care team because his poorly controlled diabetes places him at high risk of hospitalization. In David's initial occupational therapy assessment, he notes that Mr. A has difficulty performing routine diabetic foot care due to osteoarthritis in his knees. He also notes that Mr. A has significantly decreased sensation in his feet as well as excessively dry skin, callouses, and a strong odor indicating poor hygiene and self-management of diabetic foot care, placing Mr. A at high risk for wound development. David helps Mr. A to set up an appointment with his podiatrist, and he agrees to accompany him as part of one of their occupational therapy sessions. During the appointment, David notices that Mr. A appears to be having difficulty understanding what the podiatrist is telling him about the condition of his feet and the risks of not performing routine diabetic foot care. Understanding that Mr. A has limited health literacy, David breaks down the information in a way that Mr. A can appreciate. He also shares with the doctor the barriers that make routine diabetic foot care difficult for Mr. A, and explains that Mr. A values the ability to walk to his local shopping center because it allows him regular social interaction and participation in meaningful activities. David proposes that Mr. A start visiting the nail salon in the shopping center for regular pedicures, and works with the podiatrist and Mr. A to provide an educational handout for salon staff to help them identify problems requiring follow-up with Mr. A's medical team. After 1 month, Mr. A is a well-known regular at his local nail salon, and he looks forward to his weekly visits, when he gets to sit and socialize with other salon patrons. David notes that his feet appear much healthier with well-moisturized skin and no areas concerning for wound development. In his final note before discharge, David provides an objective description that indicates how his client-centered intervention improved Mr. A's performance of routine diabetic foot care, improved the condition of his feet, and decreased his risk of diabetes-related complications, all while fitting in with and maintaining Mr. A's valued routines and occupations.

## Professional Level

Advocacy at the professional level provides a necessary and important link to our daily practice and our recognition at the health systems level. This type of advocacy occurs in a variety of settings as well. Professional advocacy may occur in clinical practice when we educate potential referral sources about the role of occupational therapy in our setting. Engaging in program development to provide occupational therapy services to a specific population or group to enhance quality of life is professional advocacy. Educating insurance companies on the role of occupational therapy in certain areas can lead to decreased denials and increased payments for service, a direct result from professional advocacy efforts. Participating in coalitions in which we use our occupational therapy knowledge to promote services for individuals and populations that meet societal needs is another example of high-value professional advocacy.

**Practical Examples of Professional Level Advocacy**

- Noticing a high rate of falls in the long-term care setting where she works, an occupational therapy practitioner develops a proposal for a falls-prevention program and presents it to management
- After encountering a client who may benefit from occupational therapy services, a practitioner advocates to the client's doctor for a referral
- An occupational therapy researcher designing a study on an occupation-based intervention for dementia includes outcome measures related to cost savings to advocate for occupational therapy's value in dementia care to third-party payers and policymakers
- After receiving a denial of insurance coverage for services provided, an occupational therapy practitioner appeals with objective data and outcome measures that demonstrate that his client is benefitting from skilled occupational therapy services
- Two occupational therapy students educate a group of medical students on the role of occupational therapy in chronic disease management to advocate for occupational therapy's inclusion in a free, student-run health clinic

## Health Systems Level

The health systems level is where public policy is introduced, debated, and passed; it can influence the practice of occupational therapy and the individuals/populations that we serve. It is not always a logical process, as it is more often than not influenced by politics. This should not discourage occupational therapy professionals. Instead, this should motivate us to share our message. We, the members of the profession, are the experts in occupational therapy. Policymakers do not know or understand the profession. It is our responsibility to share the occupational therapy message with these influential individuals to ensure that laws are supportive of occupational therapy practice. There are several important points to remember regarding this health systems level of advocacy: policy affects every area of occupational therapy practice, professional associations are essential in our advancement, and occupational therapy is a wise investment in the U.S. health services system. As professionals we must understand how to articulate the distinct value of occupational therapy. "Occupational therapy's distinct value is to improve health and quality of life through facilitating participation and engagement in occupations, the meaningful, necessary, and familiar activities of everyday life. Occupational therapy is client-centered, achieves positive outcomes and is cost effective" (AOTA, 2015). AOTA is supporting occupational therapy professionals with this language to clearly, consistently articulate the value of occupational therapy. It is important to know that it does not stop at articulating the distinct value, rather it is in the demonstration of the distinct value in our daily practice that serves as one of the strongest platforms we have to advocate for the occupational therapy profession. What people know about occupational therapy is often correlated to experiences they have had. We have the power through our daily practice to affect policy by showing the value of occupational therapy to individuals and populations we serve.

Policy affects every area of occupational therapy practice, regardless of age or setting. The IDEA supports our practice in school-based settings. The ADA supports our work in accessibility design, and home and work modifications to support independence in daily life. Inclusion under Medicare laws supports occupational therapy practice in numerous settings with older adults and created a path for inclusion with other third-party reimbursement systems. The PPACA recognized the value of occupational therapy in the essential benefits package with the inclusion of rehabilitation and habilitation, as well as our roles in wellness and prevention and working with persons with mental health and substance use disorders. Recognizing the link between policy and practice is essential for every occupational therapy professional in today's context. Articulating the value of occupational therapy through grassroots advocacy efforts is the responsibility of every practitioner, educator, and researcher.

Professional associations are essential in our advancement as a profession. Having a strong national professional organization is a fundamental key to advocacy success. Without the advocacy efforts of our national association, occupational therapy may not have been included in the policies we have already discussed in this chapter. Without these policies in place, our practice would be limited. A healthy state association is equally important to the profession of occupational therapy as our national association. All politics are local. Federal law often filters down to states for implementation. It is then that our state occupational therapy associations step forward and make the occupational therapy voice heard, protecting our practice and promoting our profession. Therefore, a simple first step to being an occupational therapy advocate is to be a member of both your national and state occupational therapy associations. In doing so, you provide the associations with the necessary resources they need to protect and advance the practice of occupational therapy and the clients that we serve each day.

Occupational therapy is a part of the solution to the challenges of the U.S. health services system and a wise investment for policymakers (Rexe, Lammi, & von Zweck, 2013). In 2010, the President of the United States signed into law the PPACA, which sets forth a plan to restructure the U.S. health services system. A foundational concept of the PPACA is often referred to as the Triple Aim of health care reform (Berwick, Nolan, & Whittington, 2008) to control costs, improve quality, and increase efficiency. With occupational therapy professionals engaging in advocacy efforts, we can strategically position ourselves with the Triple Aim (Leland, Crum, Phipps, Roberts, & Gage, 2014). Occupational therapy provides the necessary services to individuals and populations (Braveman, 2015) to allow them to live, work, and play at their highest level of independence, which is valuable in controlling costs. Occupational therapy improves quality of care by utilizing evidence-based assessments and interventions to increase a person's functional status and enhance quality of life (Persch, Lamb, Metzler, & Fristad, 2015). Occupational therapy can increase the efficiency of the system by using our distinct skill set as we examine clients across the contexts in which they live, work, and play to appropriately evaluate risks, make recommendations, and engage in intervention to decrease potential unnecessary utilization of the system (Lamb & Metzler, 2014; Robinson, Fisher, & Broussard, 2016).

The engagement in grassroots advocacy is a professional obligation for all occupational therapy professionals. Toto (2012) offered practical advice for practitioners emphasizing the importance of recognizing our individual strengths and seeking advocacy opportunities for our talents; whether within an organization, a state, or at the national level, we all have a role to take. When we all participate in the process, share a consistent message, and provide the highest quality of care possible in our daily practice, our effect will be significant.

## Practical Examples of Health Systems Level Advocacy

- Be a member of both your state association and AOTA so that your membership dues support critical advocacy work at both the state and national levels
- Help your state legislative committee to advocate for occupational therapy's inclusion in key legislation and to defend occupational therapy's scope of practice from encroachment from other disciplines
- Participate in political action committees to build relationships with legislators and educate them on the value of occupational therapy
- Provide testimony to legislators on issues relevant to occupational therapy practice
- Write letters or using AOTA's Legislative Action Center to send form letters to state and federal representatives about health issues
- Draft fact sheets for policymakers about the profession's role in health care
- Invite legislators to visit your facility to provide a first-hand experience
- Share occupational therapy research with legislators and regulatory agencies to demonstrate occupational therapy's value in a changing health care environment

## Case Study 2

In April 2014, Congress passed the Protecting Access to Medicare Act (H.R. 4302), which created a demonstration program to improve community mental health services by establishing federally certified community behavioral health clinics (CCBHCs). After the bill was passed, the Department of Health and Human Services and the Substance Abuse and Mental Health Services Administration (SAMHSA) began implementation of the law by writing the rules that defined what mental health services and supports would be provided by the CCBHCs.

AOTA members and staff seized upon this historic opportunity to advocate for the distinct value of occupational therapy in providing quality community-based behavioral health services. The AOTA's federal affairs staff and President Ginny Stoffel met with SAMHSA officials to discuss why occupational therapy should be a part of the new CCBHCs. This meeting underscored the importance of having Congressional support for occupational therapy's inclusion, as well as broad support during the public comment period.

AOTA staff drafted a Congressional letter to SAMHSA supporting occupational therapy's inclusion in the staffing requirements for the new CCBHCs. With the help of 550 AOTA members who met with their legislators on Capitol Hill as part of AOTA's Annual Hill Day and many more members who participated virtually, the letter was submitted to SAMHSA signed by 18 Congressional representatives. Later, when SAMHSA announced plans for a public listening session to solicit feedback on how it would write the rules governing the new CCBHCs, AOTA's federal affairs staff mobilized massive grassroots support. Hundreds of occupational therapy practitioners and students submitted comments to SAMHSA advocating for occupational therapy's inclusion in CCBHC staffing criteria, and many spoke passionately and eloquently about the distinct value of occupational therapy in mental health services during the listening session. Because occupational therapy dominated the listening session, AOTA staff was included in all subsequent stakeholder discussions about the draft CCBHC criteria. They submitted further details to the Department of Health and Human Services related to payment and reimbursement for services.

As a result of the advocacy efforts of AOTA members and staff, SAMHSA included occupational therapy in its suggested staffing criteria for the new CCBHCs, thereby paving the way for a new, stronger role for occupational therapy in community-based behavioral health services.

# Effective Advocacy Tips

It all begins with an idea. Whether it is an idea for a new program to be developed or a policy to be introduced, it all begins at this basic point. After an idea has been generated and the science supporting it has been identified, the idea needs to become a reality. That is where advocacy comes in. Effective advocates are passionate. As occupational therapy professionals, we must be passionate about our message and the work that we do. This passion can serve as a driver for moving occupational therapy forward.

## Know Your Audience

Before you begin to advocate, you first need to know something about the decision makers you will be meeting with and the issues that they care about. Your proposal is more likely to be received favorably if you can demonstrate how it can address your audience's most pressing concerns. Policymakers may be more inclined to support your issues if it aligns with their platform (i.e., mental health reform, veterans' issues). Managers may be more receptive to your program proposal if you can demonstrate how it can improve health outcomes or reduce costs. Before a meeting, ask yourself, "What does this person care about? What kinds of problems is this person/facility/organization facing?" Then craft your message in a focused way that shows how you can contribute to a solution.

## Clearly Communicate Your Message

Prepare before meetings and plan ahead what you would like to say. The AOTA has helpful one-page fact sheets and talking points on many of the key legislative issues for occupational therapy; using and distributing such resources ensures that a consistent message is communicated from the profession. Create a talking-point guide for a laser-like focus on the essential points you want the decision maker to understand. Share only these essential points and avoid getting lost in some of the interesting but nonessential information. Do not get discouraged if you need to deliver the message more than once to decision makers. Often a message will need to be heard multiple times in alternative ways prior to action taking place. Be patient, prepared, and focused. View every meeting as an opportunity to strengthen relationships, deepen understanding, and broaden support.

## Stories Have Effect

Telling stories is a powerful way to deliver a message. The use of stories is very valuable in advocacy efforts. We become engrossed in stories. We can take a complex concept and break it down in a way that decision makers can relate to through stories. A story can paint a vivid picture and message that will be remembered long after we leave the meeting. Identify a powerful story from practice with links to the area that you are focusing your advocacy on and practice sharing that story with a colleague. Finally, when in a meeting with a decision maker, clearly and confidently share this story as a way to personalize the message that you are delivering, showcasing your occupational therapy expertise.

## Network

Networking and advocacy go hand in hand. Advocates are constantly looking to expand their network and meet new people. Develop a network with key decision makers and their staff before you need to approach them for support on an issue. Send them a congratulatory note when they win an election or take a leadership position. Attend meetings and events that they are a part of and stop to talk with them at the end. The goal of networking and building this relationship is not only for you to advance an issue but also so that they know you are a valuable resource for advice on issues in your area of expertise.

## Speak With Confidence

Remember that you are the expert in occupational therapy. You have the message they need to hear—they have a problem and you have a solution. Have confidence in the message you are sharing. Using language that is accessible to people outside of our profession is important in crafting our message to avoid misunderstandings. Using inclusive language is also important so that decision makers recognize that you intend to work with them to achieve a common goal. Finally, do not forget to tell decision makers the outcome you want from the meeting, and ask them how you can assist them with their efforts. Perhaps you want their support on a particular piece of legislation or a program you are proposing; to receive you must first ask. If you do not ask, the answer will always be no. Let the decision maker clearly know what it is that you advocate and propose possible solutions.

## Evidence-Based Research Chart

| Issue | Evidence |
|---|---|
| Foundation of advocacy | AOTA, 2006; Quiroga, 1995; West, 1968 |
| Effective advocacy | AOTA, 2012; Daly, 2011; Field, Gauld, & Laurence, 2012; Toto, 2012 |
| Future directions for advocacy | Berwick, Nolan, & Whittington, 2008; Bisognano & Kenney, 2012; Weissert & Weissert, 2012 |

### Advocacy Do's

- Establish an ongoing relationship and reputation for reliability.
- Express appreciation for the person's previous or ongoing support for your work.
- Treat the person as a friend/intelligent person.
- Be specific and know your facts.
- Provide a brief, clearly written summary of your position.
- Know your audience and frame your issue so that it aligns with the person's existing priorities.
- Request specific action.
- Be sure to express thanks for the opportunity to advocate.

### Advocacy Don'ts

- Don't try to talk with people when they are obviously in a hurry.
- Don't be argumentative or abrasive.
- Don't overload them with written material.
- Don't assume that they are familiar with your issues.
- Don't bluff if you don't know the answer to a question.
- Don't talk about too many issues at once.
- Don't be late.
- Don't threaten a legislator with votes.

## Summary

Advocacy has been foundational to occupational therapy since our inception, positioning us for success in the U.S. health care and educational systems. Advocacy is also about empowerment. Our profession is empowered by the recognition of policymakers who understand the value occupational therapy brings to the greater systems at hand. Our professionals are empowered by the contributions that they have made to improve the system and ensure access for the clients we serve. Our clients are empowered through participation in occupational therapy. Decisions being made today will drive the practice of tomorrow; the time is now for occupational therapy professionals to make their voices heard and be a part of the process.

## Electronic Resources

American Occupational Therapy Association: www.aota.org

Key search terms:
Annual Hill Day
Congressional Affairs
Federal Regulatory Affairs
Health Care Reform
Legislative Action Center
Legislative Updates
State Policy

Health Affairs: www.healthaffairs.org

Showalter Group: www.showaltergroup.com

## References


American Occupational Therapy Association. (2006). *The road to the Centennial Vision*. Retrieved from http://www.aota.org/News/Centennial.aspx

American Occupational Therapy Association. (2012). *AOTA's guide to promotion and advocacy*. Retrieved from http://www.aota.org/pubs/otp/2012-issues/otp-102912.aspx?ft=.pdf

American Occupational Therapy Association. (2015). *Articulating the distinct value of occupational therapy*. Retrieved from http://www.aota.org/Publications-News/AOTANews/2015/distinct-value-of-occupational-therapy.aspx

Americans with Disabilities Act (ADA). (1990). Pub. L. No. 101-336, 104 Stat 328.

Berwick, D. M., Nolan, T. W., & Whittington, J. (2008). The triple aim: Care, health, and cost. *Health Affairs, 27*, 759-769. PubMed http://dx.doi.org/10.1377/hlthaff.27.3.759

Bisognano, M., & Kenney, C. (2012). *Pursuing the triple aim*. San Francisco, CA: Jossey-Bass.

Braveman, B. (2015). Population health and occupational therapy. *American Journal of Occupational Therapy, 70*(1), 1-6.

Daly, J. (2011). *Advocacy: Championing ideas and influencing others*. New Haven, CT: Yale University Press.

Field, P., Gauld, R., & Laurence, M. (2012). Evidence-informed health policy: The crucial role of advocacy. *International Journal of Clinical Practice, 66*(4), 337-341.

Individuals with Disabilities Education Act. Pub. L. 101-476, 20 U.S.C., Chapter 33. (1990).

Lamb, A. J., & Metzler, C. A. (2014). Defining the value of occupational therapy: A health policy lens on research and practice. *American Journal of Occupational Therapy, 28*(1), 9-14.

Leland, N. E., Crum, K., Phipps, S., Roberts, P., & Gage, B. (2014). Advancing the value and quality of occupational therapy in health service delivery. *American Journal of Occupational Therapy, 69*(1), 1-7.

Merriam-Webster. (2016). *Advocacy.* Retrieved from http://www.m-w.com/dictionary/advocacy

Patient Protection and Affordable Care Act, Pub. L. 111–148, § 3502, 124 Stat. 119, 124 (2010).

Persch, A. C., Lamb, A. J., Metzler, C. A., & Fristad, M. A. (2015). Health policy perspectives—Healthy habits for children: Leveraging existing evidence to demonstrate value. *American Journal of Occupational Therapy, 69*, 6904090010. doi:10.5014/ajot.2015.694001

Quiroga, V. (1995). *Occupational therapy: The first 30 years—1900 to 1930.* Bethesda, MD: AOTA Press.

Rexe, K., Lammi, B. M., & von Zweck, C. (2013). Occupational therapy: Cost effective solutions for changing health system needs. *Healthcare Quarterly, 16*(1), 69-75.

Robinson, M., Fisher, T. F., & Broussard, K. (2016). Role of occupational therapy in case management and care coordination for clients with complex conditions. *American Journal of Occupational Therapy, 70*(2), 1-6.

Toto, P. (2012). Be an occupational therapy superhero. *OT Practice, 17*(7), 9-12.

Weissert, W. G., & Weissert, C. S. (2012). *Governing health: The politics of health policy.* Baltimore, MD: John Hopkins University Press.

West, W. L. (1968). The 1967 Eleanor Clarke Slagle lecture: Professional responsibility in times of change. *American Journal of Occupational Therapy, 22*(1), 9-15.

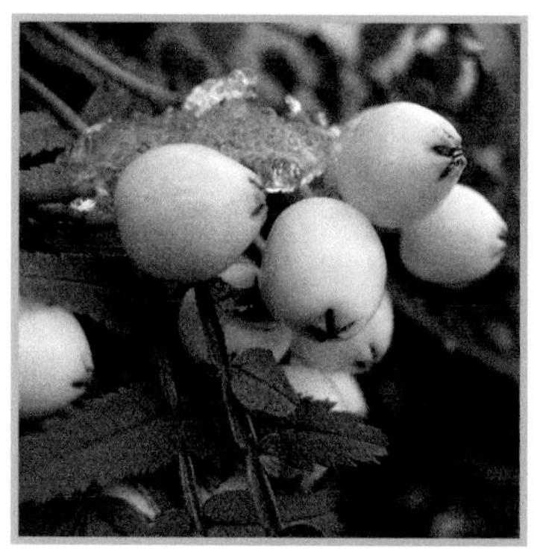

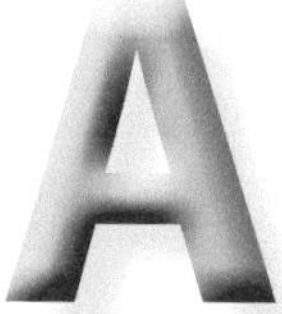

# 2011 Accreditation Council for Occupational Therapy Education Standards and Interpretive Guide

*Reprinted with permission from the American Occupational Therapy Association.*



Jacobs, K., & MacRae, N. (Eds.).
*Occupational Therapy Essentials for Clinical Competence, Third Edition* (pp. 801-844).

## 2011 Accreditation Council for Occupational Therapy Education (ACOTE®) Standards and Interpretive Guide (effective July 31, 2013)

### January 2012 Interpretive Guide Version

| STANDARD NUMBER | ACCREDITATION STANDARDS FOR A DOCTORAL-DEGREE-LEVEL EDUCATIONAL PROGRAM FOR THE OCCUPATIONAL THERAPIST | ACCREDITATION STANDARDS FOR A MASTER'S-DEGREE-LEVEL EDUCATIONAL PROGRAM FOR THE OCCUPATIONAL THERAPIST | ACCREDITATION STANDARDS FOR AN ASSOCIATE-DEGREE-LEVEL EDUCATIONAL PROGRAM FOR THE OCCUPATIONAL THERAPY ASSISTANT |
|---|---|---|---|
| | **PREAMBLE** | | |
| | The rapidly changing and dynamic nature of contemporary health and human services delivery systems provides challenging opportunities for the occupational therapist to use knowledge and skills in a practice area as a direct care provider, consultant, educator, manager, leader, researcher, and advocate for the profession and the consumer.<br><br>A graduate from an ACOTE-accredited doctoral-degree-level occupational therapy program must | The rapidly changing and dynamic nature of contemporary health and human services delivery systems requires the occupational therapist to possess basic skills as a direct care provider, consultant, educator, manager, researcher, and advocate for the profession and the consumer.<br><br>A graduate from an ACOTE-accredited master's-degree-level occupational therapy program must | The rapidly changing and dynamic nature of contemporary health and human services delivery systems requires the occupational therapy assistant to possess basic skills as a direct care provider, educator, and advocate for the profession and the consumer.<br><br>A graduate from an ACOTE-accredited associate-degree-level occupational therapy assistant program must |
| | • Have acquired, as a foundation for professional study, a breadth and depth of knowledge in the liberal arts and sciences and an understanding of issues related to diversity. | • Have acquired, as a foundation for professional study, a breadth and depth of knowledge in the liberal arts and sciences and an understanding of issues related to diversity. | • Have acquired an educational foundation in the liberal arts and sciences, including a focus on issues related to diversity. |
| | • Be educated as a generalist with a broad exposure to the delivery models and systems used in settings where occupational therapy is currently practiced and where it is emerging as a service. | • Be educated as a generalist with a broad exposure to the delivery models and systems used in settings where occupational therapy is currently practiced and where it is emerging as a service. | • Be educated as a generalist with a broad exposure to the delivery models and systems used in settings where occupational therapy is currently practiced and where it is emerging as a service. |
| | • Have achieved entry-level competence through a combination of academic and fieldwork education. | • Have achieved entry-level competence through a combination of academic and fieldwork education. | • Have achieved entry-level competence through a combination of academic and fieldwork education. |
| | • Be prepared to articulate and apply occupational therapy theory and evidence-based evaluations and interventions to achieve expected outcomes as related to occupation. | • Be prepared to articulate and apply occupational therapy theory and evidence-based evaluations and interventions to achieve expected outcomes as related to occupation. | • Be prepared to articulate and apply occupational therapy principles and intervention tools to achieve expected outcomes as related to occupation. |
| | • Be prepared to articulate and apply therapeutic use of occupations with individuals or groups for the purpose of participation in roles and situations in home, school, workplace, community, and other settings. | • Be prepared to articulate and apply therapeutic use of occupations with individuals or groups for the purpose of participation in roles and situations in home, school, workplace, community, and other settings. | • Be prepared to articulate and apply therapeutic use of occupations with individuals or groups for the purpose of participation in roles and situations in home, school, workplace, community, and other settings. |
| | • Be able to plan and apply occupational therapy interventions to address the physical, cognitive, psychosocial, sensory, and other aspects of performance in a variety of contexts and | • Be able to plan and apply occupational therapy interventions to address the physical, cognitive, psychosocial, sensory, and other aspects of performance in a variety of contexts and environments to support engagement in everyday | • Be able to apply occupational therapy interventions to address the physical, cognitive, psychosocial, sensory, and other aspects of performance in a variety of contexts and environments to support engagement in everyday |

| STANDARD NUMBER | ACCREDITATION STANDARDS FOR A DOCTORAL-DEGREE-LEVEL EDUCATIONAL PROGRAM FOR THE OCCUPATIONAL THERAPIST | ACCREDITATION STANDARDS FOR A MASTER'S-DEGREE-LEVEL EDUCATIONAL PROGRAM FOR THE OCCUPATIONAL THERAPIST | ACCREDITATION STANDARDS FOR AN ASSOCIATE-DEGREE-LEVEL EDUCATIONAL PROGRAM FOR THE OCCUPATIONAL THERAPY ASSISTANT |
|---|---|---|---|
| | environments to support engagement in everyday life activities that affect health, well-being, and quality of life.<br>• Be prepared to be a lifelong learner and keep current with evidence-based professional practice.<br>• Uphold the ethical standards, values, and attitudes of the occupational therapy profession.<br>• Understand the distinct roles and responsibilities of the occupational therapist and occupational therapy assistant in the supervisory process.<br>• Be prepared to effectively communicate and work interprofessionally with those who provide care for individuals and/or populations in order to clarify each member's responsibility in executing components of an intervention plan.<br>• Be prepared to advocate as a professional for the occupational therapy services offered and for the recipients of those services.<br>• Be prepared to be an effective consumer of the latest research and knowledge bases that support practice and contribute to the growth and dissemination of research and knowledge.<br>• Demonstrate in-depth knowledge of delivery models, policies, and systems related to the area of practice in settings where occupational therapy is currently practiced and where it is emerging as a service.<br>• Demonstrate thorough knowledge of evidence-based practice.<br>• Demonstrate active involvement in professional development, leadership, and advocacy.<br>• Relate theory to practice and demonstrate synthesis of advanced knowledge in a practice area through completion of a culminating project. | life activities that affect health, well-being, and quality of life.<br>• Be prepared to be a lifelong learner and keep current with evidence-based professional practice.<br>• Uphold the ethical standards, values, and attitudes of the occupational therapy profession.<br>• Understand the distinct roles and responsibilities of the occupational therapist and occupational therapy assistant in the supervisory process.<br>• Be prepared to effectively communicate and work interprofessionally with those who provide care for individuals and/or populations in order to clarify each member's responsibility in executing components of an intervention plan.<br>• Be prepared to advocate as a professional for the occupational therapy services offered and for the recipients of those services.<br>• Be prepared to be an effective consumer of the latest research and knowledge bases that support practice and contribute to the growth and dissemination of research and knowledge. | life activities that affect health, well-being, and quality of life.<br>• Be prepared to be a lifelong learner and keep current with the best practice.<br>• Uphold the ethical standards, values, and attitudes of the occupational therapy profession.<br>• Understand the distinct roles and responsibilities of the occupational therapist and occupational therapy assistant in the supervisory process.<br>• Be prepared to effectively communicate and work interprofessionally with those who provide care for individuals and/or populations in order to clarify each member's responsibility in executing components of an intervention plan.<br>• Be prepared to advocate as a professional for the occupational therapy services offered and for the recipients of those services. |

| STANDARD NUMBER | ACCREDITATION STANDARDS FOR A DOCTORAL-DEGREE-LEVEL EDUCATIONAL PROGRAM FOR THE OCCUPATIONAL THERAPIST | ACCREDITATION STANDARDS FOR A MASTER'S-DEGREE-LEVEL EDUCATIONAL PROGRAM FOR THE OCCUPATIONAL THERAPIST | ACCREDITATION STANDARDS FOR AN ASSOCIATE-DEGREE-LEVEL EDUCATIONAL PROGRAM FOR THE OCCUPATIONAL THERAPY ASSISTANT |
|---|---|---|---|
| | • Develop in-depth experience in one or more of the following areas through completion of a doctoral experiential component: clinical practice skills, research skills, administration, leadership, program and policy development, advocacy, education, and theory development. | | |
| | *FOR ALL STANDARDS LISTED BELOW, IF ONE COMPONENT OF THE STANDARD IS NONCOMPLIANT, THE ENTIRE STANDARD WILL BE CITED. THE PROGRAM MUST DEMONSTRATE COMPLIANCE WITH ALL COMPONENTS OF THE STANDARD IN ORDER FOR THE AREA OF NONCOMPLIANCE TO BE REMOVED.* | | |
| **SECTION A: GENERAL REQUIREMENTS** | | | |
| **A.1.0. SPONSORSHIP AND ACCREDITATION** | | | |
| A.1.1. | The sponsoring institution(s) and affiliates, if any, must be accredited by the recognized regional accrediting authority. For programs in countries other than the United States, ACOTE will determine an alternative and equivalent external review process. | The sponsoring institution(s) and affiliates, if any, must be accredited by the recognized regional accrediting authority. For programs in countries other than the United States, ACOTE will determine an alternative and equivalent external review process. | The sponsoring institution(s) and affiliates, if any, must be accredited by a recognized regional or national accrediting authority. |
| A.1.2. | Sponsoring institution(s) must be authorized under applicable law or other acceptable authority to provide a program of postsecondary education and have appropriate doctoral degree–granting authority. | Sponsoring institution(s) must be authorized under applicable law or other acceptable authority to provide a program of postsecondary education and have appropriate degree-granting authority. | Sponsoring institution(s) must be authorized under applicable law or other acceptable authority to provide a program of postsecondary education and have appropriate degree-granting authority, or the institution must be a program offered within the military services. |
| A.1.3. | Accredited occupational therapy educational programs may be established only in senior colleges, universities, or medical schools. | Accredited occupational therapy educational programs may be established only in senior colleges, universities, or medical schools. | Accredited occupational therapy assistant educational programs may be established only in community, technical, junior, and senior colleges; universities; medical schools; vocational schools or institutions; or military services. |
| A.1.4. | The sponsoring institution(s) must assume primary responsibility for appointment of faculty, admission of students, and curriculum planning at all locations where the program is offered. This would include course content, satisfactory completion of the educational program, and granting of the degree. The sponsoring institution(s) must also be responsible for the coordination of classroom teaching and supervised fieldwork practice and for providing assurance that the practice activities assigned to students in a fieldwork setting are appropriate to the program. | The sponsoring institution(s) must assume primary responsibility for appointment of faculty, admission of students, and curriculum planning at all locations where the program is offered. This would include course content, satisfactory completion of the educational program, and granting of the degree. The sponsoring institution(s) must also be responsible for the coordination of classroom teaching and supervised fieldwork practice and for providing assurance that the practice activities assigned to students in a fieldwork setting are appropriate to the program. | The sponsoring institution(s) must assume primary responsibility for appointment of faculty, admission of students, and curriculum planning at all locations where the program is offered. This would include course content, satisfactory completion of the educational program, and granting of the degree. The sponsoring institution(s) must also be responsible for the coordination of classroom teaching and supervised fieldwork practice and for providing assurance that the practice activities assigned to students in a fieldwork setting are appropriate to the program. |
| | *THE DEGREES MOST COMMONLY CONFERRED ARE THE OCCUPATIONAL THERAPY DOCTORATE (OTD) AND DOCTOR OF OCCUPATIONAL THERAPY (DrOT).* | *THE DEGREES MOST COMMONLY CONFERRED ARE THE MASTER OF OCCUPATIONAL THERAPY (MOT), MASTER OF SCIENCE IN OCCUPATIONAL THERAPY (MSOT), AND MASTER OF SCIENCE (MS). PROGRAMS OFFERING COMBINED BACCALAUREATE/MASTER'S (BS/MS OR BS/MOT) DEGREES ARE STRONGLY* | *THE DEGREES MOST COMMONLY CONFERRED ARE THE ASSOCIATE OF APPLIED SCIENCE (AAS) AND ASSOCIATE OF SCIENCE (AS).* |

| STANDARD NUMBER | ACCREDITATION STANDARDS FOR A DOCTORAL-DEGREE-LEVEL EDUCATIONAL PROGRAM FOR THE OCCUPATIONAL THERAPIST | ACCREDITATION STANDARDS FOR A MASTER'S-DEGREE-LEVEL EDUCATIONAL PROGRAM FOR THE OCCUPATIONAL THERAPIST | ACCREDITATION STANDARDS FOR AN ASSOCIATE-DEGREE-LEVEL EDUCATIONAL PROGRAM FOR THE OCCUPATIONAL THERAPY ASSISTANT |
|---|---|---|---|
| | | *ENCOURAGED TO AVOID USING "BACCALAUREATE IN OCCUPATIONAL THERAPY" AS THE BACCALAUREATE PORTION OF THE DEGREE NAME TO AVOID CONFUSING THE PUBLIC. DEGREE NAMES FOR THE BACCALAUREATE PORTION OF THE PROGRAM MOST COMMONLY USED ARE "BACCALAUREATE IN HEALTH SCIENCES," "BACCALAUREATE IN ALLIED HEALTH," "BACCALAUREATE IN OCCUPATIONAL SCIENCE," AND "BACCALAUREATE IN HEALTH STUDIES."* | |
| A.1.5. | The program must<br>• Inform ACOTE of the transfer of program sponsorship or change of the institution's name within 30 days of the transfer or change.<br>• Inform ACOTE within 30 days of the date of notification of any adverse accreditation action taken to change the sponsoring institution's accreditation status to probation or withdrawal of accreditation.<br>• Notify and receive ACOTE approval for any significant program changes prior to the admission of students into the new/changed program.<br>• Inform ACOTE within 30 days of the resignation of the program director or appointment of a new or interim program director.<br>• Pay accreditation fees within 90 days of the invoice date.<br>• Submit a Report of Self-Study and other required reports (e.g., Interim Report, Plan of Correction, Progress Report) within the period of time designated by ACOTE. All reports must be complete and contain all requested information.<br>• Agree to a site visit date before the end of the period for which accreditation was previously awarded.<br>• Demonstrate honesty and integrity in all interactions with ACOTE. | The program must<br>• Inform ACOTE of the transfer of program sponsorship or change of the institution's name within 30 days of the transfer or change.<br>• Inform ACOTE within 30 days of the date of notification of any adverse accreditation action taken to change the sponsoring institution's accreditation status to probation or withdrawal of accreditation.<br>• Notify and receive ACOTE approval for any significant program changes prior to the admission of students into the new/changed program.<br>• Inform ACOTE within 30 days of the resignation of the program director or appointment of a new or interim program director.<br>• Pay accreditation fees within 90 days of the invoice date.<br>• Submit a Report of Self-Study and other required reports (e.g., Interim Report, Plan of Correction, Progress Report) within the period of time designated by ACOTE. All reports must be complete and contain all requested information.<br>• Agree to a site visit date before the end of the period for which accreditation was previously awarded.<br>• Demonstrate honesty and integrity in all interactions with ACOTE. | The program must<br>• Inform ACOTE of the transfer of program sponsorship or change of the institution's name within 30 days of the transfer or change.<br>• Inform ACOTE within 30 days of the date of notification of any adverse accreditation action taken to change the sponsoring institution's accreditation status to probation or withdrawal of accreditation.<br>• Notify and receive ACOTE approval for any significant program changes prior to the admission of students into the new/changed program.<br>• Inform ACOTE within 30 days of the resignation of the program director or appointment of a new or interim program director.<br>• Pay accreditation fees within 90 days of the invoice date.<br>• Submit a Report of Self-Study and other required reports (e.g., Interim Report, Plan of Correction, Progress Report) within the period of time designated by ACOTE. All reports must be complete and contain all requested information.<br>• Agree to a site visit date before the end of the period for which accreditation was previously awarded.<br>• Demonstrate honesty and integrity in all interactions with ACOTE. |
| | *THE INSTITUTION AND THE ACCREDITED PROGRAM WILL BE ADVISED THAT THE PROGRAM IS ON ADMINISTRATIVE PROBATIONARY ACCREDITATION WHEN THE PROGRAM DOES NOT COMPLY WITH ONE OR MORE OF THE ABOVE ADMINISTRATIVE REQUIREMENTS FOR MAINTAINING ACCREDITATION. THE POLICIES AND PROCEDURES FOR ADMINISTRATIVE PROBATIONARY ACCREDITATION ARE DETAILED IN ACOTE POLICY IV.C., "CLASSIFICATION OF ACCREDITATION CATEGORIES."*<br><br>*THE PROGRAM IS ALSO RESPONSIBLE FOR COMPLYING WITH THE CURRENT REQUIREMENTS OF ALL ACOTE POLICIES, INCLUDING THE REQUIREMENT FOR THE PROGRAM TO SUBMIT A LETTER OF INTENT TO SEEK ACCREDITATION FOR AN ADDITIONAL LOCATION AT LEAST 12 MONTHS PRIOR TO THE PLANNED ADMISSION OF STUDENTS INTO THAT ADDITIONAL LOCATION.* | | |

| STANDARD NUMBER | ACCREDITATION STANDARDS FOR A DOCTORAL-DEGREE-LEVEL EDUCATIONAL PROGRAM FOR THE OCCUPATIONAL THERAPIST | ACCREDITATION STANDARDS FOR A MASTER'S-DEGREE-LEVEL EDUCATIONAL PROGRAM FOR THE OCCUPATIONAL THERAPIST | ACCREDITATION STANDARDS FOR AN ASSOCIATE-DEGREE-LEVEL EDUCATIONAL PROGRAM FOR THE OCCUPATIONAL THERAPY ASSISTANT |
|---|---|---|---|
| **A.2.0. ACADEMIC RESOURCES** | | | |
| A.2.1. | The program must identify an individual as the program director who is assigned to the occupational therapy educational program on a full-time basis. The director may be assigned other institutional duties that do not interfere with the management and administration of the program. The institution must document that the program director has sufficient release time to ensure that the needs of the program are being met. | The program must identify an individual as the program director who is assigned to the occupational therapy educational program on a full-time basis. The director may be assigned other institutional duties that do not interfere with the management and administration of the program. The institution must document that the program director has sufficient release time to ensure that the needs of the program are being met. | The program must identify an individual as the program director who is assigned to the occupational therapy educational program on a full-time basis. The director may be assigned other institutional duties that do not interfere with the management and administration of the program. The institution must document that the program director has sufficient release time to ensure that the needs of the program are being met. |
| . | *THE STANDARD DOES NOT ALLOW THE APPOINTMENT OF CO-DIRECTORS.* | | |
| A.2.2. | The program director must be an initially certified occupational therapist who is licensed or otherwise regulated according to regulations in the state(s) or jurisdiction(s) in which the program is located. The program director must hold a doctoral degree awarded by an institution that is accredited by a regional accrediting body recognized by the U.S. Department of Education (USDE). The doctoral degree is not limited to a doctorate in occupational therapy. | The program director must be an initially certified occupational therapist who is licensed or otherwise regulated according to regulations in the state(s) or jurisdiction(s) in which the program is located. The program director must hold a doctoral degree awarded by an institution that is accredited by a regional accrediting body recognized by the U.S. Department of Education (USDE). The doctoral degree is not limited to a doctorate in occupational therapy. | The program director must be an initially certified occupational therapist or occupational therapy assistant who is licensed or otherwise regulated according to regulations in the state(s) or jurisdiction(s) in which the program is located. The program director must hold a minimum of a master's degree awarded by an institution that is accredited by a regional or national accrediting body recognized by the U.S. Department of Education (USDE). The master's degree is not limited to a master's degree in occupational therapy. |
| | *A DOCTORAL DEGREE THAT WAS AWARDED PRIOR TO JULY 1, 2013, FROM AN INSTITUTION THAT WAS NOT REGIONALLY ACCREDITED IS CONSIDERED ACCEPTABLE TO MEET THIS STANDARD.*<br><br>*FOR DEGREES FROM INSTITUTIONS IN COUNTRIES OTHER THAN THE UNITED STATES, ACOTE WILL DETERMINE AN ALTERNATIVE AND EQUIVALENT EXTERNAL REVIEW PROCESS.* | | *A MASTER'S DEGREE THAT WAS AWARDED PRIOR TO JULY 1, 2013, FROM AN INSTITUTION THAT WAS NOT REGIONALLY OR NATIONALLY ACCREDITED IS CONSIDERED ACCEPTABLE TO MEET THIS STANDARD.*<br><br>*FOR DEGREES FROM INSTITUTIONS IN COUNTRIES OTHER THAN THE UNITED STATES, ACOTE WILL DETERMINE AN ALTERNATIVE AND EQUIVALENT EXTERNAL REVIEW PROCESS.* |
| A.2.3. | The program director must have a minimum of 8 years of documented experience in the field of occupational therapy. This experience must include<br>• Clinical practice as an occupational therapist;<br>• Administrative experience including, but not limited to, program planning and implementation, personnel management, evaluation, and budgeting;<br>• Scholarship (e.g., scholarship of application, scholarship of teaching and learning); and<br>• At least 3 years of experience in a full-time academic appointment with teaching responsibilities at the postbaccalaureate level. | The program director must have a minimum of 8 years of documented experience in the field of occupational therapy. This experience must include<br>• Clinical practice as an occupational therapist;<br>• Administrative experience including, but not limited to, program planning and implementation, personnel management, evaluation, and budgeting;<br>• Scholarship (e.g., scholarship of application, scholarship of teaching and learning); and<br>• At least 3 years of experience in a full-time academic appointment with teaching responsibilities at the postsecondary level. | The program director must have a minimum of 5 years of documented experience in the field of occupational therapy. This experience must include<br>• Clinical practice as an occupational therapist or occupational therapy assistant;<br>• Administrative experience including, but not limited to, program planning and implementation, personnel management, evaluation, and budgeting;<br>• Understanding of and experience with occupational therapy assistants; and<br>• At least 1 year of experience in a full-time academic appointment with teaching responsibilities at the postsecondary level. |

| STANDARD NUMBER | ACCREDITATION STANDARDS FOR A DOCTORAL-DEGREE-LEVEL EDUCATIONAL PROGRAM FOR THE OCCUPATIONAL THERAPIST | ACCREDITATION STANDARDS FOR A MASTER'S-DEGREE-LEVEL EDUCATIONAL PROGRAM FOR THE OCCUPATIONAL THERAPIST | ACCREDITATION STANDARDS FOR AN ASSOCIATE-DEGREE-LEVEL EDUCATIONAL PROGRAM FOR THE OCCUPATIONAL THERAPY ASSISTANT |
|---|---|---|---|
| A.2.4. | The program director must be responsible for the management and administration of the program, including planning, evaluation, budgeting, selection of faculty and staff, maintenance of accreditation, and commitment to strategies for professional development. | The program director must be responsible for the management and administration of the program, including planning, evaluation, budgeting, selection of faculty and staff, maintenance of accreditation, and commitment to strategies for professional development. | The program director must be responsible for the management and administration of the program, including planning, evaluation, budgeting, selection of faculty and staff, maintenance of accreditation, and commitment to strategies for professional development. |
| A.2.5. | *(No related Standard)* | *(No related Standard)* | In addition to the program director, the program must have at least one full-time equivalent (FTE) faculty position at each accredited location where the program is offered. This position may be shared by up to three individuals who teach as adjunct faculty. These individuals must have one or more additional responsibilities related to student advisement, supervision, committee work, program planning, evaluation, recruitment, and marketing activities. |
| A.2.6. | The program director and faculty must possess the academic and experiential qualifications and backgrounds (identified in documented descriptions of roles and responsibilities) that are necessary to meet program objectives and the mission of the institution. | The program director and faculty must possess the academic and experiential qualifications and backgrounds (identified in documented descriptions of roles and responsibilities) that are necessary to meet program objectives and the mission of the institution. | The program director and faculty must possess the academic and experiential qualifications and backgrounds (identified in documented descriptions of roles and responsibilities) that are necessary to meet program objectives and the mission of the institution. |
| A.2.7. | The program must identify an individual for the role of academic fieldwork coordinator who is specifically responsible for the program's compliance with the fieldwork requirements of Standards Section C.1.0 and is assigned to the occupational therapy educational program as a full-time faculty member as defined by ACOTE. The academic fieldwork coordinator may be assigned other institutional duties that do not interfere with the management and administration of the fieldwork program. The institution must document that the academic fieldwork coordinator has sufficient release time to ensure that the needs of the fieldwork program are being met.<br><br>This individual must be a licensed or otherwise regulated occupational therapist. Coordinators must hold a doctoral degree awarded by an institution that is accredited by a USDE-recognized regional accrediting body. | The program must identify an individual for the role of academic fieldwork coordinator who is specifically responsible for the program's compliance with the fieldwork requirements of Standards Section C.1.0 and is assigned to the occupational therapy educational program as a full-time faculty member as defined by ACOTE. The academic fieldwork coordinator may be assigned other institutional duties that do not interfere with the management and administration of the fieldwork program. The institution must document that the academic fieldwork coordinator has sufficient release time to ensure that the needs of the fieldwork program are being met.<br><br>This individual must be a licensed or otherwise regulated occupational therapist. Coordinators must hold a minimum of a master's degree awarded by an institution that is accredited by a USDE-recognized regional accrediting body. | The program must identify an individual for the role of academic fieldwork coordinator who is specifically responsible for the program's compliance with the fieldwork requirements of Standards Section C.1.0 and is assigned to the occupational therapy assistant educational program as a full-time faculty member as defined by ACOTE. The academic fieldwork coordinator may be assigned other institutional duties that do not interfere with the management and administration of the fieldwork program. The institution must document that the academic fieldwork coordinator has sufficient release time to ensure that the needs of the fieldwork program are being met.<br><br>This individual must be a licensed or otherwise regulated occupational therapist or occupational therapy assistant. Coordinators must hold a minimum of a baccalaureate degree awarded by an institution that is accredited by a USDE-recognized regional or national accrediting body. |

| STANDARD NUMBER | ACCREDITATION STANDARDS FOR A DOCTORAL-DEGREE-LEVEL EDUCATIONAL PROGRAM FOR THE OCCUPATIONAL THERAPIST | ACCREDITATION STANDARDS FOR A MASTER'S-DEGREE-LEVEL EDUCATIONAL PROGRAM FOR THE OCCUPATIONAL THERAPIST | ACCREDITATION STANDARDS FOR AN ASSOCIATE-DEGREE-LEVEL EDUCATIONAL PROGRAM FOR THE OCCUPATIONAL THERAPY ASSISTANT |
|---|---|---|---|
| | *A DOCTORAL DEGREE THAT WAS AWARDED PRIOR TO JULY 1, 2013, FROM AN INSTITUTION THAT WAS NOT REGIONALLY ACCREDITED IS CONSIDERED ACCEPTABLE TO MEET THIS STANDARD.*<br><br>*FOR DEGREES FROM INSTITUTIONS IN COUNTRIES OTHER THAN THE UNITED STATES, ACOTE WILL DETERMINE AN ALTERNATIVE AND EQUIVALENT EXTERNAL REVIEW PROCESS.* | *A MASTER'S DEGREE THAT WAS AWARDED PRIOR TO JULY 1, 2013, FROM AN INSTITUTION THAT WAS NOT REGIONALLY ACCREDITED IS CONSIDERED ACCEPTABLE TO MEET THIS STANDARD.*<br><br>*FOR DEGREES FROM INSTITUTIONS IN COUNTRIES OTHER THAN THE UNITED STATES, ACOTE WILL DETERMINE AN ALTERNATIVE AND EQUIVALENT EXTERNAL REVIEW PROCESS.* | *A BACCALAUREATE DEGREE THAT WAS AWARDED PRIOR TO JULY 1, 2013, FROM AN INSTITUTION THAT WAS NOT REGIONALLY OR NATIONALLY ACCREDITED IS CONSIDERED ACCEPTABLE TO MEET THIS STANDARD.*<br><br>*FOR DEGREES FROM INSTITUTIONS IN COUNTRIES OTHER THAN THE UNITED STATES, ACOTE WILL DETERMINE AN ALTERNATIVE AND EQUIVALENT EXTERNAL REVIEW PROCESS.* |
| A.2.8. | Core faculty who are occupational therapists or occupational therapy assistants must be currently licensed or otherwise regulated according to regulations in the state or jurisdiction in which the program is located.<br><br>Faculty in residence and teaching at additional locations must be currently licensed or otherwise regulated according to regulations in the state or jurisdiction in which the additional location is located. | Core faculty who are occupational therapists or occupational therapy assistants must be currently licensed or otherwise regulated according to regulations in the state or jurisdiction in which the program is located.<br><br>Faculty in residence and teaching at additional locations must be currently licensed or otherwise regulated according to regulations in the state or jurisdiction in which the additional location is located. | Core faculty who are occupational therapists or occupational therapy assistants must be currently licensed or otherwise regulated according to regulations in the state or jurisdiction in which the program is located.<br><br>Faculty in residence and teaching at additional locations must be currently licensed or otherwise regulated according to regulations in the state or jurisdiction in which the additional location is located. |
| A.2.9. | *(No related Standard)* | *(No related Standard)* | In programs where the program director is an occupational therapy assistant, an occupational therapist must be included on faculty and contribute to the functioning of the program through a variety of mechanisms including, but not limited to, teaching, advising, and committee work. In a program where there are only occupational therapists on faculty who have never practiced as an occupational therapy assistant, the program must demonstrate that an individual who is an occupational therapy assistant or an occupational therapist who has previously practiced as an occupational therapy assistant is involved in the program as an adjunct faculty or teaching assistant. |
| A.2.10. | All full-time faculty teaching in the program must hold a doctoral degree awarded by an institution that is accredited by a USDE-recognized regional accrediting body. The doctoral degree is not limited to a doctorate in occupational therapy. | The majority of full-time faculty who are occupational therapists or occupational therapy assistants must hold a doctoral degree. All full-time faculty must hold a minimum of a master's degree. All degrees must be awarded by an institution that is accredited by a USDE-recognized regional accrediting body. The degrees are not limited to occupational therapy.<br><br>For an even number of full-time faculty, at least half must hold doctorates. The program director is counted as a faculty member. | All occupational therapy assistant faculty who are full-time must hold a minimum of a baccalaureate degree awarded by an institution that is accredited by a USDE-recognized regional or national accrediting body. |

| STANDARD NUMBER | ACCREDITATION STANDARDS FOR A DOCTORAL-DEGREE-LEVEL EDUCATIONAL PROGRAM FOR THE OCCUPATIONAL THERAPIST | ACCREDITATION STANDARDS FOR A MASTER'S-DEGREE-LEVEL EDUCATIONAL PROGRAM FOR THE OCCUPATIONAL THERAPIST | ACCREDITATION STANDARDS FOR AN ASSOCIATE-DEGREE-LEVEL EDUCATIONAL PROGRAM FOR THE OCCUPATIONAL THERAPY ASSISTANT |
|---|---|---|---|
| | *A DOCTORAL DEGREE THAT WAS AWARDED PRIOR TO JULY 1, 2013, FROM AN INSTITUTION THAT WAS NOT REGIONALLY ACCREDITED IS CONSIDERED ACCEPTABLE TO MEET THIS STANDARD.*<br>*FOR DEGREES FROM INSTITUTIONS IN COUNTRIES OTHER THAN THE UNITED STATES, ACOTE WILL DETERMINE AN ALTERNATIVE AND EQUIVALENT EXTERNAL REVIEW PROCESS.* | *A DOCTORAL OR MASTER'S DEGREE THAT WAS AWARDED PRIOR TO JULY 1, 2013, FROM AN INSTITUTION THAT WAS NOT REGIONALLY ACCREDITED IS CONSIDERED ACCEPTABLE TO MEET THIS STANDARD.*<br>*FOR DEGREES FROM INSTITUTIONS IN COUNTRIES OTHER THAN THE UNITED STATES, ACOTE WILL DETERMINE AN ALTERNATIVE AND EQUIVALENT EXTERNAL REVIEW PROCESS.* | *A BACCALAUREATE DEGREE THAT WAS AWARDED PRIOR TO JULY 1, 2013, FROM AN INSTITUTION THAT WAS NOT REGIONALLY OR NATIONALLY ACCREDITED IS CONSIDERED ACCEPTABLE TO MEET THIS STANDARD.*<br>*FOR DEGREES FROM INSTITUTIONS IN COUNTRIES OTHER THAN THE UNITED STATES, ACOTE WILL DETERMINE AN ALTERNATIVE AND EQUIVALENT EXTERNAL REVIEW PROCESS.* |
| A.2.11. | The faculty must have documented expertise in their area(s) of teaching responsibility and knowledge of the content delivery method (e.g., distance learning). | The faculty must have documented expertise in their area(s) of teaching responsibility and knowledge of the content delivery method (e.g., distance learning). | The faculty must have documented expertise in their area(s) of teaching responsibility and knowledge of the content delivery method (e.g., distance learning). |
| | *EVIDENCE OF EXPERTISE IN TEACHING ASSIGNMENTS MIGHT INCLUDE DOCUMENTATION OF RECENT CONTINUING EDUCATION, RELEVANT EXPERIENCE, FACULTY DEVELOPMENT PLAN REFLECTING ACQUISITION OF NEW CONTENT, INCORPORATION OF FEEDBACK FROM COURSE EVALUATIONS, AND OTHER SOURCES.* | | |
| A.2.12. | For programs with additional accredited location(s), the program must identify a faculty member who is an occupational therapist as site coordinator at each location who is responsible for ensuring uniform implementation of the program and ongoing communication with the program director. | For programs with additional accredited location(s), the program must identify a faculty member who is an occupational therapist as site coordinator at each location who is responsible for ensuring uniform implementation of the program and ongoing communication with the program director. | For programs with additional accredited location(s), the program must identify a faculty member who is an occupational therapist or occupational therapy assistant as site coordinator at each location who is responsible for ensuring uniform implementation of the program and ongoing communication with the program director. |
| A.2.13. | The occupational therapy faculty at each accredited location where the program is offered must be sufficient in number and must possess the expertise necessary to ensure appropriate curriculum design, content delivery, and program evaluation. The faculty must include individuals competent to ensure delivery of the broad scope of occupational therapy practice. Multiple adjuncts, part-time faculty, or full-time faculty may be configured to meet this goal. Each accredited additional location must have at least one full-time equivalent (FTE) faculty member. | The occupational therapy faculty at each accredited location where the program is offered must be sufficient in number and must possess the expertise necessary to ensure appropriate curriculum design, content delivery, and program evaluation. The faculty must include individuals competent to ensure delivery of the broad scope of occupational therapy practice. Multiple adjuncts, part-time faculty, or full-time faculty may be configured to meet this goal. Each accredited additional location must have at least one full-time equivalent (FTE) faculty member. | The occupational therapy assistant faculty at each accredited location where the program is offered must be sufficient in number and must possess the expertise necessary to ensure appropriate curriculum design, content delivery, and program evaluation. The faculty must include individuals competent to ensure delivery of the broad scope of occupational therapy practice. Multiple adjuncts, part-time faculty, or full-time faculty may be configured to meet this goal. Each accredited additional location must have at least one full-time equivalent (FTE) faculty member. |
| A.2.14. | Faculty responsibilities must be consistent with and supportive of the mission of the institution. | Faculty responsibilities must be consistent with and supportive of the mission of the institution. | Faculty responsibilities must be consistent with and supportive of the mission of the institution. |
| A.2.15. | The faculty–student ratio must permit the achievement of the purpose and stated objectives for laboratory and lecture courses, be compatible with accepted practices of the institution for similar programs, and ensure student and consumer safety. | The faculty–student ratio must permit the achievement of the purpose and stated objectives for laboratory and lecture courses, be compatible with accepted practices of the institution for similar programs, and ensure student and consumer safety. | The faculty–student ratio must permit the achievement of the purpose and stated objectives for laboratory and lecture courses, be compatible with accepted practices of the institution for similar programs, and ensure student and consumer safety. |
| A.2.16. | Clerical and support staff must be provided to the program, consistent with institutional practice, to meet | Clerical and support staff must be provided to the program, consistent with institutional practice, to meet | Clerical and support staff must be provided to the program, consistent with institutional practice, to meet |

| STANDARD NUMBER | ACCREDITATION STANDARDS FOR A DOCTORAL-DEGREE-LEVEL EDUCATIONAL PROGRAM FOR THE OCCUPATIONAL THERAPIST | ACCREDITATION STANDARDS FOR A MASTER'S-DEGREE-LEVEL EDUCATIONAL PROGRAM FOR THE OCCUPATIONAL THERAPIST | ACCREDITATION STANDARDS FOR AN ASSOCIATE-DEGREE-LEVEL EDUCATIONAL PROGRAM FOR THE OCCUPATIONAL THERAPY ASSISTANT |
|---|---|---|---|
| | programmatic and administrative requirements, including support for any portion of the program offered by distance education. | programmatic and administrative requirements, including support for any portion of the program offered by distance education. | programmatic and administrative requirements, including support for any portion of the program offered by distance education. |
| A.2.17. | The program must be allocated a budget of regular institutional funds, not including grants, gifts, and other restricted sources, sufficient to implement and maintain the objectives of the program and to fulfill the program's obligation to matriculated and entering students. | The program must be allocated a budget of regular institutional funds, not including grants, gifts, and other restricted sources, sufficient to implement and maintain the objectives of the program and to fulfill the program's obligation to matriculated and entering students. | The program must be allocated a budget of regular institutional funds, not including grants, gifts, and other restricted sources, sufficient to implement and maintain the objectives of the program and to fulfill the program's obligation to matriculated and entering students. |
| A.2.18. | Classrooms and laboratories must be provided that are consistent with the program's educational objectives, teaching methods, number of students, and safety and health standards of the institution, and they must allow for efficient operation of the program. | Classrooms and laboratories must be provided that are consistent with the program's educational objectives, teaching methods, number of students, and safety and health standards of the institution, and they must allow for efficient operation of the program. | Classrooms and laboratories must be provided that are consistent with the program's educational objectives, teaching methods, number of students, and safety and health standards of the institution, and they must allow for efficient operation of the program. |
| A.2.19. | If the program offers distance education, it must include<br>• A process through which the program establishes that the student who registers in a distance education course or program is the same student who participates in and completes the program and receives academic credit,<br>• Technology and resources that are adequate to support a distance-learning environment, and<br>• A process to ensure that faculty are adequately trained and skilled to use distance education methodologies. | If the program offers distance education, it must include<br>• A process through which the program establishes that the student who registers in a distance education course or program is the same student who participates in and completes the program and receives academic credit,<br>• Technology and resources that are adequate to support a distance-learning environment, and<br>• A process to ensure that faculty are adequately trained and skilled to use distance education methodologies. | If the program offers distance education, it must include<br>• A process through which the program establishes that the student who registers in a distance education course or program is the same student who participates in and completes the program and receives academic credit,<br>• Technology and resources that are adequate to support a distance-learning environment, and<br>• A process to ensure that faculty are adequately trained and skilled to use distance education methodologies. |
| A.2.20. | Laboratory space provided by the institution must be assigned to the occupational therapy program on a priority basis. If laboratory space for occupational therapy lab classes is provided by another institution or agency, there must be a written and signed agreement to ensure assignment of space for program use. | Laboratory space provided by the institution must be assigned to the occupational therapy program on a priority basis. If laboratory space for occupational therapy lab classes is provided by another institution or agency, there must be a written and signed agreement to ensure assignment of space for program use. | Laboratory space provided by the institution must be assigned to the occupational therapy assistant program on a priority basis. If laboratory space for occupational therapy assistant lab classes is provided by another institution or agency, there must be a written and signed agreement to ensure assignment of space for program use. |
| A.2.21. | Adequate space must be provided to store and secure equipment and supplies. | Adequate space must be provided to store and secure equipment and supplies. | Adequate space must be provided to store and secure equipment and supplies. |
| A.2.22. | The program director and faculty must have office space consistent with institutional practice. | The program director and faculty must have office space consistent with institutional practice. | The program director and faculty must have office space consistent with institutional practice. |
| A.2.23. | Adequate space must be provided for the private advising of students. | Adequate space must be provided for the private advising of students. | Adequate space must be provided for the private advising of students. |
| A.2.24. | Appropriate and sufficient equipment and supplies must be provided by the institution for student use and for the didactic, supervised fieldwork, and | Appropriate and sufficient equipment and supplies must be provided by the institution for student use and for the didactic and supervised fieldwork | Appropriate and sufficient equipment and supplies must be provided by the institution for student use and for the didactic and supervised fieldwork |

| STANDARD NUMBER | ACCREDITATION STANDARDS FOR A DOCTORAL-DEGREE-LEVEL EDUCATIONAL PROGRAM FOR THE OCCUPATIONAL THERAPIST | ACCREDITATION STANDARDS FOR A MASTER'S-DEGREE-LEVEL EDUCATIONAL PROGRAM FOR THE OCCUPATIONAL THERAPIST | ACCREDITATION STANDARDS FOR AN ASSOCIATE-DEGREE-LEVEL EDUCATIONAL PROGRAM FOR THE OCCUPATIONAL THERAPY ASSISTANT |
|---|---|---|---|
| | experiential components of the curriculum. | components of the curriculum. | components of the curriculum. |
| A.2.25. | Students must be given access to and have the opportunity to use the evaluative and treatment methodologies that reflect both current practice and practice in the geographic area served by the program. | Students must be given access to and have the opportunity to use the evaluative and treatment methodologies that reflect both current practice and practice in the geographic area served by the program. | Students must be given access to and have the opportunity to use the evaluative and treatment methodologies that reflect both current practice and practice in the geographic area served by the program. |
| A.2.26. | Students must have ready access to a supply of current and relevant books, journals, periodicals, computers, software, and other reference materials needed for the practice areas and to meet the requirements of the curriculum. This may include, but is not limited to, libraries, online services, interlibrary loan, and resource centers. | Students must have ready access to a supply of current and relevant books, journals, periodicals, computers, software, and other reference materials needed to meet the requirements of the curriculum. This may include, but is not limited to, libraries, online services, interlibrary loan, and resource centers. | Students must have ready access to a supply of current and relevant books, journals, periodicals, computers, software, and other reference materials needed to meet the requirements of the curriculum. This may include, but is not limited to, libraries, online services, interlibrary loan, and resource centers. |
| A.2.27. | Instructional aids and technology must be available in sufficient quantity and quality to be consistent with the program objectives and teaching methods. | Instructional aids and technology must be available in sufficient quantity and quality to be consistent with the program objectives and teaching methods. | Instructional aids and technology must be available in sufficient quantity and quality to be consistent with the program objectives and teaching methods. |
| **A.3.0.** | **STUDENTS** | | |
| A.3.1. | Admission of students to the occupational therapy program must be made in accordance with the practices of the institution. There must be stated admission criteria that are clearly defined and published and reflective of the demands of the program. | Admission of students to the occupational therapy program must be made in accordance with the practices of the institution. There must be stated admission criteria that are clearly defined and published and reflective of the demands of the program. | Admission of students to the occupational therapy assistant program must be made in accordance with the practices of the institution. There must be stated admission criteria that are clearly defined and published and reflective of the demands of the program. |
| A.3.2. | Institutions must require that program applicants hold a baccalaureate degree or higher prior to admission to the program. | *(No related Standard)* | *(No related Standard)* |
| A.3.3. | Policies pertaining to standards for admission, advanced placement, transfer of credit, credit for experiential learning (if applicable), and prerequisite educational or work experience requirements must be readily accessible to prospective students and the public. | Policies pertaining to standards for admission, advanced placement, transfer of credit, credit for experiential learning (if applicable), and prerequisite educational or work experience requirements must be readily accessible to prospective students and the public. | Policies pertaining to standards for admission, advanced placement, transfer of credit, credit for experiential learning (if applicable), and prerequisite educational or work experience requirements must be readily accessible to prospective students and the public. |
| A.3.4. | Programs must document implementation of a mechanism to ensure that students receiving credit for previous courses and/or work experience have met the content requirements of the appropriate doctoral Standards. | Programs must document implementation of a mechanism to ensure that students receiving credit for previous courses and/or work experience have met the content requirements of the appropriate master's Standards. | Programs must document implementation of a mechanism to ensure that students receiving credit for previous courses and/or work experience have met the content requirements of the appropriate occupational therapy assistant Standards. |
| A.3.5. | Criteria for successful completion of each segment of the educational program and for graduation must be given in advance to each student. | Criteria for successful completion of each segment of the educational program and for graduation must be given in advance to each student. | Criteria for successful completion of each segment of the educational program and for graduation must be given in advance to each student. |

| STANDARD NUMBER | ACCREDITATION STANDARDS FOR A DOCTORAL-DEGREE-LEVEL EDUCATIONAL PROGRAM FOR THE OCCUPATIONAL THERAPIST | ACCREDITATION STANDARDS FOR A MASTER'S-DEGREE-LEVEL EDUCATIONAL PROGRAM FOR THE OCCUPATIONAL THERAPIST | ACCREDITATION STANDARDS FOR AN ASSOCIATE-DEGREE-LEVEL EDUCATIONAL PROGRAM FOR THE OCCUPATIONAL THERAPY ASSISTANT |
|---|---|---|---|
| A.3.6. | Evaluation content and methods must be consistent with the curriculum design; objectives; and competencies of the didactic, fieldwork, and experiential components of the program. | Evaluation content and methods must be consistent with the curriculum design, objectives, and competencies of the didactic and fieldwork components of the program. | Evaluation content and methods must be consistent with the curriculum design, objectives, and competencies of the didactic and fieldwork components of the program. |
| A.3.7. | Evaluation must be conducted on a regular basis to provide students and program officials with timely indications of the students' progress and academic standing. | Evaluation must be conducted on a regular basis to provide students and program officials with timely indications of the students' progress and academic standing. | Evaluation must be conducted on a regular basis to provide students and program officials with timely indications of the students' progress and academic standing. |
| A.3.8. | Students must be informed of and have access to the student support services that are provided to other students in the institution. | Students must be informed of and have access to the student support services that are provided to other students in the institution. | Students must be informed of and have access to the student support services that are provided to other students in the institution. |
| A.3.9. | Advising related to professional coursework, fieldwork education, and the experiential component of the program must be the responsibility of the occupational therapy faculty. | Advising related to professional coursework and fieldwork education must be the responsibility of the occupational therapy faculty. | Advising related to coursework in the occupational therapy assistant program and fieldwork education must be the responsibility of the occupational therapy assistant faculty. |
| **A.4.0.** | **OPERATIONAL POLICIES** | | |
| A.4.1. | All program publications and advertising—including, but not limited to, academic calendars, announcements, catalogs, handbooks, and Web sites—must accurately reflect the program offered. | All program publications and advertising—including, but not limited to, academic calendars, announcements, catalogs, handbooks, and Web sites—must accurately reflect the program offered. | All program publications and advertising—including, but not limited to, academic calendars, announcements, catalogs, handbooks, and Web sites—must accurately reflect the program offered. |
| A.4.2. | Accurate and current information regarding student and program outcomes must be readily available to the public on the program's Web page. At a minimum, the following data must be reported for the previous 3 years:<br>• Total number of program graduates<br>• Graduation rates.<br>The program must provide the direct link to the National Board for Certification in Occupational Therapy (NBCOT) program data results on the program's home page. | Accurate and current information regarding student and program outcomes must be readily available to the public on the program's Web page. At a minimum, the following data must be reported for the previous 3 years:<br>• Total number of program graduates<br>• Graduation rates.<br>The program must provide the direct link to the National Board for Certification in Occupational Therapy (NBCOT) program data results on the program's home page. | Accurate and current information regarding student and program outcomes must be readily available to the public on the program's Web page. At a minimum, the following data must be reported for the previous 3 years:<br>• Total number of program graduates,<br>• Graduation rates.<br>The program must provide the direct link to the National Board for Certification in Occupational Therapy (NBCOT) program data results on the program's home page. |
| A.4.3. | The program's accreditation status and the name, address, and telephone number of ACOTE must be published in all of the following materials used by the institution: catalog, Web site, and program-related brochures or flyers available to prospective students. A link to www.acoteonline.org must be provided on the program's home page. | The program's accreditation status and the name, address, and telephone number of ACOTE must be published in all of the following materials used by the institution: catalog, Web site, and program-related brochures or flyers available to prospective students. A link to www.acoteonline.org must be provided on the program's home page. | The program's accreditation status and the name, address, and telephone number of ACOTE must be published in all of the following materials used by the institution: catalog, Web site, and program-related brochures or flyers available to prospective students. A link to www.acoteonline.org must be provided on the program's home page. |
| | *SAMPLE WORDING: "THE OCCUPATIONAL THERAPY/OCCUPATIONAL THERAPY ASSISTANT PROGRAM IS ACCREDITED BY THE ACCREDITATION COUNCIL FOR OCCUPATIONAL THERAPY EDUCATION (ACOTE) OF THE AMERICAN OCCUPATIONAL THERAPY ASSOCIATION (AOTA), LOCATED AT 4720 MONTGOMERY LANE, PO BOX 31220, BETHESDA, MD 20824-1220. ACOTE'S TELEPHONE NUMBER, C/O AOTA, IS (301) 652-AOTA."* | | |

| STANDARD NUMBER | ACCREDITATION STANDARDS FOR A DOCTORAL-DEGREE-LEVEL EDUCATIONAL PROGRAM FOR THE OCCUPATIONAL THERAPIST | ACCREDITATION STANDARDS FOR A MASTER'S-DEGREE-LEVEL EDUCATIONAL PROGRAM FOR THE OCCUPATIONAL THERAPIST | ACCREDITATION STANDARDS FOR AN ASSOCIATE-DEGREE-LEVEL EDUCATIONAL PROGRAM FOR THE OCCUPATIONAL THERAPY ASSISTANT |
|---|---|---|---|
| A.4.4. | All practices within the institution related to faculty, staff, applicants, and students must be nondiscriminatory. | All practices within the institution related to faculty, staff, applicants, and students must be nondiscriminatory. | All practices within the institution related to faculty, staff, applicants, and students must be nondiscriminatory. |
| A.4.5. | Graduation requirements, tuition, and fees must be accurately stated, published, and made known to all applicants. When published fees are subject to change, a statement to that effect must be included. | Graduation requirements, tuition, and fees must be accurately stated, published, and made known to all applicants. When published fees are subject to change, a statement to that effect must be included. | Graduation requirements, tuition, and fees must be accurately stated, published, and made known to all applicants. When published fees are subject to change, a statement to that effect must be included. |
| A.4.6. | The program or sponsoring institution must have a defined and published policy and procedure for processing student and faculty grievances. | The program or sponsoring institution must have a defined and published policy and procedure for processing student and faculty grievances. | The program or sponsoring institution must have a defined and published policy and procedure for processing student and faculty grievances. |
| A.4.7. | Policies and procedures for handling complaints against the program must be published and made known. The program must maintain a record of student complaints that includes the nature and disposition of each complaint. | Policies and procedures for handling complaints against the program must be published and made known. The program must maintain a record of student complaints that includes the nature and disposition of each complaint. | Policies and procedures for handling complaints against the program must be published and made known. The program must maintain a record of student complaints that includes the nature and disposition of each complaint. |
| A.4.8. | Policies and processes for student withdrawal and for refunds of tuition and fees must be published and made known to all applicants. | Policies and processes for student withdrawal and for refunds of tuition and fees must be published and made known to all applicants. | Policies and processes for student withdrawal and for refunds of tuition and fees must be published and made known to all applicants. |
| A.4.9. | Policies and procedures for student probation, suspension, and dismissal must be published and made known. | Policies and procedures for student probation, suspension, and dismissal must be published and made known. | Policies and procedures for student probation, suspension, and dismissal must be published and made known. |
| A.4.10. | Policies and procedures for human-subject research protocol must be published and made known. | Policies and procedures for human-subject research protocol must be published and made known. | Policies and procedures for human-subject research protocol must be published and made known (if applicable to the program). |
| A.4.11. | Programs must make available to students written policies and procedures regarding appropriate use of equipment and supplies and for all educational activities that have implications for the health and safety of clients, students, and faculty (including infection control and evacuation procedures). | Programs must make available to students written policies and procedures regarding appropriate use of equipment and supplies and for all educational activities that have implications for the health and safety of clients, students, and faculty (including infection control and evacuation procedures). | Programs must make available to students written policies and procedures regarding appropriate use of equipment and supplies and for all educational activities that have implications for the health and safety of clients, students, and faculty (including infection control and evacuation procedures). |
| A.4.12. | A program admitting students on the basis of ability to benefit (defined by the USDE as admitting students who do not have either a high school diploma or its equivalent) must publicize its objectives, assessment measures, and means of evaluating the student's ability to benefit. | A program admitting students on the basis of ability to benefit (defined by the USDE as admitting students who do not have either a high school diploma or its equivalent) must publicize its objectives, assessment measures, and means of evaluating the student's ability to benefit. | A program admitting students on the basis of ability to benefit (defined by the USDE as admitting students who do not have either a high school diploma or its equivalent) must publicize its objectives, assessment measures, and means of evaluating the student's ability to benefit. |
| A.4.13. | Documentation of all progression, retention, graduation, certification, and credentialing requirements must be published and made known to applicants. A statement on the program's Web site about the potential impact of a felony conviction on a | Documentation of all progression, retention, graduation, certification, and credentialing requirements must be published and made known to applicants. A statement on the program's Web site about the potential impact of a felony conviction on a | Documentation of all progression, retention, graduation, certification, and credentialing requirements must be published and made known to applicants. A statement on the program's Web site about the potential impact of a felony conviction on a |

| STANDARD NUMBER | ACCREDITATION STANDARDS FOR A DOCTORAL-DEGREE-LEVEL EDUCATIONAL PROGRAM FOR THE OCCUPATIONAL THERAPIST | ACCREDITATION STANDARDS FOR A MASTER'S-DEGREE-LEVEL EDUCATIONAL PROGRAM FOR THE OCCUPATIONAL THERAPIST | ACCREDITATION STANDARDS FOR AN ASSOCIATE-DEGREE-LEVEL EDUCATIONAL PROGRAM FOR THE OCCUPATIONAL THERAPY ASSISTANT |
|---|---|---|---|
| | graduate's eligibility for certification and credentialing must be provided. | graduate's eligibility for certification and credentialing must be provided. | graduate's eligibility for certification and credentialing must be provided. |
| | *SAMPLE WORDING: "GRADUATES OF THE PROGRAM WILL BE ELIGIBLE TO SIT FOR THE NATIONAL CERTIFICATION EXAMINATION FOR THE OCCUPATIONAL THERAPIST, ADMINISTERED BY THE NATIONAL BOARD FOR CERTIFICATION IN OCCUPATIONAL THERAPY (NBCOT). AFTER SUCCESSFUL COMPLETION OF THIS EXAM, THE GRADUATE WILL BE AN OCCUPATIONAL THERAPIST, REGISTERED (OTR). IN ADDITION, MOST STATES REQUIRE LICENSURE TO PRACTICE; HOWEVER, STATE LICENSES ARE USUALLY BASED ON THE RESULTS OF THE NBCOT CERTIFICATION EXAMINATION. A FELONY CONVICTION MAY AFFECT A GRADUATE'S ABILITY TO SIT FOR THE NBCOT CERTIFICATION EXAMINATION OR ATTAIN STATE LICENSURE."* | | *SAMPLE WORDING: "GRADUATES OF THE PROGRAM WILL BE ELIGIBLE TO SIT FOR THE NATIONAL CERTIFICATION EXAMINATION FOR THE OCCUPATIONAL THERAPY ASSISTANT, ADMINISTERED BY THE NATIONAL BOARD FOR CERTIFICATION IN OCCUPATIONAL THERAPY (NBCOT). AFTER SUCCESSFUL COMPLETION OF THIS EXAM, THE GRADUATE WILL BE A CERTIFIED OCCUPATIONAL THERAPY ASSISTANT (COTA). IN ADDITION, MOST STATES REQUIRE LICENSURE TO PRACTICE; HOWEVER, STATE LICENSES ARE USUALLY BASED ON THE RESULTS OF THE NBCOT CERTIFICATION EXAMINATION. A FELONY CONVICTION MAY AFFECT A GRADUATE'S ABILITY TO SIT FOR THE NBCOT CERTIFICATION EXAMINATION OR ATTAIN STATE LICENSURE."* |
| A.4.14. | The program must have a documented and published policy to ensure that students complete all graduation, fieldwork, and experiential component requirements in a timely manner. This policy must include a statement that all Level II fieldwork and the experiential component of the program must be completed within a time frame established by the program. | The program must have a documented and published policy to ensure that students complete all graduation and fieldwork requirements in a timely manner. This policy must include a statement that all Level II fieldwork must be completed within a time frame established by the program. | The program must have a documented and published policy to ensure that students complete all graduation and fieldwork requirements in a timely manner. This policy must include a statement that all Level II fieldwork must be completed within a time frame established by the program. |
| | *SAMPLE WORDING: "STUDENTS MUST COMPLETE ALL LEVEL II FIELDWORK AND THE EXPERIENTIAL COMPONENT OF THE PROGRAM WITHIN [XX] MONTHS FOLLOWING COMPLETION OF THE DIDACTIC PORTION OF THE PROGRAM."* | *SAMPLE WORDING: "STUDENTS MUST COMPLETE ALL LEVEL II FIELDWORK WITHIN [XX] MONTHS FOLLOWING COMPLETION OF THE DIDACTIC PORTION OF THE PROGRAM."* | |
| A.4.15. | Records regarding student admission, enrollment, fieldwork, and achievement must be maintained and kept in a secure setting. Grades and credits for courses must be recorded on students' transcripts and permanently maintained by the sponsoring institution. | Records regarding student admission, enrollment, fieldwork, and achievement must be maintained and kept in a secure setting. Grades and credits for courses must be recorded on students' transcripts and permanently maintained by the sponsoring institution. | Records regarding student admission, enrollment, fieldwork, and achievement must be maintained and kept in a secure setting. Grades and credits for courses must be recorded on students' transcripts and permanently maintained by the sponsoring institution. |
| **A.5.0. STRATEGIC PLAN AND PROGRAM ASSESSMENT**<br>**For programs that are offered at more than one location, the program's strategic plan, evaluation plan, and results of ongoing evaluation must address each program location as a component of the overall plan.** | | | |
| A.5.1. | The program must document a current strategic plan that articulates the program's future vision and guides the program development (e.g., faculty recruitment and professional growth, scholarship, changes in the curriculum design, priorities in academic resources, | The program must document a current strategic plan that articulates the program's future vision and guides the program development (e.g., faculty recruitment and professional growth, scholarship, changes in the curriculum design, priorities in academic resources, | The program must document a current strategic plan that articulates the program's future vision and guides the program development (e.g., faculty recruitment and professional growth, scholarship, changes in the curriculum design, priorities in academic resources, |

| STANDARD NUMBER | ACCREDITATION STANDARDS FOR A DOCTORAL-DEGREE-LEVEL EDUCATIONAL PROGRAM FOR THE OCCUPATIONAL THERAPIST | ACCREDITATION STANDARDS FOR A MASTER'S-DEGREE-LEVEL EDUCATIONAL PROGRAM FOR THE OCCUPATIONAL THERAPIST | ACCREDITATION STANDARDS FOR AN ASSOCIATE-DEGREE-LEVEL EDUCATIONAL PROGRAM FOR THE OCCUPATIONAL THERAPY ASSISTANT |
|---|---|---|---|
| | procurement of fieldwork and experiential component sites). A program strategic plan must be for a minimum of a 3-year period and include, but need not be limited to,<br>• Evidence that the plan is based on program evaluation and an analysis of external and internal environments.<br>• Long-term goals that address the vision and mission of both the institution and the program, as well as specific needs of the program.<br>• Specific measurable action steps with expected timelines by which the program will reach its long-term goals.<br>• Person(s) responsible for action steps.<br>• Evidence of periodic updating of action steps and long-term goals as they are met or as circumstances change. | procurement of fieldwork sites). A program strategic plan must be for a minimum of a 3-year period and include, but need not be limited to,<br>• Evidence that the plan is based on program evaluation and an analysis of external and internal environments.<br>• Long-term goals that address the vision and mission of both the institution and the program, as well as specific needs of the program.<br>• Specific measurable action steps with expected timelines by which the program will reach its long-term goals.<br>• Person(s) responsible for action steps.<br>• Evidence of periodic updating of action steps and long-term goals as they are met or as circumstances change. | procurement of fieldwork sites). A program strategic plan must be for a minimum of a 3-year period and include, but need not be limited to,<br>• Evidence that the plan is based on program evaluation and an analysis of external and internal environments.<br>• Long-term goals that address the vision and mission of both the institution and the program, as well as specific needs of the program.<br>• Specific measurable action steps with expected timelines by which the program will reach its long-term goals.<br>• Person(s) responsible for action steps.<br>• Evidence of periodic updating of action steps and long-term goals as they are met or as circumstances change. |
| A.5.2. | The program director and each faculty member who teaches two or more courses must have a current written professional growth and development plan. Each plan must contain the signature of the faculty member and supervisor. At a minimum, the plan must include, but need not be limited to,<br>• Goals to enhance the faculty member's ability to fulfill designated responsibilities (e.g., goals related to currency in areas of teaching responsibility, teaching effectiveness, research, scholarly activity).<br>• Specific measurable action steps with expected timelines by which the faculty member will achieve the goals.<br>• Evidence of annual updates of action steps and goals as they are met or as circumstances change.<br>• Identification of the ways in which the faculty member's professional development plan will contribute to attaining the program's strategic goals. | The program director and each faculty member who teaches two or more courses must have a current written professional growth and development plan. Each plan must contain the signature of the faculty member and supervisor. At a minimum, the plan must include, but need not be limited to,<br>• Goals to enhance the faculty member's ability to fulfill designated responsibilities (e.g., goals related to currency in areas of teaching responsibility, teaching effectiveness, research, scholarly activity).<br>• Specific measurable action steps with expected timelines by which the faculty member will achieve the goals.<br>• Evidence of annual updates of action steps and goals as they are met or as circumstances change.<br>• Identification of the ways in which the faculty member's professional development plan will contribute to attaining the program's strategic goals. | The program director and each faculty member who teaches two or more courses must have a current written professional growth and development plan. Each plan must contain the signature of the faculty member and supervisor. At a minimum, the plan must include, but need not be limited to,<br>• Goals to enhance the faculty member's ability to fulfill designated responsibilities (e.g., goals related to currency in areas of teaching responsibility, teaching effectiveness, research, scholarly activity).<br>• Specific measurable action steps with expected timelines by which the faculty member will achieve the goals.<br>• Evidence of annual updates of action steps and goals as they are met or as circumstances change.<br>• Identification of the ways in which the faculty member's professional development plan will contribute to attaining the program's strategic goals. |
| | *THE PLAN SHOULD REFLECT THE INDIVIDUAL FACULTY MEMBER'S DESIGNATED RESPONSIBILITIES (E.G., EVERY PLAN DOES NOT NEED TO INCLUDE SCHOLARLY ACTIVITY IF THIS IS NOT PART OF THE FACULTY MEMBER'S RESPONSIBILITIES. SIMILARLY, IF THE FACULTY MEMBER'S PRIMARY ROLE IS RESEARCH, HE OR SHE MAY NOT NEED A GOAL RELATED TO TEACHING EFFECTIVENESS).* | | |
| A.5.3. | Programs must routinely secure and document sufficient qualitative and quantitative information to allow for meaningful analysis about the extent to | Programs must routinely secure and document sufficient qualitative and quantitative information to allow for meaningful analysis about the extent to | Programs must routinely secure and document sufficient qualitative and quantitative information to allow for meaningful analysis about the extent to |

| STANDARD NUMBER | ACCREDITATION STANDARDS FOR A DOCTORAL-DEGREE-LEVEL EDUCATIONAL PROGRAM FOR THE OCCUPATIONAL THERAPIST | ACCREDITATION STANDARDS FOR A MASTER'S-DEGREE-LEVEL EDUCATIONAL PROGRAM FOR THE OCCUPATIONAL THERAPIST | ACCREDITATION STANDARDS FOR AN ASSOCIATE-DEGREE-LEVEL EDUCATIONAL PROGRAM FOR THE OCCUPATIONAL THERAPY ASSISTANT |
|---|---|---|---|
| | which the program is meeting its stated goals and objectives. This must include, but need not be limited to,<br>• Faculty effectiveness in their assigned teaching responsibilities.<br>• Students' progression through the program.<br>• Student retention rates.<br>• Fieldwork and experiential component performance evaluation.<br>• Student evaluation of fieldwork and the experiential component experience.<br>• Student satisfaction with the program.<br>• Graduates' performance on the NBCOT certification exam.<br>• Graduates' job placement and performance as determined by employer satisfaction.<br>• Graduates' scholarly activity (e.g., presentations, publications, grants obtained, state and national leadership positions, awards). | which the program is meeting its stated goals and objectives. This must include, but need not be limited to,<br>• Faculty effectiveness in their assigned teaching responsibilities.<br>• Students' progression through the program.<br>• Student retention rates.<br>• Fieldwork performance evaluation.<br>• Student evaluation of fieldwork experience.<br>• Student satisfaction with the program.<br>• Graduates' performance on the NBCOT certification exam.<br>• Graduates' job placement and performance as determined by employer satisfaction. | which the program is meeting its stated goals and objectives. This must include, but need not be limited to,<br>• Faculty effectiveness in their assigned teaching responsibilities.<br>• Students' progression through the program.<br>• Student retention rates.<br>• Fieldwork performance evaluation.<br>• Student evaluation of fieldwork experience.<br>• Student satisfaction with the program.<br>• Graduates' performance on the NBCOT certification exam.<br>• Graduates' job placement and performance as determined by employer satisfaction. |
| A.5.4. | Programs must routinely and systematically analyze data to determine the extent to which the program is meeting its stated goals and objectives. An annual report summarizing analysis of data and planned action responses must be maintained. | Programs must routinely and systematically analyze data to determine the extent to which the program is meeting its stated goals and objectives. An annual report summarizing analysis of data and planned action responses must be maintained. | Programs must routinely and systematically analyze data to determine the extent to which the program is meeting its stated goals and objectives. An annual report summarizing analysis of data and planned action responses must be maintained. |
| | *THE INTENT OF STANDARD A.5.4 IS THAT PROGRAMS PREPARE AN ANNUAL REPORT THAT SUMMARIZES AN ANALYSIS OF DATA COLLECTED ABOUT THE EXTENT TO WHICH THE PROGRAM IS MEETING ITS STATED GOALS AND OBJECTIVES AS REQUIRED BY STANDARD A.5.3 (E.G., FACULTY EFFECTIVENESS IN THEIR ASSIGNED TEACHING RESPONSIBILITIES; STUDENTS' PROGRESSION THROUGH THE PROGRAM, STUDENT RETENTION RATES, FIELDWORK PERFORMANCE EVALUATION, STUDENT EVALUATION OF FIELDWORK EXPERIENCE, STUDENT SATISFACTION WITH THE PROGRAM, GRADUATES' PERFORMANCE ON THE NBCOT CERTIFICATION EXAM, GRADUATES' JOB PLACEMENT, AND PERFORMANCE AS DETERMINED BY EMPLOYER SATISFACTION).* | | |
| A.5.5. | The results of ongoing evaluation must be appropriately reflected in the program's strategic plan, curriculum and other dimensions of the program. | The results of ongoing evaluation must be appropriately reflected in the program's strategic plan, curriculum, and other dimensions of the program. | The results of ongoing evaluation must be appropriately reflected in the program's strategic plan, curriculum, and other dimensions of the program. |
| A.5.6. | The average pass rate over the 3 most recent calendar years for graduates attempting the national certification exam within 12 months of graduation from the program must be 80% or higher (regardless of the number of attempts). If a program has less than 25 test takers in the 3 most recent calendar years, the program may include test takers from additional years until it reaches 25 or until the 5 most recent calendar years are included in the total. | The average pass rate over the 3 most recent calendar years for graduates attempting the national certification exam within 12 months of graduation from the program must be 80% or higher (regardless of the number of attempts). If a program has less than 25 test takers in the 3 most recent calendar years, the program may include test takers from additional years until it reaches 25 or until the 5 most recent calendar years are included in the total. | The average pass rate over the 3 most recent calendar years for graduates attempting the national certification exam within 12 months of graduation from the program must be 80% or higher (regardless of the number of attempts). If a program has less than 25 test takers in the 3 most recent calendar years, the program may include test takers from additional years until it reaches 25 or until the 5 most recent calendar years are included in the total. |
| | *PROGRAMS THAT DID NOT HAVE CANDIDATES WHO SAT FOR THE EXAM IN EACH OF THE 3 MOST RECENT CALENDAR YEARS MUST MEET THE REQUIRED 80% PASS RATE EACH YEAR UNTIL DATA FOR 3 CALENDAR YEARS ARE AVAILABLE.* | | |

| STANDARD NUMBER | ACCREDITATION STANDARDS FOR A DOCTORAL-DEGREE-LEVEL EDUCATIONAL PROGRAM FOR THE OCCUPATIONAL THERAPIST | ACCREDITATION STANDARDS FOR A MASTER'S-DEGREE-LEVEL EDUCATIONAL PROGRAM FOR THE OCCUPATIONAL THERAPIST | ACCREDITATION STANDARDS FOR AN ASSOCIATE-DEGREE-LEVEL EDUCATIONAL PROGRAM FOR THE OCCUPATIONAL THERAPY ASSISTANT |
|---|---|---|---|
| **A.6.0. CURRICULUM FRAMEWORK**<br>**The curriculum framework is a description of the program that includes the program's mission, philosophy, and curriculum design.** | | | |
| A.6.1. | The curriculum must ensure preparation to practice as a generalist with a broad exposure to current practice settings (e.g., school, hospital, community, long-term care) and emerging practice areas (as defined by the program). The curriculum must prepare students to work with a variety of populations including, but not limited to, children, adolescents, adults, and elderly persons in areas of physical and mental health. | The curriculum must include preparation for practice as a generalist with a broad exposure to current practice settings (e.g., school, hospital, community, long-term care) and emerging practice areas (as defined by the program). The curriculum must prepare students to work with a variety of populations including, but not limited to, children, adolescents, adults, and elderly persons in areas of physical and mental health. | The curriculum must include preparation for practice as a generalist with a broad exposure to current practice settings (e.g., school, hospital, community, long-term care) and emerging practice areas (as defined by the program). The curriculum must prepare students to work with a variety of populations including, but not limited to, children, adolescents, adults, and elderly persons in areas of physical and mental health. |
| A.6.2. | The curriculum must include course objectives and learning activities demonstrating preparation beyond a generalist level in, but not limited to, practice skills, research skills, administration, professional development, leadership, advocacy, and theory. | *(No related Standard)* | *(No related Standard)* |
| A.6.3. | The occupational therapy doctoral degree must be awarded after a period of study such that the total time to the degree, including both preprofessional and professional preparation, equals at least 6 FTE academic years. The program must document a system and rationale for ensuring that the length of study of the program is appropriate to the expected learning and competence of the graduate. | The program must document a system and rationale for ensuring that the length of study of the program is appropriate to the expected learning and competence of the graduate. | The program must document a system and rationale for ensuring that the length of study of the program is appropriate to the expected learning and competence of the graduate. |
| A.6.4. | The curriculum must include application of advanced knowledge to practice through a combination of experiential activities and a culminating project. | *(No related Standard)* | *(No related Standard)* |
| A.6.5. | The statement of philosophy of the occupational therapy program must reflect the current published philosophy of the profession and must include a statement of the program's fundamental beliefs about human beings and how they learn. | The statement of philosophy of the occupational therapy program must reflect the current published philosophy of the profession and must include a statement of the program's fundamental beliefs about human beings and how they learn. | The statement of philosophy of the occupational therapy assistant program must reflect the current published philosophy of the profession and must include a statement of the program's fundamental beliefs about human beings and how they learn. |
| A.6.6. | The statement of the mission of the occupational therapy program must be consistent with and supportive of the mission of the sponsoring institution. The program's mission statement should explain the unique nature of the program and how it helps fulfill or advance the mission of the sponsoring institution, including religious missions. | The statement of the mission of the occupational therapy program must be consistent with and supportive of the mission of the sponsoring institution. The program's mission statement should explain the unique nature of the program and how it helps fulfill or advance the mission of the sponsoring institution, including religious missions. | The statement of the mission of the occupational therapy assistant program must be consistent with and supportive of the mission of the sponsoring institution. The program's mission statement should explain the unique nature of the program and how it helps fulfill or advance the mission of the sponsoring institution, including religious missions. |
| A.6.7. | The curriculum design must reflect the mission and philosophy of both the occupational therapy program and the institution and must provide the basis for | The curriculum design must reflect the mission and philosophy of both the occupational therapy program and the institution and must provide the basis for | The curriculum design must reflect the mission and philosophy of both the occupational therapy assistant program and the institution and must provide the |

| STANDARD NUMBER | ACCREDITATION STANDARDS FOR A DOCTORAL-DEGREE-LEVEL EDUCATIONAL PROGRAM FOR THE OCCUPATIONAL THERAPIST | ACCREDITATION STANDARDS FOR A MASTER'S-DEGREE-LEVEL EDUCATIONAL PROGRAM FOR THE OCCUPATIONAL THERAPIST | ACCREDITATION STANDARDS FOR AN ASSOCIATE-DEGREE-LEVEL EDUCATIONAL PROGRAM FOR THE OCCUPATIONAL THERAPY ASSISTANT |
|---|---|---|---|
| | program planning, implementation, and evaluation. The design must identify curricular threads and educational goals and describe the selection of the content, scope, and sequencing of coursework. | program planning, implementation, and evaluation. The design must identify curricular threads and educational goals and describe the selection of the content, scope, and sequencing of coursework. | basis for program planning, implementation, and evaluation. The design must identify curricular threads and educational goals and describe the selection of the content, scope, and sequencing of coursework. |
| A.6.8. | The program must have clearly documented assessment measures by which students are regularly evaluated on their acquisition of knowledge, skills attitudes, and competencies required for graduation. | The program must have clearly documented assessment measures by which students are regularly evaluated on their acquisition of knowledge, skills, attitudes, and competencies required for graduation. | The program must have clearly documented assessment measures by which students are regularly evaluated on their acquisition of knowledge, skills, attitudes, and competencies required for graduation. |
| A.6.9. | The program must have written syllabi for each course that include course objectives and learning activities that, in total, reflect all course content required by the Standards. Instructional methods (e.g., presentations, demonstrations, discussion) and materials used to accomplish course objectives must be documented. Programs must also demonstrate the consistency between course syllabi and the curriculum design. | The program must have written syllabi for each course that include course objectives and learning activities that, in total, reflect all course content required by the Standards. Instructional methods (e.g., presentations, demonstrations, discussion) and materials used to accomplish course objectives must be documented. Programs must also demonstrate the consistency between course syllabi and the curriculum design. | The program must have written syllabi for each course that include course objectives and learning activities that, in total, reflect all course content required by the Standards. Instructional methods (e.g., presentations, demonstrations, discussion) and materials used to accomplish course objectives must be documented. Programs must also demonstrate the consistency between course syllabi and the curriculum design. |
| **SECTION B: CONTENT REQUIREMENTS**<br>**The content requirements are written as expected student outcomes. Faculty are responsible for developing learning activities and evaluation methods to document that students meet these outcomes.** | | | |
| **B.1.0.** | **FOUNDATIONAL CONTENT REQUIREMENTS**<br>**Program content must be based on a broad foundation in the liberal arts and sciences. A strong foundation in the biological, physical, social, and behavioral sciences supports an understanding of occupation across the lifespan. If the content of the Standard is met through prerequisite coursework, the application of foundational content in sciences must also be evident in professional coursework. The student will be able to** | | **FOUNDATIONAL CONTENT REQUIREMENTS**<br>**Program content must be based on a broad foundation in the liberal arts and sciences.**<br>**A strong foundation in the biological, physical, social, and behavioral sciences supports an understanding of occupation across the lifespan. If the content of the Standard is met through prerequisite coursework, the application of foundational content in sciences must also be evident in professional coursework. The student will be able to** |
| B.1.1. | Demonstrate knowledge and understanding of the structure and function of the human body to include the biological and physical sciences. Course content must include, but is not limited to, biology, anatomy, physiology, neuroscience, and kinesiology or biomechanics. | Demonstrate knowledge and understanding of the structure and function of the human body to include the biological and physical sciences. Course content must include, but is not limited to, biology, anatomy, physiology, neuroscience, and kinesiology or biomechanics. | Demonstrate knowledge and understanding of the structure and function of the human body to include the biological and physical sciences. Course content must include, but is not limited to, anatomy, physiology, and biomechanics. |
| B.1.2. | Demonstrate knowledge and understanding of human development throughout the lifespan (infants, children, adolescents, adults, and older adults). Course content must include, but is not limited to, | Demonstrate knowledge and understanding of human development throughout the lifespan (infants, children, adolescents, adults, and older adults). Course content must include, but is not limited to, | Demonstrate knowledge and understanding of human development throughout the lifespan (infants, children, adolescents, adults, and older adults). Course content must include, but is not limited to, |

| STANDARD NUMBER | ACCREDITATION STANDARDS FOR A DOCTORAL-DEGREE-LEVEL EDUCATIONAL PROGRAM FOR THE OCCUPATIONAL THERAPIST | ACCREDITATION STANDARDS FOR A MASTER'S-DEGREE-LEVEL EDUCATIONAL PROGRAM FOR THE OCCUPATIONAL THERAPIST | ACCREDITATION STANDARDS FOR AN ASSOCIATE-DEGREE-LEVEL EDUCATIONAL PROGRAM FOR THE OCCUPATIONAL THERAPY ASSISTANT |
|---|---|---|---|
| | developmental psychology. | developmental psychology. | developmental psychology. |
| B.1.3. | Demonstrate knowledge and understanding of the concepts of human behavior to include the behavioral sciences, social sciences, and occupational science. Course content must include, but is not limited to, introductory psychology, abnormal psychology, and introductory sociology or introductory anthropology. | Demonstrate knowledge and understanding of the concepts of human behavior to include the behavioral sciences, social sciences, and occupational science. Course content must include, but is not limited to, introductory psychology, abnormal psychology, and introductory sociology or introductory anthropology. | Demonstrate knowledge and understanding of the concepts of human behavior to include the behavioral and social sciences (e.g., principles of psychology, sociology, abnormal psychology) and occupational science. |
| B.1.4. | Apply knowledge of the role of sociocultural, socioeconomic, and diversity factors and lifestyle choices in contemporary society to meet the needs of individuals and communities. Course content must include, but is not limited to, introductory psychology, abnormal psychology, and introductory sociology or introductory anthropology. | Demonstrate knowledge and appreciation of the role of sociocultural, socioeconomic, and diversity factors and lifestyle choices in contemporary society. Course content must include, but is not limited to, introductory psychology, abnormal psychology, and introductory sociology or introductory anthropology. | Demonstrate knowledge and appreciation of the role of sociocultural, socioeconomic, and diversity factors and lifestyle choices in contemporary society (e.g., principles of psychology, sociology, and abnormal psychology). |
| B.1.5. | Demonstrate an understanding of the ethical and practical considerations that affect the health and wellness needs of those who are experiencing or are at risk for social injustice, occupational deprivation, and disparity in the receipt of services. | Demonstrate an understanding of the ethical and practical considerations that affect the health and wellness needs of those who are experiencing or are at risk for social injustice, occupational deprivation, and disparity in the receipt of services. | Articulate the ethical and practical considerations that affect the health and wellness needs of those who are experiencing or are at risk for social injustice, occupational deprivation, and disparity in the receipt of services. |
| B.1.6. | Demonstrate knowledge of global social issues and prevailing health and welfare needs of populations with or at risk for disabilities and chronic health conditions. | Demonstrate knowledge of global social issues and prevailing health and welfare needs of populations with or at risk for disabilities and chronic health conditions. | Demonstrate knowledge of global social issues and prevailing health and welfare needs of populations with or at risk for disabilities and chronic health conditions. |
| B.1.7. | Apply quantitative statistics and qualitative analysis to interpret tests, measurements, and other data for the purpose of establishing and/or delivering evidence-based practice. | Demonstrate the ability to use statistics to interpret tests and measurements for the purpose of delivering evidence-based practice. | Articulate the importance of using statistics, tests, and measurements for the purpose of delivering evidence-based practice. |
| B.1.8. | Demonstrate an understanding of the use of technology to support performance, participation, health and well-being. This technology may include, but is not limited to, electronic documentation systems, distance communication, virtual environments, and telehealth technology. | Demonstrate an understanding of the use of technology to support performance, participation, health and well-being. This technology may include, but is not limited to, electronic documentation systems, distance communication, virtual environments, and telehealth technology., | Demonstrate an understanding of the use of technology to support performance, participation, health and well-being. This technology may include, but is not limited to, electronic documentation systems, distance communication, virtual environments, and telehealth technology. |
| **B.2.0. BASIC TENETS OF OCCUPATIONAL THERAPY**<br>**Coursework must facilitate development of the performance criteria listed below. The student will be able to** | | | |
| B.2.1. | Explain the history and philosophical base of the profession of occupational therapy and its importance in meeting society's current and future occupational needs. | Articulate an understanding of the importance of the history and philosophical base of the profession of occupational therapy. | Articulate an understanding of the importance of the history and philosophical base of the profession of occupational therapy. |
| B.2.2. | Explain the meaning and dynamics of occupation and activity, including the interaction of areas of | Explain the meaning and dynamics of occupation and activity, including the interaction of areas of | Describe the meaning and dynamics of occupation and activity, including the interaction of areas of |

| STANDARD NUMBER | ACCREDITATION STANDARDS FOR A DOCTORAL-DEGREE-LEVEL EDUCATIONAL PROGRAM FOR THE OCCUPATIONAL THERAPIST | ACCREDITATION STANDARDS FOR A MASTER'S-DEGREE-LEVEL EDUCATIONAL PROGRAM FOR THE OCCUPATIONAL THERAPIST | ACCREDITATION STANDARDS FOR AN ASSOCIATE-DEGREE-LEVEL EDUCATIONAL PROGRAM FOR THE OCCUPATIONAL THERAPY ASSISTANT |
|---|---|---|---|
| | occupation, performance skills, performance patterns, activity demands, context(s) and environments, and client factors. | occupation, performance skills, performance patterns, activity demands, context(s) and environments, and client factors. | occupation, performance skills, performance patterns, activity demands, context(s) and environments, and client factors. |
| B.2.3. | Articulate to consumers, potential employers, colleagues, third-party payers, regulatory boards, policymakers, other audiences, and the general public both the unique nature of occupation as viewed by the profession of occupational therapy and the value of occupation to support performance, participation, health, and well-being. | Articulate to consumers, potential employers, colleagues, third-party payers, regulatory boards, policymakers, other audiences, and the general public both the unique nature of occupation as viewed by the profession of occupational therapy and the value of occupation to support performance, participation, health, and well-being. | Articulate to consumers, potential employers, colleagues, third-party payers, regulatory boards, policymakers, other audiences, and the general public both the unique nature of occupation as viewed by the profession of occupational therapy and the value of occupation support performance, participation, health, and well-being. |
| B.2.4. | Articulate the importance of balancing areas of occupation with the achievement of health and wellness for the clients. | Articulate the importance of balancing areas of occupation with the achievement of health and wellness for the clients. | Articulate the importance of balancing areas of occupation with the achievement of health and wellness for the clients. |
| B.2.5. | Explain the role of occupation in the promotion of health and the prevention of disease and disability for the individual, family, and society. | Explain the role of occupation in the promotion of health and the prevention of disease and disability for the individual, family, and society. | Explain the role of occupation in the promotion of health and the prevention of disease and disability for the individual, family, and society. |
| B.2.6. | Analyze the effects of heritable diseases, genetic conditions, disability, trauma, and injury to the physical and mental health and occupational performance of the individual. | Analyze the effects of heritable diseases, genetic conditions, disability, trauma, and injury to the physical and mental health and occupational performance of the individual. | Understand the effects of heritable diseases, genetic conditions, disability, trauma, and injury to the physical and mental health and occupational performance of the individual. |
| B.2.7. | Demonstrate task analysis in areas of occupation, performance skills, performance patterns, activity demands, context(s) and environments, and client factors to formulate an intervention plan. | Demonstrate task analysis in areas of occupation, performance skills, performance patterns, activity demands, context(s) and environments, and client factors to formulate an intervention plan. | Demonstrate task analysis in areas of occupation, performance skills, performance patterns, activity demands, context(s) and environments, and client factors to implement the intervention plan. |
| B.2.8. | Use sound judgment in regard to safety of self and others and adhere to safety regulations throughout the occupational therapy process as appropriate to the setting and scope of practice. | Use sound judgment in regard to safety of self and others and adhere to safety regulations throughout the occupational therapy process as appropriate to the setting and scope of practice. | Use sound judgment in regard to safety of self and others and adhere to safety regulations throughout the occupational therapy process as appropriate to the setting and scope of practice. |
| B.2.9. | Express support for the quality of life, well-being, and occupation of the individual, group, or population to promote physical and mental health and prevention of injury and disease considering the context (e.g., cultural, personal, temporal, virtual) and environment. | Express support for the quality of life, well-being, and occupation of the individual, group, or population to promote physical and mental health and prevention of injury and disease considering the context (e.g., cultural, personal, temporal, virtual) and environment. | Express support for the quality of life, well-being, and occupation of the individual, group, or population to promote physical and mental health and prevention of injury and disease considering the context (e.g., cultural, personal, temporal, virtual) and environment. |
| B.2.10. | Use clinical reasoning to explain the rationale for and use of compensatory strategies when desired life tasks cannot be performed. | Use clinical reasoning to explain the rationale for and use of compensatory strategies when desired life tasks cannot be performed. | Explain the need for and use of compensatory strategies when desired life tasks cannot be performed. |
| B.2.11. | Analyze, synthesize, evaluate, and apply models of occupational performance. | Analyze, synthesize, and apply models of occupational performance. | Identify interventions consistent with models of occupational performance. |

| STANDARD NUMBER | ACCREDITATION STANDARDS FOR A DOCTORAL-DEGREE-LEVEL EDUCATIONAL PROGRAM FOR THE OCCUPATIONAL THERAPIST | ACCREDITATION STANDARDS FOR A MASTER'S-DEGREE-LEVEL EDUCATIONAL PROGRAM FOR THE OCCUPATIONAL THERAPIST | ACCREDITATION STANDARDS FOR AN ASSOCIATE-DEGREE-LEVEL EDUCATIONAL PROGRAM FOR THE OCCUPATIONAL THERAPY ASSISTANT |
|---|---|---|---|
| **B.3.0.** | **OCCUPATIONAL THERAPY THEORETICAL PERSPECTIVES**<br>**The program must facilitate the development of the performance criteria listed below. The student will be able to** | | |
| B.3.1. | Evaluate and apply theories that underlie the practice of occupational therapy. | Apply theories that underlie the practice of occupational therapy. | Describe basic features of the theories that underlie the practice of occupational therapy. |
| B.3.2. | Compare, contrast, and integrate a variety of models of practice and frames of reference that are used in occupational therapy. | Compare and contrast models of practice and frames of reference that are used in occupational therapy. | Describe basic features of models of practice and frames of reference that are used in occupational therapy. |
| B.3.3. | Use theories, models of practice, and frames of reference to guide and inform evaluation and intervention. | Use theories, models of practice, and frames of reference to guide and inform evaluation and intervention. | Discuss how occupational therapy history and occupational therapy theory, and the sociopolitical climate influence practice. |
| B.3.4. | Analyze and discuss how occupational therapy history, occupational therapy theory, and the sociopolitical climate influence and are influenced by practice. | Analyze and discuss how occupational therapy history, occupational therapy theory, and the sociopolitical climate influence practice. | *(No related Standard)* |
| B.3.5. | Apply theoretical constructs to evaluation and intervention with various types of clients in a variety of practice contexts and environments, including population-based approaches, to analyze and effect meaningful occupation outcomes. | Apply theoretical constructs to evaluation and intervention with various types of clients I a variety of practice contexts and environments to analyze and effect meaningful occupation outcomes. | *(No related Standard)* |
| B.3.6. | Articulate the process of theory development in occupational therapy and its desired impact and influence on society. | Discuss the process of theory development and its importance to occupational therapy. | *(No related Standard)* |
| **B.4.0.** | **SCREENING, EVALUATION, AND REFERRAL**<br>**The process of screening, evaluation, referral, and diagnosis as related to occupational performance and participation must be culturally relevant and based on theoretical perspectives, models of practice, frames of reference, and available evidence. In addition, this process must consider the continuum of need from individuals to populations. The program must facilitate development of the performance criteria listed below. The student will be able to** | **SCREENING, EVALUATION, AND REFERRAL**<br>**The process of screening, evaluation, and referral as related to occupational performance and participation must be culturally relevant and based on theoretical perspectives, models of practice, frames of reference, and available evidence. In addition, this process must consider the continuum of need from individuals to populations The program must facilitate development of the performance criteria listed below. The student will be able to** | **SCREENING AND EVALUATION**<br>**The process of screening and evaluation as related to occupational performance and participation must be conducted under the supervision of and in cooperation with the occupational therapist and must be culturally relevant and based on theoretical perspectives, models of practice, frames of reference, and available evidence. The program must facilitate development of the performance criteria listed below. The student will be able to** |
| B.4.1. | Use standardized and nonstandardized screening and assessment tools to determine the need for occupational therapy intervention. These tools include, but are not limited to, specified screening tools; assessments; skilled observations; occupational histories; consultations with other professionals; and interviews with the client, family, significant others, and community. | Use standardized and nonstandardized screening and assessment tools to determine the need for occupational therapy intervention. These tools include, but are not limited to, specified screening tools; assessments; skilled observations; occupational histories; consultations with other professionals; and interviews with the client, family, significant others, and community. | Gather and share data for the purpose of screening and evaluation using methods including, but not limited to, specified screening tools; assessments; skilled observations; occupational histories; consultations with other professionals; and interviews with the client, family, and significant others. |

| STANDARD NUMBER | ACCREDITATION STANDARDS FOR A DOCTORAL-DEGREE-LEVEL EDUCATIONAL PROGRAM FOR THE OCCUPATIONAL THERAPIST | ACCREDITATION STANDARDS FOR A MASTER'S-DEGREE-LEVEL EDUCATIONAL PROGRAM FOR THE OCCUPATIONAL THERAPIST | ACCREDITATION STANDARDS FOR AN ASSOCIATE-DEGREE-LEVEL EDUCATIONAL PROGRAM FOR THE OCCUPATIONAL THERAPY ASSISTANT |
|---|---|---|---|
| B.4.2. | Select appropriate assessment tools on the basis of client needs, contextual factors, and psychometric properties of tests. These must be culturally relevant, based on available evidence, and incorporate use of occupation in the assessment process. | Select appropriate assessment tools on the basis of client needs, contextual factors, and psychometric properties of tests. These must be culturally relevant, based on available evidence, and incorporate use of occupation in the assessment process. | Administer selected assessments using appropriate procedures and protocols (including standardized formats) and use occupation for the purpose of assessment. |
| B.4.3. | Use appropriate procedures and protocols (including standardized formats) when administering assessments. | Use appropriate procedures and protocols (including standardized formats) when administering assessments. | *(No related Standard)* |
| B.4.4. | Evaluate client(s)' occupational performance in activities of daily living (ADLs), instrumental activities of daily living (IADLs), education, work, play, rest, sleep, leisure, and social participation. Evaluation of occupational performance using standardized and nonstandardized assessment tools includes<br>• The occupational profile, including participation in activities that are meaningful and necessary for the client to carry out roles in home, work, and community environments.<br>• Client factors, including values, beliefs, spirituality, body functions (e.g., neuromuscular, sensory and pain, visual, perceptual, cognitive, mental) and body structures (e.g., cardiovascular, digestive, nervous, genitourinary, integumentary systems).<br>• Performance patterns (e.g., habits, routines, rituals, roles).<br>• Context (e.g. cultural, personal, temporal, virtual) and environment (e.g., physical, social).<br>• Performance skills, including motor and praxis skills, sensory–perceptual skills, emotional regulation skills, cognitive skills, and communication and social skills. | Evaluate client(s)' occupational performance in activities of daily living (ADLs), instrumental activities of daily living (IADLs), education, work, play, rest, sleep, leisure, and social participation. Evaluation of occupational performance using standardized and nonstandardized assessment tools includes<br>• The occupational profile, including participation in activities that are meaningful and necessary for the client to carry out roles in home, work, and community environments.<br>• Client factors, including values, beliefs, spirituality, body functions (e.g., neuromuscular, sensory and pain, visual, perceptual, cognitive, mental) and body structures (e.g., cardiovascular, digestive, nervous, genitourinary, integumentary systems).<br>• Performance patterns (e.g., habits, routines, rituals, roles).<br>• Context (e.g., cultural, personal, temporal, virtual) and environment (e.g., physical, social).<br>• Performance skills, including motor and praxis skills, sensory–perceptual skills, emotional regulation skills, cognitive skills, and communication and social skills. | Gather and share data for the purpose of evaluating client(s)' occupational performance in activities of daily living (ADLs), instrumental activities of daily living (IADLs), education, work, play, rest, sleep, leisure, and social participation. Evaluation of occupational performance includes<br>• The occupational profile, including participation in activities that are meaningful and necessary for the client to carry out roles in home, work, and community environments.<br>• Client factors, including values, beliefs, spirituality, body functions (e.g., neuromuscular, sensory and pain, visual, perceptual, cognitive, mental) and body structures (e.g., cardiovascular, digestive, nervous, genitourinary, integumentary systems).<br>• Performance patterns (e.g., habits, routines, rituals, roles).<br>• Context (e.g., cultural, personal, temporal, virtual) and environment (e.g., physical, social).<br>• Performance skills, including motor and praxis skills, sensory–perceptual skills, emotional regulation skills, cognitive skills, and communication and social skills. |
| B.4.5. | Compare and contrast the role of the occupational therapist and occupational therapy assistant in the screening and evaluation process along with the importance of and rationale for supervision and collaborative work between the occupational therapist and occupational therapy assistant in that process. | Compare and contrast the role of the occupational therapist and occupational therapy assistant in the screening and evaluation process along with the importance of and rationale for supervision and collaborative work between the occupational therapist and occupational therapy assistant in that process. | Articulate the role of the occupational therapy assistant and occupational therapist in the screening and evaluation process along with the importance of and rationale for supervision and collaborative work between the occupational therapy assistant and occupational therapist in that process. |
| B.4.6. | Interpret criterion-referenced and norm-referenced standardized test scores on the basis of an understanding of sampling, normative data, standard and criterion scores, reliability, and validity. | Interpret criterion-referenced and norm-referenced standardized test scores on the basis of an understanding of sampling, normative data, standard and criterion scores, reliability, and validity. | *(No related Standard)* |

| STANDARD NUMBER | ACCREDITATION STANDARDS FOR A DOCTORAL-DEGREE-LEVEL EDUCATIONAL PROGRAM FOR THE OCCUPATIONAL THERAPIST | ACCREDITATION STANDARDS FOR A MASTER'S-DEGREE-LEVEL EDUCATIONAL PROGRAM FOR THE OCCUPATIONAL THERAPIST | ACCREDITATION STANDARDS FOR AN ASSOCIATE-DEGREE-LEVEL EDUCATIONAL PROGRAM FOR THE OCCUPATIONAL THERAPY ASSISTANT |
|---|---|---|---|
| B.4.7. | Consider factors that might bias assessment results, such as culture, disability status, and situational variables related to the individual and context. | Consider factors that might bias assessment results, such as culture, disability status, and situational variables related to the individual and context. | *(No related Standard)* |
| B.4.8. | Interpret the evaluation data in relation to accepted terminology of the profession, relevant theoretical frameworks, and interdisciplinary knowledge. | Interpret the evaluation data in relation to accepted terminology of the profession and relevant theoretical frameworks. | *(No related Standard)* |
| B.4.9. | Evaluate appropriateness and discuss mechanisms for referring clients for additional evaluation to specialists who are internal and external to the profession. | Evaluate appropriateness and discuss mechanisms for referring clients for additional evaluation to specialists who are internal and external to the profession. | Identify when to recommend to the occupational therapist the need for referring clients for additional evaluation. |
| B.4.10. | Document occupational therapy services to ensure accountability of service provision and to meet standards for reimbursement of services, adhering to the requirements of applicable facility, local, state, federal, and reimbursement agencies. Documentation must effectively communicate the need and rationale for occupational therapy services. | Document occupational therapy services to ensure accountability of service provision and to meet standards for reimbursement of services, adhering to the requirements of applicable facility, local, state, federal, and reimbursement agencies. Documentation must effectively communicate the need and rationale for occupational therapy services. | Document occupational therapy services to ensure accountability of service provision and to meet standards for reimbursement of services, adhering to the requirements of applicable facility, local, state, federal, and reimbursement agencies. Documentation must effectively communicate the need and rationale for occupational therapy services. |
| B.4.11. | Articulate screening and evaluation processes for all practice areas. Use evidence-based reasoning to analyze, synthesize, evaluate, and diagnose problems related to occupational performance and participation | *(No related Standard)* | *(No related Standard)* |
| **B.5.0.** | **INTERVENTION PLAN: FORMULATION AND IMPLEMENTATION** **The process of formulation and implementation of the therapeutic intervention plan to facilitate occupational performance and participation must be culturally relevant; reflective of current and emerging occupational therapy practice; based on available evidence; and based on theoretical perspectives, models of practice, and frames of reference. In addition, this process must consider the continuum of need from individual- to population-based interventions. The program must facilitate development of the performance criteria listed below. The student will be able to** | **INTERVENTION PLAN: FORMULATION AND IMPLEMENTATION** **The process of formulation and implementation of the therapeutic intervention plan to facilitate occupational performance and participation must be culturally relevant; reflective of current occupational therapy practice; based on available evidence; and based on theoretical perspectives, models of practice, and frames of reference. The program must facilitate development of the performance criteria listed below. The student will be able to** | **INTERVENTION AND IMPLEMENTATION** **The process of intervention to facilitate occupational performance and participation must be done under the supervision of and in cooperation with the occupational therapist and must be culturally relevant, reflective of current occupational therapy practice, and based on available evidence. The program must facilitate development of the performance criteria listed below. The student will be able to** |
| B.5.1. | Use evaluation findings to diagnose occupational performance and participation based on appropriate theoretical approaches, models of practice, frames of reference, and interdisciplinary knowledge. Develop occupation-based intervention plans and strategies (including goals and methods to achieve them) on the basis of the stated needs of the client as well as data | Use evaluation findings based on appropriate theoretical approaches, models of practice, and frames of reference to develop occupation-based intervention plans and strategies (including goals and methods to achieve them) on the basis of the stated needs of the client as well as data gathered during the evaluation process in collaboration with the client | Assist with the development of occupation-based intervention plans and strategies (including goals and methods to achieve them) on the basis of the stated needs of the client as well as data gathered during the evaluation process in collaboration with the client and others. Intervention plans and strategies must be culturally relevant, reflective of current occupational |

| STANDARD NUMBER | ACCREDITATION STANDARDS FOR A DOCTORAL-DEGREE-LEVEL EDUCATIONAL PROGRAM FOR THE OCCUPATIONAL THERAPIST | ACCREDITATION STANDARDS FOR A MASTER'S-DEGREE-LEVEL EDUCATIONAL PROGRAM FOR THE OCCUPATIONAL THERAPIST | ACCREDITATION STANDARDS FOR AN ASSOCIATE-DEGREE-LEVEL EDUCATIONAL PROGRAM FOR THE OCCUPATIONAL THERAPY ASSISTANT |
|---|---|---|---|
| | gathered during the evaluation process in collaboration with the client and others. Intervention plans and strategies must be culturally relevant, reflective of current occupational therapy practice, and based on available evidence. Interventions address the following components:<br>• The occupational profile, including participation in activities that are meaningful and necessary for the client to carry out roles in home, work, and community environments.<br>• Client factors, including values, beliefs, spirituality, body functions (e.g., neuromuscular, sensory and pain, visual, perceptual, cognitive, mental) and body structures (e.g., cardiovascular, digestive, nervous, genitourinary, integumentary systems).<br>• Performance patterns (e.g., habits, routines, rituals, roles).<br>• Context (e.g., cultural, personal, temporal, virtual) and environment (e.g., physical, social).<br>• Performance skills, including motor and praxis skills, sensory–perceptual skills, emotional regulation skills, cognitive skills, and communication and social skills. | and others. Intervention plans and strategies must be culturally relevant, reflective of current occupational therapy practice, and based on available evidence. Interventions address the following components:<br>• The occupational profile, including participation in activities that are meaningful and necessary for the client to carry out roles in home, work, and community environments.<br>• Client factors, including values, beliefs, spirituality, body functions (e.g., neuromuscular, sensory and pain, visual, perceptual, cognitive, mental) and body structures (e.g., cardiovascular, digestive, nervous, genitourinary, integumentary systems).<br>• Performance patterns (e.g., habits, routines, rituals, roles).<br>• Context (e.g., cultural, personal, temporal, virtual) and environment (e.g., physical, social).<br>• Performance skills, including motor and praxis skills, sensory–perceptual skills, emotional regulation skills, cognitive skills, and communication and social skills. | therapy practice, and based on available evidence. Interventions address the following components:<br>• The occupational profile, including participation in activities that are meaningful and necessary for the client to carry out roles in home, work, and community environments.<br>• Client factors, including values, beliefs, spirituality, body functions (e.g., neuromuscular, sensory and pain, visual, perceptual, cognitive, mental) and body structures (e.g., cardiovascular, digestive, nervous, genitourinary, integumentary systems).<br>• Performance patterns (e.g., habits, routines, rituals, roles).<br>• Context (e.g., cultural, personal, temporal, virtual) and environment (e.g., physical, social).<br>• Performance skills, including motor and praxis skills, sensory–perceptual skills, emotional regulation skills, cognitive skills, and communication and social skills. |
| B.5.2. | Select and provide direct occupational therapy interventions and procedures to enhance safety, health and wellness, and performance in ADLs, IADLs, education, work, play, rest, sleep, leisure, and social participation. | Select and provide direct occupational therapy interventions and procedures to enhance safety, health and wellness, and performance in ADLs, IADLs, education, work, play, rest, sleep, leisure, and social participation. | Select and provide direct occupational therapy interventions and procedures to enhance safety, health and wellness, and performance in ADLs, IADLs, education, work, play, rest, sleep, leisure, and social participation. |
| B.5.3. | Provide therapeutic use of occupation, exercises, and activities (e.g., occupation-based intervention, purposeful activity, preparatory methods). | Provide therapeutic use of occupation, exercises, and activities (e.g., occupation-based intervention, purposeful activity, preparatory methods). | Provide therapeutic use of occupation, exercises, and activities (e.g., occupation-based intervention, purposeful activity, preparatory methods). |
| B.5.4. | Design and implement group interventions based on principles of group development and group dynamics across the lifespan. | Design and implement group interventions based on principles of group development and group dynamics across the lifespan. | Implement group interventions based on principles of group development and group dynamics across the lifespan. |
| B.5.5. | Provide training in self-care, self-management, health management and maintenance, home management, and community and work integration. | Provide training in self-care, self-management, health management and maintenance, home management, and community and work integration. | Provide training in self-care, self-management, health management and maintenance, home management, and community and work integration. |
| B.5.6. | Provide development, remediation, and compensation for physical, mental, cognitive, perceptual, neuromuscular, behavioral skills, and sensory functions (e.g., vision, tactile, auditory, gustatory, olfactory, pain, temperature, pressure, | Provide development, remediation, and compensation for physical, mental, cognitive, perceptual, neuromuscular, behavioral skills, and sensory functions (e.g., vision, tactile, auditory, gustatory, olfactory, pain, temperature, pressure, | Provide development, remediation, and compensation for physical, mental, cognitive, perceptual, neuromuscular, behavioral skills, and sensory functions (e.g., vision, tactile, auditory, gustatory, olfactory, pain, temperature, pressure, |

| STANDARD NUMBER | ACCREDITATION STANDARDS FOR A DOCTORAL-DEGREE-LEVEL EDUCATIONAL PROGRAM FOR THE OCCUPATIONAL THERAPIST | ACCREDITATION STANDARDS FOR A MASTER'S-DEGREE-LEVEL EDUCATIONAL PROGRAM FOR THE OCCUPATIONAL THERAPIST | ACCREDITATION STANDARDS FOR AN ASSOCIATE-DEGREE-LEVEL EDUCATIONAL PROGRAM FOR THE OCCUPATIONAL THERAPY ASSISTANT |
|---|---|---|---|
| | vestibular, proprioception). | vestibular, proprioception). | vestibular, proprioception). |
| B.5.7. | Demonstrate therapeutic use of self, including one's personality, insights, perceptions, and judgments, as part of the therapeutic process in both individual and group interaction. | Demonstrate therapeutic use of self, including one's personality, insights, perceptions, and judgments, as part of the therapeutic process in both individual and group interaction. | Demonstrate therapeutic use of self, including one's personality, insights, perceptions, and judgments, as part of the therapeutic process in both individual and group interaction. |
| B.5.8. | Develop and implement intervention strategies to remediate and/or compensate for cognitive deficits that affect occupational performance. | Develop and implement intervention strategies to remediate and/or compensate for cognitive deficits that affect occupational performance. | Implement intervention strategies to remediate and/or compensate for cognitive deficits that affect occupational performance. |
| B.5.9. | Evaluate and adapt processes or environments (e.g., home, work, school, community) applying ergonomic principles and principles of environmental modification. | Evaluate and adapt processes or environments (e.g., home, work, school, community) applying ergonomic principles and principles of environmental modification. | Adapt environments (e.g., home, work, school, community) and processes, including the application of ergonomic principles. |
| B.5.10. | Articulate principles and be able to design, fabricate, apply, fit, and train in assistive technologies and devices (e.g., electronic aids to daily living, seating and positioning systems) used to enhance occupational performance and foster participation and well-being. | Articulate principles of and be able to design, fabricate, apply, fit, and train in assistive technologies and devices (e.g., electronic aids to daily living, seating and positioning systems) used to enhance occupational performance and foster participation and well-being. | Articulate principles of and demonstrate strategies with assistive technologies and devices (e.g., electronic aids to daily living, seating and positioning systems) used to enhance occupational performance and foster participation and well-being. |
| B.5.11. | Provide design, fabrication, application, fitting, and training in orthotic devices used to enhance occupational performance and participation. Train in the use of prosthetic devices, based on scientific principles of kinesiology, biomechanics, and physics. | Provide design, fabrication, application, fitting, and training in orthotic devices used to enhance occupational performance and participation. Train in the use of prosthetic devices, based on scientific principles of kinesiology, biomechanics, and physics. | Provide fabrication, application, fitting, and training in orthotic devices used to enhance occupational performance and participation, and training in the use of prosthetic devices. |
| B.5.12. | Provide recommendations and training in techniques to enhance functional mobility, including physical transfers, wheelchair management, and mobility devices. | Provide recommendations and training in techniques to enhance functional mobility, including physical transfers, wheelchair management, and mobility devices. | Provide training in techniques to enhance functional mobility, including physical transfers, wheelchair management, and mobility devices. |
| B.5.13. | Provide recommendations and training in techniques to enhance community mobility, including public transportation, community access, and issues related to driver rehabilitation. | Provide recommendations and training in techniques to enhance community mobility, including public transportation, community access, and issues related to driver rehabilitation. | Provide training in techniques to enhance community mobility, including public transportation, community access, and issues related to driver rehabilitation. |
| B.5.14. | Provide management of feeding, eating, and swallowing to enable performance (including the process of bringing food or fluids from the plate or cup to the mouth, the ability to keep and manipulate food or fluid in the mouth, and swallowing assessment and management) and train others in precautions and techniques while considering client and contextual factors. | Provide management of feeding, eating, and swallowing to enable performance (including the process of bringing food or fluids from the plate or cup to the mouth, the ability to keep and manipulate food or fluid in the mouth, and swallowing assessment and management) and train others in precautions and techniques while considering client and contextual factors. | Enable feeding and eating performance (including the process of bringing food or fluids from the plate or cup to the mouth, the ability to keep and manipulate food or fluid in the mouth, and the initiation of swallowing) and train others in precautions and techniques while considering client and contextual factors. |

| STANDARD NUMBER | ACCREDITATION STANDARDS FOR A DOCTORAL-DEGREE-LEVEL EDUCATIONAL PROGRAM FOR THE OCCUPATIONAL THERAPIST | ACCREDITATION STANDARDS FOR A MASTER'S-DEGREE-LEVEL EDUCATIONAL PROGRAM FOR THE OCCUPATIONAL THERAPIST | ACCREDITATION STANDARDS FOR AN ASSOCIATE-DEGREE-LEVEL EDUCATIONAL PROGRAM FOR THE OCCUPATIONAL THERAPY ASSISTANT |
|---|---|---|---|
| B.5.15. | Demonstrate safe and effective application of superficial thermal and mechanical modalities as a preparatory measure to manage pain and improve occupational performance, including foundational knowledge, underlying principles, indications, contraindications, and precautions. | Demonstrate safe and effective application of superficial thermal and mechanical modalities as a preparatory measure to manage pain and improve occupational performance, including foundational knowledge, underlying principles, indications, contraindications, and precautions. | Recognize the use of superficial thermal and mechanical modalities as a preparatory measure to improve occupational performance. On the basis of the intervention plan, demonstrate safe and effective administration of superficial thermal and mechanical modalities to achieve established goals while adhering to contraindications and precautions. |
| | *SKILLS, KNOWLEDGE, AND COMPETENCIES FOR ENTRY-LEVEL PRACTICE ARE DERIVED FROM AOTA PRACTICE DOCUMENTS AND NBCOT PRACTICE ANALYSIS STUDIES. SUPERFICIAL THERMAL MODALITIES INCLUDE, BUT ARE NOT LIMITED TO, HYDROTHERAPY/WHIRLPOOL, CRYOTHERAPY (COLD PACKS, ICE), FLUIDOTHERAPY™, HOT PACKS, PARAFFIN, WATER, AND INFRARED. MECHANICAL MODALITIES INCLUDE, BUT ARE NOT LIMITED TO, VASOPNEUMATIC DEVICES AND CONTINUOUS PASSIVE MOTION.*<br>*THE WORD "DEMONSTRATE" DOES NOT REQUIRE THAT A STUDENT ACTUALLY PERFORM THE TASK TO VERIFY KNOWLEDGE AND UNDERSTANDING. THE PROGRAM MAY SELECT THE TYPES OF LEARNING ACTIVITIES AND ASSESSMENTS THAT WILL INDICATE COMPLIANCE WITH THE STANDARD.*<br>*FOR INSTITUTIONS IN STATES WHERE REGULATIONS RESTRICT THE USE OF PHYSICAL AGENT MODALITIES, IT IS RECOMMENDED THAT STUDENTS BE EXPOSED TO THE MODALITIES OFFERED IN PRACTICE TO ALLOW STUDENTS KNOWLEDGE AND EXPERIENCE WITH THE MODALITIES IN PREPARATION FOR THE NBCOT EXAMINATION AND FOR PRACTICE OUTSIDE OF THE STATE IN WHICH THE EDUCATIONAL INSTITUTION RESIDES.* | | |
| B.5.16. | Explain the use of deep thermal and electrotherapeutic modalities as a preparatory measure to improve occupational performance, including indications, contraindications, and precautions. | Explain the use of deep thermal and electrotherapeutic modalities as a preparatory measure to improve occupational performance, including indications, contraindications, and precautions. | *(No related Standard)* |
| | *SKILLS, KNOWLEDGE, AND COMPETENCIES FOR ENTRY-LEVEL PRACTICE ARE DERIVED FROM AOTA PRACTICE DOCUMENTS AND NBCOT PRACTICE ANALYSIS STUDIES. DEEP THERMAL MODALITIES INCLUDE, BUT ARE NOT LIMITED TO, THERAPEUTIC ULTRASOUND AND PHONOPHORESIS. ELECTROTHERAPEUTIC MODALITIES INCLUDE, BUT ARE NOT LIMITED TO, BIOFEEDBACK, NEUROMUSCULAR ELECTRICAL STIMULATION, FUNCTIONAL ELECTRICAL STIMULATION, TRANSCUTANEOUS ELECTRICAL NERVE STIMULATION, ELECTRICAL STIMULATION FOR TISSUE REPAIR, HIGH-VOLTAGE GALVANIC STIMULATION, AND IONTOPHORESIS.* | | |
| B.5.17. | Develop and promote the use of appropriate home and community programming to support performance in the client's natural environment and participation in all contexts relevant to the client. | Develop and promote the use of appropriate home and community programming to support performance in the client's natural environment and participation in all contexts relevant to the client. | Promote the use of appropriate home and community programming to support performance in the client's natural environment and participation in all contexts relevant to the client. |
| B.5.18. | Demonstrate an understanding of health literacy and the ability to educate and train the client, caregiver, family and significant others, and communities to facilitate skills in areas of occupation as well as prevention, health maintenance, health promotion, and safety. | Demonstrate an understanding of health literacy and the ability to educate and train the client, caregiver, family and significant others, and communities to facilitate skills in areas of occupation as well as prevention, health maintenance, health promotion, and safety. | Demonstrate an understanding of health literacy and the ability to educate and train the client, caregiver, and family and significant others to facilitate skills in areas of occupation as well as prevention, health maintenance, health promotion, and safety. |
| B.5.19. | Apply the principles of the teaching–learning process using educational methods to design experiences to address the needs of the client, family, significant others, communities, colleagues, other health providers, and the public. | Apply the principles of the teaching–learning process using educational methods to design experiences to address the needs of the client, family, significant others, colleagues, other health providers, and the public. | Use the teaching–learning process with the client, family, significant others, colleagues, other health providers, and the public. Collaborate with the occupational therapist and learner to identify appropriate educational methods. |

| STANDARD NUMBER | ACCREDITATION STANDARDS FOR A DOCTORAL-DEGREE-LEVEL EDUCATIONAL PROGRAM FOR THE OCCUPATIONAL THERAPIST | ACCREDITATION STANDARDS FOR A MASTER'S-DEGREE-LEVEL EDUCATIONAL PROGRAM FOR THE OCCUPATIONAL THERAPIST | ACCREDITATION STANDARDS FOR AN ASSOCIATE-DEGREE-LEVEL EDUCATIONAL PROGRAM FOR THE OCCUPATIONAL THERAPY ASSISTANT |
|---|---|---|---|
| B.5.20. | Effectively interact through written, oral, and nonverbal communication with the client, family, significant others, communities, colleagues, other health providers, and the public in a professionally acceptable manner. | Effectively interact through written, oral, and nonverbal communication with the client, family, significant others, colleagues, other health providers, and the public in a professionally acceptable manner. | Effectively interact through written, oral, and nonverbal communication with the client, family, significant others, colleagues, other health providers, and the public in a professionally acceptable manner. |
| B.5.21. | Effectively communicate, coordinate, and work interprofessionally with those who provide services for individuals, organizations, and/or populations in order to clarify each member's responsibility in executing components of an intervention plan. | Effectively communicate and work interprofessionally with those who provide services to individuals, organizations, and/or populations in order to clarify each member's responsibility in executing an intervention plan. | Effectively communicate and work interprofessionally with those who provide services to individuals and groups in order to clarify each member's responsibility in executing an intervention plan. |
| B.5.22. | Refer to specialists (both internal and external to the profession) for consultation and intervention. | Refer to specialists (both internal and external to the profession) for consultation and intervention. | Recognize and communicate the need to refer to specialists (both internal and external to the profession) for consultation and intervention. |
| B.5.23. | Grade and adapt the environment, tools, materials, occupations, and interventions to reflect the changing needs of the client, the sociocultural context, and technological advances. | Grade and adapt the environment, tools, materials, occupations, and interventions to reflect the changing needs of the client, the sociocultural context, and technological advances. | Grade and adapt the environment, tools, materials, occupations, and interventions to reflect the changing needs of the client and the sociocultural context. |
| B.5.24. | Select and teach compensatory strategies, such as use of technology and adaptations to the environment that support performance, participation, and well-being. | Select and teach compensatory strategies, such as use of technology and adaptations to the environment, that support performance, participation, and well-being. | Teach compensatory strategies, such as use of technology and adaptations to the environment, that support performance,-participation, and well-being. |
| B.5.25. | Identify and demonstrate techniques in skills of supervision and collaboration with occupational therapy assistants and other professionals on therapeutic interventions. | Identify and demonstrate techniques in skills of supervision and collaboration with occupational therapy assistants and other professionals on therapeutic interventions. | Demonstrate skills of collaboration with occupational therapists and other professionals on therapeutic interventions. |
| B.5.26. | Demonstrate use of the consultative process with groups, programs, organizations, or communities. | Understand when and how to use the consultative process with groups, programs, organizations, or communities. | Understand when and how to use the consultative process with specific consumers or consumer groups as directed by an occupational therapist. |
| B.5.27. | Demonstrate care coordination, case management, and transition services in traditional and emerging practice environments. | Describe the role of the occupational therapist in care coordination, case management, and transition services in traditional and emerging practice environments. | Describe the role of the occupational therapy assistant in care coordination, case management, and transition services in traditional and emerging practice environments. |
| B.5.28. | Monitor and reassess, in collaboration with the client, caregiver, family, and significant others, the effect of occupational therapy intervention and the need for continued or modified intervention. | Monitor and reassess, in collaboration with the client, caregiver, family, and significant others, the effect of occupational therapy intervention and the need for continued or modified intervention. | Monitor and reassess, in collaboration with the client, caregiver, family, and significant others, the effect of occupational therapy intervention and the need for continued or modified intervention, and communicate the identified needs to the occupational therapist. |

| STANDARD NUMBER | ACCREDITATION STANDARDS FOR A DOCTORAL-DEGREE-LEVEL EDUCATIONAL PROGRAM FOR THE OCCUPATIONAL THERAPIST | ACCREDITATION STANDARDS FOR A MASTER'S-DEGREE-LEVEL EDUCATIONAL PROGRAM FOR THE OCCUPATIONAL THERAPIST | ACCREDITATION STANDARDS FOR AN ASSOCIATE-DEGREE-LEVEL EDUCATIONAL PROGRAM FOR THE OCCUPATIONAL THERAPY ASSISTANT |
|---|---|---|---|
| B.5.29. | Plan for discharge, in collaboration with the client, by reviewing the needs of the client, caregiver, family, and significant others; available resources; and discharge environment. This process includes, but is not limited to, identification of client's current status within the continuum of care; identification of community, human, and fiscal resources; recommendations for environmental adaptations; and home programming to facilitate the client's progression along the continuum toward outcome goals. | Plan for discharge, in collaboration with the client, by reviewing the needs of the client, caregiver, family, and significant others; available resources; and discharge environment. This process includes, but is not limited to, identification of client's current status within the continuum of care; identification of community, human, and fiscal resources; recommendations for environmental adaptations; and home programming to facilitate the client's progression along the continuum toward outcome goals. | Facilitate discharge planning by reviewing the needs of the client, caregiver, family, and significant others; available resources; and discharge environment, and identify those needs to the occupational therapist, client, and others involved in discharge planning. This process includes, but is not limited to, identification of community, human, and fiscal resources; recommendations for environmental adaptations; and home programming. |
| B.5.30. | Organize, collect, and analyze data in a systematic manner for evaluation of practice outcomes. Report evaluation results and modify practice as needed to improve client outcomes. | Organize, collect, and analyze data in a systematic manner for evaluation of practice outcomes. Report evaluation results and modify practice as needed to improve client outcomes. | Under the direction of an administrator, manager, or occupational therapist, collect, organize, and report on data for evaluation of client outcomes. |
| B.5.31. | Terminate occupational therapy services when stated outcomes have been achieved or it has been determined that they cannot be achieved. This process includes developing a summary of occupational therapy outcomes, appropriate recommendations, and referrals and discussion of postdischarge needs with the client and with appropriate others. | Terminate occupational therapy services when stated outcomes have been achieved or it has been determined that they cannot be achieved. This process includes developing a summary of occupational therapy outcomes, appropriate recommendations, and referrals and discussion of post-discharge needs with the client and with appropriate others. | Recommend to the occupational therapist the need for termination of occupational therapy services when stated outcomes have been achieved or it has been determined that they cannot be achieved. Assist with developing a summary of occupational therapy outcomes, recommendations, and referrals. |
| B.5.32. | Document occupational therapy services to ensure accountability of service provision and to meet standards for reimbursement of services. Documentation must effectively communicate the need and rationale for occupational therapy services and must be appropriate to the context in which the service is delivered. | Document occupational therapy services to ensure accountability of service provision and to meet standards for reimbursement of services. Documentation must effectively communicate the need and rationale for occupational therapy services and must be appropriate to the context in which the service is delivered. | Document occupational therapy services to ensure accountability of service provision and to meet standards for reimbursement of services. Documentation must effectively communicate the need and rationale for occupational therapy services and must be appropriate to the context in which the service is delivered. |
| B.5.33. | Provide population-based occupational therapy intervention that addresses occupational needs as identified by a community. | *(No related Standard)* | *(No related Standard)* |
| **B.6.0. CONTEXT OF SERVICE DELIVERY**<br>**Context of service delivery includes the knowledge and understanding of the various contexts, such as professional, social, cultural, political, economic, and ecological, in which occupational therapy services are provided. The program must facilitate development of the performance criteria listed below. The student will be able to** | | | |
| B.6.1. | Evaluate and address the various contexts of health care, education, community, political, and social systems as they relate to the practice of occupational therapy. | Evaluate and address the various contexts of health care, education, community, political, and social systems as they relate to the practice of occupational therapy. | Describe the contexts of health care, education, community, and social systems as they relate to the practice of occupational therapy. |
| B.6.2. | Analyze the current policy issues and the social, economic, political, geographic, and demographic | Analyze the current policy issues and the social, economic, political, geographic, and demographic | Identify the potential impact of current policy issues and the social, economic, political, geographic, or |

| STANDARD NUMBER | ACCREDITATION STANDARDS FOR A DOCTORAL-DEGREE-LEVEL EDUCATIONAL PROGRAM FOR THE OCCUPATIONAL THERAPIST | ACCREDITATION STANDARDS FOR A MASTER'S-DEGREE-LEVEL EDUCATIONAL PROGRAM FOR THE OCCUPATIONAL THERAPIST | ACCREDITATION STANDARDS FOR AN ASSOCIATE-DEGREE-LEVEL EDUCATIONAL PROGRAM FOR THE OCCUPATIONAL THERAPY ASSISTANT |
|---|---|---|---|
| | factors that influence the various contexts for practice of occupational therapy. | factors that influence the various contexts for practice of occupational therapy. | demographic factors on the practice of occupational therapy. |
| B.6.3. | Integrate current social, economic, political, geographic, and demographic factors to promote policy development and the provision of occupational therapy services. | Integrate current social, economic, political, geographic, and demographic factors to promote policy development and the provision of occupational therapy services. | *(No related Standard)* |
| B.6.4. | Advocate for changes in service delivery policies, effect changes in the system, and identify opportunities to address societal needs. | Articulate the role and responsibility of the practitioner to advocate for changes in service delivery policies, to effect changes in the system, and to identify opportunities in emerging practice areas. | Identify the role and responsibility of the practitioner to advocate for changes in service delivery policies, to effect changes in the system, and to recognize opportunities in emerging practice areas. |
| B.6.5. | Analyze the trends in models of service delivery, including, but not limited to, medical, educational, community and social models, and their potential effect on the practice of occupational therapy. | Analyze the trends in models of service delivery, including, but not limited to, medical, educational, community, and social models, and their potential effect on the practice of occupational therapy. | *(No related Standard)* |
| B.6.6. | Integrate national and international resources in education, research, practice, and policy development. | Utilize national and international resources in making assessment or intervention choices and appreciate the influence of international occupational therapy contributions to education, research, and practice. | *(No related Standard)* |
| **B.7.0.** | **LEADERSHIP AND MANAGEMENT**<br>**Leadership and management skills include principles and applications of leadership and management theory. The program must facilitate development of the performance criteria listed below. The student will be able to** | **MANAGEMENT OF OCCUPATIONAL THERAPY SERVICES**<br>**Management of occupational therapy services includes the application of principles of management and systems in the provision of occupational therapy services to individuals and organizations. The program must facilitate development of the performance criteria listed below. The student will be able to** | **ASSISTANCE WITH MANAGEMENT OF OCCUPATIONAL THERAPY SERVICES**<br>**Assistance with management of occupational therapy services includes the application of principles of management and systems in the provision of occupational therapy services to individuals and organizations. The program must facilitate development of the performance criteria listed below. The student will be able to** |
| B.7.1. | Identify and evaluate the impact of contextual factors on the management and delivery of occupational therapy services for individuals and populations. | Describe and discuss the impact of contextual factors on the management and delivery of occupational therapy services. | Identify the impact of contextual factors on the management and delivery of occupational therapy services. |
| B.7.2. | Identify and evaluate the systems and structures that create federal and state legislation and regulations and their implications and effects on practice and policy. | Describe the systems and structures that create federal and state legislation and regulations and their implications and effects on practice. | Identify the systems and structures that create federal and state legislation and regulations and their implications and effects on practice. |
| B.7.3. | Demonstrate knowledge of applicable national requirements for credentialing and requirements for licensure, certification, or registration under state laws. | Demonstrate knowledge of applicable national requirements for credentialing and requirements for licensure, certification, or registration under state laws. | Demonstrate knowledge of applicable national requirements for credentialing and requirements for licensure, certification, or registration under state laws. |
| B.7.4. | Demonstrate knowledge of various reimbursement systems (e.g., federal, state, third party, private payer), appeals mechanisms, and documentation requirements that affect society and the practice of | Demonstrate knowledge of various reimbursement systems (e.g., federal, state, third party, private payer), appeals mechanisms, and documentation requirements that affect the practice of occupational | Demonstrate knowledge of various reimbursement systems (e.g., federal, state, third party, private payer) and documentation requirements that affect |

| STANDARD NUMBER | ACCREDITATION STANDARDS FOR A DOCTORAL-DEGREE-LEVEL EDUCATIONAL PROGRAM FOR THE OCCUPATIONAL THERAPIST | ACCREDITATION STANDARDS FOR A MASTER'S-DEGREE-LEVEL EDUCATIONAL PROGRAM FOR THE OCCUPATIONAL THERAPIST | ACCREDITATION STANDARDS FOR AN ASSOCIATE-DEGREE-LEVEL EDUCATIONAL PROGRAM FOR THE OCCUPATIONAL THERAPY ASSISTANT |
|---|---|---|---|
| | occupational therapy | therapy. | the practice of occupational therapy. |
| B.7.5. | Demonstrate leadership skills in the ability to plan, develop, organize, and market the delivery of services to include the determination of programmatic needs and service delivery options and formulation and management of staffing for effective service provision. | Demonstrate the ability to plan, develop, organize, and market the delivery of services to include the determination of programmatic needs and service delivery options and formulation and management of staffing for effective service provision. | Demonstrate the ability to participate in the development, marketing, and management of service delivery options. |
| B.7.6. | Demonstrate leadership skills in the ability to design ongoing processes for quality improvement (e.g., outcome studies analysis) and develop program changes as needed to ensure quality of services and to direct administrative changes. | Demonstrate the ability to design ongoing processes for quality improvement (e.g., outcome studies analysis) and develop program changes as needed to ensure quality of services and to direct administrative changes. | Participate in the documentation of ongoing processes for quality improvement and implement program changes as needed to ensure quality of services. |
| B.7.7. | Develop strategies for effective, competency-based legal and ethical supervision of occupational therapy and non–occupational therapy personnel. | Develop strategies for effective, competency-based legal and ethical supervision of occupational therapy and non–occupational therapy personnel. | Identify strategies for effective, competency-based legal and ethical supervision of nonprofessional personnel. |
| B.7.8. | Describe the ongoing professional responsibility for providing fieldwork education and the criteria for becoming a fieldwork educator. | Describe the ongoing professional responsibility for providing fieldwork education and the criteria for becoming a fieldwork educator. | Describe the ongoing professional responsibility for providing fieldwork education and the criteria for becoming a fieldwork educator. |
| B.7.9. | Demonstrate knowledge of and the ability to write program development plans for provision of occupational therapy services to individuals and populations. | *(No related Standard)* | *(No related Standard)* |
| B.7.10. | Identify and adapt existing models or develop new service provision models to respond to policy, regulatory agencies, and reimbursement and compliance standards. | *(No related Standard)* | *(No related Standard)* |
| B.7.11. | Identify and develop strategies to enable occupational therapy to respond to society's changing needs. | *(No related Standard)* | *(No related Standard)* |
| B.7.12. | Identify and implement strategies to promote staff development that are based on evaluation of the personal and professional abilities and competencies of supervised staff as they relate to job responsibilities. | *(No related Standard)* | *(No related Standard)* |
| **B.8.0. SCHOLARSHIP**<br>**Promotion of scholarly endeavors will serve to describe and interpret the scope of the profession, establish new knowledge, and interpret and apply this knowledge to practice. The program must facilitate development of the performance criteria listed below. The student will be able to** | | | |
| B.8.1. | Articulate the importance of how scholarly activities contribute to the development of a body of knowledge relevant to the profession of occupational therapy. | Articulate the importance of how scholarly activities contribute to the development of a body of knowledge relevant to the profession of occupational therapy. | Articulate the importance of how scholarly activities and literature contribute to the development of the profession. |

| STANDARD NUMBER | ACCREDITATION STANDARDS FOR A DOCTORAL-DEGREE-LEVEL EDUCATIONAL PROGRAM FOR THE OCCUPATIONAL THERAPIST | ACCREDITATION STANDARDS FOR A MASTER'S-DEGREE-LEVEL EDUCATIONAL PROGRAM FOR THE OCCUPATIONAL THERAPIST | ACCREDITATION STANDARDS FOR AN ASSOCIATE-DEGREE-LEVEL EDUCATIONAL PROGRAM FOR THE OCCUPATIONAL THERAPY ASSISTANT |
|---|---|---|---|
| B.8.2. | Effectively locate, understand, critique, and evaluate information, including the quality of evidence. | Effectively locate, understand, critique, and evaluate information, including the quality of evidence. | Effectively locate and understand information, including the quality of the source of information. |
| B.8.3. | Use scholarly literature to make evidence-based decisions. | Use scholarly literature to make evidence-based decisions. | Use professional literature to make evidence-based practice decisions in collaboration with the occupational therapist.. |
| B.8.4. | Select, apply, and interpret basic descriptive, correlational, and inferential quantitative statistics and code, analyze, and synthesize qualitative data. | Understand and use basic descriptive, correlational, and inferential quantitative statistics and code, analyze, and synthesize qualitative data. | *(No related Standard)* |
| B.8.5. | Understand and critique the validity of research studies, including their design (both quantitative and qualitative) and methodology. | Understand and critique the validity of research studies, including their design (both quantitative and qualitative) and methodology. | *(No related Standard)* |
| B.8.6. | Design a scholarly proposal that includes the research question, relevant literature, sample, design, measurement, and data analysis. | Demonstrate the skills necessary to design a scholarly proposal that includes the research question, relevant literature, sample, design, measurement, and data analysis. | *(No related Standard)* |
| B.8.7. | Implement a scholarly study that evaluates professional practice, service delivery, and/or professional issues (e.g., Scholarship of Integration, Scholarship of Application, Scholarship of Teaching and Learning). | Participate in scholarly activities that evaluate professional practice, service delivery, and/or professional issues (e.g., Scholarship of Integration, Scholarship of Application, Scholarship of Teaching and Learning). | Identify how scholarly activities can be used to evaluate professional practice, service delivery, and/or professional issues (e.g., Scholarship of Integration, Scholarship of Application, Scholarship of Teaching and Learning). |
| | | *THE INTENT OF STANDARD B.8.7 IS TO EMPHASIZE THE "DOING" PART OF THE RESEARCH PROCESS THAT CAN SUPPORT BEGINNING RESEARCH SKILLS IN A PRACTICE SETTING. SYSTEMATIC REVIEWS THAT REQUIRE ANALYSIS AND SYNTHESIS OF DATA MEET THE REQUIREMENT FOR THIS STANDARD. NARRATIVE REVIEWS DO NOT MEET THIS STANDARD.*<br><br>*A CULMINATING PROJECT RELATED TO RESEARCH IS NOT REQUIRED FOR THE MASTER'S LEVEL. IF IT IS CONSISTENT WITH THE PROGRAM'S CURRICULUM DESIGN AND GOALS, THE PROGRAM MAY CHOOSE TO REQUIRE A CULMINATING RESEARCH LEARNING ACTIVITY (E.G., SYSTEMATIC REVIEW OF LITERATURE, FACULTY-LED RESEARCH ACTIVITY, STUDENT RESEARCH PROJECT).* | |
| B.8.8. | Write scholarly reports appropriate for presentation or for publication in a peer-reviewed journal. Examples of scholarly reports would include position papers, white papers, and persuasive discussion papers. | Demonstrate skills necessary to write a scholarly report in a format for presentation or publication. | Demonstrate the skills to read and understand a scholarly report. |
| B.8.9. | Demonstrate an understanding of the process of locating and securing grants and how grants can serve as a fiscal resource for scholarly activities. | Demonstrate an understanding of the process of locating and securing grants and how grants can serve as a fiscal resource for scholarly activities. | *(No related Standard)* |

| STANDARD NUMBER | ACCREDITATION STANDARDS FOR A DOCTORAL-DEGREE-LEVEL EDUCATIONAL PROGRAM FOR THE OCCUPATIONAL THERAPIST | ACCREDITATION STANDARDS FOR A MASTER'S-DEGREE-LEVEL EDUCATIONAL PROGRAM FOR THE OCCUPATIONAL THERAPIST | ACCREDITATION STANDARDS FOR AN ASSOCIATE-DEGREE-LEVEL EDUCATIONAL PROGRAM FOR THE OCCUPATIONAL THERAPY ASSISTANT |
|---|---|---|---|
| B.8.10. | Complete a culminating project that relates theory to practice and demonstrates synthesis of advanced knowledge in a practice area. | *(No related Standard)* | *(No related Standard)* |
| **B.9.0. PROFESSIONAL ETHICS, VALUES, AND RESPONSIBILITIES**<br>**Professional ethics, values, and responsibilities include an understanding and appreciation of ethics and values of the profession of occupational therapy. The program must facilitate development of the performance criteria listed below. The student will be able to** | | | |
| B.9.1. | Demonstrate knowledge and understanding of the American Occupational Therapy Association (AOTA) *Occupational Therapy Code of Ethics and Ethics Standards* and AOTA *Standards of Practice* and use them as a guide for ethical decision making in professional interactions, client interventions, and employment settings. | Demonstrate knowledge and understanding of the American Occupational Therapy Association (AOTA) *Occupational Therapy Code of Ethics and Ethics Standards* and AOTA *Standards of Practice* and use them as a guide for ethical decision making in professional interactions, client interventions, and employment settings. | Demonstrate knowledge and understanding of the American Occupational Therapy Association (AOTA) *Occupational Therapy Code of Ethics and Ethics Standards* and AOTA *Standards of Practice* and use them as a guide for ethical decision making in professional interactions, client interventions, and employment settings. |
| B.9.2. | Discuss and justify how the role of a professional is enhanced by knowledge of and involvement in international, national, state, and local occupational therapy associations and related professional associations. | Discuss and justify how the role of a professional is enhanced by knowledge of and involvement in international, national, state, and local occupational therapy associations and related professional associations. | Explain and give examples of how the role of a professional is enhanced by knowledge of and involvement in international, national, state, and local occupational therapy associations and related professional associations. |
| B.9.3. | Promote occupational therapy by educating other professionals, service providers, consumers, third-party payers, regulatory bodies, and the public. | Promote occupational therapy by educating other professionals, service providers, consumers, third-party payers, regulatory bodies, and the public. | Promote occupational therapy by educating other professionals, service providers, consumers, third-party payers, regulatory bodies, and the public. |
| B.9.4. | Identify and develop strategies for ongoing professional development to ensure that practice is consistent with current and accepted standards. | Discuss strategies for ongoing professional development to ensure that practice is consistent with current and accepted standards. | Discuss strategies for ongoing professional development to ensure that practice is consistent with current and accepted standards. |
| B.9.5. | Discuss professional responsibilities related to liability issues under current models of service provision. | Discuss professional responsibilities related to liability issues under current models of service provision. | Identify professional responsibilities related to liability issues under current models of service provision. |
| B.9.6. | Discuss and evaluate personal and professional abilities and competencies as they relate to job responsibilities. | Discuss and evaluate personal and professional abilities and competencies as they relate to job responsibilities. | Identify personal and professional abilities and competencies as they relate to job responsibilities. |
| B.9.7. | Discuss and justify the varied roles of the occupational therapist as a practitioner, educator, researcher, policy developer, program developer, advocate, administrator, consultant, and entrepreneur. | Discuss and justify the varied roles of the occupational therapist as a practitioner, educator, researcher, consultant, and entrepreneur. | Identify and appreciate the varied roles of the occupational therapy assistant as a practitioner, educator, and research assistant. |
| B.9.8. | Explain and justify the importance of supervisory roles, responsibilities, and collaborative professional relationships between the occupational therapist and the occupational therapy assistant. | Explain and justify the importance of supervisory roles, responsibilities, and collaborative professional relationships between the occupational therapist and the occupational therapy assistant. | Identify and explain the need for supervisory roles, responsibilities, and collaborative professional relationships between the occupational therapist and the occupational therapy assistant. |

| STANDARD NUMBER | ACCREDITATION STANDARDS FOR A DOCTORAL-DEGREE-LEVEL EDUCATIONAL PROGRAM FOR THE OCCUPATIONAL THERAPIST | ACCREDITATION STANDARDS FOR A MASTER'S-DEGREE-LEVEL EDUCATIONAL PROGRAM FOR THE OCCUPATIONAL THERAPIST | ACCREDITATION STANDARDS FOR AN ASSOCIATE-DEGREE-LEVEL EDUCATIONAL PROGRAM FOR THE OCCUPATIONAL THERAPY ASSISTANT |
|---|---|---|---|
| B.9.9. | Describe and discuss professional responsibilities and issues when providing service on a contractual basis. | Describe and discuss professional responsibilities and issues when providing service on a contractual basis. | Identify professional responsibilities and issues when providing service on a contractual basis. |
| B.9.10. | Demonstrate strategies for analyzing issues and making decisions to resolve personal and organizational ethical conflicts. | Demonstrate strategies for analyzing issues and making decisions to resolve personal and organizational ethical conflicts. | Identify strategies for analyzing issues and making decisions to resolve personal and organizational ethical conflicts. |
| B.9.11. | Demonstrate a variety of informal and formal strategies for resolving ethics disputes in varying practice areas. | Explain the variety of informal and formal systems for resolving ethics disputes that have jurisdiction over occupational therapy practice. | Identify the variety of informal and formal systems for resolving ethics disputes that have jurisdiction over occupational therapy practice. |
| B.9.12. | Describe and implement strategies to assist the consumer in gaining access to occupational therapy and other health and social services. | Describe and discuss strategies to assist the consumer in gaining access to occupational therapy services. | Identify strategies to assist the consumer in gaining access to occupational therapy services. |
| B.9.13. | Demonstrate advocacy by participating in and exploring leadership positions in organizations or agencies promoting the profession (e.g., AOTA, state occupational therapy associations, World Federation of Occupational Therapists, advocacy organizations), consumer access and services, and the welfare of the community. | Demonstrate professional advocacy by participating in organizations or agencies promoting the profession (e.g., AOTA, state occupational therapy associations, advocacy organizations). | Demonstrate professional advocacy by participating in organizations or agencies promoting the profession (e.g., AOTA, state occupational therapy associations, advocacy organizations). |
| **SECTION C: FIELDWORK EDUCATION AND DOCTORAL EXPERIENTIAL COMPONENT** | | | |
| **C.1.0: FIELDWORK EDUCATION**<br>**Fieldwork education is a crucial part of professional preparation and is best integrated as a component of the curriculum design. Fieldwork experiences should be implemented and evaluated for their effectiveness by the educational institution. The experience should provide the student with the opportunity to carry out professional responsibilities under supervision of a qualified occupational therapy practitioner serving as a role model. The academic fieldwork coordinator is responsible for the program's compliance with fieldwork education requirements. The academic fieldwork coordinator will** | | | |
| C.1.1. | Ensure that the fieldwork program reflects the sequence and scope of content in the curriculum design in collaboration with faculty so that fieldwork experiences strengthen the ties between didactic and fieldwork education. | Ensure that the fieldwork program reflects the sequence and scope of content in the curriculum design in collaboration with faculty so that fieldwork experiences strengthen the ties between didactic and fieldwork education. | Ensure that the fieldwork program reflects the sequence and scope of content in the curriculum design in collaboration with faculty so that fieldwork experiences strengthen the ties between didactic and fieldwork education. |
| C.1.2. | Document the criteria and process for selecting fieldwork sites, to include maintaining memoranda of understanding, complying with all site requirements, maintaining site objectives and site data, and communicating this information to students. | Document the criteria and process for selecting fieldwork sites, to include maintaining memoranda of understanding, complying with all site requirements, maintaining site objectives and site data, and communicating this information to students. | Document the criteria and process for selecting fieldwork sites, to include maintaining memoranda of understanding, complying with all site requirements, maintaining site objectives and site data, and communicating this information to students. |
| C.1.3. | Demonstrate that academic and fieldwork educators collaborate in establishing fieldwork objectives and communicate with the student and fieldwork educator about progress and performance during fieldwork. | Demonstrate that academic and fieldwork educators collaborate in establishing fieldwork objectives and communicate with the student and fieldwork educator about progress and performance during fieldwork. | Demonstrate that academic and fieldwork educators collaborate in establishing fieldwork objectives and communicate with the student and fieldwork educator about progress and performance during fieldwork. |

| STANDARD NUMBER | ACCREDITATION STANDARDS FOR A DOCTORAL-DEGREE-LEVEL EDUCATIONAL PROGRAM FOR THE OCCUPATIONAL THERAPIST | ACCREDITATION STANDARDS FOR A MASTER'S-DEGREE-LEVEL EDUCATIONAL PROGRAM FOR THE OCCUPATIONAL THERAPIST | ACCREDITATION STANDARDS FOR AN ASSOCIATE-DEGREE-LEVEL EDUCATIONAL PROGRAM FOR THE OCCUPATIONAL THERAPY ASSISTANT |
|---|---|---|---|
| C.1.4. | Ensure that the ratio of fieldwork educators to students enables proper supervision and the ability to provide frequent assessment of student progress in achieving stated fieldwork objectives. | Ensure that the ratio of fieldwork educators to students enables proper supervision and the ability to provide frequent assessment of student progress in achieving stated fieldwork objectives. | Ensure that the ratio of fieldwork educators to students enables proper supervision and the ability to provide frequent assessment of student progress in achieving stated fieldwork objectives. |
| C.1.5. | Ensure that fieldwork agreements are sufficient in scope and number to allow completion of graduation requirements in a timely manner in accordance with the policy adopted by the program as required by Standard A.4.14. | Ensure that fieldwork agreements are sufficient in scope and number to allow completion of graduation requirements in a timely manner in accordance with the policy adopted by the program as required by Standard A.4.14. | Ensure that fieldwork agreements are sufficient in scope and number to allow completion of graduation requirements in a timely manner in accordance with the policy adopted by the program as required by Standard A.4.14. |
| C.1.6. | The program must have evidence of valid memoranda of understanding in effect and signed by both parties at the time the student is completing the Level I or Level II fieldwork experience. (Electronic memoranda of understanding and signatures are acceptable.) Responsibilities of the sponsoring institution(s) and each fieldwork site must be clearly documented in the memorandum of understanding. | The program must have evidence of valid memoranda of understanding in effect and signed by both parties at the time the student is completing the Level I or Level II fieldwork experience. (Electronic memoranda of understanding and signatures are acceptable.) Responsibilities of the sponsoring institution(s) and each fieldwork site must be clearly documented in the memorandum of understanding. | The program must have evidence of valid memoranda of understanding in effect and signed by both parties at the time the student is completing the Level I or Level II fieldwork experience. (Electronic memoranda of understanding and signatures are acceptable.) Responsibilities of the sponsoring institution(s) and each fieldwork site must be clearly documented in the memorandum of understanding. |
| | *IF A FIELD TRIP, OBSERVATION, OR SERVICE LEARNING ACTIVITY IS USED TO COUNT TOWARD PART OF LEVEL I FIELDWORK, THEN A MEMORANDUM OF UNDERSTANDING IS REQUIRED. IF A FIELD TRIP, OBSERVATION, OR SERVICE LEARNING ACTIVITY IS NOT USED TO COUNT TOWARD PART OF LEVEL I FIELDWORK, THEN NO MEMORANDUM OF UNDERSTANDING IS REQUIRED.*<br><br>*WHEN A MEMORANDUM OF UNDERSTANDING IS ESTABLISHED WITH A MULTISITE SERVICE PROVIDER (E.G., CONTRACT AGENCY, CORPORATE ENTITY), THE ACOTE STANDARDS DO NOT REQUIRE A SEPARATE MEMORANDUM OF UNDERSTANDING WITH EACH PRACTICE SITE.* | | |
| C.1.7. | Ensure that at least one fieldwork experience (either Level I or Level II) has as its focus psychological and social factors that influence engagement in occupation | Ensure that at least one fieldwork experience (either Level I or Level II) has as its focus psychological and social factors that influence engagement in occupation. | Ensure that at least one fieldwork experience (either Level I or Level II) has as its focus psychological and social factors that influence engagement in occupation. |
| **The goal of Level I fieldwork is to introduce students to the fieldwork experience, to apply knowledge to practice, and to develop understanding of the needs of clients. The program will** | | | |
| C.1.8. | Ensure that Level I fieldwork is integral to the program's curriculum design and include experiences designed to enrich didactic coursework through directed observation and participation in selected aspects of the occupational therapy process. | Ensure that Level I fieldwork is integral to the program's curriculum design and include experiences designed to enrich didactic coursework through directed observation and participation in selected aspects of the occupational therapy process. | Ensure that Level I fieldwork is integral to the program's curriculum design and include experiences designed to enrich didactic coursework through directed observation and participation in selected aspects of the occupational therapy process. |
| C.1.9. | Ensure that qualified personnel supervise Level I fieldwork. Examples may include, but are not limited to, currently licensed or otherwise regulated occupational therapists and occupational therapy assistants, psychologists, physician assistants, teachers, social workers, nurses, and physical therapists. | Ensure that qualified personnel supervise Level I fieldwork. Examples may include, but are not limited to, currently licensed or otherwise regulated occupational therapists and occupational therapy assistants, psychologists, physician assistants, teachers, social workers, nurses, and physical therapists. | Ensure that qualified personnel supervise Level I fieldwork. Examples may include, but are not limited to, currently licensed or otherwise regulated occupational therapists and occupational therapy assistants, psychologists, physician assistants, teachers, social workers, nurses, and physical therapists. |

| STANDARD NUMBER | ACCREDITATION STANDARDS FOR A DOCTORAL-DEGREE-LEVEL EDUCATIONAL PROGRAM FOR THE OCCUPATIONAL THERAPIST | ACCREDITATION STANDARDS FOR A MASTER'S-DEGREE-LEVEL EDUCATIONAL PROGRAM FOR THE OCCUPATIONAL THERAPIST | ACCREDITATION STANDARDS FOR AN ASSOCIATE-DEGREE-LEVEL EDUCATIONAL PROGRAM FOR THE OCCUPATIONAL THERAPY ASSISTANT |
|---|---|---|---|
| C.1.10. | Document all Level I fieldwork experiences that are provided to students, including mechanisms for formal evaluation of student performance. Ensure that Level I fieldwork is not substituted for any part of Level II fieldwork. | Document all Level I fieldwork experiences that are provided to students, including mechanisms for formal evaluation of student performance. Ensure that Level I fieldwork is not substituted for any part of Level II fieldwork. | Document all Level I fieldwork experiences that are provided to students, including mechanisms for formal evaluation of student performance. Ensure that Level I fieldwork is not substituted for any part of Level II fieldwork. |
| **The goal of Level II fieldwork is to develop competent, entry-level, generalist occupational therapists. Level II fieldwork must be integral to the program's curriculum design and must include an in-depth experience in delivering occupational therapy services to clients, focusing on the application of purposeful and meaningful occupation and research, administration, and management of occupational therapy services. It is recommended that the student be exposed to a variety of clients across the lifespan and to a variety of settings. The program will** | | | **The goal of Level II fieldwork is to develop competent, entry-level, generalist occupational therapy assistants. Level II fieldwork must be integral to the program's curriculum design and must include an in-depth experience in delivering occupational therapy services to clients, focusing on the application of purposeful and meaningful occupation. It is recommended that the student be exposed to a variety of clients across the lifespan and to a variety of settings. The program will** |
| C.1.11. | Ensure that the fieldwork experience is designed to promote clinical reasoning and reflective practice, to transmit the values and beliefs that enable ethical practice, and to develop professionalism and competence in career responsibilities. | Ensure that the fieldwork experience is designed to promote clinical reasoning and reflective practice, to transmit the values and beliefs that enable ethical practice, and to develop professionalism and competence in career responsibilities. | Ensure that the fieldwork experience is designed to promote clinical reasoning appropriate to the occupational therapy assistant role, to transmit the values and beliefs that enable ethical practice, and to develop professionalism and competence in career responsibilities. |
| C.1.12. | Provide Level II fieldwork in traditional and/or emerging settings, consistent with the curriculum design. In all settings, psychosocial factors influencing engagement in occupation must be understood and integrated for the development of client-centered, meaningful, occupation-based outcomes. The student can complete Level II fieldwork in a minimum of one setting if it is reflective of more than one practice area, or in a maximum of four different settings. | Provide Level II fieldwork in traditional and/or emerging settings, consistent with the curriculum design. In all settings, psychosocial factors influencing engagement in occupation must be understood and integrated for the development of client-centered, meaningful, occupation-based outcomes. The student can complete Level II fieldwork in a minimum of one setting if it is reflective of more than one practice area, or in a maximum of four different settings. | Provide Level II fieldwork in traditional and/or emerging settings, consistent with the curriculum design. In all settings, psychosocial factors influencing engagement in occupation must be understood and integrated for the development of client-centered, meaningful, occupation-based outcomes. The student can complete Level II fieldwork in a minimum of one setting if it is reflective of more than one practice area, or in a maximum of three different settings. |
| C.1.13. | Require a minimum of 24 weeks' full-time Level II fieldwork. This may be completed on a part-time basis, as defined by the fieldwork placement in accordance with the fieldwork placement's usual and customary personnel policies, as long as it is at least 50% of an FTE at that site. | Require a minimum of 24 weeks' full-time Level II fieldwork. This may be completed on a part-time basis, as defined by the fieldwork placement in accordance with the fieldwork placement's usual and customary personnel policies, as long as it is at least 50% of an FTE at that site. | Require a minimum of 16 weeks' full-time Level II fieldwork. This may be completed on a part-time basis, as defined by the fieldwork placement in accordance with the fieldwork placement's usual and customary personnel policies, as long as it is at least 50% of an FTE at that site. |

| STANDARD NUMBER | ACCREDITATION STANDARDS FOR A DOCTORAL-DEGREE-LEVEL EDUCATIONAL PROGRAM FOR THE OCCUPATIONAL THERAPIST | ACCREDITATION STANDARDS FOR A MASTER'S-DEGREE-LEVEL EDUCATIONAL PROGRAM FOR THE OCCUPATIONAL THERAPIST | ACCREDITATION STANDARDS FOR AN ASSOCIATE-DEGREE-LEVEL EDUCATIONAL PROGRAM FOR THE OCCUPATIONAL THERAPY ASSISTANT |
|---|---|---|---|
| C.1.14. | Ensure that the student is supervised by a currently licensed or otherwise regulated occupational therapist who has a minimum of 1 year full-time (or its equivalent) of practice experience subsequent to initial certification and who is adequately prepared to serve as a fieldwork educator. The supervising therapist may be engaged by the fieldwork site or by the educational program. | Ensure that the student is supervised by a currently licensed or otherwise regulated occupational therapist who has a minimum of 1 year full-time (or its equivalent) of practice experience subsequent to initial certification and who is adequately prepared to serve as a fieldwork educator. The supervising therapist may be engaged by the fieldwork site or by the educational program. | Ensure that the student is supervised by a currently licensed or otherwise regulated occupational therapist or occupational therapy assistant (under the supervision of an occupational therapist) who has a minimum of 1 year full-time (or its equivalent) of practice experience subsequent to initial certification and who is adequately prepared to serve as a fieldwork educator. The supervising therapist may be engaged by the fieldwork site or by the educational program. |
| C.1.15. | Document a mechanism for evaluating the effectiveness of supervision (e.g., student evaluation of fieldwork) and for providing resources for enhancing supervision (e.g., materials on supervisory skills, continuing education opportunities, articles on theory and practice). | Document a mechanism for evaluating the effectiveness of supervision (e.g., student evaluation of fieldwork) and for providing resources for enhancing supervision (e.g., materials on supervisory skills, continuing education opportunities, articles on theory and practice). | Document a mechanism for evaluating the effectiveness of supervision (e.g., student evaluation of fieldwork) and for providing resources for enhancing supervision (e.g., materials on supervisory skills, continuing education opportunities, articles on theory and practice). |
| C.1.16. | Ensure that supervision provides protection of consumers and opportunities for appropriate role modeling of occupational therapy practice. Initially, supervision should be direct and then decrease to less direct supervision as appropriate for the setting, the severity of the client's condition, and the ability of the student. | Ensure that supervision provides protection of consumers and opportunities for appropriate role modeling of occupational therapy practice. Initially, supervision should be direct and then decrease to less direct supervision as appropriate for the setting, the severity of the client's condition, and the ability of the student. | Ensure that supervision provides protection of consumers and opportunities for appropriate role modeling of occupational therapy practice. Initially, supervision should be direct and then decrease to less direct supervision as appropriate for the setting, the severity of the client's condition, and the ability of the student. |
| C.1.17. | Ensure that supervision provided in a setting where no occupational therapy services exist includes a documented plan for provision of occupational therapy services and supervision by a currently licensed otherwise regulated occupational therapist with at least 3 years' full-time or its equivalent of professional experience. Supervision must include a minimum of 8 hours of direct supervision each week of the fieldwork experience. An occupational therapy supervisor must be available, via a variety of contact measures, to the student during all working hours. An on-site supervisor designee of another profession must be assigned while the occupational therapy supervisor is off site. | Ensure that supervision provided in a setting where no occupational therapy services exist includes a documented plan for provision of occupational therapy services and supervision by a currently licensed or otherwise regulated occupational therapist with at least 3 years' full-time or its equivalent of professional experience. Supervision must include a minimum of 8 hours of direct supervision each week of the fieldwork experience. An occupational therapy supervisor must be available, via a variety of contact measures, to the student during all working hours. An on-site supervisor designee of another profession must be assigned while the occupational therapy supervisor is off site. | Ensure that supervision provided in a setting where no occupational therapy services exist includes a documented plan for provision of occupational therapy assistant services and supervision by a currently licensed or otherwise regulated occupational therapist or occupational therapy assistant (under the direction of an occupational therapist) with at least 3 years' full-time or its equivalent of professional experience. Supervision must include a minimum of 8 hours of direct supervision each week of the fieldwork experience. An occupational therapy supervisor must be available, via a variety of contact measures, to the student during all working hours. An on-site supervisor designee of another profession must be assigned while the occupational therapy supervisor is off site. |

| STANDARD NUMBER | ACCREDITATION STANDARDS FOR A DOCTORAL-DEGREE-LEVEL EDUCATIONAL PROGRAM FOR THE OCCUPATIONAL THERAPIST | ACCREDITATION STANDARDS FOR A MASTER'S-DEGREE-LEVEL EDUCATIONAL PROGRAM FOR THE OCCUPATIONAL THERAPIST | ACCREDITATION STANDARDS FOR AN ASSOCIATE-DEGREE-LEVEL EDUCATIONAL PROGRAM FOR THE OCCUPATIONAL THERAPY ASSISTANT |
|---|---|---|---|
| C.1.18. | Document mechanisms for requiring formal evaluation of student performance on Level II fieldwork (e.g., the AOTA *Fieldwork Performance Evaluation for the Occupational Therapy Student* or equivalent). | Document mechanisms for requiring formal evaluation of student performance on Level II fieldwork (e.g., the AOTA *Fieldwork Performance Evaluation for the Occupational Therapy Student* or equivalent). | Document mechanisms for requiring formal evaluation of student performance on Level II fieldwork (e.g., the AOTA *Fieldwork Performance Evaluation for the Occupational Therapy Assistant Student* or equivalent). |
| C.1.19. | Ensure that students attending Level II fieldwork outside the United States are supervised by an occupational therapist who graduated from a program approved by the World Federation of Occupational Therapists and has 1 year of experience in practice. | Ensure that students attending Level II fieldwork outside the United States are supervised by an occupational therapist who graduated from a program approved by the World Federation of Occupational Therapists and has 1 year of experience in practice. | Ensure that students attending Level II fieldwork outside the United States are supervised by an occupational therapist who graduated from a program approved by the World Federation of Occupational Therapists and has 1 year of experience in practice. |
| **C.2.0. DOCTORAL EXPERIENTIAL COMPONENT**<br><br>**The goal of the doctoral experiential component is to develop occupational therapists with advanced skills (those that are beyond a generalist level). The doctoral experiential component shall be an integral part of the program's curriculum design and shall include an in-depth experience in one or more of the following: clinical practice skills, research skills, administration, leadership, program and policy development, advocacy, education, or theory development.**<br><br>**The student must successfully complete all coursework and Level II fieldwork and pass a competency requirement prior to the commencement of the doctoral experiential component. The specific content and format of the competency requirement is determined by the program. Examples include a written comprehensive exam, oral exam, NBCOT certification exam readiness tool, and the NBCOT practice exams.** | | | |
| C.2.1. | Ensure that the doctoral experiential component is designed and administered by faculty and provided in setting(s) consistent with the program's curriculum design, including individualized specific objectives and plans for supervision. | *(No related Standard)* | *(No related Standard)* |
| C.2.2. | Ensure that there is a memorandum of understanding that, at a minimum, includes individualized specific objectives, plans for supervision or mentoring, and responsibilities of all parties. | *(No related Standard)* | *(No related Standard)* |
| C.2.3. | Require that the length of this doctoral experiential component be a minimum of 16 weeks (640 hours). This may be completed on a part-time basis and must be consistent with the individualized specific objectives and culminating project. No more than 20% of the 640 hours can be completed outside of | *(No related Standard)* | *(No related Standard)* |

| STANDARD NUMBER | ACCREDITATION STANDARDS FOR A DOCTORAL-DEGREE-LEVEL EDUCATIONAL PROGRAM FOR THE OCCUPATIONAL THERAPIST | ACCREDITATION STANDARDS FOR A MASTER'S-DEGREE-LEVEL EDUCATIONAL PROGRAM FOR THE OCCUPATIONAL THERAPIST | ACCREDITATION STANDARDS FOR AN ASSOCIATE-DEGREE-LEVEL EDUCATIONAL PROGRAM FOR THE OCCUPATIONAL THERAPY ASSISTANT |
|---|---|---|---|
| | the mentored practice setting(s). Prior fieldwork or work experience may not be substituted for this experiential component. | | |
| C.2.4. | Ensure that the student is mentored by an individual with expertise consistent with the student's area of focus. The mentor does not have to be an occupational therapist. | *(No related Standard)* | *(No related Standard)* |
| | *MENTORING IS DEFINED AS A RELATIONSHIP BETWEEN TWO PEOPLE IN WHICH ONE PERSON (THE MENTOR) IS DEDICATED TO THE PERSONAL AND PROFESSIONAL GROWTH OF THE OTHER (THE MENTEE). A MENTOR HAS MORE EXPERIENCE AND KNOWLEDGE THAN THE MENTEE. THE PROGRAM MUST HAVE A SYSTEM TO ENSURE THAT MENTOR HAS DEMONSTRATED EXPERTISE IN ONE OR MORE OF THE FOLLOWING AREAS IDENTIFIED AS THE STUDENT'S FOCUSED AREA OF STUDY: CLINICAL PRACTICE SKILLS, RESEARCH SKILLS, ADMINISTRATION, LEADERSHIP, PROGRAM AND POLICY DEVELOPMENT, ADVOCACY, EDUCATION, OR THEORY DEVELOPMENT.* | | |
| C.2.5. | Document a formal evaluation mechanism for objective assessment of the student's performance during and at the completion of the doctoral experiential component. | *(No related Standard)* | *(No related Standard)* |

## GLOSSARY

**Accreditation Standards for a Doctoral-Degree-Level Educational Program for the Occupational Therapist, Masters-Degree-Level Educational Program for the Occupational Therapist, and Associate-Degree-Level Educational Program for the Occupational Therapy Assistant**

***Definitions given below are for the purposes of these documents.***

**ABILITY TO BENEFIT:** A phrase that refers to a student who does not have a high school diploma or its recognized equivalent, but is eligible to receive funds under the Title IV Higher Education Act programs after taking an independently administered examination and achieving a score, specified by the Secretary of the U.S. Department of Education (USDE), indicating that the student has the ability to benefit from the education being offered.

**ACADEMIC CALENDAR:** The official institutional document that lists registration dates, semester/quarter stop and start dates, holidays, graduation dates, and other pertinent events. Generally, the academic year is divided into two major semesters, each approximately 14 to 16 weeks long. A smaller number of institutions have quarters rather than semesters. Quarters are approximately 10 weeks long; there are three major quarters and the summer session.

**ACTIVITY:** A term that describes a class of human actions that are goal directed (AOTA, 2008b).

**ADVANCED:** The stage of being beyond the elementary or introductory.

**AFFILIATE:** An entity that formally cooperates with a sponsoring institution in implementing the occupational therapy educational program.

**AREAS OF OCCUPATION:** Activities in which people engage: activities of daily living, instrumental activities of daily living, rest and sleep, education, work, play, leisure, and social participation.

**ASSIST:** To aid, help, or hold an auxiliary position.

**BODY FUNCTIONS:** The physiological functions of body systems (including psychological functions).

**BODY STRUCTURES:** Anatomical parts of the body such as organs, limbs, and their components.

**CARE COORDINATION:** The process that links clients with appropriate services and resources.

**CASE MANAGEMENT:** A system to ensure that individuals receive appropriate health care services.

**CLIENT:** The term used to name the entity that receives occupational therapy services. Clients may include (1) individuals and other persons relevant to the client's life including family, caregivers, teachers, employers, and others who may also help or be served indirectly; (2) organizations, such as businesses, industries, or agencies; and (3) populations within a community (AOTA, 2008b).

**CLIENT-CENTERED SERVICE DELIVERY:** An orientation that honors the desires and priorities of clients in designing and implementing interventions.

**CLIENT FACTORS:** Factors that reside within the client and that may affect performance in areas of occupation. Client factors include body functions and body structures.

**CLINICAL REASONING:** Complex multifaceted cognitive process used by practitioners to plan, direct, perform, and reflect on intervention.

**COLLABORATE:** To work together with a mutual sharing of thoughts and ideas.

**COMPETENT:** To have the requisite abilities/qualities and capacity to function in a professional environment.

**CONSUMER:** The direct and/or indirect recipient of educational and/or practitioner services offered.

**CONTEXT/CONTEXTUAL FACTORS AND ENVIRONMENT:**

**CONTEXT:** The variety of interrelated conditions within and surrounding the client that influence performance. Contexts include cultural, personal, temporal, and virtual aspects.

**ENVIRONMENT:** The external physical and social environment that surrounds the client and in which the client's daily life occupations occur.

**CONTEXT OF SERVICE DELIVERY:** The knowledge and understanding of the various contexts in which occupational therapy services are provided.

**CRITERION-REFERENCED:** Tests that compare the performance of an individual to that of another group, known as the *norm group*.

**CULMINATING PROJECT:** A project that is completed by a doctoral student that demonstrates the student's ability to relate theory to practice and to synthesize advanced knowledge in a practice area.

**CURRICULUM DESIGN:** An overarching set of assumptions that explains how the curriculum is planned, implemented, and evaluated. Typically, a curriculum design includes educational goals and curriculum threads and provides a clear rationale for the selection of content, the determination of scope of content, and the sequence of the content. A curriculum design is expected to be consistent with the mission and philosophy of the sponsoring institution and the program.

**CURRICULUM THREADS:** Curriculum threads, or *themes,* are identified by the program as areas of study and development that follow a path through the curriculum and represent the unique qualities of the program, as demonstrated by the program's graduates. Curriculum threads are typically based on the profession's and program's vision, mission, and philosophy (e.g., occupational needs of society, critical thinking/professional reasoning, diversity/globalization . (AOTA, 2008a).

**DIAGNOSIS:** The process of analyzing the cause or nature of a condition, situation, or problem. Diagnosis as stated in Standard B.4.0. refers to the occupational therapist's ability to analyze a problem associated with occupational performance and participation.

**DISTANCE EDUCATION:** Education that uses one or more of the technologies listed below to deliver instruction to students who are separated from the instructor and to support regular and substantive interaction between the students and the instructor, either synchronously or asynchronously. The technologies may include

- The Internet;
- One-way and two-way transmissions through open broadcast, closed circuit, cable, microwave, broadband lines, fiber optics, satellite, or wireless communications devices;
- Audio conferencing; or
- Video cassettes, DVDs, and CD-ROMs, if the cassettes, DVDs, or CD-ROMs are used in a course.

**DRIVER REHABILITATION:** Specialized evaluation and training to develop mastery of specific skills and techniques to effectively drive a motor vehicle independently and in accordance with state department of motor vehicles regulations.

**ENTRY-LEVEL OCCUPATIONAL THERAPIST:** The outcome of the occupational therapy educational and certification process; an individual prepared to begin generalist practice as an occupational therapist with less than 1 year of experience.

**ENTRY-LEVEL OCCUPATIONAL THERAPY ASSISTANT:** The outcome of the occupational therapy educational and certification process; an individual prepared to begin generalist practice as an occupational therapy assistant with less than 1 year of experience.

**FACULTY:**

**FACULTY, CORE:** Persons who are resident faculty, including the program director, appointed to and employed primarily in the occupational therapy educational program.

**FACULTY, FULL TIME:** Core faculty members who hold an appointment that are full-time, as defined by the institution, and whose job responsibilities include teaching and/or contributing to the delivery of the designed curriculum regardless of the position title (e.g., full-time instructional staff and clinical instructors would be considered faculty).

**FACULTY, PART TIME:** Core faculty members who hold an appointment that is considered by that institution to constitute less than full-time service and whose job responsibilities include teaching and/or contributing to the delivery of the designed curriculum regardless of the position title.

**FACULTY, ADJUNCT:** Persons who are responsible for teaching at least 50% of a course and are part-time, nonsalaried, non-tenure-track faculty members who are paid for each class they teach.

**FIELDWORK COORDINATOR:** Faculty member who is responsible for the development, implementation, management, and evaluation of fieldwork education.

**FRAME OF REFERENCE:** A set of interrelated, internally consistent concepts, definitions, postulates, and principles that provide a systematic description of a practitioner's interaction with clients. A frame of reference is intended to link theory to practice.

**FULL-TIME EQUIVALENT (FTE):** An equivalent position for a full-time faculty member (as defined by the institution). A full-time equivalent can be made up of no more than 3 individuals.

**GRADUATION RATE:** The total number of students who graduated from a program within 150% of the published length of the program, divided by the number of students on the roster who started in the program.

**HABITS:** "Automatic behavior that is integrated into more complex patterns that enable people to function on a day-to-day basis" (Neidstadt & Crepeau, 1998).

**HEALTH LITERACY:** Degree to which individuals have the capacity to obtain, process, and understand basic health information and services needed to make appropriate health decisions (National Network of Libraries of Medicine, 2011).

**INTERPROFESSIONAL COLLABORATIVE PRACTICE:** "Multiple health workers from different professional backgrounds working together with patients, families, careers, and communities to deliver the highest quality of care"(World Health Organization, 2010).

**MEMORANDUM OF UNDERSTANDING (MOU):** A document outlining the terms and details of an agreement between parties, including each parties' requirements and responsibilities. A memorandum of understanding may be signed by any individual who is authorized by the institution to sign fieldwork memoranda of understanding on behalf of the institution.

**MENTORING:** A relationship between two people in which one person (the mentor) is dedicated to the personal and professional growth of the other (the mentee). A mentor has more experience and knowledge than the mentee.

**MISSION:** A statement that explains the unique nature of a program or institution and how it helps fulfill or advance the goals of the sponsoring institution, including religious missions.

**MODALITIES:** Application of a therapeutic agent, usually a physical agent modality.

**DEEP THERMAL MODALITIES:** Modalities such as therapeutic ultrasound and phonophoresis.

**ELECTROTHERAPEUTIC MODALITIES:** Modalities such as biofeedback, neuromuscular electrical stimulation, functional electrical stimulation, transcutaneous electrical nerve stimulation, electrical stimulations for tissue repair, high-voltage galvanic stimulation, and iontophoresis.

**MECHANICAL MODALITIES:** Modalities such as vasopneumatic devices and continuous passive motion.

**SUPERFICIAL THERMAL MODALITIES:** Modalities such as hydrotherapy, whirlpool, cryotherapy, fluidotherapy, hot packs, paraffin, water, and infrared.

**MODEL OF PRACTICE:** The set of theories and philosophies that defines the views, beliefs, assumptions, values, and domain of concern of a particular profession or discipline. Models of practice delimit the boundaries of a profession.

**OCCUPATION:** "Activities . . . of everyday life, named, organized and given value and meaning by individuals and a culture. Occupation is everything that people do to occupy themselves, including looking after themselves . . . enjoying life . . . and contributing to the social and economic fabric of their communities" (Law, Polatajko, Baptiste, & Townsend, 1997).

**OCCUPATIONAL PROFILE:** An analysis of a client's occupational history, routines, interests, values, and needs to engage in occupations and occupational roles.

**OCCUPATIONAL THERAPY:** The art and science of applying occupation as a means to effect positive, measurable change in the health status and functional outcomes of a client by a qualified occupational therapist and/or occupational therapy assistant (as appropriate).

**OCCUPATIONAL THERAPY PRACTITIONER:** An individual who is initially credentialed as an occupational therapist or an occupational therapy assistant.

**PARTICIPATION:** Active engagement in occupations.

**PERFORMANCE PATTERNS:** Patterns of behavior related to daily life activities that are habitual or routine. Performance patterns include habits, routines, rituals, and roles.

**PERFORMANCE SKILLS:** Features of what one does, not what one has, related to observable elements of action that have implicit functional purposes. Performance skills include motor and praxis, sensory/perceptual, emotional regulation, cognitive, and communication and social skills.

**PHILOSOPHY:** The underlying belief and value structure for a program that is consistent with the sponsoring institution and which permeates the curriculum and the teaching learning process.

**POPULATION-BASED INTERVENTIONS:** Interventions focused on promoting the overall health status of the community by preventing disease, injury, disability, and premature death. A population-based health intervention can include assessment of the community's needs, health promotion and public education, disease and disability prevention, monitoring of services, and media interventions. Most interventions are tailored to reach a subset of a population, although some may be targeted toward the population at large. Populations and subsets may be defined by geography, culture, race and ethnicity, socioeconomic status, age, or other characteristics. Many of these characteristics relate to the health of the described population (Keller, Schaffer, Lia-Hoagberg, & Strohschein, 2002).

**PREPARATORY METHODS:** Intervention techniques focused on client factors to help a client's function in specific activities.

**PROGRAM DIRECTOR** (associate-degree-level occupational therapy assistant): An initially certified occupational therapist or occupational therapy assistant who is licensed or credentialed according to regulations in the state or jurisdiction in which the program is located. The program director must hold a minimum of a master's degree.

**PROGRAM DIRECTOR** (master's-degree-level occupational therapist): An initially certified occupational therapist who is licensed or credentialed according to regulations in the state or jurisdiction in which the program is located. The program director must hold a doctoral degree.

**PROGRAM DIRECTOR** (doctoral-degree-level occupational therapist): An initially certified occupational therapist who is licensed or credentialed according to regulations in the state or jurisdiction in which the program is located. The program director must hold a doctoral degree.

**PROGRAM EVALUATION:** A continuing system for routinely and systematically analyzing data to determine the extent to which the program is meeting its stated goals and objectives.

**PURPOSEFUL ACTIVITY:** "An activity used in treatment that is goal directed and that the [client] sees as meaningful or purposeful" (Low, 2002).

**RECOGNIZED REGIONAL OR NATIONAL ACCREDITING AUTHORITY:** Regional and national accrediting agencies recognized by the USDE and/or the Council for Higher Education Accreditation (CHEA) to accredit postsecondary educational programs/institutions. The purpose of recognition is to ensure that the accrediting agencies are reliable authorities for evaluating quality education or training programs in the institutions they accredit.

**Regional accrediting bodies recognized by USDE:**

- Accrediting Commission for Community and Junior Colleges, Western Association of Schools and Colleges (ACCJC/WASC)
- Accrediting Commission for Senior Colleges and Universities, Western Association of Schools and Colleges (ACSCU/WASC)
- Commission on Colleges, Southern Association of Colleges and Schools (SACS)
- Commission on Institutions of Higher Education, New England Association of Schools and Colleges (CIHE/NEASC)
- Higher Learning Commission, North Central Association of Colleges and Schools (HLC)
- Middle States Commission on Higher Education, Middle States Association of Colleges and Schools (MSCHE)
- Northwest Commission on Colleges and Universities (NWCCU)

**National accrediting bodies recognized by USDE:**

- Accrediting Bureau of Health Education Schools (ABHES)
- Accrediting Commission of Career Schools and Colleges (ACCSC)
- Accrediting Council for Continuing Education and Training (ACCET)
- Accrediting Council for Independent Colleges and Schools (ACICS)
- Council on Occupational Education (COE)
- Distance Education and Training Council Accrediting Commission (DETC)

**REFLECTIVE PRACTICE:** Thoughtful consideration of one's experiences and knowledge when applying such knowledge to practice. Reflective practice includes being coached by professionals.

**RELEASE TIME:** Period when a person is freed from regular duties, especially teaching, to allow time for other tasks or activities.

**RETENTION RATE:** A measure of the rate at which students persist in their educational program, calculated as the percentage of students on the roster, after the add period, from the beginning of the previous academic year who are again enrolled in the beginning of the subsequent academic year.

**SCHOLARSHIP:** "A systematic investigation . . . designed to develop or to contribute to generalizable knowledge" (45 CFR § 46). Scholarship is made public, subject to review, and part of the discipline or professional knowledge base (Glassick, Huber, & Maeroff, 1997). It allows others to build on it and further advance the field (AOTA, 2009).

**SCHOLARSHIP OF DISCOVERY:** Engagement in activity that leads to the development of "knowledge for its own sake." The Scholarship of Discovery encompasses original research that contributes to expanding the knowledge base of a discipline (Boyer,1990).

**SCHOLARSHIP OF INTEGRATION:** Investigations making creative connections both within and across disciplines to integrate, synthesize, interpret, and create new perspectives and theories (Boyer , 1990).

**SCHOLARSHIP OF APPLICATION:** Practitioners apply the knowledge generated by Scholarship of Discovery or Integration to address real problems at all levels of society (Boyer, 1990). In occupational therapy, an example would be the application of theoretical knowledge to practice interventions or to teaching in the classroom.

**SCHOLARSHIP OF TEACHING AND LEARNING:** ""Involves the systematic study of teaching and/or learning and the public sharing and review of such work through presentations, publications, and performances" (McKinney, 2007, p. 10).

**SKILL:** The ability to use one's knowledge effectively and readily in execution or performance.

**SPONSORING INSTITUTION:** The identified legal entity that assumes total responsibility for meeting the minimal standards for ACOTE accreditation.

**STRATEGIC PLAN:** A comprehensive plan that articulates the program's future vision and guides the program development (e.g., faculty recruitment and professional growth, changes in the curriculum design priorities in academic resources, procurement of fieldwork sites). A program's strategic plan must include, but need not be limited to,

- Evidence that the plan is based on program evaluation and an analysis of external and internal environments,
- Long-term goals that address the vision and mission of both the institution and program, as well as specific needs of the program,
- Specific measurable action steps with expected timelines by which the program will reach its long-term goals,
- Person(s) responsible for action steps, and
- Evidence of periodic updating of action steps and long-term goals as they are met or as circumstances change.

**SUPERVISE:** To direct and inspect the performance of workers or work.

**SUPERVISION, DIRECT:** Supervision that occurs in real time and offers both audio and visual capabilities to ensure opportunities for timely feedback.

**SUPERVISOR:** One who ensures that tasks assigned to others are performed correctly and efficiently.

**THEORY:** A set of interrelated concepts used to describe, explain, or predict phenomena.

**TRANSFER OF CREDIT:** A term used in higher education to award a student credit for courses earned in another institution prior to admission to the occupational therapy or occupational therapy assistant program.

---

**References**

American Occupational Therapy Association. (2008a). *Occupational therapy model curriculum.* Bethesda MD: Author. Retrieved from www.aota.org/Educate/EdRes/COE/Other-Education-Documents/CT-Model-Curriculum.aspx

American Occupational Therapy Association. (2008b). Occupational therapy practice framework: Domain and process (2nd ed.). *American Journal of Occupational Therapy*, 62, 625–683.

American Occupational Therapy Association. (2009). Scholarship in occupational therapy. *American Journal of Occupational Therapy, 63,* 790–796. http://dx.doi.org/10.5014/ajot.63.6.790

Boyer, E. L. (1990). *Scholarship reconsidered: Priorities of the professoriate*. San Francisco: Jossey-Bass.

Crepeau, E. B., Cohn, E., & Schell, B. (Eds.). (2008). *Willard and Spackman's occupational therapy* (11th ed.). Philadelphia: Lippincott Williams & Wilkins.

Glassick, C. E., Huber, M. T., & Maeroff, G. I. (1997). *Scholarship assessed: Evaluation of the professoriate.* San Francisco: Jossey-Bass.

Interprofessional Education Collaborative Expert Panel. (2011). *Core competencies for interprofessional collaborative practice: Report of an expert panel.* Washington, DC: Interprofessional Education Collaborative.

Keller, L., Schaffer, M., Lia-Hoagberg B., & Strohschein S. (2002). Assessment, program planning and evaluation in population-based public health practice. *Journal of Public Health Management and Practice, 8*(5), 30–44.

Law, M., Polatajko, H., Baptiste W., & Townsend, E. (1997). Core concepts of occupational therapy. In E. Townsend (Ed.), *Enabling occupation: An occupational therapy perspective* (pp. 29–56). Ottawa, ON: Canadian Association of Occupational Therapists.

Low, J. (2002). Historical and social foundations for practice. In C. A. Trombly & M. V. Radomski (Eds.), *Occupational therapy for physical dysfunction* (5th ed., pp. 17–30). Philadelphia: Lippincott Williams & Wilkins.

McKinney, K. (2007). *Enhancing learning through the scholarship of teaching and learning.* San Francisco: Jossey-Bass.

National Network of Libraries of Medicine. (2011). *Health literacy.* Retrieved February 3, 2012, from http://nnlm.gov/outreach/consumer/hlthlit.html

Schon, D. A. (1987). *Educating the reflective practitioner.* San Francisco: Jossey-Bass.

*Public welfare: Protection of human subjects,* 45 CFR § 46 (2005).

U.S. Department of Education (2011). *Funding Your Education: The Guide to Federal Student Aid, 2012-13.* Retrieved February 3, 2012, from http://studentaid.ed.gov/students/attachments/siteresources/12-13_Guide.pdf.

World Health Organization. (2010). *Framework for action on interprofessional education and collaborative practice.* Geneva: Author. Retrieved from http://whqlibdoc.who.int/hq/2010/WHO_HRH_HPN_10.3_eng.pdf.

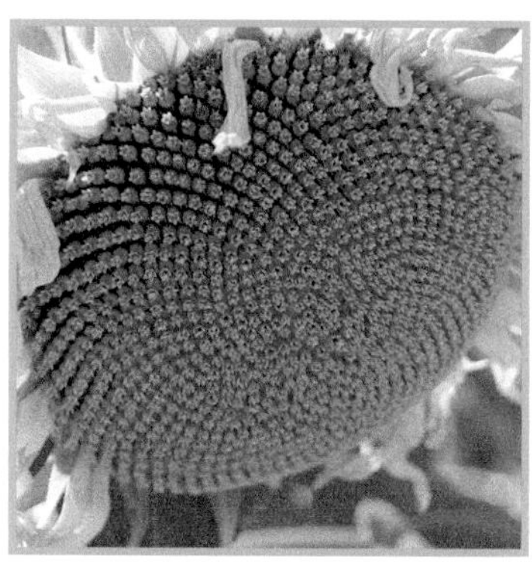

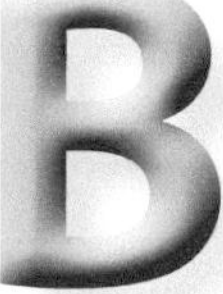

# Assessment Tool Grid



Jacobs, K., & MacRae, N. (Eds.).
*Occupational Therapy Essentials for Clinical Competence, Third Edition* (pp. 845-861).

# Assessment Tool Grid

Amy Peluso Burns

Printed with permission from the author.

| Foundations for Functional Activity | | | | | |
|---|---|---|---|---|---|
| **Name of Assessment tool, Author, and Publication date** | **Standardized** | **Validity/ Reliability** | **Setting Used** | **Areas Assessed** | **Age Group** |
| **Balance/Posture/Mobility** | | | | | |
| **Berg Scale**<br>*Measures 14 balance items. Includes sitting and standing unsupported, sit-to-stand, transfers, picking up objects from floor, and turning.* | No | Valid and Reliable | Home or clinic setting | Transfers, sitting, standing, balance | Adult/elderly |
| **Functional Reach Test**<br>*Simple way to measure standing balance. Measures the difference between arm's length and maximal forward reach.* | Yes | Valid and Reliable | Wall and tape measure needed | Reaching and balance | Adult/elderly |
| **Modified Gait Abnormality Rating Scale (GARS)**<br>*Seven item assessment of gait, stepping and arm movements, staggering foot contact, hip ROM, shoulder extension, etc.* | No | | Room to walk | Hip ROM, foot contact, staggering, arm/leg symmetry, guarding | Adult/elderly |
| **Timed Get Up and Go (TGUG)**<br>*Measures the overall time to complete a series of functionally important tasks. Helps to identify clients with balance deficits.* | No | Valid and Reliable | Room to walk 10 feet; chair | Balance, posture, mobility | Adult/elderly |
| **Tinetti**<br>*Measures a client's gait and balance.* | No | Inter-rater reliability | Room to walk 10 feet; chair | Balance and gait | Adult/elderly |
| **Cognition** | | | | | |
| **Autobiographical Memory Interview (AMI)**<br>*Interview recalling events from the clients' past including school, wedding, children, etc.* | Yes | Valid and Reliable | Quiet environment with minimal distractions | Memory, retrograde amnesia | Adult/elderly |
| **Bay Area Functional Performance Evaluation (BaFPE)**<br>*Assesses how a client might function in task-oriented settings and settings with social interaction. Uses sea shells, design blocks, and associated items.* | Yes | Valid and Reliable | Seated at table | Memory, organization, attention span | Adult/elderly |
| **Behavioral Inattention Test**<br>*Assesses unilateral visual neglect. Includes card sorting, article reading, figure/shape copying, etc.* | Yes | Valid and Reliable | Quiet environment with minimal distractions | Unilateral visual neglect, picture recalling, line crossing, article reading, phone dialing | Adult/elderly |

| | | | | | |
|---|---|---|---|---|---|
| **Brown ADD Scale**<br>*Assesses executive function impairments associated with ADD/ADHD and related problems.* | Yes | Valid and Reliable | Quiet environment with minimal distractions | Attention, listening skills | Age 3 to adult |
| **Cognitive Assessment of Minnesota (CAM)**<br>*Assesses the cognitive abilities of adults with neurological impairments.* | Yes | Valid and Reliable | Quiet room | Attention, memory, visual neglect | Ages 18 to 70 |
| **Contextual Memory Test**<br>*Assesses awareness of memory capacity, strategy use, and recall in adults with memory dysfunction.* | Yes | Valid and Reliable | Quiet room with minimal distraction | Memory, awareness of memory capacity, recall of line drawings | Adult/elderly |
| **Glasgow Coma Scale**<br>*Measures response of eyes, verbal response, and motor response in numerical levels.* | No | Reliable | In hospital | Alertness, awareness, verbal response, motor response | All ages |
| **King-Devick Test of Oculomotor Speed and Accuracy (K-D)**<br>*Assesses residual oculomotor functions in a clinical setting, and its components can also be used for vision therapy training purposes as well.* | Yes | Valid and Reliable | Quiet environment with minimal distractions | eye tracking skills, general motor skills | Ages 6 to 14 |
| **Leiter International Performance Scale - Revised (Leiter-R)**<br>*A non-verbal test to assess cognitive functions in children and adolescents.* | Yes | Valid and Reliable | Individual setting, comfortable for the client | Intellectual ability, memory, attention | Ages 2 to 20 years, 11 months |
| **Lowenstein Occupational Therapy Cognitive Assessment (LOTCA) (also LOTCA-Geriatric)**<br>*Assesses clients with neurological deficits and mental health issues. Tests orientation, visual/spatial perception, praxis, visuomotor. Includes cards, blocks, pegboard.* | Yes | Valid and Reliable | Quiet environment with minimal distractions | Orientation, perception, praxis, visuomotor, organization, thinking operations | Adult/elderly |
| **Luria-Nebraska Neuropsychological Battery**<br>*Reading numbers, writing words, differentiate hard/soft touch, sounds. Provides a pattern analysis of strengths and weakness across areas of brain function.* | Yes | Valid and Reliable | Quiet environment with minimal distractions | Numbers, reading, writing, touching | All ages |
| **Mini-Mental Status Evaluation (MMSE)**<br>*Used to assess cognitive function.* | Yes | Valid and Reliable | Seated at table | Brain injury, writing, reading, drawing | Ages 18+ |

| | | | | | |
|---|---|---|---|---|---|
| **Ranchos Los Amigos** (Developed at the Rancho Los Amigos Hospital in California by the Head Injury Treatment Team) *Medical scale, assesses the level of recovery of a client with a brain injury and those recovering from a coma.* | No | Reliable | In hospital | Alertness, awareness | All ages |
| **Rivermead Behavioral Memory Test (RBMT-II)** *Assessment of gross memory impairments encountered by clients in their everyday lives. Identifies everyday memory problems and monitors change over time.* | Yes | Valid and Reliable | Quiet environment with minimal distractions | Memory: immediate and recall | Ages 16+ |
| **Severe Impairment Battery** *Evaluates cognitive abilities at the lower end of the range (severely impaired dementia client). Allows for non-verbal and partially correct responses.* | Yes | Valid and Reliable | Quiet environment with minimal distractions | Memory, completing simple actions | Adult/elderly |
| **Test of Everyday Attention** *Measures selective attention, sustained attention, and attentional switching. Includes map search, telephone search, elevator counting, etc.* | Yes | Valid and Reliable | Quiet room; table and chairs | Everyday materials (map searching, phone skills, etc.) | Ages 18 to 80 |
| **Dexterity** | | | | | |
| **Jebsen-Taylor Hand Function Test** *Assesses a broad range of hand functions used in daily activities. A seven-part test that uses common items such as paper clips, cans, pencils, etc.* | Yes | Reliable | Seated, requires adequate lighting | Writing, page turning, lifting small/large objects, simulated feeding | Ages 20 to 94 |
| **Manipulative Aptitude Test** *Measures hand/arm/finger dexterity and speed through sorting and assembling.* | Yes | Valid and Reliable | Seated at a table or desk | Dexterity, manipulative aptitude, dominant hand | Ages 13+ |
| **Minnesota Rate of Manipulation** *Assesses unilateral and bilateral manual dexterity along with eye-hand coordination. Provides information on standing tolerance, sustained neck flexion, weight bearing, and repetitive reach.* | Yes | Valid and Reliable | Table and chair | Manual dexterity, turning, displacing | Ages 13+ |
| **Nine Hole Peg** *Client places nine dowels in nine holes while being timed.* | Yes | Valid and Reliable | Table and chair | Finger dexterity | Ages 20+ |
| **O'Connor Finger Dexterity Test** *Requires hand placement of 3 pins per hole.* | Yes | | Table and chair | Predictor of rapid manipulation | Ages 13+ |

| | | | | | |
|---|---|---|---|---|---|
| **O'Connor Tweezer Dexterity Test** *Measures the speed with which a client can puck up pins with a tweezer, one at a time, and place the pin into a small hole.* | Yes | | Table and chair | Finger dexterity, fine motor coordination, speed, eye-hand coordination | Ages 13+ |
| **Pennsylvania Bi-manual Worksample** *Assesses finger dexterity of both hands, as well as gross movements of both arms.* | Yes | Reliable | Table and chair | Finger dexterity of both hands, gross movements of both arms, eye-hand coordination | Ages 16+ |
| **Purdue Pegboard** *Assesses gross movement of hands/fingers/arms, as well as fingertip dexterity.* | Yes | Valid and Reliable | Table and chair | Gross movement of hands, fingers, and arms; fingertip dexterity | Ages 5+ |
| **Range of Motion** *Measurement of the achievable distance between the flexed position and the extended position of a particular joint or muscle group.* | Yes | Valid, not 100% reliable | Comfortable for client, chair/mat | Biomechanical | All ages |
| **Rosenbusch Test of Finger Dexterity** *Measures the speed of inter-digital manipulation of each hand separately.* | Yes | Valid and Reliable | Table and chair | Manipulation of all parts of the hand | All ages |
| **Strength Testing** *The strength of each muscle group is measured on a scale of 0/5 to 5/5.* | Yes | Valid, not 100% reliable | Comfortable for client, chair/mat | Biomechanical | All ages |
| **Motor/cognition/coping/self-help (Pediatric)** | | | | | |
| **Battelle Developmental Inventory, Second Edition, (BDI-2)** *Developmental assessment for early childhood. Screening, diagnosis, and evaluation of early development.* | Yes | Valid and Reliable | Familiar to child; little to no auditory and visual distractions | Personal-social, motor, adaptive, communication, cognitive (all with sub-domains too) | Birth to age 8 |
| **Bayley Scales of Infant Development (BIDS)** *Measures the mental and motor development and tests the behavior of infants.* | Yes | Valid and Reliable | Quiet environment with minimal distractions | Performance in occupation, performance skills, context, activity demands | Ages 1 to 42 months |
| **Behavioral-Characteristics Progression (BCP)** *Curriculum-based assessment and planning tool for use by special education professionals serving children and adults who are functioning between the developmental ages of 1 to 14 years.* | No | Valid and Reliable | Comfortable for child | Self-help, fine motor, gross motor, academic, etc. | Ages 1 to 14 |
| **Bruininks-Oseretoky of Motor Proficiency** *Comprehensive index of motor proficiency as well as separate measures of both gross and fine motor skills.* | Yes | Valid and Reliable | Gym | Motor | Ages 4.5 to 14.5 |

| | | | | | |
|---|---|---|---|---|---|
| **The Carolina Curriculum for Infants and Toddlers with Special Needs, Second Edition (CCITSN)** *Designed for children who have mild to severe special needs and who function in the birth to 24-month developmental range.* | Yes | Valid and Reliable | Comfortable for child | Cognition, communication, social adaptation, fine motor, gross motor | Birth to age 2 |
| **The Carolina Curriculum for Preschoolers with Special Needs (CCPSN)** *Designed for children who have mild to severe special needs and who function in the 2- to 5-year developmental range.* | Yes | Valid and Reliable | Comfortable for child | Cognition, communication, social adaptation, fine motor, gross motor | Ages 2 to 5 |
| **Coping-Inventory** *Assesses the behavior patterns and skills used by children and adults to meet personal needs and adapt to the demands of their environment.* | No | Self-rated and observation | Variety of environments | Two forms of coping behavior, self and environment | Ages 3+ |
| **First Step (FirstSTEp)** *Screening test for evaluating pre-schooler.* | Yes | Valid and Reliable | Public schools, public health situations, pediatrician's office | IDEA domains: cognition, communication, and motor | Ages 2 years, 9 months to 6 years, 2 months |
| **Early Coping Inventory** *Assesses the coping-related behavior of children.* | No | Observation form | Comfortable for child | Sensorimotor, reactive behavior, self-initiated behavior | Ages 4 to 36 months |
| **Hawaii Early Learning Profile (HELP)** *Test is helpful to see development of child throughout periods of time.* | Criterion referenced | Valid and Reliable | Comfortable for child | Cognition, language, gross motor, fine motor, social-emotional, self-help, regulatory, sensory organization | Birth to age 3 and preschool |
| **Infant-Toddler and Family Instrument (ITFI) and Manual** *Helps to evaluate the strengths and vulnerabilities of children and their families.* | | Valid and Reliable | Family environment, comfortable | Gross and fine motor, social and emotional, language, coping and self-help | Ages 6 months to 3 years |
| **Kent Inventory of Developmental Skills (KIDS)** *Provides a clear picture of a child's development status and relative strengths and needs.* | Yes | Valid and Reliable | Familiar to child; home | Cognitive, motor, communication, self-help, social | Birth to 15 months, or up to age 6 when severe developmental disabilities are present |
| **Mullen Scales of Early Learning** *Provides a complete picture of cognitive and motor ability.* | Yes | Valid and Reliable | Clinic and school setting | Visual, linguistic, motor, distinguish between receptive and expressive processing | Birth to 68 months |

| | | | | | |
|---|---|---|---|---|---|
| **Peabody Developmental Motor Scales, Second Edition, (PDMS-2)**<br>*Measures both gross and fine motor skills.* | Yes | Valid and Reliable | Quiet environment with minimal distractions | Motor (gross and fine) | Birth to age 7 |
| **Pediatric Evaluation of Disability Inventory (PEDI)**<br>*Assesses key functional capabilities and performance.* | Yes | Valid and Reliable | Natural environment for child | Self-care, mobility, social function | Ages 6 months to 7 years |
| **PEERAMID-2**<br>*Assesses a child's performance in five different areas of development.* | Yes | n/a | Quiet, comfortable | Fine motor/ graphomotor function, language function, gross motor function, memory function, and visual processing | School Grades 4 to 10 |
| **Pediatric Examination of Educational Readiness (PEER)**<br>*Assesses the preschooler's performance in six areas.* | Yes | n/a | Quiet, child comfortable, no parents | Orientation, gross motor, visual-fine motor, sequential, linguistic, and preacademic learning | Ages 4 to 6 |
| **Pediatric Extended Exam at Three (PEET)**<br>*Assesses a child's performance in five basic areas of development.* | Yes | n/a | Quiet, comfortable, low visual stim, supportive | Gross motor, language, visual-fine motor, memory, and intersensory integration | Age 3 |
| **Pediatric Early Elementary Exam (PEEX-2)**<br>*Assesses a child's performance in five different areas of development.* | Yes | n/a | quiet, comfortable, sit to left or right of child at table | Fine motor/ graphomotor function, language function, gross motor function, memory function, and visual processing function | Ages 6 to 9 |
| **Posture and Fine Motor Assessments (PFMAI)**<br>*Designed to identify motor delays in infants and to monitor progress in the first year of life.* | Yes | Valid and Reliable | Familiar, child only in diaper | Motor | Ages 2 to 12 months |
| **Quick Neurological Screening Test - II, Revised Edition**<br>*Designed for use in screening for early identification of disabilities* | Norms suggest cutoff scores | Some Validity and Reliability | Table and chairs, room to walk | Hand skill, discrimination, eye tracking, sound patterns, movements | Ages 5+ |
| **Temperament and Atypical Behavior Scale (TABS)**<br>*Early Childhood Indicators of Developmental Dysfunction* | Norm referenced | Valid and Reliable | Parent may be able to complete independently, or with help from professional | Sensory regulation, attachment behaviors | Ages 11 to 71 months |
| **Test of Gross Motor Development (TGMD-2)**<br>*Measures gross motor abilities that develop in early life* | Yes | Valid and Reliable | School (Open and large area) | Gross motor | Ages 3 to 10 |

| | | | | | |
|---|---|---|---|---|---|
| **Toddler Infant Motor Eval (TIME)**<br>*Evaluates children who have atypical motor development.* | Yes | Valid and Reliable | Quiet environment with minimal distractions | Motor | Birth to 42 months |
| **Play** | | | | | |
| **Adolescent Role Assessment (ARA)**<br>*Gathers information on the adolescent's occupational role involvement over time and across domains.* | No | Scores lack internal consistency | Comfortable for client | Social integration, school, roles, play, family | Ages 13 to 20 |
| **Adolesant Leisure Interest Profile**<br>*Asks adolescent to report his or her interest and/or participation in a variety of age-appropriate leisure activities.* | No | Self-report, Valid and Reliable | Comfortable for child | Sports, outdoor, summer, winter, indoor, creative | Ages 12 to 21 |
| **Infant Preschool Play Assessment Scale (I-PAS)**<br>*Systematically observes children at play and in other routines or natural environments.* | Criterion referenced | Valid and Reliable | Comfortable for child | Social, sensorimotor, memory, gross motor, communication, motivation, problem solving | Birth to 5 years |
| **Kid Play Profile**<br>*Asks child to report his or her interest and/or participation in a variety of age-appropriate leisure activities.* | No | Self-report, Valid and Reliable | Comfortable for child | Sports, outdoor, summer, winter, indoor, creative | Ages 6 to 9 |
| **Knox Preschool Play Scale (KPPS)**<br>*Preschoolers can be observed during free play, and a play age can be computed.* | Yes | Valid and Reliable | Comfortable for child, classroom setting | Space management, material management, imitation, participation | Preschoolers |
| **Preteen Play Profile**<br>*Asks preteen to report his or her interest and/or participation in a variety of age-appropriate leisure activities.* | No | Self-report, Valid and Reliable | Comfortable for child | Sports, outdoor, summer, winter, indoor, creative | Ages 9 to 12 |
| **Takata Play History (TPH)**<br>*Probes past and actual play history that relate to sensory integration function.* | No | Valid and Reliable | Comfortable for child | Sensorimotor, symbolic, dramatic, games, recreational | All children |
| **Test of Playfulness (ToP)**<br>*The information gathered provides a clue on inner drive and response to just right challenges, socialization, and play.* | No | Valid and Reliable | Indoors and outdoors | Intrinsic motivation, internal control, freedom to suspend reality | Ages 18 months+ |
| **Transdiciplinary Play-Based Assessment**<br>*Allows children to initiate and engage in play activities that are natural and enjoyable.* | Norm referenced | Valid and Reliable | Environment comfortable to child | Cognitive, social-emotional, communication, language, and sensorimotor | Infancy to age 6 |
| **Sensation/Edema** | | | | | |
| **Tactile Activity Kit**<br>*Versatile tool for sensory integration therapy.* | No | Not Valid, Not Reliable | Table-top | Tactile stimulation, discrimination, and desensitization | All ages |

| | | | | | |
|---|---|---|---|---|---|
| **Volumeter**<br>*Fill container with water, measure the displaced water of both hands.* | No | | Countertop or table; need access to water faucet | Edema, swelling of UE | All ages |
| **Sensory** | | | | | |
| **DeGangi-Berk Test of Sensory Integration (TSI)**<br>*Measures overall sensory integration, as well as postural control, bilateral motor integration, and reflex integration.* | Yes | Valid and Reliable | Environment comfortable for child | Vestibular function; postural control, bilateral motor integration, reflex integration | Ages 3 to 5 |
| **Sensory Integration and Praxis Tests (SIPT)**<br>*Measures sensory processing deficits related to learning and behavior problems.* | Yes | Valid and Reliable | Environment comfortable for child | Visual, tactile, kinesthetic perception, motor performance | Ages 4 to 8 |
| **Sensory Processing Measure** *Provides a complete picture of children's sensory processing difficulties at school and at home.* | Yes | Valid and Reliable | Home Form by caregiver in the home; School Forms by staff in multiple school environments | Sensory processing, praxis, social participation | Ages 5 to 12 |
| **Sensory Profile**<br>*Measures children's responses to sensory events in everyday life.* | Yes | Valid and Reliable | Environment comfortable for child | Modulation of sensory input across sensory systems, behavioral/emotional responses associated with sensory processing | Ages 3 to 10 |
| **Sensory Profile: Infant/Toddler**<br>*Examines patterns in children who are at risk or have specific disabilities.* | Yes | Valid and Reliable | Environment comfortable for child | Modulation of sensory input across sensory systems, behavioral/emotional responses associated with sensory processing | Birth to 36 months |
| **Sensory Profile: Adolescent/Adult**<br>*Identifies sensory processing patterns and effects on functional performance.* | Based on normative information | Valid and Reliable | Environment comfortable for child | Modulation of sensory input across sensory systems, behavioral/emotional responses associated with sensory processing | Ages 11+ |
| **Sensory Profile School Companion**<br>*Assesses children's sensory processing information related to school performance.* | Yes | Valid and Reliable | Environment comfortable for child | Classroom behavior and performance | Ages 3 to 11 |

| | | | | | |
|---|---|---|---|---|---|
| **Test of Sensory Function in Infants (TSFI)**<br>*Objective assessment to determine whether, and to what extent, an infant has sensory processing deficits.* | Yes | Valid and Reliable | Individually administered, simple interaction with the infant, infant can be seated on parent's lap | Deep pressure, visual tactile integration, adaptive motor function, ocular motor control, reactivity to vestibular stimulation | Ages 4 to 18 months |
| **Vision/Visual Perceptual** | | | | | |
| **Benton Visual Form Discrimination**<br>*Assesses the ability to discriminate between complex visual configurations. Book of line drawings.* | No | Valid | Quiet environment with minimal distractions | Neglect, neuropsycho-logical | Adult/elderly |
| **Developmental Test of Visual-Motor Integration (VMI)**<br>*Visuomotor skills are tested as the student copies a series of shapes in a test booklet.* | Yes | Valid and Reliable | Seated at desk/table, lighting, free of distraction | Visual perceptual | Ages 3+ |
| **Developmental Test of Visual Perception (DTVP-2)**<br>*Measures visual perception and motor integration skills.* | Yes | Valid and Reliable | Seated at desk/table, lighting, free of distraction | Pure visual perception (no motor response) and visual-motor integration | Ages 4 to 10 |
| **Hooper Visual Organization Test (VOT)**<br>*Ability to visually integrate information into whole perceptions through the use of line drawings arranged in puzzles.* | Yes | Valid and Reliable | Quiet environment with minimal distractions | Organization of visual stimuli | Ages 13+ |
| **McDowell Visual Screening Kit**<br>*Allows vision testing of very young or severely disabled children.* | Screening | Valid and Reliable | Comfortable for child | Distance visual acuity, near point acuity, ocular alignment, color perception, ocular function | Ages 2.5 to 5.5 |
| **Motor-Free Visual Perception Test (MVPT-3)**<br>*Assesses overall visual perceptual ability.* | Yes | Valid and Reliable | Seated at table Adequate light and free from distraction | Visual perceptual | Ages 4+ |
| **STROOP Color and Word Test**<br>*Reading aloud colored words. The words themselves are names of colors, but the actual color is different than the name.* | Yes | Valid and Reliable | Quiet environment with minimal distractions | Brain function and planning | Ages 15+ |
| **Test of Visual Motor Skills**<br>*Assesses a child's ability to transcribe geometric forms.* | Yes | Valid and Reliable | Seated at desk/table, individually or in groups | Eye-hand coordination skills | Ages 3 to 14 |
| **Test of Visual Motor Skills (UPPER)**<br>*Measures visual motor functioning using 16 geometric figures.* | Yes | Valid and Reliable | Seated at table Adequate light and free from distraction | Visual motor | Ages 12 to 40 |

| | | | | | |
|---|---|---|---|---|---|
| **Test of Visual-Perceptual Skills (non-motor) (TVPS-R)**<br>*Measures seven areas of visual-perception skills.* | Yes | Valid and Reliable | Seated at desk/table, lighting, free of distraction | Visual discrimination/ memory, visual spatial relationships, visual form-constancy, visual sequential memory, visual figure ground, visual closure | Ages 4 to 13 |
| **Warren's Brain Injury Visual Assessment Battery for Adults (biVABA)**<br>*Assessment of visual processing ability after a brain injury.* | Yes | Valid and Reliable | Comfortable for client | Visual perceptual processing, oculomotor function, how function is affected | Post CVA or head/brain injury |

| **ADLs and IADL** | | | | | |
|---|---|---|---|---|---|
| **Name of Assessment tool, Author, and Publication date** | **Standardized** | **Validity/ Reliability** | **Setting Used** | **Areas Assessed** | **Age** |
| **Allen Cognitive Level Test (ACL)**<br>*Leather lacing test.* | Yes | Valid and Reliable | Environment with minimal distractions and good lighting | Problem solving, sequencing | Adults/elderly |
| **Arnadottir Occupational Therapy Neurobehavioral Evaluation (A-one)**<br>*Determines the impact of neurobehavioral impairments on activities of daily living and mobility tasks using a five-point scale.* | Yes | Valid and Reliable | Clinic or home setting | ADLs, severity of neurobehavioral impairment, occupational performance | Adults/elderly |
| **Assessment of Motor and Process Skills (AMPS)**<br>*Observational assessment, measures the quality of a person's ADLs. Rates the effort, efficiency, safety, and independence of ADL motor/process skills. *Training required.* | Yes | Valid and Reliable | Various conditions | IADLs, motor skills and processing skills | Adults/elderly |
| **Assessment of Occupational Functioning (AOF)**<br>*Assesses the functional capacity of residents in long-term treatment settings who have physical and/or psychiatric problems.* | Yes | Valid and Reliable | Comfortable for the client | IADLs, MOHO, volition, habituation, performance | Ages 13+ |
| **Barthel Index**<br>*Assesses self-care functions in older adults.* | No | Predictive validity | Individual or group evaluation | Self-care | Adults/elderly |
| **Canadian Occupational Performance Measure (COPM)**<br>*Individualized outcome measure designed to detect changes in self-perception of occupational performance over time.* | Yes, but not norm referenced | Valid and Reliable | Comfortable for client | Occupational performances and perception | All ages |
| **Comprehensive Occupational Therapy Evaluation (COTE)**<br>*Developed in an acute psychiatric setting. Identifies 25 OT-related behaviors within three categories (general behavior, interpersonal behavior, and task behavior).* | Yes | Valid and Reliable | Quiet environment with minimal distractions | Behavior | All ages |
| **Direct Assessment of Functional Abilities (DAFA)**<br>*Direct measurement of the instrumental activities of daily living. Used to determine functional deficits in clients with mild cognitive impairment.* | Yes | Valid and Reliable | Clinic setting, cafeteria, gift shop, and exam room | IADLs | Adults/elderly |

| | | | | | |
|---|---|---|---|---|---|
| **Functional Independent Measure (FIM)**<br>*Scale (range from 1 to 7) that measures a client's ability to function with independence. Collected upon admission to rehabilitation unit, upon discharge, and after discharge.* | Yes | Valid and Reliable | Clinic or home setting | ADLs, self-care, communication, cognitive function | Adults/elderly |
| **Independent Living Scales (ILS)**<br>*Offers assessment, daily living skills, self-advocacy training, and support with issues that challenge the independence of a client.* | Yes | Valid and Reliable | Table and chairs; can be bedside | IADL, memory, orientation, money management, health, safety, etc. | Ages 65+ |
| **Index of Activities of Daily Living (ADL)**<br>*Assesses functional status as a measurement of the client's ability to perform activities of daily living independently. *No longer in print, may still be seen in some clinics.* | Yes | Valid and Reliable | Inpatient observations | ADL, biological and psychological function | Ages 65+ |
| **Kitchen Task Assessment (KTA)**<br>*Measures organization, planning, and judgment skills through common kitchen tasks.* | Yes | Valid and Reliable | Kitchen/ cooking environment | IADL, initiation, organization, sequencing, judgment, safety | Adults/elderly |
| **Klein-Bell Activities of Daily Living Scale**<br>*Assesses age-related changes in activities of daily living ability. *No longer in print, may still be seen in some clinics.* | Yes | Valid and Reliable | General rehabilitation setting | ADLs | Adults/elderly |
| **Kohlman Evaluation of Living Skills (KELS)**<br>*Ability to function in 17 basic living skills. Assesses skills in five areas: self-care, safety and health, money management, transportation/ telephone, and work/leisure.* | Yes | Valid and Reliable | Table and chairs | Self-care, safety and health, money management, transportation, telephone, work, leisure | Adults/elderly |
| **Level of Rehabilitation Scale (LORS-II)**<br>*Evaluates the success of inpatient rehabilitation programs.* | Yes | Valid and Reliable | Hospital rehabilitation units | ADLs | Adults/elderly |
| **Milwaukee Evaluation of Daily Living Skills (MEDLS)**<br>*Information from clients and families; establishes baseline behaviors necessary to develop treatment plans and guide intervention in regard to daily living skills.* | No | Valid and Reliable | Home environment | ADLs, including communication, personal care, clothing care, etc. | Adult/elderly |

| | | | | | |
|---|---|---|---|---|---|
| **Occupational Circumstances Assessment and Interview Rating Scale (OCAIRS)** *A 40-minute interview that analyzes the extent and nature of a client's occupational adaptation and participation.* | No | Valid and Reliable | Comfortable for the client | MOHO, volitional, habituation, performance | Ages 13+ |
| **Occupational Performance History Interview (OPHI-II)** *Interview that gathers the appreciation of a client's life history, the direction in which they want to take their life, as well as the impact of a disability on their life.* | Yes | Valid and Reliable | Comfortable for client | Occupational roles, daily routine, critical life events | Adolescents and adults |
| **Pre-Feeding Skills Checklist** *Manual for feeding assessment and intervention.* | No | Valid and Reliable | Quiet environment with minimal distractions | Feeding positions, types, quantity, sucking, movements | Ages 1 to 24 months |
| **Performance Assessment of Self-care Skills (PASS)** *Performance-based observation tool covering functional mobility, personal care, and IADLs. Measures short term functional change in elderly after hospitalization. *Requires 2-day training workshop.* | Criterion referenced | Valid and Reliable | Clinic and home version | IADLs | Adult/elderly |
| **Role-Checklist** *Assesses the values that clients place on their occupational roles.* | Yes | Valid and Reliable | Comfortable for client | MOHO, habituation sub-system | Ages 13+ |
| **Routine Task Inventory (RTI-II)** *Measures the level of performance in activities of daily living through observation and questioning.* | No | Valid and Reliable | Clinic or home setting | ADLs, effect of cognitive impairment on task performance | Adult/elderly |
| **Occupational Self Assessment** *This is a self-assessment of perceptions of strengths and weaknesses relative to occupational functioning.* | Yes | Valid and Reliable | Comfortable for the client | MOHO, volitional, habituation, performance | Ages 16+ |
| **Environmental Evaluations** | | | | | |
| **Enabler** *Norm-based environment assessment, developed to assess the accessibility of housing and its close surroundings.* | Yes | Valid and Reliable | Home environment and close surroundings | IADLs, neurological, musculoskeletal, psychological, movement, cognition, physical | All ages |
| **Home Observation for Measurement of the Environment** *Measures the quality and quantity of stimulation and support available to a child in the home environment.* | Yes | Valid and Reliable | Home environment | Interaction, environment | Ages 3 to 15 |

| **Education** | | | | | |
|---|---|---|---|---|---|
| **Name of Assessment tool, Author, and Publication date** | **Standardized** | **Validity/ Reliability** | **Setting Used** | **Areas Assessed** | **Age** |
| **Occupational Therapy Psychosocial Assessment of Learning (OT PAL)** *Designed to examine the environmental factors to determine the best "fit" between a child and his or her environment.* | No | Content validity | Classroom | Volition, habituation, and environmental fit within the classroom setting | Ages 6 to 12 |
| **School Function Assessment** *Measures school-related functional skills.* | Yes | Valid and Reliable | School setting | Participation, task supports, activity performance, adaptations | School grades 1 to 6 |
| **Handwriting** | | | | | |
| **Denver Handwriting Analysis (DHA)** | No | Valid and Reliable | Classroom | Fine motor, visual motor, auditory | School grades 3 to 8 |
| **Erhardt Developmental Prehension Assessment (EDPA)** *Designed for charting the prehensile development of a child.* | Yes | Valid and Reliable | Quiet environment with minimal distractions | Positional-reflexive, cognitively directed, pre-writing skills | Birth to 15 months |
| **Evaluation Tool of Children's Handwriting (ETCH)** *Evaluates six different areas of children's handwriting.* | Yes | Valid and Reliable | Quiet environment with minimal distractions | Alphabet production, numerical writing, near/far point copying, dictation, sentence composition | School grades 1 to 6 |
| **Minnesota Handwriting Assessment** *Used to analyze handwriting skills.* | Yes | Valid and Reliable | Quiet environment with minimal distractions | Legibility, form, alignment, size, spacing | 1st and 2nd grade |
| **Observation of Handwriting Skills** *Looks at the functional handwriting performance of the student in the classroom. Helps to identify areas that could impact handwriting or academic performance.* | No | Valid and Reliable | Quiet environment with minimal distractions | Gross and fine motor, visual motor, visual memory | Kindergarten and 1st grade-age |

| **Work and Retirement** | | | | | |
|---|---|---|---|---|---|
| **Name of Assessment tool, Author, and Publication date** | **Standardized** | **Validity/ Reliability** | **Setting Used** | **Areas Assessed** | **Age** |
| **Worker Environment Impact Scale (WEIS)** *Assesses environmental characteristics that facilitate successful employment experiences. Goal is to maximize the "fit" of the worker and his or her skill to the job environment.* | No | Fair Validity and Reliability | Comfortable for the client | Space-related issues, fit of environment | Ages 16+ |
| **Worker Role Interview (WRI)** *Identifies psychosocial and environmental factors that influence a client's ability to return to work.* | Yes | Valid and Reliable | Work, comfortable for client | Physical evaluation, essential job functions, psychosocial capacity to return to work | Ages 16+ |

| **Leisure (many ADL/IADL evaluations include leisure)** | | | | | |
|---|---|---|---|---|---|
| **Name of Assessment tool, Author, and Publication date** | **Standardized** | **Validity/ Reliability** | **Setting Used** | **Areas Assessed** | **Age** |
| **Adolescent Leisure Interest Profile** *Asks adolescent to report his or her interest and/or participation in a variety of age-appropriate leisure activities.* | No | Self-report, Valid and Reliable | Comfortable for the client | Sports, outdoor, summer, winter, indoor, creative | Ages 12 to 21 |
| **Adolescent Role Assessment (ARA)** *Gathers information on the adolescent's occupational role involvement over time and across domains.* | No | Scores lack internal consistency | Comfortable for the client | Social integration, school, roles, play, family | Ages 13 to 20 |

## Social Participation

| Name of Assessment tool, Author, and Publication date | Standardized | Validity/ Reliability | Setting Used | Areas Assessed | Age |
|---|---|---|---|---|---|
| **Coping Inventory** *Profiles coping styles, as well as behaviors, that facilitate or interfere with adaptive coping. Self-administered and profiled.* | No | Self-report and observation | Comfortable for the client | Sensorimotor, reactive behavior, self-initiated behavior, adaptive coping | Ages 15+ |
| **Life Satisfaction Index** *Looking at five factors that make up total life satisfaction (pleasure, meaningfulness, feeling of success, self-image, happiness).* | Yes | Valid and Reliable | Comfortable for the client | Activity, developmental theory, internal satisfaction | Ages 50 to 90 |
| **Occupational Questionnaire (OQ)** *Self-report assessment. Client documents the main activity in which he or she engages for each half-hour throughout the morning/day/evening and identifies each activity as work, ADL, recreation, or rest. Explores the meaning of leisure from the client's perspective.* | Yes | Valid and Reliable | Clinic or home setting | IADLs, volition, activity pattern, life satisfaction, interests, values, personal causation | Ages 13+ |
| **Social Profile** *Assessment of activity participation, social interaction, and membership roles in a group.* | No | Valid and Reliable; Ongoing research | Activity focused | Individualized to client choices | Adolescents and adults |
| **Volitional Questionnaire** *Observational assessment, gathers information on a client's volition.* | Yes | Valid | Observations are context specific: leisure, work, ADL environments | MOHO, volition subsystem, work, leisure, intrinsic motivation, values, interests | Ages 16+ |

## Wellness

| Name of Assessment tool, Author, and Publication date | Standardized | Validity/ Reliability | Setting Used | Areas Assessed | Age |
|---|---|---|---|---|---|
| **Engagement in Meaningful Activities Survey (EMAS)** *Clients read statements about activities, put an 'X' in the box that best describes them (never to always).* | Yes, for research purposes only | Valid and Reliable | Comfortable for the client | Activities | Adult/elderly |
| **Measure of Sub-Acute Rehabilitation Potential** *Uses a five-point rating scale to assess health status, history, hope, help, health efforts.* | No | | 90-day type clinical setting | Health status, history, hope, help, health efforts | Adult/elderly |
| **Stress Management Questionnaire (SMQ)** *Identification of symptoms linked to stress and coping strategies that aid in the reduction of stress.* | Yes | Valid and Reliable | Comfortable for the client | Coping, stressors, behavioral theory | Adult/elderly |

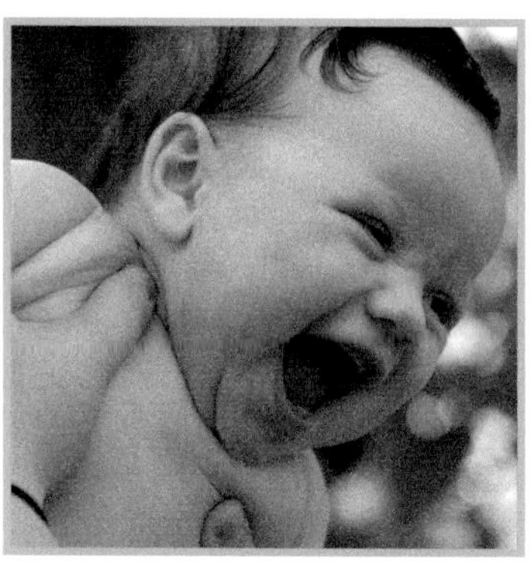

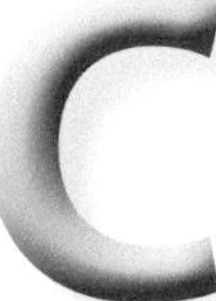

# ASSESSMENTS IN PLAY AND LEISURE



Jacobs, K., & MacRae, N. (Eds.).
*Occupational Therapy Essentials for Clinical Competence, Third Edition* (pp. 863-870).

# Play Assessments

| Child-Initiated Pretend Play Assessment | |
|---|---|
| **Ages** | Children 3 to 7 years of age |
| **Purpose** | Measures the quality of spontaneous pretend play (Bundy, 2005) |
| **Format/ Procedure** | Observation of play in two 15-minute sessions. Assesses three items—elaborate play actions, substitutions, and imitated actions. Involves imaginative play with typical toys and symbolic, unstructured play. Author recommends that the administrator should be professionally trained to work with children (Bundy, 2005) |
| **Psychometric Properties** | Scoring manual is unpublished. Internal consistency = not reported. Interrater reliability (involves use of videotapes): elaborate play actions 0.96 or 0.98; substitutions 1.00 or 0.97; imitated actions 0.98 to 1.00; Test-retest reliability: elaborate play actions $r = 0.73$ to $r = 0.85$; substitutions $r = 0.56$ to $r = 0.57$. Distribution of the remaining items was not normal. Content validity has been established via expert review, and play items were tested for developmental sensitivity and gender neutrality; Construct validity = not reported (Bundy, 2005). Interrater reliability also established at kappa 0.7 (Swindells & Stagnitti, 2006) |

| Children's Playfulness Scale | |
|---|---|
| **Ages** | Preschool- and toddler-aged children |
| **Purpose** | Measures the predisposition to be playful |
| **Format/ Procedure** | Twenty-three item instrument categorized into five areas of playfulness: physical spontaneity, social spontaneity, cognitive spontaneity, manifest joy, and sense of humor. Rater scored based on observations |
| **Psychometric Properties** | Interrater reliability ranged from 0.92 to 0.97; Test-retest reliability ranged from 0.84 to 0.88 at 1 month, 0.88 to 0.92 at 3 months, and 0.89 to 0.95 between the two intervals. Internal consistency for the scales ranged from 0.80 to 0.89 and 0.88 overall. Content validity based on playfulness research; Construct validity reported (Asher, 1996) |

| (Revised) Knox Preschool Play Scale | |
|---|---|
| **Ages** | Children 0 to 6 years of age |
| **Purpose** | Provides child's capacity for play and some information regarding play interests. Has been used for both diagnostic purposes and as an outcome measure for intervention (Bundy, 2005) |
| **Format/ Procedure** | Observation of play inside and outside in familiar settings and with familiar toys and peers. Four dimensions of play are observed: space management, material management, imitation, and participation. Administered in two 30-minute observations (Bundy, 2005; Sturgess, 1997) |
| **Psychometric Properties** | Not standardized as administration occurs in familiar environments. Internal consistency-not reported; Interrater reliability-coefficients ranged from $r = 0.88$ to $r = 0.996$; $P = 0.0001$; Test-retest reliability-coefficients range from $r = 0.91$ to $r = 0.965$; $P = 0.0001$; content validity has been established via an extensive review of the literature; Construct validity-not reported (Bundy, 2005; Rodger & Ziviani, 1999; Stagnitti, 2004) |

| Penn Interactive Peer Play Scale | |
|---|---|
| **Ages** | Preschool and kindergarten age in disadvantaged urban areas |
| **Purpose** | Developed to assess peer play interactions in disadvantaged urban children at risk for experiencing disconnection between school and home life (Fantuzzo & Hampton, 2000) |
| **Format/ Procedure** | Parallel versions of parent and teacher rating scales, with preschool and kindergarten versions. The parent versions assess play in the home and neighborhood, and the teacher version examines play in structured and unstructured school activities. Each version is composed of 32 items indicating the frequency the behavior is observed during free play within the preceding 2 months in three constructs: play interaction, play disruption, and play disconnection (Fantuzzo & Hampton) |
| **Psychometric Properties** | Each construct demonstrated a Cronbach alpha reliability of 0.90, 0.91, and 0.87. Inter-rater reliability of each construct was 0.84, 0.81, and 0.74. Content validity based on theoretical research. Congruence among test items was established (Fantuzzo & Hampton) |

| Play History | |
|---|---|
| **Ages** | 0 to 16 years |
| **Purpose** | Caregiver perspective of children's play; a tool for intervention planning |
| **Format/ Procedure** | Semi-structured interview administered to parents and/or caregivers; gather information on past play experiences and actual play; records play in five epochs—sensorimotor, symbolic, and simple constructive; dramatic; complex constructive; pre-game; and recreational. Each section is divided into four elements: materials, actions, people, and setting (Bundy, 2005; Sturgess, 1997; Taylor, Menarchek-Fetkovich, & Day, 2000) |
| **Psychometric Properties** | Test-retest reliability coefficient was 0.77 with section coefficients ranging from 0.41 to 0.78; Inter-rater reliability using videotaped interviews was 0.91 with section coefficients ranging from 0.58-0.85. Reliability was higher for typically developing children than children with disabilities (Behnke & Menarchek-Fetkovich, 1984); content validity based on theoretical research (Bundy; Taylor et al.) |

| Play in Early Childhood Education System | |
|---|---|
| **Ages** | Early childhood |
| **Purpose** | To develop a standardized procedure for assessment and coding of play in preschoolers |
| **Format/ Procedure** | Still being developed |
| **Psychometric Properties** | Relatively new assessment that is still being developed and standardized. Research is limited. However, initial studies indicate reliability of the assessment. Content validity is reported by the authors secondary to development based on empirical research (Kelly-Vance & Ryalls, 2005) |

## Symbolic Play Test

| | |
|---|---|
| **Ages** | Ages 1 to 3 |
| **Purpose** | Developed to assess functional play skills typically demonstrated in children between 12 and 36 months (Power & Radcliffe, 2000) |
| **Format/ Procedure** | Children are observed in several modes of play, including tactile exploration, self-orientation, and doll orientation. Four sets of toys are presented in a specific manner. Administration takes approximately 15 to 20 minutes, and raw scores are obtained and converted to a developmental age (Power & Radcliffe). Assesses symbolic play to determine whether language development relates to difficulties with symbolism or concept formation (Sturgess, 1997) |
| **Psychometric Properties** | Split-half reliability coefficients were corrected by the Spearman-Brown formula and ranged from 0.52 to 0.92. Reliability coefficients at the 15- and 18-month age levels were low (0.57 and 0.52, respectively), borderline at the 12-, 21-, and 36-month levels (0.74-0.79), and acceptable at the 24- and 30-month levels (greater than 0.90). Test-retest reliability was 0.72 at 3 months. Floor and ceiling effects affect validity. Normative data was obtained on 137 children, with much of the testing occurring on the same children. This included seven age ranges with small sample sizes within each range (Power & Radcliffe) |

## Test of Playfulness

| | |
|---|---|
| **Ages** | 3 months to 15 years |
| **Purpose** | Captures the four playfulness components: intrinsic motivation, internal control, freedom from some constraints of reality, and framing (Bundy, 2005) |
| **Format/ Procedure** | 29 observational items; each item is scored 0 to 3 reflecting extent, intensity, or skill. Administered during 15 to 20 minutes of free play in a familiar environment. Author urges administration in more than one environment (Bundy, 2005); The Test of Playfulness continues to be developed and researched (Stagnitti, 2004) |
| **Psychometric Properties** | Internal consistency—Cronbach's alpha was near 1.00; Interrater reliability—Rasch model goodness of fit; Test-retest reliability is being established and is not yet published; Content validity has been established via an extensive review of the literature; Construct validity—28/29 items demonstrate acceptable goodness of fit statistics using Rasch analysis (Bundy, 2005) |

The Test of Playfulness (ToP) is not commercially available, but may be obtained by contacting the author, Anita Bundy, ScD, OTR, School of Occupation and Leisure Sciences, University of Sydney, PO Box 170, Lidcombe NSW, Australia, bookspublishing@slackinc.com (Bundy, 2005).

## Transdisciplinary Play-Based Assessment, Second Edition

| | |
|---|---|
| **Ages** | Children 0 to 6 years of age |
| **Purpose** | Captures the four playfulness components: intrinsic motivation, internal control, freedom from some constraints of reality, and framing (Bundy, 2005; Linder, 2000) |
| **Format/ Procedure** | 29 observational items; each item is scored 0 to 3 reflecting extent, intensity, or skill. Administered during 15 to 20 minutes of free play in a familiar environment. Author urges administration in more than one environment (Bundy, 2005; Linder, 2000) |
| **Psychometric Properties** | Internal consistency—Cronbach's alpha was near 1.00; Interrater reliability—Rasch model goodness of fit; Test-retest reliability is being established and is not yet published; Content validity has been established via an extensive review of the literature; Construct validity—28/29 items demonstrate acceptable goodness of fit statistics using Rasch analysis (Bundy, 2005; Linder, 2000) |

# Leisure Assessments

## Activity Card Sort

| | |
|---|---|
| **Ages** | Adults with and without cognitive impairment |
| **Purpose** | Originally designed to identify activity level for adults with Alzheimer's Disease; has been used with different populations. Includes Healthy Older Adult version, Institutional version, and Recovering version (Connolly, Law, & MacGuire, 2005) |
| **Format/ Procedure** | 80 photo cards; caregiver or client sorts into categories. Categories vary depending upon version administered; Israeli version has been developed |
| **Psychometric Properties** | Test-retest reliability 0.897 (Baum & Edwards, 2001); internal consistency for Israeli version: high for IADL (0.82) and cultural activities (0.80) and moderate for low physical activities (0.66) and high physical activities (0.61) (Katz, Karpin, Lak, Furman, & Hartman-Maeir, 2003). Content and construct validity reported (Connolly et al., 2005) |

## Children's Assessment of Participation and Enjoyment

| | |
|---|---|
| **Ages** | From ages 6 to 21; should be able to sort/categorize (Connolly et al., 2005) |
| **Purpose** | Identify participation in/enjoyment of daily activities |
| **Format/ Procedure** | 55 item instrument; divided into five scales: recreational, active physical, social, skill-based, and self-improvement/educational. Can be categorized into formal and informal activities. Measures participation in five areas: diversity of activity, intensity/frequency, with whom activity occurs, where activity occurs, and enjoyment of activity. Includes two versions: self-administered and interviewer-assisted (Connolly et al.) |
| **Psychometric Properties** | Test-retest reliability ranges from 0.12 to 0.86. Internal consistency ranged from 0.32 to 0.62. Content, construct, and criterion validity are reported (Connolly et al.) |

## Interest Checklist/Activity Checklist

| | |
|---|---|
| **Ages** | Adolescent to adult |
| **Purpose** | Identify an individual's level of interest in leisure activities |
| **Format/ Procedure** | Original Interest Checklist included 80 items in five categories: manual skills, physical sports, social recreation, ADL, and cultural/educational (Matsutsuyu, 1969). Revised and renamed Activity Checklist contains 60 items in four categories: sports and physical tasks, intellectual and musical tasks, social tasks, and fine manual tasks and homemaking (Katz, 1988). Both are self-report instruments with level of interest rating. |
| **Psychometric Properties** | Test retest reliability at three weeks ranged from 0.84 to 0.92 for each category and 0.92 overall (Asher, 1996); internal consistency has not been reported. Testing on content validity has revealed mixed results (Connolly et al., 2005). |

| Leisure Activity Profile | |
|---|---|
| **Population** | Diagnosis of alcoholism |
| **Purpose** | Time use measurement of individuals with alcoholism; identifies dysfunctional patterns of leisure activities related to alcohol use (Mann & Talty, 1990) |
| **Format/ Procedure** | 38 item instrument; 19 related to alcohol consumption. Self-report or interviewer administration. Client reports time spent in activities, with whom activities occur, enjoyment, and alcohol consumption during activities |
| **Psychometric Properties** | Test retest reliability $r = 0.90$ to $r = 0.94$. Internal consistency not reported. Content and construct validity reported (Connolly et al., 2005) |

| Leisure Assessment Inventory | |
|---|---|
| **Population** | Adults with mental retardation |
| **Purpose** | Measures leisure behavior for adults with mental retardation |
| **Format/ Procedure** | Contains four indices based upon a conceptual definition of leisure: The Leisure Activity Participation Index reflects a person's leisure repertoire and involves 50 picture-cued activity cards; the Leisure Preference and Leisure Interest Indices represent 2 different aspects of choice making to assess the perceived degree of well-being, self-worth, and self-determination experienced during leisure; and the Leisure Constraints Index measures the degree in which internal and external constraints inhibit engagement in new leisure activities. Administered using a structured, three-part interview (Hawkins, Ardovino, & Hsieh, 1998) |
| **Psychometric Properties** | Reliability: Leisure Activity Participation ($r = 0.84$, $P < 0.01$), Leisure Preference ($r = 0.53$, $P < 0.01$), Leisure Interest ($r = 0.77$, $P < 0.01$), and Leisure Constraints ($r = 0.48$, $P < 0.01$); Content validity at $P < 0.01$ for each index |

| Leisure Attitude Scale | |
|---|---|
| **Population** | |
| **Purpose** | To examine leisure attitude |
| **Format/ Procedure** | 36 item instrument; three subscales assessing various aspects of attitude, including cognitive, affective, and behavioral subscales; Elderly version modified from original and includes 26 items measuring desired leisure, perceived leisure, self definition through work or leisure, affinity for leisure, and society's role in leisure planning. Can be administered as an interview or questionnaire (Teaff, Ernst, & Ernst, 1982) |
| **Psychometric Properties** | Overall reliability 0.95; subscales reliability: Cognitive 0.89; Affective 0.90; Behavioral 0.91 (Siegenthaler & O'Dell, 2000) |

| Leisure Boredom Scale | |
|---|---|
| **Ages** | Adolescents and young adults |
| **Purpose** | Assess perception of boredom relative to leisure opportunities |
| **Format/ Procedure** | 16-item self-report instrument rating relative to boredom |
| **Psychometric Properties** | Test-retest reliability $r = 0.73$ with 95% confidence interval; Moderate Cohen's Kappa for seven items (0.41 to 0.52); fair for two items (0.32 to 0.38); Internal consistency reported at 0.85; 0.86, 0.88; Construct validity reported (Connolly et al., 2005). |

## Leisure Competence Measure

| | |
|---|---|
| **Ages** | Adults |
| **Purpose** | Evaluates changes in leisure functioning |
| **Format/ Procedure** | Service provider rating based on observation, interview, and review of records; eight subscales including Leisure Awareness, Leisure Attitude, Leisure Skills, Cultural/Social Behaviors, Interpersonal Skills, Community Integration Skills, Social Contact, and Community Participation. Takes approximately 1 hour to administer |
| **Psychometric Properties** | No test-retest reliability reported; Inter-rater reliability = 0.91 overall and 0.71-0.91 for subscales; Internal consistency—Cronbach's Alpha 0.92; Content validity reported (Connolly et al., 2005) |

## Leisure Diagnostic Battery [1]

| | |
|---|---|
| **Ages** | Individuals with adapted IQ of 80 and higher; mental age 12 and older; Rancho Los Amigos level of seven and higher; mild to no orientation disability (Connolly et al., 2005) |
| **Purpose** | Identify client's leisure capacity |
| **Format/ Procedure** | Comprised of four assessments: Leisure Attitude Measure (LAM), Leisure Interest Measure (LIM), Leisure Motivation Scale (LMS), and Leisure Satisfaction Measure (LSM). Leisure Attitude Measure assesses leisure attitude on cognitive, affective, and behavioral levels; Leisure Interest Measure assesses interest in eight areas: physical, outdoor, mechanical, artistic, service, social, cultural, and reading. Leisure Motivation Scale includes 48 item Full Scale and 32 item Short Scale measuring client motivation; Leisure Satisfaction Measure assesses six satisfaction subscales: psychological, educational, social, relaxation, physiological, and aesthetic. Self report instruments |
| **Psychometric Properties** | Test-retest not reported. Internal consistency: LAM: 0.89-0.94; LIM: 0.87 overall, poor internal reliability in artistic domain, acceptable in all others; LMS: Authors report strong internal reliability (Beard & Ragheb, 1983); LSM: overall reliability 0.93; Content validity reported for all four assessments; Construct validity reported for LAM and LSM; Criterion validity reported for LAM (Connolly et al., 2005) |

## Leisure Diagnostic Battery [2]

| | |
|---|---|
| **Ages** | One version for youth with disabilities; one for adults |
| **Purpose** | Assess perception of freedom and barriers to participation in leisure |
| **Format/ Procedure** | 147 item Full Forms (A and C; youth and adults, respectively) related to control, competence, needs, playfulness, barriers, and knowledge. 25-item Short Form (B). Both forms are self-report instruments. |
| **Psychometric Properties** | Test retest (Form A) 0.72. Internal consistency 0.83 to 0.94 (Form A), 0.89 to 0.94 (Form B), and 0.90 to 0.96 (Form C). Content and construct validity reported for Form A (Connolly et al., 2005) |

## Leisure Satisfaction Scale

| | |
|---|---|
| **Ages** | Adults |
| **Purpose** | To examine leisure satisfaction and the extent in which individuals perceive their needs are being met through participation in leisure activities |
| **Format/ Procedure** | Self report measure; Original version: 51 item instrument; six subscales assessing satisfaction, including Psychological, Educational, Social, Relaxational, Physiological, and Aesthetic subscales; Short Form: 24 item instrument; same six subscales as original version |
| **Psychometric Properties** | Test-retest reliability not reported; One study reports reliability at 0.96 (Siegenthaler & O'Dell, 2000); Internal consistency ranged from 0.86 to 0.92 for subtest and overall 0.96 (original version) and 0.93 (short form). Content validity reported (Connolly et al., 2005) |

## Preferences for Activities of Children

| | |
|---|---|
| **Ages** | From ages 6 to 21; should be able to sort/categorize (Connolly et al., 2005) |
| **Purpose** | Identify activity preferences |
| **Format/ Procedure** | 55 item instrument; five activity scales: Recreational, Active Physical, Social, Skill-Based, and Self-Improvement/Educational in two domains: formal and informal activities. Can be self administered or interviewer-assisted (Connolly et al., 2005) |
| **Psychometric Properties** | Test-retest reliability not reported; Intenal consistency ranged from 0.67 to 0.84. Content validity reported; Construct validity related to participation outcome variables ($r < 0.01$); correlations with CAPE ranged from 0.22 to 0.61 (Connolly et al., 2005) |

## References


Asher, I. E. (1996). *Occupational therapy assessment tools: An annotated index* (2nd ed.). Bethesda, MD: AOTA Press.

Baum, C. M., & Edwards, D. (2001). *Activity card sort.* St. Louis, MO: Washington University at St. Louis.

Beard, J. G., & Ragheb, M. G. (1983). Measuring leisure motivation. *Journal of Leisure Research, 15*(3), 219-228.

Behnke, C. J., & Menarchek-Fetkovich, M. M. (1984). Examining the reliability and validity of the Play History. *American Journal of Occupational Therapy, 38*(2), 94-100.

Bundy, A. C. (2005). Measuring play performance. In M. Law, C. Baum, & W. Dunn (Eds.), *Measuring occupational performance: Supporting best practice in occupational therapy* (2nd ed., pp. 129-150). Thorofare, NJ: SLACK Incorporated.

Connolly, K., Law, M., & MacGuire, B. (2005). Measuring leisure performance. In M. Law, W. Dunn, & C. Baum (Eds.), *Measuring occupational performance: Supporting best practice in occupational therapy* (2nd ed., pp. 249-276). Thorofare, NJ: SLACK Incorporated.

Fantuzzo, J. W., & Hampton, V. R. (2000). Penn Interactive Peer Play Scale: A parent and teacher rating system for young children. In K. Gitlin-Weiner, S. Sandgrund, & C. Schaefer (Eds.), *Play diagnosis and assessment* (2nd ed., pp. 599-620). New York, NY: John Wiley and Sons.

Hawkins, B. A., Ardovino, P., & Hsieh, C. (1998). Validity and reliability of the Leisure Assessment Inventory. *Mental Retardation, 36*(4), 303-313.

Katz, N. (1988). Interest checklist: A factor analytical study. *Occupational Therapy in Mental Health, 8*(1), 45-55.

Katz, N., Karpin, H., Lak, A., Furman, T., & Hartman-Maeir, A. (2003). Participation in occupational performance: Reliability and validity of the Activity Card Sort. *Occupational Therapy Journal of Research, 23*(1), 10-17.

Kelly-Vance, L., & Ryalls, B. O. (2005). A systematic, reliable approach to play assessment in preschoolers. *School Psychology International, 26*(4), 398-412.

Linder, T. (2000). Transdisciplinary play-based assessment. In K. Gitlin-Weiner, S. Sandgrund, & C. Schaefer (Eds.), *Play diagnosis and assessment* (2nd ed., pp. 139-166). New York, NY: John Wiley and Sons.

Mann, W. C., & Talty, P. (1990). Leisure Activity Profile: Measuring use of leisure time by persons with alcoholism. *Occupational Therapy in Mental Health, 10*(4), 31-41.

Matsutsuyu, J. S. (1969). The Interest Checklist. *American Journal of Occupational Therapy, 23,* 323-328.

Power, T. J., & Radcliffe, J. (2000). Assessing the cognitive ability of infants and toddlers through play: The Symbolic Play Test. In K. Gitlin-Weiner, A. Sandgrund, & C. Schaefer (Eds.), *Play diagnosis and assessment* (2nd ed., pp. 58-79). New York, NY: John Wiley and Sons.

Rodger, S., & Ziviani, J. (1999). Play-based occupational therapy. *International Journal of Disability, Development, and Education, 46*(3), 337-365.

Siegenthaler, K. L., & O'Dell, I. (2000). Leisure attitude, leisure satisfaction, and perceived freedom in leisure within family dyads. *Leisure Sciences, 22*(4), 281-296.

Stagnitti, K. (2004). Understanding play: The implications for play assessment. *Australian Occupational Therapy Journal, 51,* 3-12.

Sturgess, J. L. (1997). Current trends in assessing children's play. *British Journal of Occupational Therapy, 60*(9), 410-414.

Swindells, D., & Stagnitti, K. (2006). Pretend play and parents' view of social competence: The construct validity of the Child-Initiated Pretend Play Assessment. *Australian Occupational Therapy Journal, 53,* 314-324.

Taylor, K. M., Menarchek-Fetkovich, M., & Day, C. (2000). The Play History interview. In K. Gitlin-Weiner, S. Sandgrund, & C. Schaefer (Eds.), *Play diagnosis and assessment* (2nd ed., pp. 114-138). New York, NY: John Wiley and Sons.

Teaff, J. D., Ernst, N. W., & Ernst, M. (1982). Elderly Leisure Attitude Scale. In D. J. Mangen & W. A. Peterson (Eds.), *Research instruments in social gerontology: Vol. 2. Social roles and social participation* (pp. 498-499; 535-537). Minneapolis, MN: University of Minnesota Press.

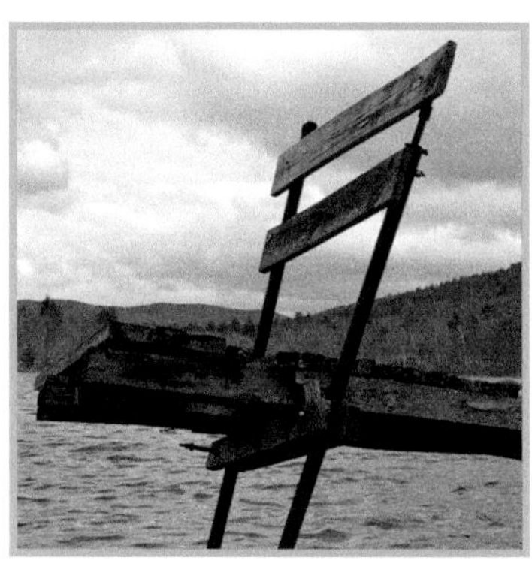

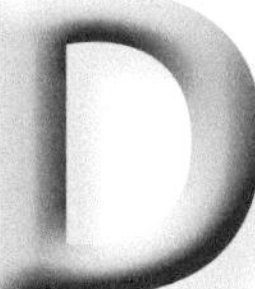

# Intervention Plan Outline



Jacobs, K., & MacRae, N. (Eds.).
*Occupational Therapy Essentials for Clinical Competence, Third Edition* (pp. 871-872).

# Intervention Plan

Client's name:
Age:
Date of plan:
How long will sessions be? Where? When?:

Diagnosis:

Background information:

Precautions:

Strengths and weaknesses:

Goals and objectives:

Frame of reference:

◊ Principles of the frame of reference that will be used to design intervention:

◊ Rationale for using frame of reference:

◊ Evidence to support using frame of reference with this type of client:

Sample activity selection:

Progression of activities—how will they be graded and adapted?:

Equipment needs:

Safety concerns:

Describe the role of the occupational therapy practitioner according to the frame of reference:

Describe what is expected of the client:

Other:

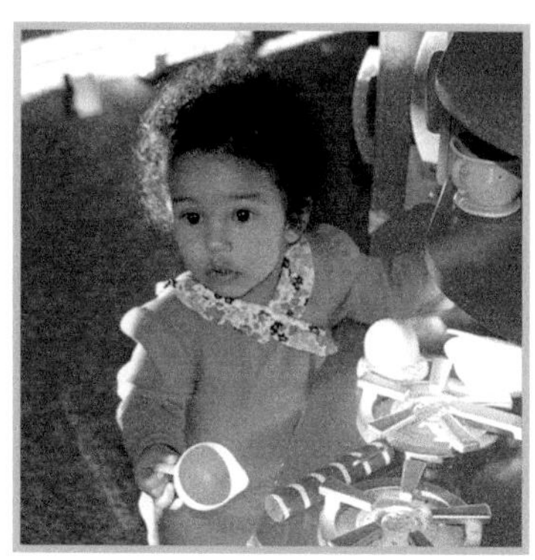

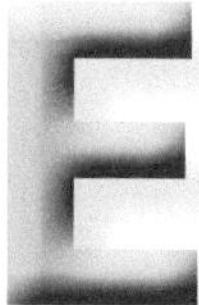

# Sample of an Individualized Education Program

Barbara J. Steva, MS, OTR/L



Jacobs, K., & MacRae, N. (Eds.).
*Occupational Therapy Essentials for Clinical Competence, Third Edition* (pp. 873-879).

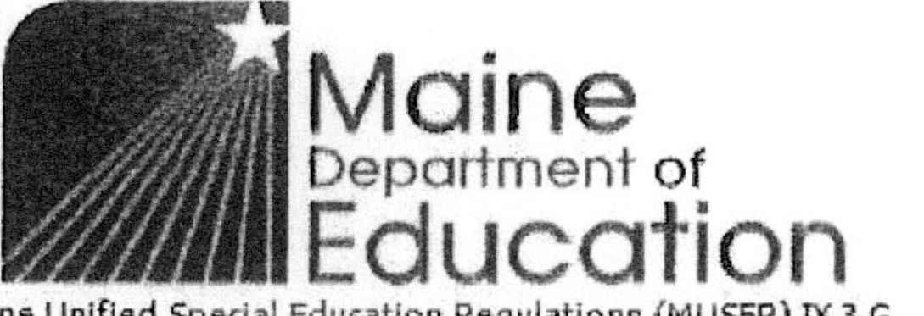


Maine Unified Special Education Regulations (MUSER) IX.3.G.

**SAU/School/Grade or CDS Placement:** Arundel, Kennebunk, Kennebunkport Regional School Unit 21 / Mildred L Day School / 01

Date IEP Sent to Parent: 5/23/2013

**INDIVIDUALIZED EDUCATION PROGRAM (IEP)**

**1. CHILD INFORMATION**

| | | | |
|---|---|---|---|
| Child's Name: | [redacted] | Date of Meeting: | 05/02/2013 |
| Date of Birth: | 8/11/2005 Age: 7 | Effective Date of IEP: | 5/6/2013 - 5/1/2014 |
| School/Program: | Mildred L Day School Grade: 01 | Date of Annual IEP Review: | 5/1/2014 |
| Parent Information: | [redacted] | Date of Re-evaluation: | 4/28/2016 |
| | | Date(s) of Amended IEP: | N/A |
| | | Case Manager: | [redacted] |

State Agency Client: Yes ☐ No ☒

**2. DISABILITY** (MUSER) VII.2

| | | |
|---|---|---|
| ☐ Autism | ☐ Deaf-Blindness | ☐ Deafness |
| ☐ Developmental Delay (ages 3-5) | ☐ Developmental Delay (Kindergarten) | ☐ Emotional Disturbance |
| ☐ Hearing Impairment | ☐ Intellectual Disability | ☐ Multiple Disabilities(list concomitant disabilities) |
| ☐ Other Health Impairment | ☐ Orthopedic Impairment | ☐ Speech/Language Impairment |
| ☒ Specific Learning Disability | ☐ Traumatic Brain Injury | ☐ Visual Impairment (Including Blindness) |

Child's Name:

## 3. CONSIDERATIONS

**In developing each child's IEP, the IEP team must consider** - MUSER IX.3.C.

A. **Concerns** of parents for enhancing the education of their child. MUSER IX.3.C.(1)(b)

is pleased with the results of the evaluation. She is happy that will be receiving services. She expressed that it is frustrating sometimes when she is unable to help him understand information. She said that he is very uncoordinated but is very active at home.

B. **Results** of the initial evaluation or most recent evaluation of the child. MUSER IX.3.C.(1)(c)

April 2013:
WISC-IV: Verbal Comprehension Composite Score 98, 45%; Perceptual Reasoning Composite Score 90, 25%; Working Memory Composite Score 83, 13%; Processing Speed Composite Score 70, 2%; Full Scale Composite Score 83, 13%.

WRMT: Readiness SS 83, 13%; Basic Skills 70, 2%; Reading Comprehension 81, 10%; Total Reading 70, 2%.

KeyMath3: Basic Concepts SS 97, 42%; Operations 90, 25%; Applications 88, 21%; Total Test Composite 89, 23%.

Peabody Picture Vocabulary Test-4: SS 140, 99.6%
Expressive Vocabulary Test-2: SS 112, 79%
CELF-4: Core Language Score SS 102, 55%; Receptive Language Index 117, 87%; Expressive Language Index 101, 53%; Language Content Index 121, 92%; Language Structure Index 106, 66%.

Beery Developmental Test of Visual Motor Integration-6: Visual Motor Integration SS 71, 3%; Visual Perception 104,61%; Motor Coordination Unable to Score.
Bruininks-Oseretsky Test of Motor Proficiency-2: Fine Motor Precision 9; Fine Motor Integration 10; Manual Dexterity 14; Upper Limb Coordination 16; Fine Manual Control 37, 10%; Manual Coordination 50, 50%; Motor Free Visual Perception Test 95, 37%.

C. **Strengths** of the child. MUSER IX.3.C.(1)(a)

has great communication skills with adults. Has strength in expressive and receptive language skills.

D. **Needs** of the child - academic, developmental, and functional. MUSER IX.3.C.(1)(d)

Academic: Due to his weaknesses in Processing Speed and Working Memory requires specially designed instruction in Reading and Writing to access tl General Education Curriculum.

Developmental: s poor muscle strength through his core muscles impacts his ability to maintain a stable base on which to build refined fine motor control needed to complete academic tasks at a level consistent with same age and grade level peers.

Functional: Due to his difficulty with forming peer relations and anxious behaviors will benefit from Social Work services to help access the general education curriculum.

Child's Name:

## Consideration of Special Factors: The IEP Team must - MUSER IX.3.C.(2)

E. In the case of a child whose behavior impedes the child's learning or that of others consider the use of positive behavioral interventions and supports and other strategies to address the behavior. MUSER IX.3.C.(2)(a)

Check if not needed [X] **If needed, indicate where it is addressed in the IEP.**

F. In the case of a child with limited English proficiency, consider the language needs of the child as those needs relate to the child's IEP. MUSER IX.3.C.(2)(b)

Check if not needed [X] **If needed, indicate where it is addressed in the IEP.**

G. In the case of a child who is blind or visually impaired, provide for instruction in Braille and the use of Braille unless the IEP Team determines, after an evaluation of the child's reading and writing skills, needs, and appropriate reading and writing media (including an evaluation of the child's future needs for instruction in Braille or the use of Braille), that instruction in Braille or the use of Braille is not appropriate for the child. MUSER IX.3.C.(2)(c)

Check if not needed [X] **If needed, indicate where it is addressed in the IEP.**

H. Consider the communication needs of the child, and in the case of a child who is deaf or hard of hearing, consider the child's language and communication needs, opportunities for direct communication with peers and professional personnel in the child's language and communication mode, academic level, and full range of needs including opportunities for direct instruction in the child's language and communication mode. MUSER IX.3.C.(2)(d)

Check if not needed [ ] **If needed, indicate where it is addressed in the IEP.**
FM System as needed in the regular education classroom only.

I. Consider whether the child needs assistive technology devices and services. MUSER IX.3.C.(2)(e)

Check if not needed [X] **If needed, indicate where it is addressed in the IEP.**

Child's Name:

## 4. PRESENT LEVELS OF ACADEMIC AND FUNCTIONAL PERFORMANCE MUSER IX.3.A.(1)(a)(i)&(ii)

A statement of Present levels of academic achievement and functional performance.

**Goal ID: 21622 Academic**
Currently, independently uses a Powerplan to initiate the writing process 15% of the time as measured by Teacher Observations.
**Goal ID: 21621 Academic**
Currently, has a grade equivalent score of <1.0 on Oral Reading Fluency as measured by the WRMT-III.
**Goal ID: 21620 Academic**
Currently, has a Basic Reading Skills grade equivalent score of <1.0 as measured by WRMT-III.
**Goal ID: 21702 OT**
Currently, uses bilateral coordination and graded motions to cut 1/16" lines, containing at least two directional changes, with no more than 2 deviations from the line, 10% of trials.
**Goal ID: 21700 OT**
Currently, demonstrates the ability to plan, sequence, and carry out a motor task, requiring right and left side and upper and lower extremity coordination, 20% of the time.
**Goal ID: 21699 OT**
Currently, independently creates and constructs projects (including gathering needed materials and sequencing of steps), involving 4 or more steps from a model, 30% of the time.
**Goal ID: 21689 OT**
Currently, writes demonstrating spontaneous letter formation 83% of the time. The expectation for the end of first grade is 96%.
Currently, writes demonstrating appropriate placement on and within the writing lines 75% of the time. The expectation for the end of first grade is 88%.
**Goal ID: 21618 PT**
runs around the gym 1 time without slowing down or stopping
**Goal ID: 21617 PT**
will accesses 5 climbing items on the playground.
**Goal ID: 21616 PT**
will sits upright on the floor and table top in a crossed legged pattern without leaning on arms for supports less than 30 seconds at a time.
**Goal ID: 21615 PT**
squats to stand 4 times without the support of his hands
**Goal ID: 21614 PT**
does not complete an exercise program.
**Goal ID: 21639 Social/Emotional**
Currently, is able to focus 50% of the time.
**Goal ID: 21637 Social/Emotional**
Based on staff reports interacts with peers appropriately 25% of the time.

How the child's disability affects the child's involvement and progress in the general education curriculum. For preschool children, as appropriate, how the disability affects the child's participation in appropriate activities.

has weaknesses in Processing Speed and Working Memory. He needs specially designed instruction in reading, writing, Physical Therapy, and Occupational Therapy in order to access the general education curriculum. has difficulty interacting with peers and making peer relationships and this adversely effects his academic setting.

Child's Name:

## 5. ANNUAL GOAL(S)

A statement of measurable annual goals, including academic and functional goals, designed to: meet the child's needs that result from the child's disability to enable the child to be involved in and make progress in the general education curriculum which must be for children 3-5 aligned with the Early Learning Guidelines and for children 5-20 aligned with the system of Maine's Learning Results; and meet each of the child's other educational needs that result from the child's disability. The IEP shall reflect the individual goals to successfully meet the content standards of the system of Maine's Learning Results in addition to any other diploma requirements applicable to all secondary children pursuant to 20-A MRSA §4722.
Include below a statement of how the child's progress toward meeting the annual goals will be measured. MUSER IX.3.A.(1)(b)&(c).

| Measurable Annual Goal | * 1, 2, 3, 4 For Pre School only | How Goal will be Measured | ** PROGRESS |
|---|---|---|---|
| **Goal ID: 21702 OT -** Given therapeutic activities, will use bilateral coordination and graded motions to cut 1/16" lines, containing at least two directional changes, with no more than 2 deviations from the line, 60% of trials, by May 2014. | N/A | Clinical data collection, informal assessment, work samples and observation of functional daily performance. | 6/20/2013<br>12/6/2013<br>3/21/2014 |
| **Goal ID: 21700 OT -** Given therapeutic activities to improve planning and dissociation of body parts, will demonstrate the ability to plan, sequence, and carry out a motor task, requiring right and left side and upper and lower extremity coordination, 60% of the time, by May 2014. | N/A | clinical data collection, informal assessment, and observation of functional daily performance | 6/20/2013<br>12/6/2013<br>3/21/2014 |
| **Goal ID: 21699 OT -** Given visual and verbal cues as needed and a completed model, will independently create and construct projects (including gathering needed materials and sequencing of steps), involving 4 or more steps from a model, 60% of the time, by May 2014. | N/A | clinical data collecdtion, informal assessment, work samples and observation of functional daily performance | 6/20/2013<br>12/6/2013<br>3/21/2014 |
| **Goal ID: 21689 OT -** Given direct intervention, will write a minimum of two sentences, demonstrating spontaneous letter formation and correct letter height, spacing and placement within the writing lines, 90% of the time, by May 2014. | N/A | clinical data collection, informal assessment, work samples, and observation of functional daily performance | 6/20/2013<br>12/6/2013<br>3/21/2014 |

Child's Name: [redacted]

## 7. SPECIAL EDUCATION AND RELATED SERVICES MUSER IX.3.A.(1)(d) & IX.3.A.(1)(g)

| Special Education Services | Position Responsible | Location | Frequency | Duration Beginning/Ending Date |
|---|---|---|---|---|
| Specially Designed Instruction Reading and Writing | Special Educator | Special ed. | 5 times per Week for 1 hour and 30 minutes | 5/6/2013 to 5/1/2014 |

| Related Services | Position Responsible | Location | Frequency | Duration Beginning/Ending Date |
|---|---|---|---|---|
| Social Work Service | Social Worker | Special ed. | 2 times per Week for 30 minutes | 5/6/2013 to 5/1/2014 |
| Occupational Therapy | Occupational Therapist | Special ed. | 2 times per Week for 30 minutes | 5/6/2013 to 5/1/2014 |
| Physical Therapy Services | Physical Therapist | Special ed. | 2 times per Week for 30 minutes | 5/6/2013 to 5/1/2014 |

## 9. LEAST RESTRICTIVE ENVIRONMENT

What percentage of time is this child with non-disabled children?

68%

An explanation of the extent, if any, to which the child will not participate with non disabled children in the regular class and in extracurricular and other nonacademic activities: MUSER IX.3.A.(1)(e)

[redacted] will participate in all regular education activities/settings with the exception of 5x1.5 hours per week of Specially Designed Instruction in Reading and Writing, 2x 30 minutes per week of Social Work, 2x30 minutes per week of Occupational Therapy, and 2x30 minutes per week of Physical Therapy.

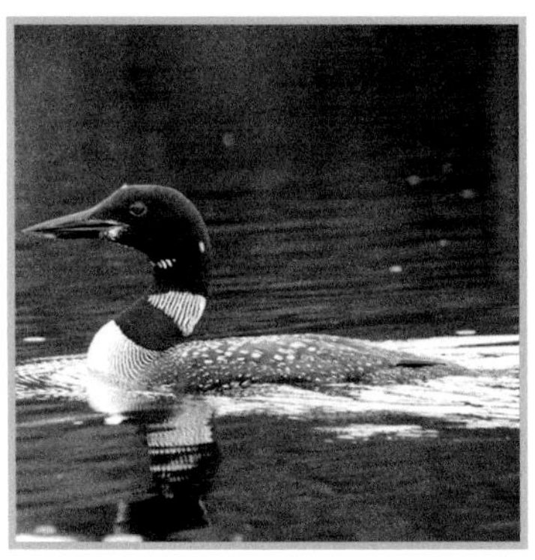

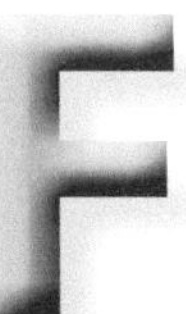


# American Occupational Therapy Association *Occupational Therapy Code of Ethics (2015)*

*Reprinted with permission from the American Occupational Therapy Association.*



Jacobs, K., & MacRae, N. (Eds.).
*Occupational Therapy Essentials for Clinical Competence, Third Edition* (pp. 881-889).

# Occupational Therapy Code of Ethics (2015)

## Preamble

The 2015 *Occupational Therapy Code of Ethics* (Code) of the American Occupational Therapy Association (AOTA) is designed to reflect the dynamic nature of the profession, the evolving health care environment, and emerging technologies that can present potential ethical concerns in research, education, and practice. AOTA members are committed to promoting inclusion, participation, safety, and well-being for all recipients in various stages of life, health, and illness and to empowering all beneficiaries of service to meet their occupational needs. Recipients of services may be individuals, groups, families, organizations, communities, or populations (AOTA, 2014b).

The Code is an AOTA Official Document and a public statement tailored to address the most prevalent ethical concerns of the occupational therapy profession. It outlines Standards of Conduct the public can expect from those in the profession. It should be applied to all areas of occupational therapy and shared with relevant stakeholders to promote ethical conduct.

The Code serves two purposes:

1. It provides aspirational Core Values that guide members toward ethical courses of action in professional and volunteer roles.
2. It delineates enforceable Principles and Standards of Conduct that apply to AOTA members.

Whereas the Code helps guide and define decision-making parameters, ethical action goes beyond rote compliance with these Principles and is a manifestation of moral character and mindful reflection. It is a commitment to benefit others, to virtuous practice of artistry and science, to genuinely good behaviors, and to noble acts of courage. Recognizing and resolving ethical issues is a systematic process that includes analyzing the complex dynamics of situations, weighing consequences, making reasoned decisions, taking action, and reflecting on outcomes. Occupational therapy personnel, including students in occupational therapy programs, are expected to abide by the Principles and Standards of Conduct within this Code. Personnel roles include clinicians (e.g., direct service, consultation, administration); educators; researchers; entrepreneurs; business owners; and those in elected, appointed, or other professional volunteer service.

The process for addressing ethics violations by AOTA members (and associate members, where applicable) is outlined in the Code's Enforcement Procedures (AOTA, 2014a).

Although the Code can be used in conjunction with licensure board regulations and laws that guide standards of practice, the Code is meant to be a free-standing document, guiding ethical dimensions of professional behavior, responsibility, practice, and decision making. This Code is not exhaustive; that is, the Principles and Standards of Conduct cannot address every possible situation. Therefore, before making complex ethical decisions that require further expertise, occupational therapy personnel should seek out resources to assist in resolving ethical issues not addressed in this document. Resources can include, but are not limited to, ethics committees, ethics officers, the AOTA Ethics Commission or Ethics Program Manager, or an ethics consultant.

## Core Values

The profession is grounded in seven long-standing Core Values: (1) Altruism, (2) Equality, (3) Freedom, (4) Justice, (5) Dignity, (6) Truth, and (7) Prudence. *Altruism* involves demonstrating concern for the welfare of others. *Equality* refers to treating all people impartially and free of bias. *Freedom* and personal choice are paramount in a profession in which the values and desires of the client guide our interventions. *Justice* expresses a state in which diverse communities are inclusive; diverse communities are organized and structured such that all members can function, flourish, and live a satisfactory life. Occupational therapy personnel, by virtue of the specific nature of the practice of occupational therapy, have a vested interest in addressing unjust inequities that limit opportunities for participation in society (Braveman & Bass-Haugen, 2009).

Inherent in the practice of occupational therapy is the promotion and preservation of the individuality and *Dignity* of the client by treating him or her with respect in all interactions. In all situations, occupational therapy personnel must provide accurate information in oral, written, and electronic forms (*Truth*). Occupational therapy personnel use their clinical and ethical reasoning skills, sound judgment, and reflection to make decisions in professional and volunteer roles (*Prudence*).

The seven Core Values provide a foundation to guide occupational therapy personnel in their interactions with others. Although the Core Values are not themselves enforceable standards, they should be considered when determining the most ethical course of action.

## Principles and Standards of Conduct

The Principles and Standards of Conduct that are enforceable for professional behavior include (1) Beneficence, (2) Nonmaleficence, (3) Autonomy, (4) Justice, (5) Veracity, and (6) Fidelity. Reflection on the historical foundations of occupational therapy and related professions resulted in the inclusion of Principles that are consistently referenced as a guideline for ethical decision making.

### BENEFICENCE

**Principle 1. Occupational therapy personnel shall demonstrate a concern for the well-being and safety of the recipients of their services.**

Beneficence includes all forms of action intended to benefit other persons. The term *beneficence* connotes acts of mercy, kindness, and charity (Beauchamp & Childress, 2013). Beneficence requires taking action by helping others, in other words, by promoting good, by preventing harm, and by removing harm. Examples of beneficence include protecting and defending the rights of others, preventing harm from occurring to others, removing conditions that will cause harm to others, helping persons with disabilities, and rescuing persons in danger (Beauchamp & Childress, 2013).

### RELATED STANDARDS OF CONDUCT

**Occupational therapy personnel shall**

A. Provide appropriate evaluation and a plan of intervention for recipients of occupational therapy services specific to their needs.

B. Reevaluate and reassess recipients of service in a timely manner to determine whether goals are being achieved and whether intervention plans should be revised.

C. Use, to the extent possible, evaluation, planning, intervention techniques, assessments, and therapeutic equipment that are evidence based, current, and within the recognized scope of occupational therapy practice.

D. Ensure that all duties delegated to other occupational therapy personnel are congruent with credentials, qualifications, experience, competency, and scope of practice with respect to service delivery, supervision, fieldwork education, and research.

E. Provide occupational therapy services, including education and training, that are within each practitioner's level of competence and scope of practice.

F. Take steps (e.g., continuing education, research, supervision, training) to ensure proficiency, use careful judgment, and weigh potential for harm when generally recognized standards do not exist in emerging technology or areas of practice.

G. Maintain competency by ongoing participation in education relevant to one's practice area.

H. Terminate occupational therapy services in collaboration with the service recipient or responsible party when the services are no longer beneficial.

I. Refer to other providers when indicated by the needs of the client.

J. Conduct and disseminate research in accordance with currently accepted ethical guidelines and standards for the protection of research participants, including determination of potential risks and benefits.

**NONMALEFICENCE**

**Principle 2. Occupational therapy personnel shall refrain from actions that cause harm.**

*Nonmaleficence* "obligates us to abstain from causing harm to others" (Beauchamp & Childress, 2013, p. 150). The Principle of *Nonmaleficence* also includes an obligation to not impose risks of harm even if the potential risk is without malicious or harmful intent. This Principle often is examined under the context of due care. The standard of *due care* "requires that the goals pursued justify the risks that must be imposed to achieve those goals" (Beauchamp & Childress, 2013, p. 154). For example, in occupational therapy practice, this standard applies to situations in which the client might feel pain from a treatment intervention; however, the acute pain is justified by potential longitudinal, evidence-based benefits of the treatment.

**RELATED STANDARDS OF CONDUCT**

**Occupational therapy personnel shall**

A. Avoid inflicting harm or injury to recipients of occupational therapy services, students, research participants, or employees.

B. Avoid abandoning the service recipient by facilitating appropriate transitions when unable to provide services for any reason.

C. Recognize and take appropriate action to remedy personal problems and limitations that might cause harm to recipients of service, colleagues, students, research participants, or others.

D. Avoid any undue influences that may impair practice and compromise the ability to safely and competently provide occupational therapy services, education, or research.

E. Address impaired practice and, when necessary, report it to the appropriate authorities.

F. Avoid dual relationships, conflicts of interest, and situations in which a practitioner, educator, student, researcher, or employer is unable to maintain clear professional boundaries or objectivity.

G. Avoid engaging in sexual activity with a recipient of service, including the client's family or significant other, student, research participant, or employee, while a professional relationship exists.

H. Avoid compromising the rights or well-being of others based on arbitrary directives (e.g., unrealistic productivity expectations, falsification of documentation, inaccurate coding) by exercising professional judgment and critical analysis.

I. Avoid exploiting any relationship established as an occupational therapy clinician, educator, or researcher to further one's own physical, emotional, financial, political, or business interests at the expense of recipients of services, students, research participants, employees, or colleagues.

J. Avoid bartering for services when there is the potential for exploitation and conflict of interest.

AUTONOMY

**Principle 3. Occupational therapy personnel shall respect the right of the individual to self-determination, privacy, confidentiality, and consent.**

The Principle of *Autonomy* expresses the concept that practitioners have a duty to treat the client according to the client's desires, within the bounds of accepted standards of care, and to protect the client's confidential information. Often, respect for Autonomy is referred to as the *self-determination principle.* However, respecting a person's autonomy goes beyond acknowledging an individual as a mere agent and also acknowledges a person's right "to hold views, to make choices, and to take actions based on [his or her] values and beliefs" (Beauchamp & Childress, 2013, p. 106). Individuals have the right to make a determination regarding care decisions that directly affect their lives. In the event that a person lacks decision-making capacity, his or her autonomy should be respected through involvement of an authorized agent or surrogate decision maker.

RELATED STANDARDS OF CONDUCT

**Occupational therapy personnel shall**

A. Respect and honor the expressed wishes of recipients of service.

B. Fully disclose the benefits, risks, and potential outcomes of any intervention; the personnel who will be providing the intervention; and any reasonable alternatives to the proposed intervention.

C. Obtain consent after disclosing appropriate information and answering any questions posed by the recipient of service or research participant to ensure voluntariness.

D. Establish a collaborative relationship with recipients of service and relevant stakeholders to promote shared decision making.

E. Respect the client's right to refuse occupational therapy services temporarily or permanently, even when that refusal has potential to result in poor outcomes.

F. Refrain from threatening, coercing, or deceiving clients to promote compliance with occupational therapy recommendations.

G. Respect a research participant's right to withdraw from a research study without penalty.

H. Maintain the confidentiality of all verbal, written, electronic, augmentative, and nonverbal communications, in compliance with applicable laws, including all aspects of privacy laws and exceptions thereto (e.g., Health Insurance Portability and Accountability Act [Pub. L. 104–191], Family Educational Rights and Privacy Act [Pub. L. 93–380]).

I. Display responsible conduct and discretion when engaging in social networking, including but not limited to refraining from posting protected health information.

J. Facilitate comprehension and address barriers to communication (e.g., aphasia; differences in language, literacy, culture) with the recipient of service (or responsible party), student, or research participant.

**JUSTICE**

**Principle 4. Occupational therapy personnel shall promote fairness and objectivity in the provision of occupational therapy services.**

The Principle of *Justice* relates to the fair, equitable, and appropriate treatment of persons (Beauchamp & Childress, 2013). Occupational therapy personnel should relate in a respectful, fair, and impartial manner to individuals and groups with whom they interact. They should also respect the applicable laws and standards related to their area of practice. Justice requires the impartial consideration and consistent following of rules to generate unbiased decisions and promote fairness. As occupational therapy personnel, we work to uphold a society in which all individuals have an equitable opportunity to achieve occupational engagement as an essential component of their life.

**RELATED STANDARDS OF CONDUCT**

**Occupational therapy personnel shall**

A. Respond to requests for occupational therapy services (e.g., a referral) in a timely manner as determined by law, regulation, or policy.

B. Assist those in need of occupational therapy services in securing access through available means.

C. Address barriers in access to occupational therapy services by offering or referring clients to financial aid, charity care, or pro bono services within the parameters of organizational policies.

D. Advocate for changes to systems and policies that are discriminatory or unfairly limit or prevent access to occupational therapy services.

E. Maintain awareness of current laws and AOTA policies and Official Documents that apply to the profession of occupational therapy.

F. Inform employers, employees, colleagues, students, and researchers of applicable policies, laws, and Official Documents.

G. Hold requisite credentials for the occupational therapy services they provide in academic, research, physical, or virtual work settings.

H. Provide appropriate supervision in accordance with AOTA Official Documents and relevant laws, regulations, policies, procedures, standards, and guidelines.

I. Obtain all necessary approvals prior to initiating research activities.

J. Refrain from accepting gifts that would unduly influence the therapeutic relationship or have the potential to blur professional boundaries, and adhere to employer policies when offered gifts.

K. Report to appropriate authorities any acts in practice, education, and research that are unethical or illegal.

L. Collaborate with employers to formulate policies and procedures in compliance with legal, regulatory, and ethical standards and work to resolve any conflicts or inconsistencies.

M. Bill and collect fees legally and justly in a manner that is fair, reasonable, and commensurate with services delivered.

N. Ensure compliance with relevant laws, and promote transparency when participating in a business arrangement as owner, stockholder, partner, or employee.

O. Ensure that documentation for reimbursement purposes is done in accordance with applicable laws, guidelines, and regulations.

P. Refrain from participating in any action resulting in unauthorized access to educational content or exams (including but not limited to sharing test questions, unauthorized use of or access to content or codes, or selling access or authorization codes).

### VERACITY

**Principle 5. Occupational therapy personnel shall provide comprehensive, accurate, and objective information when representing the profession.**

Veracity is based on the virtues of truthfulness, candor, and honesty. The Principle of *Veracity* refers to comprehensive, accurate, and objective transmission of information and includes fostering understanding of such information (Beauchamp & Childress, 2013). Veracity is based on respect owed to others, including but not limited to recipients of service, colleagues, students, researchers, and research participants.

In communicating with others, occupational therapy personnel implicitly promise to be truthful and not deceptive. When entering into a therapeutic or research relationship, the recipient of service or research participant has a right to accurate information. In addition, transmission of information is incomplete without also ensuring that the recipient or participant understands the information provided.

Concepts of veracity must be carefully balanced with other potentially competing ethical principles, cultural beliefs, and organizational policies. Veracity ultimately is valued as a means to establish trust and strengthen professional relationships. Therefore, adherence to the Principle of Veracity also requires thoughtful analysis of how full disclosure of information may affect outcomes.

### RELATED STANDARDS OF CONDUCT

**Occupational therapy personnel shall**

A. Represent credentials, qualifications, education, experience, training, roles, duties, competence, contributions, and findings accurately in all forms of communication.

B. Refrain from using or participating in the use of any form of communication that contains false, fraudulent, deceptive, misleading, or unfair statements or claims.

C. Record and report in an accurate and timely manner and in accordance with applicable regulations all information related to professional or academic documentation and activities.

D. Identify and fully disclose to all appropriate persons errors or adverse events that compromise the safety of service recipients.

E. Ensure that all marketing and advertising are truthful, accurate, and carefully presented to avoid misleading recipients of service, research participants, or the public.

F. Describe the type and duration of occupational therapy services accurately in professional contracts, including the duties and responsibilities of all involved parties.

G. Be honest, fair, accurate, respectful, and timely in gathering and reporting fact-based information regarding employee job performance and student performance.

H. Give credit and recognition when using the ideas and work of others in written, oral, or electronic media (i.e., do not plagiarize).

I. Provide students with access to accurate information regarding educational requirements and academic policies and procedures relative to the occupational therapy program or educational institution.

J. Maintain privacy and truthfulness when using telecommunication in the delivery of occupational therapy services.

**FIDELITY**

**Principle 6. Occupational therapy personnel shall treat clients, colleagues, and other professionals with respect, fairness, discretion, and integrity.**

The Principle of Fidelity comes from the Latin root *fidelis,* meaning loyal. *Fidelity* refers to the duty one has to keep a commitment once it is made (Veatch, Haddad, & English, 2010). In the health professions, this commitment refers to promises made between a provider and a client or patient based on an expectation of loyalty, staying with the client or patient in a time of need, and compliance with a code of ethics. These promises can be implied or explicit. The duty to disclose information that is potentially meaningful in making decisions is one obligation of the moral contract between provider and client or patient (Veatch et al., 2010).

Whereas respecting Fidelity requires occupational therapy personnel to meet the client's reasonable expectations, the Principle also addresses maintaining respectful collegial and organizational relationships (Purtilo & Doherty, 2011). Professional relationships are greatly influenced by the complexity of the environment in which occupational therapy personnel work. Practitioners, educators, and researchers alike must consistently balance their duties to service recipients, students, research participants, and other professionals as well as to organizations that may influence decision making and professional practice.

**RELATED STANDARDS OF CONDUCT**

**Occupational therapy personnel shall**

A. Preserve, respect, and safeguard private information about employees, colleagues, and students unless otherwise mandated or permitted by relevant laws.

B. Address incompetent, disruptive, unethical, illegal, or impaired practice that jeopardizes the safety or well-being of others and team effectiveness.

C. Avoid conflicts of interest or conflicts of commitment in employment, volunteer roles, or research.

D. Avoid using one's position (employee or volunteer) or knowledge gained from that position in such a manner as to give rise to real or perceived conflict of interest among the person, the employer, other AOTA members, or other organizations.

E. Be diligent stewards of human, financial, and material resources of their employers, and refrain from exploiting these resources for personal gain.

F. Refrain from verbal, physical, emotional, or sexual harassment of peers or colleagues.

G. Refrain from communication that is derogatory, intimidating, or disrespectful and that unduly discourages others from participating in professional dialogue.

H. Promote collaborative actions and communication as a member of interprofessional teams to facilitate quality care and safety for clients.

I. Respect the practices, competencies, roles, and responsibilities of their own and other professions to promote a collaborative environment reflective of interprofessional teams.

J. Use conflict resolution and internal and alternative dispute resolution resources as needed to resolve organizational and interpersonal conflicts, as well as perceived institutional ethics violations.

K. Abide by policies, procedures, and protocols when serving or acting on behalf of a professional organization or employer to fully and accurately represent the organization's official and authorized positions.

L. Refrain from actions that reduce the public's trust in occupational therapy.

M. Self-identify when personal, cultural, or religious values preclude, or are anticipated to negatively affect, the professional relationship or provision of services, while adhering to organizational policies when requesting an exemption from service to an individual or group on the basis of conflict of conscience.

## References

American Occupational Therapy Association. (2014a). Enforcement procedures for the *Occupational therapy code of ethics and ethics standards*. *American Journal of Occupational Therapy, 68*(Suppl. 3), S3–S15. http://dx.doi.org/10.5014/ajot.2014.686S02

American Occupational Therapy Association. (2014b). Occupational therapy practice framework: Domain and process (3rd ed.). *American Journal of Occupational Therapy, 68*(Suppl. 1), S1–S48. http://dx.doi.org/10.5014/ajot.2014.682006

Beauchamp, T. L., & Childress, J. F. (2013). *Principles of biomedical ethics* (7th ed.). New York: Oxford University Press.

Braveman, B., & Bass-Haugen, J. D. (2009). Social justice and health disparities: An evolving discourse in occupational therapy research and intervention. *American Journal of Occupational Therapy, 63,* 7–12. http://dx.doi.org/10.5014/ajot.63.1.7

Purtilo, R., & Doherty, R. (2011). *Ethical dimensions in the health professions* (5th ed.). Philadelphia: Saunders/Elsevier.

Veatch, R. M., Haddad, A. M., & English, D. C. (2010). *Case studies in biomedical ethics*. New York: Oxford University Press.

**Ethics Commission**

Yvette Hachtel, JD, OTR/L, *Chair (2013–2014)*
Lea Cheyney Brandt, OTD, MA, OTR/L, *Chair (2014–2015)*
Ann Moodey Ashe, MHS, OTR/L *(2011–2014)*
Joanne Estes, PhD, OTR/L *(2012–2015)*
Loretta Jean Foster, MS, COTA/L *(2011–2014)*
Wayne L. Winistorfer, MPA, OTR *(2014–2017)*
Linda Scheirton, PhD, RDH *(2012–2015)*
Kate Payne, JD, RN *(2013–2014)*
Margaret R. Moon, MD, MPH, FAAP *(2014–2016)*
Kimberly S. Erler, MS, OTR/L *(2014–2017)*
Kathleen McCracken, MHA, COTA/L *(2014–2017)*
Deborah Yarett Slater, MS, OT/L, FAOTA, *AOTA Ethics Program Manager*

*Adopted by the Representative Assembly 2015AprilC3.*

*Note.* This document replaces the 2010 document *Occupational Therapy Code of Ethics and Ethics Standards (2010)*, previously published and copyrighted in 2010 by the American Occupational Therapy Association in the *American Journal of Occupational Therapy, 64,* S17–S26. http://dx.doi.org/10.5014/ajot.2010.64S17



*Citation.* American Occupational Therapy Association. (2015). Occupational therapy code of ethics (2015). *American Journal of Occupational Therapy, 69*(Suppl. 3), 6913410030. http://dx.doi.org/10.5014/ajot.2015.696S03

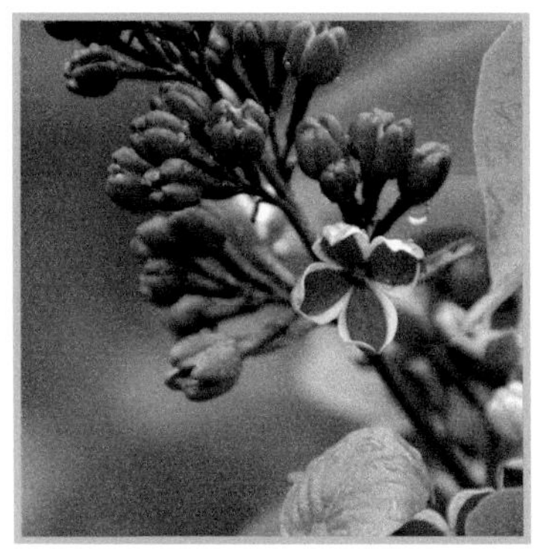

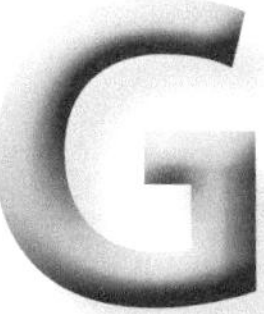

# Procedures for the Enforcement of the National Board for Certification in Occupational Therapy Candidate/Certificant Code of Conduct

*Reprinted with permission from the National Board for Certification in Occupational Therapy.*



Jacobs, K., & MacRae, N. (Eds.).
*Occupational Therapy Essentials for Clinical Competence, Third Edition* (pp. 891-898).

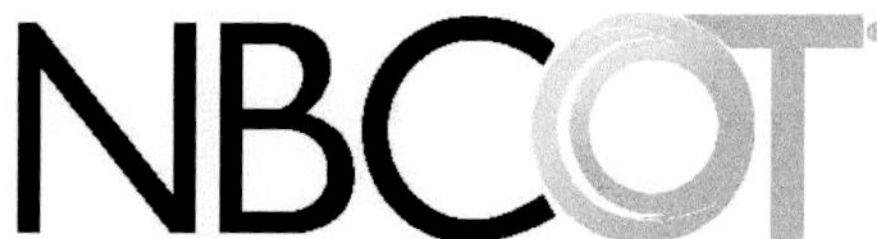

# PROCEDURES FOR THE ENFORCEMENT OF THE NBCOT® CANDIDATE/CERTIFICANT CODE OF CONDUCT

SECTION A. Preamble

In exercising its responsibility for promoting and maintaining standards of professional conduct in the practice of occupational therapy and in order to protect the public from those practitioners whose behavior falls short of these standards, the National Board for Certification in Occupational Therapy, Inc. ("NBCOT®," formerly known as "AOTCB") has adopted a Candidate/Certificant Code of Conduct. The NBCOT has adopted these procedures for resolving issues arising under the Candidate/Certificant Code of Conduct with respect to persons who have been certified by the NBCOT or who have applied for such certification. These procedures are intended to enable the NBCOT, through its Qualifications and Compliance Review Committee ("QCRC"), comprised of both professional and public members, QCRC Chair, (or Co-Chair when Chair is unavailable) and Staff to act fairly in the performance of its responsibilities to the public as a certifying agency, and to ensure that the rights of candidates and certificants are protected.

SECTION B. Basis for Sanction

A violation of the Candidate/Certificant Code of Conduct provides basis for action and sanction under these Procedures.

SECTION C. Sanctions

1. Violations of the Candidate/Certificant Code of Conduct may result in one or more of the following sanctions:

    a. Ineligibility for certification, which means that an individual is barred from becoming certified by the NBCOT, either indefinitely or for a certain duration.

    b. Reprimand, which means a formal expression of disapproval, which shall be retained in the certificant's file, but shall not be publicly announced.

    c. Censure, which means a formal expression of disapproval which is publicly announced.

    d. Probation, which means continued certification is subject to fulfillment of specified conditions, e.g., monitoring, education, supervision, and/or counseling.

    e. Suspension, which means the loss of certification for a certain duration, after which the individual may be required to apply for reinstatement.

    f. Revocation, which means permanent loss of certification.

2. All sanctions other than reprimand shall be announced publicly, in accordance with Section D.10. All sanctions other than reprimand shall be disclosed in response to inquiries in accordance with Section D.10.

SECTION D. Procedures For The Enforcement of The Candidate/Certificant Code of Conduct

1. Jurisdiction

The NBCOT has jurisdiction over all individuals who have been certified as an OCCUPATIONAL THERAPIST REGISTERED OTR (OTR®) henceforth OTR, or CERTIFIED OCCUPATIONAL THERAPY ASSISTANT COTA (COTA®) henceforth COTA, or who have applied for certification, or have applied for Occupational Therapist Eligibility Determination (OTED) to take the NBCOT Certification Examination for OTR. In addition, NBCOT has jurisdiction over all individuals who have applied for an Early Determination Review to determine eligibility to take the Certification Examination for OTR or COTA; Jurisdiction, in this case, is for the limited purpose of acting upon a request for an Early Determination.

2. Initiation of the Review Process

The NBCOT Staff ("Staff") shall initiate the process upon receipt by the NBCOT of information indicating that an individual subject to NBCOT's jurisdiction may have violated the Candidate/Certificant Code of Conduct. Receipt of such information shall be considered a complaint for the purposes of these procedures, regardless of the source.

3. Staff Investigation and Action

a. Staff shall review all complaints and investigate these complaints, as it deems appropriate.

b. Staff may review any evidence, which it deems appropriate and relevant.

i. If Staff determines that the evidence does not support the allegation(s), no file shall be opened and the complainant shall be notified of the Staff's decision.

ii. If Staff determines that the evidence does support the allegation(s) and decides to investigate, the subject of the complaint shall be notified. This notification shall be in writing and shall include a description of the complaint. The subject of the complaint shall have thirty (30) days from the date notification is sent to respond in writing to the complaint. The Staff may extend this period up to an additional thirty (30) days upon request, provided sufficient justification for the extension is given.

iii. In addition to providing a written response to the complaint and as part of the investigative process, the subject may request a telephone conference with an NBCOT representative. The purpose of this call is to give the subject an additional opportunity to verbally provide information about the case. The subject may also submit additional written information or documentation.

c. Upon the completion of its investigation, Staff shall either:

i. Dismiss the case due to insufficient evidence, the matter being insufficiently serious, or other reasons as may be warranted. The qualifications and compliance review shall be considered closed at the time such decision is made; or

ii. Present a proposed sanction to the QCRC Chair in the form of a disciplinary action agreement. At the discretion of the Chair additional members, both professional and public, may be asked to assist with the decision making process prior to taking the case to the full Committee.

4. <u>Voluntary Forfeiture</u>

The subject of a complaint may voluntarily forfeit his or her certification. This forfeiture must be submitted in writing and can be made, at any time, while the complaint is either under active investigation or when disciplinary action has been taken by the NBCOT but the terms of the sanction remain incomplete.

Staff will advise the Qualifications and Compliance Review Committee (QCRC) Chair of any voluntary forfeiture.

If the subject requests reinstatement of certification, after voluntary forfeiture, the subject must meet all of the following requirements:

a. submit reinstatement of certification request in writing
b. satisfy current certification examination eligibility requirements (including academic and fieldwork requirements) and
c. re-take and pass the national certification examination

Further, any pending investigation will be resumed upon request to regain certification.

If the subject's certification is voluntarily forfeited, public notice may be given in accordance with Section D.10 of these procedures.

5. <u>Non-Response (Noncomplaint-Inactive)</u>

If the subject does not respond to investigative inquiries, the subject's certification will be placed on Noncompliant-Inactive status in accordance with Section 9.

Staff will advise the QCRC Chair of this action.

If the subject requests reinstatement of certification, after being placed on Non Compliant-Inactive status, the subject must meet all of the following requirements:

a. submit reinstatement of certification request in writing
b. satisfy current certification renewal requirements, and
c. cooperate with and provide written response and supporting documentation to the NBCOT investigative inquiry

6. QCRC Chair Review and Procedures for Disciplinary Action Agreement

Staff shall prepare a case summary of its investigation along with the disciplinary action agreement for the QCRC Chair to consider. The report shall include the basis for Staff's findings, as well as any written responses, or other materials submitted in relation to the investigation of the complaint.

If Staff and the QCRC Chair are not able to reach agreement on the proposed sanction, the Chair will schedule a meeting of the QCRC to review and determine final conditions and terms of the disciplinary action agreement.

If the QCRC Chair and Staff are in agreement on the proposed sanction, Staff shall forward the disciplinary action agreement to the subject.

The subject may either:

a. Accept the disciplinary action agreement and thereby waive his/her right to a hearing. The disciplinary action agreement will be sent to the subject in writing. To accept the agreement, the subject must sign, date and return the agreement to NBCOT. Upon the subject's acceptance of the disciplinary action agreement, the qualifications and compliance process shall be considered closed. The public notification standards of Section D.10 are applicable if the settlement contains a sanction that warrants such announcement be made; or

b. Not accept the disciplinary action agreement and request a hearing before the QCRC. Request for a hearing must be submitted by the subject in writing.

   At the hearing:

   i. The subject of the complaint may be represented at the hearing by his/her legal counsel, or any other individual of his or her choosing.

   ii. The subject of the complaint shall be solely responsible for all of his/her own expenses related to the hearing. Hearings can be conducted via teleconference call or in person at the sole discretion of the QCRC. Should the subject cancel the hearing, he/she must notify the QCRC of the cancellation no less than fifteen (15) days prior to the hearing date. Should the subject cancel the hearing within fifteen (15) days of the hearing date or not appear at the scheduled hearing, all costs associated with the preparation of the hearing shall be paid by the subject (e.g. court reporting fees, teleconference fees, hearing manual preparation fees).

iii. The subject of the complaint shall provide the QCRC with any and all materials he/she may wish to include for the hearing no less than fifteen (15) days prior to the hearing date.

Following the hearing, Staff shall notify (in writing) the complainant and the subject of the complaint of the QCRC's decision within thirty (30) days of the decision. The decision shall take effect immediately unless otherwise provided by the QCRC.

c. If the subject fails to respond to the disciplinary action agreement, within thirty (30) days after the agreement has been sent to the subject, conditions and terms of the agreement take effect immediately.

7. <u>Appeals Process</u>

Within thirty (30) days after the notification of the QCRC's decision, any individual(s) sanctioned by the QCRC at the hearing may appeal the hearing decision to the NBCOT Directors. A notice of appeal, which must be in writing and signed by the subject, shall be sent by the subject to the NBCOT Chairperson in care of the President/Chief Executive Officer. The basis for the appeal shall be fully explained in this notice.

The Chairperson shall form an Appeals Panel within thirty (30) days after receipt of the notice of appeal. The Appeals Panel shall be comprised of three (3) NBCOT Directors and shall include at least one (1) OTR or one (1) COTA and one (1) public member. Members of the QCRC who participated in any aspect of the proceedings related to the complaint shall not serve on the Appeals Panel.

An appeal must relate to evidence, issues and procedures that are part of the record of the QCRC hearing and decision. The appeal may also address the substance of the disciplinary action. However, the Panel may in its discretion consider additional evidence.

Within fifteen (15) days after the notice of appeal is received by the Appeals Panel, the Panel shall provide the subject with an opportunity to schedule a hearing. The subject may be represented at the hearing by legal counsel or any other individual of his/her choosing. The subject shall be solely responsible for all of his/her own expenses related to the hearing.

Within fifteen (15) days after the appeals hearing or if the subject elects not to request a formal hearing, the Panel shall decide the appeal and notify the Chairperson of its decision.

The Appeals Panel may either:

a. Affirm the QCRC's disciplinary action agreement;

b. Deny the QCRC's disciplinary action agreement;

c. Refer the case back to the Staff for further investigation and resolution with full right of appeal; or

d. Modify the QCRC's disciplinary action agreement, but not in a manner that would be more adverse to the subject.

The Chairperson shall promptly notify the subject of the Appeals Panel's decision. The decision of the Appeals Panel shall be final.

8. Cooperation with NBCOT Enforcement Procedures

Failure to respond to any aspect of the Enforcement Procedures, will be considered a violation of the Candidate/Certificant Code of Conduct, Principle 2, and is sufficient grounds for the imposition of sanction by the NBCOT.

9. Noncompliant-Inactive

Individuals who do not satisfy the NBCOT certification renewal requirements by their scheduled renewal date, or who are non-responsive to NBCOT investigative inquiries are "Noncompliant-Inactive" and CANNOT a) identify themselves to the public as an OCCUPATIONAL THERAPIST REGISTERED (OTR) or CERTIFIED OCCUPATIONAL THERAPY ASSISTANT (COTA) or b) use the OTR or COTA credential after their name.

10. Announcement of Sanction

If an individual's certification status is voluntarily forfeited, suspended or revoked, or he/she is censured or placed on probation, occupational therapy state regulatory bodies shall be notified and an announcement included on its web site and in one or more publications of general circulation to persons engaged or otherwise interested in the profession of occupational therapy. The NBCOT may also disclose its final decision, including ineligibility for certification, to others as it deems appropriate, including, but not limited to, persons inquiring about the status of an individual's certification, employers, third party payers and the general public.

11. Notification

All notifications referred to in these procedures shall be in writing and if the subject does not respond, shall be by confirmation of signature, return receipt mail, unless otherwise indicated. Subjects of complaints who live outside of the U.S. may be given additional time to respond to any notifications they are sent, as determined by the Staff in its discretion.

12. Records and Reports

At the completion of this procedure, all records and reports shall be returned to the Staff. The complete files in the qualifications and compliance review proceedings shall be maintained.

13. <u>Expedited Action</u>

The NBCOT may expedite a matter by shortening any notice or response period provided for under these procedures if the responsible party determines in its sole discretion that shortening the period is appropriate in order to protect against the possibility of harm to recipients of occupational therapy services.

In matters where the severity of the allegations and evidence provided warrant such action in order to protect the public, the NBCOT may authorize immediate suspension/revocation of certification. The subject will be duly notified of the action and given fifteen (15) days to contest the suspension or revocation.

14. <u>Standard Of Proof</u>

The NBCOT shall take disciplinary action against an individual only where there is clear and convincing evidence of a violation of the Candidate/Certificant Code of Conduct.

15. <u>Special Accommodations</u>

The NBCOT recognizes the definition of disability as defined by the Americans with Disabilities Act (ADA) and acknowledges the provisions and protections of the Act. The NBCOT shall offer hearings related to qualifications and compliance review or the appeals process in a site and manner, which is architecturally accessible to persons with disabilities or offer alternative arrangements for such individuals.

An individual with a documented disability may request special accommodations for a hearing by providing reasonable advance notice to the NBCOT of his or her disability and of the modifications or aids needed at the hearing at his or her own expense.

16. <u>Amendment to Procedures</u>

These procedures may be amended at any time by the NBCOT Directors.

 

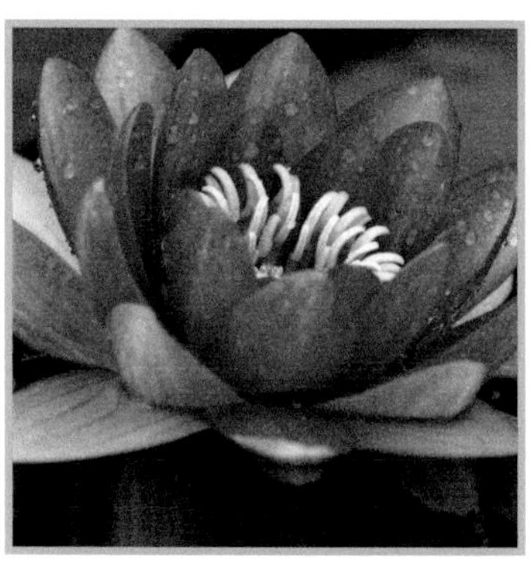

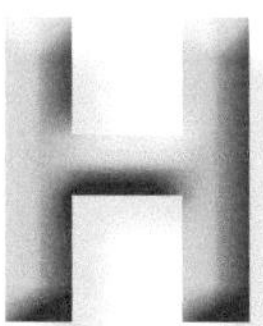

# National Board for Certification in Occupational Therapy Complaint Form

*Reprinted with permission from the National Board for Certification in Occupational Therapy.*



Jacobs, K., & MacRae, N. (Eds.).
*Occupational Therapy Essentials for Clinical Competence, Third Edition* (pp. 899-901).

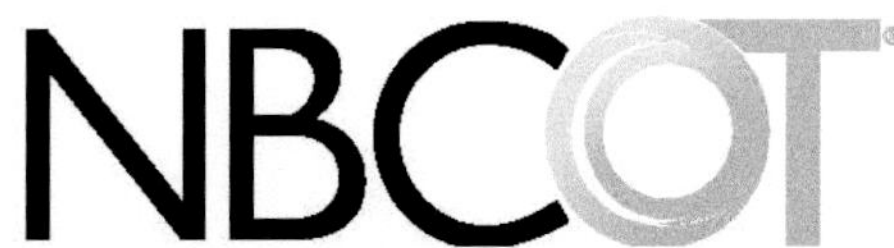

# COMPLAINT FORM

1. **Complaint is filed against:**

**Name:** ______________________________ **Telephone:** ________________

**Address:** ____________________________ **NBCOT Cert #:** ________________

2. **Person filing complaint (complainant):**

**Name:** ______________________________ **Telephone:** ________________

**Address:** ______________________________________________________

3. **Complainant's relationship with the person against whom the complaint is being filed (e.g., supervisor, co-worker, patient, etc.):**

4. **Summary of complaint (in your own words – who, what, where, when, why, and how): [Use additional sheets if needed].**

5. **Other persons with knowledge of the incident(s) giving rise to this complaint:**

**Name:** ____________________________ **Telephone:** ____________________

**Address:** ______________________________________________________

**Name:** ____________________________ **Telephone:** ____________________

**Address:** ______________________________________________________

(see reverse side)

6. **Other agencies or organizations you have submitted this complaint to (i.e., state licensing boards, Medicare, AOTA, police or other authorities, etc.):**

7. **State in your own words how this incident(s) relates to the NBCOT's "Candidate/Certificant Code of Conduct" (use additional sheets if needed):**

______________________________

______________________________

______________________________

______________________________

______________________________

______________________________

______________________________

______________________________

______________________________

______________________________

**Complainant Signature** ______________________ **Date** ______________

(Note: Complete separate form for each complaint or complainant)

Revision Date: 01/02/2013

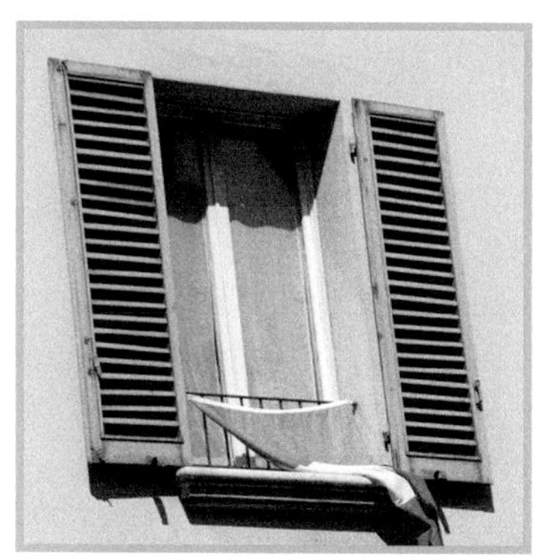

I

# World Federation of Occupational Therapists Code of Ethics

*Reprinted with permission from the World Federation of Occupational Therapists.*



Jacobs, K., & MacRae, N. (Eds.).
*Occupational Therapy Essentials for Clinical Competence, Third Edition* (pp. 903-904).

# WORLD FEDERATION of OCCUPATIONAL THERAPISTS (WFOT)

## CODE OF ETHICS

This code describes the general categories of appropriate conduct for occupational therapists in any professional circumstance. It is understood that each member association will have a detailed code of ethics particular to its needs.

### Personal Attributes

Occupational therapists demonstrate personal integrity, reliability, open-mindedness and loyalty in all aspects of their professional role.

### Responsibility towards the Recipient of Occupational Therapy Services

Occupational therapists approach all persons receiving their services with respect and have regard for their individual situations. Occupational therapists shall not discriminate against these persons on the basis of race, colour, impairment, disability, national origin, age, gender, sexual preference, religion, political beliefs or status in society.

The values, preferences and ability to participate of persons receiving occupational therapy will be taken into account in providing services.

Confidentiality of the persons' personal information is guaranteed and any personal details are passed on only with that person's consent.

### Professional Conduct in Collaborative Practice

Occupational therapists recognise the need for inter-professional collaboration and respect the unique contributions of other professions. Occupational therapists' contribution to inter-professional collaboration is based on occupational performance as it affects the health and well-being of people.

### Developing Professional Knowledge

Occupational therapists participate in professional development through life-long learning and apply their acquired knowledge and skills in their professional work which is based on the best available evidence.

When participating in research occupational therapists respect the ethical implications involved.

### Promotion and Development

Occupational therapists are committed to the improvement and development of the profession in general. They are also concerned with ethically promoting occupational therapy to the public, other professional organisations and government bodies at regional, national and international levels.

Updated IMM05

# Glossary

**ABA design:** A single case experimental design where (A) baseline data is measured, (B) intervention provided, and (C) measurement repeated.

**AbleData:** A federally sponsored website that organizes and tracks adaptive tools and provides an overview of a wide range of assistive devices across a wide spectrum of functions.

**abstract:** Summary of an article or paper containing the most important points of each subsection.

**activities of daily living (ADLs):** "Activities oriented toward taking care of one's own body (adapted from Rogers & Holm, 1994). ADLs also are referred to as basic activities of daily living (BADLs) and personal activities of daily living (PADLs). These activities are 'fundamental to living in a social world; they enable basic survival and well-being' (Christiansen & Hammecker, 2001, p. 156; see Table 1)" (AOTA, 2014, p. S41).

**activity/activities:** The execution of a task or action by an individual (WHO, 2001); "actions designed and selected to support the development of performance skills and performance patterns to enhance occupational engagement" (AOTA, 2014, p. S41).

**activity demands:** Requirements specific to the activity and independent of the person.

**ADA Amendments Act (2008) (ADAAA):** This federal act amended the Americans with Disabilities Act of 1990. The changes, which apply to both the ADA and the Rehabilitation Act, include an updated definition of the term *disability* which clarifies and broadens the words used in order to protect more people under the ADA and other Federal disability nondiscrimination laws. The definition of *major life activities* was expanded to include bodily functions, which allows many people with internal function disorders such as gastrointestinal disorders, cancer, sleep disorders, insulin-dependent diabetes, and heart disease to now be covered under the ADA. The act also required the Equal Employment Opportunity Commission (EEOC) to adopt the changes into their regulations in order to protect the rights of a greater number of employees.

**adaptation:** "Occupational therapy practitioners enable participation by modifying a task, the method of accomplishing the task, and the environment to promote engagement in occupation (James, 2008)" (AOTA, 2014, p. S41).

**adapting:** To make suitable to or fit for a specific use or situation (Dictionary.com); to change something (i.e., the demands of the activity) so that the client is successful.

**advertisement:** To make something known; to make publicly and generally known; to announce publicly especially by a printed notice or a broadcast; to call public attention to especially by emphasizing desirable qualities so as to arouse a desire to buy or patronize (Merriam-Webster, 2006).

**advertising:** "A specific communication task to be accomplished with a specific audience in mind in a specific



Jacobs, K., & MacRae, N. (Eds.).
*Occupational Therapy Essentials for Clinical Competence, Third Edition* (pp. 905-920).

target market during a specific period of time. The advertisement goals are based on achieving one of four aims: to inform, to persuade, to remind, or to reinforce" (Kotler, 2003, p. 312).

**advocacy:** To speak up for or plead the case of another.

**affordable insurance exchange:** A new transparent, competitive insurance marketplace where individuals and small businesses can purchase affordable and qualified health benefit plans.

**American Psychological Association (APA) format:** The standard format used in health science literature for in-text citation and reference information.

**Americans with Disabilities Act (ADA):** A Federal law that prevents discrimination against individuals with disabilities.

**analysis of occupational performance:** A multistep process conducted by the occupational therapist. Based on a select model and/or frame(s) of reference, the occupational therapist analyzes the occupational profile in conjunction with other occupational therapists' assessments to formulate hypotheses about which factors encourage as well as disrupt the client's successful engagement in occupations and in daily life activities.

**analysis of variance (ANOVA):** A statistical procedure used to measure differences between measurements.

**annotated bibliography:** A citation and short summary.

**autism:** A complex developmental disability that typically appears during the first 3 years of life and affects a person's ability to communicate, read facial expressions, and interact with others. Autism is defined by a certain set of behaviors including repetitive actions, self-stimulation (rocking, hand flapping, spinning, etc.), avoidance of eye contact, and echoalia. Autism is a spectrum disorder that affects individuals differently and to varying degrees. Developmental disorder characterized by a severely reduced ability to communicate and emotionally relate to other people; self-absorption.

**autistic spectrum disorders (ASDs):** Common name for a variety of autistic disorders. Autism spectrum disorders are a group of developmental disabilities that can cause significant social, communication, and behavioral challenges. ASDs affect individuals differently and the spectrum includes those who are severely affected and experience great difficulty in communicating and building relationships, in addition to those with more mild forms such as Asperger's, who mainly have difficulty with obsessive interests and social situations.

**applied research:** Research directed toward the solution of specified practical problems in delineated areas, or to achieve practical goals (Kerlinger, 1979).

**applied theory:** The results of applied research, intended to address problems of practical interest.

**Arts and Crafts Movement:** A transformation of the American lifestyle, created in response to workers and their working environments, to restore the relationship between nature and creativity.

**aspiration:** The entry of secretions, fluids, food, or any foreign substance below the vocal cords and into the lungs that may result in aspiration pneumonia and may be fatal (AOTA, 2007).

**assessment:** Specific tools, instruments, or procedures used to obtain data during the evaluative process.

**assistive technology:** Devices that augment or extend a user's ability to function in the task environment.

**associative level participation:** Consists of approaching others briefly in verbal or nonverbal interactions.

**assumptions:** Broad general statements that are taken for granted for the sake of argument.

**attitude:** Your mindset or outlook.

**backward chaining:** A technique that teaches the last part of a task first, thus ensuring success. Once the last part is learned, the next to last part is taught, until the entire task is learned.

**basic cooperative level participation:** Includes selecting longer activities or tasks of mutual interest and following the norms or rules of interaction in play or work.

**basic research:** Systematic study to test theory and to understand relations among phenomena without consideration of application of the results (Kerlinger, 1979).

**bed mobility:** Safely and effectively moving in bed for comfort, skin integrity, and function.

**behavioral response:** Ability to express oneself in a social situation using independently generated verbal and nonverbal cues.

**benchmark:** Quantifiable measures of the outcomes of a process used as comparisons to current targets for improvement (Braveman, 2006).

**body functions and structures:** Physiologic and psychological aspects of individual systems, including anatomic parts (WHO, 2001).

**body mechanics:** The utilization of appropriate muscles and positions to complete heavy work safely and efficiently (Brookside Associates, 2007).

**bolus:** Food or liquid in a mass form (AOTA, 2007).

**bullying:** Unwanted, repetitive, aggressive behavior that may involve physical, verbal, relational, and/or electronic means of exerting power over another individual.

**care coordination:** A process that facilitates the linkage of individuals and their families with appropriate services and resources in a coordinated effort to achieve good health.

**career:** A line of business or way of making a living.

**caring:** A set of feelings, attitudes, and actions that convey respect, hope, and care toward others.

**case management:** A collaborative process that assesses, plans, implements, coordinates, monitors, and evaluates the options and services required to meet the client's health and human services needs.

**case mix groups (CMGs):** A term that classifies client discharges into diagnostic categories.

**certified occupational therapy assistant:** Professional personnel who work under the supervision of an occupational therapist and deliver occupational therapy intervention in partnership with occupational therapists.

**circadian process:** The process within our body that uses environmental cues (light/dark cycle) to train the body to have the ability of knowing when to sleep even if there are no environmental cues present at a given time.

**client:** "Person or persons (including those involved in the care of a client), group (collective of individuals, e.g., families, workers, students, or community members), or population (collective of groups or individuals living in a similar locale—e.g., city, state, or country—or sharing the same or like concerns)" (AOTA, 2014, p. S41).

**client-centered care:** Therapeutic interventions where the person who is receiving services has a major role in the decision making regarding his or her care. The practitioner takes a collaborative rather than an authoritative role.

**client-centered practice:** A partnership between a client and therapist that serves to empower a client toward reaching goals of his or her own choosing; "an approach to therapy that supports a respectful partnership between therapists and clients" (Law, Baptiste, & Mills, 1995, p. 256). Client-centered practice includes the following concepts: (1) recognition of each client's unique perspective; (2) a shift in power toward the client having more say in defining and directing intervention; (3) a shift to an enablement intervention model; (4) an understanding of the importance of the influence on intervention of the client's culture, preferences, interests, roles, and environments; (5) an understanding of the importance of flexible and dynamic interventions that emphasize learning and problem solving; and (6) respect for the client's values regardless of whether these are shared by the therapist.

**client factors:** The physiological and psychological aspects that reside within a client and body structures that may affect occupational performance (AOTA, 2014).

**clinical education:** The full scope of application experiences that focus on the development of students' practice skills.

**clinical instructor:** On-site supervisor for practical experiences; assists all parties in recognizing that these individuals are part of the students' education, thus offering the title of instructor.

**clinical pathway:** A method used in health care settings as a way of organizing, evaluating, and limiting variations in expected client care secondary to diagnosis and other client-specific factors.

**clinical reasoning:** Complex cognitive process composed of various types of reasoning.

**cluster sampling:** When a researcher collects data from groups of participants.

**coalition:** Individuals or groups joining forces together for a common cause.

**code of ethics:** A collection of formal explicit statements forming a moral guide for an identified group outlining right and valued behavior, principles, and values.

**cognitive behavioral therapy:** A therapy approach that is used when a practitioner is aiming to change the way a client thinks about something; this is done using the assumption that the way in which we think about a situation controls how we feel and in turn controls our actions and the consequences to those actions.

**co-occupations:** Activities that involve the social interaction of two or more persons.

**collaboration:** Both parties have their perspectives and beliefs, but individual goals are put aside to do what is best for the situation and the organization, not what is best for the respective parties.

**community mobility:** Engaging in mobility resulting in successful participation in the community (AOTA, 2008).

**compensation:** Changing the way a person completes an activity so that they can be successful given their current situation.

**competencies:** Explicit statements defining specific areas of expertise; are related to effective or superior performance in a job (Spencer & Spencer, 1993).

**compromise:** Both parties work together and each side concedes a portion of their viewpoint in order to arrive at an agreement and to resolve the conflict.

**concept:** An idea or notion formed by mentally combining characteristics (Reed & Sanderson, 1999).

**conceptual models in occupational therapy:** Graphic or schematic representations of concepts and assumptions that explain why the profession works as it does (Reed & Sanderson, 1999).

**concurrent validity:** A form of criterion-related validity that shows differences between participants at the time of the measure.

**conditional reasoning:** Holistic approach to understanding the person, his or her illness, and intervention.

**conflict resolution:** The ability to identify conflict, to understand the various approaches, and to arrive at a resolution that is beneficial to all parties.

**confounding variable:** A factor other than the controlled variables that influences the study's results.

**construct:** Models of assembled relationships between or among two or more concepts (Depoy & Gitlin, 2005).

**construct validity:** The relationship of one construct to another, such as the relationship of the scores on two different but similar assessments.

**consultation:** The provision of advice or information; the exchange of ideas with an expert who is called on for professional advice (AOTA, 1994).

**content analysis:** Process of analyzing written words as data.

**contexts:** "Variety of interrelated conditions within and surrounding the client that influence performance, including cultural, personal, temporal, and virtual contexts" (AOTA, 2014, p. S42), the circumstances in which an event occurs; a setting (Dictionary.com); the multitude of factors that can define the situation in which leadership takes place.

**context and environment:** Contextual and environmental influences both internal and external to a client that influence occupational performance including physical and social environment and cultural, personal, temporal, and virtual context (AOTA, 2014).

**continuing competence:** Refers to an individual's ongoing or lifelong capacity to perform responsibilities as a part of one's professional role performance.

**continuing competency:** Focuses on an individual's actual performance in a particular situation compared to a standard as a part of one's current professional role performance.

**contractor:** A person who provides services on a contractual basis.

**control group:** Participants in an experimental research design who receive no intervention.

**convenient sample:** Sample of participants that is easily available to the researcher.

**correlational coefficient:** A measurement of the direction and magnitude of a relationship of two variables.

**countertransference:** When one person, usually the therapist, accepts the role the client has placed on him or her.

**criterion referenced:** The client's score can be compared to a set of specific skills or skill components of standard performance rather than a normative group.

**cultural competence:** A process of gaining self-awareness, knowledge and awareness of others, and the skills necessary to interact effectively and sensitively in communicating with diverse groups of people (Wells & Black, 2000).

**culturally competent care:** The process of interacting collaboratively and effectively with culturally diverse clients in order to provide culturally sensitive assessments and interventions.

**culture:** "Refers to learned behaviors, values, norms, and symbols that are passed from generation to generation within a society" (Loveland, 1999, p. 18).

**DAP format:** A format for documentation that includes description, assessment, and plan.

**data:** Any numerical result of research; always written in the plural form (i.e., "data are").

**decubitus ulcers:** Pressure sores due to excessive pressure on or shearing of the skin.

**deep thermal agents:** Those procedures or interventions that use a form of energy capable of raising tissue temperature to a depth of up to 5 cm.

**deglutition:** Consuming of solids or liquids in a normal sensorimotor process (Jenks & Smith, 2006, p. 610).

**deinstitutionalization:** The closing of mental hospitals and residential institutions, which resulted in mentally ill clients joining the community.

**demographics:** "Data related to the size and growth rate of populations in different cities, regions, and nations; age distribution and ethnic mix; educational levels; household patterns; and regional characteristics and movements" (Kotler, 2003, p. 100).

**dependent variable:** One or more clinical findings, behaviors, personal attributes, or internal experiences that are measured in research; the dependent variable might be hypothesized to change as the result of the independent variable or to differ between independent variable groupings.

**disability:** Medical and social construct related to the paradox of describing individual capacity (ability and impairment) and community capacity (attitudes and resources; Finkelstein, 1991).

**discharge:** The termination of therapy services.

**discontinuation note:** A note that summarizes the course of a client's intervention and includes recommendations for the future.

**disease:** "A disorder with a specific cause and recognizable signs and symptoms; any bodily abnormality or failure to function properly, except that resulting directly from physical injury" (Encyclopedia.com, 2008).

**documentation:** The legal and professional responsibility of recording occupational therapy service delivery and outcomes.

**driver rehabilitation:** A form of therapy that focuses on evaluation and intervention in the occupation of driving a vehicle.

**durable medical equipment (DME):** Medically necessary equipment that can be provided to a client to increase safety and independence in the home. Examples include hospital beds, wheelchairs, and walkers. Items such as grab bars, reachers, and long-handled sponges are not considered DME. All covered DME requires a physician prescription.

**dysphagia:** Difficulty with swallowing or the inability to swallow (Jenks & Smith, 2006).

**eating:** The ability to manipulate and swallow food and liquids (Jenks & Smith, 2006).

**education (as an intervention):** "Activities that impart knowledge and information about occupation, health, well-being, and participation, resulting in acquisition by the client of helpful behaviors, habits, and routines that may or may not require application at the time of the intervention session" (AOTA, 2014, p. S42).

**education (as an occupation):** "Activities involved in learning and participating in the educational environment" (AOTA, 2014, p. S42).

**educational activities:** Tasks that facilitate learning (i.e., reading, writing, and math).

**educator:** A faculty member in an academic setting (AOTA, 2004a).

**effect size:** Magnitude of the effect; the strength and magnitude of a relationship between two variables.

**effective communication:** The artful interplay between listening and speaking with attention to both verbal and nonverbal communication, coupled with awareness and sensitivity to human diversity.

**electrotherapeutic agent:** Those procedures or interventions that are systematically applied to modify specific client factors that may be limiting occupational performance; use of electricity and the electromagnetic spectrum to facilitate tissue healing, improve muscle strength and endurance, decrease edema, modulate pain, decrease the inflammatory process, and modify the healing process and are used as an adjunctive method to occupation (Bracciano, 2008).

**empathy:** A process of reaching for true understanding of the experiences and feelings of another person.

**employment interests and pursuits:** Identifying and selecting work opportunities based on assets, limitations, likes, and dislikes relative to work (adapted from Mosey, 1986, p. 342).

**employment seeking and acquisition:** Identifying and recruiting for job opportunities; completing, submitting, and reviewing appropriate application materials; preparing for interviews; participating in interviews and following up afterward; discussing job benefits; and finalizing negotiations.

**enteral tube feedings:** Tubes that deliver nutrition directly to the gastrointestinal system (Morris & Klein, 2000).

**entrepreneur:** Partially or fully self-employed individuals. Includes those in private practice, independent contractors, and consultants (AOTA, 2000).

**environment:** The external physical and social environment that surrounds the client and in which the client's daily life occupations occur.

**environmental factors:** Contextual factors extrinsic to the individual such as the physical, social, and attitudinal environment in which people live and conduct their lives (WHO, 2001).

**epistemology:** The dynamics of knowing (Hooper, 2006); how we know what we know.

**ergonomics:** Study of the "fit" between human and environment.

**error variance:** The variance left over after all of the studied variance is accounted for.

**ethical dilemmas:** Situations in which there are several alternatives, all of which are ethically somewhat problematic.

**ethical reasoning:** Making sure one selects the morally justifiable decisions.

**ethics:** The study of right and wrong conduct as determined by reasonable thought processes.

**evaluation:** "The process of obtaining and interpreting data necessary for intervention. This includes planning for and documenting the evaluation process and results" (Brayman et al., 2005, p. 663).

**evidence-based occupational therapy:** Intervention "based on client information and a critical review of relevant research, expert consensus, and past experience" (CAOT, 1999).

**exceptional educational need (EEN):** Determination that a student exhibits a disability or handicapping condition that prevents educational progress.

**executive skills:** High-level cognitive skills that involve planning, problem solving, cognitive flexibility, judgment/insight, and self-monitoring.

**experience sampling method:** The use of an electronic device that randomly beeps throughout the day and requires the subject to record data regarding the quality of experience, associated challenges, and kind of activity in which he or she is engaged.

**external validity:** The degree to which the study's results can be generalized to another population.

**F-test:** A statistical measure used in ANOVA.

**face validity:** The degree to which experts in the area would agree that a measurement appears to measure what it says it does. Also called *content validity*.

**feeding:** Setting up, arranging, and bringing food or fluid from a plate or a cup to the mouth (AOTA, 2007).

**fieldwork educator:** This individual assists the student's integration of classroom knowledge and application to practice. Not permitted to supervise a Level II fieldwork student until they have practiced full-time for 1 year (ACOTE, 1999).

**FIP format:** A format of documentation that includes findings, interpretation, and plan.

**flow experience:** The way people describe their state of mind when consciousness is harmoniously ordered and they want to pursue whatever they are doing for its own sake.

**formal educational participation:** Including the categories of academic (e.g., math, reading, working on a degree), nonacademic (e.g., recess, lunchroom, hallway), extracurricular (e.g., sports, band, cheerleading, dance), and vocational (prevocational and vocational) participation.

**frame of reference:** System of compatible concepts from theory which guides a plan of action within a specific occupational therapy domain of concern (Mosey, 1986); a set of ideas, in terms of which other ideas are interpreted or assigned meaning (Dictionary.com); frames of reference provide intervention guidelines and help practitioners know what to do in practice; provide information on the nature of function/dysfunction, intervention strategies, principles guiding intervention, assessments, and expected outcomes; and define who would benefit from the intervention.

**framing:** The method through which a player offers cues about how he or she wishes to be treated during play (Bateson, 1972).

**freedom to suspend reality:** The child is able to defer the restrictions of realistic play and use his or her imagination to take on new roles and identities (Bundy, 1997; Rubin, Fein, & Vandenberg, 1983); the ability to participate in make-believe activities or pretend play (Bundy, 1997).

**frequency:** Number of participants who have a specific score.

**fun:** "That which provides mirth and amusement; enjoyment; playfulness" (Parham & Fazio, 1997, p. 250).

**function:** The ability to perform meaningful activities and tasks that involve body structure, body functions, activities, and participation (WHO, 2001).

**functional mobility:** "Moving from one position to another during performance of everyday activities" (AOTA, 2008, p. 631).

**funding agencies:** Federal, state, local, or community organizations; corporations; foundations; and trusts offering monetary support to develop programs or run research projects.

**gastroesophageal reflux disease (GERD):** "Reflux of food, medication, liquids, and gastric juice from the stomach into the esophagus" (AOTA, 2007, p. 698).

**gastroesophageal scintigraphy:** Sometimes referred to as a *milk scan*, this medical test looks at stomach emptying as well as extent and severity of reflux (Morris & Klein, 2000).

**gastrostomy tube (G-tube):** Bypasses the mouth and is surgically inserted directly into the stomach.

**goal:** Outcome measure of progress.

**grading:** Changing aspects of an activity to make it easier or more difficult.

**grants:** Monies disbursed by a funding agency to another agency or person for the purpose of a specific program, research study, or products.

**grassroots advocacy:** A group effort of like-minded individuals working together to achieve a desired outcome.

**health:** "A complete state of physical, mental, and social well-being, and not just the absence of disease or infirmity" (WHO, 1947, p. 29).

**Health Insurance Portability and Accountability Act of 1996 (HIPAA):** Title I of HIPAA protects health insurance coverage for workers and their families when they change or lose their jobs. Title II of HIPAA, known as the Administrative Simplification (AS) provisions, requires the establishment of national standards for electronic health care transactions and national identifiers for providers, health insurance plans, and employers. The act gives the right to privacy to individuals from age 12 through 18. The provider must have a signed disclosure from the affected individual before giving out any information on provided health care to anyone, including parents. The administrative simplification provisions also address the security and privacy of health data.

**health literacy:** Ability to find, understand, and use information to make health-related decisions.

**health promotion:** Actions or activities that support the enhancement of health and well-being.

**high-tech:** Devices, often electronic or electric, commonly more expensive and often customized according to the user's needs.

**holistic approach:** Perceiving interrelated components as one whole unit that cannot be subdivided into parts.

**human factors engineering:** *See* ergonomics.

**humanism:** A philosophical approach recognizing the basic goodness of being human and the uniqueness of each individual.

**ideational apraxia:** A complete loss of the ability to do a task due to a perceptual disorder.

**ideomotor apraxia:** Ability to carry out a task automatically but inability to simulate the task or do it on command due to a perceptual disorder.

**impairments:** Problems in body function or structure (WHO, 2001).

**inclusion:** The act of including and providing intervention to students with disabilities in the regular education classroom; adapting the environment for persons with disabilities to be successful in occupations, roles, and activities with others.

**independent t-test:** T-test performed on independent groups of participants' scores to measure differences between the scores.

**independent variable:** A factor in research such as an intervention that can be manipulated by the investigator; also, a stable characteristic of individuals by which they can be grouped.

**Individualized Education Program (IEP):** Written, legal document developed by the individual education team, incorporating the student's strengths and need areas as well as goals and objectives for intervention.

**informal personal educational needs or interests exploration (beyond formal education):** Identifying topics and methods for obtaining topic-related information or skills.

**informal personal education participation:** "Participating in classes, programs, and activities that provide instruction or training in identified areas of interest" (AOTA, 2008, p. 632).

**instrumental activities of daily living (IADLs):** "Activities that support daily life within the home and community and that often require more complex interactions than those used in ADLs" (AOTA, 2014, p. S43).

**interactive reasoning:** Involves understanding the client as a holistic human being and looking at issues from the client's perspective.

**interdependence:** Reciprocal reliance on others.

**internal control:** The player is in control of the materials, play interactions, and some aspect of the outcome (Bundy, 1997; Connor, Williamson, & Seipp, 1978); the extent to which the child is in control of his or her actions and, to some aspect, the outcome of the activity (Bundy, 1997).

**internal validity:** The degree to which the researcher's conclusions are accurate.

***International Classification of Diseases* (ICD-10):** International framework for coding health conditions including diseases, disorders, and injuries.

***International Classification of Functioning, Disability and Health* (ICF):** International framework for coding components of health and functioning.

**interprofessional:** A group of professions whose communication is collaborative, goals are shared between members, and are all responsible for team efforts (MacRae & Dyer, 2005).

**interprofessional collaborative practice:** "When multiple health workers from different professional backgrounds work together with patients, families, carers, and communities to deliver the highest quality of care" (World Health Organization, 2010, p. 7).

**interprofessional education:** When two or more professions learn with, from, and about each other to improve collaboration and the quality of care (Center for the Advancement of Interprofessional Education, 2010).

**intervention plan:** A collaborative listing of client-oriented actions meant to enhance occupational performance with specific targeted outcomes based on select models, frames of reference, and evidence.

**intrinsic motivation:** What drives a child to participate in an activity for pleasure rather than extrinsic reward (Bundy, 1993); the self-initiation or drive to action that is rewarded by the activity itself, rather than some external reward (Bundy, 1997).

**jejunostomy tube:** Placed directly into the jejunum (the central of the three divisions of the small intestine), bypassing the stomach.

**job performance:** Including work skills and patterns; time management; relationships with co-workers, managers, and customers; creation, production, and distribution of products and services; initiation, sustainment, and completion of work; and compliance with work norms and procedures.

**judgment:** The act of deciding after consideration of alternatives.

**"just-right" challenge:** When the challenge of a task does not exceed the abilities of the client to meet the challenge.

**kinesthesia:** The sense of movement of one's body or part of one's body (e.g., joint or limb) in space.

**knowledge:** What one knows.

**leadership:** The ability to engage and influence others to facilitate and embrace meaningful change through careful consideration of individual and societal contexts in the embodiment of a shared vision.

**least restrictive environment:** An educational environment most like a regular education classroom; developing a natural environment that enhances a person's occupational performance in as self-structured a format as possible.

**legislative process:** The path through which a bill becomes a law. Involves hearings in Congressional/Statehouse committees, votes by committee members, and if passed, voting on the floor of the legislative body.

**leisure:** "A nonobligatory activity that is intrinsically motivated and engaged in during discretionary time, that is, time not committed to obligatory occupations such as work, self-care or sleep" (Parham & Fazio, 1997, p. 250).

**leisure activities:** "Nonobligatory, discretionary, and intrinsically rewarding activities" (AOTA, 2004b, p. 674).

**Level I fieldwork:** Introductory practical experiences to expose students to a variety of practice settings.

**Level II fieldwork:** Practical experiences created to develop competent entry-level occupational therapists and occupational therapy assistants.

**lobbyist:** A person who attempts to influence the legislative process by providing information.

**low-tech:** Device that is easily fabricated or obtained.

**maintenance:** Ensuring continued competence through the use of external devices, templates, or skill retraining despite expectations of potential or eventual declines in occupational performance.

**managed care:** A variety of methods of financing and organizing the delivery of health care in which costs are contained by controlling the provision of services.

**manager:** An individual often responsible for task-specific functions within an organization.

**marketing:** "The process of planning and executing the conception, price, promotion, and distribution of ideas, goods, and services to create exchanges that satisfy individual and organizational objectives" (Bennett, 1995, p. 21).

**mature level participation:** Combines basic and supportive cooperative participation, and is focused on task completion and social interaction.

**mean:** Mathematical average of a set of scores.

**meaningful occupation:** A valued activity that contributes to identity, well-being, and quality of life.

**measures of central tendency:** Frequency, mean, mode, median.

**measures of variability:** Descriptive statistics of range, variance, and standard deviation.

**median:** Middle score of a range.

**mentorship:** Defined by AOTA as a relationship between two people in which one person (the mentor) is dedicated to the personal and professional growth of the other (the mentee). The relationship is often mutually beneficial and collaborative, both parties participating willingly and knowingly in the development of the mentee.

**meta-analysis:** Statistical analysis to integrate the results of several studies on one topic.

**mode:** The most common score in a range.

**modeling:** Demonstration of behavior.

**models of practice:** A set of ideas in terms of which other ideas are interpreted or assigned meaning; provides an overview of the occupational therapy philosophy and process. Models of practice help practitioners organize thinking.

**monitoring:** The act of observing a client's response to intervention.

**moral distress:** Distress occurring when an individual knows what she or he should do but is not able to do it.

**moral residue:** Persisting feelings that arise over time from repeated experiences of moral distress.

**moral treatment:** An approach to the treatment of what was called *madness* in the middle to late 19th century that was characterized by an "optimistic view of human nature, and influenced by enlightenment humanism and pietistic evangelicalism... [which at its] core was the belief that if treated like rational beings within a rational environment, the insane would regain their reason" (Lilleleht, 2002, p. 169).

**moral treatment movement:** A theory based on the respect and dignity for all humans and their need to participate in daily occupations.

**morality:** The accepted standards of right or wrong that direct the conduct of a person or a group.

**moratorium:** A temporary freeze on the implementation of a piece of legislation.

**multiple regression analysis:** A statistical measure that allows one variable to predict another.

**narrative reasoning:** Utilized to learn about the client's life story.

**nasogastric tube:** A feeding tube inserted through the oral pharyngeal area supplying liquid nutrition by passing the mouth.

**natural environments:** The context in which an individual lives.

**naturalistic observation:** Observation of behavior as it occurs naturally without the researcher interfering.

**neuroscience-based treatment:** Founded primarily on the idea that "the brain can be studied empirically" (Cohen & Reed, 1995, p. 562). In neuroscience, the brain is considered a dynamic system that includes virtually all of the underlying physiological and neurological processes that support human performance. An understanding of these processes supports the development of occupational therapy models of practice.

**nonlinear dynamics:** A framework for analyzing unpredictable, self-organizing systems concerning people and their context.

**nonverbal communication:** Communication through eye contact, tone of voice, facial expression, body language, and posture.

**norm referenced:** Client scores can be compared to a specific "normative" group utilized during test development.

**NPO (nil per os):** Latin for "nothing by mouth"; no food, liquid, or medication is to be given orally (Avery-Smith, 2002).

**objective:** Building blocks needed to achieve a larger goal.

**occupation:** Everyday activities and occupations that people find meaningful and purposeful (Moyers & Dale, 2007); "'goal-directed pursuits that typically extend over time have meaning to the performance, and involve multiple tasks" (Christiansen, Baum, & Bass-Haugen, 2005, p. 548); "daily activities that reflect cultural values, provide structure to living, and meaning to individuals; these activities meet human needs for self-care, enjoyment, and participation in society" (Crepeau, Cohn, & Schell, 2003, p. 1031); "activities that people engage in throughout their daily lives to fulfill their time and give life meaning. Occupations involve mental abilities and skills, and may or may not have an observable physical dimension" (Hinojosa & Kramer, 1997, p. 865); "[a]ctivities...of everyday life, named, organized, and given value and meaning by individuals and a culture. Occupation is everything people do to occupy themselves including looking after themselves... enjoying life...and contributing to the social and economic fabric of their communities" (Law, Polatajko, Baptiste, & Townsend, 1997, p. 32); "a dynamic relationship among an occupational form, a person with a unique developmental structure, subjective meanings and purpose, and the resulting occupational performance" (Nelson & Jepson Thomas, 2003, p. 90); common occupations people may engage in include activities of daily living, instrumental activities of daily living, rest and sleep, education, work, play, leisure, and social participation (AOTA, 2014).

**occupation-based:** Refers to providing intervention that includes the actual occupation (activities in which the client engages, in its actual context).

**occupation-based activity:** Activity meaningful to the person, which is conducted in the actual context.

**occupation-based model:** Proposed interaction of person, environment, and occupation that guide the organization of occupational therapy practice (Cole & Tufano, 2008).

**occupational justice:** "'A justice that recognizes occupational rights to inclusive participation in everyday occupations for all persons in society, regardless of age, ability, gender, social class, or other differences' (Nilsson & Townsend, 2010, p. 58). Access to and participation in the full range of meaningful and enriching occupations afforded to others, including opportunities for social inclusion and the resources to participate in occupations to satisfy personal, health, and societal needs (adapted from Townsend & Wilcock, 2004)" (AOTA, 2014, p. S43).

**occupational performance:** "Act of doing and accomplishing a selected action (performance skill), activity, or occupation (Fisher, 2009; Fisher & Griswold, 2014; Kielhofner, 2008) that results from the dynamic transaction among the client, the context, and the activity. Improving or enabling skills and patterns in occupational performance leads to engagement in occupations or activities (adapted in part from Law et al., 1996, p. 16)" (AOTA, 2014, p. S43).

**occupational performance model:** A framework for understanding the individual's dynamic experience in daily occupations within the environment (Baum & Law, 1995).

**occupational profile:** "Summary of the client's occupational history and experiences, patterns of daily living, interests, values, and needs" (AOTA, 2014, p. S44).

**occupational therapy:** A health and wellness profession enabling people to participate in the everyday activities they want and need to do.

**occupational therapy practitioners:** Term used to encompass occupational therapists and occupational therapy assistants.

**optimal experience:** Alternate term for *flow experience.*

**organizations:** Not limited to but includes agencies, businesses, corporations, industries, for-profits, nonprofits, or practices that receive occupational therapy services or consultations.

**outlier:** An extreme score that falls far from the mean score.

***P* value:** The alpha score of the probability of a type I error.

**paired t-test:** T-test performed on paired groups of participants' scores to measure differences between the scores.

**paradigm:** A shared vision encompassing fundamental assumptions and beliefs which serves as the cultural core of the profession (Kielhofner, 2004).

**parallel level participation:** Play, activity, or work carried out side by side, without interaction, with others present.

**parenteral tube feedings:** Tubes that deliver nutrition via bypassing the gastrointestinal system to deliver nutrition into the bloodstream (Morris & Klein, 2000).

**participation:** Involvement in life situations and activities that include the capacity to execute and perform tasks (WHO, 2001).

**partnerships in health:** Collaborations with individuals and community members that have a central mission to enhance health and well-being.

**Patient Protection and Affordable Care Act (2010) (PPACA; "ObamaCare"):** This United States federal statute is aimed at decreasing the number of uninsured Americans and reducing the overall costs of health care. It includes mandates, subsidies, and tax credits to employers and individuals with the goal of increasing the coverage rate and streamlining the delivery of health care. Insurance companies are now required to cover all applicants and offer the same rates regardless of pre-existing conditions or gender. Sometimes referred to as *ObamaCare*, the act also includes telehealth provisions that create ways to promote evidence-based medicine and patient engagement, report on quality and cost measures, and coordinate care through the use of telehealth, remote patient monitoring, and other such enabling technologies. The PPACA directs the new Center for Medicare and Medicaid Innovation (CMI), to explore as a care model how to facilitate inpatient care at local hospitals through the use of electronic monitoring by specialists. The legislation also provides states with a "health home" option for chronic conditions that include the use of health information technology in providing health home services including the use of wireless patient technology to improve coordination and management of care and increased patient adherence to recommendations made by their provider.

**Pearson correlation coefficient:** The most common measure of relationships between two factors.

**peer review:** A process in which a panel of experts in the field is responsible for judging the merit of a proposal for a scholarly publication or presentation.

**performance context:** Environment in which occupational performance occurs, including the physical environment, available resources, sensory input, temporal and societal influences, or the presence or availability of caregivers.

**performance in areas of occupation:** Activities of daily living, instrumental activities of daily living, education, work, play, social participation, leisure, rest, and sleep (AOTA, 2008).

**performance patterns:** A client's habits, routines, rituals, and roles that support engagement, participation, and health (AOTA, 2014).

**performance skills:** Actions or elements of actions that can be observed when an individual participates in meaningful occupation (AOTA, 2014).

**personal factors:** Contextual factors intrinsic to the individual such as attributes of age, gender, and social status (WHO, 2001).

**persuade:** To move by argument, entreaty, or expostulation to a belief, position, or course of action; to plead with (Merriam-Webster, 2006).

**pH probe:** Medical test used to help identify the amount and severity of gastroesophageal reflux (Morris & Klein, 2000).

**philosophy:** A fundamental belief (Meyer, 1977).

**physical agent modalities:** Procedures and interventions that are systematically applied to modify specific client factors that may be limiting occupational performance and use various forms of energy in order to modulate pain; modify tissue healing; increase tissue extensibility; modify skin and scar tissue; decrease edema, inflammation, or occupational performance secondary to musculoskeletal or integumentary conditions; and are used as an adjunctive method to occupation (Bracciano, 2008).

**physical transfers:** Teaching a client who uses a wheelchair to move from one surface to another.

**pilot test:** Trial run of a study to evaluate for problems in future experiments.

**plagiarism:** The use of information that was created by another individual as though it were original.

**play:** "Any spontaneous or organized activity that provides enjoyment, entertainment, amusement or diversion" (Parham & Fazio, 1997, p. 252).

**play activities:** "Spontaneous and organized activities that promote pleasure, amusement, and diversion" (AOTA, 2004b, p. 674).

**playfulness:** "A play temperament that is comprised of intrinsic motivation, internal control, freedom to suspend reality, and framing; a behavioral or personality trait characterized by flexibility, manifest joy, and spontaneity" (Parham & Fazio, 1997, p. 252).

**policy:** Principle or rule to guide decisions and achieve outcomes.

**populations:** Groups within communities that have a commonality such as, but not limited to, brain injury, diabetes, refugees, or prisoners of war, that receive occupational therapy services.

**positioning:** Ensuring and/or placing an individual in an ergonomically correct posture, one that enables occupational performance.

**post hoc tests:** Statistical tests used to follow up significant findings.

**postulate:** A theoretical statement that suggests how two or more concepts are related (Mosey, 1986).

**practice skills:** Repetition of an ability to improve the consistency of performance; components of occupations.

**practitioner:** Provides occupational therapy services including assessments, interventions, program planning and implementation, discharge planning, and transition planning (AOTA, 2000).

**pragmatic reasoning:** Used to understand the practical issues that may have an impact on the situation with the person and the person's family.

**pragmatism:** A philosophical view that knowledge grows through change and adaptation and is best gained through practical application and experience (Breines, 1987).

**preparatory activity:** Repetitive techniques to get a client ready to perform (e.g., stretching, mental review).

**pretest sensitization:** Participants completing the pretest complicates the post-test results.

**principles:** Basic rules of conduct.

**probability:** Likelihood of finding the same results in repeated studies.

**procedural reasoning:** Focuses on client performance and diagnosis.

**profession:** An occupation requiring extensive education or specialized training.

**professional:** A person engaged in a profession.

**professional development:** Ongoing plan to ensure practice is current and based on best known practices; a process where one plans and achieves excellence or establishes expertise in seeking a change in responsibilities, or when assuming more complex professional roles.

**professional identity:** Students develop a professional identity as an occupational therapy practitioner, aligning their professional judgments and decisions with the AOTA *Standards of Practice* and the *Occupational Therapy Code of Ethics*.

**professional presentation:** An oral report of research findings or other evidence-based practice information.

**professional portfolio:** A collection of evidence demonstrating that practice is current and based on best known practices; an archival of one's self-assessment processes, learning plans, evidence of engagement in selected learning methods, reflection on the learning process, and outcomes of the application of learning to practice.

**promote:** Further the progress of (something, especially a cause, venture, or aim); support or actively encourage.

**promotion:** Advance in station, rank, or honor; to advance (a student) from one grade to the next higher grade; to contribute to the growth or prosperity of, promote international understanding; to help bring (as in an enterprise) into being; to present (merchandise) for buyer acceptance through advertising, publicity, or discounting (Merriam-Webster, 2006).

**proposal:** The collective materials used to apply for a grant, including an application and supporting documents.

**proprioception:** The sense of one's body or parts of one's body (e.g., joint or limb) in space.

**Prospective Payment System (PPS):** Created by the Balanced Budget Act of 1997 as a method for controlling costs. Payment for skilled service is made on a daily rate, chosen based on certain admission criteria indicating an estimated level of need.

**psychometrics:** The study of psychological and behavioral measurement.

**qualitative research:** Exploratory gathering of in-depth, detailed descriptions of problems or conditions from the point of view of the group or individual experiencing them in order to discover themes and their interrelationships or linkages.

**quality assessment:** A measure of quality against standards.

**quality improvement:** Management philosophy and method for structuring problem solving.

**quantitative research:** Use of the scientific method to gather data that can be expressed numerically and analyzed statistically in order to describe population characteristics and/or determine the relationship between one or more independent and dependent variables.

**range:** Measure of variability between the highest and lowest scores.

**real life:** Individuals' description and interpretation of their life.

**recreation:** Adult play or activities whose purpose is to "regenerate energy to support the worker role" (Glantz & Richman, 2001, p. 249).

**reductionistic approach:** Perceiving many individual parts that make up the whole, which may be studied and dealt with separately or interchangeably.

**referral:** Making a professional judgment to have another occupational therapy specialist, discipline, or facility evaluate the client; the practice of directing an initial request for service or changing the degree and direction of service (Agnes, 1999).

**reflection:** A useful tool in analyzing thoughts and actions that assists practitioners to justify interventions and gives practitioners the ability to learn from experience.

**reflective listening:** A process of listening to both the verbal and emotional content of a speaker and verbalizing both the feelings and attitudes sensed behind the spoken words to the speaker (Davis, 2006).

**rehabilitation movement:** Began with a change in the way society viewed those with handicaps to individuals who could become independent and contributing members of the community.

**related service:** Services that may be required for a student to benefit from special education. Service providers include occupational therapy, physical therapy, social work, and school health services.

**reliability:** Accuracy and stability of a measure; the dependability and consistency of a measurement.

**remediation:** Helping clients regain skills and abilities.

**researcher:** An individual who "find[s] the process of discovery exhilarating because they see how it enhances occupational therapy practice" (Kielhofner, 2006).

**resource utilization groups (RUG):** Categories used in PPS that describe the amount of service clients will need.

**retirement preparation and adjustment:** Determining aptitudes, developing interests and skills, and selecting appropriate avocational pursuits.

**rigor:** Close adherence to experimental research methodology; in broader usage, embedding of sound principles and practices—agreed upon by the scientific community—into each step of the quantitative or qualitative research process in order to ensure trustworthiness of results.

**safety:** Practices that reduce the risk of adverse incidents.

**sample:** A selection from a population.

**sampling error:** The difference between the sample's scores and what the whole population would have scored.

**scaffolding:** Foundation of prerequisite skills.

**scientific reasoning:** Involves the logical thinking about the nature of the client's problems and the optimal course of action in treatment.

**scholarship:** Research activities designed to build the knowledge base of occupational therapy so as to further advance practice and teaching.

**scholarly practice:** Evidence-based practice; using the knowledge base of the profession in occupational therapy practice and teaching.

**scholarly reports:** Documents that are written by reflective practitioners for the advancement of a profession.

**screening:** The process of gathering and reviewing data with the intent to determine if additional evaluative procedures are warranted.

**seating systems:** Selection and utilization of a comfortable, supportive wheelchair or chair seat that encourages symmetry, skin integrity, and occupational performance.

**self-assessment:** Provides the means to assess performance, abilities, and skills; to analyze demands and resources of the work environment; to interpret information about clients' outcomes; to reassess current learning goals; and to develop goals and plans for professional growth and continuing competence and competency.

**simulation:** Creating as realistic as possible situations to allow learners to practice and apply skills.

**site:** Facility offering clinical affiliations to students.

**SOAP note format:** Documentation format that includes four parts in documenting a client's intervention: subjective, objective, assessment, and plan.

**social participation:** A person's performance of meaningful roles and occupations within preferred social groups such as families, classrooms, work teams, organizations, and communities (Cole & Donohue, 2011); consists of verbal and interpersonal activity interactions among people.

**standard deviation:** A measurement of variability; a description of how far from the mean a score is.

**standard precautions:** A form of infection control based on the assumption that all bodily substances may transmit infectious diseases.

**statistical significance:** The likelihood that the finding is not due to error.

**suck, swallow, breathe synchrony:** The smooth coordination of sucking, swallowing, and breathing into rhythmic patterns to allow for efficient and effective eating (Case-Smith & Humphry, 2005).

**superficial thermal agent:** Those procedures or interventions that are capable of raising or decreasing the temperature of superficial tissue to a therapeutic level.

**supervisee:** One who receives direction and undergoes evaluation by a qualified practitioner.

**supervision:** A reciprocal process involving the supervisor and supervisee aimed at the improvement of performance.

**support:** The provision of services that enable clients to achieve maximum occupational performance.

**supportive cooperative level participation:** Consists of interactions that express feelings and emotions designed to foster social cohesion in a group.

**t-test:** A statistical measure of the difference between two means.

**tacit:** Involves learning and skill, but not in a way that can be written down.

**taxonomy:** A system of classification.

**technology:** "The branch of knowledge that deals with the creation and use of technical means and their interrelation with life, society, and the environment, drawing upon such subjects as industrial arts, engineering, applied science, and pure science" (Flexner, 1987, p. 1950).

**telehealth:** The delivery of health services using telecommunication technology providers who are at a distance from clients.

**test-retest reliability:** Consistency of a score of repeated measures over time.

**theoretical constructs:** Visible and nonvisible ideas and explanations that form into a concept.

**theory:** Describes, explains, and predicts behavior and/or the relationships between concepts or events.

**therapeutic use of self:** A practitioner's intuitive nature that derives from one's personality traits, self-awareness, and personal experiences; understanding of human behavior; and observations through the use of the five senses. The practitioner makes conscious use of this nature to engage and impact a therapeutic relationship and foster a meaningful experience for the client.

**transference:** When one person, usually the client, places a role on another, usually the therapist.

**transition services:** A results-oriented process that facilitates movement between settings and providers based on changing client needs. This term is most often used in the school setting but is an essential part of care coordination across the continuum.

**TriAlliance of Health and Rehabilitation Professions:** "The TriAlliance is the largest constituency of health and rehabilitation professionals representing the professions of occupational therapy, physical therapy, audiology and speech-language pathology. In 1988, informal meetings began among the Presidents and Executive Directors of the American Occupational Therapy Association (AOTA), the American Physical Therapy Association (APTA), and the American Speech-Language-Hearing Association (ASHA)" (APTA, 2000).

**type I error:** Finding that the independent variable had an effect when it did not.

**type II error:** Finding that the independent variable did not have an effect when it did.

**universal design:** Principles that seek to promote access to and use of structures and tools across the lifespan.

**utilization review:** A look-over of care/services that were provided in a particular case to ascertain necessity, efficiency, and effectiveness.

**validity:** Generalizability of a measure to the general population; the extent to which a measurement measures what it is intended to measure.

**values:** Principles that set a standard of quality or a worthwhile ideal.

**variability:** The degree to which scores differ from each other.

**variance:** An index or score of variability that explains the differences between factors.

**videofluoroscopy:** A primary imaging technique for detailed dynamic assessment of oral, pharyngeal, and upper esophageal phases of a swallow (Arvedsen, Brodsky, & Christensen, 2002); also known as *modified barium swallow*.

**volunteer exploration:** Determining community causes, organizations, or opportunities for unpaid "work" in relationship to personal skills, interests, location, and time available.

**volunteer participation:** Performing unpaid "work" activities for the benefit of identified selected causes, organizations, or facilities" (AOTA, 2008, p. 632).

**well-being:** The state of being content, comfortable, and satisfied with one's self, relationships, and quality of life.

**wellness:** A dynamic way of life that involves actions, values, and attitudes that support or improve both health and quality of life (AOTA, 2001).

**wellness programs:** A program intended to improve and promote health and fitness that is typically offered through the workplace, although insurance plans can offer them directly to their enrollees. The program allows employers or plans to offer employees premium discounts, cash rewards, gym memberships, and other incentives to participate. The Affordable Care Act creates new incentives to promote employer wellness programs and encourage opportunities to support healthier workplaces

**wheelchair management:** Selection, utilization, and functional mobility of the wheelchair.

**work:** "Includes activities needed for engaging in remunerative employment or volunteer activities" (Mosey, 1986, p. 341).

# References


Accreditation Council for Occupational Therapy Education. (1999). Standards for an accredited educational program for the occupational therapist. *American Journal of Occupational Therapy, 53*, 575-581.

Agnes, M. (Ed.). (1999). *Webster's new world college dictionary* (4th ed.). New York, NY: Macmillan.

American Occupational Therapy Association. (1994). Occupational therapy code of ethics. *American Journal of Occupational Therapy, 48*, 1037-1038.

American Occupational Therapy Association. (2000). Occupational therapy roles and career exploration and development: A companion guide to the Occupational Therapy Role Documents. In the *reference manual of the official documents of the American Occupational Therapy Association* (8th ed.). Bethesda, MD: Author.

American Occupational Therapy Association. (2001). Position paper: Occupational therapy in the promotion of health and the prevention of disease and disability statement. *American Journal of Occupational Therapy, 55*(6), 656-660.

American Occupational Therapy Association. (2004a). Role competencies for a professional-level occupational therapist faculty member in an academic setting. *American Journal of Occupational Therapy, 58*(6), 649-650.

American Occupational Therapy Association. (2004b). Scope of practice. *American Journal of Occupational Therapy, 58*(6), 673-677.

American Occupational Therapy Association. (2007). Specialized knowledge and skills in eating and feeding for occupational therapy practice. *American Journal of Occupational Therapy, 61*, 686-700.

American Occupational Therapy Association. (2008). Occupational therapy practice framework: Domain and process (2nd ed.). *American Journal of Occupational Therapy, 62*, 625-683.

American Occupational Therapy Association. (2014). Occupational therapy practice framework: Domain and process (3rd ed.). *American Journal of Occupational Therapy, 68*(Suppl. 1), S1-S48. doi:10.5014/ajot.2014.682006

American Physical Therapy Association. (2000). TriAlliance to explore Medicare alternative payment methods. Retrieved from http://www.apta.org/AM/Template.cfm?Section=Home&TEMPLATE=/CM/ContentDisplay.cfm &CONTENTID =30620

Arvedsen, J. C., Brodsky, L., & Christensen, S. (2002). Instrumental evaluation of swallowing. In J. C. Arvedsen & L. Brodsky (Eds.), *Pediatric swallowing and feeding assessment and management* (2nd ed., pp. 341-388). Albany, NY: Singular Publishing Group.

Avery-Smith, W. (2002). Dysphagia. In C. A. Trombly & M. V. Radomski (Eds.), *Occupational therapy for physical dysfunction* (pp. 1091-1109). Philadelphia, PA: Lippincott Williams and Wilkins.

Bateson, G. (1972). Toward a theory of play and fantasy. In G. Bateson (Ed.), *Steps to an ecology of the mind* (pp. 14-20). New York, NY: Bantam.

Baum, C., & Law, M. (1995). Occupational performance: Occupational therapy's definition of function. *American Journal of Occupational Therapy, 49*, 1019.

Bennett, P. D. (Ed.). (1995). *Dictionary of marketing terms* (2nd ed.). Chicago, IL: American Marketing Association.

Bracciano, A. (2008). *Physical agent modalities: Theory and application for the occupational therapist.* Thorofare, NJ: SLACK Incorporated.

Braveman, B. (2006). *Leading & managing occupational therapy services: An evidence-based approach.* Philadelphia, PA: F. A. Davis Company.

Brayman, S. J., Roley, S. S., Clark, G. F., DeLany, J. V., Garza, E. R., Radomski, M. V., et al. (2005). Standards of practice for occupational therapy. *American Journal of Occupational Therapy, 59*(6), 663-665.

Breines, E. (1987). Pragmatism as a foundation for occupational therapy curricula. *American Journal of Occupational Therapy, 47*, 522-525.

Brookside Associates. (2007). *Nursing fundamentals I.* Retrieved from http://www.brookside- press.org/Products/Nursing_Fundamentals_1/Index.htm

Bundy, A. C. (1993). Assessment of play and leisure: Delineation of the problem. *American Journal of Occupational Therapy, 47*, 217-222.

Bundy, A. C. (1997). Play and playfulness: What to look for. In L. D. Parham & L. S. Fazio (Eds.), *Play in occupational therapy for children* (pp. 52-66). St. Louis, MO: Mosby.

Canadian Association of Occupational Therapists. (1999). Joint position statement on evidence-based occupational therapy. Retrieved from http://www.caot.ca/default.asp?ChangeID =166& pageID =156

Case-Smith, J., & Humphry, R. (2005). Feeding intervention. In J. Case-Smith (Ed.), *Occupational therapy for children* (5th ed., pp. 481-520). St. Louis, MO: Elsevier Mosby.

Center for the Advancement of Interprofessional Education. (2010). *Interprofession education: A definition.* Retrieved from www.caipe.org.uk/us/defining-ipe

Cohen, H., & Reed, K. L. (1995). The historical development of neuroscience in physical rehabilitation. *American Journal of Occupational Therapy, 50*(7), 561-568.

Cole, M., & Donohue, M. (2011). *Social participation and occupation: In schools, clinics, and communities.* Thorofare, NJ: SLACK Incorporated.

Cole, M., & Tufano, R. (2008). *Applied theories in occupational therapy.* Thorofare, NJ: SLACK Incorporated.

Connor, F. P., Williamson, G. G., & Siepp, J. M. (Eds.). (1978). *Program guide for infants and toddlers with neuromotor and other developmental disabilities.* New York, NY: Teachers College.

Davis, C. M. (2006). *Patient practitioner interaction: An experiential manual for developing the art of health care* (4th ed.). Thorofare, NJ: SLACK Incorporated.

Depoy, E., & Gitlin, L. (2005). *Introduction to research: Understanding and applying multiple strategies* (3rd ed.). New York, NY: Mosby.

Dictionary.com. Retrieved from http://dictionary.reference.com

Encyclopedia.com. (2008). Disease. In *Oxford dictionary of nursing.* Oxford University Press. Retrieved from http://www.encyclopedia.com/doc/1O62-disease.html

Finkelstein, V. (1991). Disability: An administrative challenge? In M. Oliver (Ed.), *Social work: Disabled people and disabling environments* (pp. 19-39). London, England: Jessica Kingsley.

Flexner, S. B. (Ed.). (1987). *The Random House dictionary of the English language, unabridged* (2nd ed.). New York, NY: Random House.

Glantz, C. H., & Richman, N. (2001). Leisure activities. In L. W. Pedretti & M. B. Early (Eds.), *Occupational therapy practice skills for physical dysfunction* (5th ed., pp. 249-256). St. Louis, MO: Mosby.

Hooper, B. (2006). Epistemological transformation in occupational therapy: Educational implications and challenges. *Occupational Therapy Journal of Research, 26*, 15-24.

Jenks, K. N., & Smith, G. (2006). Eating and swallowing. In H. M Pendleton & W. Schultz-Krohn (Eds.), *Pedretti's occupational therapy practice skills for physical dysfunction* (6th ed., pp. 609-645). St. Louis, MO: Mosby.

Kerlinger, F. (1979). *Behavioral research: A conceptual approach.* New York, NY: Holt, Rinehart, & Winston.

Kielhofner, G. (2004). *Conceptual foundations of occupational therapy* (3rd ed.). Philadelphia, PA: F. A. Davis Company.

Kielhofner, G. (2006). *Research in occupational therapy: Methods of inquiry for enhancing practice.* Philadelphia, PA: F. A. Davis Company.

Kotler, P. (2003). *A framework for marketing management* (2nd ed.). Upper Saddle River, NJ: Prentice Hall.

Law, M., Baptiste, S., & Mills, J. (1995). Client-centered practice: What does it mean and does it make a difference? *Canadian Journal of Occupational Therapy, 62*, 250-257.

Lilleleht, E. (2002). Progress and power: Exploring the disciplinary connections between moral treatment and psychiatric rehabilitation. *Philosophy, Psychiatry, and Psychology, 9*(2), 167-182.

Loveland, C. A. (1999). The concept of culture. In R. L. Leavitt (Ed.), *Cross-cultural rehabilitation: An international perspective* (pp. 15-24). London, England: Saunders.

MacRae, N., & Dyer, J. (2005). Collaborative teaching methods for health professionals. *Occupational Therapy in Health Care, 19*(3), 93-103.

Merriam-Webster. (2006). *On-line dictionary* (10th ed.). Retrieved from http://www.merriam-webster.com

Meyer, A. (1977). The philosophy of occupational therapy. *American Journal of Occupational Therapy, 31*, 639-642. (Original work published in 1922.)

Morris, S. E., & Klein, M. D. (2000). *Pre-feeding skills: A comprehensive resource for mealtime development* (2nd ed.). Austin, TX: Therapy Skills Builders.

Mosey, A. C. (1986). *Psychosocial components of occupational therapy.* New York, NY: Raven Press.

Moyers, P. A., & Dale, L. M. (2007). *The guide to occupational therapy practice*. Bethesda, MD: AOTA Press.

Parham, L. D., & Fazio, L. S. (1997). *Play in occupational therapy for children*. St. Louis, MO: Mosby.

Reed, K., & Sanderson, S. (1999). *Concepts of occupational therapy* (4th ed.). Baltimore, MD: Lippincott Williams and Wilkins.

Rubin, K. H., Fein, G. G., & Vandenberg, B. (1983). Play. In P. H. Mussen (Ed.), *Handbook of child psychology: Socialization, personality, and social development* (4th ed., Vol. 4, pp. 693-774). New York, NY: Wiley.

Spencer, L. M., & Spencer, S. M. (1993). *Competence at work*. New York, NY: John Wiley and Sons.

Wells, S. A., & Black, R. M. (2000). *Cultural competency for health professionals*. Bethesda, MD: AOTA Press.

World Health Organization. (1947). Constitution of the World Health Organization. *Chronicle for the World Health Organization, 1*(1),29-40.

World Health Organization. (2001). *International Classification of Functioning, Disability and Health*. Geneva, Switzerland: Author.

# Financial Disclosures

*Caroline Beals* has no financial or proprietary interest in the materials presented herein.

*Diane P. Bergey* has no financial or proprietary interest in the materials presented herein.

*Caryn Birstler Husman* has no financial or proprietary interest in the materials presented herein.

*Dr. Roxie M. Black* has no financial or proprietary interest in the materials presented herein.

*Dr. Gail M. Bloom* has no financial or proprietary interest in the materials presented herein.

*Dr. Jessica J. Bolduc* has no financial or proprietary interest in the materials presented herein.

*Dr. Alfred G. Bracciano* is the cofounder of PAMPCA, provider of continuing education content.

*Dr. Susan C. Burwash* has no financial or proprietary interest in the materials presented herein.

*Dr. Jane Clifford O'Brien* has no financial or proprietary interest in the materials presented herein.

*Marilyn B. Cole* has no financial or proprietary interest in the materials presented herein.

*Dr. Jeffrey L. Crabtree* has no financial or proprietary interest in the materials presented herein.

*Elizabeth W. Crampsey* has no financial or proprietary interest in the materials presented herein.

*William R. Croninger* has no financial or proprietary interest in the materials presented herein.

*Danielle J. Cropley* has no financial or proprietary interest in the materials presented herein.

*Laura Crossley-Marra* has no financial or proprietary interest in the materials presented herein.

*Peter DaSilva* has no financial or proprietary interest in the materials presented herein.

*Hailey C. Davis* has no financial or proprietary interest in the materials presented herein.

*Betsy DeBrakeleer* has not disclosed any relevant financial relationships.

*Dr. Mary V. Donohue* has no financial or proprietary interest in the materials presented herein.

*Dr. Nancy Doyle* has no financial or proprietary interest in the materials presented herein.

*Dr. Karen Duddy* has no financial or proprietary interest in the materials presented herein.

*Dr. Verna G. Eschenfelder* has no financial or proprietary interest in the materials presented herein.

*Dr. Thomas Fisher* has no financial or proprietary interest in the materials presented herein.

*Erica A. Flagg* has no financial or proprietary interest in the materials presented herein.

*Dr. Kathleen Flecky* has no financial or proprietary interest in the materials presented herein.

*Jan Froehlich* has no financial or proprietary interest in the materials presented herein.

*Dr. Liat Gafni Lachter* has no financial or proprietary interest in the materials presented herein.

*Dr. Heather Goertz* has no financial or proprietary interest in the materials presented herein.

*Michelle Goulet* has no financial or proprietary interest in the materials presented herein.

*Elizabeth C. Hart* has no financial or proprietary interest in the materials presented herein.

*Dr. Karen Jacobs* has no financial or proprietary interest in the materials presented herein.

*Bevin Journey* has no financial or proprietary interest in the materials presented herein.

*Dr. Leanna W. Katz* has no financial or proprietary interest in the materials presented herein.

*Dr. Rosalie M. King* has no financial or proprietary interest in the materials presented herein.

*Dr. Lisa Knecht-Sabres* has no financial or proprietary interest in the materials presented herein.

*Dr. Amy Lamb* has no financial or proprietary interest in the materials presented herein.

*Barbara Larson* has no financial or proprietary interest in the materials presented herein.

*Dr. Kathryn M. Loukas* has no financial or proprietary interest in the materials presented herein.

*Nancy MacRae* has no financial or proprietary interest in the materials presented herein.

*Sarah McKinnon* has no financial or proprietary interest in the materials presented herein.

*Dr. Scott D. McNeil* has no financial or proprietary interest in the materials presented herein.

*Meghan McNierney* has no financial or proprietary interest in the materials presented herein.

*Dr. Linda Miller* has no financial or proprietary interest in the materials presented herein.

*Dr. Penelope Moyers Cleveland* has no financial or proprietary interest in the materials presented herein.

*Dr. Julie Ann Nastasi* has no financial or proprietary interest in the materials presented herein.

*Dr. Robin Newman* has no financial or proprietary interest in the materials presented herein.

*Dr. Linda H. Niemeyer* has no financial or proprietary interest in the materials presented herein.

*Dr. Claudia E. Oakes* has no financial or proprietary interest in the materials presented herein.

*Jennifer O'Connor* has no financial or proprietary interest in the materials presented herein.

*Megha Panchal* has no financial or proprietary interest in the materials presented herein.

*Mary Elizabeth Patnaude* has no financial or proprietary interest in the materials presented herein.

*Dr. Michael E. Roberts* has no financial or proprietary interest in the materials presented herein.

*Dr. Regula H. Robnett* has no financial or proprietary interest in the materials presented herein.

*Dr. Jan Rowe* has no financial or proprietary interest in the materials presented herein.

*Courtney Shufelt* has no financial or proprietary interest in the materials presented herein.

*Dr. Wendy B. Stav* has no financial or proprietary interest in the materials presented herein.

*Barbara J. Steva* has no financial or proprietary interest in the materials presented herein.

*Dr. Christine Sullivan* has no financial or proprietary interest in the materials presented herein.

*Roseanna Tufano* has no financial or proprietary interest in the materials presented herein.

*Dr. Rebecca Twinley* has no financial or proprietary interest in the materials presented herein.

*Dr. Lori Vaughn* has no financial or proprietary interest in the materials presented herein.

*Dr. John W. Vellacott* has no financial or proprietary interest in the materials presented herein.

*Dr. Nicole Villegas* has no financial or proprietary interest in the materials presented herein.

*Iris Wilbur-Kamien* has no financial or proprietary interest in the materials presented herein.

*Dr. Kristin Winston* has no financial or proprietary interest in the materials presented herein.

*Patricia A. Wisniewski* has no financial or proprietary interest in the materials presented herein.

# Index

Printed in the United States
by Baker & Taylor Publisher Services